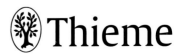

Differential Diagnosis in Computed Tomography

2nd edition

Francis A. Burgener, MD
Professor of Radiology
University of Rochester Medical Center
Rochester, New York, USA

Steven P. Meyers, MD, PhD
Professor of Radiology and Neurosurgery
University of Rochester Medical Center
Rochester, New York, USA

Christopher Herzog, MD, MBA
Department of Radiology
Rotkreuzklinikum
Munich, Germany

Wolfgang Zaunbauer, MD
Institute of Radiology
Kantonsspital St. Gallen
St. Gallen, Switzerland

In collaboration with:
Grégory Dieudonné, MD
Scott A. Mooney, MD
Richard T. White, DO

2146 illustrations

This edition includes texts and illustrations from Martti Kormano, MD, who authored Chapters 1, 2, 10, 18, 19, 20, 21, 22, 23, 24, 25, and 26 of the first edition.

Thieme
Stuttgart · New York

Library of Congress Cataloging-in-Publication Data
Burgener, Francis A., author.
Differential diagnosis in computed tomography / Francis A. Burgener, Professor of Radiology, University of Rochester Medical Center, Rochester, New York, Steven P. Meyers, MD, PhD, Professor of Radiology/Imaging Sciences, Neurosurgery Radiology, Residency Program Director, Director of the Fellowship in Magnetic Resonance Imaging, University of Rochester School of Medicine and Dentistry, Rochester, New York, Christopher Herzog, Rotkreuzklinikum, Radiologisches Institut, Munich, Germany, Wolfgang Zaunbauer, Institute for Radiology, Kantonsspital St. Gallen, St. Gallen, Switzerland. -- Second Edition.
       p. ; cm.
   Includes bibliographical references and index.
   ISBN 978-3-13-102542-5 (hardback)
   1. Tomography. 2. Diagnosis, Differential. I. Meyers, Steven P., author. II. Herzog, Christopher, author. III. Zaunbauer, Wolfgang, author. IV. Title.
   [DNLM: 1. Tomography, X-Ray Computed. 2. Diagnosis, Differential. WN 206]
   RC78.7.T6B87 2011
   616.07′572--dc22
   2010053779
   616.07′54--dc22
                    2010052679

Important note: Medicine is an ever-changing science undergoing continual development. Research and clinical experience are continually expanding our knowledge, in particular our knowledge of proper treatment and drug therapy. Insofar as this book mentions any dosage or application, readers may rest assured that the authors, editors, and publishers have made every effort to ensure that such references are in accordance with **the state of knowledge at the time of production of the book.** Nevertheless, this does not involve, imply, or express any guarantee or responsibility on the part of the publishers in respect to any dosage instructions and forms of applications stated in the book. **Every user is requested to examine carefully** the manufacturers' leaflets accompanying each drug and to check, if necessary in consultation with a physician or specialist, whether the dosage schedules mentioned therein or the contraindications stated by the manufacturers differ from the statements made in the present book. Such examination is particularly important with drugs that are either rarely used or have been newly released on the market. Every dosage schedule or every form of application used is entirely at the user's own risk and responsibility. The authors and publishers request every user to report to the publishers any discrepancies or inaccuracies noticed. If errors in this work are found after publication, errata will be posted at www.thieme.com on the product description page.

© 2012 Georg Thieme Verlag,
Rüdigerstrasse 14, 70469 Stuttgart, Germany
http://www.thieme.de
Thieme New York, 333 Seventh Avenue,
New York, NY 10001, USA
http://www.thieme.com

Cover design: Thieme Publishing Group
Typesetting by Maryland Composition, Maryland, USA

Printed by Everbest Printing Co Ltd., China

ISBN 978 3 13 102542 5   1 2 3 4 5 6

Contributors

Francis A. Burgener, MD
Professor of Radiology
University of Rochester Medical Center
Rochester, New York, USA

Christopher Herzog, MD, MBA
Institute of Radiology
Rotkreuzklinikum
Munich, Germany

Steven P. Meyers, MD, PhD
Professor of Radiology and Neurosurgery
University of Rochester Medical Center
Rochester, New York, USA

Wolfgang Zaunbauer, MD
Institute of Radiology
Kantonsspital St. Gallen
St. Gallen, Switzerland

In collaboration with:

Grégory Dieudonné, MD
Assistant Professor of Radiology
University of Rochester Medical Center
Rochester, New York, USA
—Contributed Chapter 29

Scott A. Mooney, MD
Clinical Assistant Professor of Radiology
University of Rochester Medical Center
Rochester, New York, USA
—Contributed illustrations to Chapters 11, 12, 13, 14, 15, 27, 28, and 29

Richard T. White, DO
Professor of Radiology
University of Rochester Medical Center
Rochester, New York, USA
—Contributed illustrations to Chapters 27, 28, and 29

Preface

Dr. Martti Kormano was my coauthor for the textbook *Differential Diagnosis in Conventional Radiology*, including all subsequent editions, as well as the original *Differential Diagnosis in Computed Tomography*. It was a great pleasure for me to work with him on these endeavors over two decades. Unfortunately for me, Dr. Kormano has since retired from his position as Chairman of the Diagnostic Radiology Department of the University Hospital in Turku, Finland, and because of personal commitments could not find the time and energy to be involved in the updating of this text. Because I am devoting my professional time exclusively to musculoskeletal radiology, I not only had to find new coauthors for Dr. Kormano's section of the text, but I also needed help for my original chapters outside of my area of main interest. I was fortunate to find three colleagues to completely revise Dr. Kormano's section of the original text and update some of my chapters. I believe Drs. Christopher Herzog, Steven P. Meyers, and Wolfgang Zaunbauer performed an outstanding job.

In the 15 years since the publication of the first edition, the scope of CT imaging has grown and assumed a much greater role in the field of medical imaging. Most of this growth is not related to the discovery of new disease processes but, rather, it is related to the development and refinement of CT technology. The greatly improved hardware and software in CT allows high-quality reconstruction images in various 2D and 3D planes, as well as dynamic examinations such as CT angiography and perfusion studies. These advancements result in many new indications for CT examinations such as the accurate staging of intra-articular and spinal fractures or the evaluation of vascular diseases. To account for this development, new sections have been added to every chapter and three new (Chapters 3, 4, and 15) have been included in this edition—resulting in a substantial increase in both text and illustrations. Furthermore, illustrations from the first edition have been updated with high-quality images.

CT has gained worldwide acceptance and, in addition to many new indications, has also replaced conventional radiographic techniques in many areas. CT is no longer the exclusive domain of the radiologist, but is also practiced and/or interpreted by a large number of clinicians and surgeons. With each examination, one is confronted with CT findings that require interpretation in order to arrive at a general diagnostic impression and a reasonable differential diagnosis. To assist the physician in attaining this goal, this book is based on CT findings rather than being disease-oriented like most other textbooks in radiology. Because many diseases present on CT in a variety of manifestations, some overlap in the text is unavoidable. To minimize repetition, the differential diagnosis of a CT finding is presented in tabular form whenever feasible. Most tables not only list the various diseases that may present on CT in a specific pattern, but also describe in succinct form other characteristically associated imaging findings and pertinent clinical data. The text is complemented by many CT images and drawings to visually demonstrate the image features under discussion.

I hope this revised and expanded second edition will be as well received as the original text, which was translated into eight languages. The concept of an imaging pattern approach in tabular form rather than a disease-oriented text was introduced by Dr. Kormano and myself in 1985 with the first edition of *Differential Diagnosis in Conventional Radiology* and has since been adopted by many authors. I take this as a compliment—after all, imitation is the sincerest form of flattery.

This book is meant for radiologists and physicians with some experience in the interpretation of CT examinations who wish to strengthen their diagnostic acumen. It is a comprehensive outline of CT findings and will be particularly useful to radiology residents preparing for their specialist examination. Any physician involved in the interpretation of CT examination should find this book helpful in direct proportion to his or her curiosity. It is my hope that the second edition of *Differential Diagnosis in Computed Tomography* will be as interesting as its predecessor to medical students, residents, radiologists, and physicians involved in the interpretation of CT images.

Francis A. Burgener, MD

Acknowledgments

It is impossible to thank individually all those who helped to prepare the second edition of this textbook. I wish to acknowledge the staff of our publisher, in particular, Dr. Clifford Bergman as well as Stephan Konnry and Annie Hollins, both of whom were more recently assigned by Thieme to this project to deal with, among other things, my old fashioned style relying primarily on paper, pencils, hard copies, and the telephone. Their hard work, dedication, and attention to detail for this edition are greatly appreciated. Furthermore, I am also indebted to Heidi Grauel for her editorial assistance and efficient handling of the page proofs.

I also wish to express our gratitude to the many radiologists who made this illustrative collection of computed tomography images available. Special thanks go to Drs. Allen Bernstein, Gary Hollenberg, Johnny Monu, Peter Rosella, Gwy Suk Seo, David Shrier, Charlene Varnis, Brian Webber, Eric Weinberg, and Andrea Zynda; all staff members of the University of Rochester Imaging Sciences Department; Drs. Thomas Vogl and Volkmar Jacobi, both of the Johann Wolfgang Goethe University Clinic, Frankfurt; and Drs. Tobias Hertle (Dresden), Sebastian Leschka (Zürich), Christoph Ozdoba (Bern), Reinhand Schöpf (Landeck), Nikolai Stahr (Winterthur), Björn Stinn (Zürich), and Alexander Von Hessling (Zürich).

I greatly appreciate the invaluable contribution by Dr. Patrick J. Fultz, Professor of Radiology at the University of Rochester Medical Center, who authored the original Chapter 29 of this text and graciously let us use this material in the new edition.

I wish to thank Margaret Kowaluk, Sarah Peangatelli, and Katherine Tower of the Imaging Sciences graphic services section at the University of Rochester Medical Center for their outstanding work in preparing the illustrations. The instructive new drawings were superbly executed by either Katherine Tower or Dr. Anna Zaunbauer-Womelsdorf, the daughter of one of the coauthors of this text. Their work is greatly appreciated.

Excellent secretarial support for this project was provided by Colleen Cottrell and Jill Derby for which I wish to express many thanks. The general secretarial assistance of Shirley Cappiello is also greatly appreciated. Last, but not least, I am most grateful to Alyce Norder who left the University and me after 30 years for the richness of the industry and subsequent partial retirement. She is, besides Jill Derby, the only person capable of deciphering my longhand and, as in the past, did a superb job in typing, editing, and proofreading the manuscript of the new edition of this text in her spare time, for which I am deeply grateful.

Finally, I appreciate the support of our families who have forfeited precious family time for the preparation of this text. Therefore, in appreciation of both their understanding and support, my coauthors and I dedicate this book to our wives Therese Burgener, Christine Herzog, Barbara Weber, and Isabella Zaunbauer.

Francis A. Burgener, MD

Contents

List of Tables

I Intracranial Lesions

1 Brain and Extra-axial Lesions

Steven P. Meyers

Computed tomography (CT) can provide rapid multiplanar imaging of the brain, meninges, and skull. The use of dynamic rapid data acquisition combined with bolus injection of iodinated contrast agents allows for assessment of blood perfusion rates of normal and abnormal brain tissue, as well as the generation of high-resolution CT arteriograms and venograms. CT has proven to be a powerful imaging modality in the evaluation of (1) neoplasms of the central nervous system, meninges, calvarium, and skull base; (2) traumatic lesions; (3) intracranial hemorrhage; (4) ischemia and infarction, particularly using CT perfusion studies; (5) infectious and noninfectious diseases; and (6) metabolic disorders.

The appearance of brain tissue depends on the milliampere second (mAs) and kilovolts peak (kVp) used, as well as the age of the patient imaged. Myelination of the brain begins in the fifth fetal month and progresses rapidly during the first 2 years of life. The degree of myelination affects the appearance of the brain parenchyma on CT. In adults, the cerebral cortex has intermediate attenuation that is slightly higher relative to normal white matter. For infants younger than 6 months, differentiation of white matter relative to gray matter is limited secondary to the immature myelination of brain tissue. Myelination proceeds in a predictable and characteristic pattern with regard to locations and timing. These changes are more optimally seen with magnetic resonance imaging (MRI) than with CT.

Various pathologic processes can affect the attenuation properties of the involved tissue or organ. For example, intraparenchymal hemorrhage can have variable appearances in the brain depending on the age of the hematoma, oxidation states of the iron in hemoglobin, hematocrit, protein concentration, clot formation and retraction, location, and size. Oxyhemoglobin in a hyperacute blood clot has ferrous iron. After a few hours during the acute phase of the hematoma, the oxyhemoglobin loses its oxygen to form deoxyhemoglobin. Deoxyhemoglobin also has ferrous iron, although it has unpaired electrons. Later in the early subacute phase of the hematoma, deoxyhemoglobin becomes oxidized to the ferric state, methemoglobin. Initially, red blood cells in the clot are intact. In the late subacute phase, breakdown of the membranes of the red blood cells results in extracellular methemoglobin. In the chronic phase, methemoglobin becomes further oxidized and broken down by macrophages into hemosiderin.

The CT features of subdural hematomas are variable, although the appearances can progress in patterns similar to intraparenchymal hematomas. Acute subdural hematomas often have low-intermediate attenuation.

Other lesions that can result in zones of low attenuation are dermoids (intact or ruptured), teratomas, lipomas, and cystic structures with low protein concentration or cholesterol.

Nonhemorrhagic pathologic processes tend to decrease the attenuation of the involved tissues. Such processes include ischemia, infarction, inflammation, infection, demyelination, dysmyelination, metabolic or toxic encephalopathy, trauma, neoplasms, gliosis, radiation injury, and encephalomalacic changes. Exceptions to this phenomenon include neoplasms with high nuclear to cytoplasmic ratios (e.g., medulloblastomas and small cell lymphomas), fluid collections with high protein or mineral concentrations (e.g., colloid cysts and craniopharyngiomas), and lesions with fine or clumplike calcifications (e.g., ependymomas, meningiomas, and metabolic disorders such as hypoparathyroidism and Fahr disease).

Of the various human body tissues, the brain is the least tolerant of ischemia. A lack of sufficient blood flow to the brain for approximately 5 seconds results in loss of consciousness and for several minutes can result in irreversible cerebral ischemia and infarction. For normal brain function, cerebral blood flow (CBF) must be maintained at a constant rate to deliver oxygen and glucose as well as to remove CO_2 and metabolic waste products. Maintenance of CBF is critical for neuronal function. With arterial occlusion, the loss of normal neuronal electrical activity occurs within seconds after arterial occlusion. Cellular death is dependent on the duration and magnitude of ischemia, the metabolic vulnerability of specific anatomical sites, and the oxygen content of blood. CT is important in the detection of cerebral infarction and for the presence of associated hemorrhage, which may preclude the use of thrombolytic therapy. Another clinical application of CT for stroke is a technique referred to as CT perfusion, which utilizes rapid infusion of intravenous (IV) iodinated contrast, and will be discussed at the end of this section.

Areas where there is a breakdown of the blood–brain barrier from pathologic disorders can be evaluated with iodine-based IV contrast agents. Leakage of these agents through the blood–brain barrier results in contrast enhancement localized to the involved pathologic regions. Contrast-enhanced CT images are an important portion of most imaging examinations of the head. In addition to pathologically altered intracranial tissues, contrast-enhancement can be normally seen in veins, the choroid plexus, the pituitary gland, and pineal gland. For this book, the attenuation of the various entities will be described as low, intermediate, high, or mixed and whether there is contrast enhancement or not.

Intracranial lesions are typically classified as being extra- or intra-axial. Extra-axial lesions arise from the skull, meninges, or tissues other than the brain parenchyma. They are characterized as being within epidural, subdural, or subarachnoid spaces or compartments. Lesions involving the meninges can be further categorized as involving the dura mater (e.g., with benign postoperative dural fibrosis) or involving the leptomeninges (pia and arachnoid). Abnormalities of the meninges are often best seen after the IV administration of contrast material. Dural enhancement usually has a linear configuration, whereas pathology involving the leptomeninges appears as enhancement within the sulci and basilar cisterns. Enhancement of the leptomeninges is usually related to significant pathology, such as neoplastic or inflammatory diseases.

Intra-axial lesions are located in the brain parenchyma or brainstem. Differential diagnoses of extra-axial and intra-axial masslike lesions are presented in **Tables 1.2, 1.3, 1.4, and 1.5.** Intra-axial masslike lesions are presented according to location: supra- versus infratentorial. Infratentorial neoplasms are more common in children and adolescents than adults. During childhood, intra-axial tumors such as astrocytomas, medulloblastomas, ependymomas, and brainstem gliomas are the most common neoplasms. In adults; metastatic lesions and hemangioblastomas are the most common intra-axial infratentorial tumors, and acoustic schwannomas and meningiomas are common extra-axial infratentorial neoplasms. Infratentorial lesions are discussed in **Tables 1.4 and 1.5.**

Multidetector CT is an excellent imaging modality for evaluation of the skull base, orbits, nasopharynx, oropharynx, and floor of the mouth because of its multiplanar imaging capabilities and high spatial resolution. CT is a useful method for imaging the location and extent of osseous lesions at the skull base, such as metastatic tumors, myelomas, chordomas, and chondrosarcomas.

CT can be used for the evaluation of congenital and developmental anomalies of the brain, such as semilobar holoprosencephaly, septo-optic dysplasia, schizencephaly, gray matter heterotopia, cortical dysplasia, unilateral megalencephaly, and Dandy-Walker malformation.

Diseases of white matter are classified into two major groups, dysmyelinating and demyelinating diseases. Dysmyelinating diseases, also known as leukodystrophies, are a group of disorders resulting from enzyme deficiencies that cause abnormal formation and metabolism of myelin. Demyelinating diseases are a group of disorders in which myelin is degraded or destroyed after it has formed in a normal fashion.

Abnormalities involving the lateral, third, and fourth ventricles, as well as the cerebral aqueduct, are well seen with CT because of the difference of attenuation between the brain parenchyma and cerebrospinal fluid (CSF). The production of CSF occurs in the choroid plexus within the ventricles. CSF circulates from the lateral ventricles through the foramina of Monro into the third ventricle. The third ventricle communicates with the fourth ventricle via the cerebral aqueduct. CSF from the fourth ventricle enters into the subarachnoid space through the foramina of Luschka and Magendie. Mass lesions along the CSF pathway can result in obstructive hydrocephalus with dilation of the ventricles proximal to the blockage.

Some asymmetry of the lateral ventricles can be seen normally. Altered morphology of the ventricles can result from various congenital anomalies (e.g., holoprosencephaly, septo-optic dysplasia, unilateral hemimegalencephaly, gray matter heterotopia, and Dandy-Walker malformation), as well as from distortion from intra- or extra-axial mass lesions.

The sizes of sulci can vary depending on multiple variables, such as age, congenital malformations, vascular abnormalities (e.g., cerebral infarcts, Sturge-Weber syndrome, and arteriovenous malformations [AVMs]), intra- or extra-axial mass lesions, hydrocephalus, and inflammatory diseases. Sulci should have CSF attenuation within them. The presence of contrast enhancement within the sulci and basilar cisterns is usually associated with pathology, such as inflammatory or neoplastic disease. Acute subarachnoid hemorrhage is typically seen as amorphous zones with high attenuation within the sulci and cisterns near the site of bleeding.

CT angiography (CTA) is a powerful imaging modality for evaluating normal and abnormal blood vessels. CTA has proven to be clinically useful in the evaluation of intracranial arteries, veins, and dural venous sinuses. Pathologic processes involving intracranial blood vessels, such as aneurysms, AVMs, arterial occlusions, and dural venous sinus thrombosis, can be seen with CTA.

CT perfusion is a relatively new technique using dynamic IV infusion of contrast to measure CBF, cerebral blood volume (CBV), and mean transit time (MTT) of contrast enhancement to selected volumes of interest in the brain. CT perfusion has major clinical use in the evaluation of cerebral infarcts and adjacent zones of decreased perfusion (penumbra and oligemic areas) at risk for progression to infarction. Maintenance of CBF is critical for neuronal function. With arterial occlusion, loss of normal neuronal electrical activity occurs within seconds after arterial occlusion. Cellular death is dependent on the duration and magnitude of ischemia, the metabolic vulnerability of specific anatomical sites, and the oxygen content of blood. Normal CBF ranges from 50 to 60 mL/100 g/min. When the CBF is reduced to 15 to 20 mL/100 g/min for several hours (mild to moderate hypoxia), spontaneous and evoked neuronal electrical activity decreases significantly secondary to ischemia, although it can be reversed with reperfusion with CBF > 50 mL/100 g/min. With severe hypoxia/anoxia resulting from CBF < 10 mL/100 g/min, cellular membrane depolarization and ischemia leading to brain infarction may occur in several minutes.

When thrombotic or embolic arterial occlusions occur, CBF in the involved brain tissue is usually heterogeneous, with a central core showing the greatest reductions in CBF causing irreversible cell damage and infarction and a surrounding zone (referred to as the *salvageable penumbra*) that may have moderate reduction in CBF resulting in ischemia that may be reversible with reperfusion. The penumbra typically shows loss of neuronal electrical activity without immediate anoxic depolarization, as well as loss of autoregulation. If reperfusion does not occur, the penumbra will progress to infarction. An oligemic zone of mildly reduced CBF may also be seen surrounding the penumbra, which is less vulnerable to infarction than the penumbra. Thrombolytic medication can be useful and beneficial when it results in timely reperfusion to the penumbra and oligemic zones. Estimating the sizes of the penumbra and oligemic zones can be done in the acute setting with dynamic contrast-enhanced CT. CT perfusion with iodinated contrast delivered as an IV bolus can use the linear relationship between contrast concentration and attenuation to directly calculate and quantify CBF, CBV, and MTT for sites of ischemia and infarction in the brain prior to thrombolytic treatment (**Fig. 1.1**).

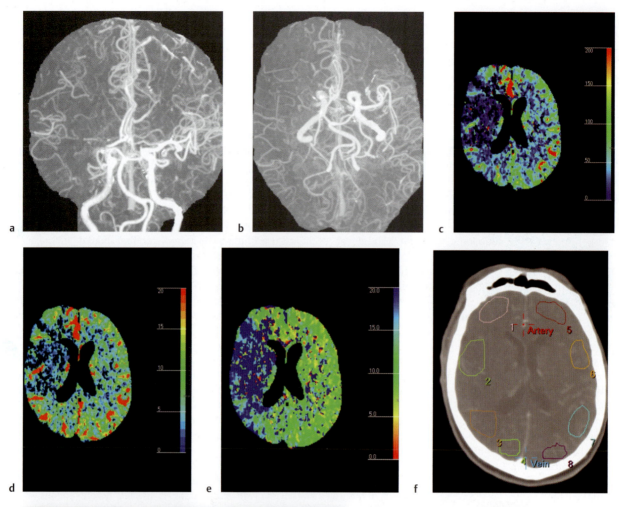

ROI Statistics for Slice 5				
ROI #	CBV (ml/100g)	CBF (ml/100g/min)	MTT (s)	TTP (s)
1	7.65	27.03	16.99	38.06
2	6.93	17.84	23.31	43.74
3	8.24	25.40	19.46	39.44
4	6.36	37.08	10.29	33.47
5	7.85	51.20	9.21	31.13
6	9.60	79.90	7.21	30.50
7	9.86	73.76	8.02	30.65
8	10.03	71.02	8.47	31.54

g

Fig. 1.1a–g   Cerebral artery embolus. Coronal (**a**) and axial (**b**) computed tomography angiogram (CTA) images show an embolus occluding nearly all blood flow through the M1 segment of the right middle cerebral artery. Cerebral blood flow (CBF) (**c**), cerebral blood volume (CBV) (**d**), and mean transit time (MTT) (**e**) are displayed qualitatively using a color scale. Locations for regions of interest are shown in (**f**), with respective quantitative values for CBF, CBV, and MTT in (**g**) showing sites of core infarction and penumbra and oligemic zones.

Table 1.1   Congenital malformations of the brain

Lesions	CT Findings	Comments
Disorders of diverticulation (formation of cerebral hemispheres and ventricles)		
Holoprosencephaly	**Alobar:** Large monoventricle with posterior midline cyst, lack of hemisphere formation with absence of falx, corpus callosum, and septum pellucidum. Fused thalami. Can be associated with facial anomalies (facial clefts, arrhinia, hypotelorism, and cyclops). ▷ *Fig. 1.2* **Semilobar:** Monoventricle with partial formation of interhemispheric fissure, occipital and temporal horns, and partially fused thalami. Absent corpus callosum and septum pellucidum. Associated with mild craniofacial anomalies. ▷ *Fig. 1.3a, b* **Lobar:** Near complete formation of interhemispheric fissure and ventricles. Fused inferior portions of frontal lobes, dysgenesis of corpus callosum with formation of posterior portion without anterior portion, malformed frontal horns of lateral ventricles, absence of septum pellucidum, separate thalami, and neuronal migration disorders. ▷ *Fig. 1.4a, b* **Syntelencephaly (middle interhemispheric variant):** Partial formation of interhemispheric fissure in the anterior and occipital regions with fusion of the portions of the upper frontal and/or parietal lobes. Genu and splenium of the corpus callosum can be observed with a focal defect in the body.	**Holoprosencephaly:** Spectrum of diverticulation disorders that occur during weeks 4 to 6 of gestation characterized by absent or partial cleavage and differentiation of the embryonic cerebrum (prosencephalon) into hemispheres and lobes. Causes include maternal diabetes, fetal genetic abnormalities such as trisomy 16 (Patau syndrome), and trisomy 18 (Edwards syndrome). Familial holoprosencephaly: mutations of *HPE1* on chromosome 21q22.3, *HPE2* on 2p21, *HPE3* on 7q36, *HPE4* on 18p, and *HPE5* on 13q32. Clinical manifestations depend on the severity of the malformation and include early death, seizures, mental retardation, facial dysmorphism, and developmental delay. Patients with syntelencephaly often have mild to moderate cognitive dysfunction, spasticity, and mild visual impairment.

(continues on page 6)

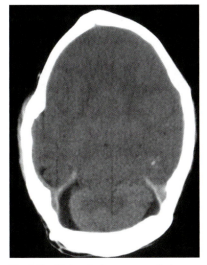

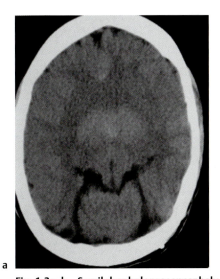

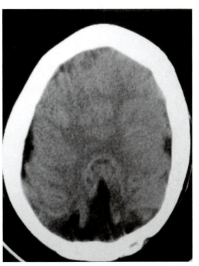

Fig. 1.2   Alobar holoprosencephaly. Axial image after ventricular shunting shows the absence of interhemispheric fissure and the lack of cerebral and cerebellar lobe formation.

Fig. 1.3a, b   Semilobar holoprosencephaly. Axial images show fusion of the anterior portion of the brain with the presence of only the posterior portion of the interhemispheric fissure.

Table 1.1   (Cont.) Congenital malformations of the brain

Lesions	CT Findings	Comments
Septo-optic dysplasia (de Morsier syndrome)	Dysgenesis/hypoplasia or agenesis of septum pellucidum, optic nerve hypoplasia, and squared frontal horns; association with schizencephaly in 50% of patients. Optic canals are often small. May be associated with schizencephaly and gray matter heterotopia.	Patients can have nystagmus, decreased visual acuity, and hypothalamic-pituitary disorders (decreased thyroid stimulating hormone and/or growth hormone). Clinical exam shows small optic discs. May be sporadic from in utero insults or from abnormal genetic expression from mutations (*HESX1* gene on chromosome 3p21.1–3p21.2) during formation of the basal prosencephalon. Some findings overlap those of mild lobar holoprosencephaly.
Arrhinia/arrhinencephaly ▷*Fig. 1.5a–d*	Absence of olfactory lobes and sulci. Other anomalies may be seen involving the corpus callosum, hypothalamus, and pituitary gland.	Arrhinia refers to the absence of nose formation; arrhinencephaly refers to the congenital absence of the olfactory lobes. Typically associated with other congenital craniofacial anomalies such as cleft palate/lip, hypertelorism, and hypoplasia of the nasal cavity. Considered to result from insult in utero or genetic mutation.
Neuronal migration disorders		
Lissencephaly (agyria or "smooth brain") ▷*Fig. 1.6a, b*	Absent or incomplete formation of gyri and sulci with shallow sylvian fissures and "figure 8" appearance of brain on axial images, abnormally thick cortex, and gray matter heterotopia with smooth gray-white matter interface.	Severe disorder of neuronal migration (occurs during weeks 7–16 of gestation) with absent or incomplete formation of gyri, sulci, and sylvian fissures. Typically in association with microcephaly (defined as head circumference 3 standard deviations below normal). Associated with severe mental retardation, developmental delay, seizures, and early death. Other associated CNS anomalies are dysgenesis of the corpus callosum, microcephaly, hypoplastic thalami, and cephaloceles. Associated with mutations at *LIS* gene at 17p13.3, chromosome 17 (Miller-Dieker syndrome); *DCX* gene at Xq22.3-q23; and *RELN* gene at 7q22.
Pachygyria (nonlissencephalic cortical dysplasia)	Thick gyri with shallow sulci involving all or portions of the brain. Thickened cortex with relatively smooth gray-white interface may have areas of low attenuation in the white matter (gliosis).	Severe disorder of neuronal migration with etiologies similar to lissencephaly. Clinical findings related to degree of extent of this malformation.

(continues on page 8)

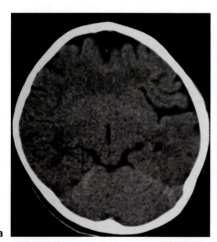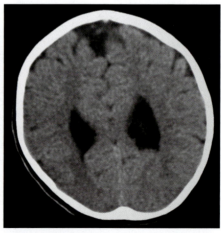

a   b

Fig. 1.4a, b   Lobar holoprosencephaly. Axial images show fusion of the inferior portions of the frontal lobes. The other portions of the frontal lobes are separated, as are the parietal and occipital lobes.

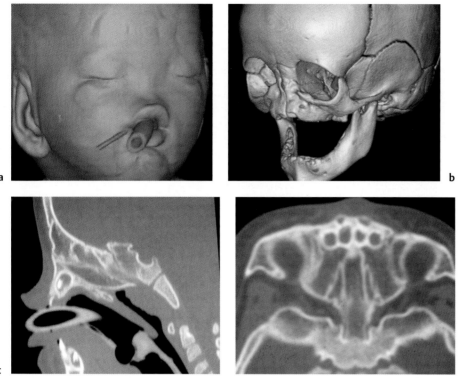

Fig. 1.5a–d   Arrhinia. Oblique coronal (**a,b**), parasagittal (**c**), and axial (**d**) images show the lack of formation of the nasal bones and severe hypoplasia of the nasal cavity.

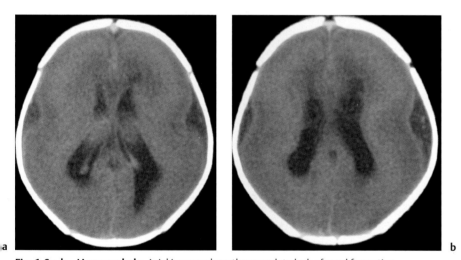

Fig. 1.6a, b   Lissencephaly. Axial images show the complete lack of gyral formation.

Table 1.1   (Cont.) Congenital malformations of the brain

Lesions	CT Findings	Comments
Gray matter heterotopia	**Laminar heterotopia** appears as a band or bands of gray matter attenuation within the cerebral white matter. ▷ *Fig. 1.7a, b* **Nodular heterotopia** appears as one or more nodules of gray matter attenuation along the ventricles or within the cerebral white matter. ▷ *Fig. 1.8* ▷ *Fig. 1.9a, b* **Focal subcortical heterotopia** can be seen as irregular nodular or multinodular masslike zones with gray matter attenuation in subcortical regions. ▷ *Fig. 1.9*	Disorder of neuronal migration (weeks 7–22 of gestation) in which a collection or layer of neurons is located between the ventricles and cerebral cortex. Can have a bandlike (laminar) or nodular appearance isodense to gray matter; may be unilateral or bilateral. Associated with seizures and schizencephaly.
Schizencephaly (split brain) ▷ *Fig. 1.10a, b*	Uni- or bilateral clefts in the brain extending from the ventricle to cortical surface lined by gray matter heterotopia, which may be polymicrogyric. The clefts may be narrow (closed lips) or wide (open lips).	Association with seizures, blindness, retardation, and other CNS anomalies (septo-optic dysplasia, etc.). Clinical manifestations related to severity of malformation. Ischemia or insult to portion or germinal matrix before hemisphere formation.
Unilateral hemimegalencephaly ▷ *Fig. 1.11*	Nodular or multinodular region of gray matter heterotopia involving all or part of a cerebral hemisphere with associated enlargement of the ipsilateral lateral ventricle and hemisphere.	Neuronal migration disorder associated with hamartomatous overgrowth of a portion of or the whole hemisphere.

(continues on page 10)

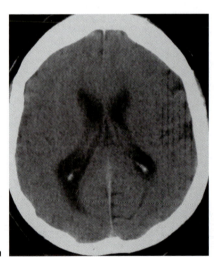 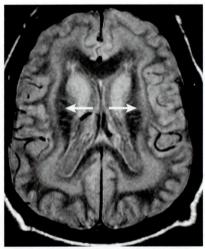 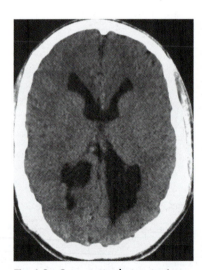

a   b

Fig. 1.7a, b   Gray matter heterotopia, band type. Axial CT (**a**) image shows a band of intermediate attenuation representing the gray matter heterotopia, which is well seen on the axial proton density-weighted magnetic resonance image (MRI) (arrows) (**b**).

Fig. 1.8   Gray matter heterotopia, nodular ependymal type. Axial image shows nodular zones with gray matter attenuation along the margins of the lateral ventricles.

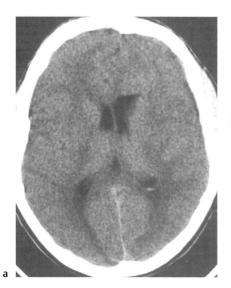
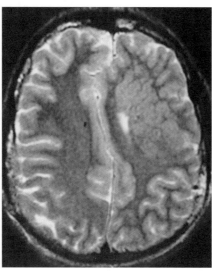

a

b

Fig. 1.9a, b   Gray matter heterotopia, subcortical masslike type. Axial CT image (**a**) shows a masslike zone with gray matter attenuation involving the anterior left frontal lobe, as seen on the axial T2-weighted MRI (**b**).

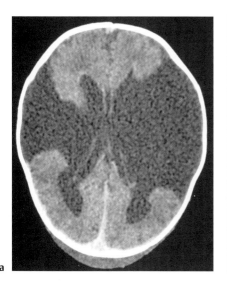
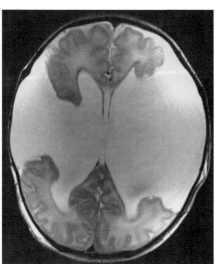

a

b

Fig. 1.10a, b   Schizencephaly, open lip type. Axial CT (**a**) and T2-weighted (**b**) images show large zones of communication between the lateral ventricles and subarachnoid space that are lined with gray matter.

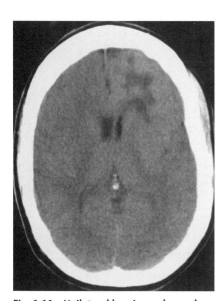

Fig. 1.11   Unilateral hemimegalencephaly. Axial image shows enlargement of the left cerebral hemisphere with abnormally thickened cerebral cortex and gyri.

Table 1.1 (Cont.) Congenital malformations of the brain

Lesions	CT Findings	Comments
Dysgenesis of the corpus callosum ▷ *Fig. 1.12 a, b* ▷ *Fig. 1.13a, b*	Spectrum of abnormalities ranging from complete to partial absence of the corpus callosum. Widely separated and parallel orientations of frontal horns and bodies of the lateral ventricles, high position of the third ventricle in relation to the interhemispheric fissure, and colpocephaly. Associated with interhemispheric cysts, lipomas, and anomalies such as Chiari II malformation, gray matter heterotopia, Dandy-Walker malformation, holoprosencephaly, azygous anterior cerebral artery, and cephaloceles.	Failure or incomplete formation of corpus callosum (7–18 wk of gestation). Axons that normally cross from one hemisphere to the other are aligned parallel along the medial walls of lateral ventricles (bundles of Probst).
Malformations in cerebral cortical development		
Polymicrogyria ▷ *Fig. 1.14a–c*	Multiple small gyri occur unilaterally (40%), bilaterally (60%), and often in the region of the sylvian fissures. On CT, the small gyri may appear as zones of thickened cortex.	Malformation in late stages of neuronal migration resulting in abnormal neuronal organization of the brain cortex. Sites involved lack a normal six-layered cerebral cortex associated with abnormal sulcation.
Focal cortical dysplasia ▷ *Fig. 1.15*	Nodular superficial zone with gray matter attenuation.	Malformation in late stages of neuronal migration resulting in a focal region of abnormal neuronal organization of the brain cortex. Can be associated with seizures.
Neural tube closure disorders		
Chiari I malformation ▷ *Fig. 1.16*	Cerebellar tonsils extend > 5 mm below the foramen magnum in adults, 6 mm in children younger than 10 y. Syringohydromyelia in 20% to 40% of cases, hydrocephalus in 25%, basilar impression in 25%. Less common association: Klippel-Feil syndrome and atlanto-occipital assimilation.	Cerebellar tonsillar ectopia. Most common anomaly of CNS. Not associated with myelomeningocele.
Chiari II malformation (Arnold-Chiari) ▷ *Fig. 1.17*	Small posterior cranial fossa with gaping foramen magnum through which there is an inferiorly positioned vermis associated with a cervicomedullary kink. Beaked dorsal margin of the tectal plate. Myelomeningoceles in all patients. Hydrocephalus and syringomyelia common. Dilated lateral ventricles posteriorly (colpocephaly).	Complex anomaly involving the cerebrum, cerebellum, brainstem, spinal cord, ventricles, skull, and dura. Failure of fetal neural folds to close properly, resulting in altered development affecting multiple sites of the CNS.
Chiari III malformation	Features of Chiari II plus lower occipital or high cervical encephalocele.	Rare anomaly associated with high mortality.

(continues on page 12)

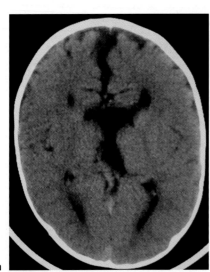 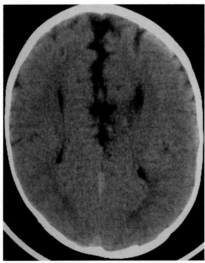

a   b

Fig. 1.12a, b Dysgenesis of the corpus callosum. Axial images show the absence of the corpus callosum with widely separated lateral ventricles.

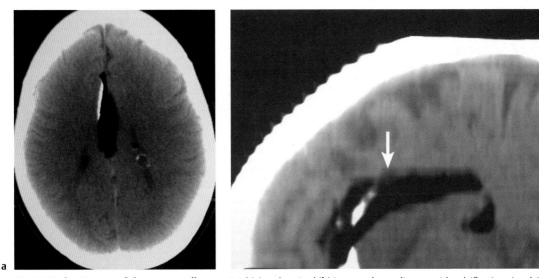

Fig. 1.13a, b   Lipoma of the corpus callosum. Axial (**a**) and sagittal (**b**) images show a lipoma with calcifications involving the anterior portion of the corpus callosum (arrow).

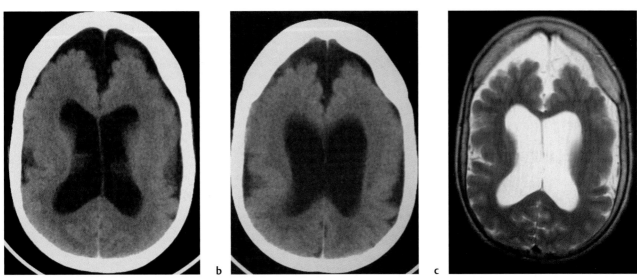

Fig. 1.14a–c   Polymicrogyria. Axial CT images (**a,b**) and axial T2-weighted MRI (**c**) show numerous small gyri.

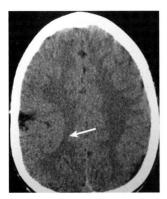

Fig. 1.15   Cortical dysplasia. Axial image shows abnormal cortical thickening involving the right frontal and parietal lobes (arrow).

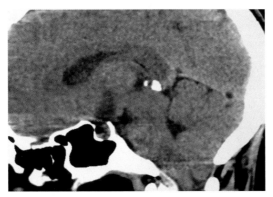

Fig. 1.16   Chiari I malformation. Sagittal image shows extension of the cerebellar tonsils below the foramen magnum to the level of the posterior arch of C1.

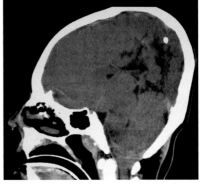

Fig. 1.17   Chiari II malformation. Sagittal image shows extension of the cerebellum through the foramen magnum, as well as a malformed fourth ventricle, dysgenesis of the corpus callosum, and a ventricular shunt catheter.

Table 1.1 (Cont.) Congenital malformations of the brain

Lesions	CT Findings	Comments
Cephaloceles (meningoceles or meningoencephaloceles) ▷ *Fig. 1.18a, b* ▷ *Fig. 1.19a, b* ▷ *Fig. 1.20*	Defect in skull through which there is either herniation of meninges and CSF (meningocele) or meninges, CSF, and brain tissue (meningoencephaloceles).	Congenital malformation involving lack of separation of neuroectoderm from surface ectoderm with resultant localized failure of bone formation. Occipital location most common in Western hemisphere, frontoethmoidal location most common site in Southeast Asians. Other sites include parietal and sphenoid bones. Cephaloceles can also result from trauma or surgery.
Cerebellar hypoplasia		
Chiari II with vanishing cerebellum	Intracranial findings of Chiari II with complete or near complete absence of the cerebellum.	Myeloceles in Chiari II malformations may rarely be associated with in utero destruction of the fetal cerebellum.
Hypoplasia of cerebellar hemisphere	Hypoplasia or absence of a cerebellar hemisphere.	In utero insult causing loss of formative cerebellar cells from ischemia or apoptosis.
Dandy-Walker malformation ▷ *Fig. 1.21a, b*	Vermian aplasia or severe hypoplasia, communication of fourth ventricle with retrocerebellar cyst, hypoplasia of cerebellar hemispheres, enlarged posterior fossa, and high position of tentorium and transverse venous sinuses. Hydrocephalus common. Associated with other anomalies, such as dysgenesis of the corpus callosum, gray matter heterotopia, schizencephaly, holoprosencephaly, and cephaloceles.	Abnormal formation of the roof of the fourth ventricle with absent or near incomplete formation of the cerebellar vermis.
Vermian hypoplasia (also referred to as "Dandy-Walker variant")	Mild vermian hypoplasia with communication of posteroinferior portion of the fourth ventricle with cisterna magna. No associated enlargement of the posterior cranial fossa.	Occasionally associated with hydrocephalus, dysgenesis of the corpus callosum, gray matter heterotopia, and other anomalies.
Cerebellar dysplastic malformations		
Joubert syndrome	Small dysplastic vermis with midline cleft between apposing cerebellar hemispheres, "molar tooth" axial appearance from small midbrain, and thickened superior cerebellar peduncles.	Malformation with hypoplasia of vermis, dysplasia and heterotopia of cerebellar nuclei, lack of decussation of superior cerebellar peduncles, and near complete absence of medullary pyramids. Clinical: ataxia, mental retardation, and abnormal eye movements.
Rhombencephalosynapsis	Dysmorphic cerebellum with no apparent separation of cerebellar hemispheres, aplasia, or severe hypoplasia of vermis.	Malformation with fusion of cerebellar hemispheres, dentate nuclei, and superior cerebellar peduncles; absent or hypoplastic vermis. Clinical: truncal ataxia, cerebral palsy, mental retardation, and seizures.
Lhermitte-Duclos disease ▷ *Fig. 1.22a, b*	Poorly defined zone of low and intermediate attenuation with laminated appearance and localized mass effect located in the cerebellum. No enhancement.	Uncommon cerebellar dysplasia with gross thickening of cerebellar folia and disorganized cellular structure.

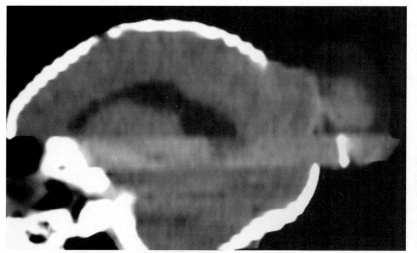
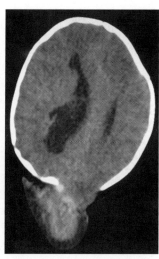

a   b

Fig. 1.18a, b   Parietal-occipital meningoencephalocele. Sagittal (**a**) and axial (**b**) images show a bone defect through which brain and meninges extend superficially.

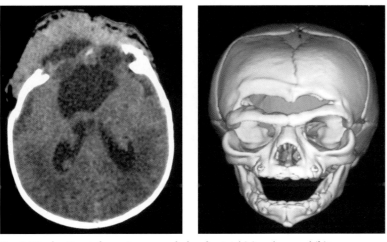

Fig. 1.19a, b Frontal meningoencephalocele. Axial (**a**) and coronal (**b**) images show a bone defect through which brain and meninges extend superficially.

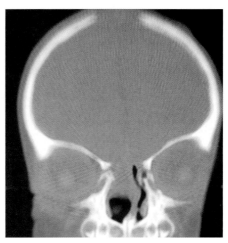

Fig. 1.20 Ethmoid meningocele. Coronal image shows a bone defect at the right cribriform plate with inferior extension of the dura.

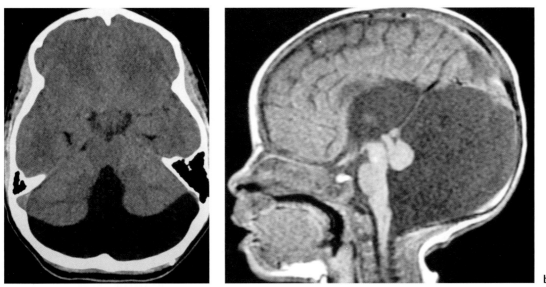

Fig. 1.21a, b Dandy-Walker malformation. Axial CT image (**a**) and sagittal T1-weighted MRI (**b**) show absence of the vermis and hypoplasia of the cerebellar hemispheres.

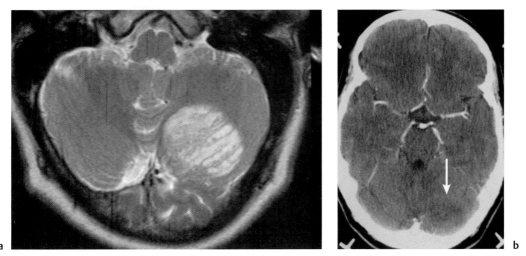

Fig. 1.22a, b Lhermitte-Duclos disease. Axial T1-weighted MRI (**a**) and axial postcontrast CT image (**b**) show a nonenhancing lesion in the left cerebellar hemisphere (arrow).

Table 1.2 Supratentorial intra-axial mass lesions

Lesions	CT Findings	Comments
Congenital		
Gray matter heterotopia	**Laminar heterotopia** appears as a band or bands of gray matter attenuation within the cerebral white matter **(see ▷ Fig. 1.7, p. 8)**. **Nodular heterotopia** appears as one or more nodules of gray matter attenuation along the ventricles **(see ▷ Fig. 1.8, p. 8)** or within the cerebral white matter **(see ▷ Fig. 1.9, p. 9)**. **Focal subcortical heterotopia** can be seen as irregular nodular or multinodular masslike zones with gray matter attenuation in subcortical regions **(see ▷ Fig. 1.9, p. 9)**.	Disorder of neuronal migration (weeks 7–22 of gestation) in which a collection or layer of neurons is located between the ventricles and cerebral cortex. Can have a bandlike (laminar) or nodular appearance isodense to gray matter; may be unilateral or bilateral. Associated with seizures and schizencephaly.
Unilateral hemimegalencephaly ▷ **Fig. 1.11, p. 9**	Nodular or multinodular region of gray matter heterotopia involving all or part of a cerebral hemisphere with associated enlargement of the ipsilateral lateral ventricle and hemisphere.	Neuronal migration disorder associated with hamartomatous overgrowth of a portion of or the whole hemisphere.
Neoplastic astrocytoma	**Low-grade astrocytoma:** Focal or diffuse mass lesion usually located in white matter with low to intermediate attenuation, with or without mild contrast enhancement. Minimal associated mass effect. ▷ **Fig. 1.23** **Juvenile pilocytic astrocytoma subtype:** Solid/cystic focal lesion with low to intermediate attenuation, usually with prominent contrast enhancement. Lesions located in the cerebellum, hypothalamus, adjacent to third or fourth ventricles, and brainstem. ▷ **Fig. 1.24** **Gliomatosis cerebri:** Infiltrative lesion with poorly defined margins with mass effect located in the white matter, with low to intermediate attenuation. Usually no contrast enhancement until late in disease. **Anaplastic astrocytoma:** Often irregularly marginated lesion located in white matter with low to intermediate attenuation, with or without contrast enhancement. ▷ **Fig. 1.25a, b**	**Low-grade astrocytoma:** Often occurs in children and adults (20–40 y). Tumors comprised of well-differentiated astrocytes. Association with neurofibromatosis type 1, 10-y survival; may become malignant. **Juvenile pilocytic astrocytoma subtype:** Common in children; usually favorable prognosis if totally resected. **Gliomatosis cerebri:** Diffusely infiltrating astrocytoma with relative preservation of underlying brain architecture. Imaging appearance may be more prognostic than histologic grade; ~2-y survival. **Anaplastic astrocytoma:** Intermediate between low-grade astrocytoma and glioblastoma multiforme; ~2-y survival.
Glioblastoma multiforme ▷ **Fig. 1.26**	Irregularly marginated mass lesion with necrosis or cyst, mixed low and intermediate attenuation, with or without hemorrhage, prominent heterogeneous contrast enhancement, peripheral edema; can cross the corpus callosum.	Most common primary central nervous system (CNS) tumor in adults, highly malignant neoplasms with necrosis and vascular proliferation, usually in patients older than 50 y; extent of lesion underestimated by CT; survival < 1 y.
Giant cell astrocytoma/ tuberous sclerosis ▷ **Fig. 1.27**	Circumscribed lesion located near the foramen of Monro with mixed low to intermediate attenuation, with or without cysts and/or calcifications, and heterogeneous contrast enhancement.	Subependymal hamartoma near the foramen of Monro; occurs in 15% of patients younger than 20 y with tuberous sclerosis. Slow-growing lesions can progressively cause obstruction of CSF flow through the foramen of Monro; long-term survival usual if resected.
Pleomorphic xanthoastrocytoma	Circumscribed supratentorial lesion involving the cerebral cortex and white matter, low to intermediate attenuation, with or without cyst(s), heterogeneous contrast enhancement, with or without enhancing mural nodule associated with cyst.	Rare type of astrocytoma occurring in young adults and children; associated with seizure history.

(continues on page 16)

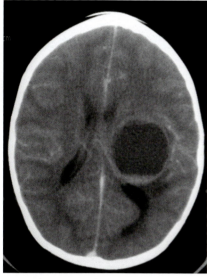

Fig. 1.23 Low-grade astrocytoma in a 5-year-old boy. Axial postcontrast image shows a circumscribed low-attenuation lesion with a thin margin of contrast enhancement in the left cerebral hemisphere.

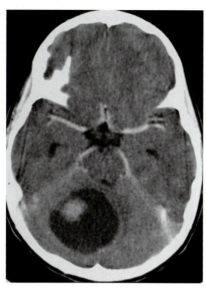

Fig. 1.24 Juvenile pilocytic astrocytoma. Axial postcontrast image shows a cystic lesion with a nodular zone of contrast enhancement in the right cerebellar hemisphere and vermis.

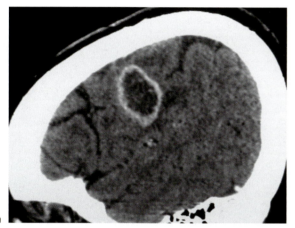

a

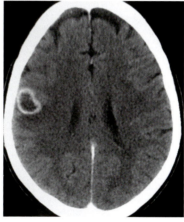

b

Fig. 1.25a, b Anaplastic astrocytoma in a 61-year-old woman. Sagittal (**a**) and axial (**b**) postcontrast images show a lesion in the right frontal lobe that has peripheral contrast enhancement.

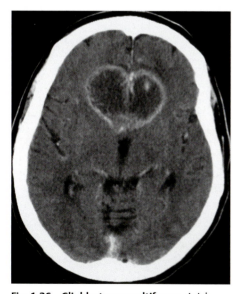

Fig. 1.26 Glioblastoma multiforme. Axial postcontrast image shows a contrast enhancing lesion involving both frontal lobes and corpus callosum.

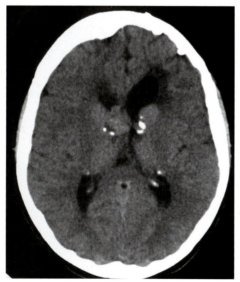

Fig. 1.27 Giant cell astrocytoma. Axial image in a patient with tuberous sclerosis shows a giant cell astrocytoma at the right foramen magnum, as well as multiple calcified ependymal hamartomas.

Table 1.2   (Cont.) Supratentorial intra-axial mass lesions

Lesions	CT Findings	Comments
Oligodendroglioma ▷ *Fig. 1.28a, b*	Circumscribed lesion with mixed low to intermediate attenuation, sites of clumplike calcification, and heterogeneous contrast enhancement; involves white matter and cerebral cortex; can cause chronic erosion of the inner table of the calvarium.	Uncommon slow-growing gliomas with usually mixed histologic patterns (astrocytoma, etc.). Usually in adults older than 35 y; 85% supratentorial. If low grade, 75% 5-y survival; higher grade lesions have a worse prognosis.
Central neurocytoma	Circumscribed lesion located at the margin of the lateral ventricle or septum pellucidum with intraventricular protrusion, heterogeneous low and intermediate attenuation, with or without calcifications and/or small cysts, heterogeneous contrast enhancement.	Rare tumors that have neuronal differentiation; imaging appearance similar to intraventricular oligodendrogliomas. Occur in young adults. Benign slow-growing lesions.
Ganglioglioma, ganglioneuroma, gangliocytoma	Circumscribed tumor, usually supratentorial, often temporal or frontal lobes, low to intermediate attenuation, with or without cysts, with or without contrast enhancement.	Ganglioglioma (contains glial and neuronal elements), ganglioneuroma (contains only ganglion cells). Uncommon tumors; seen in young adults younger than 30 y. Seizure presentation, slow-growing neoplasms. Gangliocytoma (contains only neuronal elements and dysplastic brain tissue). Favorable prognosis if completely resected.
Ependymoma ▷ *Fig. 1.29*	Circumscribed lobulated supratentorial lesion, often extraventricular, with or without cysts and/or calcifications, low to intermediate attenuation, variable contrast enhancement.	Occurs more commonly in children than adults, one third supratentorial, two-thirds infratentorial; 45% 5-y survival.
Pineal gland tumors ▷ *Fig. 1.30a, b*	Tumors often have intermediate attenuation to intermediate to slightly high attenuation, with contrast enhancement, with or without central and/or peripheral calcifications. Malignant tumors are often larger than benign pineal lesions (pineocytoma), as well as heterogeneous attenuation and contrast enhancement pattern, with or without leptomeningeal tumor.	Pineal gland tumors account for 8% of intracranial tumors in children and 1% of tumors in adults; 40% of tumors are germinomas, followed by pineoblastomas and pineocytomas, teratomas, choriocarcinomas, endodermal sinus tumors, astrocytomas, and metastatic tumors.
Hamartoma/tuberous sclerosis ▷ *Fig. 1.31*	Cortical-subcortical lesion with variable attenuation, calcifications in 50% of older children; contrast enhancement uncommon. **Subependymal hamartomas:** Small nodules located along and projecting into the lateral ventricles; calcification and contrast enhancement common.	Cortical and subependymal hamartomas are nonmalignant lesions associated with tuberous sclerosis. Tuberous sclerosis is an autosomal dominant disorder associated with hamartomas in multiple organs.
Hypothalamic hamartoma ▷ *Fig. 1.32a–c*	Sessile or pedunculated lesions at the tuber cinereum of the hypothalamus; often intermediate attenuation similar to gray matter; typically no contrast enhancement; rarely contain cystic and/or fatty portions.	Usually occur in children with isosexual precocious puberty (0–8 y) or seizures (gelastic or partial complex) in second decade; congenital/developmental heterotopia/hamartoma (nonneoplastic lesions).

(continues on page 18)

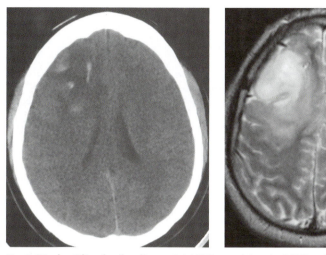

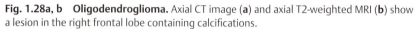

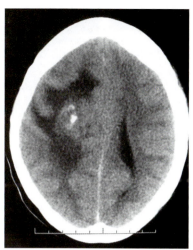

Fig. 1.28a, b   Oligodendroglioma. Axial CT image (**a**) and axial T2-weighted MRI (**b**) show a lesion in the right frontal lobe containing calcifications.

Fig. 1.29   Ependymoma. Axial image shows a lesion in the right frontal lobe that contains calcifications and is associated with adjacent axonal edema.

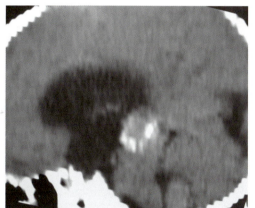

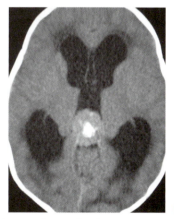

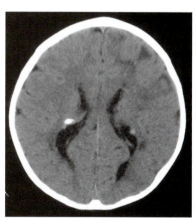

Fig. 1.30a, b   Pineoblastoma. Sagittal (**a**) and axial (**b**) images show a pineal tumor containing calcifications.

Fig. 1.31   Hamartoma. Axial image in a child with tuberous sclerosis shows multiple calcified and noncalcified ependymal hamartomas, as well as cortical tubers and zones of low attenuation in the white matter.

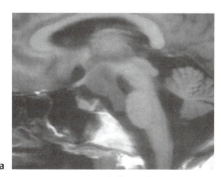

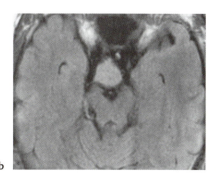

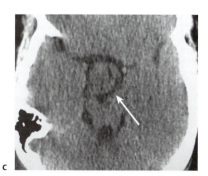

Fig. 1.32a–c   Hypothalamic hamartoma. Sagittal T1-weighted MRI (**a**), axial FLAIR MRI (**b**), and axial CT image (**c**) show a lesion involving the hypothalamus that extends inferiorly (arrow).

Table 1.2 (Cont.) Supratentorial intra-axial mass lesions

Lesions	CT Findings	Comments
Lipoma ▷ *Fig. 1.33*	**CT:** Lipomas have low attenuation equal to fat elsewhere in the field of view. **MRI:** Lipomas have signal isointense to subcutaneous fat on T1-weighted images (high signal) and on T2-weighted signals; signal suppression occurs with frequency-selective fat saturation techniques or with a short time to inversion recovery (STIR) method; typically no gadolinium contrast enhancement or peripheral edema. Lipomas can be nodular or curvilinear. Lipomas can occur in many locations, commonly the corpus callosum, cerebellopontine angle cistern, and tectal plate.	Benign fatty lesions resulting from congenital malformation often located in or near the midline; may contain calcifications and/or traversing blood vessels.
Primitive neuroectodermal tumor ▷ *Fig. 1.34a, b*	Circumscribed or invasive lesions, low to intermediate attenuation; variable contrast enhancement, frequent dissemination into the leptomeninges.	Highly malignant tumors located in the cerebrum, pineal gland, and cerebellum that frequently disseminate along CSF pathways.
Dysembryoplastic neuroepithelial tumor ▷ *Fig. 1.35a, b*	Circumscribed lesions involving the cerebral cortex and subcortical white matter, low to intermediate attenuation, with or without small cysts; usually no contrast enhancement.	Benign superficial lesions commonly located in the temporal or frontal lobes.
Lymphoma ▷ *Fig. 1.36*	**Primary CNS lymphoma:** Focal or infiltrating lesion located in the basal ganglia, periventricular regions, or posterior fossa/brainstem; low to intermediate attenuation; with or without hemorrhage/necrosis in immunocompromised patients; usually show contrast enhancement. Diffuse leptomeningeal contrast enhancement is another pattern of intracranial lymphoma.	Primary CNS lymphoma more common than secondary, usually in adults older than 40 y. B-cell lymphoma is more common than T-cell lymphoma. Increasing incidence related to the number of immunocompromised patients in the population. CT imaging features of primary and secondary lymphoma of brain overlap. Intracranial lymphoma can involve the leptomeninges in secondary lymphoma > primary lymphoma.
Hemangioblastoma	Circumscribed tumors usually located in the cerebellum and/or brainstem; small contrast-enhancing nodule with or without cyst or larger lesion with prominent heterogeneous enhancement with or without contrast-enhancing vessels within the lesion or at the periphery, Occasionally lesions have evidence of recent or remote hemorrhage.	Rarely occurs in cerebral hemispheres; occurs in adolescents and young and middle-aged adults. Lesions are typically multiple in patients with von Hippel-Lindau disease.
Metastases ▷ *Fig. 1.37a, b*	Circumscribed spheroid lesions in the brain; can have various intra-axial locations, often at gray-white matter junctions; usually low to intermediate attenuation; with or without hemorrhage, calcifications, or cysts; variable contrast enhancement. Often associated with adjacent low attenuation from axonal edema.	Represent ~33% of intracranial tumors, usually from extracranial primary neoplasm in adults older than 40 y. Primary tumor source: lung > breast > gastrointestinal (GI) > genitourinary (GU) > melanoma.
Neurocutaneous melanosis	Extra- or intra-axial lesions usually < 3 cm in diameter with irregular margins in the leptomeninges or brain parenchyma/brainstem (anterior temporal lobes, cerebellum, thalami, and inferior frontal lobes). **CT:** May show subtle hyperdensity secondary to increased melanin, with or without vermian hypoplasia, with or without arachnoid cysts, with or without Dandy-Walker malformation. **MRI:** Zones with intermediate to slightly high signal on T1-weighted images secondary to increased melanin, with gadolinium contrast enhancement; with or without vermian hypoplasia, with or without arachnoid cysts, with or without Dandy-Walker malformation.	Neuroectodermal dysplasia with proliferation of melanocytes in leptomeninges associated with large and/or numerous cutaneous nevi. May change into CNS melanoma.

(continues on page 20)

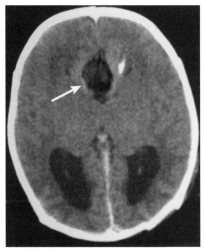

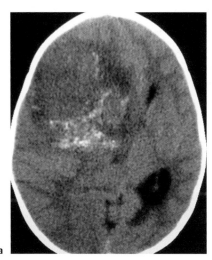

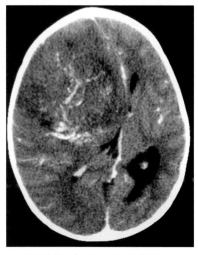

Fig. 1.33   Lipoma. Axial image shows a lipoma involving the anterior portion of the corpus callosum (arrow).

Fig. 1.34a, b   Primitive neuroectodermal tumor. Pre- (**a**) and postcontrast (**b**) images show a large tumor involving the anterior right frontal lobe containing calcifications that has associated mass effect and subfalcine herniation leftward. The lesion shows heterogeneous contrast enhancement.

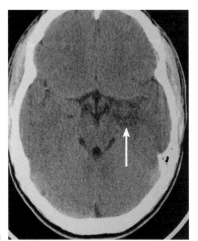

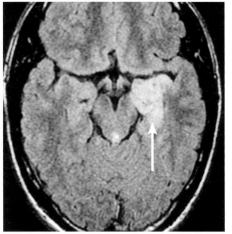

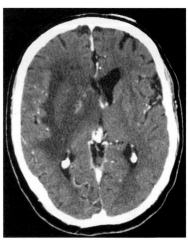

Fig. 1.35a, b   Dysembryoplastic neuroepithelial tumor. Axial CT image (**a**) and axial T2-weighted MRI (**b**) show a low-attenuation lesion with high T2 signal in the anteromedial left temporal lobe (arrows).

Fig. 1.36   Lymphoma. Axial postcontrast image shows a heterogeneous enhancing lesion in the right basal ganglia with associated mass effect.

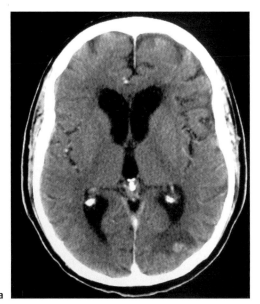

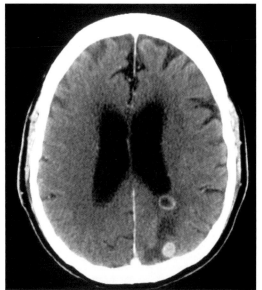

Fig. 1.37a, b   Metastases. Axial postcontrast images show ring and nodular enhancing metastatic lesions.

Table 1.2 (Cont.) Supratentorial intra-axial mass lesions

Lesions	CT Findings	Comments
Inflammatory		
Cerebritis ▷*Fig. 1.38a–c*	Poorly defined zone or focal area of decreased attenuation, minimal or no contrast enhancement; involves cerebral cortex and white matter for bacterial and fungal infections.	Focal infection/inflammation of brain tissue from bacteria or fungi, secondary to sinusitis, meningitis, surgery, hematogenous source (cardiac and other vascular shunts), and/or immunocompromised status. Can progress to abscess formation.
Pyogenic brain abscess ▷*Fig. 1.39a, b*	Circumscribed lesion with a central zone of low attenuation (with or without air-fluid level) surrounded by a thin rim of intermediate attenuation; peripheral poorly defined zone of decreased attenuation representing edema; ringlike contrast enhancement that is sometimes thicker laterally than medially.	Formation of brain abscess occurs 2 weeks after cerebritis with liquefaction and necrosis centrally surrounded by a capsule and peripheral edema. Can be multiple. Complication from meningitis and/or sinusitis, septicemia, trauma, surgery, or cardiac shunt.
Fungal brain abscess ▷*Fig. 1.40*	Findings can vary depending on organism; lesions occur in meninges and brain parenchyma; solid or cystic-appearing lesions with decreased attenuation, nodular or ring pattern of contrast enhancement, peripheral zone with decreased attenuation in brain lesions (edema).	Occur in immunocompromised or diabetic patients with resultant granulomas in meninges and brain parenchyma. *Cryptococcus* involves the basal meninges and extends along perivascular spaces into the basal ganglia; *Aspergillus* and *Mucor* spread via direct extension through the paranasal sinuses or hematogenously and invade blood vessels, resulting in hemorrhagic lesions and/or cerebral infarcts. Coccidioidomycosis usually involves the basal meninges.
Encephalitis ▷*Fig. 1.41*	Poorly defined zone or zones of decreased attenuation, minimal or no contrast enhancement; involves the cerebral cortex and/or white matter; minimal localized mass effect. Herpes simplex typically involves the temporal lobes/limbic system with or without hemorrhage; cytomegalovirus (CMV) usually in periventricular/subependymal locations. HIV often involves periatrial white matter.	Infection/inflammation of brain tissue from viruses, often seen in immunocompromised patients (e.g., herpes simplex, CMV, HIV, and progressive multifocal leukoencephalopathy) or immunocompetent patients (e.g., St. Louis encephalitis, eastern or western equine encephalitis, and Epstein-Barr virus).
Tuberculoma ▷*Fig. 1.42*	Intra-axial lesions in cerebral hemispheres, basal ganglia, and brainstem (adults) and cerebellum (children). Lesions can have decreased attenuation, central zone of low attenuation with a thin peripheral rim of intermediate attenuation; with solid or rim pattern of contrast enhancement; with or without calcification. **Meningeal lesions:** Nodular or cystic zones of basilar meningeal enhancement.	Occurs in immunocompromised patients and inhabitants of developing countries. Caseating intracranial granulomas via hematogenous dissemination; meninges > brain lesions.
Parasitic brain lesions		
Toxoplasmosis ▷*Fig. 1.43*	Single or multiple solid and/or cystic-appearing lesions located in basal ganglia and/or corticomedullary junctions in cerebral hemispheres, low to intermediate attenuation; nodular or rim pattern of contrast enhancement; with or without mild peripheral low attenuation (edema). Chronic phase: calcified granulomas.	Most common opportunistic CNS infection in patients with AIDS; caused by ingestion of food contaminated with parasites (*Toxoplasma gondii*). Can be seen as a congenital or neonatal infection (TORCH syndrome: toxoplasmosis, other agents, rubella, cytomegalovirus, herpes simplex).

(continues on page 22)

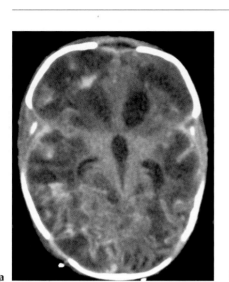
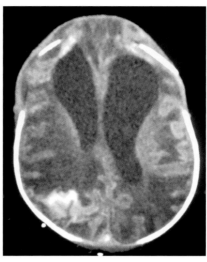
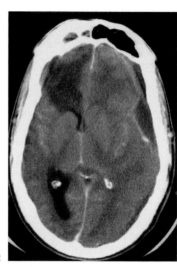

Fig. 1.38a–c Cerebritis. Postcontrast axial images (**a,b**) in a neonate show poorly defined zones of contrast enhancement involving the superficial portions of the brain with localized destruction and calcification. Axial postcontrast image (**c**) in a 35-year-old man shows cerebritis with low attenuation involving the right frontal lobe, as well as a left subdural empyema and right frontal sinusitis.

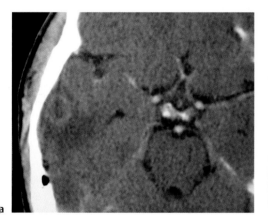
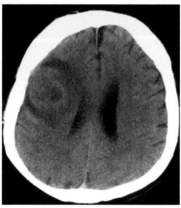
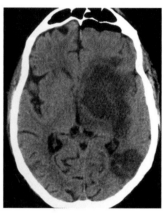

Fig. 1.39a, b Brain abscess, pyogenic. Axial postcontrast image (**a**) shows a ring-enhancing lesion in the right temporal lobe. Axial image (**b**) shows a ring-shaped lesion with low attenuation centrally and axonal edema peripheral to the abscess rim.

Fig. 1.40 Fungal brain abscess, *Aspergillus.* Axial image shows a poorly defined zone of decreased attenuation involving the left cerebral hemisphere.

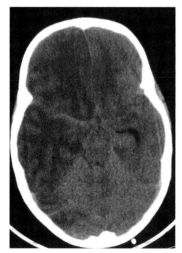
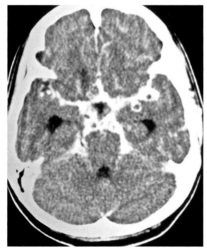
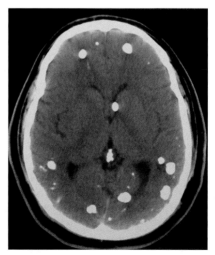

Fig. 1.41 Encephalitis, herpes type 1. Axial image shows poorly defined zones of decreased attenuation in the frontal and temporal lobes.

Fig. 1.42 Tuberculoma. Axial postcontrast image shows diffuse contrast enhancement in the basal meninges (basal meningitis), as well as a ring-enhancing lesion (tuberculoma) in the anterior left temporal lobe.

Fig. 1.43 Toxoplasmosis. Axial image shows multiple calcified (healed) granulomas.

Table 1.2 (Cont.) Supratentorial intra-axial mass lesions

Lesions	CT Findings	Comments
Cysticercosis ▷ *Fig. 1.44a, b*	Single or multiple cystic-appearing lesions in brain or meninges; acute/subacute phase: Low to intermediate attenuation, rim with or without nodular pattern of contrast enhancement, with or without peripheral low attenuation (edema). Chronic phase: calcified granulomas.	Caused by ingestion of ova (*Taenia solium*) in contaminated food (undercooked pork); involves meninges > brain parenchyma > ventricles.
Hydatid cyst	***Echinococcus granulosus:*** Single or rarely multiple cystic-appearing lesions with low attenuation surrounded by a thin wall; typically no contrast enhancement or peripheral edema unless superinfected; often located in vascular territory of the middle cerebral artery. ***Echinococcus multilocularis:*** Cystic (with or without multilocular) and/or solid lesions, central zone of intermediate attenuation surrounded by a slightly thickened rim, with contrast enhancement; peripheral zone of decreased attenuation (edema) and calcifications are common.	Caused by parasites *E. granulosus* (South America, Middle East, Australia, and New Zealand) and *E. multilocularis* (North America, Europe, Turkey, and China). CNS involvement in 2% of cases of hydatid infestation.
Inflammatory disorders		
Radiation necrosis	Focal lesion with or without mass effect or poorly defined zone of low to intermediate attenuation, with or without contrast enhancement involving tissue (gray matter and/or white matter) in field of treatment.	Usually occurs from 4 to 6 months to 10 y after radiation treatment; may be difficult to distinguish from neoplasm. Positron emission tomography (PET) and magnetic resonance spectroscopy might be helpful for evaluation.
Demyelinating disease: multiple sclerosis, acute disseminated encephalomyelitis (ADEM) ▷ *Fig. 1.45a–c*	Lesions located in cerebral or cerebellar white matter, brainstem, or basal ganglia; lesions usually have low to intermediate attenuation on CT. Zones of active demyelination may show contrast enhancement and mild localized swelling. **MRI:** Zones of low to intermediate signal on T1-weighted images and high signal on fluid attenuation inversion recovery (FLAIR) and T2-weighted images; with or without gadolinium contrast enhancement. Contrast enhancement can be ringlike or nodular, usually in acute/early subacute phase of demyelination. Lesions rarely can have associated mass effect simulating neoplasms.	Multiple sclerosis is the most common acquired demyelinating disease usually affecting women (peak age 20–40 y). Other demyelinating diseases include acute disseminated encephalomyelitis/immune mediated demyelination after viral infection; toxins (exogenous from environmental exposure or ingestion of alcohol, solvents, etc., or endogenous from metabolic disorders, e.g., leukodystrophies and mitochondrial encephalopathies), radiation injury, trauma, and vascular disease.
Sarcoidosis	Poorly marginated intra-axial zone with low to intermediate attenuation; usually shows contrast enhancement with localized mass effect and peripheral edema. Often associated with contrast enhancement in the leptomeninges.	Multisystem noncaseating granulomatous disease of uncertain cause that can involve the CNS in 5% to 15% of cases. Associated with severe neurologic deficits if untreated.

(continues on page 24)

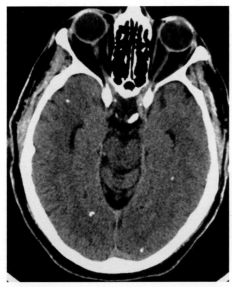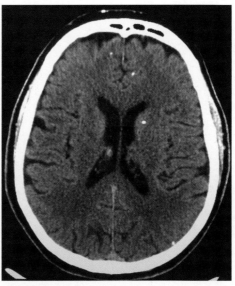

Fig. 1.44a, b Cysticercosis. Axial images show multiple calcified (healed) granulomas.

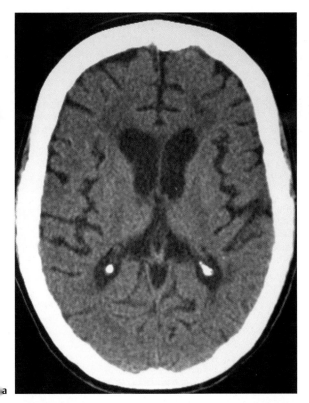

a

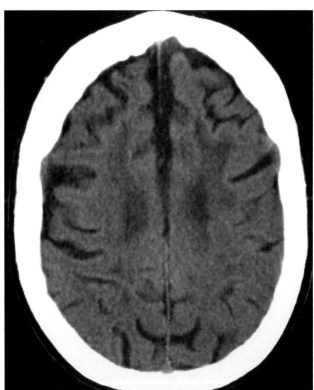

b

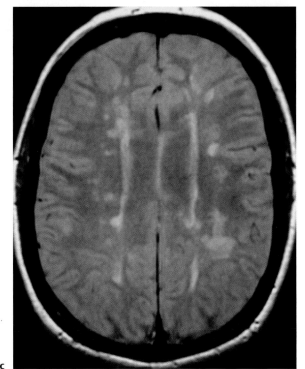

c

Fig. 1.45a–c   Multiple sclerosis. Axial CT images (**a,b**) and axial fluid attenuation inversion recovery (FLAIR) MRI (**c**) show multiple zones of decreased CT attenuation and increased T2 signal in the cerebral white matter.

Table 1.2   (Cont.) Supratentorial intra-axial mass lesions

Lesions	CT Findings	Comments
Hemorrhage		
Intracerebral hemorrhage/ hematoma	Attenuation of the hematoma depends on its age, size, location, hematocrit, hemoglobin oxidation state, clot retraction, and extent of edema. **Hyperacute phase (4–6 h):** Hemoglobin primarily as diamagnetic oxyhemoglobin (iron Fe^{2+} state). **CT:** High attenuation on CT. **MRI:** Intermediate signal on T1-weighted images and slightly high signal on T2-weighted images. **Acute phase (12–48 h):** Hemoglobin primarily as paramagnetic deoxyhemoglobin (iron, Fe^{2+} state). **CT:** High attenuation in acute clot directly related to hematocrit, hemoglobin concentration, and high protein concentration. Hematocrit in acute clot approaches 90%. ▷ *Fig. 1.46* ▷ *Fig. 1.47* ▷ *Fig. 1.48* ▷ *Fig. 1.49, p. 27* **MRI:** Intermediate signal on T1-weighted images, low signal on T2-weighted images, surrounded by a peripheral zone of high T2 signal (edema). **Early subacute phase (> 2 d):** Hemoglobin becomes oxidized to the iron Fe^{3+} state, methemoglobin, which is strongly paramagnetic. **CT:** High attenuation. **MRI:** When methemoglobin is initially intracellular, the hematoma has high signal on T1-weighted images progressing from peripheral to central and low signal on T2-weighted images, surrounded by a zone of high T2 signal (edema). When methemoglobin eventually becomes primarily extra-cellular, the hematoma has high signal on T1-weighted images and high signal on T2-weighted images. **Late subacute phase (> 7 d to 6 wk):** Intracerebral hematomas decrease 1.5 HU per day. Hematomas become isodense to hypodense; peripheral contrast enhancement from blood–brain barrier breakdown and vascularized capsule. **Chronic phase:** Hemoglobin as extracellular methemoglobin is progressively degraded to hemosiderin. **CT:** Chronic hematomas have low attenuation with localized encephalomalacia. Zones with high attenuation represent new sites of rebleeding. **MRI:** Hematoma progresses from a lesion with high signal on T1- and T2-weighted images, with a peripheral rim of low signal on T2-weighted images (hemosiderin), to predominant hemosiderin composition and low signal on T2-weighted images.	Can result from trauma, ruptured aneurysms or vascular malformations, coagulopathy, hypertension, adverse drug reaction, amyloid angiopathy, hemorrhagic transformation of cerebral infarction, metastases, abscesses, and viral infections (herpes simplex, CMV).
Cerebral contusions ▷ *Fig. 1.47*	**CT:** Appearance of contusions is initially one of focal hemorrhage involving the cerebral cortex and subcortical white matter. Contusions eventually appear as focal superficial encephalomalacia zones.	Contusions are superficial brain injuries involving the cerebral cortex and subcortical white matter that result from skull fracture and/or acceleration/deceleration trauma to the inner table of the skull. Often involve the anterior portions of the temporal and frontal lobes and inferior portions of the frontal lobes.
Metastases ▷ *Fig. 1.48a, b*	The CT appearance of a hemorrhagic metastatic lesion is one of an intracerebral hematoma involving a portion or all of the neoplasm, usually associated with peripheral edema (decreased attenuation), often multiple; with contrast enhancement in nonhemorrhagic portions of lesions.	Metastatic intra-axial tumors associated with hemorrhage include bronchogenic carcinoma, renal cell carcinoma, melanoma, choriocarcinoma, and thyroid carcinoma. May be difficult to distinguish from hemorrhage related to other etiologies, such as vascular malformations and amyloid angiopathy.

(continues on page 26)

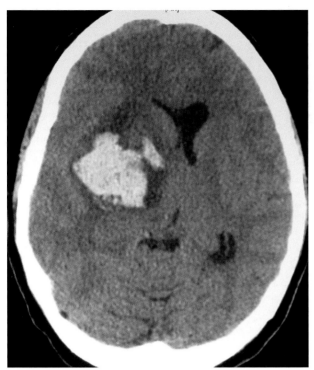

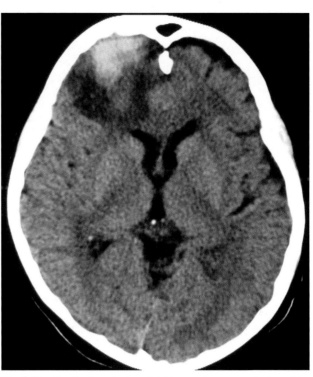

Fig. 1.46   Intracerebral hematoma. Axial image shows an acute hypertensive-related hemorrhage with high attenuation in the right basal ganglia.

Fig. 1.47   Cerebral contusion. Axial image shows a contusion with high-attenuation hemorrhage involving the anterior portion of the right frontal lobe.

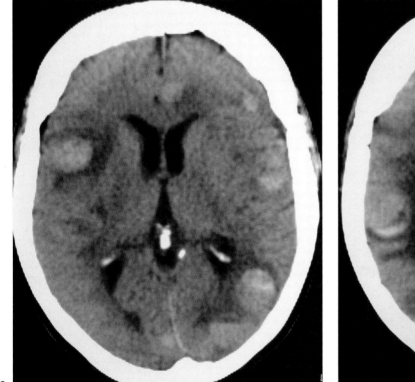

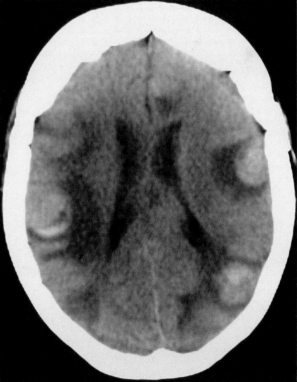

a

b

Fig. 1.48a, b   Hemorrhagic metastases from melanoma. Axial images show multiple hemorrhagic metastases.

Table 1.2   (Cont.) Supratentorial intra-axial mass lesions

Lesions	CT Findings	Comments
Vascular		
Arteriovenous malformation (AVM)	Lesions with irregular margins that can be located in the brain parenchyma (pia, dura, or both locations). **CT:** AVMs contain multiple tortuous tubular vessels that have intermediate or slightly increased attenuation that shows contrast enhancement. Calcifications occur in 30% of cases. Computed tomography angiography (CTA) shows arteries, veins, and nidus of AVM even when there is an intra-axial hemorrhage. ▷ *Fig. 1.49a, b* **MRI:** Serpiginous flow voids on T1- and T2-weighted images secondary to patent arteries with high blood flow, as well as thrombosed vessels with variable signal, areas of hemorrhage in various phases, calcifications, and gliosis. The venous portions often show gadolinium enhancement. Gradient echo MRI shows flow-related enhancement (high signal) in patent arteries and veins of the AVM. MRA using time of flight (TOF) or phase contrast techniques can provide additional detailed information about the nidus, feeding arteries and draining veins, and presence of associated aneurysms. Usually not associated with mass effect unless there is recent hemorrhage or venous occlusion.	Supratentorial AVMs occur more frequently (80%–90%) than infratentorial AVMs (10%–20%). Annual risk of hemorrhage. AVMs can be sporadic, congenital, or associated with a history of trauma. Multiple AVMs can be seen in syndromes: Rendu-Osler-Weber (AVMs in brain and lungs, and mucosal, capillary telangiectasias); Wyburn-Mason (AVMs in brain and retina, with cutaneous nevi).
Cavernous hemangioma	Single or multiple multilobulated intra-axial lesions. **CT:** Lesions have intermediate to slightly increased attenuation, with or without calcifications.	Supratentorial cavernous angiomas occur more frequently than infratentorial lesions. Can be located in many different locations, multiple lesions > 50%.
Venous angioma	**CT:** No abnormality or small, slightly hyperdense zone prior to contrast administration. Contrast enhancement seen in a slightly prominent vein draining a collection of small veins. **MRI:** On postcontrast T1-weighted images, venous angiomas are seen as a gadolinium contrast-enhancing transcortical vein draining a collection of small medullary veins (caput medusae). The draining vein can be seen as a signal void on T2-weighted images.	Considered an anomalous venous formation typically not associated with hemorrhage; usually an incidental finding except when associated with cavernous hemangioma.
Neuroepithelial cyst	**CT:** Well-circumscribed cysts with low attenuation, no contrast enhancement. **MRI:** Cysts have low signal on T1-weighted images and high signal on T2-weighted images, thin walls, no gadolinium contrast enhancement or peripheral edema.	Cyst walls have histopathologic features similar to epithelium, neuroepithelial cysts; located in choroid plexus > choroidal fissure > ventricles > brain parenchyma.
Porencephalic cyst ▷ *Fig. 1.50*	**CT:** Irregular, relatively well-circumscribed zone with low attenuation, no contrast enhancement. **MRI:** Zone of low signal on T1-weighted images and high signal on T2-weighted images similar to CSF, surrounded by poorly defined thin zone of high T2 signal in adjacent brain tissue; no gadolinium contrast enhancement or peripheral edema.	Cysts represent remote sites of brain injury (trauma, infarction, infection, or hemorrhage) with evolution into a cystic zone with CSF attenuation and MRI signal characteristics surrounded by gliosis in adjacent brain parenchyma. Gliosis (high T2 signal) allows differentiation from schizencephaly.

(continues on page 28)

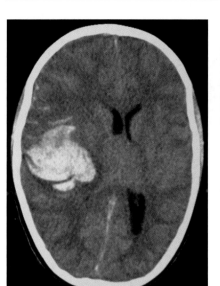

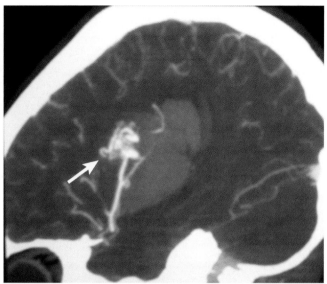

a

b

Fig. 1.49a, b Hemorrhage from an arteriovenous malformation (AVM). Axial CT image (**a**) shows an intra-axial hemorrhage in the right cerebral hemisphere. CTA image (**b**) shows an AVM as the cause of the hemorrhage (arrow).

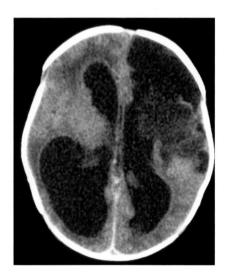

Fig. 1.50 Porencephalic cyst. Axial CT image in a neonate shows a porencephalic cyst in the anterior left frontal lobe that developed from a hemorrhage in this region.

Table 1.2   (Cont.) Supratentorial intra-axial mass lesions

Lesions	CT Findings	Comments
Cerebral infarction related to occlusion of large vessels	CT and MRI features of cerebral and cerebellar infarcts depend on the age of the infarct relative to the time of examination. **Hyperacute (< 12 h):** **CT:** No abnormality (50%); decreased attenuation and blurring of lentiform nuclei; hyperdense artery up to 50%. **MRI:** Localized edema; usually isointense signal to normal brain on T1- and T2-weighted images. Diffusion-weighted images can show positive findings related to decreased apparent diffusion coefficients secondary to cytotoxic edema, absence of arterial flow void, or arterial enhancement in the vascular distribution of the infarct. **Acute (12–24 h):** **CT:** Zones with decreased attenuation in basal ganglia, blurring of junction between cerebral cortex and white matter, sulcal effacement. **MRI:** Intermediate signal on T1-weighted images, high signal on T2-weighted images, localized edema. Signal abnormalities commonly involve the cerebral cortex and subcortical white matter and/or basal ganglia. **Early subacute (24 h–3 d):** **CT:** Localized swelling at sites with low attenuation involving gray and white matter (often wedge shaped), with or without hemorrhage **MRI:** Zones with low to intermediate signal on T1-weighted images, high signal on T2-weighted images, localized edema, with or without hemorrhage, with or without gadolinium contrast enhancement. **Late subacute (4 d–2 wk):** **CT:** Localized swelling increases and then decreases; low attenuation at lesion can become more prominent; with or without gyral contrast enhancement. **MRI:** Low to intermediate signal on T1-weighted images, high signal on T2-weighted images, edema/mass effect diminishing, with or without hemorrhage, with or without contrast enhancement. **2 weeks to 2 months:** **CT:** with or without Gyral contrast enhancement, localized mass effect resolves. **MRI:** Low to intermediate signal on T1-weighted images, high signal on T2-weighted images; edema resolves; with or without hemorrhage, with or without enhancement eventually declines. **> 2 months:** **CT:** Zone of low attenuation associated with encephalomalacia. **MRI:** Low signal on T1-weighted images, high signal on T2-weighted images, encephalomalacic changes, with or without calcification, hemosiderin. ▷ *Fig. 1.51a–d*	Cerebral infarcts usually result from occlusive vascular disease involving large, medium, or small arteries. Vascular occlusion may be secondary to atheromatous arterial disease, cardiogenic emboli, neoplastic encasement, hypercoagulable states, dissection, or congenital anomalies. Cerebral infarcts usually result from arterial occlusion involving specific vascular territories, although they occasionally occur from metabolic disorders (mitochondrial encephalopathies, etc.) or intracranial venous occlusion (thrombophlebitis, hypercoagulable states, dehydration, etc.), which do not correspond to arterial distributions.

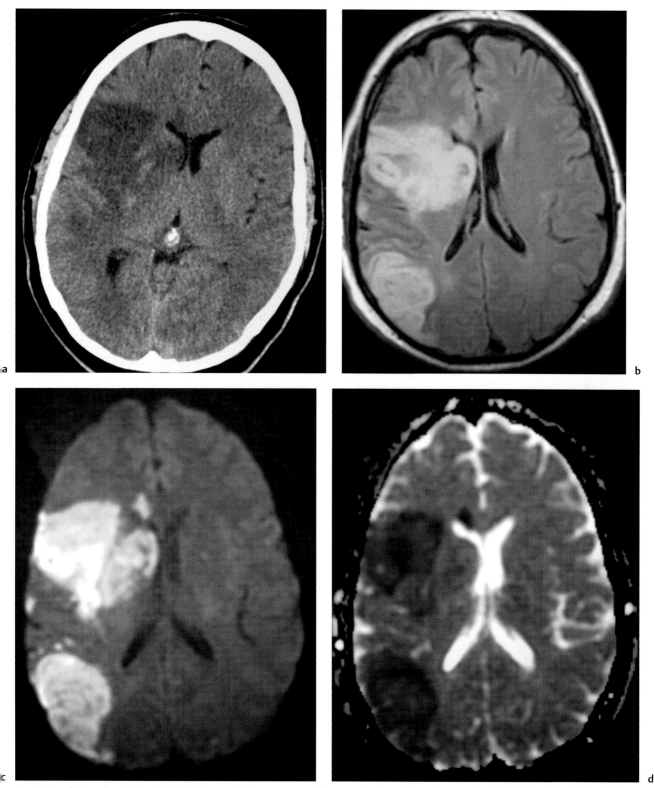

Fig. 1.51a–d   Cerebral infarct. Axial CT image (**a**) shows a zone of decreased attenuation in the vascular distribution of the right middle cerebral artery. Axial FLAIR MRI (**b**), axial diffusion-weighted MRI (**c**), and apparent diffusion coefficient (ADC) map (**d**) show high T2 signal and restricted diffusion at the site of a recent cerebral infarct.

Table 1.3   Supratentorial extra-axial lesions

Lesions	CT Findings	Comments
Neoplastic		
Meningioma ▷ *Fig. 1.52a–c*	Extra-axial dural-based lesions, well-circumscribed, supra->infratentorial, parasagittal > convexity > sphenoid ridge > parasellar > posterior fossa > optic nerve sheath > intraventricular; intermediate attenuation, usually prominent contrast enhancement; with or without calcifications, with or without hyperostosis of adjacent bone.	Most common extra-axial tumor, usually benign neoplasms; typically occurs in adults (> 40 y), women > men; multiple meningiomas seen with neurofibromatosis type II; can result in compression of adjacent brain parenchyma, encasement of arteries, and compression of dural venous sinuses; rarely invasive/malignant types.
Hemangiopericytoma ▷ *Fig. 1.53a, b*	Extra-axial mass lesions, often well circumscribed; intermediate attenuation, prominent contrast enhancement (may resemble meningiomas); with or without associated erosive bone changes, with or without calcifications.	Rare neoplasms in young adults (men > women); sometimes referred to as angioblastic meningioma or meningeal hemangiopericytoma; arise from vascular cells/pericytes; frequency of metastases > meningiomas.
Metastatic tumor ▷ *Fig. 1.54*	Single or multiple well-circumscribed or poorly defined lesions involving the skull, dura, leptomeninges, and/or choroid plexus; usually radiolucent in bone; may also be sclerotic, with or without extraosseous tumor extension, usually with contrast enhancement, with or without compression of neural tissue or vessels. Leptomeningeal tumor often best seen on postcontrast images.	Metastatic tumor may have variable destructive or infiltrative changes involving single or multiple sites of involvement.
Neurocutaneous melanosis	Extra- or intra-axial lesions usually < 3 cm in diameter with irregular margins in the leptomeninges or brain parenchyma/brainstem (anterior temporal lobes, cerebellum, thalami, and inferior frontal lobes) with isodense or slightly increased attenuation secondary to increased melanin; with or without vermian hypoplasia, with or without arachnoid cysts, with or without Dandy-Walker malformation.	Neuroectodermal dysplasia with proliferation of melanocytes in leptomeninges associated with large and/or numerous cutaneous nevi. May change into CNS melanoma.
Germinoma ▷ *Fig. 1.55a, b*	Circumscribed tumors with or without disseminated disease; pineal region > suprasellar region > third ventricle/basal ganglia; low to intermediate attenuation, with or without cystic-like regions; usually with contrast enhancement of tumor and leptomeninges (if disseminated).	Most common type of germ cell tumor, occurs in males > females (10–30 y); usually midline neoplasms.

(continues on page 32)

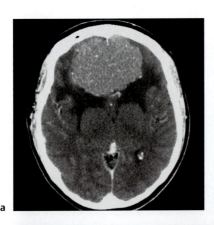
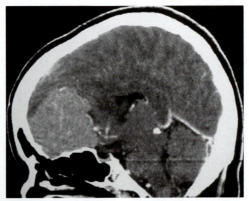

a   b

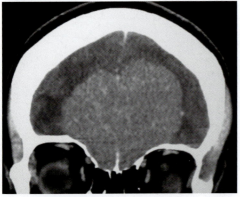

c

Fig. 1.52a–c   Meningioma. Axial (**a**), sagittal (**b**), and coronal (**c**) postcontrast images show a large contrast-enhancing extra-axial lesion arising from the dura along the olfactory groove.

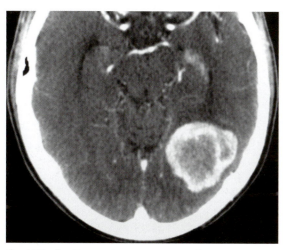
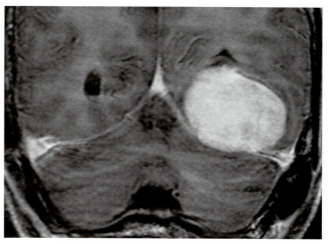

Fig. 1.53a, b Hemangiopericytoma. Axial postcontrast CT image (**a**) and coronal postcontrast T1-weighted image (**b**) show a contrast-enhancing lesion from the left tentorium.

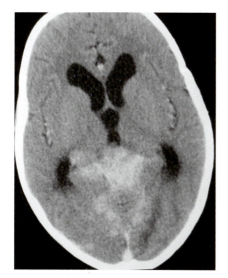

Fig. 1.54 Metastases. Pineoblastoma in a 4-year-old girl. Axial image shows abnormal contrast enhancement in the pineal recess and leptomeninges from tumor dissemination.

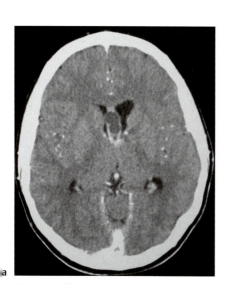
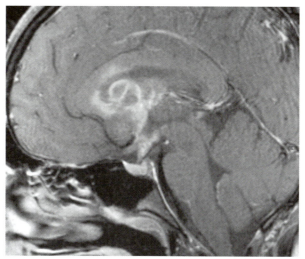

Fig. 1.55a, b Germinoma. Axial CT image (**a**) and sagittal postcontrast T1-weighted MRI (**b**) image show a poorly defined contrast-enhancing lesion in the suprasellar cistern and third and lateral ventricles.

Table 1.3 (Cont.) Supratentorial extra-axial lesions

Lesions	CT Findings	Comments
Teratoma ▷ *Fig. 1.56*	Circumscribed lesions; pineal region > suprasellar region > third ventricle; variable low, intermediate, and/or high attenuation; with or without contrast enhancement. May contain calcifications, as well as fatty components that can cause chemical meningitis if ruptured.	Second most common type of germ cell tumors; occurs in children, males > females; benign or malignant types, composed of derivatives of ectoderm, mesoderm, and/or endoderm.
Pituitary adenoma ▷ *Fig. 1.57a, b*	**Microadenomas (< 10 mm):** Commonly have low to intermediate attenuation; with or without cyst; with or without hemorrhage; with or without necrosis; typically enhance less than normal pituitary tissue; often best seen with dynamic early phase imaging. **Macroadenomas (> 10 mm):** Commonly have intermediate attenuation, with or without necrosis, with or without cyst, with or without hemorrhage; usually show contrast enhancement, extension into suprasellar cistern with waist at diaphragma sella, with or without extension into cavernous sinus; occasionally invades skull base.	Common benign slow-growing tumors representing ~50% of sellar/parasellar neoplasms in adults. Can be associated with endocrine abnormalities related to oversecretion of hormones (prolactin > nonsecretory type > growth hormone > ACTH > others). Prolactinomas: women > men; growth hormone tumors: men > women.
Craniopharyngioma ▷ *Fig. 1.58a, b*	Circumscribed lobulated lesions; both suprasellar and intrasellar location > suprasellar > intrasellar; variable low, intermediate, and/or high attenuation; with or without nodular or rim contrast enhancement. May contain cysts, lipid components, and calcifications.	Usually histologically benign but locally aggressive lesions arising from squamous epithelial rests along the Rathke cleft, occurs in children (peak age 5–15 y) and adults (> 40 y), males = females.
Choroid plexus papilloma or carcinoma ▷ *Fig. 1.59* ▷ *Fig. 1.60*	Circumscribed and/or lobulated lesions with papillary projections, intermediate attenuation, usually prominent contrast enhancement, with or without calcifications. Locations: atrium of lateral ventricle (children) > fourth ventricle (adults), rarely other locations such as third ventricle; associated with hydrocephalus.	Rare intracranial neoplasms; CT features of choroid plexus carcinoma and papilloma may overlap; both histologic types can disseminate along CSF pathways. Carcinomas often invade brain tissue and are usually larger than papillomas. Carcinomas may have heterogeneous mixed attenuation, with or without hemorrhage, with or without brain invasion.
Lymphoma	Single or multiple well-circumscribed or poorly defined lesions involving the skull, dura, and/or leptomeninges; low to intermediate attenuation; usually with contrast enhancement, with or without bone destruction. Leptomeningeal tumor often best seen on postcontrast images.	Extra-axial lymphoma may have variable destructive or infiltrative changes involving single or multiple sites of involvement.
Myeloma/plasmacytoma	Multiple (myeloma) or single (plasmacytoma) well-circumscribed or poorly defined lesions involving the skull and dura; low to intermediate attenuation; usually with contrast enhancement, with bone destruction.	Myeloma may have variable destructive or infiltrative changes involving the axial and/or appendicular skeleton.
Chordoma	Well-circumscribed lobulated lesions along the dorsal surface of the clivus, vertebral bodies, or sacrum, with localized bone destruction. **CT:** Lesions have low to intermediate attenuation, with or without calcifications from destroyed bone carried away by tumor, with contrast enhancement.	Rare, slow-growing tumors. Detailed anatomical display of extension of chordomas by CT and MRI is important for planning of surgical approaches.

(continues on page 34)

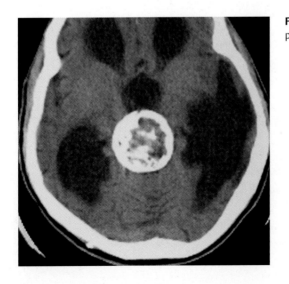

Fig. 1.56 Teratoma. Axial image shows a calcified lesion involving the pineal gland.

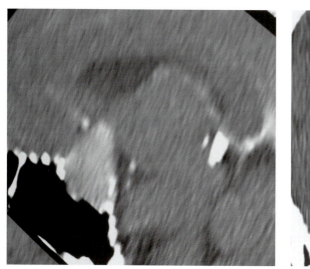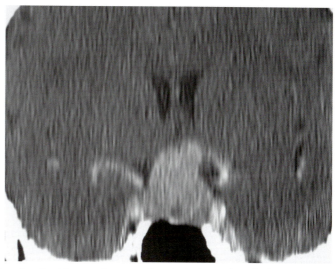

Fig. 1.57a, b Pituitary adenoma. Sagittal (**a**) and coronal (**b**) postcontrast images show an enhancing lesion in the sella that extends into the suprasellar cistern.

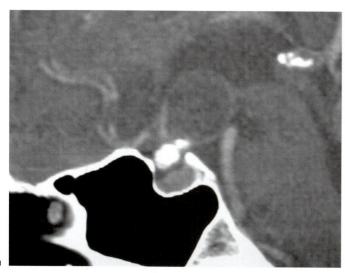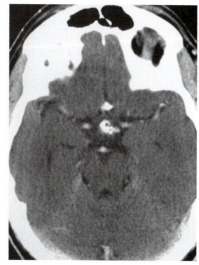

Fig. 1.58a, b Craniopharyngioma. Sagittal (**a**) and axial (**b**) postcontrast images show a lesion in the suprasellar cistern that contains soft tissue attenuation, cystic zones, and calcifications.

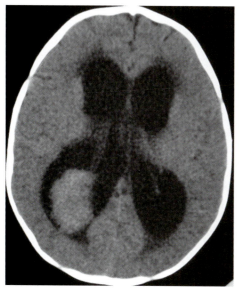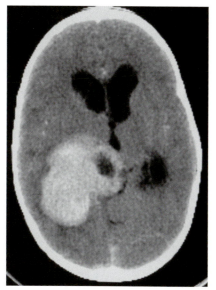

Fig. 1.59 Choroid plexus papilloma in a 3-year-old girl. Axial image shows a lobulated lesion in the right lateral ventricle.

Fig. 1.60 Choroid plexus carcinoma in a 17-month-old girl. Axial postcontrast image shows a large enhancing lesion in the right lateral ventricle.

Table 1.3 (Cont.) Supratentorial extra-axial lesions

Lesions	CT Findings	Comments
	MRI: Lesions have low to intermediate signal on T1-weighted images, high signal on T2-weighted images, with gadolinium enhancement (usually heterogeneous); locally invasive associated with bone erosion/destruction, encasement of vessels and nerves; skull base–clivus common location, usually in the midline. ▷ *Fig. 1.61a–d*	
Chondrosarcoma	Lobulated lesions with bone destruction at synchondroses. **CT:** Lesions have low-intermediate attenuation associated with localized bone destruction, with or without chondroid matrix calcifications, with contrast enhancement. **MRI:** Lesions have low to intermediate signal on T1-weighted images, high signal on T2-weighted images with or without matrix mineralization, low signal on T2-weighted images with gadolinium enhancement (usually heterogeneous); locally invasive associated with bone erosion/destruction, encasement of vessels and nerves; skull base–petro-occipital synchondrosis common location, usually off midline. ▷ *Fig. 1.62*	Rare, slow-growing tumors. Detailed anatomical display of extension of chondrosarcomas by CT and MRI is important for planning of surgical approaches.
Osteogenic sarcoma	Destructive bone lesions involving the skull base. **CT:** Lesions have low to intermediate attenuation associated with localized bone destruction, with or without osteoid matrix calcifications, with contrast enhancement. **MRI:** Lesions have low to intermediate signal on T1-weighted images, mixed low, intermediate, or high signal on T2-weighted images usually with matrix mineralization/ossification; low signal on T2-weighted images with gadolinium-enhancement (usually heterogeneous). ▷ *Fig. 1.63a–c*	Rare lesions involving the endochondral bone-forming portions of the skull base; more common than chondrosarcomas and Ewing sarcoma; locally invasive, high metastatic potential. Occurs in children as primary tumors and adults (associated with Paget disease, irradiated bone, chronic osteomyelitis, osteoblastoma, giant cell tumor, and fibrous dysplasia).

(continues on page 36)

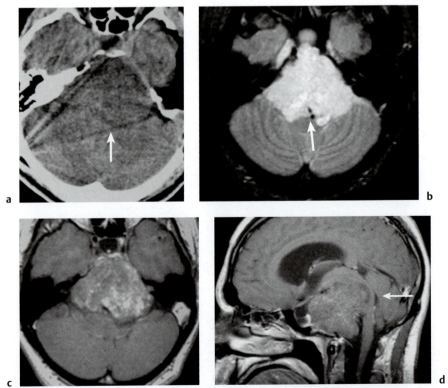

Fig. 1.61a–d Chordoma. Axial CT image (**a**) shows a large lesion along the endocranial surface of the clivus that has high signal on the T2-weighted MRI (**b**) and shows heterogeneous contrast enhancement on the axial (**c**) and sagittal (**d**) T1-weighted MRI (arrows).

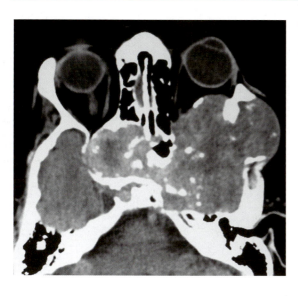

Fig. 1.62 Chondrosarcoma. Axial image shows a large destructive lesion involving the skull base and orbits that contains ring- and arc-shaped chondroid calcifications.

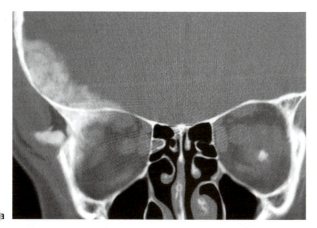

a

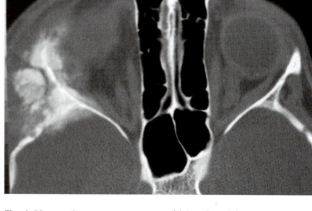

b

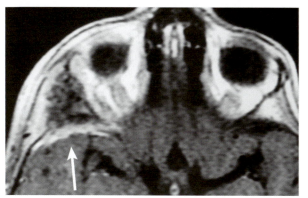

c

Fig. 1.63a–c Osteosarcoma. Coronal (**a**) and axial (**b**) CT images show a destructive lesion involving the right frontal bone associated with extraosseous tumor containing malignant ossifications. The lesion shows heterogeneous contrast enhancement on the postcontrast axial T1-weighted image (**c**) (arrow).

Table 1.3   (Cont.) Supratentorial extra-axial lesions

Lesions	CT Findings	Comments
Ewing sarcoma	Destructive lesions involving the skull base; low to intermediate attenuation, with or without matrix mineralization, with contrast enhancement (usually heterogeneous).	Rare lesions involving the skull base; usually occur between the ages of 5 and 30 y, males > females; locally invasive; high metastatic potential.
Sinonasal squamous cell carcinoma ▷ *Fig. 1.64a, b*	Destructive lesions in the nasal cavity, paranasal sinuses, and nasopharynx; with or without intracranial extension via bone destruction or perineural spread; intermediate attenuation; mild contrast enhancement; large lesions (with or without necrosis and/or hemorrhage).	Occurs in adults usually older than 55 y, males > females; associated with occupational or other exposure to nickel, chromium, mustard gas, radium, and manufacture of wood products.
Adenoid cystic carcinoma	Destructive lesions in the paranasal sinuses, nasal cavity, and nasopharynx, with or without intracranial extension via bone destruction or perineural spread; intermediate attenuation; variable mild, moderate, or prominent contrast enhancement.	Lesions account for 10% of sinonasal tumors; arise in any location within sinonasal cavities; usually occur in adults older than 30 y.
Esthesioneuroblastoma	Locally destructive lesions with low to intermediate attenuation, with prominent contrast enhancement. Location: superior nasal cavity and ethmoid air cells with occasional extension into the other paranasal sinuses, orbits, anterior cranial fossa, and cavernous sinuses.	Tumors also referred to as olfactory neuroblastoma; arise from olfactory epithelium in the superior nasal cavity. Occurs in adolescents and adults, males > females.
Hemorrhagic		
Epidural hematoma	Biconvex extra-axial hematoma located between the skull and dura; displaced dura has intermediate attenuation. The attenuation of the hematoma itself depends on its age, size, hematocrit, and oxygen tension; with or without edema involving the displaced brain parenchyma; with or without subfalcine, uncal herniation. **Hyperacute hematoma:** Biconvex hematoma with high or mixed intermediate and high attenuation. **Acute hematoma:** High or mixed intermediate and high attenuation. ▷ *Fig. 1.65a, b* **Subacute hematoma:** High, or mixed low, intermediate, and high attenuation.	Epidural hematomas usually result from trauma/tearing of an epidural artery (often the middle meningeal artery) or dural venous sinus; epidural hematomas do not cross cranial sutures; with or without skull fracture.
Subdural hematoma	Crescentic extra-axial hematoma located in the potential space between the inner margin of the dura and outer margin of the arachnoid membrane. The attenuation of the hematoma depends on its age, size, hematocrit, and oxygen tension; with or without edema involving the displaced brain parenchyma; with or without subfalcine, uncal herniation. **Hyperacute hematoma:** High and/or high and intermediate attenuation. **Acute hematoma:** High and/or high and intermediate attenuation. ▷ *Fig. 1.66* **Subacute hematoma:** Intermediate attenuation; may be isodense to brain; with or without contrast enhancement of organizing neomembrane and adjacent blood vessels. **Chronic hematoma:** Variable, often low to intermediate attenuation; with or without contrast enhancement of organizing neomembrane. Mixed intermediate to high attenuation can result if rebleeding occurs into chronic collection.	Subdural hematomas usually result from trauma/stretching/tearing of cortical veins where they enter the subdural space to drain into dural venous sinuses; subdural hematomas do cross sites of cranial sutures; with or without skull fracture.
Subarachnoid hemorrhage	**CT:** Acute subarachnoid hemorrhage typically appears as poorly defined zone with high attenuation in the leptomeninges within the sulci and basal cisterns. Usually becomes isodense or hypodense after 1 week unless there is rebleeding. ▷ *Fig. 1.67a, b* **MRI:** May not be seen on T1- or T2-weighted images, although it may have intermediate to slightly high signal on FLAIR images.	Extravasated blood in the subarachnoid space can result from ruptured arterial aneurysms or dural venous sinuses, vascular malformations, hypertensive hemorrhages, trauma, cerebral infarcts, coagulopathy, etc.

(continues on page 38)

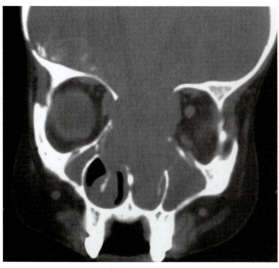
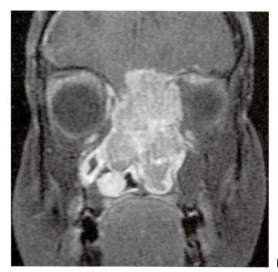

Fig. 1.64a, b Sinonasal squamous cell carcinoma. Coronal CT image (**a**) and coronal postcontrast T1-weighted fat-suppressed MRI (**b**) show a destructive lesion involving the nasal cavity, ethmoid sinuses, skull base, and dura.

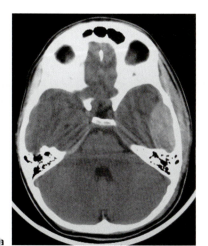
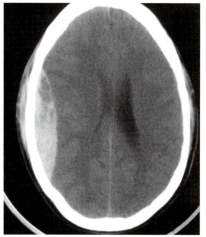
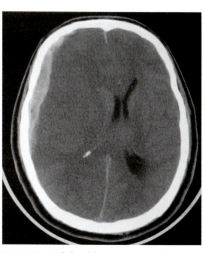

Fig. 1.65a, b Epidural hematoma. Axial images show an epidural hematoma on the left (**a**) and another example of one on the right (**b**).

Fig. 1.66 Subdural hematoma. Axial image showing right-sided subdural hematoma with mass effect causing subfalcine herniation to the left.

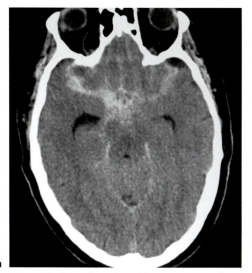
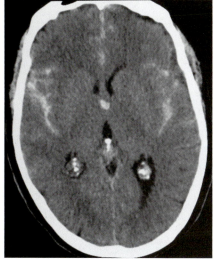

Fig. 1.67a, b Subarachnoid hematoma. Axial images show diffuse high attenuation in the subarachnoid space.

Table 1.3   (Cont.) Supratentorial extra-axial lesions

Lesions	CT Findings	Comments
Inflammatory		
Subdural/epidural abscess, empyema ▷ *Fig. 1.68* ▷ *Fig. 1.69a, b*	Epidural or subdural collections with low attenuation, linear peripheral zones of contrast enhancement.	Often results from complications related to sinusitis (usually frontal), meningitis, otitis media, ventricular shunts, or surgery. Can be associated with venous sinus thrombosis and venous cerebral or cerebellar infarctions, cerebritis, or brain abscess; mortality 30%.
Leptomeningeal infection/ inflammation ▷ *Fig. 1.70a, b*	Single or multiple nodular enhancing lesions and/or focal or diffuse abnormal subarachnoid enhancement. Leptomeningeal inflammation often best seen on postcontrast images.	Contrast enhancement in the intracranial subarachnoid space (leptomeninges) usually is associated with significant pathology (inflammation and/or infection vs neoplasm). Inflammation and/ or infection of the leptomeninges can result from pyogenic, fungal, or parasitic diseases as well as tuberculosis. Neurosarcoid results in granulomatous disease in the leptomeninges producing similar patterns of subarachnoid enhancement.
Eosinophilic granuloma ▷ *Fig. 1.71a–c*	Single or multiple circumscribed soft tissue lesions in the marrow of the skull associated with focal bony destruction/erosion with extension extracranially, intracranially, or both. Lesions usually have low to intermediate attenuation, with contrast enhancement, with or without enhancement of the adjacent dura.	Single lesion commonly seen in males > females younger than 20 y; proliferation of histiocytes in medullary cavity with localized destruction of bone with extension in adjacent soft tissues. Multiple lesions associated with syndromes such as Letterer-Siwe disease (lymphadenopathy hepatosplenomegaly), in children younger than 2 y; Hand-Schüller-Christian disease (lymphadenopathy, exophthalmos, diabetes insipidus) in children 5 to 10 y old.
Sarcoidosis	Poorly marginated nodular and/or diffuse contrast enhancement in the leptomeninges; may be associated with intra-axial lesions with contrast enhancement, edema, and localized mass effect.	Multisystem noncaseating granulomatous disease of uncertain cause that can involve the CNS in 5% to 15% of cases. Associated with severe neurologic deficits if untreated.

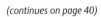

(continues on page 40)

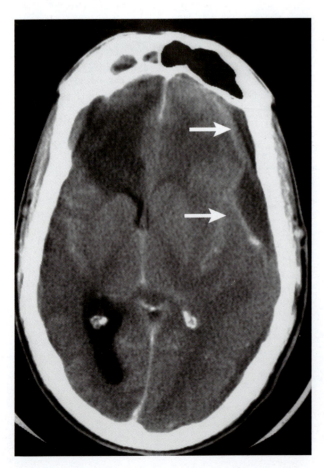

Fig. 1.68   Subdural empyema. Axial postcontrast CT image shows a left subdural empyema (arrows) and low attenuation in the right frontal lobe from cerebritis.

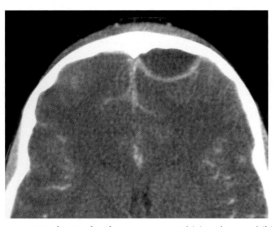
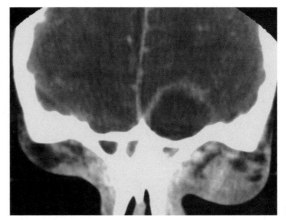

Fig. 1.69a, b **Epidural empyema.** Axial (**a**) and coronal (**b**) postcontrast images show a left frontal epidural empyema.

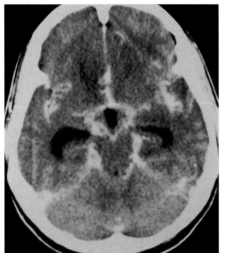
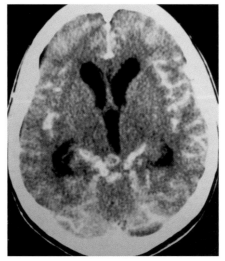

Fig. 1.70a, b **Leptomeningeal infection, tuberculosis.** Axial postcontrast images show diffuse contrast enhancement in the subarachnoid space from meningitis.

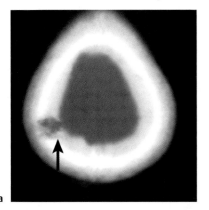
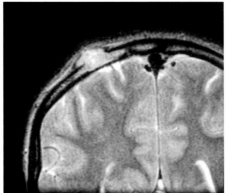

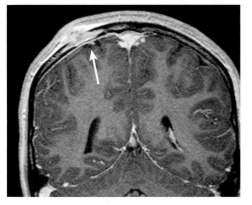

Fig. 1.71a–c **Eosinophilic granuloma.** Axial CT image (**a**) shows an osteolytic skull lesion. Coronal T2-weighted MRI (**b**) shows a destructive lesion involving the marrow and both inner and outer tables of the skull. The lesion shows contrast enhancement with dural involvement on the coronal postcontrast T1-weighted MRI (**c**) (arrows).

Table 1.3 (Cont.) Supratentorial extra-axial lesions

Lesions	CT Findings	Comments
Other		
Vascular		
Arterial aneurysm	**Saccular aneurysm:** Focal, well-circumscribed zone of intermediate to high attenuation; with contrast enhancement in nonthrombosed portion of aneurysm; easily visualized on CTA. ▷ *Fig 1.72a, b* **Giant aneurysm:** Focal, well-circumscribed structure with layers of low, intermediate, and/or high attenuation secondary to layers of thrombus of different ages, as well as a zone of contrast enhancement representing a patent lumen if present; with or without wall calcifications present. ▷ *Fig. 1.73a, b* **Fusiform aneurysm:** Elongated and ectatic arteries with intermediate attenuation, with or without calcifications, variable contrast enhancement related to turbulent or slowed blood flow or partial/complete thrombosis. **Dissecting aneurysms:** The involved arterial wall is thickened and has intermediate to high attenuation, and the lumen may be occluded or narrowed. CTA shows contrast enhancement of the patent narrowed lumen.	Abnormal fusiform or focal dilation of artery secondary to acquired/degenerative etiology, polycystic disease, connective tissue disease, atherosclerosis, trauma, infection (mycotic), oncotic, AVM, vasculitis, and drugs. Focal aneurysms are also referred to as saccular aneurysms, which typically occur at arterial bifurcations, and are multiple in 20% of cases. Saccular aneurysms > 2.5 cm in diameter are referred to as giant aneurysms. Fusiform aneurysms are often related to atherosclerosis or collagen vascular disease (e.g., Marfan syndrome and Ehlers-Danlos syndrome). Dissecting aneurysms: hemorrhage occurs in the arterial wall from incidental or significant trauma.
Dural AVM	Dural AVMs contain multiple tortuous contrast-enhancing vessels on CTA at the site of a recanalizing thrombosed dural venous sinus. Usually not associated with mass effect unless there is recent hemorrhage or venous occlusion.	Dural AVMs are usually acquired lesions resulting from thrombosis or occlusion of an intracranial venous sinus with subsequent recanalization resulting in direct arterial to venous sinus communications. Transverse, sigmoid venous sinuses > cavernous sinuses > straight, superior sagittal sinuses.
Vein of Galen aneurysm ▷ *Fig. 1.74*	Multiple tortuous contrast-enhancing vessels involving choroidal and thalamoperforate arteries, internal cerebral veins, vein of Galen (aneurysmal formation), straight and transverse venous sinuses, and other adjacent veins and arteries. The venous portions often show contrast enhancement. CTA shows contrast enhancement in patent portions of the vascular malformation.	Heterogeneous group of vascular malformations with arteriovenous shunts and dilated deep venous structures draining into and from an enlarged vein of Galen, with or without hydrocephalus, with or without hemorrhage, with or without macrocephaly, with or without parenchymal vascular malformation components, with or without seizures, high-output congestive heart failure in neonates.

(continues on page 42)

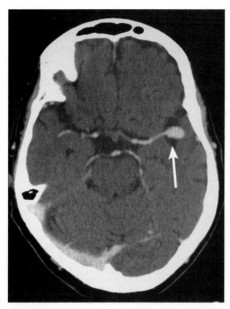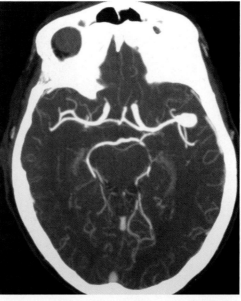

Fig. 1.72a, b Saccular arterial aneurysm. Axial postcontrast image (**a**) shows a nodular zone of enhancement at the lateral portion of the left middle cerebral artery (arrow) that is also seen on the CTA image (**b**).

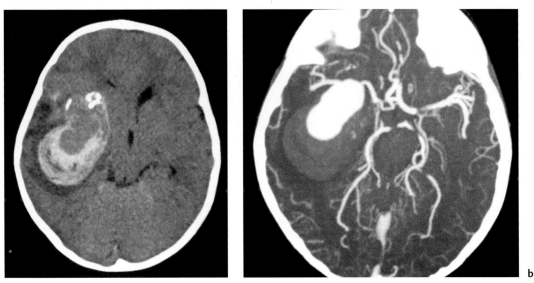

Fig. 1.73a, b   Giant aneurysm. Axial precontrast image (**a**) shows a large lesion with mural hemorrhage at the lateral portion of the right middle cerebral artery. The CTA image (**b**) shows the patent enhancing portion of the giant aneurysm.

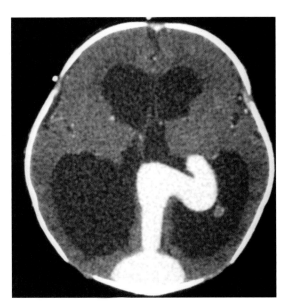

Fig. 1.74   Vein of Galen aneurysm. Axial postcontrast image shows an abnormally enlarged enhancing vein of Galen and confluence of the straight, superior sagittal, and transverse venous sinuses.

Table 1.3 (Cont.) Supratentorial extra-axial lesions

Lesions	CT Findings	Comments
Nonneoplastic lesions		
Arachnoid cyst ▷ *Fig. 1.75a–c*	Well-circumscribed extra-axial lesions with low attenuation, no contrast enhancement. Commonly located in the anterior middle cranial fossa > suprasellar/quadrigeminal > frontal convexities > posterior cranial fossa.	Nonneoplastic congenital, developmental, or acquired extra-axial lesions filled with CSF; usually mild mass effect on adjacent brain; supratentorial > infratentorial locations; males > females; with or without related clinical symptoms.
Rathke cleft cyst	Well-circumscribed lesion with variable low, intermediate, or high attenuation, no contrast enhancement; 25% have intermediate MRI signal, without gadolinium contrast enhancement centrally, with or without thin peripheral enhancement. Lesion locations: 50% intrasellar, 25% suprasellar, 25% intra- and suprasellar.	Uncommon sella/juxtasellar benign cystic lesion containing fluid with variable amounts of protein, mucopolysaccharide, and/or cholesterol; arise from epithelial rests of the craniopharyngeal duct.
Leptomeningeal cyst	Well-circumscribed extra-axial lesions with low attenuation similar to CSF, no contrast enhancement. Associated with erosion of the adjacent skull.	Nonneoplastic extra-axial lesions filled with CSF thought to be secondary to trauma with dural tear/skull fracture, usually mild mass effect on adjacent brain with progressive erosion of adjacent skull; occasionally presents as a scalp lesion; occurs in children > adults.
Pineal cyst ▷ *Fig. 1.76*	Well-circumscribed extra-axial lesions with low attenuation similar to CSF; no central enhancement, thin linear peripheral contrast enhancement; rarely atypical appearance with proteinaceous contents; intermediate, slightly high attenuation.	Common and usually incidental nonneoplastic cyst in pineal gland.
Colloid cyst ▷ *Fig. 1.77*	Well-circumscribed spheroid lesions located at the anterior portion of the third ventricle; variable attenuation (low, intermediate or high), no contrast enhancement.	Common presentation of headaches and intermittent hydrocephalus, removal leads to cure.
Lipoma	Lipomas have CT attenuation similar to subcutaneous fat; typically no contrast enhancement or peripheral edema.	Benign fatty lesions resulting from congenital malformation often located in or near the midline; may contain calcifications and/or traversing blood vessels.
Epidermoid ▷ *Fig. 1.78a–c*	Well-circumscribed spheroid or multilobulated extra-axial ectodermal inclusion cystic lesions with low to intermediate attenuation that is often similar to CSF. Often insinuate along CSF pathways; chronic deformation of adjacent neural tissue (brainstem, brain parenchyma). Commonly located in posterior cranial fossa (cerebellopontine angle cistern) > parasellar/middle cranial fossa.	Nonneoplastic congenital or acquired extra-axial off-midline lesions filled with desquamated cells and keratinaceous debris; usually mild mass effect on adjacent brain, infratentorial > supratentorial locations. Adults: men = women; with or without related clinical symptoms.
Dermoid	Well-circumscribed spheroid or multilobulated extra-axial lesions, usually with low attenuation, with or without fat/fluid or fluid/debris levels. Can cause chemical meningitis if dermoid cyst ruptures into the subarachnoid space. Commonly located at or near midline; supratentorial > infratentorial.	Nonneoplastic congenital or acquired ectodermal inclusion cystic lesions filled with lipid material, cholesterol, desquamated cells, and keratinaceous debris; usually mild mass effect on adjacent brain. Adults: men slightly > women; with or without related clinical symptoms.

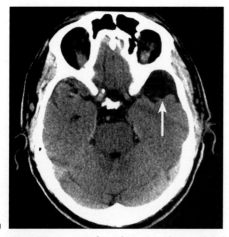 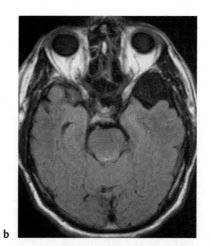 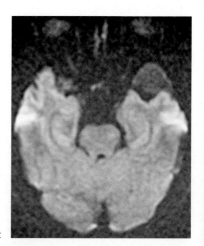

a   b   c

Fig. 1.75a–c Arachnoid cyst. Axial image (**a**) show an extra-axial zone with cerebrospinal fluid (CSF) attenuation in the anterior portion of the left middle cranial fossa (arrow), which has low signal on the axial FLAIR image (**b**) and diffusion-weighted MRI (**c**).

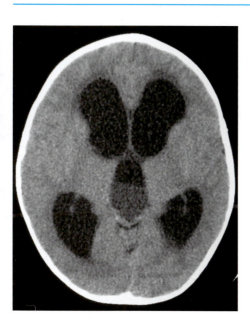

Fig. 1.76   Pineal cyst. Axial image shows a large pineal cyst causing hydrocephalus.

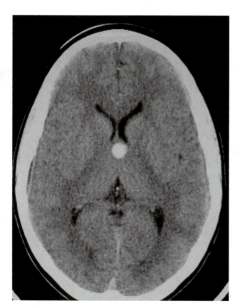

Fig. 1.77   Colloid cyst. Axial image shows a small nodular lesion in the anterior portion of the third ventricle that has high attenuation.

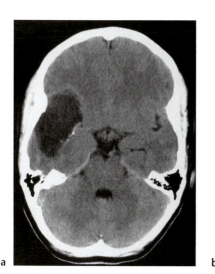

a

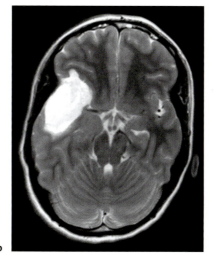

b

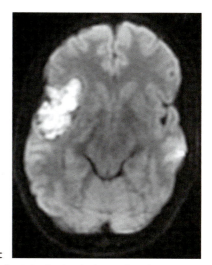

c

Fig. 1.78a–c   Epidermoid. Axial image (**a**) shows an extra-axial lesion with low attenuation on the right that has high signal on the T2-weighted MRI (**b**) and axial diffusion-weighted MRI (**c**).

Table 1.4   Intra-axial lesions in the posterior cranial fossa (infratentorial)

Lesions	CT Findings	Comments
Congenital		
Chiari I malformation ▷ *Fig. 1.16, p. 11*	Cerebellar tonsils extend > 5 mm below the foramen magnum in adults, 6 mm in children younger than 10 y. Syringohydromyelia in 20% to 40%, hydrocephalus in 25%, basilar impression in 25%. Less common association: Klippel-Feil syndrome, atlanto-occipital assimilation.	Cerebellar tonsillar ectopia. Most common anomaly of CNS. Not associated with myelomeningocele.
Chiari II malformation (Arnold-Chiari) ▷ *Fig. 1.17, p. 11*	Small posterior cranial fossa with gaping foramen magnum through which there is an inferiorly positioned vermis associated with a cervicomedullary kink. Beaked dorsal margin of the tectal plate. Myelomeningoceles in nearly all patients. Hydrocephalus and syringomyelia common. Dilated lateral ventricles posteriorly (colpocephaly).	Complex malformation of the hindbrain and posterior cranial fossa related to disorder of neural tube closure at the lumbosacral region where there is either a myelocele or a myelomeningocele.
Dandy-Walker malformation ▷ *Fig. 1.21, p. 13*	Vermian aplasia or severe hypoplasia, communication of fourth ventricle with retrocerebellar cyst, enlarged posterior fossa, high position of tentorium and transverse venous sinuses. Hydrocephalus common. Associated with other anomalies such as dysgenesis of the corpus callosum, gray matter heterotopia, schizencephaly, holoprosencephaly, and cephaloceles.	Abnormal formation of roof of fourth ventricle with absent or near incomplete formation of cerebellar vermis.
Dandy-Walker variant	Mild vermian hypoplasia with communication of posteroinferior portion of the fourth ventricle with cisterna magna. No associated enlargement of the posterior cranial fossa.	Occasionally associated with hydrocephalus, dysgenesis of corpus callosum, gray matter heterotopia, and other anomalies.
Lhermitte-Duclos disease ▷ *Fig. 1.22, p. 13*	**CT:** Poorly defined zone with low to intermediate attenuation, no contrast enhancement. **MRI:** Poorly defined zone of low T1 signal, high T2 signal with laminated appearance and localized mass effect located in the cerebellum. No contrast enhancement.	Uncommon cerebellar dysplasia with gross thickening of cerebellar folia and disorganized cellular structure. Also known as dysplastic gangliocytoma.
Joubert syndrome	Small dysplastic vermis with midline cleft between apposing cerebellar hemispheres; "molar tooth" axial appearance from small midbrain and thickened superior cerebellar peduncles.	Malformation with hypoplasia of vermis, dysplasia and heterotopia of cerebellar nuclei, lack of decussation of superior cerebellar peduncles, and near complete absence of medullary pyramids. Clinical: ataxia, mental retardation, and abnormal eye movements.
Rhombencephalosynapsis	Dysmorphic cerebellum with no apparent separation of cerebellar hemispheres, aplasia, or severe hypoplasia of vermis.	Malformation with fusion of cerebellar hemispheres, dentate nuclei, and superior cerebellar peduncles; absent or hypoplastic vermis. Clinical: truncal ataxia, cerebral palsy, mental retardation, and seizures.
Lipoma	Lipomas have CT attenuation similar to fat and MRI signal isointense to subcutaneous fat on T1-weighted images (high signal), and T2-weighted images; signal suppression occurs with frequency on selective fat saturation techniques or with a STIR method, typically no gadolinium enhancement or peripheral edema. Lipomas can be nodular or curvilinear. Common locations in the posterior cranial fossa include cerebellopontine angle cisterns and tectal plate.	Benign fatty lesions resulting from congenital malformation often located in or near the midline; may contain calcifications and/or traversing blood vessels.
Neoplastic		
Intra-axial lesions		
Astrocytoma	**Low-grade astrocytoma:** Focal or diffuse mass lesion usually located in cerebellar white matter or brainstem. **CT:** Low to intermediate attenuation lesion; with or without contrast enhancement. ▷ *Fig. 1.79a–c* **MRI:** Lesion with low to intermediate signal on T1-weighted images, high signal on T2-weighted images, with or without mild gadolinium contrast enhancement. Minimal associated mass effect.	**Low-grade astrocytoma:** Often occurs in children and adults (20–40 y). Tumors comprised of well-differentiated astrocytes. Association with neurofibromatosis type 1; 10-y survival; may become malignant.

(continues on page 46)

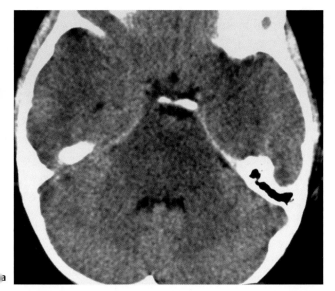

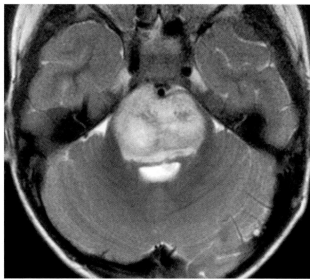

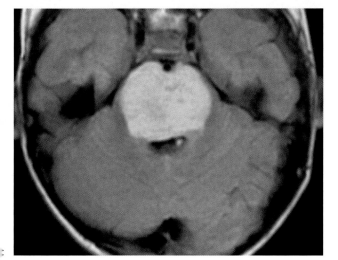

Fig. 1.79a–c   Pontine glioma. Axial CT image (**a**) shows the tumor in the pons to have decreased attenuation. High signal is seen on the axial T2-weighted MRI (**b**) and FLAIR MRI (**c**).

Table 1.4   (Cont.) Intra-axial lesions in the posterior cranial fossa (infratentorial)

Lesions	CT Findings	Comments
	Juvenile pilocytic astrocytoma, subtype: **CT:** Solid/cystic focal lesion with low to intermediate attenuation, with contrast enhancement. ▷ *Fig. 1.80* **MRI:** Low to intermediate signal on T1-weighted images, high signal on T2-weighted images, usually with prominent gadolinium contrast enhancement. Lesions located in cerebellum, brainstem.	**Juvenile pilocytic astrocytoma, subtype:** Common in children; usually favorable prognosis if totally resected.
	Gliomatosis cerebri: **CT:** Infiltrative lesions with low to intermediate attenuation and poorly defined margins with mass effect, located in the white matter. **MRI:** Lesion has low to intermediate signal on T1-weighted images and high signal on T2-weighted images; usually no gadolinium-contrast enhancement until late in disease.	**Gliomatosis cerebri:** Diffusely infiltrating astrocytoma with relative preservation of underlying brain architecture. Imaging appearance may be more prognostic than histologic grade; ~2-y survival.
	Anaplastic astrocytoma: **CT:** Irregularly marginated lesions located in white matter with low to intermediate attenuation, mass effect, with or without contrast enhancement. **MRI:** Lesions often have low to intermediate signal on T1-weighted images, high signal on T2-weighted images, with or without gadolinium-contrast enhancement. ▷ *Fig. 1.81a–c*	**Anaplastic astrocytoma:** Intermediate between low-grade astrocytoma and glioblastoma multiforme; ~2-y survival.
Medulloblastoma (primitive neuroectodermal tumor of the cerebellum) ▷ *Fig. 1.82a–d*	**CT:** Circumscribed or invasive lesions, intermediate to slightly increased attenuation, variable contrast enhancement. **MRI:** Circumscribed or invasive lesions, low to intermediate signal on T1-weighted images, intermediate to high signal on T2-weighted images; variable gadolinium contrast enhancement; frequent dissemination into the leptomeninges.	Highly malignant tumors that frequently disseminate along CSF pathways.

(continues on page 48)

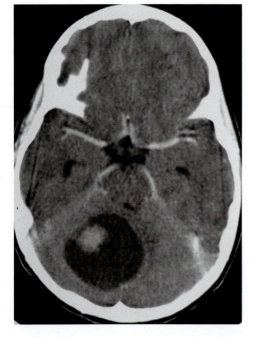

Fig. 1.80   Juvenile pilocytic astrocytoma. Axial postcontrast image shows a cystic lesion with a contrast-enhancing mural nodule in the right cerebellar hemisphere and vermis.

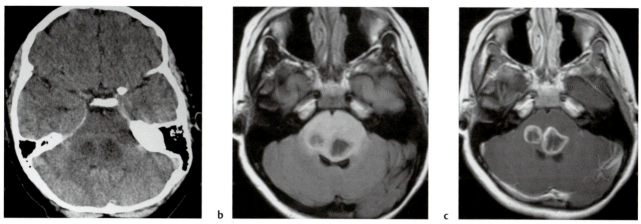

Fig. 1.81a–c Anaplastic astrocytoma. Axial CT image (**a**) shows the pontine tumor to have decreased attenuation, with heterogeneous high signal on the axial FLAIR MRI (**b**). The lesion shows irregular ring patterns of contrast enhancement on the axial T1-weighted MRI (**c**).

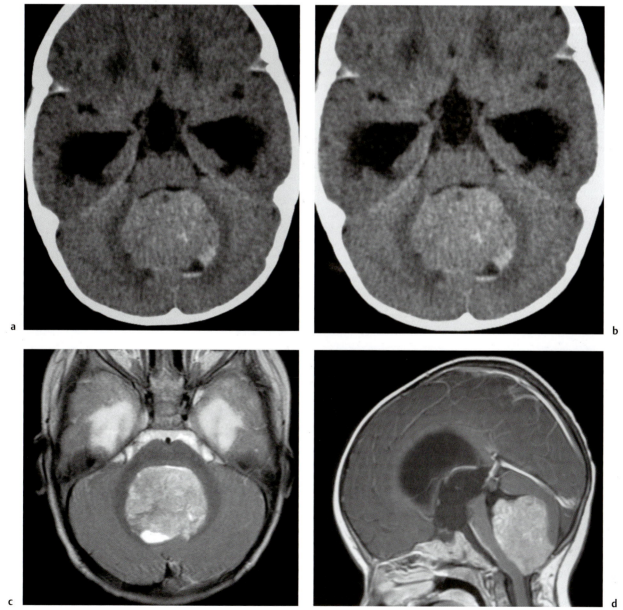

Fig. 1.82a–d Medulloblastoma. Precontrast axial image (**a**) shows a tumor in the vermis with slightly high attenuation causing compression of the fourth ventricle and resulting in hydrocephalus. The tumor shows contrast enhancement on the CT image (**b**), has high signal on the axial T2-weighted MRI (**c**), and shows contrast enhancement on the sagittal T1-weighted MRI (**d**).

Table 1.4   (Cont.) Intra-axial lesions in the posterior cranial fossa (infratentorial)

Lesions	CT Findings	Comments
Ependymoma ▷ *Fig. 1.83a, b*	**CT:** Circumscribed spheroid or lobulated infratentorial lesion, usually in the fourth ventricle, with or without cysts and/or calcifications, low to intermediate attenuation, variable contrast enhancement. **MRI:** Circumscribed spheroid or lobulated infratentorial lesion, usually in the fourth ventricle, with or without cysts and/or calcifications; low to intermediate signal on T1-weighted images, intermediate to high signal on T2-weighted images; variable gadolinium contrast enhancement, with or without extension through the foramina of Luschka and Magendie.	Occurs more commonly in children than adults; two thirds infratentorial, one third supratentorial.
Atypical teratoid/ rhabdoid tumors ▷ *Fig. 1.84a, b*	**CT:** Circumscribed or poorly defined mass lesions with intermediate attenuation, with or without zones of high attenuation from hemorrhage, usually prominent contrast enhancement with or without heterogeneous pattern. **MRI:** Circumscribed mass lesions with intermediate signal on T1-weighted images, with or without zones of high signal from hemorrhage on T1-weighted images; variable mixed low, intermediate, and/or high signal on T2-weighted images; usually prominent gadolinium enhancement with or without heterogeneous pattern.	Rare malignant tumors involving the CNS usually occurring in the first decade. Histologically appear as solid tumors with or without necrotic areas, similar to malignant rhabdoid tumors of the kidney. Associated with a poor prognosis.
Metastases ▷ *Fig. 1.85a, b*	**CT:** Spheroid lesions in brain; can have various intra-axial locations often at gray-white matter junctions; usually low to intermediate attenuation, with or without hemorrhage, calcifications, cysts; variable contrast enhancement, often low attenuation peripheral to nodular-enhancing lesion representing axonal edema. **MRI:** Circumscribed spheroid lesions in brain; can have various intra-axial locations, often at gray-white matter junctions; usually low to intermediate signal on T1-weighted images, intermediate to high signal on T2-weighted images; with or without hemorrhage, calcifications, cysts; variable gadolinium enhancement; often high signal on T2-weighted images peripheral to nodular peripheral to nodular-enhancing lesion representing axonal edema.	Represents ~33% of intracranial tumors, usually from extracranial primary neoplasm in adults older than 40 y. Primary tumor source: lung > breast > GI > GU > melanoma. Metastatic lesions in the cerebellum can present with obstructive hydrocephalus/neurosurgical emergency.
Lymphoma	**Primary CNS lymphoma:** Focal or infiltrating lesion located in the basal ganglia, posterior fossa/brainstem. **CT:** Low to intermediate attenuation, with or without hemorrhage/necrosis in immunocompromised patients; usually show contrast enhancement. **MRI:** Low to intermediate signal on T1-weighted images, intermediate to slightly high signal on T2-weighted images, with or without hemorrhage/necrosis in immunocompromised patients; usually show gadolinium contrast enhancement. Diffuse leptomeningeal enhancement is another pattern of intracranial lymphoma.	Primary CNS lymphoma more common than secondary, usually in adults older than 40 y; B-cell lymphoma more common than T-cell lymphoma; increasing incidence related to number of immunocompromised patients in population. CT and MRI imaging features of primary and secondary lymphoma of brain overlap. Intracranial lymphoma can involve the leptomeninges in secondary lymphoma > primary lymphoma.
Hemangioblastoma ▷ *Fig. 1.86*	Circumscribed tumors usually located in the cerebellum and/or brainstem; **CT:** Small contrast-enhancing nodule with or without cyst, or larger lesion with prominent heterogeneous enhancement, with or without hemorrhage. **MRI:** Small gadolinium-enhancing nodule with or without cyst, or larger lesion with prominent heterogeneous enhancement with or without flow voids within lesion or at the periphery; intermediate signal on T1-weighted images, intermediate to high signal on T2-weighted images; occasionally lesions have evidence of recent or remote hemorrhage.	Occurs in adolescents, young and middle-aged adults. Lesions are typically multiple in patients with von Hippel-Lindau disease.
Neurocutaneous melanosis	Extra- or intra-axial lesions usually < 3 cm in diameter with irregular margins in the leptomeninges or brain parenchyma/brainstem (anterior temporal lobes, cerebellum, thalami, and inferior frontal lobes). **CT:** May show subtle hyperdensity secondary to increased melanin, with or without vermian hypoplasia, with or without arachnoid cysts, with or without Dandy-Walker malformation. **MRI:** Zones with intermediate to slightly high signal on T1-weighted images secondary to increased melanin, with gadolinium contrast enhancement, with or without vermian hypoplasia, with or without arachnoid cysts, with or without Dandy-Walker malformation.	Rare neuroectodermal dysplasia with proliferation of melanocytes in leptomeninges associated with large and/or numerous cutaneous nevi. May change into CNS melanoma.

(continues on page 50)

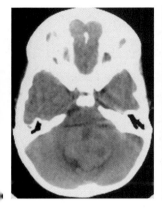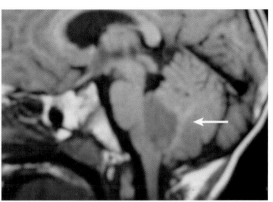

Fig. 1.83a, b   Ependymoma. Axial CT image (**a**) shows a tumor within the fourth ventricle that has mixed intermediate and low attenuation. The tumor has intermediate signal on the sagittal T1-weighted MRI (**b**) (arrow).

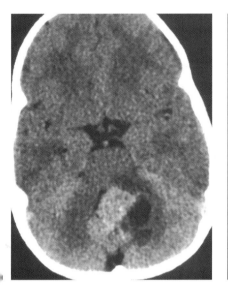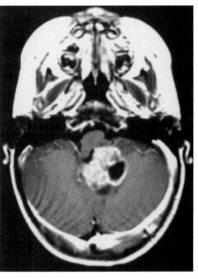

Fig. 1.84a, b   Atypical teratoid/rhabdoid tumor. Axial CT image (**a**) shows the tumor involving the vermis and fourth ventricle with mixed low, intermediate, and slightly high attenuation. The lesion shows heterogeneous contrast enhancement on the axial T1-weighted MRI (**b**).

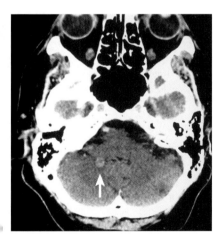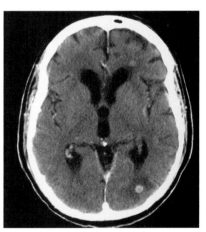

Fig. 1.85a, b   Metastases. Postcontrast axial images show enhancing lesions in the right cerebellar hemisphere (arrow) (**a**) and cerebrum (**b**).

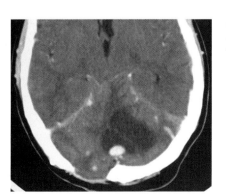

Fig. 1.86   Hemangioblastoma. Postcontrast axial image in a patient with von Hippel-Lindau disease shows enhancing tumors in the cerebellum, the largest of which has an associated tumoral cyst.

Table 1.4   (Cont.) Intra-axial lesions in the posterior cranial fossa (infratentorial)

Lesions	CT Findings	Comments
Inflammatory lesions		
Cerebellitis	**CT:** Poorly defined zone or focal area of low to intermediate attenuation, minimal or no contrast enhancement; involves cerebellar cortex and white matter. Edema may result in hydrocephalus from compression of fourth ventricle. **MRI:** Poorly defined zone or focal area of low to intermediate signal on T1-weighted images, intermediate to high signal on T2-weighted images, minimal or no gadolinium contrast enhancement; involves cerebellar cortex and white matter. Edema may result in hydrocephalus from compression of fourth ventricle.	Focal infection/inflammation of brain tissue from bacteria or fungi, secondary to sinusitis, meningitis, surgery, hematogenous source (cardiac and other vascular shunts), and/or immunocompromised status. Can progress to abscess formation. Childhood illnesses (coxsackievirus, rubella, typhoid fever, polio virus, pertussis, diphtheria, varicella zoster, and Epstein-Barr virus) can cause acute cerebellitis.
Pyogenic brain abscess ▷ *Fig. 1.87a, b*	**CT:** Circumscribed lesion with a central zone of low attenuation (with or without air-fluid level) surrounded by a thin rim of intermediate attenuation; peripheral poorly defined zone of decreased attenuation representing edema; ringlike contrast enhancement that is sometimes thicker laterally than medially. **MRI:** Circumscribed lesion with low signal on T1-weighted images, central zone of high signal on T2-weighted images (with or without air-fluid level) surrounded by a thin rim of low T2 signal; peripheral poorly defined zone of high signal on T2-weighted images representing edema; ringlike gadolinium contrast enhancement.	Formation of brain abscess occurs 2 weeks after cerebritis with liquefaction and necrosis centrally surrounded by a capsule and peripheral edema. Can be multiple. Complication from meningitis and/or sinusitis, septicemia, trauma, surgery, or cardiac shunt.
Fungal brain abscess	Vary depending on organism, lesions occur in meninges and brain parenchyma. **CT:** Solid or cystic-appearing lesions with decreased attenuation, nodular or ring pattern of contrast enhancement, peripheral zone with decreased attenuation in brain lesions (edema). **MRI:** Solid or cystic lesions with low to intermediate signal on T2-weighted images, high signal on T2-weighted images, nodular or ring enhancement, peripheral high signal in brain lesions on T2-weighted images (edema).	Occur in immunocompromised or diabetic patients with resultant granulomas in meninges and brain parenchyma.
Encephalitis	**CT:** Poorly defined zone or zones of decreased attenuation, minimal or no contrast enhancement; involves cerebral cortex and/or white matter; minimal localized mass effect. **MRI:** Poorly defined zone or zones of low to intermediate signal on T1-weighted images, intermediate to high signal on T2-weighted images, minimal or no gadolinium contrast enhancement; involves cerebellar cortex and/or white matter; minimal localized mass effect.	Encephalitis: infection/inflammation of brain tissue from viruses, often seen in immunocompromised patients (e.g., herpes simplex, CMV, HIV, and progressive multifocal leukoencephalopathy) or immunocompetent patients (e.g., St. Louis encephalitis, eastern or western equine encephalitis, and Epstein-Barr virus).
Tuberculoma ▷ *Fig. 1.88a–c*	**CT:** Intra-axial lesions in cerebral hemispheres and basal ganglia (adults) or cerebellum (children). Lesions can have decreased attenuation, central zone of low attenuation with a thin peripheral rim of intermediate attenuation; with solid or rim pattern of contrast enhancement; with or without calcification. **Meningeal lesions:** Nodular or cystic zones of basilar meningeal enhancement. **MRI:** Lesions often have low to intermediate signal on T1-weighted images, central zone of high signal on T2-weighted images with a thin peripheral rim of low signal, occasionally low signal on T2-weighted images; with solid or rim gadolinium contrast enhancement; with or without calcification. Meningeal lesions: nodular or cystic zones of basilar meningeal enhancement.	Occurs in immunocompromised patients and in inhabitants of developing countries. Caseating intracranial granulomas via hematogenous dissemination; meninges > brain lesions.

(continues on page 52)

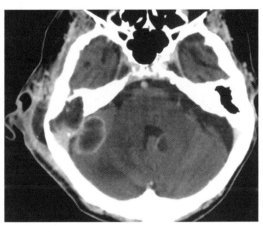
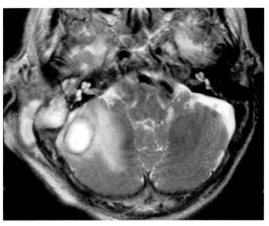

Fig. 1.87a, b   Pyogenic abscess. Postcontrast axial CT image (**a**) shows a ring-enhancing lesion in the lateral portion of the right cerebellar hemisphere, as well as findings of osteomyelitis at the right mastoid bone. Similar findings are seen on the axial T2-weighted MRI (**b**).

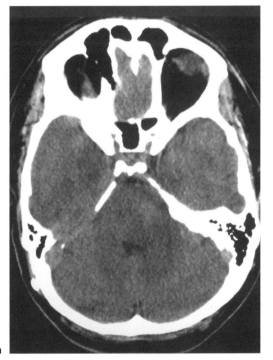
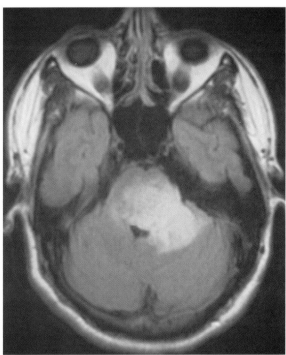

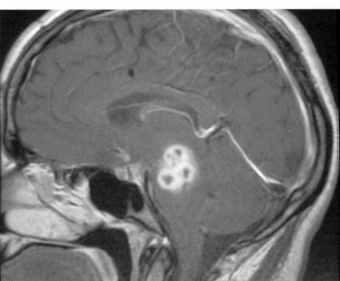

Fig. 1.88a–c   Tuberculoma. Axial CT image (**a**) shows a poorly defined lesion with decreased attenuation involving the left side of the pons and the left middle cerebellar peduncle. The lesion has corresponding high signal on the axial FLAIR MRI (**b**) and shows contrast enhancement on the sagittal T1-weighted MRI (**c**).

Table 1.4 (Cont.) Intra-axial lesions in the posterior cranial fossa (infratentorial)

Lesions	CT Findings	Comments
Parasitic brain lesions		
Toxoplasmosis	**CT:** Single or multiple solid and/or cystic-appearing lesions with low to intermediate, nodular or rim pattern of contrast enhancement, with or without mild peripheral low attenuation (edema). Chronic phase: calcified granulomas. **MRI:** Single or multiple solid and/or cystic lesions, low to intermediate signal on T1-weighted images, high signal on T2-weighted images, nodular or rim pattern of gadolinium contrast enhancement, with or without peripheral high T2 signal (edema).	Most common opportunistic CNS infection in AIDS patients; caused by ingestion of food contaminated with parasites (*Toxoplasma gondii*).
Cysticercosis	**CT:** Single or multiple cystic-appearing lesions in brain or meninges. **Acute/subacute phase:** Low to intermediate attenuation, rim with or without nodular pattern of contrast enhancement, with or without peripheral low attenuation (edema). **Chronic phase:** Calcified granulomas. **MRI:** Single or multiple cystic lesions in brain or meninges. **Acute/subacute phase:** Low to intermediate signal on T1-weighted images, high signal on T2-weighted images, rim with or without nodular pattern of gadolinium contrast enhancement, with or without peripheral high T2 signal (edema). **Chronic phase:** Calcified granulomas.	Caused by ingestion of ova (*Taenia solium*) in contaminated food (undercooked pork); involves meninges > brain parenchyma > ventricles.
Hydatid cyst	***Echinococcus granulosus:*** **CT:** Single or rarely multiple cystic-appearing lesions with low attenuation surrounded by a thin wall; typically no contrast enhancement or peripheral edema unless superinfected; often located in vascular territory of the middle cerebral artery. **MRI:** Single or rarely multiple cystic lesions with low signal on T1-weighted images and high signal on T2-weighted images with a thin wall with low signal; typically no gadolinium contrast enhancement or peripheral edema unless superinfected; often located in vascular territory of the middle cerebral artery. ***Echinococcus multilocularis:*** **CT:** Cystic (with or without multilocular) and/or solid lesions, central zone of intermediate attenuation surrounded by a slightly thickened rim, with contrast enhancement; peripheral zone of decreased attenuation (edema) and calcifications are common. **MRI:** Cystic (with or without multilocular) and/or solid lesions, central zone of intermediate signal on T1-weighted images surrounded by a slightly thickened rim of low signal on T2-eighted images, with gadolinium enhancement; peripheral zone of high signal on T2-weighted images (edema) and calcifications are common.	Caused by parasites *E. granulosus* (South America, Middle East, Australia, and New Zealand) and *E. multilocularis* (North America, Europe, Turkey, and China). CNS involvement in 2% of cases of hydatid infestation.
Radiation injury/necrosis	**CT:** Focal lesion with or without mass effect or poorly defined zone of low to intermediate attenuation, with or without contrast enhancement involving tissue (gray matter and/or white matter) in field of treatment. **MRI:** Focal lesion with or without mass effect or poorly defined zone of low to intermediate signal on T1-weighted images, intermediate to high signal on T2-weighted images, with or without gadolinium contrast enhancement involving tissue (gray matter and/or white matter) in field of treatment.	Usually occurs from 4 to 6 months to 10 y after radiation treatment; may be difficult to distinguish from neoplasm. PET and magnetic resonance spectroscopy might be helpful for evaluation.

(continues on page 53)

Table 1.4   (Cont.) Intra-axial lesions in the posterior cranial fossa (infratentorial)

Lesions	CT Findings	Comments
Acute demyelinating Disease: Multiple sclerosis, ADEM	Lesions located in cerebellar white matter and/or brainstem. **CT:** Lesions usually have low to intermediate attenuation. Zones of active demyelination may show contrast enhancement and mild localized swelling. **MRI:** Zones of low to intermediate signal on T1-weighted images and high signal on FLAIR and T2-weighted images; with or without gadolinium contrast enhancement. Contrast enhancement can be ringlike or nodular, usually in acute/early subacute phase of demyelination. Lesions rarely can have associated mass effect simulating neoplasms.	Multiple sclerosis is the most common acquired demyelinating disease usually affecting women (peak ages 20–40 y). Other demyelinating diseases are acute disseminated encephalomyelitis, immune mediated demyelination after viral infection; toxins (exogenous from environmental exposure or ingestion of alcohol, solvents, etc.; or endogenous from metabolic disorder, e.g., leukodystrophies, and mitochondrial encephalopathies), radiation injury, trauma, and vascular disease.
Sarcoidosis	Poorly marginated intra-axial zone with low to intermediate attenuation; usually shows contrast enhancement, with localized mass effect and peripheral edema. Often associated with contrast enhancement in the leptomeninges.	Multisystem noncaseating granulomatous disease of uncertain cause that can involve the CNS in 5% to 15% of cases. Associated with severe neurologic deficits if untreated.
Hemorrhage		
Cerebellar hemorrhage	The attenuation of the hematoma depends on its age, size, location, hematocrit, hemoglobin oxidation state, clot retraction, and extent of edema. **Hyperacute phase (4–6 h):** Hemoglobin primarily as diamagnetic oxyhemoglobin (iron Fe^{2+} state). **CT:** Zone with high attenuation. **MRI:** Intermediate signal on T1-weighted images, slightly high signal on T2-weighted images. **Acute phase (12–48 h):** Hemoglobin primarily as paramagnetic deoxyhemoglobin (iron, Fe^{2+} state). **CT:** High attenuation in acute clot directly related to hematocrit, hemoglobin concentration, and high protein concentration. Hematocrit in acute clot approaches 90%. ▷ *Fig. 1.89a, b, p. 55* **MRI:** Intermediate signal on T1-weighted images, low signal on T2-weighted images, surrounded by a peripheral zone of high T2 signal (edema).The signal of the hematoma depends on its age, size, location, hematocrit, hemoglobin oxidation state, clot retraction, and extent of edema. **Early subacute phase (> 2 d):** Hemoglobin becomes oxidized to the iron Fe^{3+} state, methemoglobin, which is strongly paramagnetic. **CT:** Zone with high attenuation; **MRI:** When methemoglobin is initially intracellular, the hematoma has high signal on T1-weighted images progressing from peripheral to central and low signal on T2-weighted images, surrounded by a zone of high T2 signal (edema). When methemoglobin eventually becomes primarily extracellular, the hematoma has high signal on T1-weighted images and high signal on T2-weighted images. **Late subacute phase (> 7 d–6 w):** Intracerebral hematomas decrease 1.5 HU per day. Hematomas become isodense to hypodense, peripheral contrast enhancement from blood–brain barrier breakdown and vascularized capsule. **Chronic phase:** Hemoglobin as extracellular methemoglobin is progressively degraded to hemosiderin. **CT:** Chronic hematomas have low attenuation with localized encephalomalacia. Zone with high attenuation represent new sites of rebleeding. **MRI:** The hematoma progresses from a lesion with high signal on T1- and T2-weighted images with a peripheral rim of low signal on T2-weighted images (hemosiderin) to predominant hemosiderin composition with low signal on T2-weighted images.	Can result from trauma, ruptured aneurysms or vascular malformations, coagulopathy, hypertension, adverse drug reaction, amyloid angiopathy, hemorrhagic transformation of cerebral infarction, metastases, abscesses, and viral infections (e.g., herpes simplex and CMV).

(continues on page 54)

Table 1.4   (Cont.) Intra-axial lesions in the posterior cranial fossa (infratentorial)

Lesions	CT Findings	Comments
Cerebellar contusions	**CT:** Appearance of contusions is initially one of focal hemorrhage involving the cerebral cortex and subcortical white matter. Contusions eventually appear as focal superficial encephalomalacia zones. **MRI:** Appearance of contusions is initially one of focal hemorrhage involving the cerebellar cortex and subcortical white matter. The MRI signal of the contusion depends on its age and presence of oxyhemoglobin, deoxyhemoglobin, methemoglobin, hemosiderin, etc. Contusions eventually appear as focal superficial encephalomalacic zones with high signal on T2-weighted images, with or without small zones of low signal on T2-weighted images from hemosiderin.	Contusions are superficial brain injuries involving the cerebellar cortex and subcortical white matter that result from skull fracture and/or acceleration deceleration trauma to the inner table of the skull.
Metastases	**CT:** Intracerebral hematoma involving a portion or all of the neoplasm; usually associated with peripheral edema (decreased attenuation); often multiple with contrast enhancement in nonhemorrhagic portions of lesions. **MRI:** Intracerebral hematoma involving a portion or all of the neoplasm; usually associated with peripheral edema (high signal on T2-weighted images); often multiple.	Metastatic intra-axial tumors associated with hemorrhage include bronchogenic carcinoma, renal cell carcinoma, melanoma, choriocarcinoma, and thyroid carcinoma. May be difficult to distinguish from hemorrhage related to other etiologies.
Vascular		
AVM ▷ *Fig. 1.89a, b*	Lesions with irregular margins that can be located in the brain parenchyma (pia, dura, or both locations). **CT:** AVMs contain multiple tortuous tubular vessels that have intermediate or slightly increased attenuation that show contrast enhancement. Calcifications occur in 30% of cases. CTA shows arteries, veins, and nidus of AVM even when there is an intra-axial hemorrhage. **MRI:** Serpiginous flow voids on T1- and T2-weighted images secondary to patent arteries with high blood flow, as well as thrombosed vessels with variable signal, areas of hemorrhage in various phases, calcifications, and gliosis. The venous portions often show gadolinium contrast enhancement. Gradient echo MRI shows flow-related enhancement (high signal) in patent arteries and veins of the AVM. MRA using TOF with or without IV contrast, or phase contrast techniques can provide additional detailed information about the nidus, feeding arteries, and draining veins, as well as presence of associated aneurysms. Usually not associated with mass effect unless there is recent hemorrhage or venous occlusion.	Infratentorial AVMs much less common than supratentorial AVMs.
Cavernous hemangioma ▷ *Fig. 1.90a, b*	Single or multiple multilobulated intra-axial lesions. **CT:** Lesions have intermediate to slightly increased attenuation, with or without calcifications, variable contrast enhancement (most show no or minimal enhancement, few show more prominent enhancement). **MRI:** Peripheral rim or irregular zone of low signal on T2-weighted images secondary to hemosiderin, surrounding a central zone of variable signal (low, intermediate, high, or mixed) on T1- and T2-weighted images depending on ages of hemorrhagic portions. Gradient echo techniques useful for detecting multiple lesions.	Infratentorial lesions less common than supratentorial locations. Can be seen in many different locations; multiple lesions > 50%. Association with venous angiomas and risk of hemorrhage.

(continues on page 56)

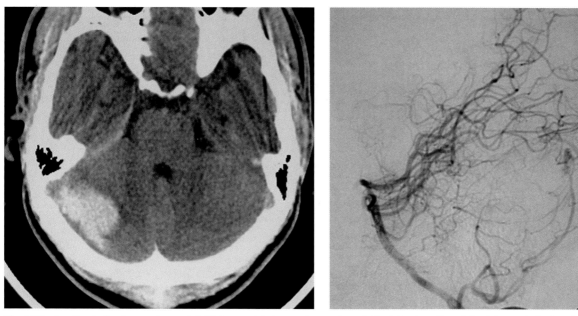

Fig. 1.89a, b   Cerebellar hemorrhage. Axial CT image (**a**) shows a hemorrhage in the lateral portion of the right cerebellar hemisphere from an AVM as seen on the conventional arteriogram (**b**).

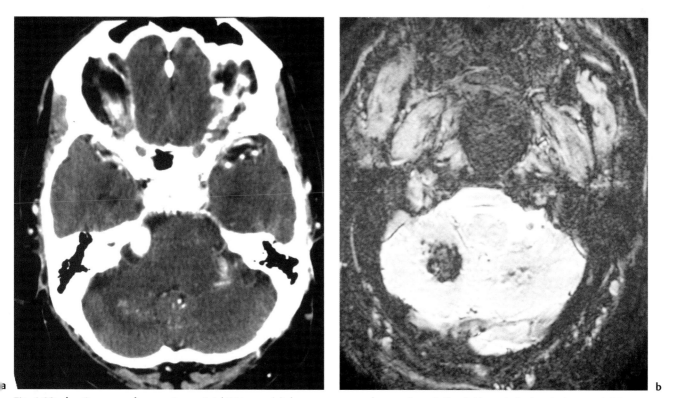

Fig. 1.90a, b   Cavernous hemangioma. Axial CT image (**a**) shows a cavernous hemangioma in the right cerebellar hemisphere containing calcifications. The lesion has low signal on the axial gradient echo MRI (**b**).

Table 1.4 (Cont.) Intra-axial lesions in the posterior cranial fossa (infratentorial)

Lesions	CT Findings	Comments
Venous angioma ▷ *Fig. 1.91*	**CT:** No abnormality or small slightly hyperdense zone prior to contrast administration. Contrast enhancement seen in a slightly prominent vein draining a collection of small veins. **MRI:** On postcontrast T1-weighted images, venous angiomas are seen as a gadolinium contrast-enhancing transcortical vein draining a collection of small medullary veins (caput medusae). The draining vein can be seen as a signal void on T2-weighted images.	Considered an anomalous venous formation typically not associated with hemorrhage; usually an incidental finding except when associated with cavernous hemangioma.
Cerebellar/brainstem infarction ▷ *Fig. 1.92a–c*	CT and MRI features of cerebral, cerebellar, and brainstem infarcts depend on age of infarct relative to time of examination. **Hyperacute (< 12 h):** **CT:** No abnormality (50%), decreased attenuation and blurring of lentiform nuclei, hyperdense artery in up to 50% of cases. **MRI:** Localized edema, usually isointense signal to normal brain on T1- and T2-weighted images. Diffusion-weighted images can show positive findings related to decreased apparent diffusion coefficients secondary to cytotoxic edema, absence of arterial flow void, or arterial enhancement in the vascular distribution of the infarct. **Acute phase (12–24 h):** **CT:** Zones with decreased attenuation in brainstem, blurring of junction between cerebellar cortex and white matter, sulcal effacement. **MRI:** Intermediate signal on T1-weighted images, high signal on T2-weighted images, localized edema. Signal abnormalities commonly involve the cerebellar cortex and subcortical white matter and/or basal ganglia. **Early subacute phase (24 h–3 d):** **CT:** Localized swelling at sites with low attenuation involving gray and white matter (often wedge shaped), with or without hemorrhage. **MRI:** Zones with low to intermediate signal on T1-weighted images, high signal on T2-weighted images, localized edema, with or without hemorrhage, with or without gadolinium contrast enhancement. **Late subacute phase (4 d–2 wk):** **CT:** Localized swelling increases and then decreases; low attenuation at lesion can become more prominent, with or without gyral contrast enhancement. **MRI:** Low to intermediate signal on T1-weighted images, high signal on T2-weighted images, edema/mass effect diminishing, with or without hemorrhage, with or without contrast enhancement. **2 weeks to 2 months:** **CT:** With or without gyral contrast enhancement; localized mass effect resolves. **MRI:** Low to intermediate signal on T1-weighted images, high signal on T2-weighted images; edema resolves; with or without hemorrhage; with or without enhancement eventually declines. **> 2 months:** **CT:** Zone of low attenuation associated with encephalomalacia. **MRI:** Low signal on T1-weighted images, high signal on T2-weighted images, encephalomalacic changes, with or without calcification, hemosiderin.	Cerebellar and brainstem infarcts usually result from occlusive vascular disease involving branches from the basilar artery (posteroinferior cerebellar artery [PICA], anteroinferior cerebellar artery [AICA], perforating arteries). Vascular occlusion may be secondary to atheromatous arterial disease, cardiogenic emboli, neoplastic encasement, hypercoagulable states, dissection, or congenital anomalies. Cerebellar infarcts usually result from arterial occlusion involving specific vascular territories, although they occasionally occur from metabolic disorders (mitochondrial encephalopathies, etc.) or intracranial venous occlusion (thrombophlebitis, hypercoagulable states, dehydration, etc., which do not correspond to arterial distributions.

(continues on page 58)

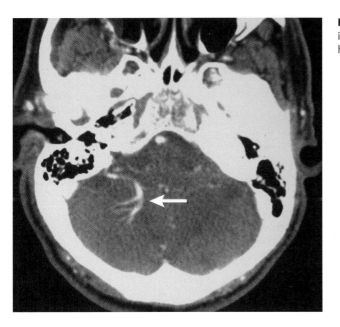

Fig. 1.91   Venous angioma. Postcontrast image shows an enhancing venous angioma in the anterior portion of the right cerebellar hemisphere (arrow).

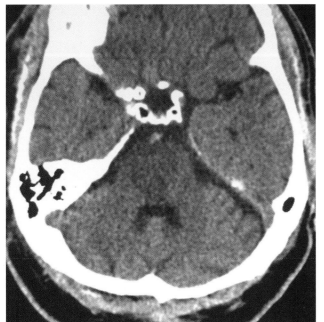

a

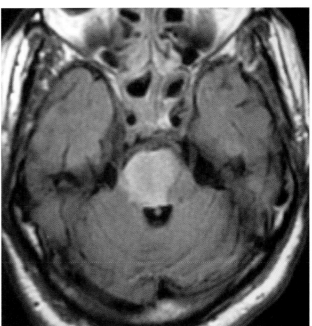

b

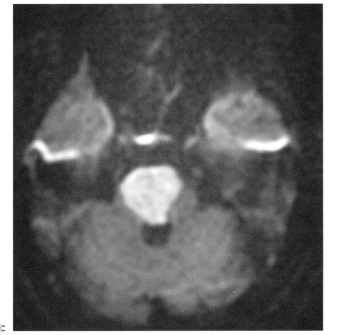

c

Fig. 1.92a–c   Brainstem infarction. Axial CT image (**a**) shows an infarct with decreased attenuation in the pons. High signal is seen on the axial FLAIR MRI (**b**) and diffusion-weighted image (**c**).

Table 1.4   (Cont.) Intra-axial lesions in the posterior cranial fossa (infratentorial)

Lesions	CT Findings	Comments
Wallerian degeneration ▷ *Fig. 1.93a, b*	Corticospinal tract involvement from infarct or injury at motor cortex or posterior limb of internal capsule can result in the following: **CT:** Hemiatrophy of brainstem (midbrain, pons) ipsilateral to cerebral lesion. **MRI:** Linear zone of high signal on T2-weighted images in ipsilateral corticospinal tract of brainstem (high signal on T2-weighted images 5–12 wk after). Injury results from edema (> 12 weeks secondary to gliosis), with or without associated atrophy in brainstem at ipsilateral corticospinal tract. Extensive unilateral cerebral cortical atrophy can result in atrophy of the contralateral middle cerebellar peduncle and cerebellum from interruption of the corti-copontocerebellar pathway (which connects the cerebral cortex to the contralateral middle cerebellar peduncle via pontine nuclei).	Refers to pathologic changes (degeneration, myelin degradation, atrophy) in axons secondary to injuries involving the cell bodies of neurons (hemorrhage, cerebral infarction, contusion, surgery, etc.).

Table 1.5   Extra-axial lesions in the posterior cranial fossa (infratentorial)

Lesions	CT Findings	Comments
Neoplastic		
Metastatic tumor ▷ *Fig. 1.94a, b* ▷ *Fig. 1.95*	Single or multiple well-circumscribed or poorly defined lesions involving the skull, dura, leptomeninges, and/or choroid plexus; low to intermediate attenuation, usually with contrast enhancement, with or without bone destruction, with or without compression of neural tissue or vessels. Leptomeningeal tumor often best seen on postcontrast images.	Metastatic tumor may have variable destructive or infiltrative changes involving single or multiple sites of involvement.

(continues on page 60)

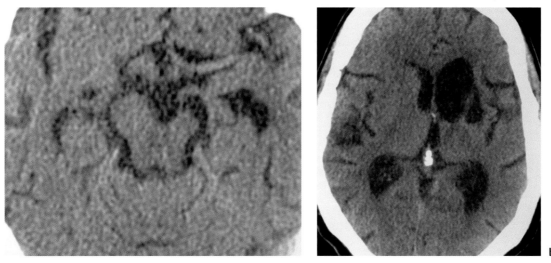

Fig. 1.93a, b   Wallerian degeneration. Atrophy of the left cerebral peduncle (**a**) is seen on MRI related to prior infarction involving the left basal ganglia (**b**).

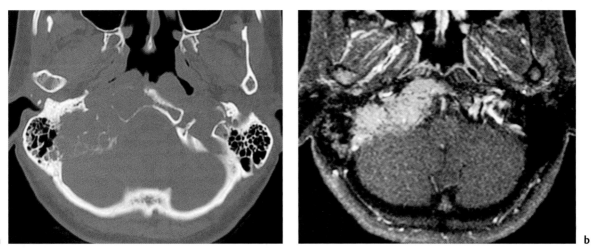

Fig. 1.94a, b   Metastatic tumor, breast carcinoma. Axial CT image (**a**) shows a destructive lesion involving the right occipital and temporal bones. The lesion shows contrast enhancement on the axial fat-suppressed, T1-weighted MRI (**b**), as well as dural involvement.

Fig. 1.95   Metastatic tumor, leptomeninges. Postcontrast image shows diffuse tumoral enhancement in the leptomeninges from a pineoblastoma.

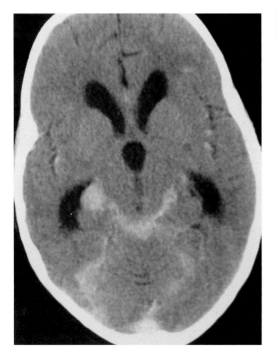

Table 1.5   (Cont.) Extra-axial lesions in the posterior cranial fossa (infratentorial)

Lesions	CT Findings	Comments
Schwannoma (neurinoma): acoustic, trigeminal, etc. ▷ *Fig. 1.96* ▷ *Fig. 1.97a, b*	Circumscribed or lobulated extra-axial lesions, low to intermediate attenuation, with contrast enhancement. Attenuation and contrast enhancement can be heterogeneous in large lesions.	Acoustic (vestibular nerve) schwannomas account for 90% of intracranial schwannomas and represent 75% of lesions in the cerebellopontine angle cisterns; trigeminal schwannomas are the next most common intracranial schwannomas, followed by facial nerve schwannomas and multiple schwannomas seen with neurofibromatosis type 2.
Meningioma ▷ *Fig. 1.98a, b* ▷ *Fig. 1.99a, b*	Extra-axial dural-based lesions, well-circumscribed; supra- > infratentorial; intermediate attenuation signal, usually with contrast enhancement, with or without calcifications.	Most common extra-axial tumors, usually benign neoplasms, typically occur in adults (older than 40 y), women > men; multiple meningiomas seen with neurofibromatosis type 2; can result in compression of adjacent brain parenchyma, encasement of arteries, and compression of dural venous sinuses; rarely invasive/malignant types.
Hemangiopericytoma	Extra-axial mass lesions, often well circumscribed; intermediate attenuation, with contrast enhancement (may resemble meningiomas), with or without associated erosive bone changes.	Rare neoplasms in young adults (men > women) sometimes referred to as angioblastic meningioma or meningeal hemangiopericytoma; arise from vascular cells/pericytes; frequency of metastases > meningiomas.
Paraganglioma glomus jugulare ▷ *Fig. 1.100a–c*	Extra-axial mass lesions located in jugular foramen, often well circumscribed; intermediate attenuation, with contrast enhancement; often associated with erosive bone changes and expansion of jugular foramen.	Lesions, also referred to as chemodectomas, arise from paraganglia in multiple sites in the body and are named accordingly (glomus jugular, tympanicum, vagale, etc.).

(continues on page 62)

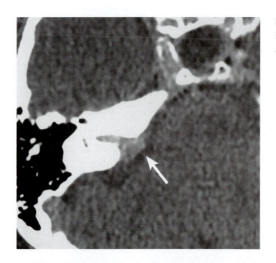

Fig. 1.96   Schwannoma, eighth cranial nerve. Postcontrast image shows an enhancing lesion in the right cerebellopontine angle cistern that extends into the right internal auditory canal (arrow).

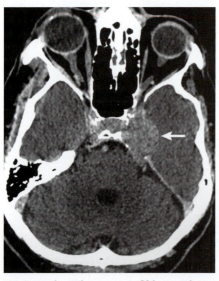

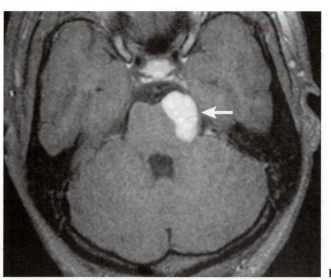

a   b

Fig. 1.97a, b   Schwannoma, fifth cranial nerve. Postcontrast axial CT image (**a**) shows enhancement of the schwannoma involving the left trigeminal nerve. Similar findings are seen on the postcontrast axial fat-suppressed MRI (arrows) (**b**).

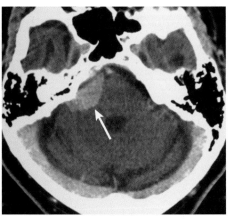 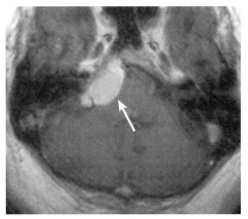

b

Fig. 1.98a, b Meningioma along the petrous bone. Postcontrast axial CT image (**a**) shows enhancement of the meningioma along the endocranial surface of the right petrous bone and clivus. Similar findings are seen on the postcontrast axial MRI (**b**) (arrows).

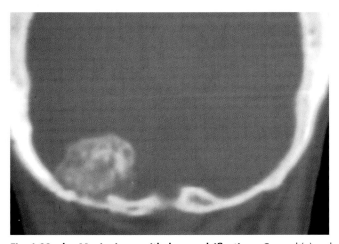 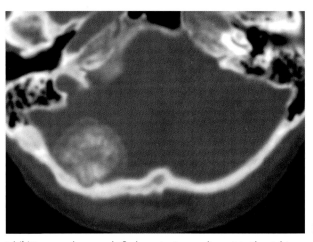

b

Fig. 1.99a, b Meningioma with dense calcifications. Coronal (**a**) and axial (**b**) images show a calcified meningioma adjacent to the right occipital bone.

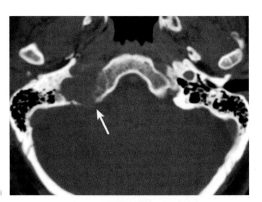 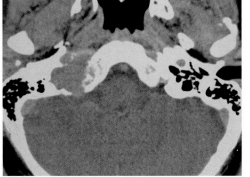

b

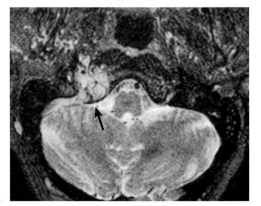

Fig. 1.100a–c Paraganglioma/glomus tumor. Axial CT images (**a,b**) show a soft tissue tumor eroding the right jugular foramen. The tumor has mostly high signal on the axial fat-suppressed, T2-weighted MRI (**c**), as well as small foci of a low-signal, "salt and pepper" pattern (arrows).

Table 1.5 (Cont.) Extra-axial lesions in the posterior cranial fossa (infratentorial)

Lesions	CT Findings	Comments
Choroid plexus papilloma or carcinoma ▷ *Fig. 1.101a, b* ▷ *Fig. 1.102a, b*	Circumscribed and/or lobulated lesions with papillary projections, intermediate attenuation, usually prominent contrast enhancement, with or without calcifications. Locations: atrium of lateral ventricle (children) > fourth ventricle (adults), rarely other locations such as third ventricle. Associated with hydrocephalus.	Rare intracranial neoplasms. CT features of choroid plexus carcinoma and papilloma may overlap; both histologic types can disseminate along CSF pathways. Carcinomas tend to be larger, have greater degrees of mixed/heterogeneous attenuation than papillomas. Carcinomas often show invasion of adjacent brain, whereas papillomas often do not.
Lymphoma	Single or multiple well-circumscribed or poorly defined lesions involving the skull, dura, and/or leptomeninges; low to intermediate attenuation usually with contrast enhancement, with or without bone destruction. Leptomeningeal tumor often best seen on postcontrast images.	Extra-axial lymphoma may have variable destructive or infiltrative changes involving single or multiple sites of involvement.
Neurocutaneous melanosis	Extra- or intra-axial lesions usually < 3 cm in diameter with irregular margins in the leptomeninges or brain parenchyma/brainstem (anterior temporal lobes, cerebellum, thalami, and inferior frontal lobes); may show no abnormalities on CT, occasionally show zones with intermediate to slightly high attenuation secondary to increased melanin, with or without contrast enhancement. With or without vermian hypoplasia, with or without arachnoid cysts, with or without Dandy-Walker malformation.	Neuroectodermal dysplasia with proliferation of melanocytes in leptomeninges associated with large and/or numerous cutaneous nevi. May change into CNS melanoma.
Myeloma/plasmacytoma	Multiple (myeloma) or single (plasmacytoma) well-circumscribed or poorly defined lesions involving the skull and dura; low to intermediate attenuation, with or without contrast enhancement, with bone destruction.	Myeloma may have variable destructive or infiltrative changes involving the axial and/or appendicular skeleton.
Chordoma ▷ *Fig. 1.103a–c*	Well-circumscribed lobulated lesions, low to intermediate attenuation, with contrast enhancement (usually heterogeneous); locally invasive associated with bone erosion/destruction, encasement of vessels and nerves; skull base–clivus common location, usually in the midline.	Rare, slow-growing, malignant cartilaginous tumors derived from notochordal remnants. Detailed anatomical display of extension of chordomas by CT and MRI is important for planning of surgical approaches.
Chondrosarcoma ▷ *Fig. 1.104a, b*	Lobulated lesions, low to intermediate attenuation, with or without chondroid matrix mineralization, with contrast/enhancement (usually heterogeneous); locally invasive associated with bone erosion/destruction, encasement of vessels and nerves; skull base petro-occipital synchondrosis common location, usually off midline.	Rare, slow-growing tumors. Detailed anatomical display of extension of chondrosarcomas by CT and MRI is important for planning of surgical approaches.
Osteogenic sarcoma	Destructive lesions involving the skull base; low to intermediate attenuation, usually with matrix mineralization/ossification, with contrast enhancement (usually heterogeneous).	Rare lesions involving the skull base and calvarium; more common than chondrosarcomas and Ewing sarcoma; locally invasive; high metastatic potential. Occurs in children as primary tumors and adults (associated with Paget disease, irradiated bone, chronic osteomyelitis, osteoblastoma, giant cell tumor, and fibrous dysplasia).

(continues on page 64)

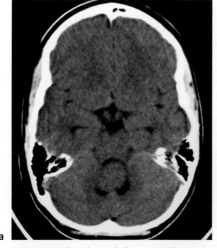
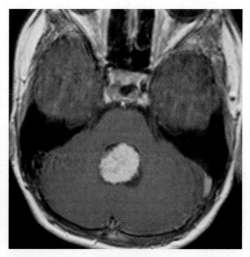

a   b

Fig. 1.101a, b Choroid plexus papilloma. Axial CT image (**a**) shows an intraventricular lesion in the fourth ventricle, which shows contrast enhancement on the axial T1-weighted MRI (**b**).

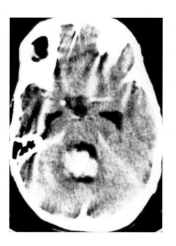 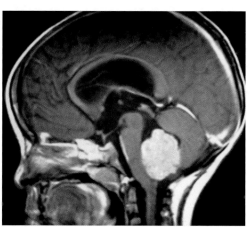

Fig. 1.102a, b   Choroid plexus carcinoma. Postcontrast axial CT image (**a**) shows an enhancing intraventricular lesion in the fourth ventricle, which shows contrast enhancement on the sagittal T1-weighted MRI (**b**).

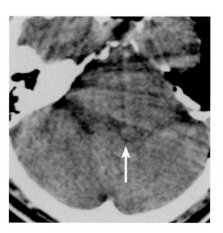 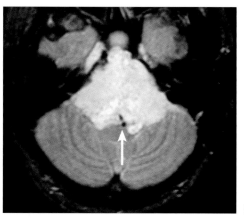

Fig. 1.103a–c   Chordoma. Axial CT image (**a**) shows the chordoma along the endocranial surface of the clivus causing posterior displacement of the brainstem. The tumor has high signal on the axial fat-suppressed, T2-weighted image (**b**) and shows heterogeneous contrast enhancement on the axial T1-weighted image (**c**) (arrows).

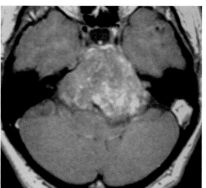

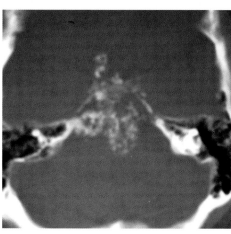 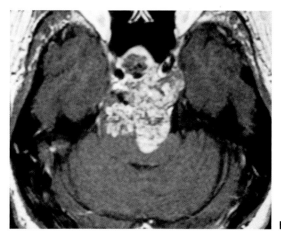

Fig. 1.104a, b   Chondrosarcoma. Axial CT image (**a**) shows the tumor destroying the clivus and causing posterior displacement of the brainstem. The tumor contains chondroid calcifications and shows heterogeneous contrast enhancement on the axial T1-weighted image (**b**).

Table 1.5 (Cont.) Extra-axial lesions in the posterior cranial fossa (infratentorial)

Lesions	CT Findings	Comments
Ewing sarcoma	Destructive lesions involving the skull base; low to intermediate attenuation; usually lack matrix mineralization, with contrast enhancement (usually heterogeneous).	Rare lesions involving the skull base; usually occur between the ages of 5 and 30 y, males > females; locally invasive; high metastatic potential.
Sinonasal squamous cell carcinoma	Destructive lesions in the nasal cavity, paranasal sinuses, and nasopharynx; with or without intracranial extension via bone destruction or perineural spread; intermediate attenuation; mild contrast enhancement; large lesions (with or without necrosis and/or hemorrhage).	Occurs in adults usually > 55 y, men > women; associated with occupational or other exposure to nickel, chromium, mustard gas, radium, and manufacture of wood products.
Adenoid cystic carcinoma	Destructive lesions in the paranasal sinuses, nasal cavity, and nasopharynx, with or without intracranial extension via bone destruction or perineural spread; intermediate attenuation; variable degrees of contrast enhancement.	Account for 10% of sinonasal tumors; arise from any location within the sinonasal cavities; usually occur in adults older than 30 y.
Arachnoid cyst ▷ *Fig. 1.105a–d*	Well-circumscribed extra-axial lesions with low attenuation equivalent to CSF, no contrast enhancement. Commonly located in the anterior middle cranial fossa > suprasellar/quadrigeminal > frontal convexities > posterior cranial fossa.	Nonneoplastic congenital, developmental, or acquired extra-axial lesions filled with CSF, usually mild mass effect on adjacent brain; supratentorial > infratentorial locations; men > women; with or without related clinical symptoms
Lipoma	Lipomas have CT attenuation similar to subcutaneous fat; typically no contrast enhancement or peripheral edema.	Benign fatty lesions resulting from congenital malformation often located in or near the midline; may contain calcifications and/or traversing blood vessels.
Epidermoid cyst ▷ *Fig. 1.106a, b*	Well-circumscribed spheroid or multilobulated, extra-axial ectodermal inclusion cystic lesions with low to intermediate attenuation, no contrast enhancement, with or without bone erosion/destruction. Often insinuate along CSF pathways; chronic deformation of adjacent neural tissue (brainstem, brain parenchyma). Commonly located in the posterior cranial fossa (cerebellopontine angle cistern) > parasellar/middle cranial fossa.	Nonneoplastic congenital or acquired extra-axial off-midline lesions filled with desquamated cells and keratinaceous debris; usually mild mass effect on adjacent brain; infratentorial > supratentorial locations. Adults: men = women, with or without related clinical symptoms.
Dermoid	Well-circumscribed spheroid or multilobulated extra-axial lesions with variable low, intermediate, and/or high attenuation, contrast enhancement, with or without fluid/fluid or fluid/debris levels. Can cause chemical meningitis if dermoid cyst ruptures into the subarachnoid space. Commonly located: at or near the midline; supratentorial > infratentorial.	Nonneoplastic congenital or acquired ectodermal inclusion cystic lesions filled with lipid material, cholesterol, desquamated cells, and keratinaceous debris; usually mild mass effect on adjacent brain. Adults: men slightly > women; with or without related clinical symptoms.
Fibrous dysplasia ▷ *Fig. 1.107*	Expansile process involving the skull base and calvarium with mixed intermediate attenuation with "ground glass" appearance, heterogeneous contrast enhancement.	Usually seen in adolescents and young adults; can result in narrowing of neuroforamina with cranial nerve compression, facial deformities, mono- and polyostotic forms (with or without endocrine abnormalities, such as with McCune-Albright syndrome, precocious puberty).
Paget disease ▷ *Fig. 1.108*	Expansile sclerotic/lytic process involving the skull with mixed intermediate and high attenuation. Irregular/indistinct borders between marrow and inner margins of the outer and inner tables of the skull.	Usually seen in older adults; can result in narrowing of neuroforamina with cranial nerve compression, basilar impression with or without compression of brainstem.

(continues on page 66)

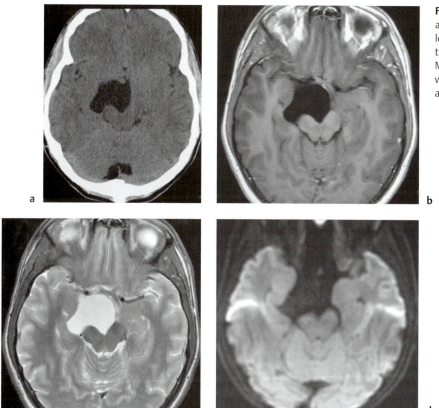

Fig. 1.105a–d Arachnoid cyst. (**a**) The arachnoid cyst with CSF attenuation is located anterior to the brainstem and medial to the right temporal lobe. The cyst has an MRI signal similar to CSF on the axial T1-weighted MRI (**b**), axial T2-weighted MRI (**c**), and diffusion-weighted image (**d**).

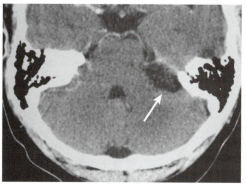
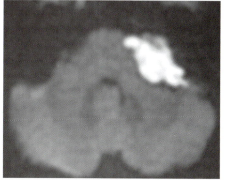

Fig. 1.106a, b Epidermoid. The lesion is located anterior to the left middle cerebellar peduncle and left cerebellar hemisphere and has low attenuation on the axial CT image (arrow) (**a**). The epidermoid has high signal from restricted diffusion on the diffusion-weighted image (**b**).

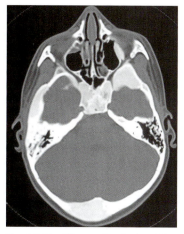
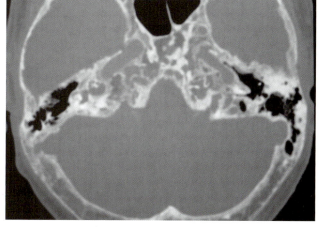

Fig. 1.107 Fibrous dysplasia. Multifocal sites of skull thickening with a "ground glass" appearance are seen in this patient with polyostotic fibrous dysplasia.

Fig. 1.108 Paget disease. Axial image shows thickening of the skull with blurring of the margins between the diploic space and the inner and outer tables of the skull.

Table 1.5 (Cont.) Extra-axial lesions in the posterior cranial fossa (infratentorial)

Lesions	CT Findings	Comments
Inflammatory		
Subdural/epidural abscess, empyema	Epidural or subdural collections with low attenuation, thin linear peripheral zones of contrast enhancement.	Often results from complications related to sinusitis (usually frontal), meningitis, otitis media, ventricular shunts, or surgery. Can be associated with venous sinus thrombosis and venous cerebral or cerebellar infarctions, cerebritis, brain abscess; mortality 30%.
Leptomeningeal infection/ inflammation ▷ *Fig. 1.109*	Single or multiple nodular-enhancing lesions and/or focal or diffuse abnormal subarachnoid enhancement. Leptomeningeal inflammation often best seen on postcontrast images.	Contrast enhancement in the intracranial subarachnoid space (leptomeninges) usually is associated with significant pathology (inflammation and/or infection vs neoplasm). Inflammation and/or infection of the leptomeninges can result from pyogenic, fungal, or parasitic diseases, as well as tuberculosis. Neurosarcoid results in granulomatous disease in the leptomeninges producing similar patterns of subarachnoid enhancement.
Eosinophilic granuloma ▷ *Fig. 1.110*	Single or multiple circumscribed soft tissue lesions in the marrow of the skull associated with focal bony destruction/erosion with extension extracranially, intracranially, or both. Lesions usually have low to intermediate attenuation, with contrast enhancement, with or without enhancement of the adjacent dura.	Single lesion commonly seen in males > females younger than 20 y; proliferation of histiocytes in medullary cavity with localized destruction of bone with extension in adjacent soft tissues. Multiple lesions with syndromes such as Letterer-Siwe disease (lymphadenopathy hepatosplenomegaly), children younger than 2 y; Hand-Schüller-Christian disease (lymphadenopathy, exophthalmos, diabetes insipidus) children 5 to 10 y.
Sarcoidosis	Poorly marginated nodular and/or diffuse contrast enhancement in the leptomeninges; may be associated with intra-axial lesions with contrast enhancement, edema, and localized mass effect.	Multisystem noncaseating granulomatous disease of uncertain cause that can involve the CNS in 5% to 15% of cases. Associated with severe neurologic deficits if untreated.
Other		
Vascular **AVM** ▷ *Fig. 1.111a, b*	Lesions with irregular margins that can be located in the brain parenchyma, (pia, dura, or both locations). AVMs contain multiple tortuous vessels. The venous portions often show contrast enhancement. Usually not associated with mass effect unless there is recent hemorrhage or venous occlusion. CTA can show the arterial, nidus, and venous portions of the AVMs.	Supratentorial AVMs occur more frequently (80%–90%) than infratentorial AVMs (10%–20%). Annual risk of hemorrhage. AVMs can be sporadic, congenital, or associated with a history of trauma.
Dural AVM	Dural AVMs contain multiple tortuous small vessels at the site of a recanalized thrombosed dural venous sinus. Usually not associated with mass effect unless there is recent hemorrhage or venous occlusion.	Dural AVMs are usually acquired lesions resulting from thrombosis or occlusion of an intracranial venous sinus with subsequent recanalization resulting in direct arterial to venous sinus communications. Transverse, sigmoid venous sinuses > cavernous sinuses > straight, superior sagittal sinuses.
Aneurysm ▷ *Fig. 1.112a, b*	**Saccular aneurysm:** Focal, well-circumscribed zone of soft tissue attenuation, with or without wall calcifications; usually shows contrast enhancement. **Fusiform aneurysm:** Tubular dilation of the involved artery.	Abnormal fusiform or focal saccular dilation of the artery secondary to acquired/degenerative etiology, polycystic disease, connective tissue disease, atherosclerosis, trauma, infection (mycotic), oncotic, AVM, vasculitis, and drugs. Focal aneurysms, also referred to as saccular aneurysms, typically occur at arterial bifurcations and are multiple in 20% of cases. The chance of rupture of a saccular aneurysm causing subarachnoid hemorrhage is related to the size of the aneurysm. Saccular aneurysms > 2.5 cm in diameter are referred to as giant aneurysms. Fusiform aneurysms are often related to atherosclerosis or collagen vascular disease.

(continues on page 68)

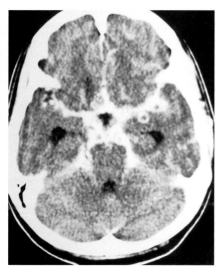

Fig. 1.109   Leptomeningeal infection, tubercular meningitis. Axial postcontrast image shows diffuse abnormal contrast enhancement in the basal meninges and sylvian and interhemispheric fissures.

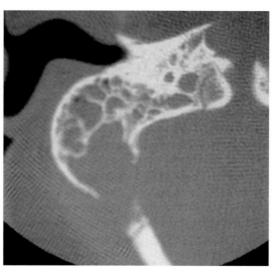

Fig. 1.110   Eosinophilic granuloma. Axial image shows a destructive lesion involving the mastoid portion of the right temporal bone and adjacent right occipital bone.

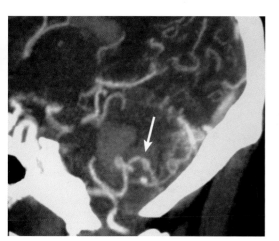
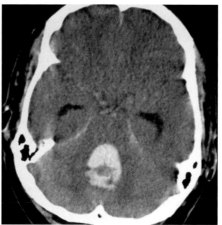

b

Fig. 1.111a, b   AVM. Sagittal CTA image (**a**) shows an abnormal collection of vessels involving the cerebellum (arrow) that is associated with an intraventricular hemorrhage (**b**).

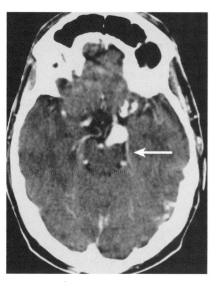
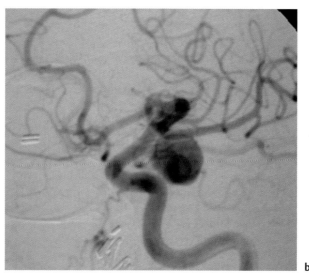

b

Fig. 1.112a, b   Aneurysm. Postcontrast axial CT image (**a**) shows the enhancing posterior communicating artery aneurysm indenting the left cerebral peduncle (arrow), as also seen on conventional angiography (**b**).

Table 1.5 (Cont.) Extra-axial lesions in the posterior cranial fossa (infratentorial)

Lesions	CT Findings	Comments
Hemorrhagic **Epidural hematoma**	Biconvex extra-axial hematoma located between the skull and dura; displaced dura has high attenuation. The CT attenuation and MRI signal of the hematoma depend on its age, size, hematocrit, and oxygen tension; with or without edema (low attenuation on CT and high signal on T2-weighted images) involving the displaced brain parenchyma; with or without subfalcine, uncal herniation. **Hyperacute hematoma:** **CT:** Can have high and/or mixed high and intermediate attenuation. **MRI:** Intermediate signal on T1-weighted images, intermediate to high signal on T2-weighted images. **Acute hematoma:** **CT:** Can have high and/or mixed high and intermediate attenuation. **MRI:** Low to intermediate signal on T1-weighted images, high signal on T2-weighted images. **Subacute hematoma:** **CT:** Can have high and/or mixed high and intermediate attenuation. **MRI:** High signal on T1- and T2-weighted images.	Epidural hematomas usually result from trauma/tearing of an epidural artery or dural venous sinus; epidural hematomas do not cross cranial sutures; with or without skull fracture.
Subdural hematoma	Crescentic extra-axial hematoma located in the potential space between the inner margin of the dura and the outer margin of the arachnoid membrane. The CT attenuation and MRI signal of the hematoma depend on its age, size, hematocrit, and oxygen tension; with or without edema (low attenuation on CT and high signal on T2-weighted images) involving the displaced brain parenchyma; with or without subfalcine, uncal herniation. **Hyperacute hematoma:** **CT:** Can have high or mixed high, intermediate, and/or low attenuation. **MRI:** Intermediate signal on T1-weighted images, intermediate to high signal on T2-weighted images. **Acute hematoma:** **CT:** Can have high or mixed high, intermediate, and/or low attenuation. **MRI:** Low to intermediate signal on T1-weighted images, low signal on T2-weighted images. **Subacute hematoma:** **CT:** Can have intermediate attenuation (isodense to brain) and/or low to intermediate attenuation. **MRI:** High signal on T1- and T2-weighted images. **Chronic hematoma:** **CT:** Usually have low attenuation (hypodense to brain). **MRI:** Variable, often low to intermediate signal on T1-weighted images, high signal on T2-weighted images, with or without enhancement of collection and organizing neomembrane. Mixed MRI signal can result if rebleeding occurs into chronic collection.	Subdural hematomas usually result from trauma/stretching/tearing of cortical veins where they enter the subdural space to drain into dural venous sinuses; subdural hematomas do cross sites of cranial sutures; with or without skull fracture.
Subarachnoid hemorrhage ▷ *Fig. 1.67a, b, p. 37*	**CT:** Acute subarachnoid hemorrhage typically appears as poorly defined zones with high attenuation in the leptomeninges within the sulci and basal cisterns. Usually becomes isodense or hypodense after 1 week unless there is rebleeding. **MRI:** May not be seen on T1- or T2-weighted images, although it may have intermediate to slightly high signal on FLAIR images.	Extravasated blood in the subarachnoid space can result from ruptured arterial aneurysms or dural venous sinuses, vascular malformations, hypertensive hemorrhages, trauma, cerebral infarcts, coagulopathy, etc.

Table 1.6   Cystic, cystlike, and cyst-containing intracranial lesions

Lesions	CT Findings	Comments
Intra-axial		
Astrocytoma	**Low-grade astrocytoma:** Focal or diffuse mass lesion usually located in the white matter with low to intermediate attenuation, with or without mild contrast enhancement, with or without cysts. Minimal associated mass effect. ▷ *Fig. 1.113a, b*	Often occurs in children and adults (20–40 y). Tumors comprised of well-differentiated astrocytes. Association with neurofibromatosis type 1; 10-y survival; may become malignant.
	Juvenile pilocytic astrocytoma, subtype: Solid/cystic focal lesion with low to intermediate attenuation, usually with prominent contrast enhancement. Lesions located in cerebellum, hypothalamus, adjacent to third or fourth ventricles, and brainstem. ▷ *Fig. 1.114*	Common in children; usually favorable prognosis if totally resected.
	Anaplastic astrocytoma: Often irregularly marginated lesion located in the white matter with low to intermediate attenuation, with or without contrast enhancement, with or without cysts.	Intermediate between low-grade astrocytoma and glioblastoma multiforme; ~2-y survival.
Glioblastoma multiforme ▷ *Fig. 1.115a, b*	Irregularly marginated mass lesion with necrosis or cyst, mixed attenuation, with or without hemorrhage, heterogeneous contrast enhancement, peripheral edema; can cross corpus callosum.	Most common primary CNS tumor; highly malignant neoplasms with necrosis and vascular proliferation; usually seen in patients older than 50 y; extent of lesion underestimated by CT; survival < 1 y.

(continues on page 70)

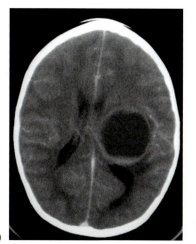 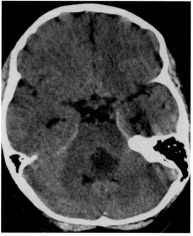

b

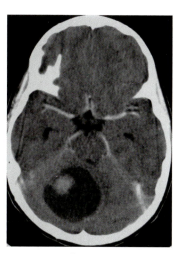

Fig. 1.113a, b   Low-grade astrocytoma. Axial postcontrast image (**a**) shows a circumscribed cystic astrocytoma in the left cerebral hemisphere that has a thin peripheral rim of enhancement. Axial image (**b**) shows an astrocytoma in the pons containing a low-attenuation cystic-appearing region.

Fig. 1.114   Pilocytic astrocytoma. Axial postcontrast CT image shows the tumor to contain a cyst with a nodular-enhancing portion.

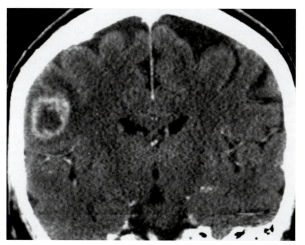 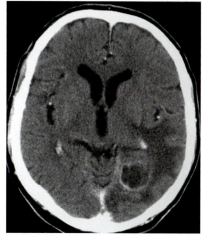

b

Fig. 1.115a, b   Glioblastoma multiforme. Coronal (**a**) and axial (**b**) postcontrast images in two different patients show peripherally enhancing tumors containing low-attenuation centers representing cystic necrotic regions. Decreased attenuation in the brain surrounding the enhancing portions of the tumors can represent axonal edema and/or tumor extension.

Table 1.6   (Cont.) Cystic, cystlike, and cyst-containing intracranial lesions

Lesions	CT Findings	Comments
Oligodendroglioma	Circumscribed lesion with mixed low to intermediate attenuation, clumplike calcifications, heterogeneous contrast enhancement; involves white matter and cerebral cortex, with or without cysts; can cause chronic erosion of inner table of calvarium.	Uncommon slow-growing gliomas with usually mixed histologic patterns (e.g., astrocytomas). Usually seen in adults older than 35 y; 85% supratentorial. If low grade, 75% 5-y survival; higher grade lesions have a worse prognosis.
Central neurocytoma	Circumscribed lesion located at the margin of the lateral ventricle or septum pellucidum with intraventricular protrusion, heterogeneous intermediate attenuation signal, with or without calcifications and/or small cysts; heterogeneous contrast enhancement.	Rare tumors that have neuronal differentiation; imaging appearance similar to intraventricular oligodendrogliomas; occur in young adults; benign slow-growing lesions.
Ganglioglioma, ganglioneuroma, gangliocytoma	Circumscribed tumor, usually supratentorial, often temporal or frontal lobes; low to intermediate attenuation; with or without cysts, with or without contrast enhancement.	Ganglioglioma (contains glial and neuronal elements), ganglioneuroma (contains only ganglion cells). Uncommon tumors seen in patients younger than 30 y; seizure presentation; slow-growing neoplasms. Gangliocytomas contain only neuronal elements, dysplastic brain tissue. Favorable prognosis if completely resected.
Dysembryoplastic neuroepithelial tumor	Circumscribed lesions involving the cerebral cortex and subcortical white matter, low to intermediate attenuation, with or without small cysts, usually no contrast enhancement.	Benign superficial lesions commonly located in the temporal or frontal lobes.
Pleomorphic xanthoastrocytoma	Circumscribed supratentorial lesion involving the cerebral cortex and white matter, low to intermediate attenuation, with or without cyst(s), heterogeneous contrast enhancement, with or without enhancing mural nodule associated with cyst.	Rare type of astrocytoma occurring in young adults and children; associated with seizure history.
Primitive neuroectodermal tumor	Circumscribed or invasive lesions, low to intermediate attenuation signal; variable contrast enhancement, with or without cysts; frequent dissemination into the leptomeninges.	Highly malignant tumors that frequently disseminate along CSF pathways.
Ependymoma ▷ *Fig. 1.116*	Circumscribed lobulated supratentorial lesion, often extraventricular, with or without cysts and/or calcifications; low to intermediate attenuation, variable contrast enhancement.	Occurs more commonly in children than adults; one third supratentorial, two thirds infratentorial; 45% 5-y survival
Hemangioblastoma ▷ *Fig. 1.117*	Circumscribed tumors usually located in the cerebellum and/or brainstem; contrast-enhancing nodule with or without cyst, or larger lesion with prominent heterogeneous enhancement with or without vessels within lesion or at the periphery; intermediate attenuation; occasionally lesions have evidence of recent or remote hemorrhage.	Occurs in adolescents, young and middle-aged adults. Lesions are typically multiple in patients with von Hippel-Lindau disease.
Metastases	Circumscribed spheroid lesions in brain can have various intra-axial locations, often at gray-white matter junctions, usually low to intermediate attenuation; with or without hemorrhage, calcifications, cysts; variable contrast enhancement, often low attenuation peripheral to nodular-enhancing lesion representing axonal edema.	Represent ~33% of intracranial tumors, usually from extracranial primary neoplasm in adults older than 40 y.
Pyogenic brain abscess ▷ *Fig. 1.118a, b*	Circumscribed lesion with low attenuation (with or without air-fluid level) surrounded by a thin rim of low to intermediate attenuation that shows ringlike contrast enhancement, as well as a peripheral poorly defined zone of low attenuation representing edema.	Formation of brain abscess occurs 2 weeks after cerebritis with liquefaction and necrosis centrally surrounded by a capsule and peripheral edema. Can be multiple. Complication from meningitis and/or sinusitis, septicemia, trauma, surgery, and cardiac shunt.
Fungal brain abscess ▷ *Fig. 1.119a, b*	Vary depending on organism; lesions occur in meninges and brain parenchyma, solid or cystic lesions with low to intermediate attenuation, nodular or ring contrast enhancement, peripheral low attenuation in adjacent brain tissue.	Occur in immunocompromised or diabetic patients with resultant granulomas in meninges and brain parenchyma. Abscess formation can occur.

(continues on page 72)

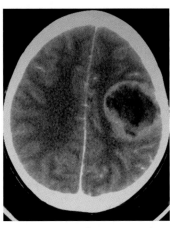

Fig. 1.116 Ependymoma. Axial postcontrast image shows a peripherally enhancing tumor surrounding a low-attenuation central portion.

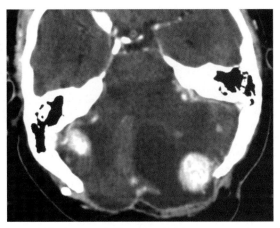

Fig. 1.117 Hemangioblastoma. Axial postcontrast image in a patient with von Hippel-Lindau disease shows a nodular-enhancing lesion in the left cerebellar hemisphere associated with a cyst. Smaller nodular-enhancing hemangioblastomas are also seen in the cerebellum.

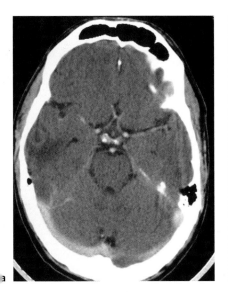

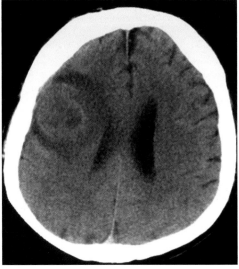

Fig. 1.118a, b Pyogenic brain abscess. Axial postcontrast images in two different patients show peripherally enhancing abscesses surrounding a low-attenuation central portion. Decreased attenuation in the brain surrounding the abscess represents axonal edema.

a

b

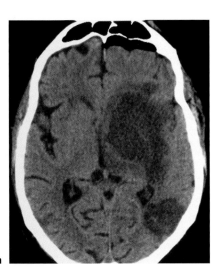

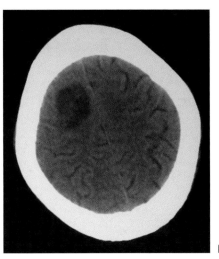

Fig. 1.119a, b Fungal brain abscess. Axial images in two different patients show poorly defined zones with low attenuation in the left cerebral hemisphere from *Aspergillus* infection (**a**) and in the upper right frontal lobe from *Mucor* infection (**b**).

a

b

Table 1.6   (Cont.) Cystic, cystlike, and cyst-containing intracranial lesions

Lesions	CT Findings	Comments
Tuberculoma ▷ *Fig. 1.120*	Intra-axial lesions in cerebral hemispheres, basal ganglia, and brainstem (adults), and cerebellum (children). Lesions can have decreased attenuation, central zone of low attenuation with a thin peripheral rim of intermediate attenuation, with solid or rim pattern of contrast enhancement, with or without calcification. **Meningeal lesions:** Nodular or ring-shaped zones of basilar meningeal enhancement.	Occurs in immunocompromised patients and in inhabitants of developing countries. Caseating intracranial granulomas via hematogenous dissemination; meninges > brain lesions.
Toxoplasmosis	Single or multiple solid and/or ring-shaped lesions located in basal ganglia and/or corticomedullary junctions in cerebral hemispheres, low to intermediate attenuation, nodular or rim pattern of contrast enhancement, with or without peripheral low attenuation (edema).	Most common opportunistic CNS infection in AIDS patients; caused by ingestion of food contaminated with parasites (*Toxoplasma gondii*).
Cysticercosis	Single or multiple cystic lesions in brain or meninges. **Acute/subacute phase:** Low to intermediate attenuation, rim with or without nodular pattern of contrast enhancement, with or without peripheral low attenuation (edema). **Chronic phase:** Calcified granulomas.	Caused by ingestion of ova (*Taenia solium*) in contaminated food (undercooked pork); involves meninges > brain parenchyma > ventricles.
Hydatid cyst	*Echinococcus granulosus:* Single or rarely multiple cystic lesions with low attenuation with a thin wall with low to intermediate attenuation; typically no contrast enhancement or peripheral edema unless superinfected; often located in vascular territory of the middle cerebral artery. *Echinococcus multilocularis:* Cystic (with or without multilocular) and/or solid lesions; central zone of intermediate attenuation surrounded by a slightly thickened rim of low to intermediate attenuation, with contrast enhancement; peripheral zone of low attenuation (edema) and calcifications are common.	Caused by parasites *E. granulosus* (South America, Middle East, Australia, and New Zealand) and *E. multilocularis* (North America, Europe, Turkey, and China). CNS involvement in 2% of cases of hydatid infestation.
Demyelinating disease: ADEM, multiple sclerosis	Demyelinating lesions rarely can have a cystlike appearance. Lesions can be located in the cerebral or cerebellar white matter, brainstem, and basal ganglia; Contrast enhancement can be ringlike; usually in acute/early subacute phase of demyelination.	Multiple sclerosis is the most common acquired demyelinating disease. Other demyelinating diseases are acute disseminated encephalomyelitis/immune mediated demyelination after viral infection, toxins, or metabolic disorders.
Radiation necrosis	Focal lesion with or without mass effect or poorly defined zone of low to intermediate attenuation, with or without contrast enhancement involving tissue (gray matter and/or white matter) in field of treatment.	Usually occurs from 4 to 6 months to 10 y after radiation treatment; may be difficult to distinguish from neoplasm. PET and magnetic resonance hydrogen spectroscopy might be helpful for evaluation.
Porencephalic cyst ▷ *Fig. 1.121*	Irregular, relatively well-circumscribed zone with low attenuation similar to CSF, surrounded by poorly defined thin zone of low to intermediate attenuation in the adjacent brain tissue; no contrast enhancement or peripheral edema.	Represent remote sites of brain injury (trauma, infarction, infection, hemorrhage) with evolution into a cystic zone with CSF attenuation surrounded by gliosis in adjacent brain parenchyma. Gliosis (low to intermediate attenuation) allows differentiation from schizencephaly.
Neuroepithelial cyst	Well-circumscribed cysts with low attenuation signal, thin walls; no contrast enhancement or peripheral edema.	Cyst walls have histopathologic features similar to epithelium, neuroepithelial cysts located in choroid plexus > choroidal fissure > ventricles > brain parenchyma.
Extra-axial		
Craniopharyngioma ▷ *Fig. 1.122*	Circumscribed lobulated lesions; variable low, intermediate, and/or high attenuation; with or without nodular or rim patterns of contrast enhancement. May contain cysts, lipid components, and calcifications.	Usually histologically benign but locally aggressive lesions arising from squamous epithelial rests along the Rathke cleft; occur in children (10 y) and adults (> 40 y), males = females.
Germinoma ▷ *Fig. 1.123a, b*	Circumscribed tumors with or without disseminated disease; pineal region > suprasellar region > third ventricle/basal ganglia; low to intermediate attenuation; with contrast enhancement of tumor and leptomeninges if disseminated.	Most common type of germ cell tumor; occurs in males > females (10–30 y), usually midline neoplasms.

(continues on page 74)

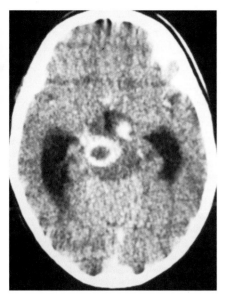

Fig. 1.120   Tuberculoma. Axial postcontrast image shows a ring-enhancing tuberculous abscess involving the brainstem, as well as a nodular-enhancing lesion in the basal meninges.

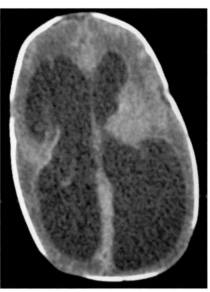

Fig. 1.121   Porencephalic cyst. Axial image shows a cyst adjacent to the frontal horn of the right lateral ventricle in a patient with hydrocephalus and periventricular leukoencephalopathy.

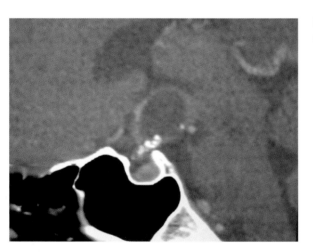

Fig. 1.122   Craniopharyngioma. Postcontrast sagittal image shows a complex cystic and solid lesion in the suprasellar cistern.

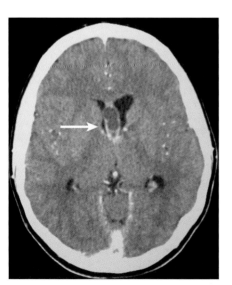

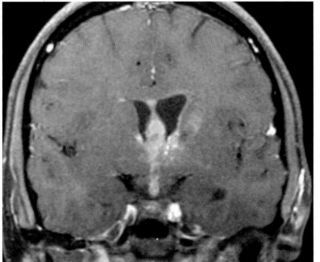

b

Fig. 1.123a, b   Germinoma. Axial postcontrast CT image (**a**) shows a peripherally enhancing lesion involving the septum pellucidum surrounding a low-attenuation central portion (arrow). Coronal postcontrast fat-suppressed, T1-weighted image (**b**) shows abnormal tumoral enhancement in the suprasellar cistern and third and lateral ventricles, as well as the septum pellucidum.

Table 1.6 (Cont.) Cystic, cystlike, and cyst-containing intracranial lesions

Lesions	CT Findings	Comments
Teratoma	Circumscribed lesions; pineal region > suprasellar region > third ventricle; variable low to intermediate attenuation; with or without contrast enhancement. May contain calcifications, cysts, as well as fatty components, which can cause chemical meningitis if ruptured.	Second most common type of germ cell tumors; occur in children, males > females; benign or malignant types, composed of derivatives of ectoderm, mesoderm, and/or endoderm.
Pineal cyst ▷ *Fig. 1.124a, b*	Well-circumscribed, extra-axial lesions with low attenuation signal similar to CSF; no central enhancement, thin linear peripheral contrast enhancement; rarely atypical appearance with proteinaceous contents; intermediate, slightly high attenuation.	Common usually incidental nonneoplastic cyst in pineal gland.
Arachnoid cyst ▷ *Fig. 1.125*	Well-circumscribed, extra-axial lesions with low attenuation similar to CSF; no contrast enhancement. Commonly located in the anterior middle cranial fossa > suprasellar/quadrigeminal > frontal convexities > posterior cranial fossa.	Nonneoplastic congenital, developmental, or acquired extra-axial lesions filled with CSF; usually mild mass effect on adjacent brain; supratentorial > infratentorial locations; males > females; with or without related clinical symptoms.
Leptomeningeal cyst	Well-circumscribed, extra-axial lesions with low attenuation similar to CSF, no contrast enhancement. Associated with erosion of the adjacent skull.	Nonneoplastic extra-axial lesions filled with CSF; thought to be secondary to trauma with dural tear/skull fracture; usually mild mass effect on adjacent brain with progressive erosion of adjacent skull; occasionally presents as a scalp lesion; occurs in children > adults.
Colloid cyst	Well-circumscribed spheroid lesions located at the anterior portion of the third ventricle; variable attenuation (low, intermediate, or high), no contrast enhancement.	Common presentation of headaches and intermittent hydrocephalus; removal leads to cure.
Choroid plexus cysts	Low-attenuation cystic structure similar to CSF attenuation within the choroid plexus. On MRI, cysts within the choroid plexus have signal similar to CSF, whereas xanthogranulomatous cysts often have high signal on T2-weighted images and intermediate signal on FLAIR. Xanthogranulomatous cysts have restricted diffusion on diffusion-weighted images as well as apparent diffusion coefficient (ADC) maps.	The choroid plexus can contain incidental simple cysts or xanthogranulomatous cystic lesions.
Epidermoid ▷ *Fig. 1.126*	Well-circumscribed spheroid or multilobulated extra-axial ectodermal inclusion cystic lesions with low to intermediate attenuation that may be similar to CSF; no contrast enhancement. Often insinuate along CSF pathways; chronic deformation of adjacent neural tissue (brainstem, brain parenchyma). Commonly located in the posterior cranial fossa (cerebellopontine angle cistern) > parasellar/middle cranial fossa.	Nonneoplastic congenital or acquired extra-axial off-midline lesions filled with desquamated cells and keratinaceous debris; usually mild mass effect on adjacent brain; infratentorial > supratentorial locations. Adults: men = women; with or without related clinical symptoms.
Dermoid	Well-circumscribed spheroid or multilobulated extra-axial lesions, usually with low attenuation, no contrast enhancement. With or without fluid/fluid or fluid/debris levels. Can cause chemical meningitis if dermoid cyst ruptures into the subarachnoid space. Commonly located at or near the midline; supratentorial > infratentorial.	Congenital or acquired ectodermal inclusion cystic lesions filled with lipid material, cholesterol, desquamated cells, and keratinaceous debris; usually mild mass effect on adjacent brain. Adults: men slightly > women; with or without related clinical symptoms.
Rathke cleft cyst	Well-circumscribed lesion with variable low or intermediate attenuation, no central contrast enhancement, with or without thin peripheral contrast enhancement. Lesion locations: 50% intrasellar, 25% suprasellar, 25% intra- and suprasellar.	Uncommon sella/juxtasellar benign cystic lesion containing fluid with variable amounts of protein, mucopolysaccharide, and/or cholesterol; arise from epithelial rests of the craniopharyngeal duct.
Epidural/subdural empyema ▷ *Fig. 1.127a, b*	Epidural or subdural collections with low attenuation, linear peripheral zones of contrast enhancement.	Often results from complications related to sinusitis (usually frontal), meningitis, otitis media, ventricular shunts, or surgery. Can be associated with venous sinus thrombosis and venous cerebral or cerebellar infarctions, cerebritis, and brain abscess; mortality 30%.
Meningitis ▷ *Fig. 1.128*	Single or multiple nodular-enhancing lesions and/or focal or diffuse abnormal subarachnoid enhancement. Leptomeningeal inflammation often best seen on postcontrast images.	Contrast enhancement in the intracranial subarachnoid space (leptomeninges) usually is associated with significant pathology (inflammation and/or infection vs neoplasm). Inflammation and/or infection of the leptomeninges can result from pyogenic, fungal, or parasitic diseases, as well as tuberculosis. Neurosarcoid results in granulomatous disease in the leptomeninges, producing similar patterns of subarachnoid enhancement.

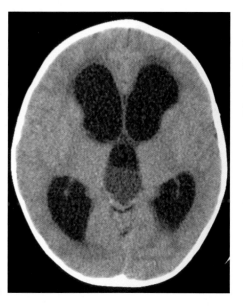

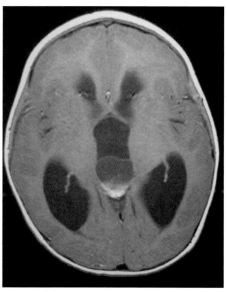

Fig. 1.124a, b Pineal cyst. Axial CT image (**a**) shows a large pineal cyst causing hydrocephalus. Postcontrast axial T1-weighted MRI (**b**) shows thin peripheral enhancement of the pineal cyst.

a

b

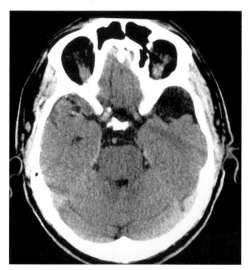

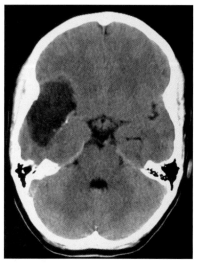

Fig. 1.125 Arachnoid cyst. Axial image shows an arachnoid cyst in the anterior portion of the left middle cranial fossa.

Fig. 1.126 Epidermoid. Axial image shows an extra-axial low-attenuation lesion indenting the right temporal and frontal lobes.

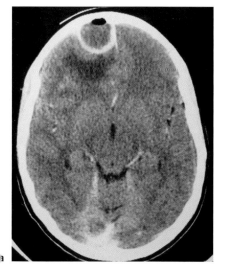

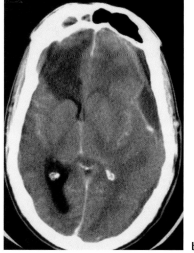

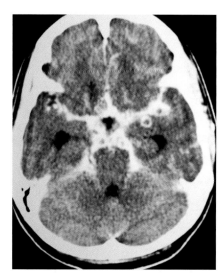

a

b

Fig. 1.127a, b Epidural/subdural abscess. Axial postcontrast images in two different patients show extra-axial lesions with low attenuation with enhancing rims from an epidural abscess (**a**) and subdural abscess on the left (**b**).

Fig. 1.128 Meningitis. Axial postcontrast image in a patient with tubercular meningitis shows thick leptomeningeal enhancement in the subarachnoid space and basal cisterns, as well as two ring-enhancing lesions with central low attenuation.

Table 1.7 Abnormalities and lesions of the basal ganglia

Lesions	CT Findings	Comments
Neoplasms		
Astrocytoma ▷ *Fig. 1.129a–c*	**Low-grade astrocytoma:** Focal or diffuse mass lesion with low to intermediate attenuation, with or without mild contrast enhancement. Minimal associated mass effect. **Juvenile pilocytic astrocytoma, subtype:** Solid/cystic focal lesion with low to intermediate attenuation signal, usually with contrast enhancement. Lesions located in the cerebellum, hypothalamus, adjacent to third or fourth ventricles, brainstem. **Gliomatosis cerebri:** Infiltrative lesion with poorly defined margins with mass effect located in the white matter that can extend into the basal ganglia, with low to intermediate attenuation, usually no contrast enhancement until late in disease. **Anaplastic astrocytoma:** Often irregularly marginated lesion located in the white matter and extending into the basal ganglia with low to intermediate attenuation, with or without contrast enhancement.	Often occurs in children and adults (20–40 y). Tumors comprised of well-differentiated astrocytes. Association with neurofibromatosis type 1; 10-y survival; may become malignant. Common in children, usually favorable prognosis if totally resected. Diffusely infiltrating astrocytoma with relative preservation of underlying brain architecture. Imaging appearance may be more prognostic than histologic grade; ~2 y survival. Intermediate between low-grade astrocytoma and glioblastoma multiforme; ~2- y survival.
Glioblastoma multiforme ▷ *Fig. 1.130*	Irregularly marginated mass lesion with necrosis or cyst, mixed attenuation images, heterogeneous, with or without hemorrhage, prominent heterogeneous contrast enhancement; peripheral edema; can cross the corpus callosum.	Most common primary CNS tumor, highly malignant neoplasms with necrosis and vascular proliferation; usually seen in patients older than 50 y; extent of lesion underestimated by CT and MRI; survival < 1 y.
Giant cell astrocytoma/ tuberous sclerosis ▷ *Fig. 1.131*	Circumscribed lesion located near the foramen of Monro with mixed low to intermediate attenuation with or without cysts and/or calcifications, with heterogeneous contrast enhancement.	Subependymal hamartoma near the foramen of Monro; occurs in 15% of patients with tuberous sclerosis < 20 y; slow-growing lesions can progressively cause obstruction of CSF flow through the foramen of Monro. Long-term survival usual if resected.
Hamartoma/tuberous sclerosis ▷ *Fig. 1.132*	Cortical-subcortical lesion with variable attenuation; calcifications in 50% of older children; contrast enhancement uncommon. **Subependymal hamartomas:** Small nodules located along and projecting into the lateral ventricles; calcification and contrast enhancement common.	Cortical and subependymal hamartomas are nonmalignant lesions associated with tuberous sclerosis. Tuberous sclerosis is an autosomal dominant disorder associated with hamartomas in multiple organs.
Pleomorphic xanthoastrocytoma	Circumscribed supratentorial lesion; low to intermediate attenuation, heterogeneous contrast enhancement, with or without enhancing mural nodule associated with cyst.	Rare type of astrocytoma occurring in young adults and children; associated with seizure history.
Oligodendroglioma	Circumscribed lesion with mixed low to intermediate attenuation; with or without areas of clumplike calcification, heterogeneous contrast enhancement.	Uncommon slow-growing gliomas with usually mixed histologic patterns (e.g., astrocytomas). Usually in adults older than 35 y; 85% supratentorial. If low grade, 75% 5-y survival; higher grade lesions have a worse prognosis.
Ganglioglioma, ganglioneuroma, gangliocytoma	Circumscribed tumor, usually supratentorial, often temporal or frontal lobes; low to intermediate attenuation, with or without cysts, with or without contrast enhancement.	Ganglioglioma (contains glial and neuronal elements), ganglioneuroma (contains only ganglion cells). Uncommon tumors, < 30 y, seizure presentation, slow-growing neoplasms. Gangliocytoma (contains only neuronal elements, dysplastic brain tissue). Favorable prognosis if completely resected.
Ependymoma	Circumscribed lobulated supratentorial lesion, often extraventricular, with or without cysts and/or calcifications, variable contrast enhancement.	Occurs more commonly in children than adults; one third supratentorial, two thirds infratentorial; 45% 5-y survival.
Lymphoma ▷ *Fig. 1.133*	**Primary CNS lymphoma:** Focal or infiltrating lesion located in the basal ganglia, periventricular regions, posterior fossa/brainstem; low to intermediate attenuation, with or without hemorrhage/necrosis in immunocompromised patients; usually show contrast enhancement. Diffuse leptomeningeal enhancement is another pattern of intracranial lymphoma.	Primary CNS lymphoma more common than secondary, usually in adults older than 40 y. B-cell lymphoma more common than T-cell lymphoma; increasing incidence related to number of immunocompromised patients in population. CT and MRI imaging features of primary and secondary lymphoma of brain overlap. Intracranial lymphoma can involve the leptomeninges in secondary lymphoma > primary lymphoma.

(continues on page 78)

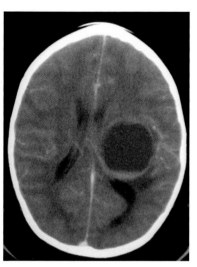
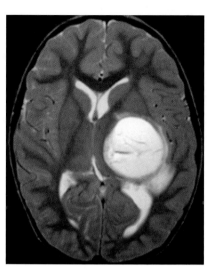
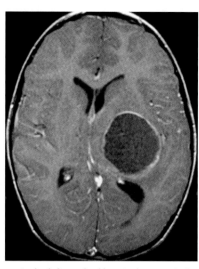

Fig. 1.129a–c   Astrocytoma. Axial postcontrast image (**a**) shows a circumscribed cystic astrocytoma in the left cerebral hemisphere, including the basal ganglia, which has a thin peripheral rim of enhancement. The tumor has high signal on the axial T2-weighted MRI (**b**) and low signal with rim enhancement on the axial T1-weighted MRI (**c**).

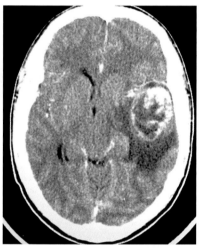
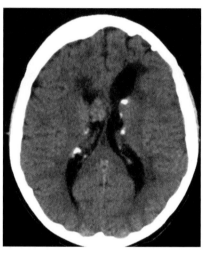
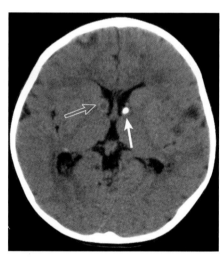

Fig. 1.130   Glioblastoma multiforme. Axial postcontrast image shows a peripherally enhancing tumor in the left cerebral hemisphere extending into the basal ganglia. Poorly defined low attenuation is seen adjacent to the enhancing portion of the tumor and may represent tumor and/ or edema.

Fig. 1.131   Giant cell astrocytoma/ tuberous sclerosis. Axial image shows a nodular lesion at the right foramen of Monro, as well as multiple small calcified ependymal hamartomas.

Fig. 1.132   Hamartoma, tuberous sclerosis. Axial image shows a calcified ependymal hamartoma at the left foramen of Monro (arrow) and a noncalcified hamartoma at the right foramen of Monro (open arrow).

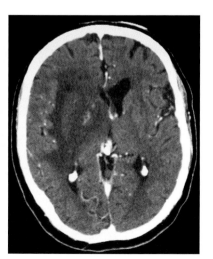

Fig. 1.133   B-cell lymphoma. Axial postcontrast image shows a tumor involving the right basal ganglia with mass effect and compression of the third ventricle. Only a small portion of the tumor shows contrast enhancement.

Table 1.7 (Cont.) Abnormalities and lesions of the basal ganglia

Lesions	CT Findings	Comments
Metastases	Circumscribed spheroid lesions in the brain, usually low to intermediate attenuation with or without hemorrhage, calcifications, cysts; variable contrast enhancement, often low attenuation peripheral to nodular-enhancing lesion representing axonal edema.	Represent ~33% of intracranial tumors, usually from extracranial primary neoplasm in adults older than 40 y. Primary tumor source: lung > breast > GI > GU > melanoma.
Tumorlike lesions		
Neuroepithelial cyst	Well-circumscribed cysts with low attenuation similar to CSF; thin walls; no contrast enhancement or peripheral edema.	Cyst walls have histopathologic features similar to epithelium; neuroepithelial cysts located in choroid plexus > choroidal fissure > ventricles > brain parenchyma.
Perivascular spaces	Focus or foci with attenuation similar to CSF, no contrast enhancement; located in the basal ganglia, high subcortical white matter/centrum semiovale.	Pial-lined spaces filled with CSF containing arteries supplying brain parenchyma; also referred to as Virchow-Robin spaces. Perivascular spaces increase in size and number with aging.
Infections		
Cerebritis ▷ *Fig. 1.134*	Poorly defined zone or focal area of low to intermediate attenuation signal; minimal or no contrast enhancement; involves cerebral cortex and white matter for bacterial and fungal infections.	Focal infection/inflammation of brain tissue from bacteria or fungi; secondary to sinusitis, meningitis, surgery, hematogenous source (cardiac and other vascular shunts), and/or immunocompromised status. Can progress to abscess formation.
Pyogenic brain abscess	Circumscribed lesion with low attenuation signal (with or without air-fluid level) surrounded by a thin rim of low to intermediate attenuation that shows contrast enhancement surrounded by a peripheral poorly defined zone of low attenuation representing edema; ringlike zone of contrast enhancement is sometimes thicker laterally than medially.	Formation of brain abscess occurs 2 weeks after cerebritis with liquefaction and necrosis centrally surrounded by a capsule and peripheral edema. Can be multiple. Complication from meningitis and/or sinusitis, septicemia, trauma, surgery, and cardiac shunt.
Fungal brain infection/Abscess ▷ *Fig. 1.135*	Vary depending on organism; lesions occur in meninges and brain parenchyma, solid or cystic lesions with low to intermediate attenuation, nodular or ring enhancement, peripheral low attenuation in brain representing edema.	Occur in immunocompromised or diabetic patients with resultant granulomas in meninges and brain parenchyma. *Cryptococcus* involves the basal meninges and extends along perivascular spaces into the basal ganglia; *Aspergillus* and *Mucor* spread via direct extension through paranasal sinuses or hematogenously, invade blood vessels resulting in hemorrhagic lesions and/or cerebral infarcts; coccidioidomycosis usually involves the basal meninges.
Tuberculoma	**Intra-axial lesions** in cerebral hemispheres and basal ganglia (adults) and cerebellum (children): low to intermediate attenuation; with solid or rim pattern of contrast enhancement; with or without calcification. **Meningeal lesions:** Nodular or cystic-appearing zones of basilar meningeal contrast enhancement.	Occurs in immunocompromised patients and in inhabitants in developing countries. Caseating intracranial granulomas via hematogenous dissemination; meninges > brain lesions.
Encephalitis ▷ *Fig. 1.136*	Poorly defined zone of low to intermediate attenuation. Minimal or no contrast enhancement; involves cerebral cortex and/or white matter; minimal localized mass effect. Herpes simplex typically involves the temporal lobes/limbic system with or without hemorrhage; CMV usually in periventricular location.	Infection/inflammation of brain tissue from viruses, often in immunocompromised patients (e.g., herpes simplex, CMV, and progressive multifocal leukoencephalopathy) or immunocompetent patients (e.g., St. Louis encephalitis, eastern or western equine encephalitis, and Epstein-Barr virus).
Rasmussen encephalitis	Progressive atrophy of one cerebral hemisphere with poorly defined zones of low attenuation involving the white matter, basal ganglia, and cortex; usually no contrast enhancement.	Usually seen in children younger than 10 y; severe and progressive epilepsy and unilateral neurologic deficits (hemiplegia, psychomotor deterioration, chronic slow viral infectious process possibly caused by CMV or Epstein-Barr virus). Treatment: hemispherectomy.
Creutzfeldt-Jakob disease	Progressive cerebral atrophy. Typically no contrast enhancement.	Spongiform encephalopathy caused by slow infection from prion (proteinaceous infectious particle); usually seen in adults 40 to 80 y, progressive dementia, <10% survive more than 2 y.

(continues on page 80)

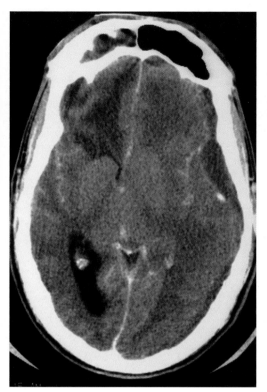

Fig. 1.134   Cerebritis. Axial postcontrast image shows decreased attenuation involving the right frontal lobe extending into the right basal ganglia, as well as the left subdural empyema.

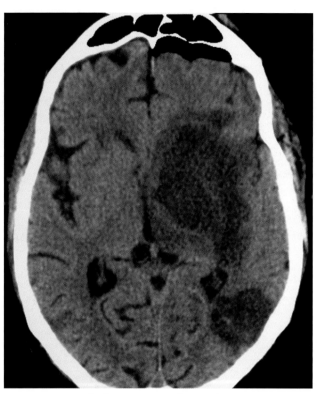

Fig. 1.135   Fungal infection, *Aspergillus.* Axial image shows zones of decreased attenuation involving the left cerebral hemisphere, including the left basal ganglia, from fungal infection.

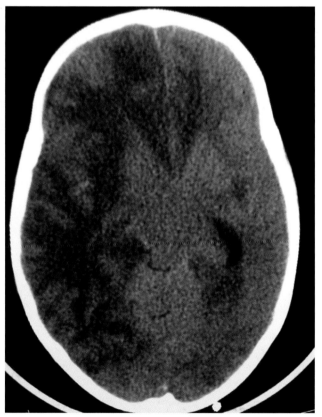

Fig. 1.136   Encephalitis, herpes. Axial image shows an extensive poorly defined zone of decreased attenuation involving the right cerebral hemisphere.

Table 1.7   (Cont.) Abnormalities and lesions of the basal ganglia

Lesions	CT Findings	Comments
Parasitic brain lesions		
Toxoplasmosis ▷ *Fig. 1.137*	Single or multiple solid and/or cystic-appearing lesions located in basal ganglia and/or corticomedullary junctions in cerebral hemispheres, low to intermediate attenuation; nodular or rim pattern of contrast enhancement, with or without peripheral low attenuation (edema).	Most common opportunistic CNS infection in AIDS patients; caused by ingestion of food contaminated with parasites (*Toxoplasma gondii*).
Cysticercosis	Single or multiple cystic-appearing lesions in brain or meninges. **Acute/subacute phase:** Low to intermediate attenuation, with or without rim and/or nodular pattern of contrast enhancement, with or without peripheral low attenuation (edema). **Chronic phase:** Calcified granulomas.	Caused by ingestion of ova (*Taenia solium*) in contaminated food (undercooked pork); involves meninges > brain parenchyma > ventricles.
Hydatid cyst	***Echinococcus granulosus:*** Single or rarely multiple cystic lesions with low attenuation with a thin wall with intermediate attenuation; typically no contrast enhancement or peripheral edema unless superinfected; often located in vascular territory of the middle cerebral artery. ***Echinococcus multilocularis:*** Cystic (with or without multilocular) and/or solid lesions; central zone of low attenuation surrounded by a slightly thickened rim of intermediate attenuation, with contrast enhancement; peripheral zone of low attenuation (edema) and calcifications are common.	Caused by parasites *E. granulosus* (South America, Middle East, Australia, and New Zealand) and *E. multilocularis* (North America, Europe, Turkey, and China). CNS involvement in 2% of cases of hydatid infestation.
Inflammatory lesions		
Demyelinating Disease: **multiple sclerosis, ADEM**	Lesions located in cerebral or cerebellar white matter, brainstem, and basal ganglia; lesions usually have low to intermediate attenuation. With or without contrast enhancement. Contrast enhancement can be ringlike or nodular, usually in acute/early subacute phase of demyelination. Lesions rarely can have associated mass effect simulating neoplasms.	Multiple sclerosis is the most common acquired demyelinating disease usually affecting women (peak ages 20–40 y). Other demyelinating diseases are acute disseminated encephalomyelitis/immune mediated demyelination after viral infection; toxins (exogenous from environmental exposure or ingestion of alcohol, solvents, etc.) or endogenous from metabolic disorder (leukodystrophies, mitochondrial encephalopathies, etc.), radiation injury, trauma, or vascular disease.
Sarcoidosis ▷ *Fig. 1.138a–c*	Poorly marginated intra-axial zone with low to intermediate attenuation, usually shows contrast enhancement, with localized mass effect and peripheral edema. Often associated with contrast enhancement in the leptomeninges.	Multisystem noncaseating granulomatous disease of uncertain cause that can involve the CNS in 5% to 15% of cases. Associated with severe neurologic deficits if untreated.
Radiation Necrosis	Focal lesion with or without mass effect or poorly defined zone of low to intermediate attenuation, with or without contrast enhancement involving tissue (gray matter and/or white matter) in field of treatment.	Usually occurs from 4 to 6 months to 10 y after radiation treatment; may be difficult to distinguish from neoplasm. PET and magnetic resonance hydrogen spectroscopy might be helpful for evaluation.

(continues on page 82)

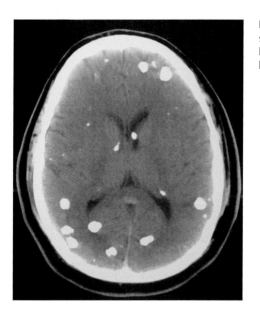

Fig. 1.137   Toxoplasmosis. Axial image shows multiple healed and calcified granulomas from prior infection in both cerebral hemispheres.

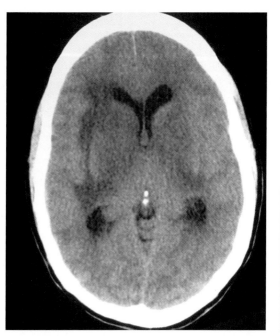

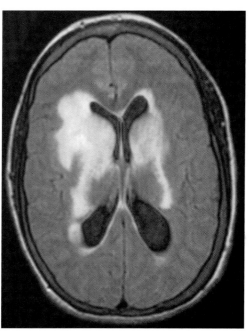

b

Fig. 1.138a–c   Sarcoidosis. Axial CT image (**a**) shows poorly defied zones with decreased attenuation involving both basal ganglia, which show corresponding high signal on the axial FLAIR MRI (**b**). Postcontrast axial T1-weighted MRI (**c**) shows multiple zones of abnormal enhancement in the cerebral hemispheres.

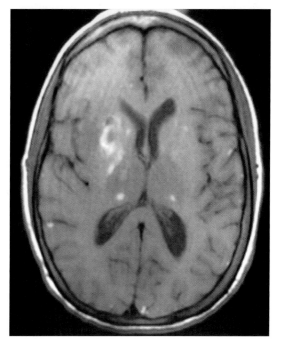

Table 1.7   (Cont.) Abnormalities and lesions of the basal ganglia

Lesions	CT Findings	Comments
Vascular lesions		
Cerebral infarction	**Ischemic anoxic or lacunar infarcts:** CT features of cerebral infarcts depend on age of infarct relative to time of examination. **Hyperacute phase (< 12 h):** **CT:** No abnormality (50%), decreased attenuation and blurring of lentiform nuclei; hyperdense artery in up to 50% of cases. **MRI:** Localized edema, usually isointense signal to normal brain on T1- and T2-weighted images. Diffusion-weighted images can show positive findings related to decreased apparent diffusion coefficients secondary to cytotoxic edema, absence of arterial flow void, or arterial enhancement in the vascular distribution of the infarct. **Acute (12–24 h):** **CT:** Zones with decreased attenuation in basal ganglia, blurring of junction between cerebral cortex and white matter, sulcal effacement. **MRI:** Intermediate signal on T1-weighted images, high signal on T2-weighted images, localized edema. Signal abnormalities commonly involve the basal ganglia. **Early subacute phase (24 h–3 d):** **CT:** Localized swelling at sites with low attenuation involving gray and white matter (often wedge shaped), with or without hemorrhage. ▷ *Fig. 1.139a* **MRI:** Zones with low to intermediate signal on T1-weighted images, high signal on T2-weighted images, localized edema, with or without hemorrhage, with or without gadolinium contrast enhancement. **Late subacute phase (4 d–2 wk):** **CT:** Localized swelling increases and then decreases; low attenuation at lesion can become more prominent, with or without gyral contrast enhancement. ▷ *Fig. 1.139b* **MRI:** Low to intermediate signal on T1-weighted images, high signal on T2-weighted images; edema/mass effect diminishing, with or without hemorrhage, with or without enhancement. **2 weeks to 2 months:** **CT:** With or without gyral contrast enhancement; localized mass effect resolves. ▷ *Fig. 1.139c* **MRI:** Low to intermediate signal on T1-weighted images, high signal on T2-weighted images; edema resolves; with or without hemorrhage, with or without enhancement; eventually declines. **> 2 months:** **CT:** Zone of low attenuation associated with encephalomalacia. ▷ *Fig. 1.139d* **MRI:** Low signal on T1-weighted images, high signal on T2-weighted images; encephalomalacic changes; with or without calcification, hemosiderin.	Cerebral infarcts usually result from occlusive vascular disease involving large, medium, or small arteries. Vascular occlusion may be secondary to atheromatous arterial disease, hypertension, cardiogenic emboli, neoplastic encasement, hypercoagulable states, dissection, congenital anomalies or inherited disorders, such as cerebral autosomal dominant arteriopathy with subcortical infarcts and leukoencephalopathy (CADASIL). Cerebral infarcts usually result from arterial occlusion involving specific vascular territories, although occasionally they occur from metabolic disorders (mitochondrial encephalopathies, etc.) or intracranial venous occlusion (thrombophlebitis, hypercoagulable states, dehydration, etc., which do not correspond to arterial distributions).

(continues on page 84)

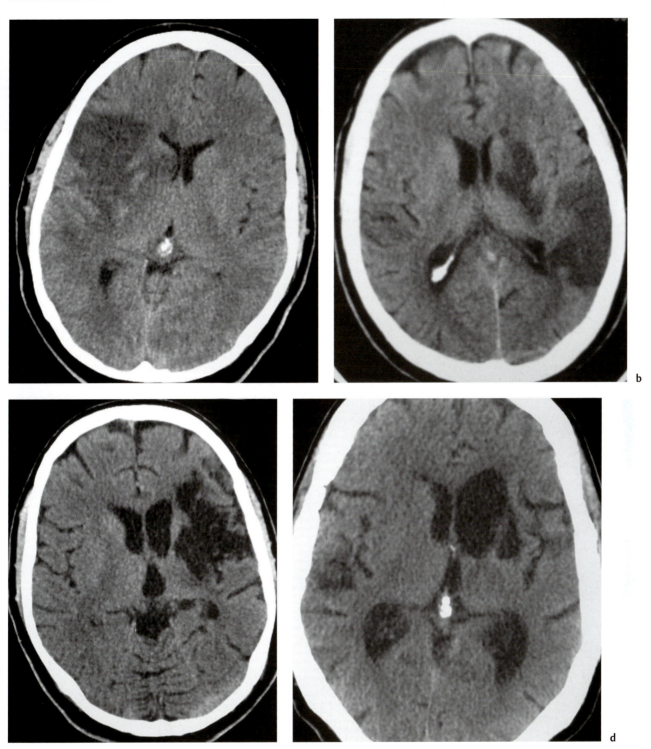

Fig. 1.139a–d   Cerebral ischemia/infarction of different ages/phases in four patients. Axial image (**a**) shows a cerebral infarct (early subacute phase) in the vascular distribution of the right middle cerebral artery. Axial images in three other patients show cerebral infarcts in the vascular distribution of the left middle cerebral artery which are in the late subacute phase of less than 2 weeks (**b**), late phase from 2 weeks to 2 months (**c**), and chronic phase of 2 months (**d**).

Table 1.7 (Cont.) Abnormalities and lesions of the basal ganglia

Lesions	CT Findings	Comments
Hypoxic ischemic encephalopathy ▷ *Fig. 1.140*	Bilateral zones of low attenuation in the basal ganglia, caudate nuclei, thalami, brainstem, and/or perisylvian cerebral cortex.	Prolonged hypotension and anoxia results in ischemia and infarction in portions of the brain with selective vulnerability to hypoxia and impairment of aerobic metabolism. Can result from drowning, asphyxiation, or cardiac arrest.
AVM ▷ *Fig. 1.141*	Lesions with irregular margins that can be located in the brain parenchyma (pia, dura, or both locations). AVMs contain multiple tortuous tubular vessels consisting of patent arteries with high blood flow, as well as thrombosed vessels, areas of hemorrhage in various phases, calcifications, and gliosis. The patent arterial and venous portions often show contrast enhancement on CTAs. CTAs can provide additional detailed information about the nidus, feeding arteries, and draining veins, as well as the presence of associated aneurysms. Usually not associated with mass effect unless there is recent hemorrhage or venous occlusion.	Infratentorial AVMs much less common than supratentorial AVMs.
Cavernous hemangioma ▷ *Fig. 1.142*	Single or multiple multilobulated intra-axial lesions. **CT:** Lesions have intermediate to slightly increased attenuation, with or without calcifications, variable contrast enhancement (most show no or minimal enhancement, few show more prominent enhancement). **MRI:** Peripheral rim or irregular zone of low signal on T2-weighted images secondary to hemosiderin, surrounding a central zone of variable signal (low, intermediate, high, or mixed) on T1- and T2-weighted images depending on ages of hemorrhagic portions. Gradient echo techniques useful for detecting multiple lesions.	Intra-axial lesions composed of endothelial sinusoidal vessels under low pressure. Can be located in many different locations; multiple lesions > 50%. Association with venous angiomas and risk of hemorrhage causing seizures.
Venous angioma	On postcontrast images, venous angiomas are seen as a contrast-enhancing transcortical vein draining a collection of small medullary veins (caput medusae).	Considered an anomalous venous formation typically not associated with hemorrhage; usually an incidental finding except when associated with cavernous hemangioma.
Moyamoya	Multiple tortuous tubular vessels seen in the basal ganglia and thalami secondary to dilated collateral arteries, with contrast enhancement of these arteries related to slow flow within these collateral arteries versus normal-sized arteries. Often with contrast enhancement of the leptomeninges related to pial collateral vessels. Decreased or absent caliber of contrast-enhanced supraclinoid portions of the internal carotid arteries and proximal middle and anterior cerebral arteries. CTA shows stenosis and occlusion of the distal internal carotid arteries with collateral arteries (lenticulostriate, thalamoperforate, and leptomeningeal); best seen after contrast administration enabling detection of slow blood flow.	Progressive occlusive disease of the intracranial portions of the internal carotid arteries with resultant numerous dilated collateral arteries arising from the lenticulostriate and thalamoperforate arteries, as well as other parenchymal, leptomeningeal, and transdural arterial anastomoses. Term translated as "puff of smoke," referring to the angiographic appearance of the collateral arteries (lenticulostriate, thalamoperforate). Usually nonspecific etiology but can be associated with neurofibromatosis, radiation-angiopathy, atherosclerosis, and sickle cell disease; usually children > adults in Asia.

(continues on page 86)

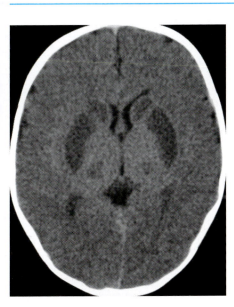

Fig. 1.140   Hypoxic ischemic encephalopathy in a 2-month-old infant. Axial image shows bilateral zones of decreased attenuation involving the basal ganglia.

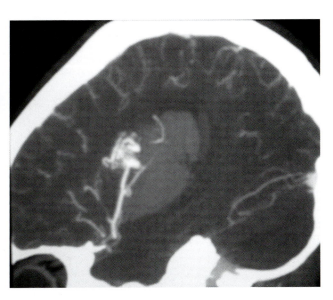

Fig. 1.141   AVM. Sagittal CTA shows an abnormal cluster of arteries involving a branch of the middle cerebral artery associated with an intra-axial hematoma.

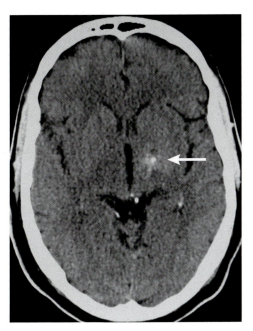

Fig. 1.142   Cavernous hemangioma. Axial image shows a lesion with slightly increased attenuation in the left basal ganglia region containing several small calcifications (arrow).

Table 1.7 (Cont.) Abnormalities and lesions of the basal ganglia

Lesions	CT Findings	Comments
Hematoma	The attenuation of the hematoma depends on its age, size, location, hematocrit, hemoglobin oxidation state, clot retraction, and extent of edema. **Hyperacute phase (4–6 h):** Hemoglobin primarily as diamagnetic oxyhemoglobin (iron Fe^{2+} state). **CT:** High attenuation on CT. ▷ *Fig. 1.143a* **MRI:** Intermediate signal on T1-weighted images, slightly high signal on T2-weighted images. **Acute phase (12–48 h):** Hemoglobin primarily as paramagnetic deoxyhemoglobin (iron, Fe^{2+} state). ▷ *Fig. 1.143b* **CT:** High attenuation in acute clot directly related to hematocrit, hemoglobin concentration, and high protein concentration. Hematocrit in acute clot approaches 90%. **MRI:** Intermediate signal on T1-weighted images, low signal on T2-weighted images, surrounded by a peripheral zone of high T2 signal (edema). **Early subacute phase (> 2 d):** Hemoglobin becomes oxidized to the iron Fe^{3+} state, methemoglobin, which is strongly paramagnetic. **CT:** High attenuation. ▷ *Fig. 1.143c* **MRI:** When methemoglobin is initially intracellular, the hematoma has high signal on T1-weighted images progressing from peripheral to central and low signal on T2-weighted images, surrounded by a zone of high T2 signal (edema). When methemoglobin eventually becomes primarily extracellular, the hematoma has high signal on T1-weighted images and high signal on T2-weighted images. **Late subacute phase (> 7 d–6 wk):** Intracerebral hematomas decrease 1.5 HU per day. Hematomas become isodense to hypodense; peripheral contrast enhancement from blood–brain barrier breakdown and vascularized capsule. **Chronic phase:** Hemoglobin as extracellular methemoglobin is progressively degraded to hemosiderin. **CT:** Chronic hematomas have low attenuation with localized encephalomalacia. Zone with high attenuation represents new sites of rebleeding. **MRI:** The hematoma progresses from a lesion with high signal on T1- and T2-weighted images with a peripheral rim of low signal on T2-weighted images (hemosiderin) to predominant hemosiderin composition with low signal on T2-weighted images.	Can result from trauma, ruptured aneurysms or vascular malformations, coagulopathy, hypertension, adverse drug reaction, amyloid angiopathy, hemorrhagic transformation of cerebral infarction, metastases, abscesses, and viral infections (herpes simplex, CMV).

(continues on page 88)

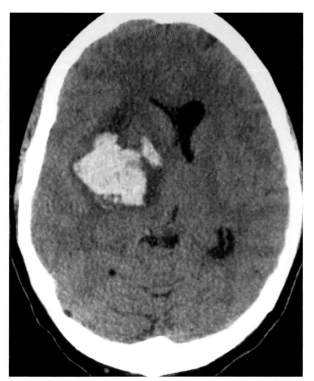

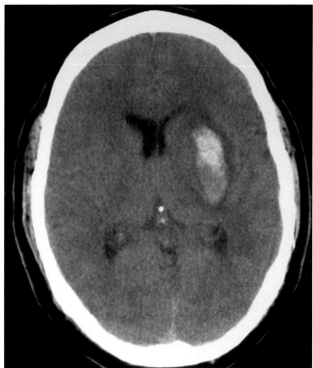

b

Fig. 1.143a–c   Hematoma. Axial images from three different patients show acute hematomas with high attenuation in the right basal ganglia (**a**) and left basal ganglia (**b,c**) with varying degrees of associated mass effect.

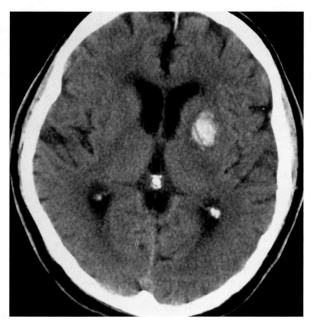

Table 1.7   (Cont.) Abnormalities and lesions of the basal ganglia

Lesions	CT Findings	Comments
Toxic/metabolic abnormalities		
Carbon monoxide poisoning ▷ *Fig. 1.144*	**CT:** Acute poisoning shows symmetric decreased attenuation in the globus pallidi. **MRI:** Low signal on T1-weighted images and high signal on T2-weighted images in the putamen and globus pallidus bilaterally, with or without patchy contrast enhancement in necrotic zones. Diffusion-weighted images show restricted diffusion from acute necrosis. Similar but less pronounced findings are seen in the brainstem and cerebellum.	Toxic effects of CO result in selective necrosis of basal ganglia bilaterally and also to a lesser degree the brainstem and cerebellum. Atrophic changes involving the brain can be seen later that may be associated with cognitive impairment. The binding of CO to the heme protein is 250 times greater than oxygen, resulting in tissue hypoxia.
Methanol intoxication	**CT:** Acute poisoning shows symmetric decreased attenuation in the basal ganglia and subcortical white matter, with or without hemorrhage. **MRI:** High signal on T2-weighted images in the putamen and globus pallidus bilaterally, with or without hemorrhage, with or without contrast enhancement.	Toxic effects result in selective necrosis of basal ganglia/putamina bilaterally and subcortical white matter 12 to 24 hours after ingestion secondary to metabolic conversion by hepatic alcohol dehydrogenase to the toxin formic acid.
Mitochondrial encephalopathy, lactic acidosis, and strokelike events (MELAS) and myoclonic epilepsy, ragged red fiber (MERRF) syndromes	**CT:** Symmetric zones of low attenuation in the basal ganglia and cerebral infarction that is not limited to one vascular distribution. **MRI:** High T2 signal in basal ganglia usually symmetric, as well as high T2 signal in cerebral and cerebellar cortex and subcortical white matter not corresponding to a specific large arterial vascular territory. Signal abnormalities may resolve and reappear.	MELAS is a maternally inherited disease affecting transfer RNA in mitochondria. MERRF is a mitochondrial encephalopathy associated with muscle weakness and myoclonic epilepsy, short stature, ophthalmoplegia, and cardiac disease.
Leigh disease ▷ *Fig. 1.145*	**CT:** Zones of low attenuation in both caudate nuclei and putamina, with or without decreased attenuation in white matter; typically no contrast enhancement. **MRI:** Symmetric high signal on T2-weighted images in the globus pallidus, putamen, and caudate, as well as high signal on T2-weighted images in the thalami, cerebral and cerebellar white matter, cerebellar cortex, brainstem, and spinal cord gray matter; typically no gadolinium contrast enhancement.	Autosomal recessive disorder, also referred to as subacute necrotizing encephalopathy, occurs in three forms (infantile, juvenile, and adult onset); etiology related to abnormalities in oxidative metabolism in mitochondria from one of several defective enzymes; progressive neurodegenerative disease. Lesions in brainstem are associated with loss of respiratory control.
Kearns-Sayre syndrome ▷ *Fig. 1.146*	**CT:** Zones of low attenuation in both caudate nuclei and putamina, with or without decreased attenuation in white matter, with or without calcifications of basal ganglia, thalami, and dentate nuclei. **MRI:** Symmetric high signal on T2-weighted images in the globus pallidus, putamen, and caudate; high signal on T2-weighted images in the thalami, cerebral and cerebellar white matter, cerebellar cortex, and brainstem; typically no gadolinium enhancement.	Mitochondrial disorder associated with external ophthalmoplegia, retinitis pigmentosa, and onset of clinical muscular and neurologic signs in patients younger than 20 y.
Cockayne syndrome ▷ *Fig. 1.147*	**CT:** Calcifications in basal ganglia and dentate nuclei, zones of low attenuation in cerebral white matter. **MRI:** High signal on T2-weighted images involving the periventricular white matter, basal ganglia, and dentate nuclei, with calcifications in basal ganglia and dentate nuclei, progressive cerebral and cerebellar atrophy, microcephaly.	Autosomal recessive disorder with deficient repair mechanisms for DNA; presents in first decade with progressive neurologic dysfunction, cataracts, cutaneous photosensitivity, optic atrophy, and dwarfism.
Wilson disease	**CT:** Zones of low attenuation in the basal ganglia and thalami. No abnormal contrast enhancement seen. Progressive atrophy of the cerebrum, cerebellum, and brainstem. **MRI:** High signal on T2-weighted images in the putamen bilaterally, as well as in the thalami, caudate nuclei, dentate nuclei, and brainstem (periaqueductal zone). Low signal on T2-weighted images can also be seen in the caudate and putamen. Progressive atrophy of the cerebrum, cerebellum, and brainstem.	Autosomal recessive disease manifest by decreased functional serum ceruloplasmin levels and altered copper metabolism with increased urinary excretion of copper. Usually presents in childhood with abnormal toxic copper deposition in tissues, resulting in cirrhosis and degenerative changes in the basal ganglia (lentiform nuclei) and brainstem.

(continues on page 90)

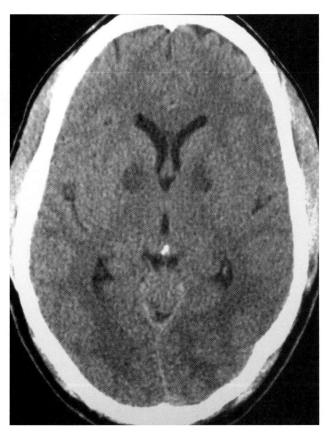

Fig. 1.144   Carbon monoxide poisoning. Axial image shows abnormal decreased attenuation in the globus pallidus regions bilaterally from necrosis.

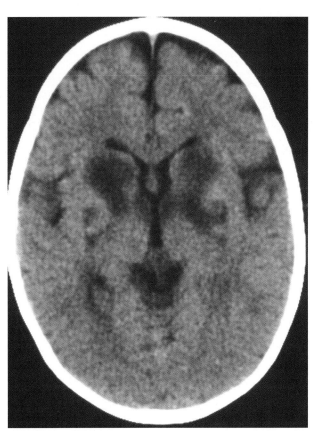

Fig. 1.145   Leigh disease. Axial image shows decreased attenuation in both basal ganglia regions.

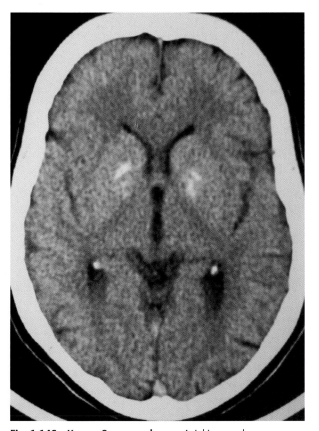

Fig. 1.146   Kearns-Sayre syndrome. Axial image shows calcifications in both basal ganglia regions.

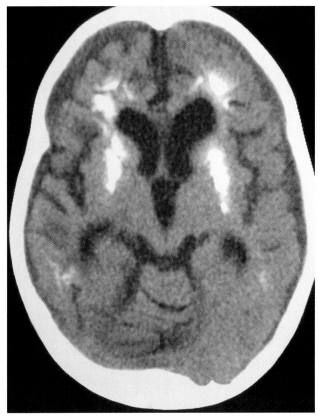

Fig. 1.147   Cockayne syndrome. Axial image shows calcifications in the basal ganglia regions and within the cerebral white matter bilaterally.

Table 1.7 (Cont.) Abnormalities and lesions of the basal ganglia

Lesions	CT Findings	Comments
Shy-Drager syndrome	**CT:** Progressive atrophy of the brainstem and cerebellum. **MRI:** Low signal on T2-weighted images in putamen nuclei equal to or more pronounced than in the globus pallidus. Atrophy of the brainstem and cerebellum.	Autonomic dysfunction in adults with orthostatic hypotension; cerebellar and extrapyramidal clinical signs.
Neurodegeneration with brain iron accumulation	**CT:** Zones of low attenuation in the globus pallidus bilaterally. **MRI:** Low signal with or without areas of high signal on T2-weighted images in the globus pallidus bilaterally; no gadolinium enhancement.	Rare autosomal recessive metabolic disorder from mutations in the pantothenate kinase 2 *(PANK2)* gene with onset usually in childhood with progressive limb rigidity and gait dysfunction, dysarthria, and mental deterioration. Increased iron deposition and destruction of globus pallidus and substantia nigra bilaterally.
Pelizaeus-Merzbacher disease	**CT:** Cerebral and cerebellar atrophy, slightly decreased attenuation in the cerebral white matter. **MRI:** Heterogeneous or diffuse high signal on T2-weighted images in cerebral white matter, with or without involvement of the cerebellum, brainstem; with or without low signal on T2-weighted images in basal ganglia, thalami; without gadolinium contrast enhancement; progressive cerebral and cerebellar atrophy.	X-linked (type 1) or autosomal recessive (type 2) leukodystrophy; five subtypes; deficiency of proteolipid component of myelin; presentation during neonatal period (type 2)/infancy (type 1) with abnormal eye movements, nystagmus, delayed psychomotor development; death in first decade; males > females.
Lysosomal enzyme defects ▷ *Fig. 1.148*	**Tay-Sachs disease:** **CT:** Increased attenuation in the thalami and decreased attenuation in the white matter; progressive cerebral and cerebellar atrophy. **MRI:** Slightly increased signal on T2-weighted images in caudate nuclei, putamen, and thalami, with or without slightly increased signal on T2-weighted images in cerebral white matter. Slightly reduced diffusion in ventral thalamic nucleus, progressive cerebral and cerebellar atrophy. **Neuronal ceroid lipofuscinosis:** **CT:** Progressive cerebral and cerebellar atrophy. **MRI:** With or without low or high signal on T2-weighted images in caudate, putamen, and thalami; with or without high signal on T2-weighted images in white matter; typically without gadolinium contrast enhancement. Progressive cerebral and cerebellar atrophy. **Mucopolysaccharidoses:** **CT:** Zones of decreased attenuation in the cerebral white matter, with or without foci of low attenuation in the corpus callosum, cerebral white matter, and basal ganglia. **MRI:** Foci or diffuse zones of high signal on T2-weighted images in cerebral white matter; with or without foci of high signal on T2-weighted images in the corpus callosum and basal ganglia; perivascular spaces, cerebral cortical/subcortical infarcts, progressive cerebral atrophy, with or without macrocephaly, with or without communicating hydrocephalus, with or without meningeal thickening.	Functional defects (usually autosomal recessive) involving lysosomal catabolic enzymes. Tay-Sachs disease: functional hexosaminidase deficiency; neuronal ceroid-lipofuscinosis: lipofuscin deposits in cytosomes; mucopolysaccharidoses: autosomal recessive or X-linked disorders related to abnormal metabolism of mucopolysaccharides (Hurler, Hunter, Sanfilippo, and Morquio syndromes). Result in axonal loss and demyelination related to the accumulation of abnormal metabolites within cells.
Disorders of amino acid metabolism	**Phenylketonuria, propionic acidemia, methylmalonic aciduria, homocystinuria, ornithine transcarbamylase deficiency, leucinosis ("maple syrup" urine disease), and glutaric acidemia:** **CT:** Zones with decreased attenuation in the cerebral and/or cerebellar white matter, with or without zones with decreased attenuation in the globus pallidi, putamina, caudate nuclei, thalami, and brainstem. **MRI:** High signal on T2-weighted images in cerebral and/or cerebellar white matter, with or without high signal on T2-weighted images in globus pallidi, putamina, caudate nuclei, thalami, and brainstem.	Autosomal recessive disorders involving defective enzymes regulating amino acid metabolism and mitochondrial function. These enzymatic defects can cause significant alteration of normal formation and maintenance of myelin.

(continues on page 91)

Table 1.7   (Cont.) Abnormalities and lesions of the basal ganglia

Lesions	CT Findings	Comments
Basal ganglia calcifications ▷ *Fig. 1.149* ▷ *Fig. 1.150*	**CT:** Idiopathic calcifications in the basal ganglia can be seen in adults older than 30 y. Calcifications involving the basal ganglia in patients younger than or older than 30 y may be seen with hypoparathyroidism, pseudohypoparathyroidism, pseudo-pseudo-hypoparathyroidism, hyperparathyroidism, hypothyroidism, lead toxicity, Fahr disease, and neurodegeneration with brain iron accumulation. **MRI:** Low, intermediate, or high signal on T1- and T2-weighted images in basal ganglia; no abnormal contrast enhancement.	Signal of calcium deposition can vary depending on the size and configuration of deposits. Calcifications can also occur in basal ganglia secondary to endocrine abnormalities involving calcium (hypoparathyroidism), hypothyroidism, iron metabolism (neurodegeneration with brain iron accumulation), prior inflammatory disease (toxoplasmosis, tuberculosis, cysticercosis, etc.), prior ischemic disease or prior toxic exposure (lead intoxication, carbon monoxide, etc.), and Fahr disease.
Acquired hepatocerebral degeneration	**CT:** No zones with definite abnormal attenuation seen in the basal ganglia, with or without cerebral and cerebellar atrophy. **MRI:** High signal on T1-weighted images in basal ganglia; no abnormal contrast enhancement.	Signal abnormality related to hepatic dysfunction (alcoholic cirrhosis, hepatitis, portal-systemic shunts) possibly related to increased serum ammonia and manganese levels. The signal hyperintensity may reverse after liver transplantation.
Huntington disease	Disproportionate atrophy of basal ganglia (caudate > putamen > cerebellum/brainstem). **CT:** Progressive atrophy of caudate and putamen bilaterally. **MRI:** Variable low signal (iron deposition) or high signal (gliosis) changes on T2-weighted images involving the putamen bilaterally; usually no abnormal contrast enhancement.	**Adults:** Autosomal dominant neurodegenerative disease related to abnormal segment (CAG repeats) of DNA on chromosome 4 involving the Huntington gene. Usually presents after age 40 y with progressive movement disorders (choreoathetosis, rigidity, hypokinesia); behavioral and progressive mental dysfunction/dementia. Juvenile Huntington disease also occurs in a small number of patients in the second decade. Patients present with rigidity, hypokinesia, seizures, and/or progressive mental dysfunction.

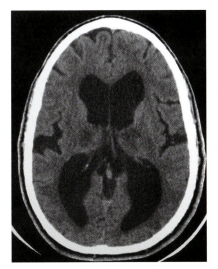

Fig. 1.148   Hurler-Scheie syndrome. Axial image shows zones of decreased attenuation in the thalami and to a lesser extent in the basal ganglia.

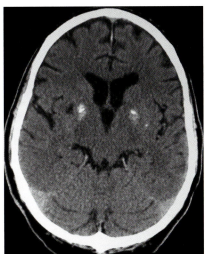

Fig. 1.149   Basal ganglia calcifications, idiopathic. Axial image shows small calcifications in both basal ganglia regions.

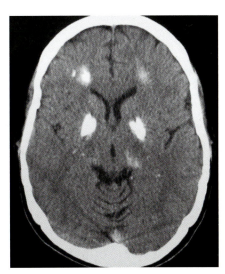

Fig. 1.150   Basal ganglia calcifications, Fahr disease. Axial image shows bilateral calcifications in the basal ganglia, thalami, and cerebral white matter.

Table 1.8 Multiple or diffuse lesions involving white matter

Lesions	CT Findings	Comments
Congenital neuronal migration disorders		
Lissencephaly ▷ *Fig. 1.6, p. 7*	Absent or incomplete formation of gyri and sulci with shallow sylvian fissures and "figure 8" appearance of brain on axial images, abnormally thick cortex, gray matter heterotopia with smooth gray-white matter interface.	Severe disorder of neuronal migration (weeks 7–16 of gestation) with absent or incomplete formation of gyri, sulci, and sylvian fissures. Associated with severe mental retardation and seizures, early death. Other associated CNS anomalies are dysgenesis of the corpus callosum, microcephaly, hypoplastic thalami, and cephaloceles.
Pachygyria (nonlissencephalic cortical dysplasia)	Thick gyri with shallow sulci involving all or portions of the brain. Thickened cortex with relatively smooth gray-white interface may have areas of decreased attenuation in the white matter (gliosis).	Severe disorder of neuronal migration. Clinical findings related to degree of extent of this malformation.
Gray matter heterotopia	Laminar heterotopia appears as a band or bands of gray matter within the cerebral white matter *(Fig. 1.7, p. 8)*. Nodular heterotopia appears as one or more nodules of gray matter along the ventricles *(Fig 1.8, p. 8)* or within the cerebral white matter *(Fig. 1.9, p. 9)*.	Disorder of neuronal migration (weeks 7–22 of gestation) in which a collection or layer of neurons is located between the ventricles and cerebral cortex. Can have a bandlike (laminar) or nodular appearance isodense to gray matter; may be unilateral or bilateral. Associated with seizures and schizencephaly.
Schizencephaly (split brain) ▷ *Fig. 1.10, p. 9*	Cleft in brain extending from the ventricle to cortical surface lined by heterotopic gray matter. The cleft may be narrow (closed lip) or wide (open lip).	Association with seizures, blindness, retardation, and other CNS anomalies (septo-optic dysplasia, etc.). Clinical manifestations related to severity of malformation. Ischemia or insult to portion of germinal matrix seen before hemisphere formation.
Unilateral hemimegalencephaly ▷ *Fig. 1.11, p. 9*	Nodular or multinodular region of gray matter heterotopia involving all or part of a cerebral hemisphere with associated enlargement of the ipsilateral lateral ventricle and hemisphere.	Neuronal migration disorder associated with hamartomatous overgrowth of the involved hemisphere.
Tuberous sclerosis	Foci and/or confluent zones of decreased attenuation in cerebral white matter.	Nonmalignant lesions in white matter associated with tuberous sclerosis, consisting of areas of demyelination and/or dysplastic white matter along pathways of radial glial fibers during neuronal migration.
Congenital dysmyelinating disorders		
Alexander disease ▷ *Fig. 1.151a–c*	Zones with decreased attenuation involving the peripheral frontal white matter with progressive involvement of the white matter posteriorly and centrally (internal and external capsules); can show a marginal pattern of contrast enhancement; can be associated with increases in size and weight of brain tissue.	Sporadic leukoencephalopathy, also referred to as fibrinoid leukoencephalopathy, presents in first year of life with macrocephaly, progressive psychomotor retardation, resulting often in death during early childhood; also juvenile and adult forms. Caused by mutation of gene on chromosome 17q21 resulting in abnormal function and levels of the filament protein (glial fibrillary acidic protein [GFAP]).

(continues on page 94)

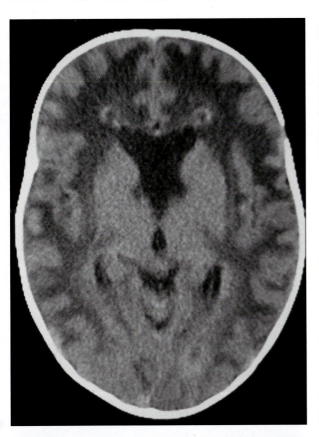

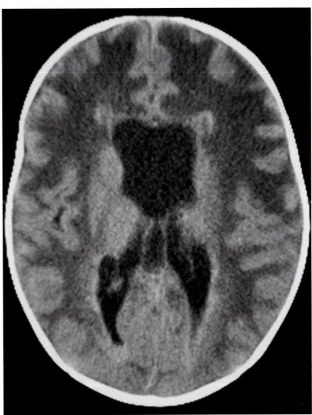

b

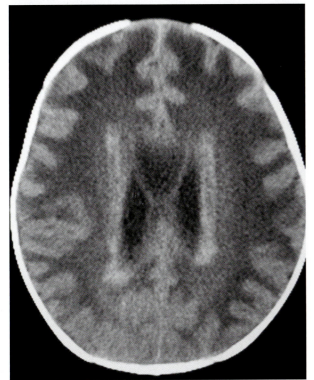

Fig. 1.151a–c   Alexander disease. Axial postcontrast images in an 11-month-old girl show zones of low attenuation in the white matter of both cerebral hemispheres, most prominently in the frontal lobes. Small zones of contrast enhancement are seen at sites of active demyelination.

Table 1.8   (Cont.) Multiple or diffuse lesions involving white matter

Lesions	CT Findings	Comments
Canavan–van Bogaert–Bertrand disease	Zones with decreased attenuation involving the peripheral cerebral and cerebellar white matter diffusely with progressive involvement of the white matter centrally and subsequent atrophy, with or without involvement of the globus pallidus; typically no contrast enhancement; associated with increases in size and weight of brain tissue, enlarged N-acetylaspartate (NAA) peak on magnetic resonance hydrogen spectroscopy.	Autosomal recessive (usually occurs in Ashkenazi Jews), spongy degeneration disorder of the brain caused by deficiency of aspartoacylase (from abnormal locus on chromosome 17-short arm) resulting in N-acetylaspartic aciduria and deposits in brain and plasma; presents in infancy with macrocephaly, hypotonia, seizures, spasticity, and optic atrophy; death often occurs in second year.
Pelizaeus–Merzbacher disease	Heterogeneous or diffuse decreased attenuation in cerebral white matter; initially involves the subcortical white matter with progression to the other remaining white matter; with or without involvement of cerebellum and brainstem; no contrast enhancement; progressive cerebral and cerebellar atrophy.	X-linked (type 1) or autosomal recessive (type 2) leukodystrophy; five subtypes; deficiency of proteolipid component of myelin; abnormality on chromosome Xq22; presentation during neonatal period (type 2)/ infancy (type 1) with abnormal eye movements, nystagmus, and delayed psychomotor development; death in first decade; males > females.
Metachromatic leukodystrophy	Symmetric diffuse zones of decreased attenuation in deep cerebral/periventricular white matter with progression of abnormal attenuation peripherally to involve the subcortical white matter; decreased attenuation involving the cerebellar white matter; no contrast enhancement; progressive atrophy.	Autosomal recessive disease involving the ARSA gene on chromosome 22q13.31-qter with deficiency of arylsulfatase A in lysosomes resulting in toxic accumulation of ceramide sulfatide (myelin breakdown product) in macrophages and Schwann cells. Three subtypes depending on onset: late infantile form (80%), juvenile form, and adult form. Progressive neurologic deterioration with peripheral neuropathy, gait disorders, and cognitive dysfunction leading to death.
Childhood adrenoleukodystrophy	Zones with decreased attenuation usually in parieto-occipital periventricular white matter and corpus callosum; progression of abnormality to the remaining cerebral white matter, with or without contrast enhancement at regions of active demyelination/ inflammation.	X-linked recessive leukodystrophy (males) involving chromosome Xq28 with functional deficiency of the peroxisomal enzyme acyl- coenzyme A (CoA) synthetase, resulting in abnormal metabolism and breakdown of very long chain fatty acids. These fatty acids accumulate in many tissues, including brain, with resultant demyelination, inflammation, gliosis, and necrosis. Onset 3 to 10 y, with psychomotor retardation, seizures, hypotonia, facial dysmorphism, progressive and deterioration. Also other subtypes: neonatal onset and adult onset.
Krabbe disease	Symmetric confluent zones of decreased attenuation involving the periventricular white matter with progressive involvement toward the subcortical white matter; cerebral white matter involved > cerebellar white matter; no contrast enhancement; progressive cerebral atrophy.	Also known as globoid cell leukodystrophy, autosomal recessive disorder involving chromosome 14q24.3-32.1 with deficiency of lysosomal enzyme galactosyl-ceramide β-galactosidase, resulting in destruction of oligodendrocytes/myelin production. Three subtypes: infantile (most common), late infantile, and adult onset. Seizures, psychomotor dysfunction, optic atrophy, and progressive neurologic deterioration leading to death.
Vanishing white matter disease ▷ *Fig. 1.152a–c*	Symmetric diffuse zones of decreased attenuation involving the cerebral white matter with progressive involvement toward the subcortical white matter; cerebral white matter involved > cerebellar white matter; no contrast enhancement; associated with increased brain size followed by progressive cerebral and cerebellar atrophy.	Also referred to as childhood ataxia with diffuse CNS hypomyelination; familial disease involving the translation initiation factor on chromosome 3q27. Progressive neurologic deterioration begins in childhood.

(continues on page 95)

Table 1.8 (Cont.) Multiple or diffuse lesions involving white matter

Lesions	CT Findings	Comments
Inherited metabolic disorders		
Lysosomal enzyme defects ▷ *Fig. 1.153 a–c*	**Tay-Sachs and Sandhoff diseases:** Increased slightly high attenuation in the thalami and decreased attenuation in the cerebral white matter followed by progressive cerebral and cerebellar atrophy. **Neuronal ceroid-lipofuscinosis:** Progressive cerebral and cerebellar atrophy; with or without zones of decreased attenuation in white matter; typically no contrast enhancement. **Mucopolysaccharidoses:** Poorly defined zones of decreased attenuation in white matter; cerebral and cerebellar atrophy, with or without foci of low attenuation in corpus callosum and basal ganglia (prominent perivascular spaces), cerebral cortical/subcortical infarcts, with or without macrocephaly, with or without communicating hydrocephalus, with or without meningeal thickening.	Functional defects (usually autosomal recessive) involving lysosomal catabolic enzymes. Tay-Sachs: functional *N*-acetyl hexosaminidase A deficiency; from mutation at *HEXA* gene on chromosome 15q-23-24. Sandhoff disease: functional *N*-acetyl hexosaminidase A and B deficiency; from mutation at *HEXB* gene on chromosome 5q-13. Neuronal ceroid-lipofuscinosis is a relatively common progressive type of encephalopathy in children 125 000 births with lipofuscin deposits in cytosomes causing cerebral and cerebellar atrophy. Mucopolysaccharidoses: autosomal recessive or X-linked disorders related to abnormal metabolism of mucopolysaccharides (Hurler, Hunter, Sanfilippo, and Morquio syndromes) result in axonal loss and demyelination related to the accumulation of abnormal mucopolysaccharide (glycosaminoglycans) metabolites within cells of various organs.

(continues on page 96)

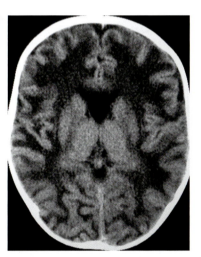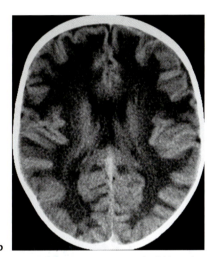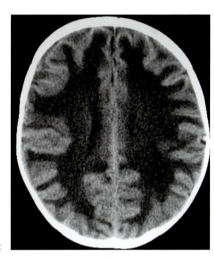

Fig. 1.152a–c Vanishing white matter disease. Axial images in a 10-month-old boy show diffuse abnormal decreased attenuation in the cerebral white matter and abnormal increased brain size.

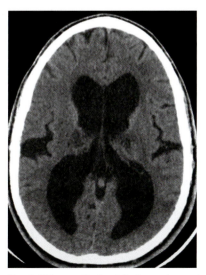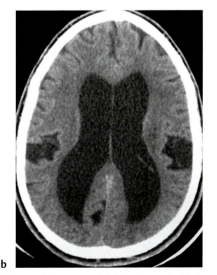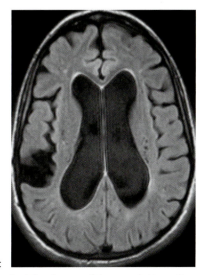

Fig. 1.153a–c Hurler-Scheie syndrome in a 24-year-old woman. Axial CT images (**a,b**) show poorly defined zones of decreased attenuation in white matter and basal ganglia, as well as cerebral atrophy. Axial FLAIR MRI (**c**) also shows cerebral atrophy.

Table 1.8   (Cont.) Multiple or diffuse lesions involving white matter

Lesions	CT Findings	Comments
Disorders of amino acid metabolism	**Phenylketonuria, propionic acidemia, methylmalonic aciduria, homocystinuria, ornithine transcarbamylase deficiency, citrullinemia, arginosuccinic aciduria, leucinosis ("maple syrup" urine disease, and glutaric aciduria):** Zones with decreased attenuation in cerebral and/or cerebellar white matter, with or without zones with decreased attenuation in globus pallidi, putamen, caudate, thalami, and brainstem.	Autosomal recessive disorders involving defective enzymes regulating amino acid metabolism and mitochondrial function. These enzymatic defects can cause significant alteration of myelin formation.
Mitochondrial metabolic disorders	**MELAS and MERRF syndromes:** Zones with decreased attenuation in the basal ganglia, usually symmetric, with or without decreased attenuation involving cerebral and cerebellar cortex; subcortical white matter abnormalities do not correspond to a specific large arterial vascular territory.	MELAS is a maternally inherited disease involving abnormal transfer of RNA-Leu from a mutation in mitochondrial DNA. MERRF is a mitochondrial encephalopathy associated with muscle weakness and myoclonic epilepsy, short stature, ophthalmoplegia, and cardiac disease.
Leigh disease	Zones of low attenuation in both caudate nuclei and putamina, with or without decreased attenuation in white matter and cerebral cortex; typically no contrast enhancement.	Autosomal recessive disorder also referred to as subacute necrotizing encephalopathy; occurs in three forms: infantile, juvenile, and adult onset. Etiology related to abnormalities in oxidative metabolism in mitochondria from one of several defective enzymes (pyruvate dehydrogenase complex, cytochrome oxidase respiratory chain, adenosinetriphosphatase [ATPase], or complex I); progressive neurodegenerative disease. Lesions in brainstem are associated with loss of respiratory control.
Kearns-Sayre syndrome	Zones of low attenuation in both caudate nuclei and putamina, with or without decreased attenuation in white matter, with or without calcifications in basal ganglia, thalami, and dentate nuclei; typically no contrast enhancement.	Mitochondrial disorder associated with external ophthalmoplegia, retinitis pigmentosa, and onset of clinical muscular and neurologic signs < 20 y.
Cockayne syndrome ▷ **Fig. 1.154a, b**	Zones with decreased attenuation involving the periventricular white matter, basal ganglia, and dentate nuclei, with calcifications in basal ganglia and dentate nuclei, progressive cerebral and cerebellar atrophy, microcephaly.	Autosomal recessive disorder with deficient repair mechanisms for DNA; presents in first decade with progressive neurologic dysfunction, cataracts, cutaneous photosensitivity, optic atrophy, and dwarfism.
Toxic/metabolic		
Marchiafava-Bignami disease	Variable mixed low, intermediate, and/or high attenuation involving the corpus callosum, with or without other sites in cerebral white matter, with or without enhancement depending on stage of demyelination (acute, subacute vs chronic).	Acquired disorder associated with alcoholism and malnourishment, with demyelination, necrosis, or hemorrhage involving the corpus callosum, as well as other commissures and cerebral white matter. Symptoms include seizures, altered consciousness, ataxia, dysarthria, and hypertonia.
Central pontine and extrapontine myelinolysis (osmotic myelinolysis)	Poorly defined zone of decreased attenuation involving the central portion of the pons (central pontine myelinolysis), Extrapontine myelinolysis occurs as zones with decreased attenuation in the cerebral white matter, external capsules, basal ganglia, thalami, midbrain, and middle cerebellar peduncles with or without occasional contrast enhancement.	Demyelinating disorder resulting from rapid correction of hyponatremia in chronically ill, malnourished, or alcoholic patients. Associated with diabetes mellitus, hepatitis, and chronic disease of the lungs, liver, and/or kidneys.
Hypertensive encephalopathy (reversible posterior leukoencephalopathy) ▷ **Fig. 1.155a, b**	Foci and/or confluent zones of decreased attenuation in subcortical white matter, with or without cerebral cortex, with or without contrast enhancement. Findings can be reversed if eliciting cause is corrected.	Occurs with elevations in blood pressure above the upper limit in cerebral vascular autoregulation resulting in capillary leakage of fluid in the brain often in arterial boundary zones. Associated with immunosuppressant drugs (e.g., tacrolimus/FK506 and cyclosporine), chemotherapy (e.g., cisplatin, and l-asparaginase), acute onset of hypertension, preeclampsia, eclampsia, renal dysfunction, and fluid overload. Neurologic symptoms include confusion, headaches, seizures, visual loss, dysarthria, and coma. Cortical abnormalities may be related to cortical laminar necrosis and hypoperfusion injury.

(continues on page 98)

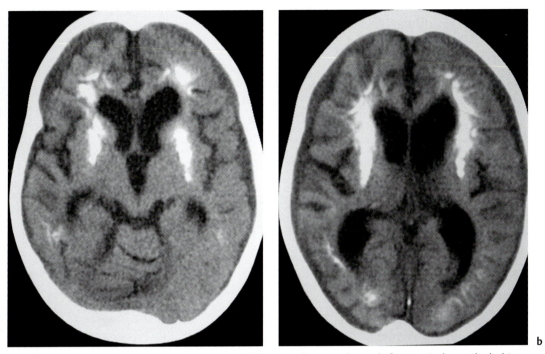

b

Fig. 1.154a, b   Cockayne syndrome in an 11-year-old boy. Axial images show calcifications in the cerebral white matter and basal ganglia.

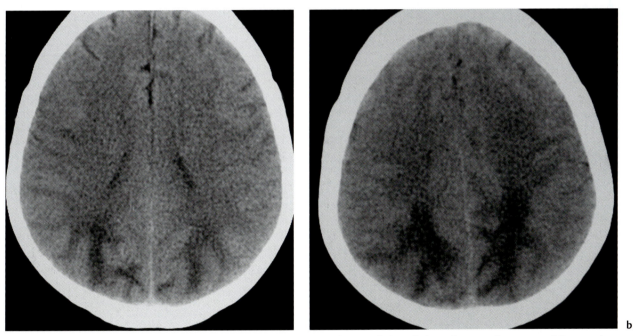

b

Fig. 1.155a, b   Hypertensive encephalopathy (reversible posterior leukoencephalopathy). Axial images show zones of decreased attenuation in the white matter of the posterior portions of both parietal lobes.

Table 1.8   (Cont.) Multiple or diffuse lesions involving white matter

Lesions	CT Findings	Comments
Vascular		
Intracerebral hemorrhage	The attenuation of the hematoma depends on its age, size, location, hematocrit, hemoglobin oxidation state, clot retraction, and extent of edema. **Hyperacute phase (4–6 h):** Hemoglobin primarily as diamagnetic oxyhemoglobin (iron Fe^{2+} state). **CT:** High attenuation. **Acute phase (12–48 h):** Hemoglobin primarily as paramagnetic deoxyhemoglobin (iron Fe^{2+} state). **CT:** High attenuation in acute clot directly related to hematocrit, hemoglobin concentration, and high protein concentration. Hematocrit in acute clot approaches 90%. ▷ *Fig. 1.156* **Early subacute phase (> 2 d):** Hemoglobin becomes oxidized to iron Fe^{3+} state, methemoglobin, which is strongly paramagnetic. **CT:** High attenuation. **Late subacute phase (> 7 d–6 wk):** Intracerebral hematomas decrease 1.5 HU per day. Hematomas become isodense to hypodense; peripheral contrast enhancement from blood–brain barrier breakdown and vascularized capsule. **Chronic phase:** Hemoglobin as extracellular methemoglobin is progressively degraded to hemosiderin. **CT:** Chronic hematomas have low attenuation with localized encephalomalacia. Zones with high attenuation represent new sites of rebleeding.	Can result from trauma, ruptured aneurysms or vascular malformations, coagulopathy, hypertension, adverse drug reaction, amyloid angiopathy, hemorrhagic transformation of cerebral infarction, metastases, abscesses, viral infections (herpes simplex and CMV).
Diffuse axonal injury ▷ *Fig. 1.157a–c*	For acute injuries, one or multiple sites of hemorrhage are seen with high attenuation; commonly occur at the corpus callosum; cerebral cortical–white matter junctions, basal ganglia, and brainstem.	Brain injury caused by deceleration and rotational shear forces that results in disruption of axons and blood vessels. The greater the degree of axonal injury, the poorer the prognosis.
Posthemorrhagic lesions	Zone or zones with decreased attenuation secondary to gliosis and encephalomalacia involving cerebral or cerebellar white matter, basal ganglia, thalami, and/or cerebral or cerebellar cortex; typically no contrast enhancement.	Sites of prior hemorrhage can have variable appearance depending on the relative ratios of gliosis, encephalomalacia, and blood breakdown products (methemoglobin, hemosiderin, etc.).
AVM ▷ *Fig. 1.158a, b*	Lesions with irregular margins that can be located in the brain parenchyma (pia, dura, or both locations). AVMs contain multiple tortuous vessels with or without calcifications. The venous portions often show contrast enhancement. Usually not associated with mass effect unless there is recent hemorrhage or venous occlusion. CTA can show the arterial, nidus, and venous portions of the AVMs.	Supratentorial AVMs occur more frequently (80%–90%) than infratentorial AVMs (10%–20%). Annual risk of hemorrhage. AVMs can be sporadic, congenital, or associated with a history of trauma. Multiple AVMs can be seen in syndromes Rendu-Osler-Weber (AVMs in brain and lungs and mucosal capillary telangiectasias) and Wyburn-Mason (AVMs in brain and retina with cutaneous nevi).

(continues on page 100)

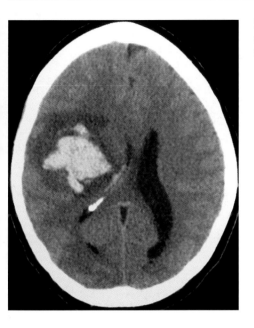

Fig. 1.156 Hypertensive acute intracerebral hematoma. Axial image shows an acute hematoma with high attenuation in the right cerebral hemisphere with mass effect and subfalcine herniation leftward.

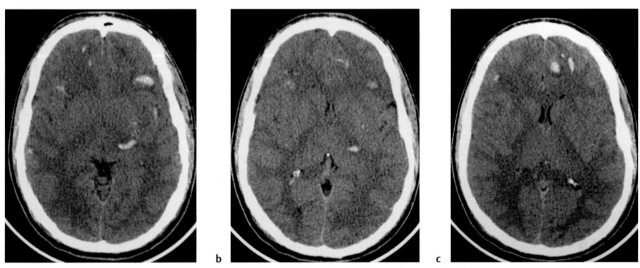

Fig. 1.157a–c Diffuse axonal injuries. Axial images show multiple small foci of hemorrhage with high attenuation in the cerebral white matter.

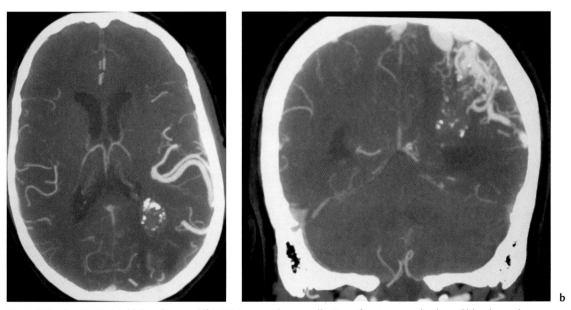

Fig. 1.158a, b AVM. Axial (**a**) and coronal (**b**) CTA images show a collection of tortuous and enlarged blood vessels in the left cerebral hemisphere representing an AVM.

Table 1.8   (Cont.) Multiple or diffuse lesions involving white matter

Lesions	CT Findings	Comments
Cavernous hemangioma ▷ *Fig. 1.159a–c*	Single or multiple multilobulated intra-axial lesions with intermediate to slightly high attenuation, with or without calcification; typically show no contrast enhancement unless associated with a venous angioma.	Intra-axial vascular malformation composed of low-pressure endovascular-lined sinusoidal spaces often associated with sites of recent and/or prior hemorrhage; 80% are supratentorial. Can present with headache and/or seizures. Can be multiple in inherited syndromes. Supratentorial cavernous angiomas occur more frequently than infratentorial lesions. Can be located in many different locations; multiple lesions > 50%. Associated with venous angiomas and risk of hemorrhage.
Venous angioma ▷ *Fig. 1.160*	No abnormality or small, slightly hyperdense zone on CT prior to contrast administration. Contrast enhancement seen in a slightly prominent vein draining a collection of small veins.	Considered an anomalous venous formation typically not associated with hemorrhage; usually an incidental finding except when associated with cavernous hemangioma.
Ischemic disease related to occlusion of large vessels	CT features of cerebral and cerebellar infarcts depend on age of infarct relative to time of examination. **Hyperacute phase (< 12 h):** **CT:** No abnormality (50%); decreased attenuation and blurring of lentiform nuclei; hyperdense artery in up to 50% of cases. **Acute phase (12–24 h):** **CT:** Zones with decreased attenuation in basal ganglia, blurring of junction between cerebral cortex and white matter, sulcal effacement. **Early subacute phase (24 h–3 d):** **CT:** Localized swelling at sites with low attenuation involving gray and white matter (often wedge shaped), with or without hemorrhage. ▷ *Fig. 1.161a* **Late subacute phase (4 d–2 wk):** **CT:** Localized swelling increases, then decreases; low attenuation at lesion can become more prominent; with or without gyral contrast enhancement. **2 weeks to 2 months:** **CT:** With or without gyral contrast enhancement; localized mass effect resolves. **> 2 months:** **CT:** Zone of low attenuation associated with encephalomalacia. ▷ *Fig. 1.161b*	Vascular occlusion of large arteries may be secondary to atheromatous arterial disease, cardiogenic emboli, neoplastic encasement, hypercoagulable states, dissection, or congenital anomalies. Cerebral infarcts usually result from arterial occlusion involving specific vascular territories, although occasionally they occur from metabolic disorders (mitochondrial encephalopathies, etc.) or intracranial venous occlusion (thrombophlebitis, hypercoagulable states, dehydration, etc.) that do not correspond to arterial distributions.
Ischemic disease related to occlusion of small vessels ▷ *Fig. 1.162a, b*	Multiple foci and/or confluent zones of decreased attenuation involving the subcortical and periventricular cerebral white matter, basal ganglia, and brainstem; no associated mass effect; typically no contrast enhancement.	Lesions in white matter and/or brainstem related to occlusive disease involving perforating arteries associated with hypertension, atherosclerosis, diabetes, vasculitis, and aging. Unlike multiple sclerosis, ischemic small vessel disease does not usually involve the corpus callosum because of its abundant blood supply from multiple branches arising from the adjacent pericallosal arteries.

(continues on page 102)

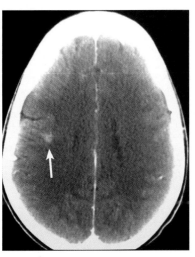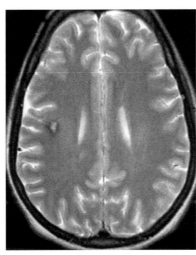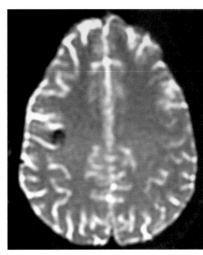

Fig. 1.159a–c   Cavernous hemangioma. Axial postcontrast CT image (**a**) shows a small lesion with increased attenuation in the right cerebral hemisphere (arrow), which has low peripheral signal peripherally surrounding a central zone with high signal on the axial T2-weighted MRI (**b**) and low T2-weighted signal on an axial two-dimensional gradient echo MRI (**c**).

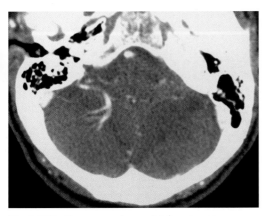

Fig. 1.160   Venous angioma. Axial contrast image shows a slightly prominent vein draining a collection of small veins in the right cerebellar hemisphere.

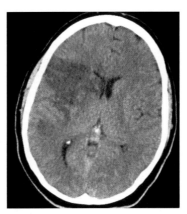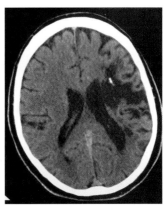

Fig. 1.161a, b   Acute and old cerebral infarctions. Axial image (**a**) shows a zone of decreased attenuation involving the right cerebral hemisphere representing an acute infarct in the vascular distribution of the right middle cerebral artery. Axial image (**b**) shows zones of decreased attenuation and encephalomalacia involving the left cerebral hemisphere representing an old cerebral infarct.

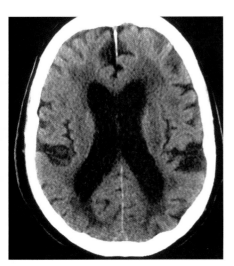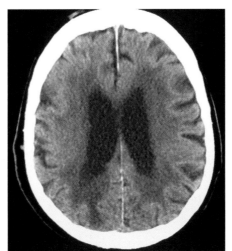

Fig. 1.162a, b   Small vessel ischemic disease in an 82-year-old man. Axial images show poorly defined zones of decreased attenuation in the cerebral white matter bilaterally.

Table 1.8 (Cont.) Multiple or diffuse lesions involving white matter

Lesions	CT Findings	Comments
Periventricular leukomalacia ▷ *Fig. 1.163a, b*	Multiple foci and/or confluent zones of decreased attenuation involving the subcortical and periventricular white matter, basal ganglia, and brainstem; no associated mass effect; no contrast enhancement; irregular ventricular margins and ventricular enlargement related to cerebral volume loss.	Ischemic injury involving fetal brain/premature infants with gliosis and resultant encephalomalacic changes involving periventricular white matter (fetal watershed vascular zones). Associated with neurologic deficits depending on severity of injuries and cerebral palsy.
CADASIL ▷ *Fig. 1.164a, b*	Multiple zones of decreased attenuation involving the subcortical and periventricular white matter, basal ganglia, thalami, and brainstem; no associated mass effect; no contrast enhancement.	CADASIL is an inherited abnormality involving chromosome 19q12, which results in angiopathy of small and medium-sized arteries. Symptoms and signs begin in the fourth decade with headaches, transient ischemic attacks, strokes, and subcortical dementia.
Susac syndrome	Multiple zones (usually < 10 mm) with decreased attenuation in the cerebral white matter and within the central portion of the corpus callosum. Zones of low attenuation may also occur in the basal ganglia (two thirds of patients). Leptomeningeal contrast enhancement may be seen in one third of patients.	Small vessel vasculitis of unknown etiology resulting in arteriolar occlusion and microinfarction involving cerebral white matter, retina, and cochlea. Patients often have headaches, cognitive changes, confusion, and memory impairment. Female/male ratio 3:1; age range 16 to 58 y.
Radiation injury/necrosis ▷ *Fig. 1.165a, b*	Focal lesion with or without mass effect or poorly defined zone of low to intermediate attenuation, with or without contrast enhancement involving tissue (gray matter and/or white matter) in field of treatment.	Usually occurs from 4 to 6 months to 10 y after radiation treatment; may be difficult to distinguish from neoplasm. PET and magnetic resonance spectroscopy might be helpful for evaluation. Radiation treatment in combination with intrathecal methotrexate may also result in necrotizing leukoencephalopathy.

(continues on page 104)

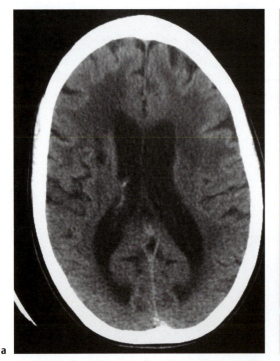 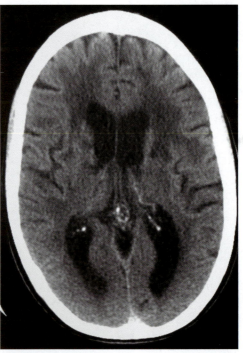

Fig. 1.163a, b Periventricular leukomalacia. Axial images show poorly defined zones of decreased attenuation in the cerebral white matter bilaterally associated with cerebral volume loss.

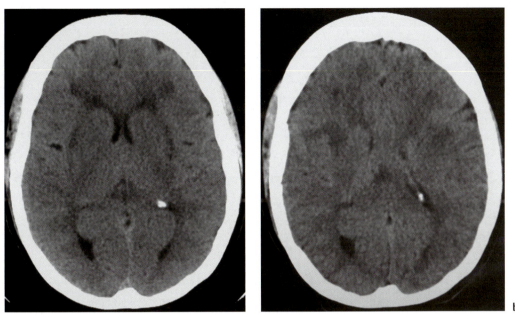

Fig. 1.164a, b Cerebral autosomal dominant arteriopathy with subcortical infarcts and leukoenceph-alopathy (CADASIL). Axial images show poorly defined zones of decreased attenuation in the cerebral white matter bilaterally.

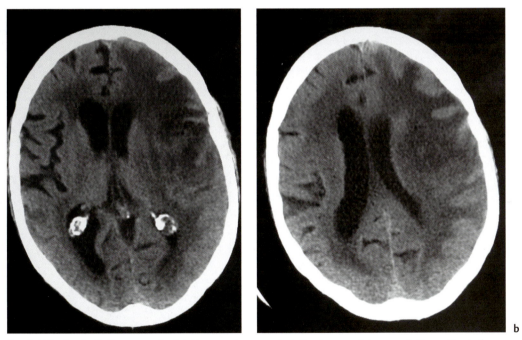

Fig. 1.165a, b Radiation necrosis. Axial images show poorly defined zones of decreased attenuation in the cerebral white matter bilaterally, greater on the left than the right. A zone of low attenuation is seen in the left frontal lobe with localized mass effect.

Table 1.8   (Cont.) Multiple or diffuse lesions involving white matter

Lesions	CT Findings	Comments
Inflammation		
Demyelinating Disease: multiple sclerosis, ADEM ▷ *Fig. 1.166a–e*	Lesions located in cerebral or cerebellar white matter, corpus callosum, brainstem, and middle cerebellar peduncles. Lesions usually have low to intermediate attenuation with or without contrast enhancement. Contrast enhancement can be ringlike or nodular, usually in acute/early subacute phase of demyelination. Lesions rarely can have associated mass effect simulating neoplasms.	Multiple sclerosis is the most common acquired demyelinating disease usually affecting women (peak ages 20–40 y). Other demyelinating diseases are acute disseminated encephalomyelitis/immune mediated demyelination after viral infection; toxins (exogenous from environmental exposure or ingestion of alcohol, solvents, etc.); or endogenous from metabolic disorders (leukodystrophies, mitochondrial encephalopathies, etc.), radiation injury, trauma, or vascular disease.
Sarcoidosis ▷ *Fig. 1.167a, b*	Poorly marginated intra-axial zone with low to intermediate attenuation; usually shows contrast enhancement, with localized mass effect and peripheral edema. Often associated with contrast enhancement in the leptomeninges.	Multisystem noncaseating granulomatous disease of uncertain cause that can involve the CNS in 5% to 15%. Associated with severe neurologic deficits if untreated.
Infection		
Cerebritis	Poorly defined zone or focal area of low to intermediate attenuation, minimal or no contrast enhancement; involves cerebral cortex and white matter in bacterial and fungal infections.	Focal infection/inflammation of brain tissue from bacteria or fungi, secondary to sinusitis, meningitis, surgery, hematogenous source (cardiac and other vascular shunts), and/or immunocompromised status. Can progress to abscess formation.
Pyogenic brain abscess ▷ *Fig. 1.168a–d*	Circumscribed lesion with low-attenuation central zone surrounded by a thin rim of intermediate attenuation representing the wall of the abscess, as well as a peripheral, poorly defined zone of low attenuation representing edema; ringlike contrast enhancement is seen at the wall of the abscess, which is sometimes thicker laterally than medially.	Formation of brain abscess occurs 2 weeks after cerebritis with liquefaction and necrosis centrally surrounded by a capsule and peripheral edema. Can be multiple. Complication from meningitis and/or sinusitis, septicemia, trauma, surgery, or cardiac shunt.

(continues on page 106)

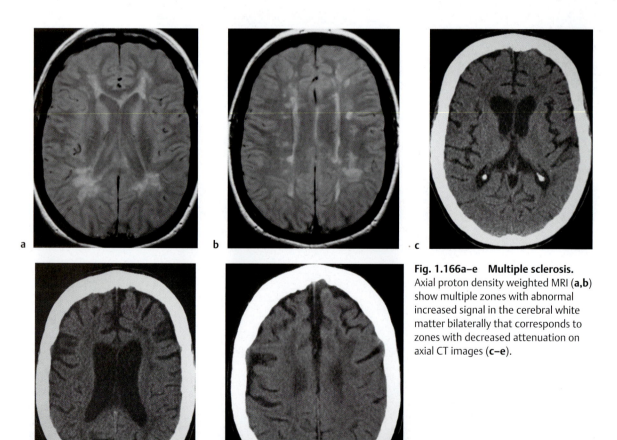

a   b   c

d   e

Fig. 1.166a–e   Multiple sclerosis.
Axial proton density weighted MRI (**a,b**) show multiple zones with abnormal increased signal in the cerebral white matter bilaterally that corresponds to zones with decreased attenuation on axial CT images (**c–e**).

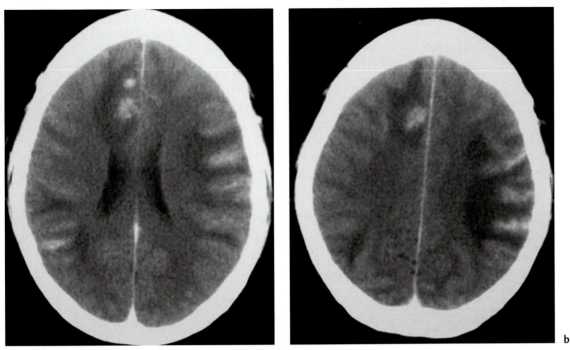

Fig. 1.167a, b   Sarcoidosis. Axial postcontrast images show zones of enhancement with adjacent low-attenuation edema in both cerebral hemispheres.

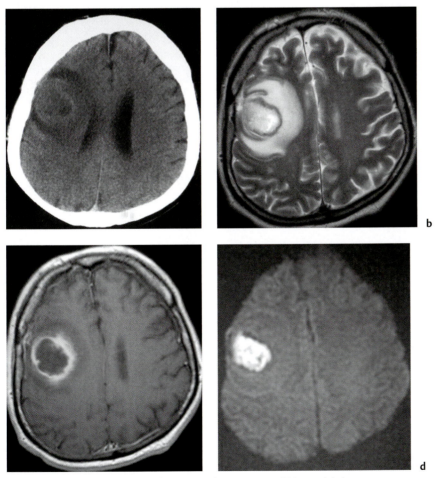

Fig. 1.168a–d   Pyogenic brain abscess. Axial postcontrast CT image (**a**) shows an abscess in the right frontal lobe with adjacent axonal edema. Axial T2-weighted MRI (**b**) shows the abscess to contain high signal with a thin peripheral rim, the latter of which shows contrast enhancement on the axial T1-weighted MRI (**c**). The abscess has high signal/restricted diffusion on the axial diffusion-weighted MRI (**d**).

Table 1.8   (Cont.) Multiple or diffuse lesions involving white matter

Lesions	CT Findings	Comments
Fungal brain abscess	Vary depending on organism; lesions occur in meninges and brain parenchyma; solid or cystic-appearing lesions with low to intermediate attenuation, nodular or ring pattern of contrast enhancement; peripheral low-attenuation edema in adjacent brain tissue.	Occurs in immunocompromised or diabetic patients with resultant granulomas in meninges and brain parenchyma. *Cryptococcus* involves the basal meninges and extends along perivascular spaces into the basal ganglia. *Aspergillus* and *Mucor* spread via direct extension through paranasal sinuses or hematogenously and invade blood vessels, resulting in hemorrhagic lesions and/or cerebral infarcts. Coccidioidomycosis usually involves the basal meninges.
Encephalitis ▷ *Fig. 1.169*	Poorly defined zone or zones of low to intermediate attenuation, minimal or no contrast enhancement; involves cerebral cortex and/or white matter; minimal localized mass effect. Herpes simplex typically involves the temporal lobes/limbic system with or without hemorrhage; CMV usually in periventricular locations. HIV often involves the periatrial/periventricular white matter.	Infection/inflammation of brain tissue from viruses, often seen in immunocompromised patients (e.g., herpes simplex, CMV, HIV, and progressive multifocal leukoencephalopathy) or immunocompetent patients (e.g., St. Louis encephalitis, eastern or western equine encephalitis, and Epstein-Barr virus).
Rasmussen encephalitis	Progressive atrophy of one cerebral hemisphere with poorly defined zones of decreased attenuation involving the white matter, basal ganglia, and cortex; usually no contrast enhancement.	Usually seen in children younger than 10 y; severe and progressive epilepsy and unilateral neurologic deficits: hemiplegia, psychomotor deterioration. Etiology: chronic slow viral infectious process possibly caused by CMV or Epstein-Barr virus. Treatment: hemispherectomy.
Creutzfeldt-Jakob disease	Zones of decreased attenuation in putamen and caudate nuclei bilaterally, with or without zones of decreased attenuation in white matter and cortex. Typically no contrast enhancement; progressive cerebral atrophy.	Spongiform encephalopathy caused by slow infection from prion (proteinaceous infectious particle); usually seen in adults age 40 to 80 y; progressive dementia; < 10% survive more than 2 y.
Reye syndrome	With or without diffuse edematous low attenuation involving basal ganglia, white matter, and cortex bilaterally.	Disorder of unknown etiology occurring in children usually younger than 16 y. Symptoms (vomiting, lethargy, seizures, and sometimes coma leading to death) occur during recovery from viral-like illness. Mortality ~20%.
Lyme disease	Foci and/or confluent zones of decreased attenuation in cerebral and/or cerebellar white matter, with or without contrast enhancement.	CNS manifestations presumed to occur from immune-related demyelination from Lyme disease (infection by spirochete *Borrelia burgdorferi*) transmitted by ticks.
Tuberculoma ▷ *Fig. 1.170a–c*	**Intra-axial lesions** in cerebral hemispheres and basal ganglia (adults) and cerebellum (children): low to intermediate attenuation, central zone of low attenuation with a thin peripheral rim of intermediate attenuation; with solid or rim pattern of contrast enhancement; with or without calcification. **Meningeal lesions:** Nodular or cystic zones of basilar meningeal contrast enhancement.	Occurs in immunocompromised patients and in inhabitants of developing countries. Caseating intracranial granulomas via hematogenous dissemination; meninges > brain lesions.
Toxoplasmosis	Single or multiple solid and/or cystic lesions located in basal ganglia and/or corticomedullary junctions in cerebral hemispheres, low to intermediate attenuation, nodular or rim pattern of contrast enhancement; with or without peripheral edema.	Most common opportunistic CNS infection in AIDS patients, caused by ingestion of food contaminated with parasites (*Toxoplasma gondii*).

(continues on page 108)

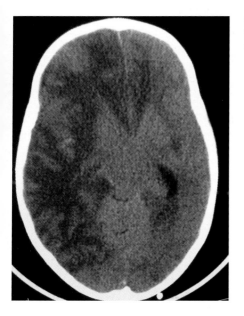

Fig. 1.169   Herpes encephalitis. Axial image shows diffuse decreased attenuation involving most of the right cerebral hemisphere and to a lesser extent in the anterior left frontal lobe.

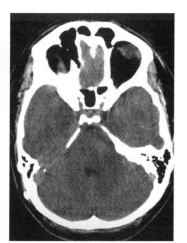
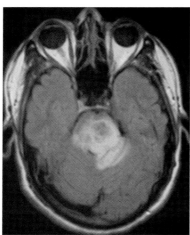

b

Fig. 1.170a–c   Tuberculoma. Axial CT image (**a**) shows a poorly defined lesion with decreased attenuation in the pons and left middle cerebellar peduncle, which shows high signal on axial FLAIR MRI (**b**) and contrast enhancement on the sagittal T1-weighted MRI (**c**).

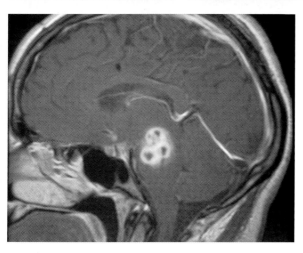

Table 1.8   (Cont.) Multiple or diffuse lesions involving white matter

Lesions	CT Findings	Comments
Parasitic brain lesions		
Cysticercosis	Single or multiple cystic lesions in brain or meninges. **Acute/subacute phase:** Low to intermediate attenuation, rim with or without nodular pattern of contrast enhancement; with or without peripheral edema. **Chronic phase:** Calcified granulomas.	Caused by ingestion of ova (*Taenia solium*) in contaminated food (undercooked pork); involves meninges > brain parenchyma > ventricles.
Hydatid cyst	*Echinococcus granulosus:* Single or rarely multiple cystic lesions with low attenuation with a thin wall with low to intermediate attenuation; typically no contrast enhancement or peripheral edema unless superinfected; often located in vascular territory of the middle cerebral artery. *Echinococcus multilocularis:* Cystic (with or without multilocular) and/or solid lesions; central zone of intermediate attenuation surrounded by a slightly thickened rim of low to intermediate attenuation; with contrast enhancement. Peripheral zone of low attenuation (edema) and calcifications are common.	Caused by parasites *E. granulosus* (South America, Middle East, Australia, and New Zealand) and *E. multilocularis* (North America, Europe, Turkey, and China). CNS involvement in 2% of cases of hydatid infestation.
Neoplastic		
Astrocytoma	**Low-grade astrocytoma:** Focal or diffuse mass lesion usually located in white matter with low to intermediate attenuation, with or without mild contrast enhancement. Minimal associated mass effect. **Juvenile pilocytic astrocytoma subtype:** Solid/cystic focal lesion with low to intermediate attenuation, usually with prominent contrast enhancement. Lesions located in cerebellum, hypothalamus, adjacent to third or fourth ventricle, brainstem. ▷ *Fig. 1.171* **Gliomatosis cerebri:** Infiltrative lesion with poorly defined margins with mass effect located in the white matter, with low to intermediate attenuation; usually no contrast enhancement until late in disease. **Anaplastic astrocytoma:** Often irregularly marginated lesion located in white matter with low to intermediate attenuation, with or without contrast enhancement. ▷ *Fig. 1.172*	Often occurs in children and adults (age 20–40 y). Tumors comprised of well-differentiated astrocytes. Association with neurofibromatosis type 1, 10-y survival; may become malignant. Common in children; usually favorable prognosis if totally resected. Diffusely infiltrating astrocytoma with relative preservation of underlying brain architecture. Imaging appearance may be more prognostic than histologic grade; ~2-y survival. Intermediate between low-grade astrocytoma and glioblastoma multiforme; ~2-y survival.
Glioblastoma multiforme ▷ *Fig. 1.173*	Irregularly marginated mass lesion with necrosis or cyst, mixed low and intermediate attenuation, with or without hemorrhage, prominent heterogeneous contrast enhancement, peripheral edema; can cross corpus callosum.	Most common primary CNS tumor; highly malignant neoplasms with necrosis and vascular proliferation, usually seen in patients older than 50 y; extent of lesion underestimated by CT; survival < 1 y.
Giant cell astrocytoma/ tuberous sclerosis ▷ *Fig. 1.174a–c*	Circumscribed lesion located near the foramen of Monro with mixed low to intermediate attenuation, with or without cysts and/or calcifications, with heterogeneous contrast enhancement. Poorly defined zones of decreased attenuation in the cerebral white matter, often in the periatrial regions.	Subependymal hamartoma near the foramen of Monro; occurs in 15% of patients with tuberous sclerosis < 20 y; slow-growing lesions that can progressively cause obstruction of CSF flow through the foramen of Monro; long-term survival usual if resected.
Pleomorphic xanthoastrocytoma	Circumscribed supratentorial lesion involving the cerebral cortex and white matter; low to intermediate attenuation, with or without cyst(s), heterogeneous contrast enhancement, with or without enhancing mural nodule associated with cyst.	Rare type of astrocytoma occurring in young adults and children, associated with seizure history.

(continues on page 110)

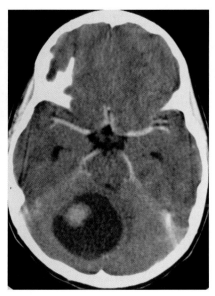

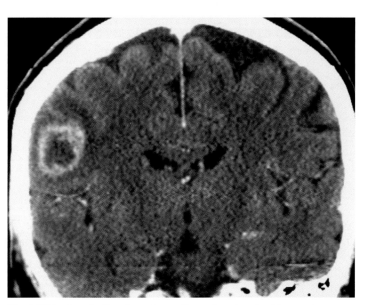

Fig. 1.171   Pilocytic astrocytoma. Axial postcontrast image shows the tumor has an enhancing nodule with a tumoral cyst in the cerebellum.

Fig. 1.172   Anaplastic astrocytoma. Coronal postcontrast image shows the tumor in the right cerebral hemisphere to have a peripheral zone of enhancement.

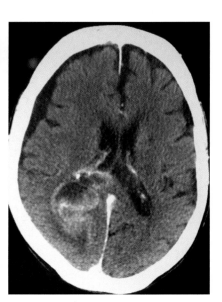

Fig. 1.173   Glioblastoma multiforme. Axial postcontrast image in an 82-year-old man shows the contrast-enhancing tumor in the right occipital lobe extending into the corpus callosum.

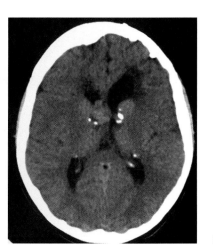
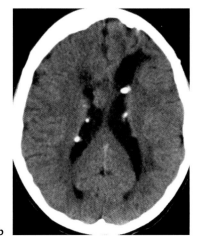
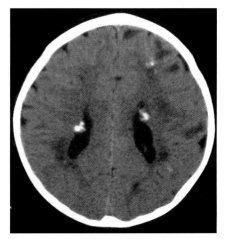

Fig. 1.174a–c   Tuberous sclerosis. Axial images show a giant cell astrocytoma at the right foramen of Monro (**a,b**), calcified ependymal hamartomas (**a–c**), zones with decreased attenuation in the cerebral white matter (**b,c**), and cortical tubers (**c**).

Table 1.8   (Cont.) Multiple or diffuse lesions involving white matter

Lesions	CT Findings	Comments
Oligodendroglioma ▷ *Fig. 1.175*	Circumscribed lesion with mixed low to intermediate attenuation; sites of clumplike calcification, heterogeneous contrast enhancement; involves white matter and cerebral cortex; can cause chronic erosion of inner table of calvarium.	Uncommon slow-growing gliomas with usually mixed histologic patterns (astrocytomas, etc.). Usually seen in adults older than 35 y; 85% supratentorial. If low grade, 75% 5-y survival; higher grade lesions have a worse prognosis.
Ganglioglioma, ganglioneuroma, gangliocytoma	Circumscribed tumor, usually supratentorial, often temporal or frontal lobes; low to intermediate attenuation; with or without cysts, with or without contrast enhancement.	Ganglioglioma (contains glial and neuronal elements); ganglioneuroma (contains only ganglion cells). Uncommon tumors, < 30 y, seizure presentation, slow-growing neoplasms. Gangliocytoma (contains only neuronal elements, dysplastic brain tissue). Favorable prognosis if completely resected.
Ependymoma ▷ *Fig. 1.176*	Circumscribed lobulated supratentorial lesion, often extraventricular, with or without cysts and/or calcifications; low to intermediate attenuation; variable contrast enhancement.	Occurs more commonly in children than adults; one third supratentorial, two thirds infratentorial; 45% 5-y survival.
Hamartoma/tuberous sclerosis ▷ *Fig. 1.174a–c, p. 109*	**Cortical/ subcortical lesions with variable attenuation:** calcifications in 50% of older children; contrast enhancement uncommon. **Subependymal hamartomas:** Small nodules located along and projecting into the lateral ventricles; calcifications and contrast enhancement are common.	Cortical and subependymal hamartomas are nonmalignant lesions associated with tuberous sclerosis.
Primitive neuroectodermal tumor ▷ *Fig. 1.177*	Circumscribed or invasive lesions; low to intermediate attenuation; variable contrast enhancement; frequent dissemination into the leptomeninges.	Highly malignant tumors located in the cerebrum, pineal gland, and cerebellum that frequently disseminate along CSF pathways.
Dysembryoplastic neuroepithelial tumor	Circumscribed lesions involving the cerebral cortex and subcortical white matter; low to intermediate attenuation; with or without small cysts; usually no contrast enhancement.	Benign superficial lesions commonly located in the temporal or frontal lobes.
Lymphoma ▷ *Fig. 1.178* ▷ *Fig. 1.179*	**Primary CNS lymphoma:** Focal or infiltrating lesion located in the basal ganglia, periventricular regions, and posterior fossa/brainstem; low to intermediate attenuation; with or without hemorrhage/necrosis in immunocompromised patients; usually show contrast enhancement. Diffuse leptomeningeal contrast enhancement is another pattern of intracranial lymphoma.	Primary CNS lymphoma more common than secondary, usually in adults older than 40 y; B-cell lymphoma more common than T-cell lymphoma; increasing incidence related to number of immunocompromised patients in population. CT features of primary and secondary lymphoma of brain overlap. Intracranial lymphoma can involve the leptomeninges in secondary lymphoma > primary lymphoma.
Metastases ▷ *Fig. 1.180*	Circumscribed spheroid lesions in brain; can have various intra-axial locations, often at gray-white matter junctions; usually low to intermediate attenuation; with or without hemorrhage, calcifications, and cysts; variable contrast enhancement, often associated with low attenuation from axonal edema.	Represent ~33% of intracranial tumors, usually from extracranial primary neoplasm in adults older than 40 y. Primary tumor source: lung > breast > GI > GU > melanoma.

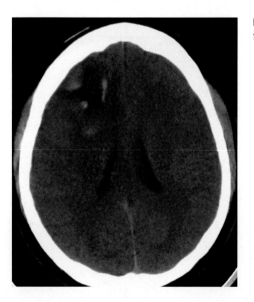

Fig. 1.175   Oligodendroglioma. Axial image shows the tumor in the anterior right frontal lobe containing calcifications.

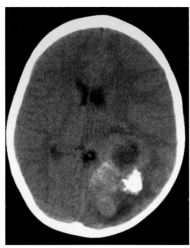

Fig. 1.176   Ependymoma. Axial postcontrast image shows the tumor in the left occipital lobe with zones of enhancement, cystic change, and calcifications.

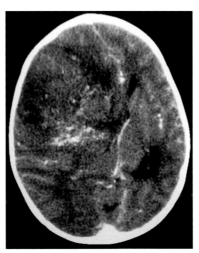

Fig. 1.177   Primitive neuroectodermal tumor. Axial postcontrast image in a 1-year-old girl shows a large mass lesion in the right cerebral hemisphere with mixed attenuation, irregular zones of enhancement, and calcifications.

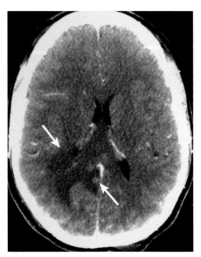

Fig. 1.178   Lymphoma. Axial postcontrast image shows lymphoma with mostly decreased attenuation in the right cerebral hemisphere extending into the corpus callosum (arrows).

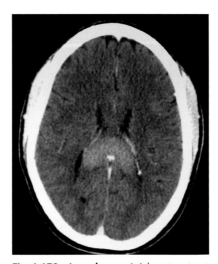

Fig. 1.179   Lymphoma. Axial postcontrast image shows a contrast-enhancing tumor involving the corpus callosum.

Fig. 1.180   Metastatic lesions. Axial postcontrast image shows two nodular-enhancing lesions in the left cerebral hemisphere with surrounding low-attenuation edema.

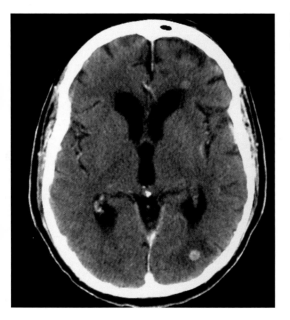

Table 1.9   Intracranial hemorrhage

Lesions	CT Findings	Comments
Hematoma		
Intra-axial hemorrhage in brain	Attenuation of the hematoma depends on its age, size, location, hematocrit, hemoglobin oxidation state, clot retraction, and extent of edema. **Hyperacute phase (4–6 h):** Hemoglobin primarily as diamagnetic oxyhemoglobin (iron Fe^{2+} state). **CT:** High attenuation on CT. **MRI:** Intermediate signal on T1-weighted images, slightly high signal on T2-weighted images. **Acute phase (12–48 h):** Hemoglobin primarily as paramagnetic deoxyhemoglobin (iron Fe^{2+} state). **CT:** High attenuation in acute clot directly related to hematocrit, hemoglobin concentration, and high protein concentration. Hematocrit in acute clot approaches 90%. ▷ *Fig. 1.181* **MRI:** Intermediate signal on T1-weighted images, low signal on T2-weighted images (deoxyhemoglobin), surrounded by a peripheral zone of high T2 signal (edema). **Early subacute phase (> 2 d):** Hemoglobin becomes oxidized to the iron Fe^{3+} state, methemoglobin, which is strongly paramagnetic. **CT:** Lesion with high attenuation. ▷ *Fig. 1.182* **MRI:** When methemoglobin is initially intracellular, the hematoma has high signal on T1-weighted images progressing from peripheral to central and low signal on T2-weighted images, surrounded by a zone of high T2 signal (edema). When methemoglobin eventually becomes primarily extracellular, the hematoma has high signal on T1-weighted images and high signal on T2-weighted images. **Late subacute phase (> 7 d–6 wk):** Intracerebral hematomas decrease 1.5 HU per day. Hematomas become isodense to hypodense; peripheral contrast enhancement from blood–brain barrier breakdown and vascularized capsule. **Chronic phase:** Hemoglobin as extracellular methemoglobin is progressively degraded to hemosiderin. **CT:** Chronic hematomas have low attenuation with localized encephalomalacia. Zones with high attenuation represent new sites of rebleeding. **MRI:** Hematoma progresses from a lesion with high signal on T1- and T2-weighted images with a peripheral rim of low signal on T2-weighted images (hemosiderin) to predominant hemosiderin composition and low signal on T2-weighted images.	Can result from trauma, ruptured aneurysms or vascular malformations, coagulopathy, hypertension, adverse drug reaction, amyloid angiopathy, hemorrhagic transformation of cerebral infarction from arterial or venous sinus occlusion, metastases, abscesses, and viral infections (e.g., herpes simplex and CMV).
Traumatic lesions		
Cerebral contusions ▷ *Fig. 1.183*	CT appearance of contusions is initially one of focal hemorrhage involving the cerebral cortex and subcortical white matter. Contusions eventually appear as focal superficial encephalomalacia zones.	Contusions are superficial brain injuries involving the cerebral cortex and subcortical white matter that result from skull fracture and/or acceleration/deceleration trauma to the inner table of the skull. Often involve the anterior portions of the temporal and frontal lobes and inferior portions of the frontal lobes.
Diffuse axonal injury ▷ *Fig. 1.184a, b*	**CT:** For acute injuries, one or multiple sites of hemorrhage are seen with high attenuation; commonly occur at the corpus callosum; cerebral cortical–white matter junctions, basal ganglia, and brainstem. **MRI:** One or multiple sites within the brain with intermediate or high signal on T1-weighted images, low, intermediate, and/or high signal on T2-weighted images, and low signal on gradient echo imaging.	Brain injury caused by deceleration and rotational shear forces that result in disruption of axons and blood vessels. The greater the degree of axonal injury, the poorer the prognosis.

(continues on page 114)

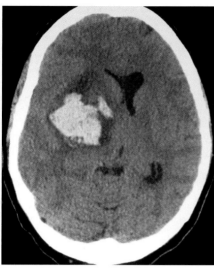

Fig. 1.181   Acute intra-axial hematoma. Axial image shows the hematoma with high attenuation in the right basal ganglia with mass effect and subfalcine herniation leftward.

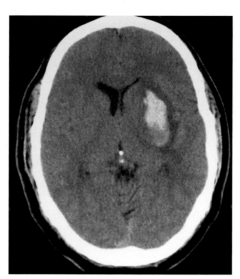

Fig. 1.182   Early subacute intra-axial hematoma. Axial image shows the hematoma with high attenuation in the left basal ganglia with minimal localized mass effect.

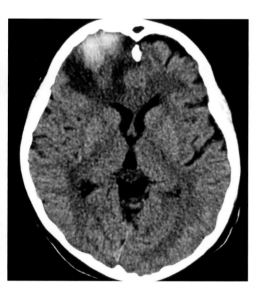

Fig. 1.183   Cerebral contusion. Axial image shows the hematoma with high attenuation in the anterior right frontal lobe with adjacent low-attenuation edema and localized mass effect.

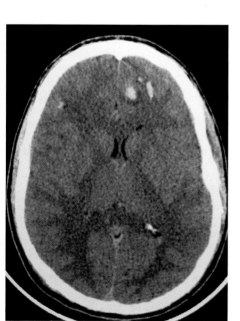

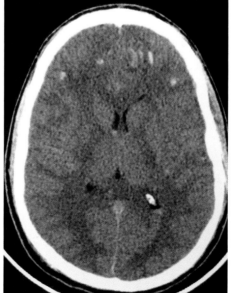

b

Fig. 1.184a, b   Diffuse axonal injuries. Axial images show multiple small zones of hemorrhage in the cerebral white matter bilaterally from axonal shear injuries.

Table 1.9   (Cont.) Intracranial hemorrhage

Lesions	CT Findings	Comments
Neoplasms		
Metastatic tumor ▷ *Fig. 1.185* ▷ *Fig. 1.186a, b*	Single or multiple well-circumscribed or poorly defined lesions involving the brain, dura, leptomeninges, choroid plexus, and /or skull with low to intermediate attenuation, usually with contrast enhancement, with or without bone destruction, with or without compression of neural tissue or vessels, with or without hemorrhage. Leptomeningeal tumor often best seen on postcontrast images.	Metastatic tumor may have variable destructive or infiltrative changes involving single or multiple sites of involvement in the brain, meninges, and/or skull. Metastatic lesions associated with hemorrhage include melanoma; carcinomas of the lung, breast, or kidney; and choriocarcinoma.
Primary brain neoplasms ▷ *Fig. 1.187a, b*	Intra-axial lesions that may have mixed attenuation with low, intermediate, and/or high attenuation, with axonal edema; usually with contrast enhancement in nonhemorrhagic portions; often multiple.	Up to 15% of primary tumors contain sites of hemorrhage. Primary brain tumors with hemorrhage include glioblastoma multiforme, anaplastic astrocytoma, oligodendrogliomas, ependymomas, lymphoma associated with HIV infection, hemangioblastomas, medulloblastomas, and atypical teratoid rhabdoid tumors.
Pituitary adenoma	Pituitary lesions with associated high attenuation from recent hemorrhage.	Pituitary adenomas are the most common intracranial tumor to be associated with hemorrhage.
Choroid plexus papilloma or carcinoma	Circumscribed and/or lobulated lesions with papillary projections, intermediate attenuation, usually prominent contrast enhancement, with or without calcifications. Locations: atrium of lateral ventricle (children) > fourth ventricle (adults), rarely other locations such as third ventricle; associated with hydrocephalus.	Rare intracranial neoplasms. CT features of choroid plexus carcinoma and papilloma may overlap; both histologic types can disseminate along CSF pathways. Carcinomas tend to be larger and have greater degrees of mixed/heterogeneous attenuation than papillomas. Carcinomas often show invasion of adjacent brain, whereas papillomas often do not.
Neurocutaneous melanosis/melanoma	Extra- or intra-axial lesions usually < 3 cm in diameter with irregular margins in the leptomeninges or brain parenchyma/brainstem (anterior temporal lobes, cerebellum, thalami, and inferior frontal lobes); may show no abnormalities on CT, occasionally show zones with intermediate to slightly high attenuation secondary to increased melanin; with or without contrast enhancement. With or without vermian hypoplasia, with or without arachnoid cysts, with or without Dandy-Walker malformation. Hemorrhage can be seen in melanomas that commonly occur in this disorder.	Neuroectodermal dysplasia with proliferation of melanocytes in leptomeninges associated with large and/or numerous cutaneous nevi. May change into CNS melanoma.
Vascular lesions		
Cerebral/cerebellar Infarction ▷ *Fig. 1.188*	CT and MRI features of cerebral and cerebellar infarcts depend on the age of the infarct relative to the time of examination. **CT:** Localized swelling at sites with low attenuation involving gray and white matter (often wedge shaped), with or without hemorrhage. **MRI:** Zones with low to intermediate signal on T1-weighted images, high signal on T2-weighted images; localized edema; with or without hemorrhage, with or without gadolinium contrast enhancement.	Cerebral infarcts usually result from occlusive vascular disease involving large, medium, or small arteries. Early subacute infarcts (24 h–3 d) can be associated with hemorrhagic transformation in which reperfusion occurs at ischemic zone with damaged endothelium. Hemorrhagic transformation usually occurs with embolic infarcts. Hemorrhages can range from petechia to large hematomas.
AVM ▷ *Fig. 1.189a–c*	Lesions with irregular margins that can be located in the brain parenchyma (pia, dura, or both locations). AVMs contain multiple tortuous vessels. The venous portions often show contrast enhancement. Usually not associated with mass effect unless there is recent hemorrhage or venous occlusion. CTA can show the arterial, nidus, and venous portions of the AVMs.	Supratentorial AVMs occur more frequently (80%–90%) than infratentorial AVMs (10%–20%). Annual risk of hemorrhage. AVMs can be sporadic, congenital, or associated with a history of trauma.
Dural AVM	Dural AVMs contain multiple tortuous small vessels at the site of a recanalized thrombosed dural venous sinus. Usually not associated with mass effect unless there is recent hemorrhage or venous occlusion.	Dural AVMs are usually acquired lesions resulting from thrombosis or occlusion of an intracranial venous sinus with subsequent recanalization resulting in direct arterial to venous sinus communications. Transverse, sigmoid venous sinuses > cavernous sinus > straight, superior sagittal sinuses.

(continues on page 116)

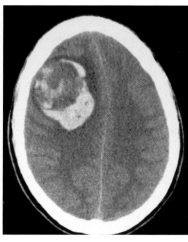

Fig. 1.185   Metastatic disease in a 16-year-old male patient with embryonal yolk sac tumor. Axial image shows a hemorrhagic metastatic lesion in the anterior right frontal lobe.

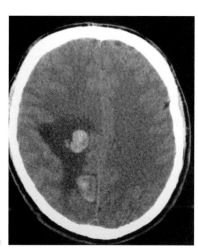
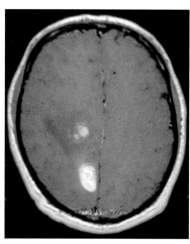

Fig. 1.186a, b   Metastatic lesions in a patient with renal cell carcinoma. Axial CT image (**a**) shows two hemorrhagic metastatic lesions with high attenuation and axonal edema in the medial portion of the right cerebral hemisphere that has high signal on the axial T1-weighted image (**b**).

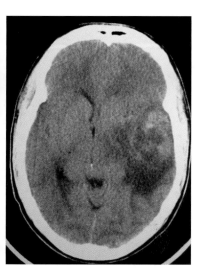
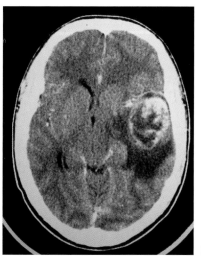

Fig. 1.187a, b   Primary intra-axial tumor. Axial image (**a**) shows a malignant glioma in the left temporal lobe containing a portion with high attenuation from hemorrhage. The tumor shows irregular enhancement on an axial postcontrast image (**b**).

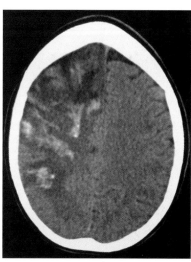

Fig. 1.188   Hemorrhagic cerebral infarction. Axial image shows an infarct in the right cerebral hemisphere that shows sites of hemorrhage.

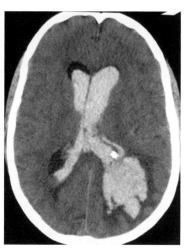
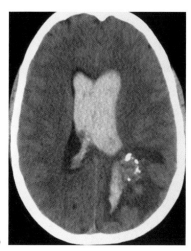
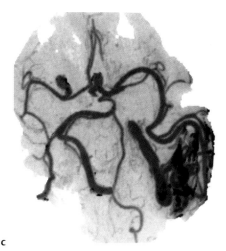

Fig. 1.189a–c   AVM. Axial CT images show intraventricular hemorrhage from an AVM, as seen on the CT angiogram (**c**).

Table 1.9   (Cont.) Intracranial hemorrhage

Lesions	CT Findings	Comments
Cavernous hemangioma	**CT:** Intermediate to slightly high attenuation, with or without calcification; typically shows no contrast enhancement unless associated with a venous angioma. **MRI:** "Popcorn"-shaped lesion with a low signal rim on T2 and gradient echo imaging surrounding a central zone with mixed low, intermediate, and/or high signal on T1 and T2; typically no contrast enhancement.	Intra-axial vascular malformation composed of low-pressure endovascular-lined sinusoidal spaces often associated with sites of recent and/or prior hemorrhage; 80% are supratentorial. Can present with headache and/or seizures. Can be multiple in inherited syndromes.
Giant aneurysm ▷ *Fig. 1.190a, b*	Bulbous extra-axial lesions with contents that can have low, intermediate, and/or high attenuation.	Giant aneurysms are > 2.5 cm in diameter and typically contain layers of clotted blood, as well as intramural hemorrhage.
Dissecting aneurysm	**Dissecting aneurysms (intramural hematoma):** The involved arterial wall is thickened in a circumferential or semilunar configuration and has intermediate attenuation. Lumen may be narrowed or occluded.	Accumulation of blood within the arterial wall secondary to a tear of the intima and internal elastic lamina.
Pseudoaneurysm	Involved arterial wall is thickened and surrounded by a localized hematoma with intermediate to high attenuation.	Rupture of involved artery with localized encapsulation of perivascular hematoma.

Inflammatory lesions

Lesions	CT Findings	Comments
Arteritis	Zones of arterial occlusion and/or foci of stenosis and post-stenotic dilation. May involve large, medium-sized, or small intra- and extracranial arteries. With or without cerebral and/or cerebellar infarcts, with or without hemorrhage.	Uncommon mixed group of inflammatory diseases/disorders involving the walls of cerebral blood vessels. Can result from noninfectious etiology (polyarteritis nodosa, Wegener granulomatosis, giant cell arteritis, Takayasu arteritis, sarcoid, drug-induced, etc.) or be related to infectious cause (bacteria, fungi, tuberculosis [TB], syphilis, or viral).

Infections

Lesions	CT Findings	Comments
Fungal infection	Fungal infections such as from *Aspergillus* and *Mucor* often invade blood vessels, causing vasculitis, vascular occlusions, with or without hemorrhagic cerebral or cerebellar infarctions, cerebritis and fungal abscess formation.	Infection from fungi can occur in immunocompetent patients (*Coccidioides, Histoplasma, Blastomyces*) and immunocompromised patients (*Cryptococcus, Aspergillus, Candida, Mucor*). Infection can occur from direct extension from the orbits and paranasal sinuses or hematogenously.
Viral infection	Herpes infections can cause necrotizing meningoencephalitis with tissue necrosis and hemorrhage.	Viral infections can result in meningitis and cerebritis. Viruses associated with intracranial infections include herpes types 1 and 2, CMV, HIV, progressive multifocal leukoencephalopathy (PML), papovaviruses, Epstein-Barr virus, varicella, rubella.

Hematoma, extra-axial

Lesions	CT Findings	Comments
Epidural hematoma	Biconvex extra-axial hematoma located between the skull and dura; displaced dura has high attenuation. CT attenuation and MRI signal of the hematoma depend on its age, size, hematocrit, and oxygen tension. With or without edema (low attenuation on CT and high signal on T2-weighted images) involving the displaced brain parenchyma. With or without subfalcine, uncal herniation. **Hyperacute hematomas:** **CT:** Can have high and/or mixed high and intermediate attenuation. **MRI:** Intermediate signal on T1-weighted images, intermediate to high signal on T2-weighted images. **Acute hematoma:** **CT:** Can have high and/or mixed high and intermediate attenuation. ▷ *Fig 1.191a, b* **MRI:** Low to intermediate signal on T1-weighted images, high signal on T2-weighted images. **Subacute hematoma:** **CT:** Can have high and/or mixed high and intermediate attenuation. **MRI:** High signal on T1- and T2-weighted images.	Epidural hematomas usually result from trauma/tearing of an epidural artery or dural venous sinus; epidural hematomas do not cross cranial sutures; with or without skull fracture.

(continues on page 118)

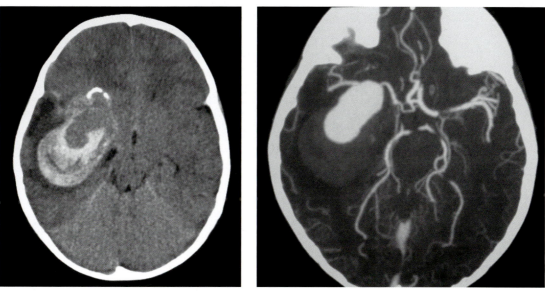

b

Fig. 1.190a, b   Giant aneurysm. Axial image (**a**) shows a large aneurysm containing mural thrombus with high attenuation. Axial CT angiogram (**b**) shows enhancement of the patent lumen of the aneurysm.

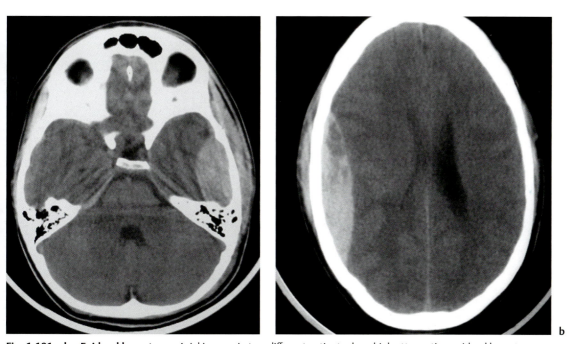

b

Fig. 1.191a, b   Epidural hematoma. Axial images in two different patients show high-attenuation epidural hematomas on the left (**a**) and right (**b**).

Table 1.9   (Cont.) Intracranial hemorrhage

Lesions	CT Findings	Comments
Subdural hematoma	Crescentic extra-axial hematoma located in the potential space between the inner margin of the dura and outer margin of the arachnoid membrane. CT attenuation and MRI signal of the hematoma depend on its age, size, hematocrit, and oxygen tension. with or without edema (low attenuation on CT and high signal on T2-weighted images) involving the displaced brain parenchyma. With or without subfalcine, uncal herniation. **Hyperacute hematoma:** **CT:** Can have high or mixed high, intermediate, and/or low attenuation. **MRI:** Intermediate signal on T1-weighted images, intermediate to high signal on T2-weighted images. **Acute hematoma:** **CT:** Can have high or mixed high, intermediate, and/or low attenuation. ▷ *Fig. 1.192* **MRI:** Low to intermediate signal on T1-weighted images, low signal on T2-weighted images. **Subacute hematoma:** **CT:** Can have intermediate attenuation (isodense to brain) and/or low to intermediate attenuation. ▷ *Fig. 1.193a, b* **MRI:** High signal on T1- and T2-weighted images. **Chronic hematoma:** **CT:** Usually has low attenuation (hypodense to brain). ▷ *Fig. 1.194* **MRI:** Variable, often low to intermediate signal on T1-weighted images, high signal on T2-weighted images; with or without enhancement of collection and organizing neomembrane. Mixed MRI signal can result if rebleeding occurs into chronic collection.	Subdural hematomas usually result from trauma/ stretching/tearing of cortical veins where they enter the subdural space to drain into dural venous sinuses; subdural hematomas do cross sites of cranial sutures; with or without skull fracture.
Subarachnoid hemorrhage ▷ *Fig. 1.195a, b*	**CT:** Acute subarachnoid hemorrhage typically appears as poorly defined zones with high attenuation in the leptomeninges within the sulci and basal cisterns. Usually becomes isodense or hypodense after 1 week unless there is rebleeding. **MRI:** May not be seen on T1- or T2-weighted images, although it may have intermediate to slightly high signal on FLAIR images.	Extravasated blood in the subarachnoid space can result from ruptured arterial aneurysms or dural venous sinuses, vascular malformations, hypertensive hemorrhages, trauma, cerebral infarcts, coagulopathy, etc.

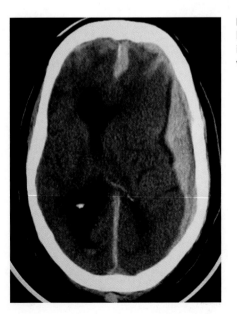

Fig. 1.192   Acute subdural hematoma. Axial image shows a subdural hematoma on the left with high attenuation and mass effect with subfalcine herniation rightward. Also seen is a subarachnoid hemorrhage anteriorly and blood in the posterior portions of the lateral ventricles from head trauma.

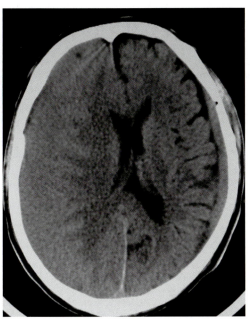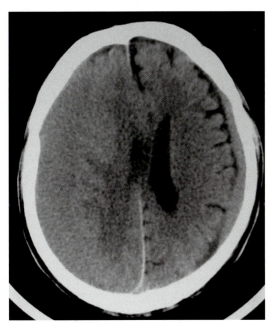

b

Fig. 1.193a, b   Isodense/subacute subdural hematoma. Axial images show a large isodense subdural hematoma on the right with subfalcine herniation leftward.

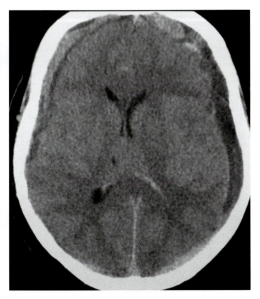

Fig. 1.194   Late subacute subdural hematoma. Axial image shows bilateral subdural hematomas with mixed low, intermediate, and slightly high attenuation. The zones with slightly increased attenuation can occur as the result of recent rebleeding.

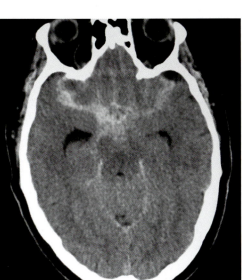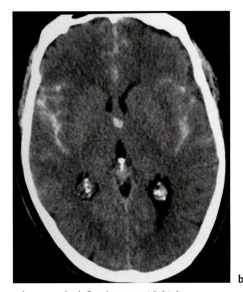

b

Fig. 1.195a, b   Subarachnoid hemorrhage. Axial images show poorly defined zones with high attenuation in the subarachnoid space from acute hemorrhage.

Table 1.10   Intracranial calcifications

Lesions	CT Findings	Comments
Normal variants		
Choroid plexus calcifications ▷ *Fig. 1.196a, b*	Calcifications occur in the choroid plexus (lateral ventricles, atria, third and fourth ventricles, and foramina of Luschka).	The choroid plexuses are invaginated folds of pia mater covered by cuboidal or low columnar epithelium of neural tube origin that extend into the ventricles. The epithelial cells of the choroid plexus secrete CSF into the ventricles. Normal physiologic calcifications in the choroid plexus begin in the pediatric population, 10% in the first 2 decades, and progressively increase in frequency with aging.
Pineal calcification ▷ *Fig. 1.196a*	Incidental calcifications commonly occur in the pineal gland.	Normal physiologic calcifications in the pineal gland occur in the pediatric population and progressively increase in frequency with aging. Calcifications usually measure < 1 cm in diameter. Can be seen in up to 40% of patients by age 20 y.
Habenula ▷ *Fig. 1.196a*	Calcifications commonly occur in the habenula, which is located anterior to the pineal gland.	The habenula is a small nuclear structure that is part of the epithalamus and is located anterior to the pineal gland. It receives input from the septal nucleus and thalamus from the stria medullaris and sends output to the interpeduncular nucleus. Normal physiologic calcifications in the habenula begin in the pediatric population and progressively increase in frequency with aging.
Falcine/dural calcifications ▷ *Fig. 1.197a, b*	Calcifications can occur as incidental findings in various intracranial dural locations in adults. Dural calcifications in children may be associated with a dural tumor or genetic abnormality, such as basal cell nevus syndrome.	The dura mater is the external layer of the meninges composed of dense connective tissue that is continuous with the inner periosteum of the skull. Metaplastic ossification changes in the dura commonly occur in adults.
Arachnoid granulation	Normal physiologic calcifications can be seen in the arachnoid granulations in adults, particularly within the transverse and sigmoid venous sinuses.	Arachnoid granulations or villi are protrusions of the arachnoid (composed of connective tissue lacking blood vessels covered by squamous epithelium) into the dural venous sinuses. The function of the arachnoid granulations is to transfer CSF from the subarachnoid space into the blood of the venous sinuses.
Idiopathic basal ganglia calcifications ▷ *Fig. 1.198*	Punctate calcifications in the caudate nuclei, thalami, putamina, and/or globus pallidi bilaterally.	The basal ganglia are involved in the initiation and modulation of movement. Physiologic and nonpathologic calcifications involving the caudate nuclei, putamen, and/or globus pallidus bilaterally occur in adults older than age 30 y. Occur in 1% to 2% of the population, usually in adults; increase in frequency with age. Idiopathic calcifications account for 75% of basal ganglia calcifications. Calcifications in these locations can also occur with disorders of calcium and phosphate metabolism (hypoparathyroidism, pseudohypoparathyroidism, pseudopseudohypoparathyroidism, hyperparathyroidism, and carbonic anhydrase II deficiency).
Dentate nuclei calcifications ▷ *Fig. 1.199*	Calcifications in the dentate nuclei of the cerebellar hemispheres.	The dentate nuclei are the most lateral of the deep cerebellar nuclei. They receive input from the lateral cerebellar hemispheres and send output via the superior cerebellar peduncles. Physiologic and nonpathologic calcifications involving the dentate nuclei occur in adults usually older than age 30 y.

(continues on page 122)

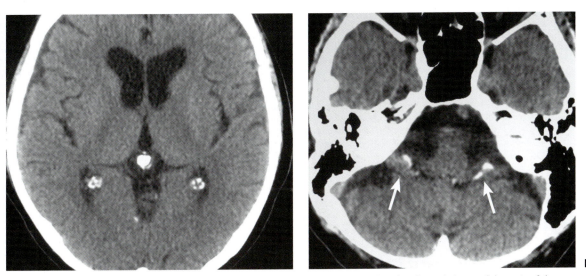

Fig. 1.196a, b Choroid plexus calcifications. Axial images show calcifications within the choroid plexus of the atria of the lateral ventricles and pineal gland (**a**) and foramina of Luschka (arrows) (**b**).

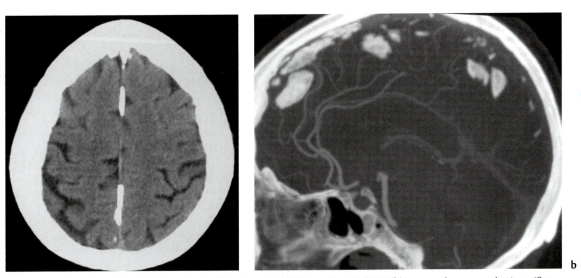

Fig. 1.197a, b Falcine dural calcification/ossification. Axial CT (**a**) and sagittal CTA (**b**) images show metaplastic ossifications involving the falx cerebri.

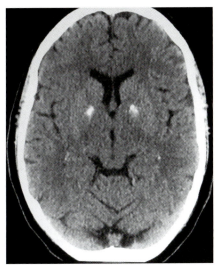

Fig. 1.198 Basal ganglia calcifications, idiopathic. Axial image shows calcifications in the basal ganglia bilaterally.

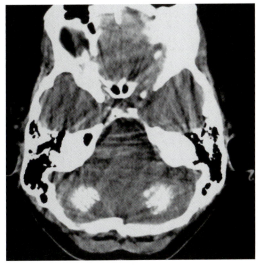

Fig. 1.199 Dentate nuclei calcifications. Axial image shows dense calcifications in the dentate nuclei.

Table 1.10   (Cont.) Intracranial calcifications

Lesions	CT Findings	Comments
Vascular		
Atherosclerotic calcifications ▷ *Fig. 1.200*	Calcified and/or soft atherosclerotic plaques in the walls of arteries in adults. Common intracranial sites include the cavernous and supraclinoid portions of the internal carotid arteries and upper vertebral arteries and basilar artery.	Commonly seen with older adults secondary to atherosclerotic arterial disease.
AVM ▷ *Fig. 1.201a, b*	Lesions with irregular margins that can be located in the brain parenchyma or meninges (pia, dura, or both locations). AVMs contain multiple tortuous enhancing blood vessels secondary to patent arteries with high blood flow, as well as thrombosed vessels with variable attenuation, areas of hemorrhage in various phases, calcifications, and gliosis. The venous portions often show contrast enhancement. CTA can provide additional detailed information about the nidus, feeding arteries, and draining veins, as well as the presence of associated aneurysms. Usually not associated with mass effect unless there is recent hemorrhage or venous occlusion.	Supratentorial AVMs occur more frequently (80%–90%) than infratentorial AVMs (10%–20%). Annual risk of hemorrhage. AVMs can be sporadic, congenital, or associated with a history of trauma. Multiple AVMs can be seen in syndromes: Rendu-Osler-Weber (AVMs in brain and lungs and mucosal capillary telangiectasias) and Wyburn-Mason (AVMs in brain and retina with cutaneous nevi).
Cavernous angioma ▷ *Fig. 1.202*	Single or multiple multilobulated intra-axial lesions that have intermediate to slightly increased attenuation; minimal or no contrast enhancement; with or without calcifications.	Cavernous angiomas can be located in many different locations; multiple lesions > 50%. Associated with venous angiomas and risk of hemorrhage.
Giant aneurysm ▷ *Fig. 1.203*	Focal, well-circumscribed structure with layers of low, intermediate, and/or high attenuation secondary to layers of thrombus of different ages, as well a zone of contrast enhancement representing a patent lumen if present. With or without wall calcifications.	Saccular aneurysms > 2.5 cm in diameter are referred to as giant aneurysms. Fusiform aneurysms are often related to atherosclerosis or collagen vascular disease (Marfan syndrome, Ehlers-Danlos syndrome, etc.). Dissecting aneurysms: hemorrhage occurs in the arterial wall from incidental or significant trauma.
Dystrophic calcifications ▷ *Fig. 1.204*	Dystrophic calcifications can occur at sites of prior cerebral and cerebellar infarction, intracerebral and extra-axial hematomas, and radiation treatment, as well as from chemotherapy.	Dystrophic calcifications result from mineralizing microangiopathy involving small arteries and arterioles causing calcifications in the basal ganglia and subcortical white matter. Necrotizing leukoencephalopathy is another cause of dystrophic calcifications in white matter.
Sturge-Weber syndrome ▷ *Fig. 1.205a–c*	Prominent localized unilateral leptomeningeal enhancement usually in parietal and/or occipital regions in children; with or without gyral enhancement; mild localized atrophic changes in brain adjacent to the pial angioma; with or without prominent medullary and/or subependymal veins; with or without ipsilateral prominence of choroid plexus. Gyral calcifications > 2 y, progressive cerebral atrophy in region of pial angioma.	Also known as encephalotrigeminal angiomatosis; neurocutaneous syndrome associated with ipsilateral "port wine" cutaneous lesion and seizures; results from persistence of primitive leptomeningeal venous drainage (pial angioma) and developmental lack of normal cortical veins producing chronic venous congestion and ischemia.

(continues on page 124)

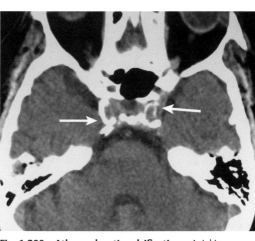

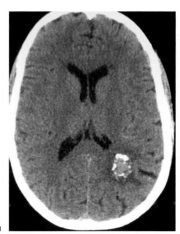 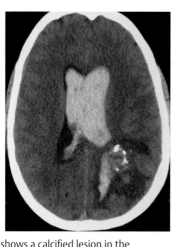

a

b

Fig. 1.200 Atherosclerotic calcifications. Axial image shows atherosclerotic calcifications involving the cavernous portions of both internal carotid arteries (arrows).

Fig. 1.201a, b AVM. Axial image (**a**) shows a calcified lesion in the posterior left cerebral hemisphere. Axial CT image 1 year later (**b**) shows intraventricular hemorrhage from the AVM.

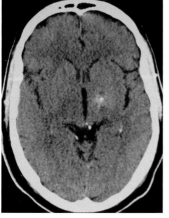 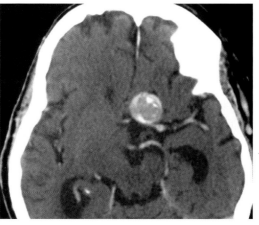 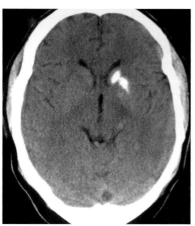

Fig. 1.202 Cavernous angioma/ hemangioma. Axial image shows a small lesion with calcifications in the left thalamus.

Fig. 1.203 Giant aneurysm. Axial postcontrast image shows a large supraclinoid aneurysm on the left side with mural calcifications.

Fig. 1.204 Dystrophic calcifications. Axial image shows dystrophic calcifications involving the left caudate head and putamen from prior ischemic injury.

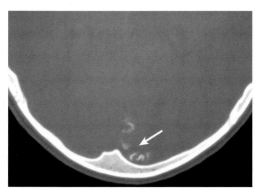 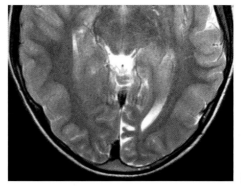

b

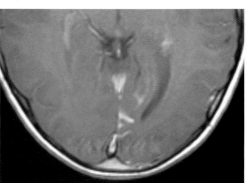

Fig. 1.205a–c Sturge-Weber syndrome. Axial CT image (**a**) shows curvilinear calcifications along the gyri of the posterior medial left occipital lobe (arrow). Axial T2-weighted MRI (**b**) shows gyral atrophy in this region. Axial postcontrast T1-weighted MRI (**c**) shows gyriform enhancement in the subarachnoid space.

Table 1.10   (Cont.) Intracranial calcifications

Lesions	CT Findings	Comments
Inflammation/infection		
Parasites (toxoplasmosis, cysticercosis, hydatid, *Paragonimus*), viruses (CMV, herpes), syphilis, and tuberculosis		
Toxoplasmosis ▷*Fig. 1.206*	Single or multiple solid and/or cystic-appearing lesions located in basal ganglia and/or corticomedullary junctions in cerebral hemispheres; low to intermediate attenuation, nodular or rim pattern of contrast enhancement, with or without mild peripheral low attenuation (edema). **Chronic phase:** Calcified granulomas.	Most common opportunistic CNS infection in AIDS patients, caused by ingestion of food contaminated with parasites (*Toxoplasma gondii*). Can also occur as congenital or neonatal infection (TORCH: *Toxoplasma, rubella,* CMV, herpes).
Cysticercosis ▷*Fig. 1.207a–c*	Single or multiple cystic-appearing lesions in brain or meninges. **Acute/subacute phase:** Low to intermediate attenuation, rim with or without nodular pattern of contrast enhancement, with or without peripheral low attenuation (edema). **Chronic phase:** Calcified granulomas.	Caused by ingestion of ova (*Taenia solium*) in contaminated food (undercooked pork); involves meninges > brain parenchyma > ventricles.
Hydatid cyst	***Echinococcus granulosus:*** Single or rarely multiple cystic-appearing lesions with low attenuation surrounded by a thin wall; typically no contrast enhancement or peripheral edema unless superinfected; often located in the vascular territory of the middle cerebral artery. ***Echinococcus multilocularis:*** Cystic (with or without multilocular) and/or solid lesions; central zone of intermediate attenuation surrounded by a slightly thickened rim, with contrast enhancement. Peripheral zone of decreased attenuation (edema) and calcifications are common.	Caused by parasites *E. granulosus* (South America, Middle East, Australia, and New Zealand) and *E. multilocularis* (North America, Europe, Turkey, and China). CNS involvement in 2% of cases of hydatid infestation.
Benign neoplasms		
Meningioma ▷*Fig. 1.208a, b*	Extra-axial dural-based lesions, well-circumscribed; supratentorial > infratentorial, parasagittal > convexity > sphenoid ridge > parasellar > posterior fossa > optic nerve sheath > intraventricular; intermediate attenuation, usually prominent contrast enhancement; with or without calcifications, with or without hyperostosis of adjacent bone.	Most common extra-axial tumor, usually benign neoplasms, typically occurs in adults (older than 40 y), women > men; multiple meningiomas seen with neurofibromatosis type II. Can result in compression of adjacent brain parenchyma, encasement of arteries, and compression of dural venous sinuses; rarely invasive/malignant types.
Lipoma of the corpus callosum ▷*Fig. 1.209a, b*	Lipomas have CT attenuation similar to subcutaneous fat, with or without calcifications; typically no contrast enhancement or peripheral edema.	Benign fatty lesions resulting from congenital malformation often located in or near the midline; may contain calcifications and/or traversing blood vessels; may be associated with dysplasia/hypoplasia of the corpus callosum.

(continues on page 126)

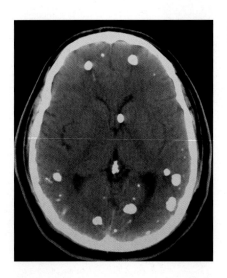

Fig. 1.206   Toxoplasmosis. Axial image shows multiple calcified healed granulomas within the brain, left lateral ventricle, and sulci.

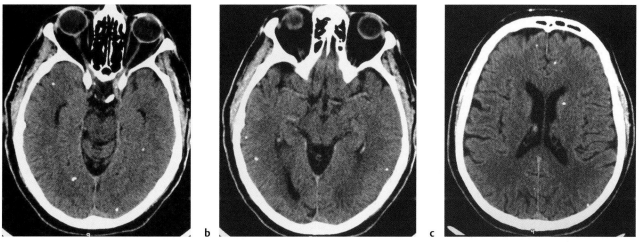

Fig. 1.207a–c **Cysticercosis.** Axial images (**a–c**) show multiple small calcified healed granulomas within the brain.

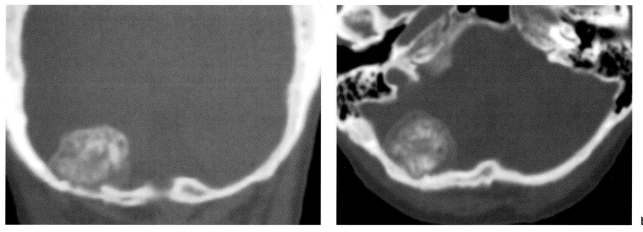

Fig. 1.208a, b **Meningioma.** Coronal (**a**) and axial (**b**) images show a calcified meningioma along the floor of the right side of the posterior cranial fossa.

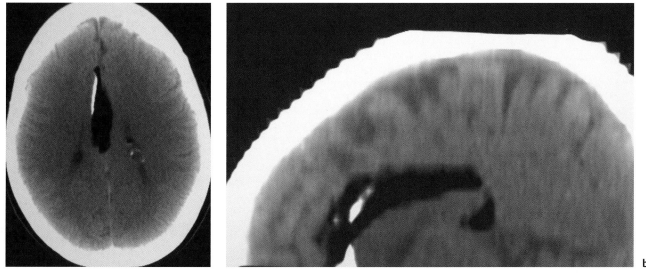

Fig. 1.209a, b **Lipoma corpus callosum.** Axial (**a**) and sagittal (**b**) images show a lipoma with low attenuation as well as calcifications at the anterior portion of the corpus callosum.

Table 1.10   (Cont.) Intracranial calcifications

Lesions	CT Findings	Comments
Choroid plexus papilloma	Circumscribed and/or lobulated lesions with papillary projections, intermediate attenuation, usually prominent contrast enhancement, with or without calcifications. Locations: atrium of lateral ventricle (children) > fourth ventricle (adults), rarely other locations, such as third ventricle. Associated with hydrocephalus.	Rare intracranial neoplasms, choroid plexus papillomas may rarely disseminate along CSF pathways.
Central neurocytoma	Circumscribed lesion located at the margin of the lateral ventricle or septum pellucidum with intraventricular protrusion, heterogeneous low and intermediate attenuation, with or without calcifications and/or small cysts; heterogeneous contrast enhancement.	Rare tumors that have neuronal differentiation, imaging appearance similar to intraventricular oligodendrogliomas; occur in young adults; benign, slow-growing lesions.
Ganglioglioma/ ganglioneuroma	Circumscribed tumor, usually supratentorial; often temporal or frontal lobes; low to intermediate attenuation; with or without cysts, with or without calcifications, with or without contrast enhancement.	Ganglioglioma (contains glial and neuronal elements), ganglioneuroma (contains only ganglion cells). Uncommon tumors, < 30 y, seizure presentation, slow-growing neoplasms. Gangliocytoma (contains only neuronal elements, dysplastic brain tissue). Favorable prognosis if completely resected.
Craniopharyngioma ▷ *Fig. 1.210a–c*	Circumscribed lobulated lesions; both suprasellar and intrasellar location > suprasellar > intrasellar; variable low, intermediate, and/or high attenuation; with or without nodular or rim contrast enhancement. May contain cysts, lipid components, and calcifications.	Usually histologically benign but locally aggressive lesions arising from squamous epithelial rests along the Rathke cleft; occurs in children (peak range, 5–15 y) and adults (> 40 y), males = females.
Osteoma	Well-circumscribed lesions involving the skull with high attenuation similar to cortical bone; typically show no contrast enhancement.	Benign proliferation of dense bone located in the skull or paranasal sinuses (frontal > ethmoid > maxillary > sphenoid).
Tuberous sclerosis ▷ *Fig. 1.211*	**Cortical/subcortical lesion with variable attenuation:** Calcifications in 50% of older children; contrast enhancement uncommon. **Subependymal hamartomas:** Small nodules located along and projecting into the lateral ventricles; calcifications and contrast enhancement are common.	Cortical and subependymal hamartomas are nonmalignant lesions associated with tuberous sclerosis. Tuberous sclerosis is an autosomal dominant disorder associated with hamartomas in multiple organs.
Giant cell astrocytoma/ tuberous sclerosis ▷ *Fig. 1.212a, b*	Circumscribed lesion located near the foramen of Monro with mixed low to intermediate attenuation, with or without cysts and/or calcifications, with heterogeneous contrast enhancement.	Subependymal hamartoma near the foramen of Monro; occurs in 15% of patients with tuberous sclerosis younger than 20 y; slow-growing lesions that can progressively cause obstruction of CSF flow through the foramen of Monro; long-term survival usual if resected.
Malignant tumors		
Metastatic disease	Circumscribed spheroid lesions in brain; can have various intra-axial locations, often at gray-white matter junctions; usually low to intermediate attenuation; with or without hemorrhage, calcifications, cysts; variable contrast enhancement, often associated with adjacent low attenuation from axonal edema.	Represent ~33% of intracranial tumors, usually from extracranial primary neoplasm in adults older than 40 y. Primary tumor source: lung > breast > GI > GU > melanoma. Metastatic lesions associated with calcifications include osteosarcoma, mucinous adenocarcinoma, and renal cell carcinoma.
Oligodendroglioma ▷ *Fig. 1.213*	Circumscribed lesion with mixed low to intermediate attenuation; sites of clumplike calcification; heterogeneous contrast enhancement; involves white matter and cerebral cortex; can cause chronic erosion of the inner table of the calvarium.	Uncommon slow-growing gliomas with usually mixed histologic patterns (astrocytomas, etc.). Usually seen in adults older than 35 y; 85% supratentorial. If low grade, 75% 5-y survival; higher grade lesions have a worse prognosis.
Ependymoma ▷ *Fig. 1.214a, b*	Circumscribed lobulated supratentorial lesion, often extraventricular; with or without cysts and/or calcifications; low to intermediate attenuation; variable contrast enhancement.	Tumors occur more commonly in children than adults; one third supratentorial, two thirds infratentorial; 45% 5-y survival.

(continues on page 128)

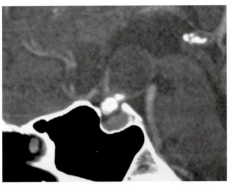
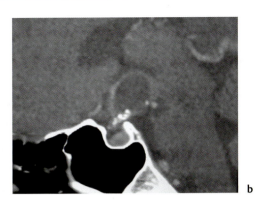

b

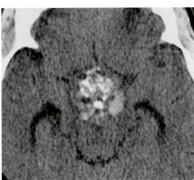

Fig. 1.210a–c   Craniopharyngioma. Sagittal images
(**a, b**) show a complex solid and cystic lesion with
calcifications in the suprasellar cistern. Axial image
(**c**) in another patient shows multiple calcifications within
a craniopharyngioma.

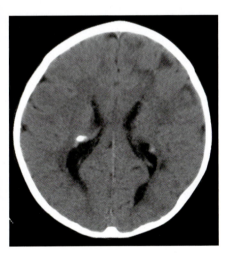

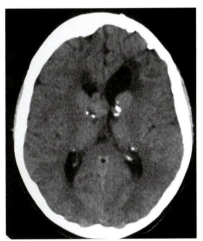

a

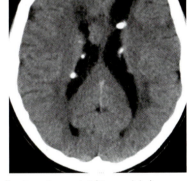

b

Fig. 1.211   Tuberous sclerosis. Axial image
shows multiple ependymal hamartomas with
calcifications.

Fig. 1.212a, b   Tuberous sclerosis, giant cell astrocytoma. Axial image (**a**) shows
a giant cell astrocytoma at the foramen of Monro. Also seen are multiple ependymal
hamartomas with calcifications (**b**).

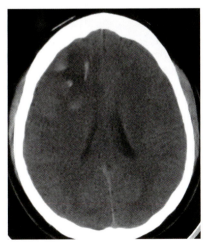

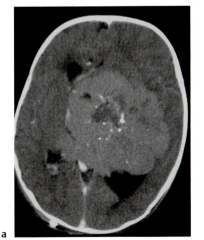

a

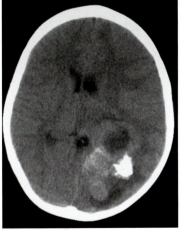

b

Fig. 1.213   Oligodendroglioma. Axial
image shows the tumor in the anterior
right frontal lobe containing calcifications.

Fig. 1.214a, b   Ependymoma. Axial image (**a**) shows a large ependymoma
containing calcifications in a neonate. Axial image (**b**) in another patient shows an
ependymoma involving the left occipital lobe with mixed low, intermediate, and
slightly high attenuation as well as calcifications.

Table 1.10   (Cont.) Intracranial calcifications

Lesions	CT Findings	Comments
Primitive neuroectodermal tumors ▷ *Fig. 1.215*	Circumscribed or invasive lesions, low to intermediate attenuation; variable contrast enhancement, with or without cysts, with or without calcifications; frequent dissemination into the leptomeninges.	Highly malignant tumors that frequently disseminate along CSF pathways.
Atypical teratoid/rhabdoid tumor ▷ *Fig. 1.216a, b*	Circumscribed or poorly defined mass lesions with intermediate attenuation, with or without zones of high attenuation from hemorrhage; usually prominent contrast enhancement with or without heterogeneous pattern.	Rare malignant tumors involving the CNS usually occurring in the first decade. Histologically appear as solid tumors with or without necrotic areas; similar to malignant rhabdoid tumors of the kidney. Associated with a poor prognosis.
Choroid plexus carcinoma ▷ *Fig. 1.217a, b*	Circumscribed and/or lobulated lesions with papillary projections; intermediate attenuation, usually prominent contrast enhancement, with or without calcifications. Locations: atrium of lateral ventricle (children) > fourth ventricle (adults); rarely other locations, such as third ventricle; associated with hydrocephalus.	Rare intracranial neoplasms, choroid plexus carcinomas frequently disseminate along CSF pathways and invade brain tissue. Carcinomas are often larger than papillomas. Carcinomas may have heterogeneous mixed attenuation, with or without hemorrhage, with or without calcifications, with or without brain invasion.
Hemangiopericytoma	Extra-axial mass lesions, often well circumscribed, intermediate attenuation, prominent contrast enhancement (may resemble meningiomas), with or without associated erosive bone changes, with or without calcifications.	Rare neoplasms in young adults (men > women) sometimes referred to as angioblastic meningioma or meningeal hemangiopericytoma; arise from vascular cells and pericytes; frequency of metastases > meningiomas.
Malignant meningioma	Extra-axial dural-based lesions, supratentorial > infratentorial; heterogeneous mixed attenuation, usually prominent heterogeneous contrast enhancement, irregular margins with invasion of adjacent brain, with or without calcifications, with or without hyperostosis of adjacent bone.	Extra-axial tumor that typically occurs in adults older than 40 y, women > men; occasionally occurs in children. Multiple meningiomas seen with neurofibromatosis type 2; can result in compression of adjacent brain parenchyma, encasement of arteries, and compression of dural venous sinuses. Malignant meningiomas often invade adjacent tissues.
Teratoma ▷ *Fig. 1.218a, b*	Circumscribed lesions; pineal region > suprasellar region > third ventricle; variable low, intermediate, and/or high attenuation; with or without contrast enhancement. May contain calcifications, as well as fatty components, which can cause chemical meningitis if ruptured.	Second most common type of germ cell tumor; occurs in children, males > females; benign or malignant types; composed of derivatives of ectoderm, mesoderm, and/or endoderm.

(continues on page 130)

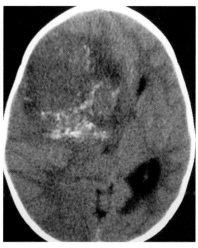 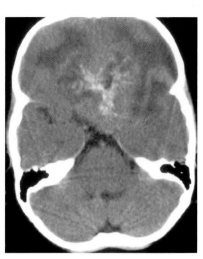 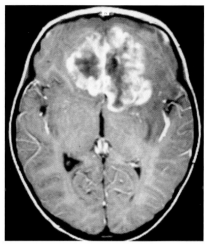

Fig. 1.215   Primitive neuroectodermal tumor. Axial image shows a large tumor in the right frontal lobe with multiple calcifications.

Fig. 1.216a, b   Atypical teratoid/rhabdoid tumor. Axial CT image (**a**) shows a large tumor involving the anterior frontal lobes and corpus callosum. The tumor shows heterogeneous contrast enhancement on the axial T1-weighted MRI (**b**).

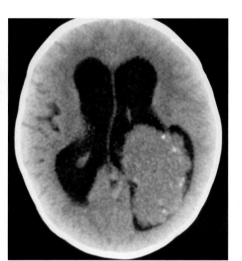 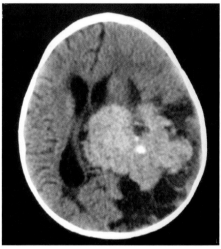

Fig. 1.217a, b   Choroid plexus carcinoma. Axial image (**a**) shows a large intraventricular tumor with high attenuation and calcifications. Axial image (**b**) in another patient shows the tumor invading the adjacent brain tissue, where there is also axonal edema.

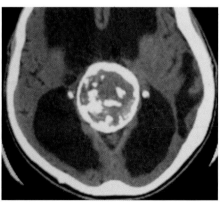 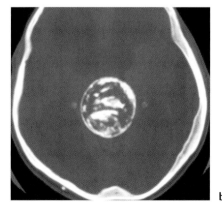

Fig. 1.218a, b   Teratoma. Axial images show dense calcifications in a teratoma involving the pineal gland.

Table 1.10   (Cont.) Intracranial calcifications

Lesions	CT Findings	Comments
Pineal gland tumors ▷ *Fig. 1.219a, b*	Tumors often have intermediate attenuation to intermediate to slightly high attenuation, with contrast enhancement, with or without central and/or peripheral calcifications. Malignant tumors are often larger than benign pineal lesions (pineocytoma), as well as heterogeneous attenuation and contrast enhancement pattern. With or without leptomeningeal tumor.	Pineal gland tumors account for 8% of intracranial tumors in children and 1% of tumors in adults; 40% of tumors are germinomas, followed by pineoblastomas and pineocytomas, teratomas, choriocarcinomas, endodermal sinus tumors, astrocytomas, and metastatic tumors.
Chordoma	Well-circumscribed, lobulated lesions destroying bone along the dorsal surface of the clivus, vertebral bodies, or sacrum. **CT:** Low to intermediate attenuation, with or without calcifications from destroyed bone carried away by tumor, with contrast enhancement. **MRI:** Lesions have low to intermediate signal on T1-weighted images, high signal on T2-weighted images, with gadolinium enhancement (usually heterogeneous); locally invasive associated with bone erosion/destruction, encasement of vessels and nerves; skull base/clivus common location, usually in the midline.	Rare, slow-growing, destructive tumors derived from notochordal remnants; detailed anatomical display of extension of chordomas by CT and MRI is important for planning of surgical approaches.
Chondrosarcoma ▷ *Fig. 1.220*	Lobulated lesions, low to intermediate attenuation, with or without chondroid matrix mineralization, with contrast enhancement (usually heterogeneous); locally invasive associated with bone erosion/destruction, encasement of vessels and nerves, skull base petrooccipital synchondrosis common location, usually off midline.	Rare, slow-growing, malignant cartilaginous tumors; detailed anatomical display of extension of chondrosarcomas by CT and MRI is important for planning of surgical approaches.
Osteosarcoma ▷ *Fig. 1.221*	Destructive lesions involving the skull base, low to intermediate attenuation, usually with matrix mineralization/ossification, with contrast enhancement (usually heterogeneous).	Rare lesions involving the endochondral bone-forming portions of the skull base or membranous-bone forming calcarium; more common than chondrosarcomas and Ewing sarcoma; locally invasive, high metastatic potential. Occurs in children as primary tumors and adults (associated with Paget disease, irradiated bone, chronic osteomyelitis, osteoblastoma, giant cell tumor, and fibrous dysplasia).
Metabolic/idiopathic		
Hypothyroidism	Punctate calcifications in the caudate nuclei, thalami, putamina, and/or globus pallidi bilaterally.	Disorder from insufficient amount of thyroid hormone that can be congenital; associated with developmental abnormalities (cretinism) or from loss of thyroid tissue (autoimmune diseases that produce antithyroid antibodies or antibodies that block the thyroid-stimulating hormone [TSH] receptor, surgery, or radioiodine ablation for treatment of Graves disease).
Hyperparathyroidism	Punctate calcifications in the caudate nuclei, thalami, putamina, and/or globus pallidi bilaterally.	Primary type results from excess production of parathyroid hormone (PTH) from hyperplasia or adenomas involving the parathyroid gland(s). PTH regulates calcium and phosphate blood levels. Excessive PTH secretion results in hypercalcemia and hypophosphatemia. Secondary hyperparathyroidism occurs with elevated PTH levels in response to low calcium levels from disorders such as chronic renal disease and vitamin D deficiency. Calcium levels in blood are low or normal, and phosphate levels are usually elevated.
Hypoparathyroidism	Punctate calcifications in the caudate nuclei, thalami, putamina, and/or globus pallidi bilaterally.	Hypoparathyroidism occurs when there is a deficiency in formation of PTH, which regulates metabolism of calcium, phosphorus, and vitamin D. Deficiency of PTH from the parathyroid glands results in decreased blood calcium levels and elevated blood phosphorus levels. Can result from injury to the parathyroid glands during head and neck surgery or radioactive iodine treatment for hyperthyroidism. DiGeorge syndrome of hypoparathyroidism occurs because of congenital absence of the parathyroid glands. Familial hypoparathyroidism occurs with other endocrine diseases, such as adrenal insufficiency, in a syndrome called type I polyglandular autoimmune syndrome.

(continues on page 132)

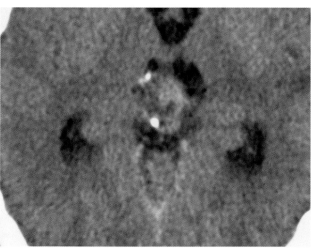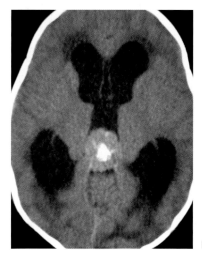

b

Fig. 1.219a, b   Pineal gland tumors. Axial images show a germinoma with several calcifications (**a**) and a pineoblastoma containing calcifications (**b**).

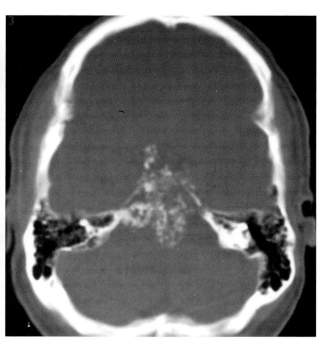

Fig. 1.220   Chondrosarcoma. Axial image shows the chondrosarcoma along the endocranial surface of the clivus containing multiple ring and arc chondroid calcifications. The tumor erodes the clivus and extends into the sphenoid sinus.

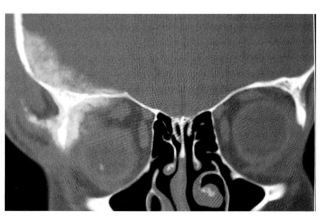

Fig. 1.221   Osteosarcoma. Coronal image shows the osteosarcoma involving the right frontal bone with malignant ossified tumor matrix.

Table 1.10   (Cont.) Intracranial calcifications

Lesions	CT Findings	Comments
Pseudohypoparathyroidism	Punctate calcifications in the caudate nuclei, thalami, putamina, and/or globus pallidi bilaterally	Pseudohypoparathyroidism is a rare syndrome in which there is resistance to the effects of PTH in the body resulting in low blood calcium levels and high blood phosphate levels. Associated with dysfunctional G proteins: G_s-a subunit, mutation in *GNAS1* gene. PTH levels are often elevated. Type Ia is autosomal dominant and results in short stature, round face, and short fourth and fifth metacarpal bones; is also called Albright hereditary osteodystrophy. Associated with abnormal *GNAS1* gene. Type Ib involves resistance to PTH only in the kidneys and is associated with a methylation defect; lacks the physical features of type I. Type II is very similar to type I, but the events that take place in the kidneys are different. Type II pseudohypoparathyroidism is associated with low blood calcium and high blood phosphate levels, although there is absence of the physical characteristics associated with type I.
Pseudo-pseudohypoparathyroidism (pseudo-PHP)	Punctate calcifications in the caudate nuclei, thalami, putamina, and/or globus pallidi bilaterally	Inherited disorder with symptoms and phenotypic appearance of pseudohypoparathyroidism type 1. Caused by a defect on the corresponding maternal chromosome as pseudo-PHP 1. Pseudo-PHP presents only with the skeletal defects of PHP, although patients have normal blood levels of calcium, phosphate, and PTH.
MELAS and MERRF syndromes	**CT:** Symmetric zones of low attenuation in the basal ganglia, along with cerebral infarction that is not limited to one vascular distribution. With or without dystrophic calcifications in basal ganglia. **MRI:** High T2 signal in basal ganglia usually symmetric; high T2 signal in cerebral and cerebellar cortex and subcortical white matter not corresponding to a specific large arterial vascular territory. Signal abnormalities may resolve and reappear.	MELAS is a maternally inherited disease affecting transfer RNA in mitochondria. MERRF is a mitochondrial encephalopathy associated with muscle weakness and myoclonic epilepsy, short stature, ophthalmoplegia, and cardiac disease.
Fahr disease ▷ *Fig. 1.222a–d*	Intra-axial calcifications occur in the basal ganglia, dentate nuclei, and cerebral white matter.	Fahr disease, also known as familial cerebrovascular ferrocalcinosis, is a group of disorders with deposition of calcification in the brain.
Cockayne syndrome ▷ *Fig. 1.223a–c*	Calcifications occur in the basal ganglia and dentate nuclei. Cerebral and cerebellar atrophy is also seen.	Autosomal recessive disease in children with cutaneous photosensitivity, progressive neurologic impairment, optic atrophy, cataracts, dwarfism, and thoracic kyphosis.
Neuronal ceroid lipofuscinosis	Progressive cerebral and cerebellar atrophy with or without calcifications in the brain.	Inherited progressive neurodegenerative disorders consisting of multiple types: infantile, late infantile, juvenile (Batten disease), early juvenile, adult dominant, adult recessive, and progressive epilepsy with mental retardation. The different types have similar clinical features of visual dysfunction, seizures, impairment of speech and motor function, and progressive dementia.

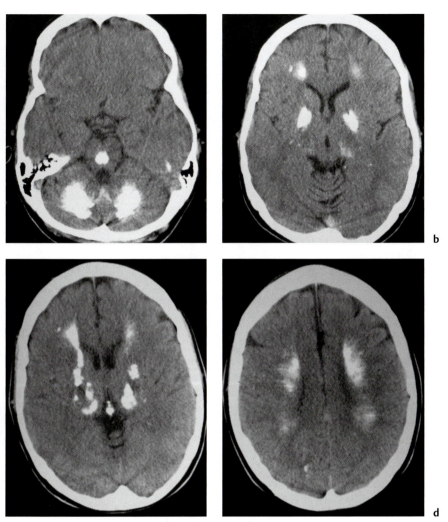

Fig. 1.222a–d   Fahr disease. Axial images show prominent calcifications in the (**a**) brainstem, (**b**) cerebellum, (**c**) basal ganglia, (**d**) thalami, and cerebral white matter.

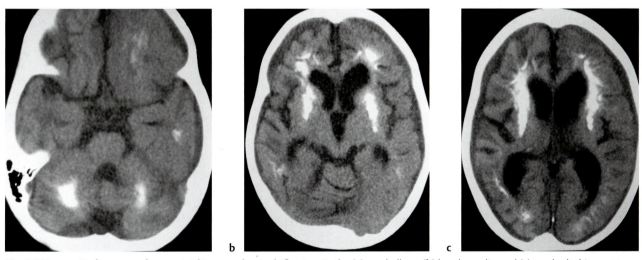

Fig. 1.223a–c   Cockayne syndrome. Axial images show calcifications in the (**a**) cerebellum, (**b**) basal ganglia, and (**c**) cerebral white matter.

2 Ventricles and Cisterns

Steven P. Meyers

The embryologic development of the ventricles begins with three expansions (primary vesicles) of the rostral neural tube (weeks 4–5 of gestation), which are referred to as the forebrain (prosencephalon), midbrain (mesencephalon), and hindbrain (rhombencephalon). The primary vesicles subsequently expand and bend with localized constrictions to form the five secondary vesicles (approximately week 7 of gestation). The forebrain gives rise to the telencephalon (eventual cerebral hemispheres and lateral ventricles) and diencephalon (thalamus, hypothalamus, and third ventricle). The midbrain eventually forms the secondary vesicle, also referred to as the mesencephalon, which eventually forms the tectum, midbrain portion of the brainstem, and cerebral aqueduct. The hindbrain gives rise to the metencephalon (eventual pons, cerebellum, and upper portion of the fourth ventricle) and myelencephalon (eventual medulla and lower portion of the fourth ventricle).

Abnormalities in development of the cerebral vesicles result in congenital anomalies, such as the holoprosencephalies, lissencephaly/pachygyria, and Dandy-Walker malformations. Abnormalities in the closure of the caudal neural tube with altered internal pressure dynamics have been proposed as a mechanism in the malformation of the ventricles and other anomalies associated with Chiari II malformations.

The normal lateral ventricles are bilateral elongated C-shaped structures, each containing a contiguous frontal horn, body, atrium (trigone), occipital horn, and temporal horn. The lateral ventricles are often symmetric, but varying degrees of asymmetry are not uncommon. The anterior portions of the lateral ventricles are normally separated by the septum pellucidum.

The third ventricle appears as a slitlike compartment filled with cerebrospinal fluid (CSF) between the thalami. The inferior border of the third ventricle is the hypothalamus, and the upper border is the choroid tela (fusion of the pia and ependymal lining of ventricle) and choroid plexus. The anterior border is the lamina terminalis and anterior commissure. The posterior border includes the pineal gland and recess, as well as the posterior commissure. The third ventricle communicates with the lateral ventricles via the foramina of Monro located anterolaterally. The third ventricle communicates with the fourth via the cerebral aqueduct posteroinferiorly.

The fourth ventricle has a pyramidal shape in the sagittal plane and an inverted C shape/inverted kidney bean shape in the axial plane. The fourth ventricle is located dorsal to the pons with its roof comprised of the cerebellar vermis. It communicates with the cerebral aqueduct at its upper margin, the cisterna magna of the subarachnoid space, via the foramen of Magendie and the paired foramina of Luschka.

CSF fills the ventricles and is produced by the choroid plexus located within the lateral, third, and fourth ventricles, as well as the foramina of Luschka and Magendie. The choroid plexus typically enhances after intravenous contrast administration because of its lack of a blood–brain barrier. CSF from the ventricles communicates with the subarachnoid space adjacent to the brain and spinal cord through the foramina of Luschka and Magendie. The primary function of CSF is to protect the brain and spinal cord from trauma and rapid changes in venous pressure. It represents ~10% of the intracranial and intraspinal spaces. A total of ~150 mL of CSF is present within the ventricles and intracranial and spinal subarachnoid spaces. The choroid plexus forms 500 mL of CSF daily, allowing turnover four or five times daily. More than 90% of the CSF is normally resorbed by arachnoid villi or granulations (grouping of villi) that penetrate the dura, with resultant emptying of fluid into the intracranial venous sinuses. The remaining small amount of fluid is resorbed through the ependymal linings of the ventricles.

Obstruction of outflow of CSF from the ventricles results in dilation of the ventricles proximal to the site of blockage. The obstruction can result from congenital malformations (e.g., Chiari II), neoplasms/other intracranial mass lesions (e.g., colloid cyst), inflammatory lesions, hemorrhage, and brain edema/swelling (ischemia and trauma). In addition to ventricular dilation, transependymal leakage of fluid can be seen with computed tomography (CT). Obstructive or noncommunicating hydrocephalus can result, if untreated, in abnormal increased intracranial pressure, intracranial herniation, and death.

Communicating hydrocephalus occurs when there is overproduction of CSF (choroid plexus papilloma/carcinoma), impaired resorption of CSF through the arachnoid villi, and/or obstruction of CSF flow through the cisterns and sulci. With communicating hydrocephalus, the ventricles are disproportionately more prominent than the sulci. Subependymal edema may be seen with CT due to the impaired resorption of CSF. Patients with communicating hydrocephalus (normal pressure hydrocephalus) may also have clinical features of gait disturbance, incontinence, and/or progressive impairment of mental function.

Ventricular enlargement can also result from cerebral infarction, cerebral atrophy, or various neurodegenerative diseases. With these disorders, sulcal prominence is usually evident with CT.

Sulci normally vary in size, although typically they increase in size with aging. Sulcal enlargement can also be seen in a child with dehydration. Congenital malformations such as lissencephaly and pachygyria result in the absence of sulci or few shallow sulci, respectively. Sulci may be asymmetrically prominent at sites of prior cerebral or cerebellar infarction, prior intra-axial hemorrhage, contusion, inflammation, and radiation injury.

The basal cisterns represent the subarachnoid compartment adjacent to the pial margins of the inferior portions of the brain and brainstem. The cisterns are named according to the adjacent neural structures. The larger of the cisterns include the cisterna magna (dorsal and inferior to the cerebellar vermis) and superior cerebellar cistern.

Approximately 10% of neoplasms in the central nervous system extend into or are completely within the ventricles. The age of the patient and the location of the tumor influence the differential diagnosis of lesions.

Common Lesions in the Third Ventricle

Table 2.1   Lateral ventricles: common mass lesions

Age	Foramen of Monro	Trigone and Atrium	Lateral Ventricle, Body
Adult	Colloid cyst Cysticercosis	Meningioma Choroid plexus cyst Neuroepithelial cyst Central neurocytoma Metastasis Neuroepithelial cyst Cysticercosis	Ependymoma Glioblastoma Metastasis Central neurocytoma Cysticercosis
Child (> 5 y)	Giant cell astrocytoma Pilocytic astrocytoma Cysticercosis	Ependymoma Choroid plexus cyst Choroid plexus papilloma Choroid plexus carcinoma Hamartoma/tuberous sclerosis Gray matter heterotopia Cysticercosis	Ependymoma Pilocytic astrocytoma Hamartoma/tuberous sclerosis Gray matter heterotopia Cysticercosis
Child (< 5 y)	Giant cell astrocytoma Pilocytic astrocytoma Cysticercosis	Choroid plexus papilloma Choroid plexus carcinoma Cysticercosis	Choroid plexus papilloma Choroid plexus carcinoma Primitive neuroectodermal tumor (PNET) Teratoma Cysticercosis

Table 2.2   Common lesions in the third ventricle

Age	Foramen of Monro	Anterior Recess	Third Ventricle, Body	Third Ventricle, Posterior
Adult	Colloid cyst Metastases Cysticercosis	Pituitary adenoma Meningioma Metastasis Aneurysm Craniopharyngioma Lymphoma Cysticercosis	Glioma Cysticercosis	Pineal tumor Glioma Vascular malformation Cysticercosis
Child	Giant cell astrocytoma Pilocytic astrocytoma Cysticercosis	Germ cell tumor Langerhans cell histiocytosis Glioma Craniopharyngioma Cysticercosis	Choroid plexus papilloma Glioma Cysticercosis	Pineal tumor Glioma Vascular malformation Cysticercosis

Table 2.3   Lesions in the fourth ventricle

Lesions	CT Findings	Comments
Child		
Astrocytoma	**Low-grade astrocytoma:** Focal or diffuse mass lesion usually located in the cerebellar white matter or brainstem with low to intermediate attenuation, with or without mild contrast enhancement. Minimal associated mass effect. May extend into ventricles.	Often occurs in children and adults (age 20–40 y). Tumors comprised of well-differentiated astrocytes. Association with neurofibromatosis type 1; 10-y survival common; may become malignant.
	Juvenile pilocytic astrocytoma subtype: Solid/cystic focal lesion with low to intermediate attenuation, usually with prominent contrast enhancement. Lesions located in the cerebellum and brainstem. May extend into ventricles.	Common in children; usually favorable prognosis if totally resected.
	Gliomatosis cerebri: Infiltrative lesion with poorly defined margins with mass effect located in the white matter, with low to intermediate attenuation; usually no contrast enhancement until late in disease.	Diffusely infiltrating astrocytoma with relative preservation of underlying brain architecture. Imaging appearance may be more prognostic than histologic grade; ~2-y survival.
	Anaplastic astrocytoma: Often irregularly marginated lesion located in white matter with low to intermediate attenuation, with or without contrast enhancement. May extend into ventricles ▷ *Fig. 2.1*	Intermediate between low-grade astrocytoma and glioblastoma multiforme; ~2-y survival.
Medulloblastoma (primitive neuroectodermal tumor of the cerebellum) ▷ *Fig. 2.2*	Circumscribed or invasive lesions; low to intermediate and/or slightly high attenuation; variable contrast enhancement; frequent dissemination into the leptomeninges and/or ventricles.	Highly malignant tumors that frequently disseminate along CSF pathways.
Ependymoma ▷ *Fig. 2.3*	Circumscribed spheroid or lobulated infratentorial lesion, usually in the fourth ventricle, with or without cysts and/or calcifications; low to intermediate attenuation; variable contrast enhancement; with or without extension through the foramina of Luschka and Magendie.	Occurs more commonly in children than adults; two thirds infratentorial, one third supratentorial.
Metastatic tumor	Single or multiple well-circumscribed or poorly defined lesions involving the brain stem and cerebellum, skull, dura, leptomeninges, ventricles, choroid plexus, or pituitary gland; low to intermediate attenuation, usually with contrast enhancement, with or without bone destruction, with or without compression of neural tissue or vessels. Leptomeningeal tumor-drop metastasis often best seen on postcontrast images.	May have variable destructive or infiltrative changes involving single or multiple sites of involvement.
Hemangioblastoma ▷ *Fig. 2.4*	Circumscribed tumors usually located in the cerebellum and/or brainstem; small contrast-enhancing nodule with or without cyst, or larger lesion with prominent heterogeneous enhancement with or without vessels within lesion or at the periphery; intermediate attenuation; occasionally lesions have evidence of recent or remote hemorrhage. May extend into ventricles.	Multiple lesions occur in adolescents with von Hippel-Lindau disease.

(continues on page 138)

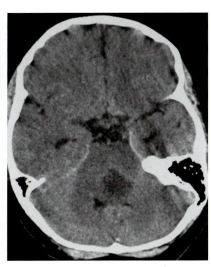

Fig. 2.1   Astrocytoma. Axial image shows the tumor within the pons.

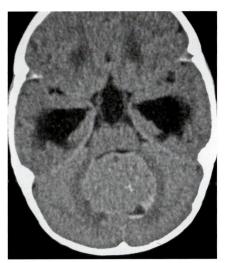

Fig. 2.2   Medulloblastoma. Axial image shows the tumor involving the vermis with extension into the fourth ventricle, resulting in obstructive hydrocephalus. The tumor has slightly high attenuation.

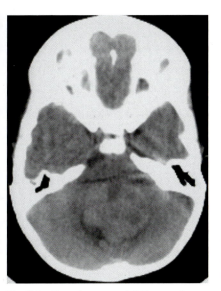

Fig. 2.3   Ependymoma. Axial image shows a tumor in the fourth ventricle that has mostly intermediate attenuation, as well as a small zone with low attenuation.

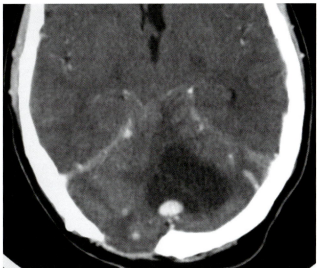

Fig. 2.4   Hemangioblastoma, von Hippel-Lindau disease. Axial postcontrast image shows multiple enhancing nodular hemangioblastomas in the cerebellum, the largest of which is associated with a tumoral cyst.

Table 2.3   (Cont.) Lesions in the fourth ventricle

Lesions	CT Findings	Comments
Choroid plexus papilloma or carcinoma ▷ *Fig. 2.5*	Circumscribed and/or lobulated lesions with papillary projections, intermediate attenuation, usually prominent contrast enhancement, with or without calcifications. Locations: atrium of lateral ventricle (children) > fourth ventricle (adults), rarely other locations such as third ventricle; associated with hydrocephalus.	Rare intracranial neoplasms, Magnetic resonance imaging (MRI) features of choroid plexus carcinoma and papilloma overlap; both histologic types can disseminate along CSF pathways and invade brain tissue.

Adult		
Metastatic tumor	Single or multiple well-circumscribed or poorly defined lesions involving the skull, dura, leptomeninges, brainstem, cerebellum, ventricles, choroid plexus, or pituitary gland; low to intermediate attenuation, usually with contrast enhancement, with or without bone destruction, with or without compression of neural tissue or vessels. Leptomeningeal tumor often best seen on postcontrast images.	May have variable destructive or infiltrative changes involving single or multiple sites of involvement.
Hemangioblastoma	Circumscribed tumors usually located in the cerebellum and/or brainstem; small contrast-enhancing nodule with or without cyst, or larger lesion with prominent heterogeneous enhancement with or without vessels within lesion or at the periphery; occasionally lesions have evidence of recent or remote hemorrhage; may extend into ventricle.	Occurs in adolescents, young and middle-aged adults. Lesions are typically multiple in patients with von Hippel-Lindau disease.
Astrocytoma	**Low-grade astrocytoma:** Focal or diffuse mass lesion usually located in the cerebellum or brainstem with low to intermediate attenuation, with or without mild contrast enhancement. Minimal associated mass effect. May extend into ventricles. **Anaplastic astrocytoma:** Often irregularly marginated lesion located in the cerebellum or brainstem with low to intermediate attenuation, with or without contrast enhancement. May extend into ventricles.	Often occurs in children and adults (age 20–40 y). Tumors comprised of well-differentiated astrocytes. Association with neurofibromatosis type 1; 10-y survival common; may become malignant. Intermediate between low grade astrocytoma and glioblastoma multiforme; ~2-y survival.
Ependymoma	Circumscribed spheroid or lobulated infratentorial lesion, usually in the fourth ventricle, with or without cysts and/or calcifications; low to intermediate attenuation, variable contrast enhancement; with or without extension through the foramina of Luschka and Magendie.	Occurs more commonly in children than adults; two thirds infratentorial, one third supratentorial.
Choroid plexus papilloma or carcinoma ▷ *Fig. 2.6a, b*	Circumscribed and/or lobulated lesions with papillary projections, intermediate attenuation, usually prominent contrast enhancement, with or without calcifications. Locations: atrium of lateral ventricle (children) > fourth ventricle (adults), rarely other locations such as third ventricle; associated with hydrocephalus.	Rare intracranial neoplasms; CT and MRI features of choroid plexus carcinoma and papilloma overlap; both histologic types can disseminate along CSF pathways and invade brain tissue.
Epidermoid	Well-circumscribed spheroid or multilobulated, extra-axial ectodermal inclusion cystic lesions with low to intermediate attenuation, no contrast enhancement, with or without bone erosion/destruction. Often insinuate along CSF pathways; chronic deformation of adjacent neural tissue (brainstem, brain parenchyma). Commonly located in posterior cranial fossa (cerebellopontine angle cistern, fourth ventricle) > parasellar/middle cranial fossa.	Nonneoplastic congenital or acquired extra-axial off-midline lesions filled with desquamated cells and keratinaceous debris; usually mild mass effect on adjacent brain; infratentorial > supratentorial locations. Adults: men = women; with or without related clinical symptoms.
Cysticercosis	Single or multiple cystic lesions in the brain, meninges, or ventricles. **Acute/subacute phase:** Low to intermediate attenuation, rim with or without nodular pattern of contrast enhancement, with or without peripheral edema. **Chronic phase:** Calcified granulomas.	Caused by ingestion of ova (*Taenia solium*) in contaminated food (undercooked pork); involves meninges > brain parenchyma > ventricles.

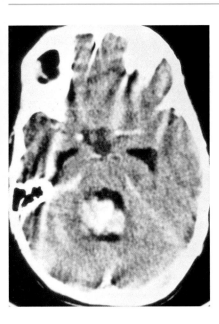

Fig. 2.5   Choroid plexus carcinoma. Postcontrast image shows an enhancing tumor in the fourth ventricle.

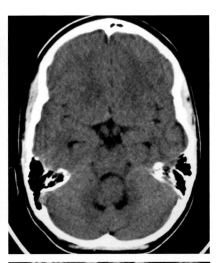

Fig. 2.6a, b   Choroid plexus papilloma. Axial CT image (**a**) reveals a lesion in the fourth ventricle that shows contrast enhancement on axial T1-weighted magnetic resonance imaging (**b**).

Table 2.4 Excessively small ventricles

Lesions	CT Findings	Comments
Normal variant	Small ventricles with normal appearance of brain parenchyma and presence of CSF in subarachnoid spaces and cisterns.	Normal variation.
Postshunt/overshunting	Small, slitlike ventricles (with or without shunt tube present).	Small ventricular size can result from acute or chronic overdrainage of ventricles with shunts.
Increased intracranial pressure	Small ventricles with effacement of subarachnoid spaces, with or without decreased attenuation in brain parenchyma; cerebral edema.	Ventricular size usually does not correlate well with intracranial pressure.
Pseudotumor cerebri	Normal shape but small ventricles, with or without mild prominence of intracranial subarachnoid spaces, with or without prominence of fluid in optic nerve sheath complex.	CT with contrast provides a role in excluding intracranial tumors involving the brain or leptomeninges.

Table 2.5 Dilated ventricles

Lesions	CT Findings	Comments
Normal variant	Mild ventricular enlargement can occur without associated cerebral or cerebellar abnormality.	Ventricular size usually increases with age, most pronounced after age 60 y.
Aqueductal stenosis	Dilation of lateral and third ventricles with normal-sized fourth ventricle, with or without dilation of only the upper portion of cerebral aqueduct and not the lower portion, with or without discrete or poorly defined lesion in midbrain.	Aqueductal stenosis can result from a small lesion/neoplasm in the midbrain, debris or adhesions from hemorrhage, or inflammatory diseases. CT and MRI can exclude other lesions, causing obstruction of CSF flow through the aqueduct, such as lesions in the posterior third ventricle or posterior cranial fossa.
Chiari I malformation	Cerebellar tonsils extend > 5 mm below the foramen magnum in adults, 6 mm in children younger than 10 y. Syringohydromyelia in 20% to 40%, hydrocephalus in 25%. Basilar impression in 25%. Less common association: Klippel-Feil syndrome; atlanto-occipital assimilation.	Cerebellar tonsillar ectopia. Most common anomaly of central nervous system (CNS). Not associated with myelomeningocele.
Chiari II malformation (Arnold-Chiari malformation) ▷ Fig. 2.7a, b	Small posterior cranial fossa with gaping foramen magnum through which there is an inferiorly positioned vermis associated with a cervicomedullary kink. Beaked dorsal margin of the tectal plate. Myelomeningoceles in nearly all patients. Hydrocephalus and syringomyelia common. Dilated lateral ventricles posteriorly (colpocephaly).	Complex anomaly involving the cerebrum, cerebellum, brainstem, spinal cord, ventricles, skull, and dura. Failure of fetal neural tube to develop properly, resulting in altered development affecting multiple sites of the CNS.
Chiari III malformation	Features of Chiari II plus lower occipital or high cervical encephalocele.	Rare anomaly associated with high mortality.
Dandy-Walker malformation ▷ Fig. 2.8	Vermian aplasia or severe hypoplasia, communication of fourth ventricle with retrocerebellar cyst, enlarged posterior fossa, high position of tentorium, and transverse venous sinuses. Hydrocephalus common. Associated with other anomalies, such as dysgenesis of the corpus callosum, gray matter heterotopia, schizencephaly, holoprosencephaly, and cephaloceles.	Abnormal formation of the roof of the fourth ventricle with absent or near incomplete formation of the cerebellar vermis.
Dandy-Walker variant	Mild vermian hypoplasia with communication of the posteroinferior portion of the fourth ventricle with the cisterna magna. No associated enlargement of the posterior cranial fossa.	Occasionally associated with hydrocephalus, dysgenesis of the corpus callosum, gray matter heterotopia, and other anomalies.
Colpocephaly ▷ Fig. 2.9	Asymmetric enlargement of the occipital horns of the lateral ventricles.	Associated with Chiari II malformations and dysgenesis of the corpus callosum.

(continues on page 142)

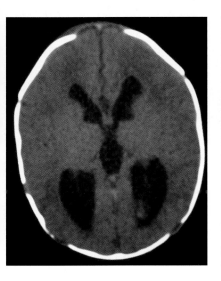 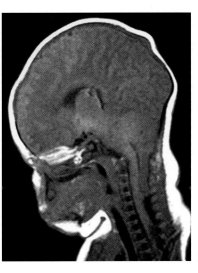

Fig. 2.7a, b   Chiari II malformation. Axial (**a**) and sagittal (**b**) images show enlarged ventricles from hydrocephalus-related herniation of the cerebellum through the foramen magnum related to the Chiari II malformation.

b

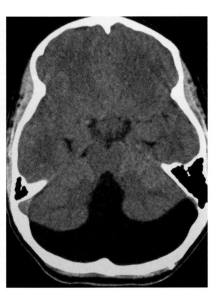

Fig. 2.8   Dandy-Walker malformation. Axial image shows the absence of the cerebellar vermis, enlarged unroofed fourth ventricle, and hypoplasia of the cerebellar hemispheres.

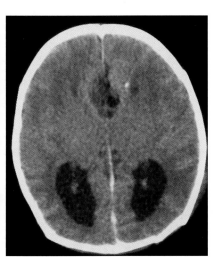

Fig. 2.9   Colpocephaly. Axial image in a young child with dysgenesis of the corpus callosum and enlarged occipital horns of the lateral ventricles.

Table 2.5   (Cont.) Dilated ventricles

Lesions	CT Findings	Comments
Neoplasms (causing obstructive hydrocephalus)		
Metastatic tumor	Single or multiple well-circumscribed or poorly defined lesions involving the brain, skull, dura, leptomeninges, ventricles, choroid plexus, or pituitary gland; low to intermediate attenuation; usually with contrast enhancement, with or without bone destruction, with or without compression of neural tissue or vessels. Leptomeningeal tumor often best seen on postcontrast images.	Metastatic tumor may have variable destructive or infiltrative changes involving single or multiple sites of involvement.
Intra-axial primary tumors		
Astrocytoma	**Low-grade astrocytoma:** Focal or diffuse mass lesion usually located in the cerebellar white matter or brainstem with low to intermediate attenuation, with or without mild contrast enhancement. Minimal associated mass effect.	Often occurs in children and adults (age 20–40 y). Tumors comprised of well-differentiated astrocytes. Association with neurofibromatosis type 1; 10-y survival; may become malignant.
	Juvenile pilocytic astrocytoma-subtype: Solid/cystic focal lesion with low to intermediate attenuation, usually with prominent contrast enhancement. Lesions located in cerebellum and brainstem.	Common in children; usually favorable prognosis if totally resected.
	Gliomatosis cerebri: Infiltrative lesion with poorly defined margins with mass effect located in the white matter, with low to intermediate attenuation; usually no contrast enhancement until late in disease.	Diffusely infiltrating astrocytoma with relative preservation of underlying brain architecture. Imaging appearance may be more prognostic than histologic grade; ~2-y survival.
	Anaplastic astrocytoma: Often irregularly marginated lesion located in the white matter with low to intermediate attenuation, with or without contrast enhancement.	Intermediate between low-grade astrocytoma and glioblastoma multiforme; ~2-y survival.
Giant cell astrocytoma (tuberous sclerosis)	Circumscribed lesion located near the foramen of Monro with mixed low to intermediate attenuation, with or without cysts and/or calcifications, with heterogeneous contrast enhancement.	Subependymal hamartoma near the foramen of Monro; occurs in 15% of patients with tuberous sclerosis younger than 20 y; slow-growing lesions can progressively cause obstruction of CSF flow through the foramen of Monro; long-term survival usual if resected.
Medulloblastoma (primitive neuroectodermal tumor of the cerebellum) ▷ *Fig. 2.10*	Circumscribed or invasive lesions, low to intermediate and/or slightly high; variable contrast enhancement; frequent dissemination into the leptomeninges.	Highly malignant tumors that frequently disseminate along CSF pathways.
Ependymoma	Circumscribed spheroid or lobulated infratentorial lesion, usually in the fourth ventricle, with or without cysts and/or calcifications; low to intermediate attenuation, variable contrast enhancement, with or without extension through the foramina of Luschka and Magendie.	Occurs more commonly in children than adults; two thirds infratentorial, one third supratentorial.
Hemangioblastoma	Circumscribed tumors usually located in the cerebellum and/or brainstem; small contrast-enhancing nodule with or without cyst, or larger lesion with prominent heterogeneous enhancement with or without vessels within lesion or at the periphery; occasionally lesions have evidence of recent or remote hemorrhage.	Multiple lesions occur in adolescents with von Hippel-Lindau disease.
Intraventricular tumors		
Choroid plexus carcinoma or papilloma ▷ *Fig. 2.11a, b* ▷ *Fig. 2.12*	Circumscribed and/or lobulated lesions with papillary projections, intermediate attenuation, usually prominent contrast enhancement, with or without calcifications. Locations: atrium of lateral ventricle (children) > fourth ventricle (adults), rarely other locations such as third ventricle; associated with hydrocephalus.	Rare intracranial neoplasms, CT and MRI features of choroid plexus carcinoma and papilloma overlap; both histologic types can disseminate along CSF pathways and invade brain tissue.

(continues on page 144)

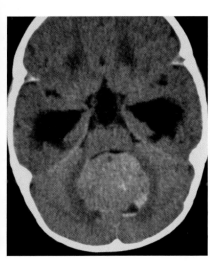

Fig. 2.10   Medulloblastoma. Axial image shows the tumor extending from the vermis into the fourth ventricle, resulting in hydrocephalus.

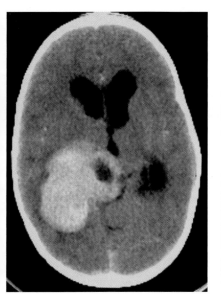 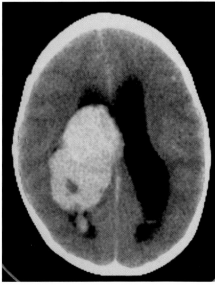

b

Fig. 2.11a, b   Choroid plexus carcinoma. Axial postcontrast images show a large enhancing tumor in the right lateral ventricle associated with ventricular dilation.

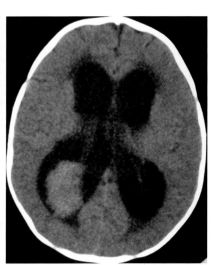

Fig. 2.12   Choroid plexus papilloma. Axial image in a 3-year-old boy shows the tumor in the right lateral ventricle associated with ventricular dilation from overproduction of cerebrospinal fluid (CSF) by the tumor.

Table 2.5 (Cont.) Dilated ventricles

Lesions	CT Findings	Comments
Meningioma	Well-circumscribed intraventricular lesions; intermediate attenuation; usually prominent contrast enhancement, with or without calcifications.	Usually benign neoplasms; typically occurs in adults (> 40 y), women > men. Multiple meningiomas seen with neurofibromatosis type 2; can result in compression of adjacent brain parenchyma, encasement of arteries, and compression of dural venous sinuses; hydrocephalus; rarely invasive/malignant types.
Hemangiopericytoma	Extra-axial mass lesions, often well circumscribed; intermediate attenuation, prominent contrast enhancement (may resemble meningiomas); with or without associated erosive bone changes.	Rare neoplasms in young adults (males > females) sometimes referred to as angioblastic meningioma or meningeal hemangiopericytoma; arise from vascular cells/pericytes; frequency of metastases > meningiomas.
Central neurocytoma	Circumscribed lesion located at margin of lateral ventricle or septum pellucidum with intraventricular protrusion, heterogeneous intermediate attenuation, with or without calcifications and/or small cysts; heterogeneous contrast enhancement.	Rare tumors that have neuronal differentiation; imaging appearance similar to intraventricular oligodendrogliomas; occur in young adults; benign slow-growing lesions.
Atypical teratoid rhabdoid tumors	Circumscribed mass lesions with intermediate attenuation, with or without zones of hemorrhage, cysts, calcifications; usually prominent contrast enhancement with or without heterogeneous pattern.	Rare malignant tumors involving the CNS usually occurring in the first decade. Histologically appear as solid tumors with or without necrotic areas, similar to malignant rhabdoid tumors of the kidney. Associated with CSF tumor dissemination and poor prognosis.
Intraventricular lesions		
Colloid cyst	Well-circumscribed spheroid lesions located at the anterior portion of the third ventricle; variable attenuation (low, intermediate, or high); no contrast enhancement.	Benign epithelial-lined cyst; common presentation of headaches and intermittent hydrocephalus; removal leads to cure.
Neuroepithelial cyst	Well-circumscribed cysts with low attenuation, thin walls; no contrast enhancement or peripheral edema.	Cyst walls have histopathologic features similar to epithelium; neuroepithelial cysts located in choroid plexus > choroidal fissure > ventricles > brain parenchyma.
Intraventricular arachnoid cyst ▷ *Fig. 2.13a, b*	Well-circumscribed cysts with low attenuation equal to CSF, thin walls; no contrast enhancement or peripheral edema.	Cyst walls have histopathologic features of arachnoid, can arise from choroid plexus or extension of arachnoid from choroidal fissure into ventricles.
Inflammation/infection		
Ependymitis/ventriculitis ▷ *Fig. 2.14a–d*	Curvilinear and/or nodular gadolinium enhancement along ventricular/ependymal margins with resultant communicating or noncommunicating types of hydrocephalus.	Complications of intracranial inflammatory processes, such as infections from bacteria, fungi, tuberculosis, viruses (cytomegalovirus [CMV]), and parasites. Noninfectious diseases such as sarcoid can result in a similar pattern.
Cysticercosis	Single or multiple cystic lesions in brain or meninges. **Acute/subacute phase:** low to intermediate attenuation; rim with or without nodular pattern of contrast enhancement, with or without peripheral edema. **Chronic phase:** Calcified granulomas.	Caused by ingestion of ova (*Taenia solium*) in contaminated food (undercooked pork); involves meninges > brain parenchyma > ventricles.
Hydatid cyst	**Echinococcus granulosus:** Single or rarely multiple cystic lesions with low attenuation, thin walls; typically no contrast enhancement or peripheral edema unless superinfected; often located in vascular territory of the middle cerebral artery. **Echinococcus multilocularis:** Cystic (with or without multilocular) and/or solid lesions; central zone of intermediate attenuation surrounded by a slightly thickened rim, with contrast enhancement; peripheral zone of edema and calcifications are common.	Caused by parasites *E. granulosus* (South America, Middle East, Australia, and New Zealand) and *E. multilocularis* (North America, Europe, Turkey, and China). CNS involvement in 2% of cases of hydatid infestation.
Rasmussen encephalitis	Progressive atrophy of one cerebral hemisphere involving the white matter, basal ganglia, and cortex, usually without enhancement; ipsilateral dilated lateral ventricle.	Usually seen in children younger than 10 y; severe and progressive epilepsy and unilateral neurologic deficits: hemiplegia, psychomotor deterioration, chronic slow viral infectious process possibly caused by CMV or Epstein-Barr virus. Treatment: hemispherectomy.

(continues on page 146)

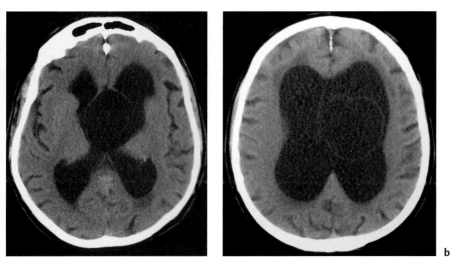

Fig. 2.13a, b   Intraventricular arachnoid cyst. Axial images show the arachnoid cyst in the third and left lateral ventricles associated with hydrocephalus.

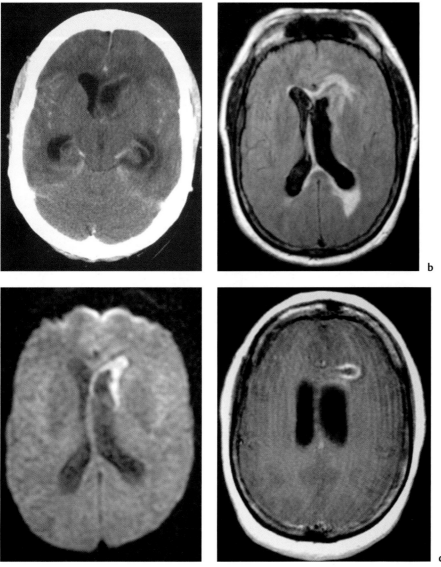

Fig. 2.14a–d   Ventriculitis. Axial postcontrast CT image (**a**) shows abnormal enhancement along the frontal horn of the left lateral ventricle. Abnormal high signal on axial fluid attenuation inversion recovery (FLAIR) MRI (**b**), restricted diffusion on axial diffusion-weighted MRI (**c**), and abnormal contrast enhancement on axial T1-weighted MRI (**d**) are seen along the ependymal margin of the left lateral ventricle.

Table 2.5   (Cont.) Dilated ventricles

Lesions	CT Findings	Comments
Intraventricular hemorrhage ▷ *Fig. 2.15*	Dilation of ventricles containing hemorrhage.	Intraventricular hemorrhage from trauma, aneurysm, arteriovenous malformation (AVM), or extension of intra-axial hematoma can result in acute and/or chronic dilation of the ventricles.
Hydranencephaly	Replacement of substantial portions of cerebral tissue with thin-walled sacs containing CSF; inferomedial portions of frontal and temporal lobes often preserved; cerebellum and thalami usually have a normal appearance.	In utero destruction of cerebral parenchyma from injury (vascular or infectious, e.g., CMV and toxoplasmosis). Patients may be normo-, micro-, or macrocephalic. Children developmentally delayed.
Porencephalic cyst ▷ *Fig. 2.16*	Irregular, relatively well-circumscribed zone with low attenuation similar to CSF, surrounded by poorly defined thin zone of decreased attenuation in adjacent brain tissue; no contrast enhancement or peripheral edema.	Represents remote sites of brain injury (trauma, infarction, infection, or hemorrhage) occurring in late second trimester with evolution by an encephaloclastic process into a cystic zone with CSF. MRI signal characteristics surrounded by zones of gliosis in adjacent brain parenchyma. Gliosis (high T2 signal) allows differentiation from schizencephaly.
Encephalomalacia ▷ *Fig. 2.17* ▷ *Fig. 2.18*	Poorly defined zone of decreased attenuation in brain tissue (gray and or white matter) with localized volume loss and compensatory dilation of adjacent ventricle.	Damaged residual brain tissue characterized by astrocytic proliferation related to prior infarct, hemorrhage, inflammation, infection, and trauma, with compensatory ipsilateral ventricular dilation resulting from localized volume loss. Encephalomalacia can occur during late gestation, postnatal period, or with mature brain when an astrocytic proliferation response is possible.
Dyke-Davidoff-Masson syndrome	Atrophy/encephalomalacia of one cerebral hemisphere with compensatory dilation of the ipsilateral lateral ventricle; unilateral ipsilateral decrease in size of cranial fossa associated with thickened calvarium, with or without enlargement of ipsilateral paranasal sinuses.	Prenatal, congenital, or acquired ischemic disorder resulting in unilateral atrophy of one cerebral hemisphere; rare disorder in adolescents presenting with seizures, mental retardation, and hemiparesis.
Alzheimer disease ▷ *Fig. 2.19*	Brain atrophy often most pronounced in temporal lobes; sulcal and ventricular prominence. Cortical atrophic changes common.	Most common form of progressive dementia with neurofibrillary tangles, senile plaques, neuronal loss, amyloid angiopathy, gliosis.
Pick's disease ▷ *Fig. 2.20*	Brain atrophy often most pronounced in frontal and temporal lobes; sulcal and ventricular prominence. Cortical atrophic changes common.	Acquired dementia much less common than Alzheimer disease. Histopathologic findings or neuronal loss and cytoplasmic inclusion bodies (Pick bodies).
Huntington disease	Disproportionate atrophy of basal ganglia (caudate > putamen > cerebellum/brainstem); variable decreased attenuation involving the putamen bilaterally; usually no contrast enhancement.	Autosomal dominant neurodegenerative disease usually presenting after age 40 y with progressive movement disorders and behavioral and mental dysfunction.
Normal pressure hydrocephalus ▷ *Fig. 2.21a, b*	Disproportionately greater prominence of the ventricles relative to the sulci.	Dilation of the ventricles with transependymal egress of CSF thought to be secondary to impaired resorption of CSF through arachnoid granulations. Associated with progressive memory impairment, urinary incontinence, and gait disorders.
Ventricular shunt failure ▷ *Fig. 2.22*	Enlargement of ventricles above site of obstruction to CSF flow.	Blockage of ventricular shunt catheters can result in progressive ventricular dilation.

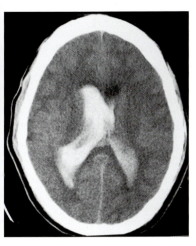

Fig. 2.15 Intraventricular hemorrhage.
Axial image shows high attenuation from acute hemorrhage within dilated lateral ventricles.

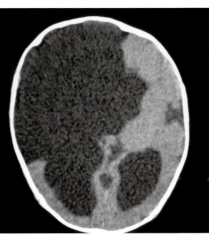

Fig. 2.16 Porencephaly. Axial image shows dilated lateral ventricles and a porencephalic cyst on the right.

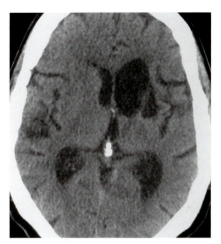

Fig. 2.17 Encephalomalacia. Dilation of the left lateral ventricle secondary to encephalomalacia from old infarction in the vascular distribution of the left middle cerebral artery.

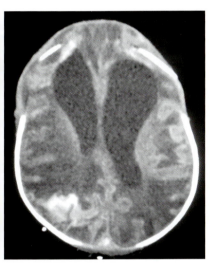

Fig. 2.18 Encephalomalacia, cerebritis.
Dilation of the lateral ventricles in a neonate secondary to encephalomalacia from destructive changes of cerebritis.

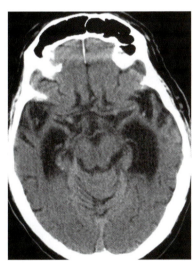

Fig. 2.19 Alzheimer disease. Axial image shows asymmetric cerebral atrophy involving the frontal and temporal lobes with compensatory dilation of the ventricles.

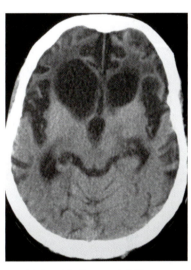

Fig. 2.20 Pick disease. Axial image shows asymmetric cerebral atrophy involving the frontal lobes with compensatory dilation of the ventricles.

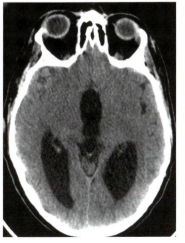

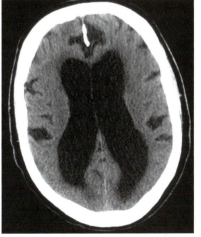

b

Fig. 2.21a, b Normal pressure hydrocephalus. Axial images show asymmetric prominence of the ventricles relative to the sulci.

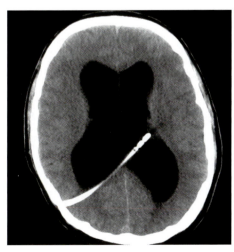

Fig. 2.22 Ventricular shunt failure. Axial image shows an intraventricular shunt with abnormally dilated ventricles.

Table 2.6   Abnormal or altered configurations of the ventricles

Lesions	CT Findings	Comments
Congenital, developmental, or acquired		
Cephaloceles (meningoceles or meningoencephaloceles) ▷ *Fig. 2.23*	Defect in skull through which there is either herniation of meninges and CSF (meningocele) or meninges, CSF, and brain tissue (meningoencephaloceles).	Congenital malformation involving lack of separation of neuroectoderm from surface ectoderm with resultant localized failure of bone formation. Occipital location most common in Western hemisphere, frontoethmoidal location most common site in Southeast Asians. Other sites include parietal and sphenoid bones. Cephaloceles can also result from trauma or surgery.
Holoprosencephaly ▷ *Fig. 2.24a, b*	**Alobar:** Large monoventricle with posterior midline cyst; lack of hemisphere formation with absence of falx, corpus callosum, and septum pellucidum. Fused thalami. **Semilobar:** Monoventricle with partial formation of interhemispheric fissure, occipital and temporal horns, partially fused thalami. Absent corpus callosum and septum pellucidum. Associated with mild craniofacial anomalies. **Lobar:** Near complete formation of interhemispheric fissure and ventricles. Fused inferior portions of frontal lobes, dysgenesis of corpus callosum, absence of septum pellucidum, separate thalami, neuronal migration disorders. **Septo-optic dysplasia (de Morsier syndrome):** Mild form of lobar holoprosencephaly. Dysgenesis or agenesis of septum pellucidum, optic nerve hypoplasia, squared frontal horns; association with schizencephaly in 50%.	**Holoprosencephaly:** Disorders of diverticulation (weeks 4–6 of gestation) characterized by absent or partial cleavage and differentiation of the embryonic cerebrum (prosencephalon) into hemispheres and lobes.
Lissencephaly ▷ *Fig. 2.25*	Absent or incomplete formation of gyri and sulci with shallow sylvian fissures and "figure 8" appearance of brain on axial images, abnormally thick cortex, gray matter heterotopia with smooth gray-white matter interface.	Severe disorder of neuronal migration (occurs during weeks 7–16 of gestation) with absent or incomplete formation of gyri, sulci, and sylvian fissures. Typically in association with microcephaly (defined as head circumference 3 standard deviations below normal). Associated with severe mental retardation, developmental delay, seizures, and early death.
Gray matter heterotopia ▷ *Fig. 2.26*	**Nodular heterotopia** appears as one or more nodules of isodense gray matter along the ventricles or within the cerebral white matter.	Disorder of neuronal migration (weeks 7–22 of gestation) in which a collection or layer of neurons is located between the ventricles and cerebral cortex. Can have a bandlike (laminar) or nodular appearance isointense to gray matter; may be unilateral or bilateral. Associated with seizures, schizencephaly.
Schizencephaly (split brain) ▷ *Fig. 2.27a, b*	Cleft in the brain extending from the ventricle to cortical surface lined by heterotopic gray matter; may be narrow (closed lip) or wide (open lip).	Association with seizures, blindness, retardation, and other CNS anomalies (septo-optic dysplasia, etc.). Clinical manifestations related to severity of malformation. Ischemia or insult to portion or germinal matrix before hemisphere formation.
Unilateral hemimegalencephaly ▷ *Fig. 2.28*	Nodular or multinodular region of gray matter heterotopia involving all or part of a cerebral hemisphere with associated enlargement of the ipsilateral lateral ventricle and hemisphere.	Neuronal migration disorder associated with hamartomatous overgrowth of the involved hemisphere.

(continues on page 150)

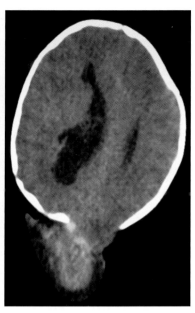

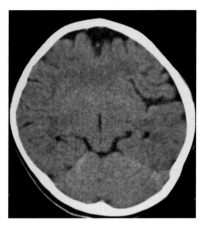

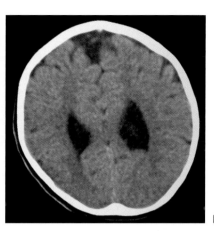

a

b

Fig. 2.24a, b   Lobar holoprosencephaly. Axial images show fusion of the anteroinferior portions of the frontal lobes (**a**) with separation of the upper portions of the frontal lobes (**b**) with an interhemispheric fissure.

Fig. 2.23   Meningoencephalocele. Axial image shows a parietal meningo-encephalocele.

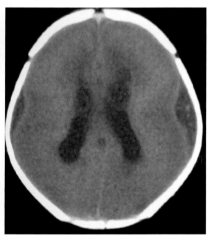

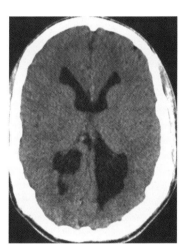

Fig. 2.26   Nodular gray matter heterotopia. Axial image shows nodular zones with intermediate attenuation along the margins of the lateral ventricles representing gray matter heterotopia.

Fig. 2.25   Lissencephaly. Axial image shows the absence of gyri and sulci and the lack of normal gray-white matter demarcation.

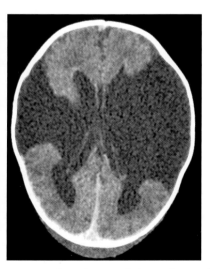

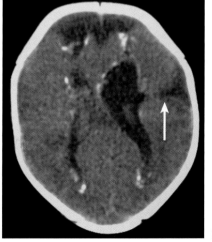

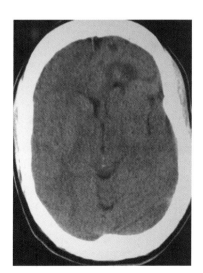

b

Fig. 2.28   Unilateral hemimegalencephaly. Axial image shows enlargement of the left cerebral hemisphere with abnormal gyral configuration and zones of decreased attenuation in the left frontal lobe.

Fig. 2.27a, b   Schizencephaly. Axial image (**a**) shows open lip schizencephaly lined by gray matter along the margins. Axial image (**b**) in a young child with congenital toxoplasmosis with closed lip schizencephaly on the left, dystrophic calcifications at sites of prior infection, and encephaloclastic changes (arrow).

Table 2.6   (Cont.) Abnormal or altered configurations of the ventricles

Lesions	CT Findings	Comments
Chiari II malformation (Arnold-Chiari malformation) ▷ *Fig. 2.29a–c*	Small posterior cranial fossa with gaping foramen magnum through which there is an inferiorly positioned vermis associated with a cervicomedullary kink. Beaked dorsal margin of the tectal plate. Myelomeningoceles in nearly all patients. Hydrocephalus and syringomyelia are common. Dilated lateral ventricles posteriorly (colpocephaly).	Complex anomaly involving the cerebrum, cerebellum, brainstem, spinal cord, ventricles, skull, and dura. Failure of fetal neural tube to develop properly results in altered development affecting multiple sites of the CNS.
Dandy-Walker malformation ▷ *Fig. 2.30a, b*	Vermian aplasia or severe hypoplasia; communication of fourth ventricle with retrocerebellar cyst; enlarged posterior fossa, high position of tentorium and transverse venous sinuses. Hydrocephalus common. Associated with other anomalies such as dysgenesis of the corpus callosum, gray matter heterotopia, schizencephaly, holoprosencephaly, and cephaloceles.	Abnormal formation of the roof of the fourth ventricle with absent or near incomplete formation of cerebellar vermis.
Dysgenesis of the corpus callosum ▷ *Fig. 2.31a, b*	Spectrum of abnormalities ranging from complete to partial absence of the corpus callosum. Widely separated and parallel orientations of frontal horns and bodies of lateral ventricles; high position of third ventricle in relation to interhemispheric fissure, colpocephaly. Associated with interhemispheric cysts, lipomas, and anomalies such as Chiari II malformation, gray matter heterotopia, Dandy-Walker malformations, holoprosencephaly, azygous anterior cerebral artery, and cephaloceles.	Failure or incomplete formation of corpus callosum (weeks 7–18 of gestation). Axons that normally cross from one hemisphere to the other are aligned parallel along the medial walls of the lateral ventricles (bundles of Probst).
Porencephalic cyst ▷ *Fig. 2.32*	Irregular, relatively well-circumscribed zone with low attenuation similar to CSF, surrounded by poorly defined thin zone of decreased attenuation in adjacent brain tissue; no contrast enhancement or peripheral edema.	Represents remote sites of brain injury (trauma, infarction, infection, or hemorrhage) with evolution into a cystic zone with CSF surrounded by gliosis in adjacent brain parenchyma.
Neuroepithelial cyst	Well-circumscribed cysts with low attenuation, thin walls; no contrast enhancement or peripheral edema.	Cyst walls have histopathologic features similar to epithelium; neuroepithelial cysts located in choroid plexus > choroidal fissure > ventricles > brain parenchyma.
Hamartoma/tuberous sclerosis ▷ *Fig. 2.33*	**Subependymal hamartomas:** Small nodules located along and projecting into the lateral ventricles with or without calcifications; MRI signal on T1- and T2-weighted images similar to cortical tubers; gadolinium enhancement common.	Cortical and subependymal hamartomas are nonmalignant lesions associated with tuberous sclerosis.

(continues on page 152)

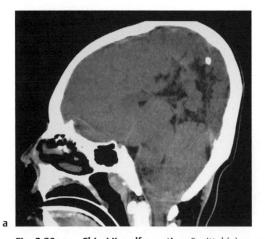
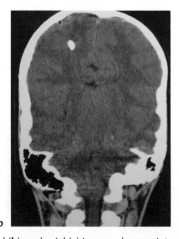
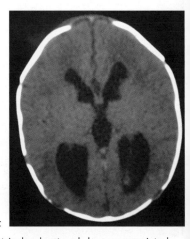

a   b   c

Fig. 2.29a–c   Chiari II malformation. Sagittal (**a**), coronal (**b**), and axial (**c**) images show an intraventricular shunt and changes associated with a Chiari II malformation, as well as an abnormally shaped fourth ventricle. Axial image in another patient shows colpocephaly.

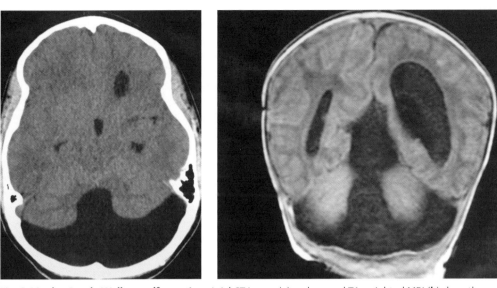

b

Fig. 2.30a, b Dandy-Walker malformation. Axial CT image (**a**) and coronal T1-weighted MRI (**b**) show the absence of the vermis and hypoplasia of the cerebellar hemispheres with altered shape of the fourth ventricle.

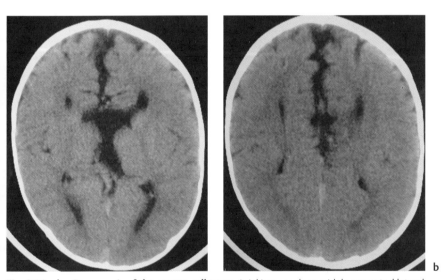

b

Fig. 2.31a, b Dysgenesis of the corpus callosum. Axial images show widely separated lateral ventricles related to bundles of Probst.

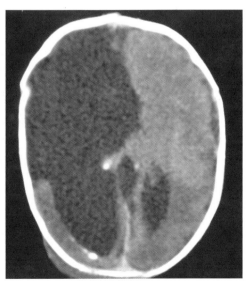

Fig. 2.32 Porencephalic cyst. Axial image shows abnormal enlargement of the right lateral ventricle from prior infection and localized brain destruction with dystrophic calcifications and a porencephalic cyst.

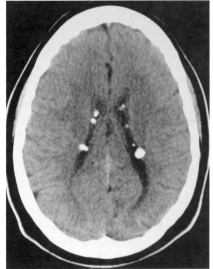

Fig. 2.33 Hamartomas, tuberous sclerosis. Axial image shows multiple calcified ependymal hamartomas.

Table 2.6 (Cont.) Abnormal or altered configurations of the ventricles

Lesions	CT Findings	Comments
Subfalcine herniation ▷ *Fig. 2.34*	Compression and shift of the lateral and third ventricles under the falx cerebri to the other side, with or without dilation of contralateral lateral ventricle because of CSF outflow obstruction from compression at the contralateral foramen of Monro; with or without displacement of ipsilateral anterior cerebral artery and subependymal veins.	Most often occurs from primary or metastatic intra-axial tumor or hemorrhage.
Transtentorial herniation ▷ *Fig. 2.35*	**Ascending type:** Upward herniation of cerebellar vermis and hemispheres through the tentorial incisura, resulting in compression and displacement of the cerebral aqueduct and posterior portion of the third ventricle, effacement of superior vermian cistern, compression and anterior displacement of the fourth ventricle; with or without obstructive hydrocephalus. **Descending type:** Medial and inferior displacement of uncus and parahippocampal gyrus below the tentorium; progressive effacement of suprasellar cistern and basal cisterns, compression of ipsilateral portion of the midbrain that is displaced toward contralateral side; with or without Kernohan notch; with or without Duret hemorrhage; with or without inferior displacement and/or compression of anterior choroidal, posterior communicating, and posterior cerebral arteries, as well as perforating branches of the basilar artery, resulting in cerebral, cerebellar, and/or brainstem infarcts. Often results in death.	Descending type more common than ascending type. Typically results from a focal mass lesion or hemorrhage, causing displacement of brain tissue across tentorium.
Cavum septum pellucidum/ cavum vergae ▷ *Fig. 2.36*	**Cavum septum pellucidum:** CSF-containing zone between two septal leaves. **Cavum vergae:** Same as cavum septum pellucidum with posterior extension of fluid-containing zone between septal leaves.	Developmental anomalies with lack of normal involution of fetal cavities separating the two septal leaves; occurs in 3% of normal adults; no clinical significance.

Table 2.7 Intraventricular mass lesions

Lesions	CT Findings	Comments
Congenital or developmental		
Pineal cyst ▷ *Fig. 2.37*	Well-circumscribed extra-axial lesions with low attenuation signal similar to CSF; no central enhancement, thin linear peripheral contrast enhancement; rarely atypical appearance with proteinaceous contents: intermediate, slightly high attenuation.	Common usually incidental nonneoplastic cyst in pineal gland.
Colloid cyst ▷ *Fig. 2.38a, b*	Well-circumscribed spheroid lesions located at the anterior portion of the third ventricle; variable attenuation (low, intermediate, or high); usually no contrast enhancement.	Benign epithelial-lined cysts; common presentation of headaches and intermittent hydrocephalus; removal leads to cure.
Neuroepithelial cyst	Well-circumscribed cysts with low attenuation, thin walls; no contrast enhancement or peripheral edema.	Cyst walls have histopathologic features similar to epithelium; neuroepithelial cysts located in choroid plexus > choroidal fissure > ventricles > brain parenchyma.

(continues on page 154)

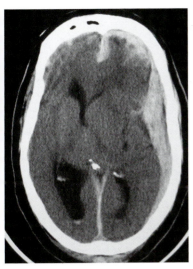

Fig. 2.34 Subfalcine herniation. Axial image shows a left-sided subdural hematoma with subfalcine herniation rightward.

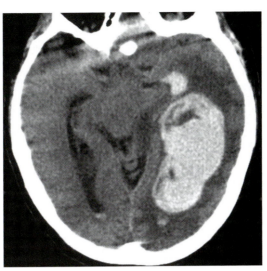

Fig. 2.35 Transtentorial herniation. Axial image shows a large hematoma in the left temporal lobe extending into the left lateral ventricle associated with mass effect causing counterclockwise rotation of the midbrain and transtentorial/uncal herniation.

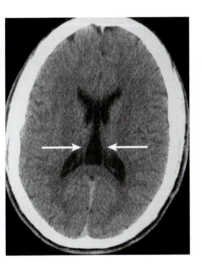

Fig. 2.36 Cavum vergae. Axial image shows separation of the two leaves of the septum pellucidum extending posteriorly (arrows).

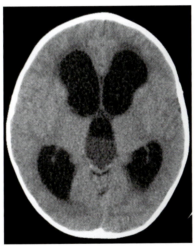

Fig. 2.37 Pineal cyst. Axial image shows a pineal cyst causing hydrocephalus.

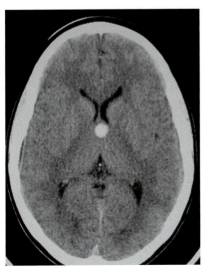

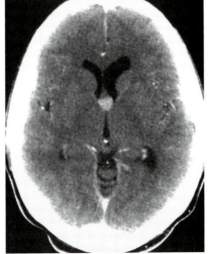

b

Fig. 2.38a, b Colloid cyst. Axial pre- (**a**) and postcontrast (**b**) images show a colloid cyst with high attenuation in the anterior upper portion of the third ventricle.

Table 2.7   (Cont.) Intraventricular mass lesions

Lesions	CT Findings	Comments
Intraventricular arachnoid cyst ▷ *Fig. 2.39a–d*	Well-circumscribed cysts with low attenuation equal to CSF; thin walls; no contrast enhancement or peripheral edema.	Cyst walls have histopathologic features of arachnoid; can arise from choroid plexus or extension of arachnoid from choroidal fissure into ventricles.
Intraventricular epidermoid	Well-circumscribed spheroid or multilobulated, extra-axial ectodermal inclusion cystic lesions with low to intermediate attenuation, no contrast enhancement, with or without bone erosion/destruction. Often insinuate along CSF pathways; chronic deformation of adjacent neural tissue.	Nonneoplastic congenital or acquired extra-axial off-midline lesions filled with desquamated cells and keratinaceous debris; usually mild mass effect on adjacent brain; infratentorial > supratentorial locations. Adults: men = women; with or without related clinical symptoms.
Gray matter heterotopia ▷ *Fig. 2.40*	**Nodular heterotopia** appears as one or more nodules of gray matter attenuation along the ventricles or within the cerebral white matter.	Disorder of neuronal migration (weeks 7–22 of gestation) in which a collection or layer of neurons is located between the ventricles and cerebral cortex. Can have a bandlike (laminar) or nodular appearance with attenuation similar to gray matter; may be unilateral or bilateral. Associated with seizures, schizencephaly.
Hamartoma/tuberous sclerosis ▷ *Fig. 2.41*	**Subependymal hamartomas:** Small nodules located along and projecting into the lateral ventricles; calcification and contrast enhancement common.	Cortical and subependymal hamartomas are nonmalignant lesions associated with tuberous sclerosis.
Neoplastic		
Metastatic tumor ▷ *Fig. 2.42a,b*	Single or multiple well-circumscribed or poorly defined lesions involving the brain, skull, dura, leptomeninges, choroid plexus/ventricles, or pituitary gland; low to intermediate attenuation usually with contrast enhancement, with or without bone destruction, with or without compression of neural tissue or vessels. Leptomeningeal tumor often best seen on postcontrast images.	Metastatic tumor may have variable destructive or infiltrative changes involving single or multiple sites of involvement. Disseminated tumor within the ventricles can result from primary CNS tumors or extraneural primary neoplasms.

(continues on page 156)

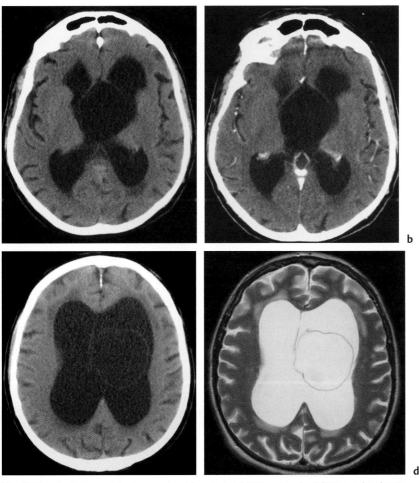

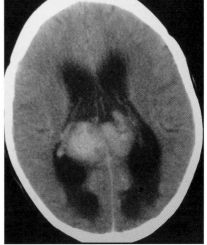

Fig. 2.40   Gray matter heterotopia. Axial image shows multiple nodular zones of gray matter heterotopia along the lateral ventricles.

Fig. 2.39a–d   Intraventricular arachnoid cyst. Axial CT (**a–c**) and axial T2-weighted MRI (**d**) images show an arachnoid cyst in the third and left lateral ventricles causing hydrocephalus.

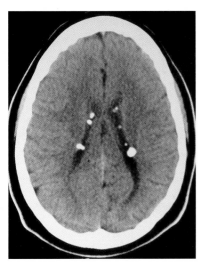

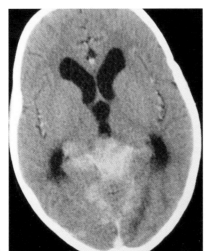

Fig. 2.41   Tuberous sclerosis, ependymal hamartomas. Axial image shows multiple calcified ependymal hamartomas.

Fig. 2.42a, b   Metastatic tumor. Axial postcontrast images show enhancing subarachnoid and intraventricular tumor from pineoblastoma.

Table 2.7   (Cont.) Intraventricular mass lesions

Lesions	CT Findings	Comments
Meningioma ▷ *Fig. 2.43*	Extra-axial dural-based lesions, well-circumscribed; supratentorial > infratentorial, parasagittal > convexity > sphenoid ridge > parasellar > posterior fossa > optic nerve sheath > intraventricular; intermediate attenuation, usually prominent contrast enhancement, with or without calcifications.	Most common extra-axial tumor; usually benign neoplasms; typically occurs in adults (> 40 y), women > men. Multiple meningiomas seen with neurofibromatosis type 2; can result in compression of adjacent brain parenchyma, encasement of arteries, and compression of dural venous sinuses; rarely invasive/malignant types.
Hemangiopericytoma ▷ *Fig. 2.44*	Extra-axial mass lesions, often well circumscribed; intermediate attenuation, prominent contrast enhancement (may resemble meningiomas), with or without associated erosive bone changes.	Rare neoplasms in young adults (males > females) sometimes referred to as angioblastic meningioma or meningeal hemangiopericytoma; arise from vascular cells/pericytes; frequency of metastases > meningiomas.
Central neurocytoma	Circumscribed lesion located at the margin of the lateral ventricle or septum pellucidum with intraventricular protrusion, heterogeneous intermediate attenuation; with or without calcifications and/or small cysts; heterogeneous contrast enhancement.	Rare tumors that have neuronal differentiation; imaging appearance similar to intraventricular oligodendrogliomas; occur in young adults; benign slow-growing lesions.
Astrocytoma	**Low-grade astrocytoma:** Focal or diffuse mass lesion usually located in cerebral or cerebellar white matter or brainstem with low to intermediate attenuation, with or without mild contrast enhancement. Minimal associated mass effect. May extend into ventricles. **Juvenile pilocytic astrocytoma subtype:** Solid/cystic focal lesion with low to intermediate attenuation, usually with prominent contrast enhancement. Lesions located in the cerebellum and brainstem. May extend into ventricles. **Gliomatosis cerebri:** Infiltrative lesion with poorly defined margins with mass effect located in the white matter, with low to intermediate attenuation; usually no contrast enhancement until late in disease. May extend into ventricles. **Anaplastic astrocytoma:** Often irregularly marginated lesion located in the white matter with low to intermediate attenuation, with or without contrast enhancement. May extend into ventricles. **Glioblastoma multiforme:** Irregularly marginated mass lesion with necrosis or cyst; mixed low and intermediate attenuation, with or without hemorrhage; prominent heterogeneous contrast enhancement, peripheral edema; can cross corpus callosum. ▷ *Fig. 2.45*	Often occur in children and adults (age 20–40 y). Tumors comprised of well-differentiated astrocytes. Association with neurofibromatosis type 1; 10-y survival common; may become malignant. Common in children; usually favorable prognosis if totally resected. Diffusely infiltrating astrocytoma with relative preservation of underlying brain architecture. Imaging appearance may be more prognostic than histologic grade; ~2-y survival. Intermediate between low-grade astrocytoma and glioblastoma multiforme; ~2-y survival. Most common primary CNS tumor; highly malignant neoplasms with necrosis and vascular proliferation, usually seen in patients older than 50 y; extent of lesion underestimated by CT; survival < 1 y.
Giant cell astrocytoma/ tuberous sclerosis ▷ *Fig. 2.46*	Circumscribed lesion located near the foramen of Monro with mixed low to intermediate attenuation, with or without cysts and/or calcifications, with heterogeneous contrast enhancement.	Subependymal hamartoma near the foramen of Monro; occurs in 15% of patients with tuberous sclerosis younger than 20 y; slow-growing lesions that can progressively cause obstruction of CSF flow through the foramen of Monro; long-term survival usual if resected.
Craniopharyngioma ▷ *Fig. 2.47*	Circumscribed, lobulated lesions; both suprasellar and intrasellar location > suprasellar > intrasellar; can extend into the third ventricle; variable low, intermediate, and/or high attenuation; with or without nodular or rim contrast enhancement. May contain cysts, lipid components, and calcifications.	Usually histologically benign but locally aggressive lesions arising from squamous epithelial rests along the Rathke cleft; occurs in children (5–15 y) and adults (> 40 y), males = females.
Medulloblastoma (primitive neuroectodermal tumor of the cerebellum) ▷ *Fig. 2.48*	Circumscribed or invasive lesions, low to intermediate attenuation; variable contrast enhancement; frequent dissemination into the leptomeninges.	Highly malignant tumors that frequently disseminate along CSF pathways.

(continues on page 158)

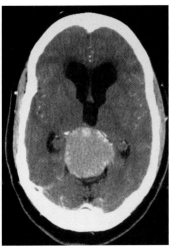

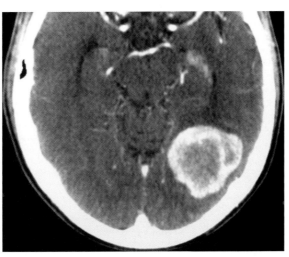

Fig. 2.43 Meningioma. Axial postcontrast image shows an enhancing tumor involving the posterior portion of the third ventricle.

Fig. 2.44 Hemangiopericytoma. Axial postcontrast image shows an enhancing lesion involving the posterior portion of the left lateral ventricle.

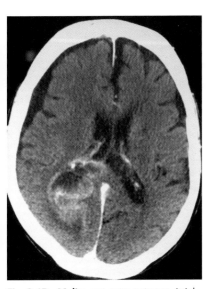

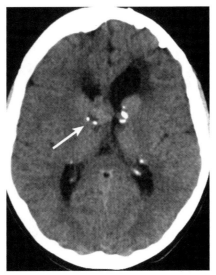

Fig. 2.45 Malignant astrocytoma. Axial postcontrast image shows an enhancing lesion in the right occipital lobe extending into the splenium of the corpus callosum.

Fig. 2.46 Giant cell astrocytoma, tuberous sclerosis. Axial image shows a tumor at the right foramen of Monro (arrow), as well as multiple calcified ependymal hamartomas.

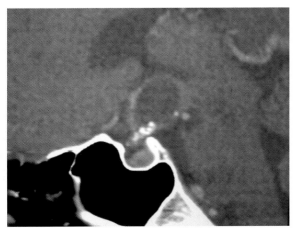

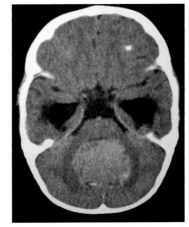

Fig. 2.47 Craniopharyngioma. Sagittal postcontrast image shows a complex lesion in the suprasellar cistern involving the third ventricle.

Fig. 2.48 Medulloblastoma. Axial image shows the tumor in the vermis extending into the fourth ventricle, causing hydrocephalus.

Table 2.7   (Cont.) Intraventricular mass lesions

Lesions	CT Findings	Comments
Ependymoma ▷ *Fig. 2.49a, b*	Circumscribed spheroid or lobulated infratentorial lesion, usually in the fourth ventricle, with or without cysts and/or calcifications; low or intermediate attenuation, variable contrast enhancement, with or without extension through the foramina of Luschka and Magendie.	Occurs more commonly in children than adults; two thirds infratentorial, one third supratentorial.
Subependymoma ▷ *Fig. 2.50*	Circumscribed intraventricular lesions with intermediate attenuation, typically no contrast enhancement; can occasionally cause obstructive hydrocephalus.	Rare benign (World Health Organization [WHO] grade 1) lesions consisting of astrocytes and ependymal cells arising from below the ventricular lining with protrusion into the ventricles (fourth > lateral > third ventricles); can involve the septum pellucidum. Usually occurs in adults, male/female ratio of 2.3:1.
Oligodendroglioma	Circumscribed lesion with mixed low to intermediate attenuation; may have areas of clumplike calcification; heterogeneous contrast enhancement; involves white matter and cerebral cortex; can cause chronic erosion of inner table of calvarium; also occurs within ventricles.	Uncommon slow-growing gliomas with usually mixed histologic patterns (astrocytoma, etc.). Usually seen in adults older than 35 y; 85% supratentorial. If low-grade, 75% 5-y survival; higher grade lesions have a worse prognosis.
Pineal gland tumors ▷ *Fig. 2.51a, b*	Tumors often have intermediate attenuation to intermediate to slightly high attenuation, with contrast enhancement, with or without central and/or peripheral calcifications. Malignant tumors are often larger than benign pineal lesions (pineocytoma), as well as heterogeneous attenuation and contrast enhancement pattern; with or without leptomeningeal tumor.	Pineal gland tumors account for 8% of intracranial tumors in children and 1% of tumors in adults; 40% of tumors are germinomas, followed by pineoblastoma and pineocytoma, teratoma, choriocarcinoma, endodermal sinus tumor, astrocytoma, and metastatic tumor.
Germinomas ▷ *Fig. 2.52*	Circumscribed tumors with or without disseminated disease; pineal region > suprasellar region > third ventricle/basal ganglia; low to intermediate attenuation, with or without cystic like regions; usually with contrast enhancement of tumor and leptomeninges (if disseminated).	Most common type of germ cell tumor; occurs in males > females (age 10–30 y); usually midline neoplasms.
Choroid plexus papilloma and carcinoma ▷ *Fig. 2.53a, b* ▷ *Fig. 2.54*	Circumscribed and/or lobulated lesions with papillary projections; intermediate attenuation; usually prominent contrast enhancement, with or without calcifications. Locations: atrium of lateral ventricle (children) > fourth ventricle (adults), rarely other locations such as the third ventricle; associated with hydrocephalus.	Rare intracranial neoplasms; CT features of choroid plexus carcinoma and papilloma overlap; both histologic types can disseminate along CSF pathways and invade brain tissue.
Atypical teratoid/rhabdoid tumors ▷ *Fig. 2.55*	Circumscribed mass lesions with intermediate attenuation, with or without zones of high attenuation from hemorrhage and/or calcifications; usually show contrast enhancement.	Rare malignant tumors involving the CNS usually occurring in the first decade. Histologically appear as solid tumors with or without necrotic areas, similar to malignant rhabdoid tumors of the kidney. Associated with a poor prognosis.

(continues on page 160)

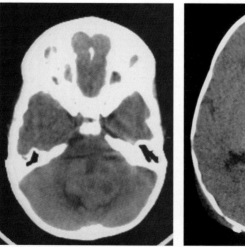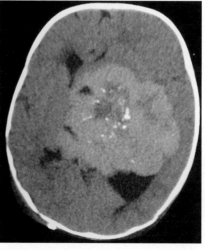

Fig. 2.49a, b   Ependymoma. Axial images in two different patients show ependymomas in the fourth ventricle (**a**) and left lateral ventricle (**b**).

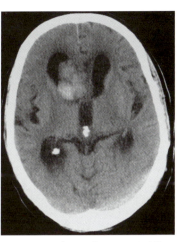

Fig. 2.50 Subependymoma. Axial image shows a tumor in the frontal horn of the right lateral ventricle.

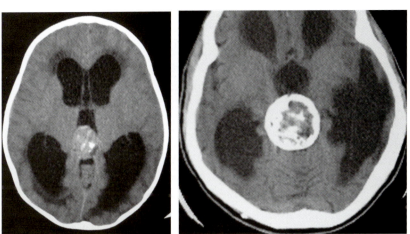

Fig. 2.51a, b Pineal gland tumors. Axial images show a pineoblastoma (**a**) and pineal teratoma (**b**) associated with dilated ventricles.

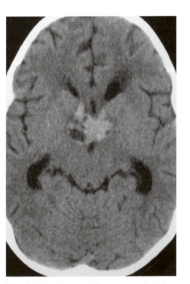

Fig. 2.52 Germ cell tumors. Axial image shows a germinoma in the third ventricle.

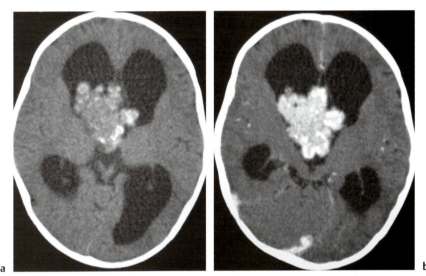

Fig. 2.53a, b Choroid plexus papilloma. Axial pre- (**a**) and postcontrast (**b**) images show an enhancing tumor in the third ventricle.

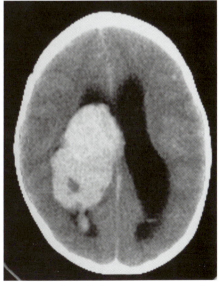

Fig. 2.54 Choroid plexus carcinoma. Axial postcontrast image shows a large enhancing tumor in the right lateral ventricle.

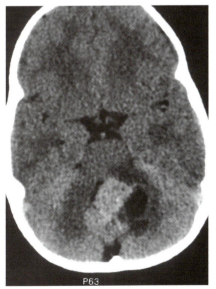

Fig. 2.55 Atypical teratoid/rhabdoid tumor. Axial postcontrast image shows a complex enhancing solid and cystic lesion in the fourth ventricle.

Table 2.7 (Cont.) Intraventricular mass lesions

Lesions	CT Findings	Comments
Inflammatory		
Tuberculosis: leptomeningeal/ cisternal/intraventricular involvement	Solid, linear, and or ringlike extra-axial contrast enhancement in basal cisterns, leptomeninges, and/or ventricles.	Occurs in immunocompromised patients and in inhabitants of developing countries. Caseating intracranial granulomas via hematogenous dissemination.
Parasitic brain lesions		
Toxoplasmosis ▷ *Fig. 2.56a, b*	Single or multiple solid and/or cystic lesions located in basal ganglia and/or corticomedullary junctions in cerebral hemispheres, rarely in ventricles; low to intermediate attenuation; nodular or rim pattern of contrast enhancement; with or without peripheral edema.	Most common opportunistic CNS infection in AIDS patients; caused by ingestion of food contaminated with parasites (*Toxoplasma gondii*).
Cysticercosis	Single or multiple cystic lesions in brain, meninges, occasionally in ventricles. **Acute/subacute phase:** Low to intermediate attenuation; with or without nodular pattern of contrast enhancement; with or without peripheral edema. **Chronic phase:** Calcified granulomas.	Caused by ingestion of ova (*Taenia solium*) in contaminated food (undercooked pork); involves meninges > brain parenchyma > ventricles.
Hydatid cyst	**Echinococcus granulosus:** Single or rarely multiple cystic lesions with a thin wall with low attenuation; typically no contrast enhancement or peripheral edema unless superinfected; often located in vascular territory of the middle cerebral artery. **Echinococcus multilocularis:** Cystic (with or without multilocular) and/or solid lesions; central zone of intermediate attenuation surrounded by a slightly thickened rim, with contrast enhancement; peripheral zone of edema and calcifications are common.	Caused by parasites *E. granulosus* (South America, Middle East, Australia, and New Zealand) or *E. multilocularis* (North America, Europe, Turkey, and China). CNS involvement in 2% of cases of hydatid infestation.
Sarcoid ▷ *Fig. 2.57a–c*	Poorly marginated extra-axial lesion with low to intermediate attenuation; usually shows contrast enhancement, with localized mass effect and peripheral edema. Often associated with contrast enhancement in the leptomeninges with or without ventricles.	Multisystem noncaseating granulomatous disease of uncertain cause that can involve the CNS in 5% to 15% of cases. Associated with severe neurologic deficits if untreated.
Vascular lesions		
AVM ▷ *Fig. 2.58a, b*	Lesions with irregular margins that can be located in the brain parenchyma, dura, and/or ventricles. **CT:** AVMs contain multiple tortuous tubular vessels that have intermediate or slightly increased attenuation that show contrast enhancement. Calcifications occur in 30%. Computed tomography angiography (CTA) shows arteries, veins, and nidus of AVM even when there is hemorrhage.	Supratentorial AVMs occur more frequently (80%–90%) than infratentorial AVMs (10%–20%). Annual risk of hemorrhage. AVMs can be sporadic, congenital, or associated with a history of trauma. Multiple AVMs can be seen in syndromes: Rendu-Osler-Weber (AVMs in brain and lungs and mucosal, capillary telangiectasias) and Wyburn-Mason (AVMs in brain and retina, with cutaneous nevi).

(continues on page 162)

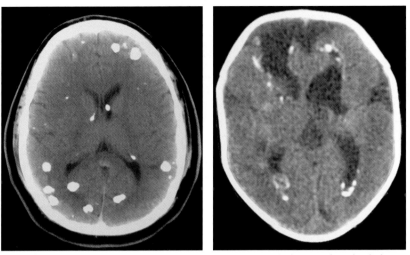

Fig. 2.56a, b   Toxoplasmosis. Axial images show multiple calcifications from healed granulomas in two different patients.

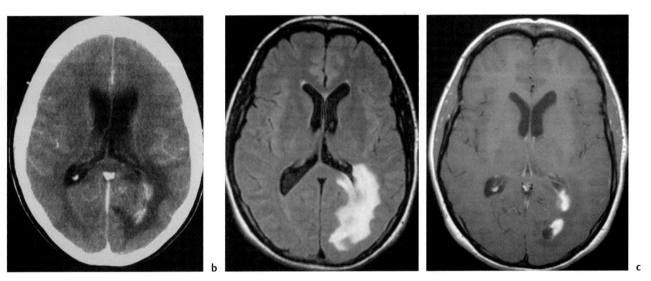

Fig. 2.57a–c   Sarcoid. Axial postcontrast CT image (**a**) shows enhancement along the atrium and occipital horn of the left lateral ventricle. Corresponding abnormal increased signal and contrast enhancement are seen on an axial FLAIR MRI (**b**) and an axial T1-weighted image (**c**), respectively.

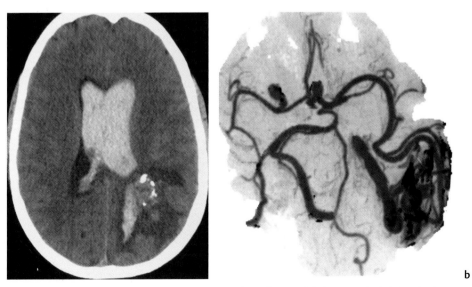

Fig. 2.58a, b   Arteriovenous malformation (AVM). Axial image (**a**) shows a calcified AVM in the left cerebral hemisphere with hemorrhage into the ventricles. Axial computed tomography angiography (CTA) image (**b**) shows the abnormal collection of vessels of the AVM.

Table 2.7   (Cont.) Intraventricular mass lesions

Lesions	CT Findings	Comments
Vein of Galen aneurysm ▷ *Fig. 2.59*	Multiple tortuous blood vessels involving choroidal and thalamoperforate arteries, internal cerebral veins, vein of Galen (aneurysmal formation), straight and transverse venous sinuses, and other adjacent veins and arteries. The venous portions often show contrast enhancement. CTA can show patent portions of the vascular malformation.	Heterogeneous group of vascular malformations with arteriovenous shunts and dilated deep venous structures draining into and from an enlarged vein of Galen, with or without hydrocephalus, with or without hemorrhage, with or without macrocephaly, with or without parenchymal vascular malformation components, with or without seizures; high-output congestive heart failure in neonates.
Sturge-Weber syndrome ▷ *Fig. 2.60*	Prominent localized unilateral leptomeningeal enhancement usually in parietal and/or occipital regions in children; with or without gyral enhancement; mild localized atrophic changes in brain adjacent to the pial angioma; with or without prominent medullary and/or subependymal veins; with or without ipsilateral prominence of choroid plexus. Gyral calcifications > 2 y; progressive cerebral atrophy in region of pial angioma.	Also known as encephalotrigeminal angiomatosis, neurocutaneous syndrome associated with ipsilateral "port wine" cutaneous lesion and seizures; results from persistence of primitive leptomeningeal venous drainage (pial angioma) and developmental lack of normal cortical veins, producing chronic venous congestion and ischemia.

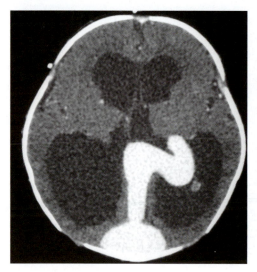

Fig. 2.59   Vein of Galen aneurysm. Axial postcontrast image shows an abnormally enlarged enhancing vein of Galen and straight venous sinus.

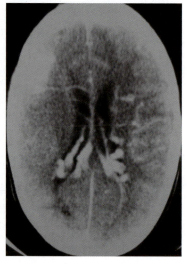

Fig. 2.60   Sturge-Weber syndrome. Axial postcontrast image shows enlarged enhancing medullary and ependymal veins.

3 Lesions Involving the Meninges and Skull

Steven P. Meyers

The cranial and spinal meninges represent three concentric contiguous membranes (dura mater, arachnoid, and pia mater) surrounding the central nervous system (CNS). The outer intracranial meningeal layer is the dura mater (pachymeninx). The outermost layer of the dura mater is a richly vascularized layer with elongated fibroblasts and large intercellular spaces that contain arteries and veins; this layer represents the periosteum of the inner table of the calvaria. The arteries and veins here form impressions on the inner table of the skull. The outer layer of the dura mater terminates at the foramen magnum. An inner layer of the dura arises from the meninx and consists of epithelial cells. This inner layer of the dura mater is contiguous with the spinal dura mater. The layers of the cranial dura separate at sites where there are large venous sinuses. Reflections of dura form the falx cerebri and tentorium cerebelli, which provide support of the normal positions of the cerebrum and cerebellum.

The arachnoid and pia mater comprise the leptomeninges. The arachnoid membrane is immediately adjacent to the inner surface of the dura. A potential space exists between the dura and the arachnoid, referred to as the subdural space. The arachnoid is thinner over the convexities than at the base of the skull. Deep to the arachnoid membrane is the subarachnoid space, which contains cerebrospinal fluid (CSF). The inner boundary of the subarachnoid space is the cranial pia mater. The cranial pia mater is a thin layer adjacent to the surface of the brain extending along the sulci. The cranial pia mater contains elastic fibers internally and collagenous fibers peripherally. Thin connective tissue strands and cellular septa extend across the arachnoid membrane to the pia except at the base of the brain, where the arachnoid membrane and pia are widely separated. These regions are referred to as the basal subarachnoid cisterns. The spinal pia mater is thicker and more adherent to the nervous tissue than the cranial pia.

The meninges (dura, arachnoid, and pia) form the extra-axial compartments of the CNS. The epidural space exists when the dura is detached from the inner table, usually from trauma/fracture and injury to a meningeal artery/epidural hematoma or occasionally from neoplasms involving the skull. The subdural space forms when a pathologic process is present, such as a subdural hematoma from trauma/skull fracture and injury of large veins, inflammatory/infectious disease, or neoplasm. Unlike the epi- and subdural compartment, the subarachnoid space exists without the presence of a pathologic process. The presence of extravascular blood in the subarachnoid space usually is associated with a ruptured intracranial aneurysm, vascular malformation, or trauma. Contrast enhancement of the dura can occur as a result of various causes, including neoplasms (primary and metastatic); inflammation/infection; and benign dural fibrosis secondary to intracranial surgery, transient hypotension (secondary to lumbar puncture), or evolving subdural hematoma. The dural enhancement follows the inner contour of the calvaria without extension into the sulci.

Contrast enhancement in the intracranial subarachnoid space (leptomeninges) is nearly always associated with significant pathology (inflammation and/or infection vs neoplasm). Inflammation and/or infection of the leptomeninges can result from pyogenic, fungal, or parasitic diseases, as well as tuberculosis. Complications of infectious meningitis include cerebritis, intra-axial abscess, ventriculitis, hydrocephalus, and venous sinus thrombosis/venous cerebral infarction. Neurosarcoid results in granulomatous disease in the leptomeninges producing similar patterns of subarachnoid enhancement. Disseminated or metastatic disease involving the leptomeninges can result from CNS tumors or primary tumors outside the CNS. Lymphoma and leukemia can also result in a similar pattern of leptomeningeal enhancement. Rarely, transient leptomeningeal enhancement can occur from chemical irritation resulting from subarachnoid blood.

Skull

The skull is comprised of two major components, the neurocranium and viscerocranium. The viscerocranium represents the facial bony structures. The neurocranium is the portion that encloses the brain and includes the skull base (chondrocranium, endochondral bone formation) and calvarium (membranous bone formation). Chondrocranial bones of the skull base include the sphenoid bone, most of the occipital bone, petrous bones, and ethmoid bone. Sites where the chondrocranial bones of the skull base fuse are referred to as synchondroses. The calvarium originates from ossification centers derived from membranous bone. Growth of the calvarium is directly dependent on growth of the immediately subadjacent dura. The orientation of the dural fibers is related to the position of five chondrocranial structures of the skull base (both petrous crests, crista galli, and both lesser sphenoid wings). Calvarial bones include frontal bones (two), parietal bones (two), a small portion of the occipital bone, and squamous portions of temporal bones (two).

Membranous borders between calvarial bones are referred to as sutures. The coronal suture is located between the frontal and parietal bones, the sagittal suture between the parietal bones, the lambdoid suture between the parietal and occipital bones, and the metopic suture between the frontal bones. The metopic suture normally closes approximately 7 months after birth. Junction regions where three or more calvarial bones meet are referred to as fontanelles. The largest is the anterior fontanelle, which is located between the frontal and parietal bones. The other fontanelles are considerably smaller and include the posterior, posterolateral (mastoid), and anterolateral (sphenoid) fontanelles. The size of the calvarial portion of the skull is dependent on growth of the intracranial contents (brain and ventricles). Patients with microcephalic brains have small-sized calvarial vaults, and those with enlarged brains (e.g., neoplasms, Alexander and Canavan diseases, and/or hydrocephalus) have enlarged calvaria. Premature closure of one or more sutures (craniosynostosis) results in various deformities of the calvaria depending on which suture is involved.

Growth of the chondrocranial bones of the skull base are less dependent on brain growth as is the calvarium. Disorders of skull base development are usually on a genetic basis (e.g., achondroplasia). Anomalies in brain formation can also affect development of the skull base. Examples include Chiari II malformations and cephaloceles. Chiari II malformations result in a small posterior cranial fossa and an enlarged foramen magnum. Cephaloceles are congenital defects in the skull through which there is herniation of the meninges and CSF or the meninges, CSF/ventricles, and brain tissue. The occipital cephalocele is the most common type in the Western hemisphere, and the frontoethmoidal type is most common in Southeast Asia. Other cephalocele locations are the parietal and sphenoid bones. Cephaloceles can also result from trauma and surgery.

Pathologic processes involving the skull can result by direct extension from adjacent anatomical structures (sinusitis resulting in osteomyelitis, intracranial neoplasm or inflammation eventually involving the skull, etc.), hematogenous seeding of infection or neoplasm into the diploic compartment, or systemic disorders (myeloma, thalassemia, sickle cell disease, hyperparathyroidism, renal osteodystrophy, etc.). Primary pathologic conditions involving the skull include craniosynostosis, Paget disease, trauma/fracture, neoplasm, infection/inflammation, nonmalignant lesions (epidermoid, hemangioma, etc.), and dermal sinus and vascular abnormalities (e.g., sinus pericranii).

Table 3.1   Abnormalities involving the meninges

Lesions	CT Findings	Comments
Developmental		
Cephaloceles (meningoceles or meningoencephaloceles) ▷ *Fig. 3.1a, b*	Defect in skull through which there is herniation of meninges and CSF (meningocele) or meninges, CSF/ventricles, and brain tissue (meningoencephaloceles).	Congenital malformation involving lack of separation of neuroectoderm from surface ectoderm with resultant localized failure of bone formation. Occipital location most common in Western hemisphere, frontoethmoidal location most common site in Southeast Asians. Other sites include parietal and sphenoid bones. Cephaloceles can also result from trauma or surgery.
Neurofibromatosis type 1 (NF1) osseous dysplasia/ meningeal ectasia ▷ *Fig. 3.2*	NF1 associated with focal ectasia of intracranial dura, widening of internal auditory canals from dural ectasia, and dural and temporal lobe protrusion into orbit through a bony defect (bony hypoplasia of the greater sphenoid wing).	Autosomal dominant disorder (1/2500 births) representing the most common type of neurocutaneous syndromes, associated with neoplasms of the central and peripheral nervous systems and skin. Also associated with meningeal and skull dysplasias.
Neoplastic		
Meningioma ▷ *Fig. 3.3a, b*	Extra-axial dural-based lesions, well circumscribed; supratentorial > infratentorial, parasagittal > convexity > sphenoid ridge > parasellar > posterior fossa > optic nerve sheath > intraventricular; intermediate attenuation; usually prominent contrast enhancement, with or without calcifications, adjacent skull hyperostosis.	Most common extra-axial tumor, usually benign; typically occurs in adults older than age 40 y; women > men. Multiple meningiomas seen with neurofibromatosis type 2; can result in compression of adjacent brain parenchyma, encasement of arteries, and compression of dural venous sinuses; rarely invasive/malignant types.

(continues on page 166)

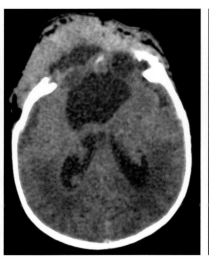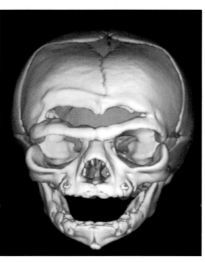

b

Fig. 3.1a, b   Cephalocele. Axial computed tomography (CT) image (**a**) shows a frontal meningoencephalocele that traverses a skull defect, as seen on the coronal CT image (**b**).

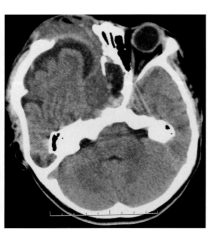

Fig. 3.2   Dural ectasia/osseous dysplasia. Axial CT image in a patient with neurofibromatosis type 1 shows the absence of the right greater sphenoid wing with protrusion of the meninges and right temporal lobe into the right orbit.

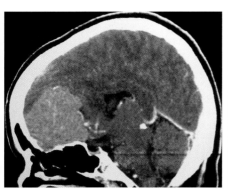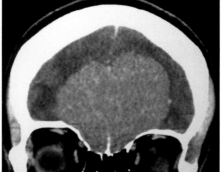

b

Fig. 3.3a, b   Meningioma. Sagittal (**a**) and coronal (**b**) postcontrast images show an enhancing meningioma along the olfactory groove.

Table 3.1 (Cont.) Abnormalities involving the meninges

Lesions	CT Findings	Comments
Hemangiopericytoma ▷ *Fig. 3.4a, b*	Extra-axial mass lesions, often well circumscribed; intermediate attenuation; prominent contrast enhancement (may resemble meningiomas); with or without associated erosive bone changes.	Rare neoplasms in young adults (males > females) sometimes referred to as angioblastic meningioma or meningeal hemangiopericytoma; arise from vascular cells/pericytes; frequency of metastases > meningiomas.
Metastatic tumor ▷ *Fig. 3.5a, b*	Single or multiple well-circumscribed or poorly defined lesions involving the skull, dura, leptomeninges, brain, and/or choroid plexus; low to intermediate attenuation; usually with contrast enhancement, with or without bone destruction, with or without compression of neural tissue or vessels. Leptomeningeal tumor often best seen on postcontrast images.	Metastatic tumor may have variable destructive or infiltrative changes involving single or multiple sites of involvement. Primary tumors can be within or outside the CNS. Metastatic disease can result from hematogenous dissemination, direct extension from bone lesions, or via the CSF pathways.
Lymphoma	Single or multiple well-circumscribed or poorly defined lesions involving the skull, dura, and/or leptomeninges; low to intermediate attenuation; usually with contrast enhancement, with or without bone destruction. Leptomeningeal tumor often best seen on postcontrast images.	Extra-axial lymphoma may have variable destructive or infiltrative changes involving single or multiple sites of involvement.
Vascular		
Arterial aneurysm ▷ *Fig. 3.6*	**Saccular aneurysm:** Focal, well-circumscribed zone of low to intermediate attenuation; variable mixed attenuation if thrombosed; with or without calcifications. CTA shows contrast enhancement of the nonthrombosed aneurysm. **Giant aneurysm:** Focal, well-circumscribed structure with layers of low, intermediate, and high attenuation secondary to layers of thrombus of different ages, as well as a contrast-enhancing patent lumen if present. **Fusiform aneurysm:** Elongated and ectatic arteries; variable low to intermediate attenuation. **Dissecting aneurysms:** The involved arterial wall is thickened and has intermediate attenuation. CTA shows the narrowing or occlusion of the vessel lumen.	Abnormal fusiform or focal dilation of artery secondary to acquired/degenerative etiology, polycystic disease, connective tissue disease, atherosclerosis, trauma, infection (mycotic), oncotic, arteriovenous malformation (AVM), vasculitis, and drugs. Focal aneurysms are also referred to as saccular aneurysms, which typically occur at arterial bifurcations and are multiple in 20% of patients. Saccular aneurysms > 2.5 cm in diameter are referred to as giant aneurysms. Fusiform aneurysms are often related to atherosclerosis or collagen vascular disease (e.g., Marfan and Ehlers-Danlos syndromes). Dissecting aneurysms: hemorrhage occurs in the arterial wall from incidental or significant trauma.
AVM ▷ *Fig. 3.7a, b*	Lesions with irregular margins that can be located in the brain parenchyma (pia, dura, or both locations). AVMs contain multiple tubular vessels from patent arteries, as well as thrombosed vessels, areas of hemorrhage in various phases, calcifications, and gliosis. The venous portions often show contrast enhancement. CTA can provide additional detailed information about the nidus, feeding arteries, and draining veins, as well as the presence of associated aneurysms. Usually not associated with mass effect unless there is recent hemorrhage or venous occlusion.	Supratentorial AVMs occur more frequently (80%–90%) than infratentorial AVMs (10%–20%). Annual risk of hemorrhage. AVMs can be sporadic, congenital, or associated with a history of trauma. Multiple AVMs can be seen in syndromes: Rendu-Osler-Weber (AVMs in the brain and lungs and mucosal capillary telangiectasias) and Wyburn-Mason (AVMs in the brain and retina with cutaneous nevi).
Dural AVM	Dural AVMs contain multiple tortuous tubular vessels. The venous portions often show contrast enhancement. CTA can show patent portions of the vascular malformation and areas of venous sinus occlusion or recanalization. Usually not associated with mass effect unless there is recent hemorrhage or venous occlusion.	Dural AVMs are usually acquired lesions resulting from thrombosis or occlusion of an intracranial venous sinus with subsequent recanalization resulting in direct arterial to venous sinus communications. Transverse, sigmoid venous sinuses > cavernous sinus > straight, superior sagittal sinuses.

(continues on page 168)

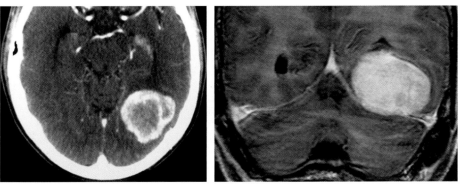

Fig. 3.4a, b   Hemangiopericytoma. Axial postcontrast CT image (**a**) and coronal postcontrast T1-weighted magnetic resonance imaging (MRI) (**b**) shows an enhancing extra-axial tumor.

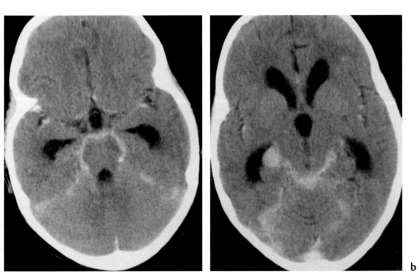

Fig. 3.5a, b   Metastatic tumor. Axial postcontrast images show an enhancing disseminated subarachnoid tumor from a pineoblastoma.

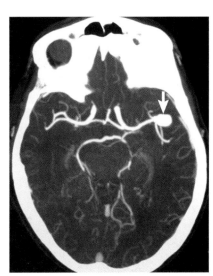

Fig. 3.6   Aneurysm. Axial computed tomography angiography (CTA) image shows an enhancing aneurysm at the lateral M1 portion of the left middle cerebral artery (arrow).

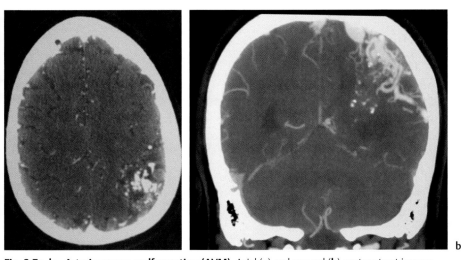

Fig. 3.7a, b   Arteriovenous malformation (AVM). Axial (**a**) and coronal (**b**) postcontrast images show a collection of tortuous enhancing blood vessels in the upper posterior left parietal lobe representing an AVM.

Table 3.1 (Cont.) Abnormalities involving the meninges

Lesions	CT Findings	Comments
Moyamoya ▷ *Fig. 3.8a, b*	Multiple tortuous tubular vessels can be seen in the basal ganglia and thalami secondary to dilated collateral arteries, with enhancement of these arteries. Often with contrast enhancement of the leptomeninges related to pial collateral vessels. Decreased or absent contrast enhancement of the supraclinoid portions of the internal carotid arteries and proximal middle and anterior cerebral arteries. CTA shows stenosis and occlusion of the distal internal carotid arteries with collateral arteries (lenticulostriate, thalamoperforate, and leptomeningeal) best seen after contrast administration enabling detection of slow blood flow.	Progressive occlusive disease of the intracranial portions of the internal carotid arteries with resultant numerous dilated collateral arteries arising from the lenticulostriate and thalamoperforate arteries, as well as other parenchymal, leptomeningeal, and transdural arterial anastomoses. Term translated as "puff of smoke," referring to the angiographic appearance of the collateral arteries (lenticulostriate, thalamoperforate). Usually nonspecific etiology, but can be associated with neurofibromatosis, radiation angiopathy, atherosclerosis, and sickle cell disease; usually children > adults in Asia.
Sturge-Weber syndrome ▷ *Fig. 3.9a–c*	Prominent localized unilateral leptomeningeal contrast enhancement usually in parietal and/or occipital regions in children; with or without gyral enhancement; mild localized atrophic changes in the brain adjacent to the pial angioma; with or without prominent medullary and/or subependymal veins; with or without ipsilateral prominence of choroid plexus. Gyral calcifications > 2 y; progressive cerebral atrophy in region of pial angioma.	Also known as encephalotrigeminal angiomatosis, neurocutaneous syndrome associated with ipsilateral "port wine" cutaneous lesion and seizures; results from persistence of primitive leptomeningeal venous drainage (pial angioma) and developmental lack of normal cortical veins, producing chronic venous congestion and ischemia.

Hemorrhagic (trauma, vascular malformation, or aneurysm)

Lesions	CT Findings	Comments
Epidural hematoma	Biconvex extra-axial hematoma located between the skull and dura; displaced dura has high attenuation. The CT attenuation of the hematoma depends on its age, size, hematocrit, and oxygen tension. With or without edema (low attenuation on CT) involving the displaced brain parenchyma; with or without subfalcine, uncal herniation. **Hyperacute hematomas:** **CT:** Can have high and/or mixed high and intermediate attenuation. **Acute hematoma:** **CT:** Can have high and/or mixed high and intermediate attenuation. ▷ *Fig. 3.10* **Subacute hematoma:** **CT:** Can have high and/or mixed high and intermediate attenuation.	Epidural hematomas usually result from trauma/tearing of an epidural artery (often the middle meningeal artery) or dural venous sinus; epidural hematomas do not cross cranial sutures; with or without skull fracture.

Hemorrhagic lesion

Lesions	CT Findings	Comments
Subdural hematoma	Crescentic extra-axial hematoma located in the potential space between the inner margin of the dura and outer margin of the arachnoid membrane. The CT attenuation of the hematoma depends on its age, size, hematocrit, and oxygen tension. With or without edema (low attenuation on CT) involving the displaced brain parenchyma; with or without subfalcine, uncal herniation. **Hyperacute hematoma:** **CT:** Can have high or mixed high, intermediate, and/or low attenuation. **Acute hematoma:** **CT:** Can have high or mixed high, intermediate, and/or low attenuation. ▷ *Fig. 3.11* **Subacute hematoma:** **CT:** Can have intermediate attenuation (isodense to brain) and/or low to intermediate attenuation.	Subdural hematomas usually result from trauma/stretching/tearing of cortical veins where they enter the subdural space to drain into dural venous sinuses; subdural hematomas do cross sites of cranial sutures; with or without skull fracture.
Subarachnoid hemorrhage ▷ *Fig. 3.12*	**Chronic hematoma:** **CT:** Acute subarachnoid hemorrhage typically appears as poorly defined zones with high attenuation in the leptomeninges within the sulci and basal cisterns. Usually become isodense or hypodense after 1 week unless there is rebleeding.	Extravasated blood in the subarachnoid space can result from ruptured arterial aneurysms or dural venous sinuses, vascular malformations, hypertensive hemorrhages, trauma, cerebral infarcts, coagulopathy, etc.

(continues on page 170)

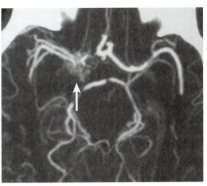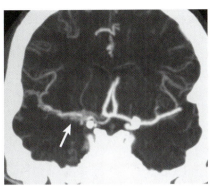

Fig. 3.8a, b Moyamoya. Axial (**a**) and coronal (**b**) CTA images show severe stenosis of the upper right internal carotid artery with collateral leptomeningeal and lenticulostriate vessels around the M1 segment of the right middle cerebral artery (arrows).

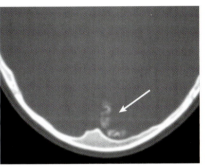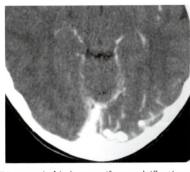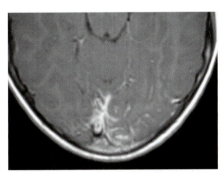

Fig. 3.9a–c Sturge-Weber syndrome. Axial CT images (**a,b**) show gyriform calcifications and an enhancing pial angioma in the left occipital region, the latter of which is also seen (arrow) on a postcontrast axial T1-weighted MRI (**c**).

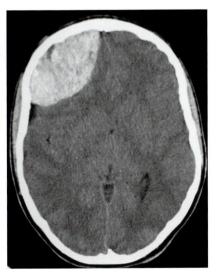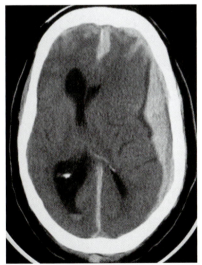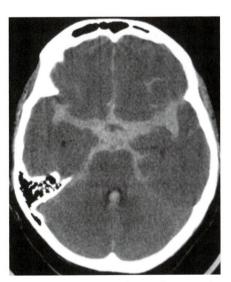

Fig. 3.10 Epidural hematoma. Acute epidural hematoma with high attenuation is seen in the right frontal region with compression of the right frontal lobe.

Fig. 3.11 Subdural hematoma. Subdural hematoma on the left is seen associated with subfalcine herniation rightward.

Fig. 3.12 Subarachnoid hemorrhage. Axial image shows diffuse high attenuation in the basal cisterns and subarachnoid space from acute hemorrhage.

Table 3.1   (Cont.) Abnormalities involving the meninges

Lesions	CT Findings	Comments
Inflammatory		
Epidural/subdural abscess/empyema ▷ *Fig. 3.13* ▷ *Fig. 3.14*	Epidural or subdural collections with low attenuation and thin linear peripheral zones of contrast enhancement.	Often results from complications related to sinusitis (usually frontal), meningitis, otitis media, ventricular shunts, or surgery. Can be associated with venous sinus thrombosis and venous cerebral or cerebellar infarctions, cerebritis, and brain abscess; mortality 30%.
Leptomeningeal infection/inflammation ▷ *Fig. 3.15* ▷ *Fig. 3.16a, b*	Single or multiple nodular contrast-enhancing lesions and/or focal or diffuse abnormal subarachnoid contrast enhancement. Leptomeningeal inflammation often best seen on postcontrast images.	Contrast enhancement in the intracranial subarachnoid space (leptomeninges) usually is associated with significant pathology (inflammation and/or infection vs neoplasm). Inflammation and/or infection of the leptomeninges can result from pyogenic, fungal, or parasitic diseases, as well as tuberculosis. Neurosarcoid results in granulomatous disease in the leptomeninges, producing similar patterns of subarachnoid enhancement.
Postsurgical pseudomeningocele ▷ *Fig. 3.17*	CSF-filled collection contiguous with the subarachnoid space with or without herniated brain tissue protruding through a surgical bony defect.	Usually not clinically significant unless it becomes large or infected.

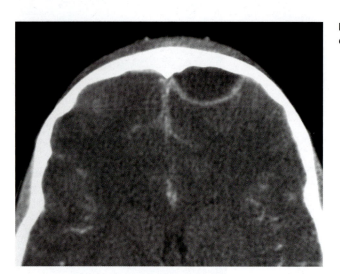

Fig. 3.13   Epidural empyema. Postcontrast axial image shows an epidural empyema in the left frontal region.

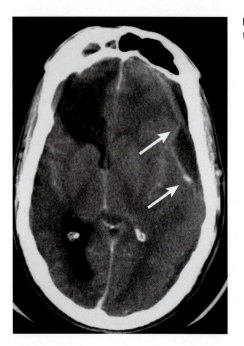

Fig. 3.14   Subdural empyema. Postcontrast axial image shows a subdural empyema on the left (arrows) and low attenuation of the anterior right frontal lobe from cerebritis.

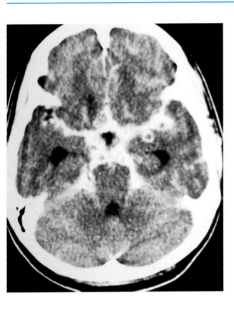

Fig. 3.15   Leptomeningeal infection/tuberculosis. Axial postcontrast image shows diffuse abnormal contrast enhancement of the basal meninges and subarachnoid space, as well as several ring-enhancing lesions.

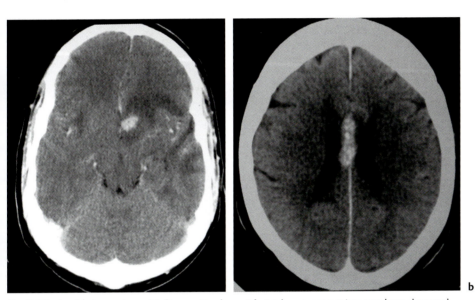

b

Fig. 3.16a, b   Leptomeningeal inflammation/sarcoid. Axial postcontrast images show abnormal enhancement involving the brain and falx from sarcoid granulomas.

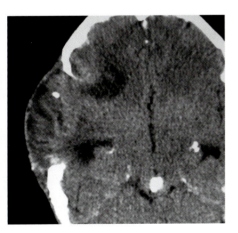

Fig. 3.17   Postsurgical pseudomeningoencephalocele. Axial image shows a right craniectomy defect through which the brain and meninges have herniated.

Table 3.2 Lesions involving the skull

Tumor/Tumorlike Lesion	CT Findings	Comments
Malignant neoplasms		
Metastatic tumor ▷ *Fig. 3.18*	Single or multiple well-circumscribed or poorly defined lesions involving the skull, dura, leptomeninges, brain, and/or choroid plexus; often show contrast enhancement, with or without bone destruction, with or without compression of neural tissue or vessels. Leptomeningeal tumor often best seen on postcontrast images.	May have variable destructive or infiltrative changes involving single or multiple sites of involvement. Primary tumors are usually from outside CNS.
Myeloma/plasmacytoma	Multiple (myeloma) or single (plasmacytoma) well-circumscribed or poorly defined lesions involving the skull and dura; low to intermediate attenuation; usually show contrast enhancement, with bone destruction.	Malignant plasma cell tumor; may have variable destructive or infiltrative changes involving the axial and/or appendicular skeleton.
Lymphoma	Single or multiple well-circumscribed or poorly defined lesions involving the skull, dura, and/or leptomeninges; low to intermediate attenuation; may show contrast enhancement, with or without bone destruction. Leptomeningeal tumor often best seen on postcontrast images.	Extra-axial lymphoma may have variable destructive or infiltrative changes involving single or multiple sites of involvement.
Leukemia	Single or multiple well-circumscribed or poorly defined lesions involving the skull, dura, and/or leptomeninges; low to intermediate attenuation; may show contrast enhancement, with or without bone destruction. Leptomeningeal tumor often best seen on postcontrast images.	Extra-axial lymphoma may have variable destructive or infiltrative changes involving single or multiple sites of involvement.
Chordoma ▷ *Fig. 3.19a–c*	Well-circumscribed, lobulated lesions; low to intermediate attenuation; usually shows contrast enhancement (usually heterogeneous); locally invasive associated with bone erosion/destruction, encasement of vessels and nerves; skull base/clivus common location, usually in the midline.	Rare, slow-growing tumors at the skull base; detailed anatomical display of extension of chordomas by CT and MRI is important for planning of surgical approaches.
Chondrosarcoma ▷ *Fig. 3.20a–c*	Lobulated lesions, low to intermediate attenuation, with or without matrix mineralization; can show contrast enhancement (often heterogeneous); locally invasive associated with bone erosion/destruction, encasement of vessels and nerves, skull base/petrous/occipital synchondrosis common location, usually off midline.	Rare, slow-growing, malignant cartilaginous tumors; detailed anatomical display of extension of chondrosarcomas by CT and MRI is important for planning of surgical approaches.
Osteogenic sarcoma ▷ *Fig. 3.21a, b*	Destructive lesions involving the skull base and calvarium; low to intermediate attenuation, usually with matrix mineralization/ossification; often shows contrast enhancement (usually heterogeneous).	Rare lesions involving the skull base and calvarium; more common than chondrosarcomas and Ewing sarcoma; locally invasive, high metastatic potential. Occurs in children as primary tumors and adults (associated with Paget disease, irradiated bone, chronic osteomyelitis, osteoblastoma, giant cell tumor, and fibrous dysplasia).

(continues on page 174)

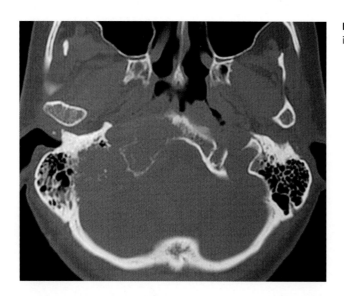

Fig. 3.18 Metastatic disease. Axial image shows a destructive tumor involving the right occipital bone and condyle and right mastoid bone.

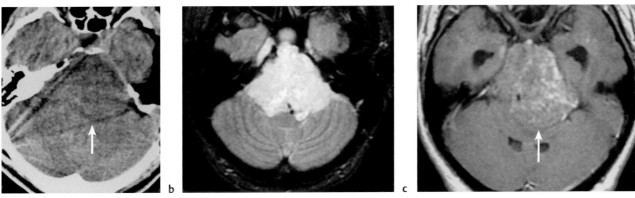

Fig. 3.19a–c   Chordoma. Axial CT image (**a**) shows the tumor along the endocranial surface of the clivus, which has high signal on axial fat-suppressed T2-weighted MRI (**b**) and shows heterogeneous contrast enhancement on axial T1-weighted MRI (**c**) (arrows).

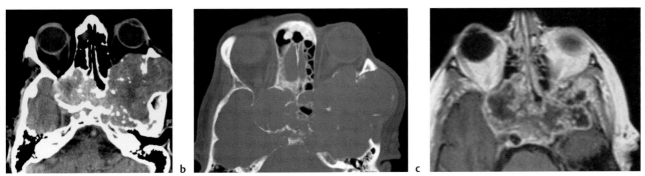

Fig. 3.20a–c   Chondrosarcoma. Axial CT images (**a,b**) show a destructive tumor involving the skull base and left orbit containing chondroid calcifications. The tumor shows a heterogeneous and lobular pattern of contrast enhancement on axial T1-weighted MRI (**c**).

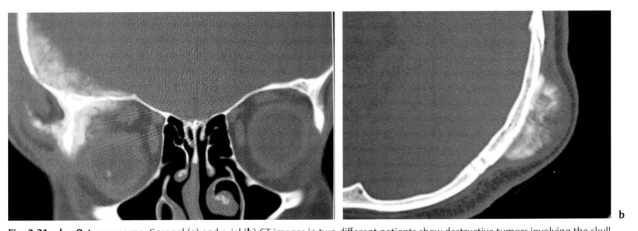

Fig. 3.21a, b   Osteosarcoma. Coronal (**a**) and axial (**b**) CT images in two different patients show destructive tumors involving the skull with extraosseous tumor containing malignant ossified matrix.

Table 3.2   (Cont.) Lesions involving the skull

Tumor/Tumorlike Lesion	CT Findings	Comments
Ewing sarcoma ▷ *Fig. 3.22*	Destructive lesions involving the skull base and calvarium; low to intermediate attenuation; can show contrast enhancement (usually heterogeneous).	Malignant bone tumors that usually occur between the ages of 5 and 30, males > females; rare lesions involving the skull base; locally invasive, high metastatic potential.
Sinonasal/nasopharyngeal carcinoma ▷ *Fig. 3.23a–c*	Destructive lesions in the nasal cavity, paranasal sinuses, nasopharynx; with or without intracranial extension via bone destruction or perineural spread; intermediate attenuation, can show contrast enhancement; large lesions (with or without necrosis and/or hemorrhage).	Occurs in adults usually older than age 55 y, men > women; associated with occupational or other exposure to nickel, chromium, mustard gas, radium, and manufacture of wood products.
Adenoid cystic carcinoma	Destructive lesions in the paranasal sinuses, nasal cavity, nasopharynx; with or without intracranial extension via bone destruction or perineural spread; intermediate attenuation, variable degrees of contrast enhancement.	Account for 10% of sinonasal tumors; arise in any location within sinonasal cavities; usually occurs in adults older than age 30 y.
Esthesioneuroblastoma	Locally destructive lesions with low to intermediate attenuation; usually shows contrast enhancement. Location: superior nasal cavity, ethmoid air cells with occasional extension into the other paranasal sinuses, orbits, anterior cranial fossa, cavernous sinuses.	Malignant tumors also referred to as olfactory neuroblastoma arise from olfactory epithelium in the superior nasal cavity. Occur in adolescents and adults, men > women.
Rhabdomyosarcoma	Lesions have low to intermediate attenuation with circumscribed and/or poorly defined margins. Areas of hemorrhage may be present. Lesions may have heterogeneous attenuation. Zones of edema may occur in the adjacent soft tissues. Tumors can be associated with destructive changes of adjacent bone; show variable degrees and patterns of contrast enhancement.	Malignant mesenchymal tumors with rhabdomyoblastic differentiation that occur primarily in soft tissue and only very rarely in bone. Occur most frequently in children.
Hemangiopericytoma	Extra-axial mass lesions, often well circumscribed; intermediate attenuation; usually show prominent contrast enhancement (may resemble meningiomas); with or without associated erosive bone changes.	Rare neoplasms in young adults (males > females) sometimes referred to as angioblastic meningioma or meningeal hemangiopericytoma; arise from vascular cells/pericytes; frequency of metastases > meningiomas.
Meningioma ▷ *Fig. 3.24a, b*	Extra-axial dural-based lesions, well-circumscribed; supratentorial > infratentorial; parasagittal > convexity > sphenoid ridge > parasellar > posterior fossa > optic nerve sheath > intraventricular; intermediate attenuation; typically show prominent contrast enhancement, with or without calcifications, with or without hyperostosis and/or invasion of adjacent skull.	Most common extra-axial tumors; usually benign neoplasms; typically occur in adults (> 40 y), women > men; multiple meningiomas seen with neurofibromatosis type II; can result in compression of adjacent brain parenchyma, encasement of arteries, and compression of dural venous sinuses; rarely invasive/malignant types.
Hemangioma ▷ *Fig. 3.25*	Circumscribed or poorly marginated structures (< 4 cm in diameter) in marrow of skull (often frontal bone) with intermediate attenuation; prominent bone trabeculae may be seen; typically show contrast enhancement, with or without widening of diploic compartment.	Benign skull lesions, adults (> 30 y).
Ossifying hemangioma ▷ *Fig. 3.26a–c*	Zone with low to intermediate attenuation; usually show prominent contrast enhancement.	Benign lesions within the temporal bone that involve the facial nerve and on CT are usually radiolucent, containing bone spicules. Lesions can be associated with slowly progressive or recurrent facial paralysis.

(continues on page 176)

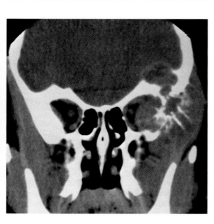

Fig. 3.22   Ewing sarcoma. Coronal image shows a destructive tumor involving the left frontal bone with extraosseous tumor extension with malignant periosteal reaction.

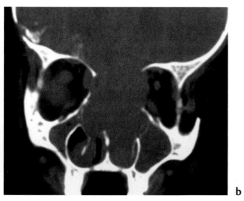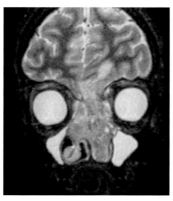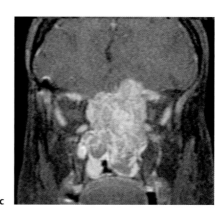

Fig. 3.23a–c   Sinonasal carcinoma. Coronal CT image (**a**) shows a tumor in the nasal cavity and ethmoid sinuses extending superiorly and laterally through zones of bone destruction. The tumor has high signal on coronal fat-suppresed T2-weighted MRI (**b**) and shows contrast enhancement on coronal fat-suppressed T1-weighted MRI (**c**).

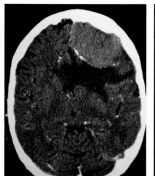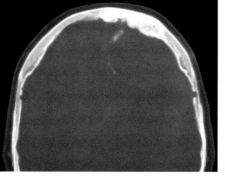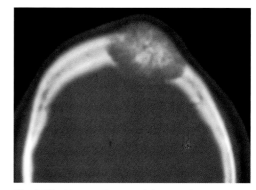

Fig. 3.24a, b   Meningioma. Axial postcontrast image (**a**) shows an enhancing meningioma in the left frontal region that has associated hyperostotic reaction involving the adjacent left frontal bone (**b**).

Fig. 3.25   Hemangioma. Axial image shows a circumscribed expansile lesion in the left frontal bone with prominent bone trabeculae.

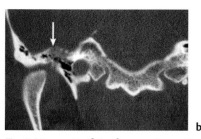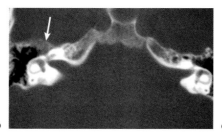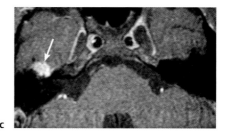

Fig. 3.26a–c   Ossifying hemangioma. Coronal (**a,b**) and axial (**c**) images show a small radiolucent lesion containing small bone spicules in the right temporal bone near the location of the geniculate ganglion of the seventh cranial nerve (arrows).

Table 3.2   (Cont.) Lesions involving the skull

Tumor/Tumorlike Lesion	CT Findings	Comments
Osteoid osteoma ▷ *Fig. 3.27*	Intraosseous circumscribed radiolucent lesion < 1.5 cm in diameter surrounded by bone sclerosis. Lesions often have low to intermediate attenuation centrally; often show contrast enhancement, surrounded by a peripheral rim of increased attenuation from associated bone sclerosis.	Benign osseous lesion containing a nidus of vascularized osteoid trabeculae surrounded by osteoblastic sclerosis that rarely occurs in the skull. Usually occurs between the ages of 5 and 25 y, males > females. Focal pain and tenderness associated with lesion that is often worse at night, relieved with aspirin.
Osteoblastoma	Expansile radiolucent lesion often > 1.5 cm surrounded by bone sclerosis. Lesions can show contrast enhancement.	Rare benign bone neoplasm (2% of bone tumors) usually occurs between the ages of 6 and 30 y; rarely involves the skull.
Enchondroma ▷ *Fig. 3.28a–c*	Lobulated intramedullary lesion that usually has low to intermediate attenuation and contains areas of chondroid matrix mineralization and fibrous strands. Lesions can show contrast enhancement.	Benign intramedullary lesions composed of hyaline cartilage; represent <10% of benign bone tumors. Enchondromas can be solitary (88%) or multiple (12%).
Chondroblastoma	Tumors often have fine lobular margins and typically have low to intermediate attenuation containing chondroid matrix mineralization (50%); contrast enhancement may be seen. Cortical destruction is uncommon.	Benign cartilaginous tumors with chondroblast-like cells and areas of chondroid matrix formation that rarely occur in the craniofacial bones. The squamous portion of the temporal bone is the most common location.
Pituitary adenoma ▷ *Fig. 3.29a, b*	**Macroadenomas (> 10 mm):** Commonly have intermediate attenuation, with or without necrosis, with or without cyst, with or without hemorrhage; usually show contrast enhancement, extension into suprasellar cistern with waist at diaphragma sella, with or without extension into cavernous sinus; occasionally invades skull base.	Common benign, slow-growing tumors representing <50% of sellar/parasellar neoplasms in adults. Can be associated with endocrine abnormalities related to oversecretion of hormones (prolactin > nonsecretory type > growth hormone > adrenocorticotropic hormone [ACTH]). Prolactinomas: women > men; growth hormone tumors: men > women.
Paraganglioma/glomus jugulare ▷ *Fig. 3.30a–c*	Ovoid or fusiform lesions with low to intermediate attenuation. Lesions can show contrast enhancement; often erode adjacent bone.	Benign encapsulated neuroendocrine tumors that arise from neural crest cells associated with autonomic ganglia (paraganglia) throughout the body. Lesions, also referred to as chemodectomas, are named according to location (glomus jugulare, tympanicum, vagale).

(continues on page 178)

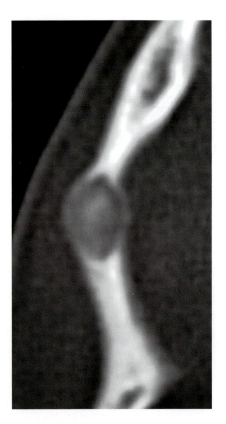

Fig. 3.27   Osteoid osteoma. Axial image shows an intraosseous circumscribed radiolucent lesion < 1.5 cm in diameter surrounded by bone sclerosis in the right frontal bone.

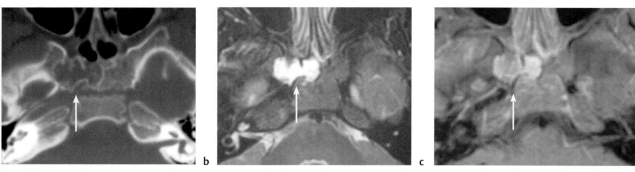

Fig. 3.28a–c   Enchondroma. Axial CT image (**a**) shows a lobulated radiolucent lesion in the right sphenoid bone that has high signal on axial T2-weighted MRI (**b**). The lesion shows contrast enhancement on axial fat-suppresed T1-weighted MRI (**c**) (arrows).

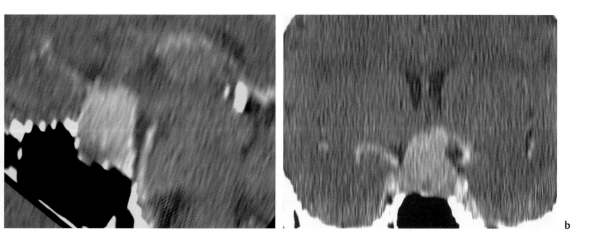

Fig. 3.29a, b   Pituitary adenoma. Sagittal (**a**) and coronal (**b**) postcontrast images show an enhancing pituitary macroadenoma that expands, remodels, and erodes the sella and sphenoid bone portion of the clivus.

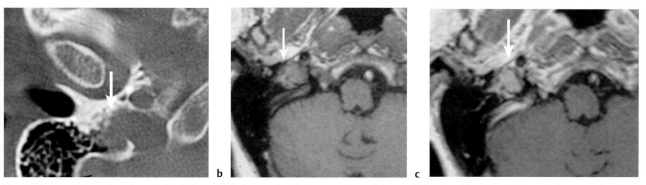

Fig. 3.30a–c   Glomus jugulare. Axial CT image (**a**) shows a locally destructive radiolucent lesion involving the right jugular foramen that has intermediate signal on axial T1-weighted MRI (**b**) and shows contrast enhancement on axial T1-weighted MRI (**c**) (arrows).

Table 3.2   (Cont.) Lesions involving the skull

Tumor/Tumorlike Lesion	CT Findings	Comments
Endolymphatic sac cystadenoma	Extra-axial retrolabyrinthine lesions involving the posterior petrous bone extending into the cerebellopontine angle cistern. Lesions can have low to intermediate attenuation and can show contrast enhancement. May contain blood products.	Rare solid and/or cystic benign or malignant papillary adenomatous tumors arising from the endolymphatic sac in children and adults. Tumors are slow growing and rarely metastasize; may be sporadic or associated with von Hippel-Lindau disease.
Other lesions		
Osteoma ▷ *Fig. 3.31a–c*	Well-circumscribed lesions involving the skull with high attenuation; typically show no contrast enhancement.	Benign proliferation of bone located in the skull or paranasal sinuses (frontal > ethmoid > maxillary > sphenoid).
Epidermoid ▷ *Fig. 3.32a–c*	Well-circumscribed, spheroid ectodermal inclusion cystic lesions in the skull associated with chronic bone erosion; low to intermediate attenuation; no contrast enhancement.	Nonneoplastic lesions filled with desquamated cells and keratinaceous debris involving the skull.
Dermoid	Well-circumscribed, spheroid lesions in the skull associated with chronic bone erosion; usually with low attenuation, no contrast enhancement, with or without fluid–fluid or fluid–debris levels.	Nonneoplastic ectodermal inclusion cystic lesions involving the skull filled with lipid material, cholesterol, desquamated cells, and keratinaceous debris.
Aneurysmal bone cyst ▷ *Fig. 3.33a, b*	Circumscribed extradural vertebral lesion usually involving the posterior elements with or without involvement of the vertebral body; with variable low, intermediate, or high attenuation; with or without lobulations, with or without one or multiple fluid/fluid levels.	Expansile blood/debris-filled lesions that may be primary or occur secondary to other bone lesions, such as giant cell tumor, fibrous dysplasia, and chondroblastoma. Most occur in patients older than 30 y. These lesions rarely involve the skull.
Giant cell reparative granuloma	Lesions are radiolucent and can have heterogeneous low to intermediate attenuation.	Giant cell reparative granulomas are also referred to as solid aneurysmal bone cysts (ABCs). Histologic appearance resembles brown tumors.
Arachnoid cyst	Well-circumscribed, extra-axial lesions with low attenuation similar to CSF; no contrast enhancement. Chronic erosive changes can be seen at the adjacent skull.	Nonneoplastic acquired, developmental, or congenital extra-axial cysts filled with CSF. Cysts can be small or large, asymptomatic or symptomatic.
Inflammatory lesions		
Pyogenic osteomyelitis ▷ *Fig. 3.34a, b*	Zones of abnormal decreased attenuation, focal sites of bone destruction, with or without complications including subgaleal empyema, epidural empyema, subdural empyema, meningitis, cerebritis, intra-axial abscess, and venous sinus thrombosis.	Osteomyelitis of the skull can result from surgery, trauma, hematogenous dissemination from another source of infection, or direct extension of infection from an adjacent site, such as the paranasal sinuses.
Eosinophilic granuloma ▷ *Fig. 3.35*	Single or multiple circumscribed soft tissue lesions in the marrow of the skull associated with focal bony destruction/erosion with extension extracranially, intracranially, or both. Lesions usually have low to intermediate attenuation; can show contrast enhancement, with or without enhancement of the adjacent dura.	Single lesions commonly seen in males > females younger than age 20 y; proliferation of histiocytes in medullary cavity with localized destruction of bone with extension in adjacent soft tissues. Multiple lesions associated with Letterer-Siwe disease (lymphadenopathy hepatosplenomegaly), children younger than 2 y; Hand-Schüller-Christian disease (lymphadenopathy, exophthalmos, diabetes insipidus), children ages 5 to 10 y.

(continues on page 180)

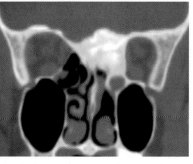
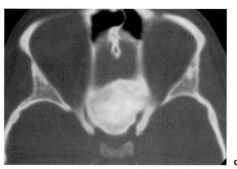
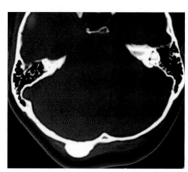

Fig. 3.31a–c Osteoma. Coronal (**a**) and axial (**b**) images show an osteoma involving the planum sphenoidale and ethmoid bone. Axial image in another patient (**c**) shows an osteoma at the outer table of the right occipital bone.

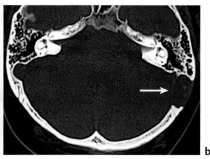
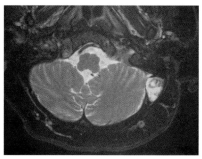
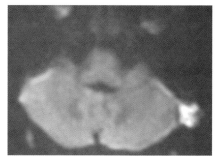

Fig. 3.32a–c Epidermoid. Axial CT image (**a**) shows a radiolucent lesion at the left occipital bone near the junction with the mastoid portion of the left temporal bone (arrow). The lesion has high signal on axial T2-weighted MRI (**b**) and axial diffusion-weighted MRI (**c**).

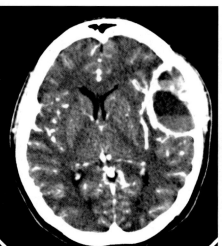
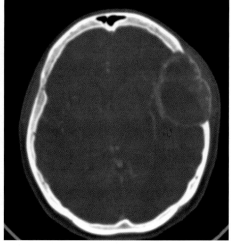

Fig. 3.33a, b Aneurysmal bone cyst. Axial images (**a,b**) show an expansile radiolucent lesion involving the left side of the skull containing fluid–fluid levels.

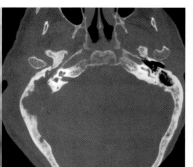
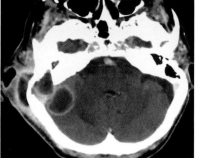

Fig. 3.34a, b Pyogenic abscess. Axial image (**a**) shows a destructive radiolucent lesion involving the right mastoid bone. Postcontrast CT image (**b**) shows an abscess in the lateral portion of the right cerebellar hemisphere, as well as abscesses in the mastoid bone and superficial soft tissues.

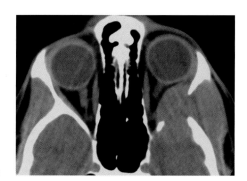

Fig. 3.35 Eosinophilic granuloma. Axial image shows a soft tissue lesion associated with bone destruction involving the left orbit and anterior portion of the left middle cranial fossa.

Table 3.2   (Cont.) Lesions involving the skull

Lesions	CT Findings	Comments
Sarcoidosis	Sarcoid lesions within marrow can be multiple or solitary, with or without bone expansion and/or erosions or areas of destruction of the inner and/or outer tables with extension intracranially or into the extracranial soft tissues. Lesions can have circumscribed and/or indistinct margins and usually have low to intermediate attenuation signal; can show variable degrees of contrast enhancement.	Chronic systemic granulomatous disease of unknown etiology in which noncaseating granulomas occur in various tissues and organs, including bone.
Paranasal sinus mucocele ▷ *Fig. 3.36a, b*	Circumscribed expansile lesion within a paranasal sinus that has variable low, intermediate, and/or high attenuation depending on contents of mucus, inspissated mucus, and protein concentration.	Lesions occurring from chronic obstruction of a paranasal sinus ostium that results in outward expansion of the osseous margins from remodeling secondary to increased pressure from accumulated secretions from the sinus mucosa. Mucoceles occur most commonly in the frontal sinuses, followed by the ethmoid, maxillary, and sphenoid sinuses.
Cholesterol granuloma ▷ *Fig. 3.37a, b*	Circumscribed lesion measuring between 2 and 4 cm in the marrow of the petrous bone often associated with mild bone expansion. Lesions usually have low attenuation.	Lesions seen in young and middle-aged adults and occur when there is obstruction of mucosal-lined air cells in the petrous bone. Multiple cycles of hemorrhage and granulomatous reaction result in accumulation of cyst contents with cholesterol granules, chronic inflammatory cells, red blood cells, hemosiderin, fibrous tissue, and debris.
Acquired		
Aneurysm	Focal, circumscribed lesion with low to intermediate and/or high attenuation. CTA shows contrast enhancement of nonthrombosed portions of lumens of aneurysms.	Abnormal dilation of artery secondary to acquired/degenerative cause, connective tissue disease, atherosclerosis, trauma, infection (mycotic), AVM, drugs, and vasculitis.
Postsurgical pseudomeningocele ▷ *Fig. 3.38*	CSF-filled collection contiguous with the subarachnoid space protruding through a surgical bony defect. Gliotic brain tissue may also accompany the dural protrusion.	Usually not clinically significant unless it becomes large or infected.
Paget disease ▷ *Fig. 3.39*	Expansile sclerotic/lytic process involving the skull with mixed intermediate to high attenuation. Irregular/indistinct borders are seen between marrow and inner margins of the outer and inner tables of the skull.	Usually seen in older adult;, can result in narrowing of neuroforamina with cranial nerve compression, basilar impression, with or without compression of brainstem.
Fibrous dysplasia ▷ *Fig. 3.40*	Expansile process involving the skull with mixed intermediate and high attenuation, often in a "ground glass" appearance; can show contrast enhancement.	Usually seen in adolescents and young adults; can result in narrowing of neuroforamina with cranial nerve compression, facial deformities, mono- and polyostotic forms with or without endocrine abnormalities, such as with McCune-Albright syndrome (precocious puberty).
Hematopoietic disorders	Enlargement of the diploic space with red marrow hyperplasia and thinning of the inner and outer tables.	Thickening of diploic space related to erythroid hyperplasia from anemia related to sickle cell disease, thalassemia major, and hereditary spherocytosis. Similar findings of red marrow expansion can be seen with polycythemia rubra.

(continues on page 182)

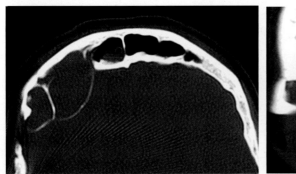
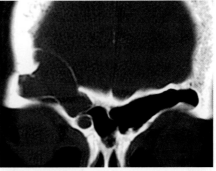

Fig. 3.36a, b   Paranasal mucocele. Axial (**a**) and coronal (**b**) images show expansion and thinning of the inner table of the skull from a mucus-containing obstructed right frontal sinus.

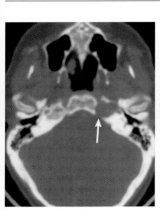 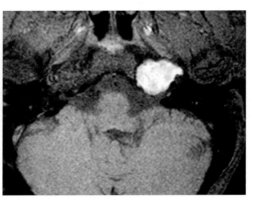

b

Fig. 3.37a, b   Cholesterol granuloma. Axial CT image (**a**) shows a radiolucent lesion in the left petrous apex (arrow) that has high signal on axial fat-suppressed T1-weighted MRI (**b**).

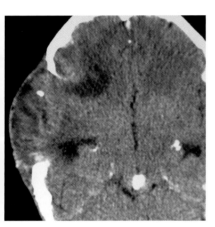

Fig. 3.38   Postsurgical meningocele. Axial image shows a right craniectomy defect through which the brain and meninges have herniated.

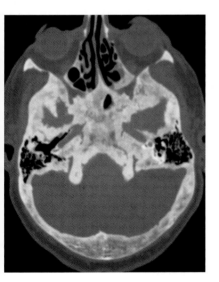

Fig. 3.39   Paget disease. Axial image in an 84-year-old man shows enlargement of the occipital bone and skull base with blurring of the margins of the inner and outer tables with the diploic space.

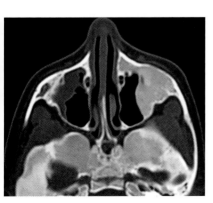

Fig. 3.40   Fibrous dysplasia. Axial image in a patient with polyostotic fibrous dysplasia shows expansile bone abnormalities with a "ground glass" appearance involving the skull base and left maxilla.

Table 3.2   (Cont.) Lesions involving the skull

Lesions	CT Findings	Comments
Osteopetrosis ▷ *Fig. 3.41a, b*	Findings include generalized bone sclerosis, hyperostosis resulting in thickening of the skull, as well as narrowing of the foramina and optic canals.	Heterogeneous group of bone disorders with defective resorption of primary spongiosa and mineralized cartilage from osteoclast dysfunction. Results in failure of conversion of immature woven bone into strong lamellar bone and pathologic fractures. In the severe autosomal recessive form, medullary crowding from immature sclerotic bone can result in anemia, thrombocytopenia, and immune dysfunction leading to death.
Hyperostosis frontalis ▷ *Fig. 3.42*	Expansion of the medullary portion of the upper frontal bone extending intracranially with well-defined cortical margin of the inner table of the skull.	Benign bilateral bone overgrowth involving the inner table of the frontal bone; most often seen in elderly women.
Trauma		
Cephalohematoma ▷ *Fig. 3.43a, b*	Hematoma located beneath periosteum of outer table; does not cross suture lines; with or without skull fracture; with or without subdural hematoma.	Results from birth trauma (complication of forceps delivery); associated with 1% of births.
Fracture ▷ *Fig. 3.44*	**Nondisplaced/nondepressed skull fractures:** With or without subgaleal hematoma, with or without epidural hematoma, with or without subdural hematoma, with or without subarachnoid hemorrhage. **Depressed skull fracture:** Angulation and internal displacement of fractured skull, with or without subgaleal hematoma, with or without epidural hematoma, with or without subdural hematoma, with or without subarachnoid hemorrhage.	Traumatic fractures of the skull can involve the calvarium or skull base; significant complications that can result include epidural hematoma, subdural hematoma, subarachnoid hemorrhage, CSF leakage/rhinorrhea, and otorrhea.
Congenital abnormalities		
Cephaloceles (meningoceles or meningoencephaloceles) ▷ *Fig. 3.45a, b*	Defect in skull through which there is herniation of meninges and CSF (meningocele) or meninges, CSF/ventricles, and brain tissue (meningoencephaloceles).	Congenital malformation involving lack of separation of neuroectoderm from surface ectoderm with resultant localized failure of bone formation. Occipital location most common in Western hemisphere; frontoethmoidal location most common site in Southeast Asians. Other sites are parietal and sphenoid bones. Cephaloceles can also result from trauma or surgery.
Chiari II malformation/lückenschädel skull ▷ *Fig. 3.46a, b*	Multifocal scalloping at the inner table of the skull.	Also referred to as lacunar skull or craniolacunae, dysplasia of membranous skull/calvarium in Chiari II with multifocal thinning of the inner table from nonossified fibrous bone from abnormal collagen development and ossification.

(continues on page 184)

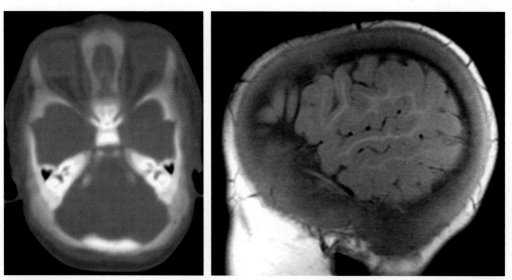

a   b

Fig. 3.41a, b   Osteopetrosis. Axial CT image (**a**) shows hyperostosis resulting in thickening of the skull. Sagittal T1-weighted MRI (**b**) shows expansion of the marrow spaces of the skull.

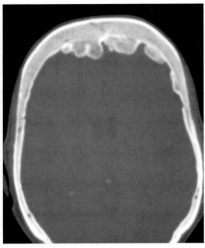

Fig. 3.42   Hyperostosis frontalis. Axial image shows expansion of the medullary portion of the upper frontal bone extending intracranially.

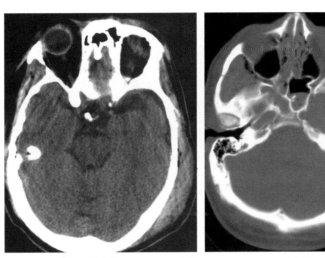

Fig. 3.43a, b   Cephalohematoma. Axial images show a superficial hematoma on the left.

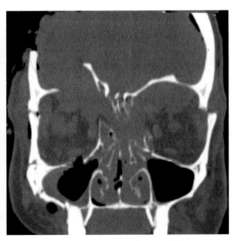

Fig. 3.44   Fracture. Coronal image shows comminuted fractures involving both frontal bones, orbits, and maxilla (Le Fort type III).

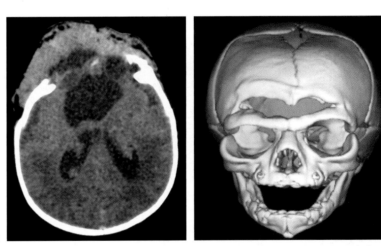

Fig. 3.45a, b   Cephalocele. Axial CT image (**a**) shows a frontal meningoencephalocele that traverses a skull defect, as seen on the coronal CT image (**b**).

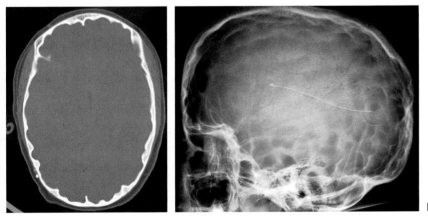

Fig. 3.46a, b   Lückenschädel. Axial CT image (**a**) and lateral radiograph (**b**) in a patient with a Chiari II malformation show multifocal scalloping at the inner table of the skull.

Table 3.2   (Cont.) Lesions involving the skull

Lesions	CT Findings	Comments
Craniosynostosis ▷ *Fig. 3.47a, b* ▷ *Fig. 3.48a–c* ▷ *Fig. 3.49a, b*	Premature closure; metopic suture results in trigonocephaly (wedge-shaped skull), sagittal suture results in scaphocephaly (long, narrow-shaped skull), coronal or lambdoid suture results in oxycephaly, and unilateral closure of coronal or lambdoid sutures result in plagiocephaly.	Premature closure of the cranial sutures results in abnormal skull shape. Can be primary from abnormal development or secondary from external forces of intrauterine compression, lack of brain growth, and/or teratogens; 15% are associated with other anomalies; 80% involve one suture. Closure of multiple sutures is often associated with genetic etiology.
Achondroplasia ▷ *Fig. 3.50*	The calvarium/skull vault is enlarged in association with a small skull base and narrow foramen magnum. Cervicomedullary myelopathy and/or hydrocephalus can result from a narrowed foramen magnum.	Autosomal dominant mutation (fibroblast growth factor gene 3; 1/10 000 births) in which the mutated gene impairs endochondral bone formation, resulting in decreased longitudinal lengthening of long bones.
Basiocciput hypoplasia ▷ *Fig. 3.51*	Hypoplasia of the lower clivus results in primary basilar invagination.	The lower clivus is a portion of the occipital bone (basiocciput) that is composed of four fused sclerotomes. Failure of formation of one or more of these sclerotomes results in a shortened clivus and primary basilar invagination (dens extending > 5 mm above the Chamberlain line).

(continues on page 186)

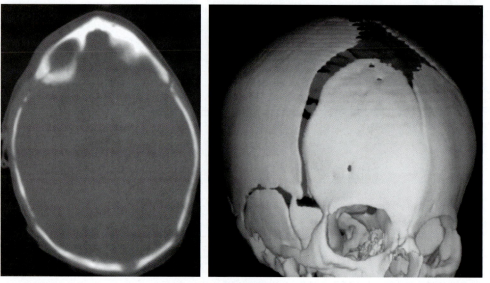

Fig. 3.47a, b   Craniosynostosis, trigonocephaly in a 15-day-old male infant. Axial (**a**) and oblique volume-rendered CT (**b**) images show premature fusion of the metopic suture with a wedge-shaped skull.

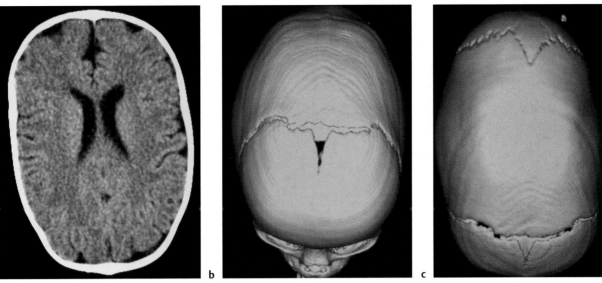

Fig. 3.48a–c   Craniosynostosis, dolichocephaly in a 3-year-old female infant. Axial (**a**) and volume-rendered CT (**b,c**) images show scaphocephaly (long, narrow-shaped skull) from premature fusion of the sagittal suture.

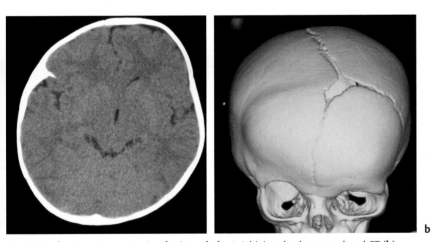

Fig. 3.49a, b   Craniosynostosis, plagiocephaly. Axial (**a**) and volume-rendered CT (**b**) images show an asymmetric head shape from premature closure of one side of the coronal suture.

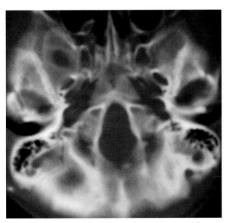

Fig. 3.50   Achondroplasia in a 7-year-old boy. Axial image shows an abnormally small foramen magnum.

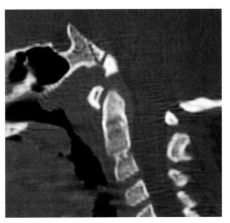

Fig. 3.51   Basiocciput hypoplasia in an 8-year-old boy. Sagittal image shows only rudimentary formation of the occipital portion of the clivus below the spheno-occipital synchondrosis resulting in basilar invagination.

Table 3.2   (Cont.) Lesions involving the skull

Lesions	CT Findings	Comments
Condylus tertius ▷ *Fig. 3.52*	Ossicle seen between the lower portion of a shortened basiocciput and the dens/atlas.	Condylus tertius or third occipital condyle results from lack of fusion of the lowermost fourth sclerotome (proatlas) with the adjacent portions of the clivus. This third occipital condyle can form a pseudojoint with the anterior arch of C1 and/or dens and can be associated with decreased range of movement.
Atlanto-occipital assimilation	Often seen as fusion of the occipital condyle with one or both lateral masses of C1.	Occurs from failure of segmentation of the occipital condyle and the C1 vertebra.
Neurofibromatosis type 1 (NF1) ▷ *Fig. 3.53a, b*	NF1 associated with focal ectasia of intracranial dura, widening of internal auditory canals from dural ectasia, dural and temporal lobe protrusion into orbit through bony defect (bony hypoplasia of greater sphenoid wing), bone malformation, or erosion from plexiform neurofibromas.	Autosomal dominant disorder (1/2500 births) representing the most common type of neurocutaneous syndromes; associated with neoplasms of central and peripheral nervous systems and skin. Also associated with meningeal and skull dysplasias.

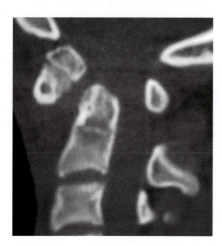

Fig. 3.52   Condylus tertius. Sagittal image shows an ossicle seen between the lower portion of a shortened basiocciput adjacent to the dens and atlas.

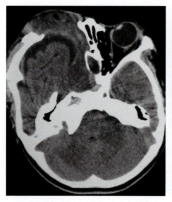
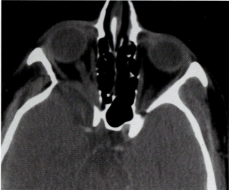

a   b

Fig. 3.53a, b   Neurofibromatosis type 1, dural ectasia/osseous dysplasia. Axial images in two patients show bone dysplasia at the greater sphenoid wings on the right with protrusion of the meninges and brain into the right orbits.

4 Vascular Lesions

Steven P. Meyers

Contrast-enhanced computed tomographic (CT) imaging is a useful imaging modality for evaluating normal and abnormal blood vessels. The appearance of blood vessels on contrast-enhanced CT images depends on various factors, such as the size of the blood vessel; the concentration of contrast material within the vessels; and the size, shape, and orientation of the vessels relative to the image plane.

By employing rapid acquisition of CT data timed to when intravenous contrast is within the blood vessels of interest using multidetector CT scanners, assessments can be made of the sizes and shapes of arterial lumens, as well as the wall thicknesses and the presence of fatty and/or calcified atherosclerotic plaques. CT angiography (CTA) can also be used to evaluate patency or occlusion of intracranial venous sinuses and veins. The acquired image data from this method can be postprocessed with computer algorithms to generate the CTA images in a display format similar to conventional arteriograms and venograms. Two commercially available types of postprocessing are the maximum intensity projection (MIP) technique and surface-rendering/three-dimensional (3D) volume imaging. The MIP CTA images can be displayed in any plane of obliquity on film or as a movie loop. Surface rendering is another postprocessing method for CTA that shows 3D relationships by giving the displayed vessels shadowing and perspective. The 3D CTA images are projected in a similar fashion to the MIP method. Surface rendering has been shown to be useful in showing spatial relationships between vessels on a single coronal image, allowing differentiation of adjacent and overlapping vessels.

CTA has proven to be clinically useful in the evaluation of the carotid arteries in the neck, intracranial arteries, veins, and dural venous sinuses. Disorders such as aneurysms, arteriovenous malformations, arterial occlusions, and dural venous sinus thromboses can be seen with CTA.

Table 4.1 Congenital/developmental vascular anomalies/variants

Lesions	CTA Findings	Comments
Persistent fetal origin of posterior cerebral artery ▷ *Fig. 4.1*	Large posterior communicating artery supplying the posterior cerebral artery; associated with hypoplasia or absence of connection between the basilar artery and the ipsilateral posterior cerebral artery.	Represents persistence of embryonic configuration; common vascular variant seen in ~20% of arteriograms.
Hypoplasia of the A1 segment of the anterior cerebral artery	Hypoplasia or absent A1 segment associated with a patent anterior communicating artery supplying blood to the ipsilateral A2 segment.	Anatomical variant seen in ~10% of arteriograms.
Persistent trigeminal artery ▷ *Fig. 4.2a, b*	Anomalous anastomosis connecting the internal carotid artery in the cavernous sinus to the basilar artery at the level of the trigeminal nerve; basilar artery below anastomosis and vertebral arteries are usually small.	Most common type of anomalous carotid/basilar anastomosis (0.5% of cerebral arteriograms); failure of involution of persistent embryonic circulatory configuration. Associated with increased incidence of aneurysms and vascular malformations. Other less common types of anomalous carotid/basilar anastomoses include persistent hypoglossal artery (adjacent to cranial nerve XII), persistent otic artery, and proatlantal intersegment artery.
Duplications of cerebral, carotid, vertebral, or basilar arteries ▷ *Fig. 4.3*	Duplication of arteries usually occurs as two parallel arteries from two separate origins, as seen on CTA, MRA, and conventional angiography.	Duplicated arteries have two origins and variable courses with or without eventual fusion. Duplication of intracranial or cervical arteries is an infrequent type of vascular variant compared with anomalies involving other intracranial arteries. Other less common types of variants include fenestrations and accessory arteries.
Arterial fenestration ▷ *Fig. 4.4a–c*	Duplication of a portion of an artery whose main trunk is derived from a single origin, as seen on CTA, MRA, and conventional angiography.	Developmental variation when there are double segments involving portions of the vertebral, basilar, or carotid arteries. With arterial fenestration, a vessel with a single origin divides into two parallel segments along its course.
Vein of Galen aneurysm ▷ *Fig. 4.5a–c*	Multiple tortuous contrast-enhancing vessels involving choroidal and thalamoperforate arteries, internal cerebral veins, vein of Galen (aneurysmal formation), straight and transverse venous sinuses, and other adjacent veins and arteries. The venous portions often show contrast enhancement. CTA shows contrast enhancement in patent portions of the vascular malformation.	Heterogeneous group of vascular malformations with arteriovenous shunts and dilated deep venous structures draining into and from an enlarged vein of Galen, with or without hydrocephalus, with or without hemorrhage, with or without macrocephaly, with or without parenchymal vascular malformation components, with or without seizures, high-output congestive heart failure in neonates.

(continues on page 190)

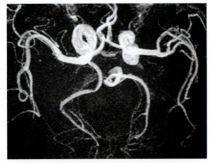

Fig. 4.1 Persistent fetal origin of the right posterior cerebral artery. Axial magnetic resonance angiography (MRA) image shows the right posterior cerebral artery receiving its blood flow from the right posterior communicating artery.

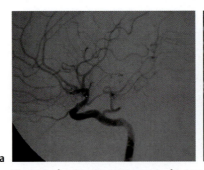
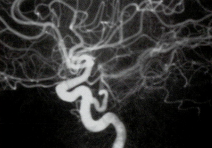

a

Fig. 4.2a, b Persistent trigeminal artery. Conventional angiograms show an arterial anastomosis connecting the internal carotid artery in the posterior portion of the cavernous sinus to the basilar artery at the level of the trigeminal nerve.

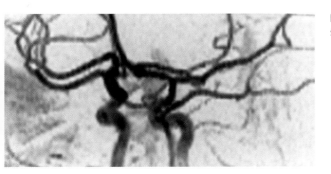

Fig. 4.3   Duplications of the middle cerebral arteries. MRA image shows duplications of both middle cerebral arteries.

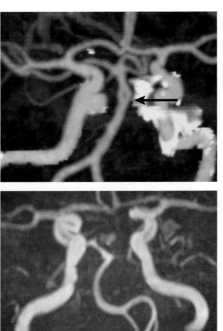
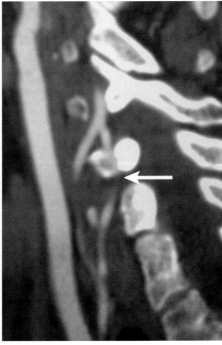

Fig. 4.4a–c   Arterial fenestration. Coronal computed tomography angiography (CTA) images in two different patients show fenestrations at the upper basilar artery (**a**) and upper left vertebral artery (**b,c**) (arrows).

c

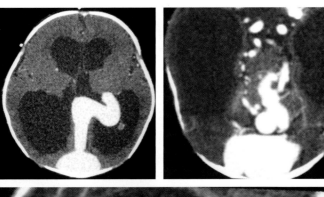
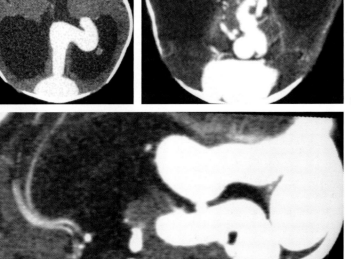

Fig. 4.5a–c   Vein of Galen aneurysm. Postcontrast axial image (**a**) in a neonate shows abnormal enlargement of the vein of Galen, straight venous sinus, and torcula Herophili. Sagittal (**b**) and axial (**c**) CTA images show the vein of Galen malformation with multiple dilated vessels adjacent to the brainstem.

c

Table 4.1   (Cont.) Congenital/developmental vascular anomalies/variants

Lesions	CTA Findings	Comments
Venous angioma (developmental venous anomaly) ▷ *Fig. 4.6*	No abnormality or small, slightly hyperdense zone prior to contrast administration. Contrast enhancement seen in a slightly prominent vein draining a collection of small veins.	Considered an anomalous venous formation typically not associated with hemorrhage; usually an incidental finding except when associated with cavernous hemangioma.
Sturge-Weber syndrome ▷ *Fig. 4.7a, b*	Prominent localized unilateral leptomeningeal enhancement usually in parietal and/or occipital regions in children, with or without gyral enhancement; mild localized atrophic changes in brain adjacent to the pial angioma, with or without prominent medullary and/or subependymal veins, with or without ipsilateral prominence of choroid plexus. Gyral calcifications > 2 y, progressive cerebral atrophy in region of pial angioma.	Also known as encephalotrigeminal angiomatosis, neurocutaneous syndrome associated with ipsilateral "port wine" cutaneous lesion and seizures; results from persistence of primitive leptomeningeal venous drainage (pial angioma) and developmental lack of normal cortical veins, producing chronic venous congestion and ischemia.
Moyamoya ▷ *Fig. 4.8a, b*	Multiple tortuous, small, enhancing vessels may be seen in the basal ganglia and thalami secondary to dilated collateral arteries, with enhancement of these arteries related to slow flow within these collateral arteries versus normal-sized arteries. Contrast enhancement of the leptomeninges related to pial collateral vessels; decreased or absent contrast enhancement in the supraclinoid portions of the internal carotid arteries and proximal middle and anterior cerebral arteries. CTA shows stenosis and occlusion of the distal internal carotid arteries with collateral arteries (lenticulostriate, thalamoperforate, and leptomeningeal); best seen after contrast administration enabling detection of slow blood flow.	Progressive occlusive disease of the intracranial portions of the internal carotid arteries with resultant numerous dilated collateral arteries arising from the lenticulostriate and thalamoperforate arteries, as well as other parenchymal, leptomeningeal, and transdural arterial anastomoses; term translated as "puff of smoke," referring to the angiographic appearance of the collateral arteries (lenticulostriate, thalamoperforate); usually nonspecific etiology, but can be associated with neurofibromatosis, radiation angiopathy, atherosclerosis, and sickle cell disease; usually children > adults in Asia.
Thoracic outlet syndrome (TOS) ▷ *Fig. 4.9a–c*	Cervical ribs or fibrous bands located adjacent to the subclavian artery, subclavian vein, and/or brachial plexus.	Signs and symptoms of TOS occur from compression of the brachial plexus (neurogenic TOS), subclavian artery (arterial TOS), and/or subclavian vein (venous TOS). Neurogenic TOS accounts for ~90% of TOS cases. Compression of the thoracic outlet structures can be static or positional. Causes of the compression include cervical ribs, fibrous bands, hypertrophy, and anomalies involving the scalene muscles.

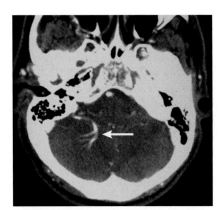

Fig. 4.6   Venous angioma. Axial postcontrast image shows an enhancing venous angioma in the right cerebellar hemisphere (arrow).

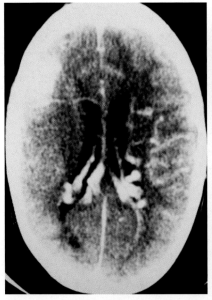
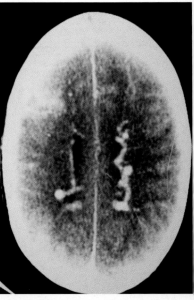

a

Fig. 4.7a, b   Sturge-Weber syndrome. Postcontrast axial images show dilated enhancing medullary and ependymal veins.

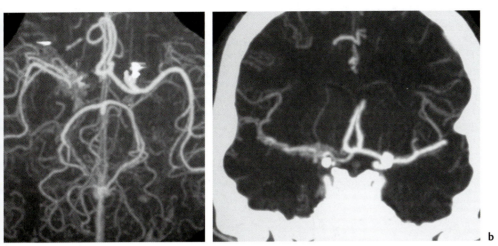

Fig. 4.8a, b   Moyamoya. Axial (**a**) and coronal (**b**) CTA images show severe stenosis of the upper right internal carotid artery with collateral leptomeningeal and lenticulostriate vessels around the M1 segment of the right middle cerebral artery.

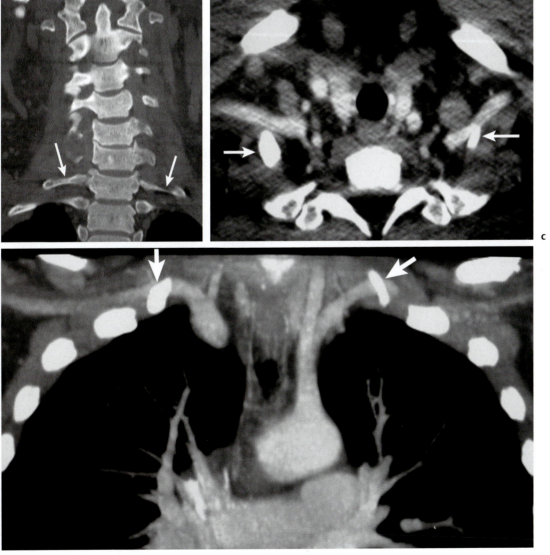

Fig. 4.9a–c   Thoracic outlet syndrome. Coronal image (**a**) shows bilateral cervical ribs that impress on the subclavian arteries, as seen on postcontrast computed tomography (CT) images (**b,c**) (arrows).

Table 4.2 Acquired vascular disease

Lesions	CTA Findings	Comments
Stenosis/occlusive vascular disease		
Arterial stenosis/occlusion ▷ *Fig. 4.10* ▷ *Fig. 4.11* ▷ *Fig. 4.12* ▷ *Fig. 4.13* ▷ *Fig. 4.14a, b*	Focal narrowing (stenosis) or absence (occlusion) of luminal contrast enhancement on CTA in artery, with or without narrowing of flow signal distal to site of stenosis.	Arterial stenosis or occlusion may result from atherosclerosis, emboli, fibromuscular disease/dysplasia, collagen vascular disease, coagulopathy, encasement by neoplasm, surgery, or radiation injury.
Subclavian steal syndrome ▷ *Fig. 4.15a–c*	CTA shows occlusion of the proximal subclavian artery with reconstitution beyond the occlusion via reversed blood flow from the ipsilateral vertebral artery.	Stenosis or occlusion of the proximal subclavian artery can cause reversal of blood flow of the ipsilateral vertebral artery to supply the subclavian artery distal to the stenosis. The reversed blood flow can result in signs of vertebrobasilar insufficiency (syncope, nausea, ataxia, vertigo, diplopia, headaches, etc.) elicited with exercise of the upper extremity on the same side where the stenosis/occlusion of the subclavian artery occurs.

(continues on page 194)

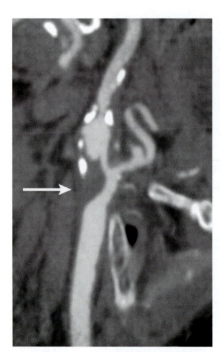

Fig. 4.10 Arterial stenosis. Sagittal CTA image shows a mostly fatty atherosclerotic plaque at the upper common carotid artery resulting in severe narrowing of the proximal internal carotid artery (arrow).

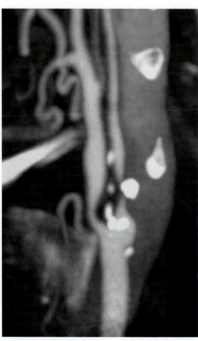

Fig. 4.11 Arterial stenosis. Sagittal CTA image shows a mixed fatty and calcified plaque causing severe stenosis of the proximal internal carotid artery.

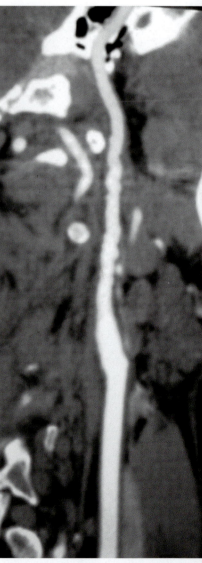

Fig. 4.12 Arterial stenosis. Sagittal CTA shows multifocal irregular wall thickening of the internal carotid artery from fibromuscular dysplasia.

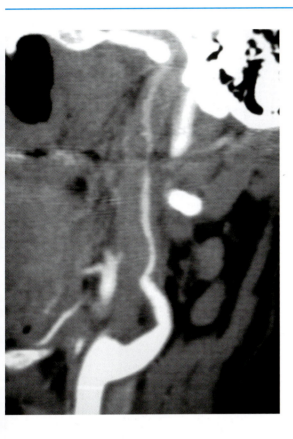

Fig. 4.13   Arterial stenosis. Sagittal CTA image shows marked narrowing of the lumen of the internal carotid artery ("string" sign) from dissection secondary to fibromuscular dysplasia.

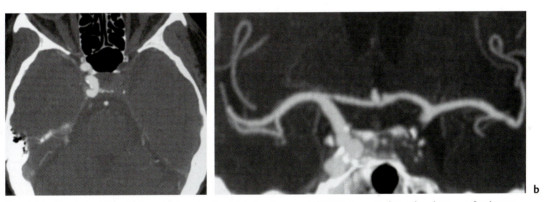

b

Fig. 4.14a, b   Arterial occlusion. Postcontrast axial (**a**) and coronal (**b**) CTA images show the absence of enhancement of the cavernous portion of the left internal carotid artery secondary to occlusion.

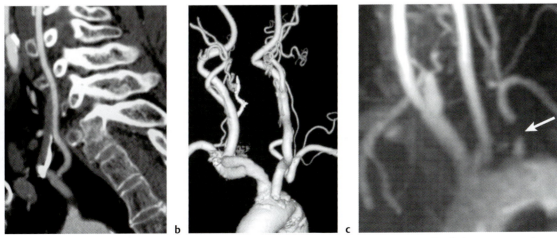

b   c

Fig. 4.15a–c   Subclavian steal syndrome. CTA images (**a,b**) show occlusion of the proximal left subclavian artery with retrograde blood flow from the vertebral artery, as also seen on the MRA image (**c**) (arrow).

Table 4.2   (Cont.) Acquired vascular disease

Lesions	CTA Findings	Comments
Arterial dissection ▷ *Fig. 4.16a–d*	The involved arterial wall is thickened in a circumferential or semilunar configuration and has intermediate attenuation. Lumen may be narrowed or occluded.	Arterial dissections can be related to trauma, collagen, vascular disease (e.g., Marfan and Ehlers-Danlos syndromes), or idiopathic. Hemorrhage occurs in the arterial wall and can cause stenosis, occlusion, and stroke.
Vasculitis ▷ *Fig. 4.17a–f*	Zones of arterial occlusion, and/or foci of stenosis and post-stenotic dilation. May involve large, medium, or small intracranial and extracranial arteries. with or without cerebral and/or cerebellar infarcts.	Uncommon mixed group of inflammatory diseases/disorders involving the walls of cerebral blood vessels. Can result from noninfectious etiology (polyarteritis nodosa, Wegener granulomatosis, giant cell arteritis, Takayasu arteritis, sarcoid, drug-induced, etc.) or be related to infectious causes (bacteria, fungi, TB, syphilis, viral).

(continues on page 196)

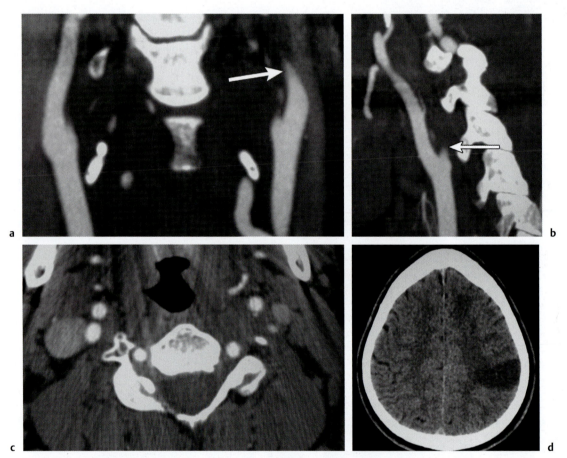

Fig. 4.16a–d   Arterial dissection. Coronal (**a**) and sagittal (**b**) CTA images show abrupt tapering of the proximal left internal carotid artery from an intramural hematoma/dissection (arrows). Axial postcontrast image (**c**) shows contrast enhancement in the left external carotid artery and absence of enhancement of the left internal carotid artery secondary to occlusion from the dissection. Axial CT image (**d**) shows a cerebral infarct in the vascular distribution of the left internal carotid artery.

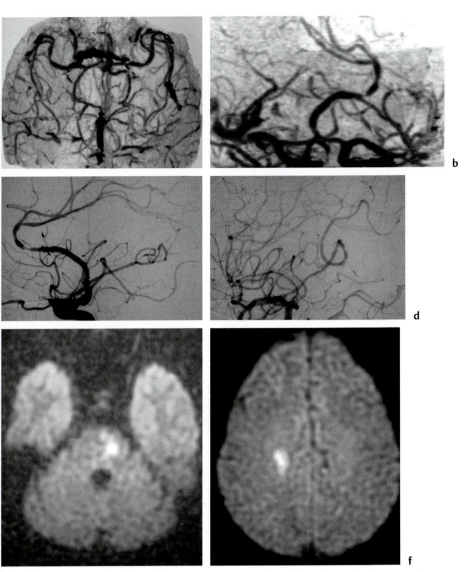

Fig. 4.17a–f   Vasculitis. Axial (**a**) and oblique coronal (**b**) CTA images show multiple zones of narrowing of the middle and anterior cerebral arteries from vasculitis, as seen on a conventional arteriogram image (**c,d**). Axial diffusion-weighted magnetic resonance imaging (MRI) shows high signal from restricted diffusion and acute ischemia in the pons (**e**) and right cerebral hemisphere (**f**).

Table 4.2   (Cont.) Acquired vascular disease

Lesions	CTA Findings	Comments
Intracranial venous sinus thrombosis ▷ *Fig. 4.18a-d*	CTA shows patent veins and venous sinuses to have high attenuation compared with zones of thrombus with lower attenuation.	Venous sinus occlusion may result from coagulopathies, encasement or invasion by neoplasm, dehydration, and adjacent infectious/inflammatory processes.
Aneurysms		
Arterial aneurysm ▷ *Fig. 4.19a, b* ▷ *Fig. 4.20a, b* ▷ *Fig. 4.21a–c*	**Saccular aneurysm:** Focal, well-circumscribed zone of contrast enhancement. **Fusiform aneurysm:** Tubular dilation of involved artery. **Dissecting aneurysms (intramural hematoma):** Initially, the involved arterial wall is thickened in a circumferential or semilunar configuration and has intermediate attenuation with luminal narrowing. Evolution of the intramural hematoma can lead to focal dilation of the arterial wall hematoma.	Abnormal fusiform or focal saccular dilation of artery secondary to acquired/degenerative etiology, polycystic disease, connective tissue disease, atherosclerosis, trauma, infection (mycotic, oncotic), AVM, vasculitis, and drugs. Focal aneurysms are also referred to as saccular aneurysms, which typically occur at arterial bifurcations and are multiple in 20%. The chance of rupture of a saccular aneurysm causing subarachnoid hemorrhage is related to the size of the aneurysm. Saccular aneurysms > 2.5 cm in diameter are referred to as giant aneurysms. Fusiform aneurysms are often related to atherosclerosis or collagen vascular disease (e.g., Marfan and Ehlers-Danlos syndromes). Dissecting aneurysms: hemorrhage occurs in the arterial wall from incidental or significant trauma.

(continues on page 198)

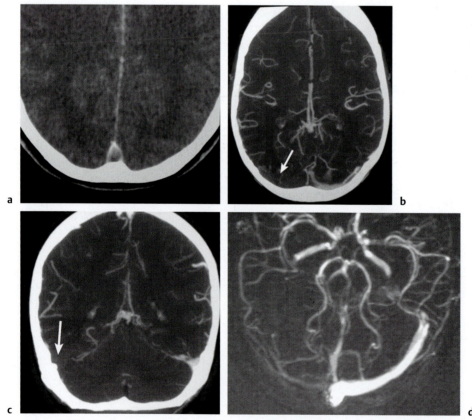

Fig. 4.18a–d   Intracranial venous thrombosis. Axial postcontrast image (**a**) shows nonenhancing thrombus in the sagittal venous sinus ("empty delta" sign). Axial (**b**) and coronal (**c**) CTA images show absence of enhancement of the right transverse venous sinus from the thrombus, as seen on axial MRA image (**d**) (arrows).

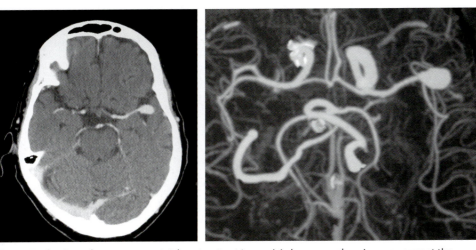

Fig. 4.19a, b Saccular aneurysm. Axial postcontrast image (**a**) shows an enhancing aneurysm at the lateral M1 portion of the left middle cerebral artery, as seen on an axial CTA image (**b**).

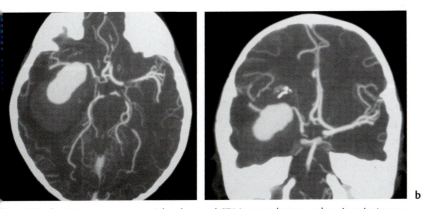

Fig. 4.20a, b Giant aneurysm. Axial and coronal CTA images show an enhancing giant aneurysm with mural thrombus involving the M1 portion of the right middle cerebral artery.

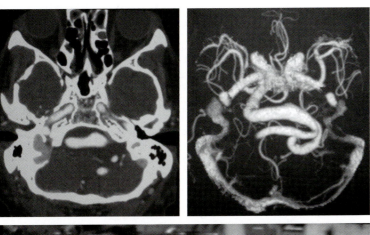

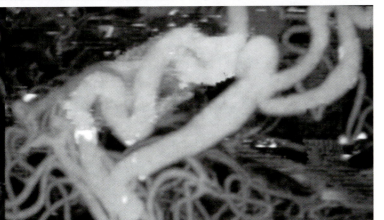

Fig. 4.21a–c Fusiform aneurysm. Postcontrast axial image (**a**) shows a tortuous and dilated basilar artery representing a fusiform aneurysm, as seen on CTA (**b**) and axial MRA (**c**) images.

Table 4.2   (Cont.) Acquired vascular disease

Lesions	CTA Findings	Comments
Vascular malformations		
AVM ▷ *Fig. 4.22a, b* ▷ *Fig. 4.23a–c*	Lesions with irregular margins that can be located in the brain parenchyma (pia, dura, or both locations). AVMs contain multiple tortuous enhancing blood vessels secondary to patent arteries with high blood flow, as well as thrombosed vessels with variable attenuation, areas of hemorrhage in various phases, calcifications, and gliosis. The venous portions often show contrast enhancement. CTA can provide additional detailed information about the nidus, feeding arteries, and draining veins, as well as the presence of associated aneurysms. Usually not associated with mass effect unless there is recent hemorrhage or venous occlusion.	Supratentorial AVMs occur more frequently (80%–90%) than infratentorial AVMs (10%–20%). Annual risk of hemorrhage. AVMs can be sporadic, congenital, or associated with a history of trauma. Multiple AVMs can be seen in syndromes: Rendu-Osler-Weber (AVMs in brain and lungs and mucosal capillary telangiectasias) and Wyburn-Mason (AVMs in brain and retina, with cutaneous nevi).
Vein of Galen aneurysm ▷ *Fig. 4.24a, b*	Multiple tortuous blood vessels involving choroidal and thalamoperforate arteries, internal cerebral veins, vein of Galen (aneurysmal formation), straight and transverse venous sinuses, and other adjacent veins and arteries. The venous portions often show contrast enhancement. CTA can show patent portions of the vascular malformation.	Heterogeneous group of vascular malformations with arteriovenous shunts and dilated deep venous structures draining into and from an enlarged vein of Galen; with or without hydrocephalus, with or without hemorrhage, with or without macrocephaly, with or without parenchymal vascular malformation components, with or without seizures, high-output congestive heart failure in neonates.
Dural AVM	Dural AVMs contain multiple tortuous tubular blood vessels. The venous portions often show contrast enhancement. CTA can show patent portions of the vascular malformation and areas of venous sinus occlusion or recanalization. Usually not associated with mass effect unless there is recent hemorrhage or venous occlusion. With or without venous brain infarction.	Dural AVMs are usually acquired lesions resulting from thrombosis or occlusion of an intracranial venous sinus with subsequent recanalization resulting in direct arterial to venous sinus communications. Transverse, sigmoid venous sinuses > cavernous sinus > straight, superior sagittal sinuses.
Carotid cavernous fistula ▷ *Fig. 4.25a–d*	CTA shows marked dilation of the cavernous sinuses, as well as the superior and inferior ophthalmic veins and facial veins.	Carotid artery to cavernous sinus fistulas usually occur as a result of blunt trauma causing dissection or laceration of the cavernous portion of the internal carotid artery. Patients can present with pulsating exophthalmos.
Cavernous hemangioma	Single or multiple multilobulated intra-axial lesions that have intermediate to slightly increased attenuation, minimal or no contrast enhancement, with or without calcifications.	Supratentorial cavernous angiomas occur more frequently than infratentorial lesions. Can be located in many different locations, multiple lesions > 50%. Association with venous angiomas and risk of hemorrhage.
Venous angioma ▷ *Fig. 4.26*	On postcontrast images, venous angiomas are seen as a contrast-enhancing transcortical vein draining a collection of small medullary veins (caput medusae).	Considered an anomalous venous formation typically not associated with hemorrhage; usually an incidental finding except when associated with cavernous hemangioma.
Capillary telangiectasia	No apparent findings on noncontrast enhanced CT; may be seen as small poorly defined zones of contrast enhancement, no abnormal mass effect.	Small venous malformations consisting of collections of dilated capillaries lacking smooth muscle and elastic fibers in walls; located in pons > other portions of brainstem, brain; typically show no enlargement over time.

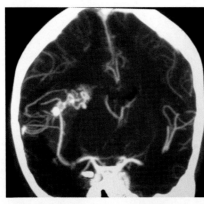
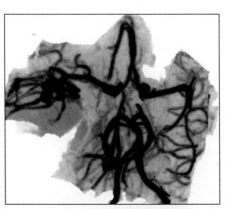

Fig. 4.22a, b   Arteriovenous malformation (AVM). Coronal (**a**) and axial (**b**) CTA images show an AVM involving the right middle cerebral artery.

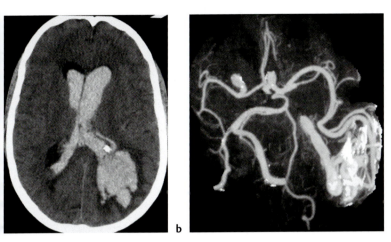
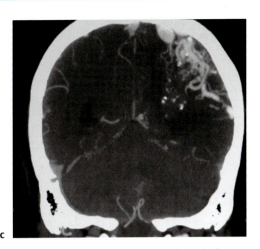

Fig. 4.23a–c   AVM with hemorrhage. Axial CT image (**a**) shows intraventricular hemorrhage from an AVM in the posterior left cerebral hemisphere, as seen on CTA images (**b,c**).

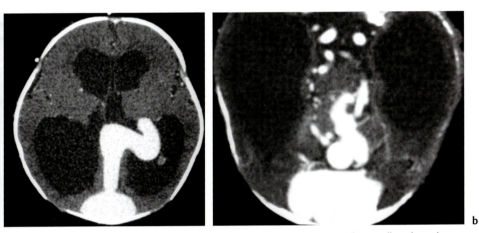

Fig. 4.24a, b   Vein of Galen aneurysm. Axial postcontrast images show an abnormally enlarged enhancing vein of Galen, straight venous sinus, and torcula Herophili.

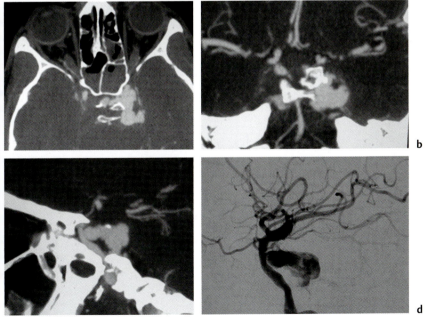

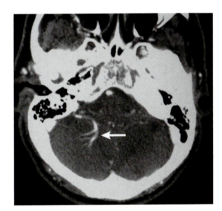

Fig. 4.26   Venous angioma. Axial postcontrast image shows an enhancing venous angioma in the right cerebellar hemisphere (arrow).

Fig. 4.25a–d   Cavernous carotid artery fistula. Axial postcontrast image (**a**) in a 20-year-old man with severe traumatic injuries shows abnormal enlargement and contrast enhancement involving the left cavernous sinus from a tear of the cavernous portion of the left internal carotid artery, as seen on coronal (**b**) and sagittal (**c**) CTA images, as well as a conventional arteriogram (**d**).

II Head and Neck

5 Skull Base and Temporal Bone

Wolfgang Zaunbauer and Francis A. Burgener

The *anterior skull base* consists of the cribriform plate of the ethmoid bone centrally, the orbital plates of the frontal bone laterally, the lesser wings of the sphenoid bone, and the planum sphenoidale (presphenoid) posteriorly. The superior surface of the anterior skull base forms the floor of the anterior cranial fossa; the inferior surface constitutes the roof of the nasal cavity, frontal and ethmoid sinuses (fovea ethmoidalis), and orbits. In addition to the frontal, ethmoid, and sphenoid bones, the undersurface of the anterior skull base is formed by the maxilla, vomer, palatine, zygomatic bones, and paired pterygoid processes, extending inferiorly from the sphenoid body. The cribriform plate contains multiple perforations through which the sensory nerve fibers of the olfactory nerve (cranial nerve [CN] I) and ethmoid arteries pass. The anterior ethmoidal foramen is located just anterior to the cribriform foramina and transmits the anterior ethmoidal artery, vein, and nerve. The posterior ethmoidal foramen is located just posterior to the cribriform foramina and transmits the posterior ethmoidal artery, vein, and nerve. The foramen cecum, located in the midline, anterior to the crista galli, transmits small vessels and is occasionally the starting point of cephaloceles or nasal gliomas.

The *central skull base* is formed by the sphenoid bone (basisphenoid and greater wings of the sphenoid) and the paired temporal bones. The middle cranial fossa extends from the lesser wings of the sphenoid and the frontal bones to the dorsum sellae and posterior clinoid processes medially and the superior margin of the petrous ridges laterally. Superior relationships of the middle cranial fossa are the temporal lobes, pituitary gland, cavernous sinus, Meckel cave, and CN II to VI. The floor of the sphenoid sinus and the basisphenoid form the anterior roof of the pharyngeal mucosal space. The deep facial spaces that abut the exocranial surface of the central skull base are the retropharyngeal space and the perivertebral space and the paired parapharyngeal space, masticator space, carotid space, and parotid space.

The *optic canal* is a round aperture within the lesser wing of the sphenoid at its junction with the sphenoid body, which transmits the optic nerve and ophthalmic artery, both of which are contained in a dural sheath. Inferolaterally, the canal is separated from the superior orbital fissure by the inferior root of the lesser wing ("optic strut").

The *superior orbital fissure,* formed by the cleft between the greater sphenoid wing inferolaterally and the lesser sphenoid wing superolaterally and the sphenoid body medially, transmits CN III, IV, V_1, and VI, recurrent branches of the lacrimal artery, the orbital branch of the middle meningeal artery, and the superior ophthalmic vein.

The *inferior orbital fissure,* which transmits the infraorbital artery, vein, and nerve, is formed by the cleft between the body of the maxilla and the greater wing of the sphenoid bone. The inferior orbital fissure communicates inferiorly with the pterygopalatine fossa.

The *foramen rotundum,* actually a canal in the base of the greater sphenoid wing, just inferiorly and laterally to the superior orbital fissure and superolaterally to the vidian canal, transmits CN V_2, the artery of the foramen rotundum, and emissary veins. The foramen rotundum empties anteriorly into the pterygopalatine fossa, which connects laterally with the masticator space through the pterygomaxillary fissure. Malignant tumors of the skin of the cheek, orbit, and sinonasal area may all use CN V_2 as a perineural route to gain intracranial access.

The *foramen ovale,* which lies completely within the greater wing of the sphenoid, transmits CN V_3 (from the middle cranial fossa to the masticator space), the lesser petrosal nerve, the accessory meningeal branch of the maxillary artery, and the emissary vein. Endocranially, the foramen ovale lies anteromedial to the foramen spinosum and posterolateral to the foramen rotundum. Exocranially, the foramen ovale is located at the base of the lateral pterygoid plate. Perineural tumor extension on the mandibular division of the trigeminal nerve in the masticator space may traverse the skull base through the foramen ovale, spread intracranially through Meckel cave and the preganglionic segment of the trigeminal nerve, and finally reach the pons at the root entry zone.

The *foramen spinosum,* located at the posteromedial aspect of the greater sphenoid wing, endocranially posterolateral to the foramen ovale, and exocranially anterior and lateral to the eustachian tube, transmits the middle meningeal artery and vein, as well as the meningeal branch of CN V_3.

The *vidian canal,* situated in the body of the pterygoid plates below and inferomedial to the foramen rotundum in the body of the sphenoid bone, connects the pterygopalatine fossa anteriorly to the foramen lacerum posteriorly and transmits the vidian artery and nerve.

The *foramen lacerum,* located at the base of the medial pterygoid plate, bound anterolaterally by the greater wing of the sphenoid bone, posteriorly by the petrous apex, and medially by the sphenoid body and basiocciput, is not a true foramen but is a canal largely filled with fibrocartilage. It represents the cartilaginous floor of the anteromedial horizontal segment of the petrous internal carotid artery canal. An inconstant meningeal branch of the ascending pharyngeal artery and the vidian nerve may pierce the cartilage.

The *sphenopalatine foramen,* located in the high posterolateral wall of the nose, connects the lateral nasal cavity with the pterygopalatine fossa. The foramen transmits the lateral nasal and nasopalatine nerves and vessels. Nasal infection and tumors can access the intracranial space, orbit, and masticator space through this escape hatch.

The *posterior skull base* is made up of the sphenoid bone, temporal bones posterior to the petrous ridge, and occipital bones. The anterior portion of the posterior cranial fossa is formed by the clivus, which is derived from the fusion of the basisphenoid and the basiocciput. It extends from the dorsum sellae to the foramen magnum. The lateral wall of the posterior cranial fossa is formed superiorly by the posterior surface of the petrous temporal bone and inferiorly by the condylar part of the occipital bone. The posterior portion of the posterior cranial fossa is made up of the mastoid portion of the temporal bone and the squamous portion of the occipital bone. The superior surface of the posterior skull base forms the floor of the posterior cranial fossa; the inferior surface constitutes the posterior roof of the pharyngeal mucosal space; the carotid, parotid, retropharyngeal, and perivertebral spaces; and the cervical spine.

The *foramen magnum* is bound by the four segments of the occipital bone: the basiocciput anteriorly, the two parts of the exocciput laterally, and the supraocciput posteriorly. The bones surrounding the foramen magnum serve as a site of attachment for numerous ligaments (apical, dental, and alar ligaments, the upper band of the cruciform ligament, the posterior longitudinal ligament, and the tectorial membrane) that stabilize the craniocervical junction. Through the foramen magnum pass the medulla oblongata, the meninges, the vertebral arteries, the anterior and posterior spinal arteries, the spinal accessory nerve (CN XI), and the veins that communicate with the internal vertebral venous plexus.

The *hypoglossal canal* traverses the occipital condyle anterolaterally while transmitting the hypoglossal nerve (CN XII), a meningeal branch of the ascending pharyngeal artery, and a venous plexus. The canal also transmits the rare persistent hypoglossal artery when it is present.

The common skull base apertures and their contents are summarized in **Table 5.1.** Diseases of the skull base can be intrinsic to the area or affect the skull base from either above or below. All these lesions are covered in other sections of this text: intracranial lesions that involve the skull base from above ("top-down" lesions) are discussed in Section I (Brain), lesions originating in the skull base in Section IV (Musculoskeletal System), and extracranial lesions affecting the skull base from below ("bottom-up" lesions) in Chapter 7 (Nasal Cavity and Paranasal Sinuses) and Chapter 8 (Suprahyoid Neck) of this section. All major lesions involving the skull base, with emphasis on intrinsic lesions, are summarized in **Table 5.2.**

II Head and Neck

Table 5.1 Skull base apertures and their content

Aperture	Location	Content
Cribriform plate	Medial floor of anterior cranial fossa	Olfactory nerve (CN I) Ethmoid arteries
Optic canal	Lesser wing of sphenoid bone	Optic nerve (CN II) Ophthalmic artery Subarachnoid space, CSF, dura by optic nerve
Superior orbital fissure	Between lesser and greater sphenoid wings	Oculomotor nerve (CN III) Trochlear nerve (CN IV) Ophthalmic division of trigeminal nerve (CN V_1) Abducens nerve (CN VI) Superior ophthalmic vein
Inferior orbital fissure	Between body of maxilla and greater wing of sphenoid	Infraorbital artery, vein, and nerve
Foramen rotundum	Medial cranial fossa floor inferior to the superior orbital fissure	Maxillary division of trigeminal nerve (CN V_2) Emissary veins Artery of foramen rotundum
Foramen ovale	Floor of middle cranial fossa lateral to sella turcica	Mandibular division of trigeminal nerve (CN V_3) Accessory meningeal branch of maxillary artery Emissary veins from cavernous sinus to pterygoid plexus
Foramen spinosum	Posterolateral to foramen ovale	Middle meningeal artery Recurrent meningeal branch of the mandibular nerve (CN V_3)
Foramen lacerum	Between sphenoid body and greater wing of sphenoid bone at petrous apex	Meningeal branches of ascending pharyngeal artery
Vidian (pterygoid) canal	In sphenoid bone inferomedial to foramen rotundum	Vidian artery Vidian nerve
Carotid canal	Within petrous temporal bone	Internal carotid artery Sympathetic plexus

Jugular foramen	Posterolateral to carotid canal, between petrous temporal bone and occipital bone	Pars nervosa (anteromedial)
		    Inferior petrosal sinus
		    Glossopharyngeal nerve (CN IX)
		    Jacobson nerve
		Pars vascularis (posterolateral)
		    Internal jugular vein
		    Vagus nerve (CN X)
		    Accessory nerve (CN XI)
		    Arnold nerve
		    Small meningeal branches of ascending pharyngeal and occipital arteries

Stylomastoid foramen	Behind styloid process	Facial nerve (CN VII)
Hypoglossal canal	Base of occipital condyles	Hypoglossal nerve (CN XII)
Foramen magnum	Floor of posterior fossa	Medulla and its meninges Spinal segment of accessory nerve (CN XI) Vertebral arteries and veins Anterior and posterior spinal arteries

Table 5.2   Skull base lesions

Disease	CT Findings	Comments
Temporal bone lesions	See **Tables 5.3** to **5.7**	
Intrinsic lesions of the skull base		A lesion is judged to be intrinsic to the skull base if the volume of the mass is centered in the plane of the skull base.

Congenital/developmental lesions

Disease	CT Findings	Comments
Primary cholesteatoma (epidermoid cyst)	Intraosseous congenital cholesteatomas are bone-expanding and bone-destructive lesions. They appear as low-density, unenhanced masses. Cholesteatoma that contains compacted squamous debris may appear heterogeneous. In rare cases, calcifications may be seen, either within or at the periphery of the cholesteatoma.	Squamous epithelial rest of embryonal origin. Occurs in the temporal bone (i.e., petrous apex, middle ear/mastoid), other skull bones, within the meninges or brain, or any other part of the body. Within the skull base, this lesion is referred to as congenital cholesteatoma; when found in the cisterns, the term *epidermoid cyst* is applied.
Cephalocele	Heterogeneous, mixed density mass due to variable amounts of CSF and brain tissue extending through a defect in the base of skull, contiguous with intracranial brain parenchyma. The apertura is smooth and defined by a rim of cortical bone. The instillation of a low dose of intrathecal contrast before CT may aid in distinguishing a simple meningocele from an encephalocele (although MRI is the best modality for confirming the presence of brain tissue in a cephalocele). Occipital cephaloceles consist of cervico-occipital, low occipital (involving the foramen magnum), and high occipital lesions (above the intact foramen magnum). Frontoethmoidal cephaloceles are subdivided into frontonasal, nasoethmoidal, and naso-orbital cephaloceles. Transethmoidal, sphenoethmoidal, transsphenoidal, spheno-orbital, and sphenomaxillary encephaloceles are types of basal cephaloceles.	A cephalocele is the protrusion of intracranial contents, including meninges and brain matter, through a defect in the skull base. Cephaloceles may be congenital or acquired secondary to surgery or trauma or due to spontaneous causes. Cephaloceles are most commonly found in the midline, at the occiput, skull base, or vertex. Frontoethmoidal (sincipital) encephaloceles occur as extranasal masses. Associated abnormalities are callosal hypogenesis, interhemispheric lipomas, neuronal migration anomalies, colloid cysts, midline craniofacial dysraphisms, hypertelorism, microcephaly, microphthalmos, and hydrocephalus.

Inflammatory/infectious conditions

Disease	CT Findings	Comments
Osteomyelitis	Poorly defined areas of osteolysis in contiguity with the focus of infection. Intracranial extension may lead to cavernous sinus thrombosis, meningitis, epidural or subdural empyemas, cerebritis, and cerebral abscess formation.	Skull base osteomyelitis is uncommon, and most cases arise from contiguous spread of ear infections. Skull base osteomyelitis infrequently complicates sinonasal infection. Odontogenic cellulitis and abscess may spread into the suprazygomatic and nasopharyngeal masticator spaces, causing osteomyelitis of the skull base. It typically occurs in a diabetic or immunosuppressed patient incompletely treated for necrotizing otitis externa. *Pseudomonas aeruginosa* is the usual pathogen. Less frequently, *Aspergillus*, *Salmonella*, *Staphylococcus*, *Mycobacterium tuberculosis*, or *Mucormycosis* is implicated.

Benign neoplasms

Disease	CT Findings	Comments
Meningioma ▷ *Fig. 5.1* ▷ *Fig. 5.2*	Meningiomas usually grow as an extra-axial, sessile, or globose, well-marginated bulky mass, dural-based at an obtuse angle. En plaque meningiomas grow as a flattened plate or sheet, especially at the sphenoid ridge, or less commonly at the superior or posterior surfaces of petrous bone. The rare intraosseus meningioma is usually sclerotic, occasionally lytic, and can mimic fibrous dysplasia or Paget disease. Most meningiomas are homogeneously hyperdense, some isodense, and a few hypodense compared with gray matter. Marked enhancement is typical. Cysts, necrosis, and hemorrhage appear as hypodense, nonenhancing areas; < 20% reveal psammomatous, nodular, or rimlike calcifications. Bony remodeling and hyperostosis may be evident. Invasion through the skull base may be present, either through natural foramina or by bone destruction.	Meningiomas represent 15% to 20% of intracranial neoplasms, have a peak incidence of 60 y, and affect predominantly female patients (F:M = 3:1). Meningiomas in childhood are rare and frequently associated with neurofibromatosis 2. Thirty-three percent arise along the dura of the skull base (sphenoid wing, sellar, and parasellar area, olfactory groove) and posterior fossa (clivus, petrous bone, foramen magnum, and jugular foramen). Because of the relatively slow tumor growth, the symptoms are often minimal and may include headache, anosmia, visual disturbance, or other cranial nerve palsies.

(continues on page 205)

Table 5.2   (Cont.) Skull base lesions

Disease	CT Findings	Comments
Malignant neoplasms		
Metastases ▷ *Fig. 5.3* ▷ *Fig. 5.4*	Focal, multifocal, or diffuse involvement of the skull base with osteolytic, osteoblastic, or mixed-type lesions. The extraosseous soft tissue extension is usually small.	Metastatic tumors are the most common malignancy of the skull base resulting from direct extension or hematogenous spread. Breast and lung, kidney, prostate, uterus, and colon carcinoma and head and neck malignancies frequently involve the skull base, especially in the late stage of tumor evolution. Multiple lesions are common. Primary neoplasms are often known at time of presentation. In children, leukemia, neuroblastoma, Wilms tumor, and Ewing sarcoma are the most common primary sites.
Malignant lymphoma	Invasive central skull base lesion, with homogeneously enhancing soft tissue density. Permeation of the tumor through the bone with preserved cortical outlines, with tumor present on both sides of the skull base and infiltration of the tumor along the dural surfaces, similar to "dural tail" without hyperostotic reaction, may be present.	Occurs usually in patients with systemic non-Hodgkin lymphoma and patients with AIDS. Primary non-Hodgkin lymphoma of the skull base without any nodal or lymphatic lesion is a very rare condition and with a different clinical presentation from other extranodal sinonasal and nasopharyngeal lymphoma: cranial nerve palsy, including ophthalmoplegia, visual loss, and hearing loss are most common presenting symptoms.

(continues on page 206)

II Head and Neck

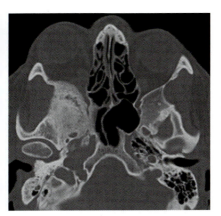

Fig. 5.1   Meningioma (en plaque). Axial bone computed tomography (CT) image shows marked hyperostotic changes of the right wings and body of the sphenoid bone, narrowing of the right optic canal and inferior orbital fissure, and proptosis of the right eye.

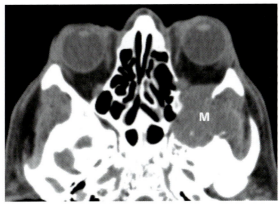

Fig. 5.2   Meningioma (globose). Axial contrast-enhanced CT image reveals a moderate enhancing soft tissue mass (M) arising from the left middle cranial fossa and expanding into the orbit and masticator space. Also seen is osteolytic destruction of the left greater wing of the sphenoid.

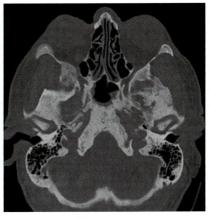

Fig. 5.3   Osteoblastic metastases from prostatic carcinoma. Axial bone CT demonstrates a diffuse sclerotic involvement of the middle cranial fossa and posterior skull base.

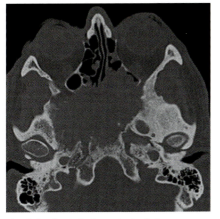

Fig. 5.4   Osteolytic metastasis from adenoid cystic carcinoma. Axial bone CT shows a large destructive soft tissue mass in the central skull base.

Table 5.2   (Cont.) Skull base lesions

Disease	CT Findings	Comments
Plasmacytoma	Solitary intraosseous expansile osteolytic lesion with scalloped, poorly marginated, nonsclerotic margins. The soft tissue mass is usually homogeneous, iso- to mildly hyperdense relative to brain, with mild to moderate homogeneous enhancement. No tumoral calcification, but peripherally displaced osseous fragments may be seen. May have both exocranial and endocranial extraosseous soft tissue components. Multiple myeloma presents similarly to hematogenous metastases. It can have lytic lesions, which may also demonstrate diffuse osteopenia, and rarely sclerosis.	Intraosseous plasmacytoma rarely manifests as primary skull base tumor. Especially sphenoid body, clivus, periorbital, and petrous temporal bone may be affected. Most present in the fifth to ninth decade with male predilection. Local pain, headache, and cranial neuropathies are most common symptoms. Progression to multiple myeloma is common.
Chordoma ▷ *Fig. 5.5*	Expansile, multilobulated, well-circumscribed midline mass involving the clivus. Chordomas cause lytic bone destruction without sclerosis. Bony sequestra within the tumor mass are frequently seen. The soft tissue mass is iso- to hypodense relative to the brain, with low to moderate contrast enhancement. The enhancement pattern is inhomogeneous secondary to areas of cystic necrosis and/or myxoid material. Expanding tumor invades or displaces cavernous sinus and sella superiorly, jugular foramen and petrous apex laterally, basilar artery and brainstem posteriorly, basisphenoid, sphenoid, and ethmoid sinuses anteriorly, nasopharynx anteroinferiorly, jugular foramen and foramen magnum posteroinferiorly.	Thirty-five percent of all chordomas arise in the skull base around spheno-occipital synchondrosis (50% are sacrococcygeal, 15% arise from vertebral bodies). Other rare locations are sellar region, sphenoid sinus, nasopharynx, maxilla, paranasal sinuses, and intradural. Most commonly occurs between the age of 30 and 50 y (2:1 male predilection) with gradual onset of ophthalmoplegia and orbitofrontal headache. Large chordoma may affect optic nerve, chiasm, and optic tracts, CN VII or VIII, and CN IX to XII with consequent cranial nerve abnormalities. Chordomas rarely metastasize (lymph nodes, lung, skeleton).
Chondrosarcoma ▷ *Fig. 5.6*	Tends to arise off midline in the petroclival fissure, petro-occipital synchondrosis, parasellar region, at the sphenoethmoid junction, and at the junction of the sphenoethmoid sinuses and vomer. Characteristically involves the clivus and prepontine region, the cerebellopontine angle, or the parasellar region. Bone destruction may be extensive, and sequestrations may form. Most tumors show prominent enhancement of the soft tissue portions. Chondroid calcification (45%–60%) may appear as arcs, rings, snowflakes, or coarse amorphous calcifications.	Chondrosarcomas of the skull base are rare and occur from childhood through old age (mean age: 43 y) without sex predilection. Commonly present with cranial nerve findings (abducens palsy; other cranial nerve palsies CN 2–5; CN 9,11,12). Late symptoms of tumor progression include increased intracranial pressure accompanied by headache or nausea and vomiting. Osteosarcoma and Ewing sarcoma originate infrequently in the skull base.
Rhabdomyosarcoma	Osteolytic bone destruction of the central skull base, often with a large, bulky intra- and extracranial soft tissue mass.	Rhabdomyosarcoma occurs almost exclusively in the pediatric age group, with the origin of the tumor in the nasopharynx, orbit, paranasal sinuses, and middle ear. A cranial neuropathy is possible.
Metabolic/dysplastic lesions		
Fibrous dysplasia ▷ *Fig. 5.7*	Expanded thickened bone with heterogeneous decreased ("ground glass") bone density is typical, with abrupt transition zone between lesion and normal bone. Involvement by fibrous dysplasia is usually unilateral, which leads to asymmetry. May have cystic regions in the early, active phase of the disease, with centrally lucent lesions and thinned but sclerotic borders. The pagetoid (mixed) pattern of fibrous dysplasia shows mixed radiopacity and radiolucency. The base of the skull is preferentially involved by diffuse areas of sclerosis. Obstructs osseous canals, foramina, pneumatic system, and sinuses. Contrast enhancement is often difficult to appreciate except in areas of lucent bone.	Benign, developmental skeletal disorder, most common in the axial skeleton. The skull is frequently affected (craniofacial region, clivus, posterior skull base). The medullary cavity of the affected bone fills and expands with fibrous tissue. The fibrous tissue then variably ossifies. Can be monostotic (75%) or polyostotic. Typically seen in adolescents and young adults. McCune-Albright syndrome is a subtype of polyostotic fibrous dysplasia (usually unilateral) with endocrine dysfunction (precocious puberty) and cutaneous hyperpigmentation (café-au-lait spots). Other skeletal dysplasias affecting the skull base are neurofibromatosis type 1, achondroplasia, osteogenesis imperfecta, and craniotubular dysplasia. Diffuse skull base involvement also occurs with mucopolysaccharidosis and severe anemias. Other fibro-osseous lesions, such as ossifying fibroma, intraosseous hemangioma, osteoma, osteoblastoma, osteoclastoma, chondroblastoma, chondromyxoid tumors, hemangiopericytoma, chondroma, and aneurysmal bone cyst, are unusual entities and very rarely found in the skull base.

(continues on page 207)

Table 5.2   (Cont.) Skull base lesions

Disease	CT Findings	Comments
Paget disease ▷ *Fig. 5.8*	Demineralization, "cotton wool" appearance, or marked sclerosis and bony enlargement with diploic widening and inner and outer table thickening of the osseous skull base are apparent. Often more diffuse and symmetric than fibrous dysplasia. Involvement of the skull base may lead to bone softening and result in basilar impression with the tip of the odontoid and anterior atlas arch above Chamberlain's line. Sarcomatous degeneration, an uncommon sequela, presents with cortical destruction, masslike marrow replacement, and soft tissue masses.	Involves temporal bone and calvarium more frequently than the craniofacial area. Usually an incidental finding in individuals older than 40 y with male predominance. Headache, ataxic gait, cranial nerve palsies, myelopathy, and hydrocephalus may be clinical manifestations. Sclerosis and thickening of the base of the skull, including the petrous bone bilaterally with stenosis or obliteration of the internal auditory canal, facial nerve canal, and otic capsule, are signs associated with a variety of congenital disorders, including osteopetrosis, pyknodysostosis, craniometaphyseal dysplasia, cleidocranial dysplasia, Camurati-Engelmann disease, and osteopathia striata. Other conditions that can cause bony sclerosis are myelofibrosis, fluorosis, mastocytosis, sickle cell disease, and tuberous sclerosis.

(continues on page 208)

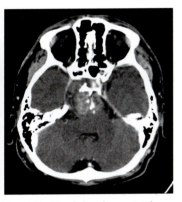

Fig. 5.5   Clival chordoma. Axial contrast-enhanced CT image reveals a heterogeneously enhancing clival mass, which invades the right cavernous sinus and displaces the brainstem posteriorly. (Courtesy of Dr. A. von Hessling, Zurich.)

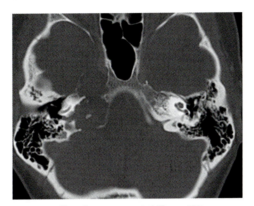

Fig. 5.6   Chondrosarcoma. Axial bone CT image demonstrates a skull base expansile mass centered on the right petro-occipital fissure. Also seen is associated bone destruction of the right petrous apex and petroclival junction with a sharp, narrow, nonsclerotic transition zone adjacent to normal bone. Notice the small bony fragments/calcifications in the tumor matrix. (Courtesy of Dr. A. von Hessling, Zurich.)

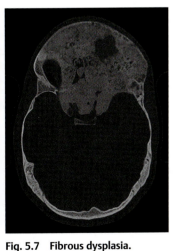

Fig. 5.7   Fibrous dysplasia. Axial bone CT image reveals diffuse "ground glass" expansion of the skull base, facial bones, and calvarium, as well as an abrupt transition zone between the lesion and normal bone. Note the obliteration of the frontal, ethmoid, and sphenoid sinuses.

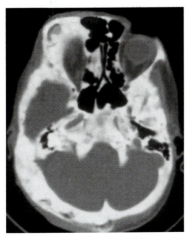

Fig. 5.8   Paget disease. Axial bone CT image reveals asymmetric, polyostotic, marked irregular thickening with both sclerotic and lytic changes of the skull base, facial bones, and both tables and diploic space of the cranial vault.

Table 5.2   (Cont.) Skull base lesions

Disease	CT Findings	Comments
Trauma		
Skull base fracture	Linear lucency with irregular borders representing fracture line, traversing the skull base, with or without separation and displacement of the fragments. It is generally associated with a dural tear. Indirect fracture signs, such as incorrectly located air (pneumocephalus, air in the labyrinth) or soft tissue densities (air–fluid levels in the tympanic cavity, mastoid cells, or sinus; meningoencephalocele), can provide additional diagnostic assistance. In fractures of the base of the skull, the temporal bone is usually involved. Fractures in the anterior fossa are of a cribriform, frontoethmoidal, lateral frontal, or complex type. Fractures resulting from temporal blows tend to propagate medially along a course parallel to the long axis of the petrous pyramid. They usually terminate in the floor of the middle fossa or in the sphenoid base. Some extend across the midline to be continuous with a contralateral temporal bone fracture. A minority extend anteriorly to exit the cranium through the anterior fossa floor laterally or through the midline and the cribriform plate. Strong occipital blows characteristically produce a fracture that disrupts the foramen magnum ring and then propagates anteriorly across the petrous pyramid at right angles to its long axis, passing to the floor of the middle fossa. The fracture may pass lateral to, through, or medial to the otic capsule. Occipital condylar fracture results from a high-energy blunt trauma with axial compression, lateral bending, or rotational injury to the alar ligament. Fractures of the clivus are subdivided into longitudinal, transverse, and oblique types. The site of the leak in CSF otorrhea and rhinorrhea can be detected accurately using CT water-soluble iodinated contrast cisternography.	Skull base fractures represent 19% to 21% of all skull fractures. The skull base is prone to fracture following severe head trauma at the thin squamous temporal and parietal bones over the temples and the foramen magnum, the petrous temporal ridge, the sphenoid sinus, and the inner parts of the sphenoid wings at the skull base. The middle cranial fossa is the weakest, with thin bones and multiple foramina. Other places prone to fracture are the cribriform plate and the roof of the orbits in the anterior cranial fossa and the areas between the mastoid and dural sinuses in the posterior cranial fossa. Skull base fractures are usually the result of extension of a vault fracture. The most important complications of these fractures are CSF leakage (otorrhea, rhinorrhea), related infection, and pneumocephalus with fistula, extracerebral and intracerebral hemorrhages, and cranial nerve and intracranial major vessel injury. Anterior and middle cranial base fractures generally cause upper cranial nerve injuries (CN I, II, III, IV, V, and VI) and vascular injuries to the carotid artery and middle cerebral artery. Posterior cranial base fractures are associated with injury to the lower cranial nerves (CN IX, X, XI, and XII) and major venous sinuses. Laterobasal fractures, including those of the petrous bone, are usually associated with deficits of facial and vestibulocochlear nerves (CN VII and VIII). Other clinical signs of a skull base fracture occurring after craniocerebral trauma are bleeding from the nose and ears, perilymphatic fistula, periorbital ecchymosis (raccoon eyes), and ecchymosis of the mastoid process of the temporal bone (Battle sign).
Miscellaneous lesions		
Langerhans cell histiocytosis	Single (eosinophilic granuloma) or multiple areas of pure osteolysis in the skull base, temporal bone, or calvarium. Well-marginated lytic bone destruction may be extensive. A heterogeneously enhancing soft tissue mass may be associated. Fragments of bone within the soft tissue component are common.	Poorly understood, nonneoplastic disease. Children and young adults primarily are affected (F:M = 1:2). Most common signs with temporal bone lesion are otalgia, otorrhea, conductive or sensorineural hearing loss, facial nerve palsy, vertigo, and postauricular swelling.

The paired *temporal bones* each form part of the middle and posterior cranial fossae and contribute to the skull base. They are composed of five parts: the squamous bone, the mastoid bone, the petrous bone, the tympanic bone, and the styloid process.

The *squamous part of the temporal bone* is broad and flat and serves as the lateral wall of the middle cranial fossa and as the bony floor of the suprazygomatic masticator space. A portion contributes to the fossa of the temporomandibular joint and the roof of the external auditory canal. The zygomatic process projects from its lower surface.

Both the petrous and the squamous portions of the temporal bone form the mastoid segment. The mastoid antrum is the large central mastoid air cell. The aditus ad antrum connects the epitympanum to the mastoid antrum. Körner septum is part of the petrosquamosal suture that runs posterolaterally through the mastoid air cells and serves as a barrier to the extension of infection from the lateral mastoid air cells to the medial mastoid air cells.

The pyramidal-shaped *petrous bone* has three surfaces: the anterior, which is close to the temporal lobe; the posterior, which is close to the brainstem and cerebellum; and the inferior surface, an area that helps to form the carotid canal and jugular foramen. The posterior surface of the petrous bone contains the porus acusticus, the vestibular aqueduct (which transmits the endolymphatic duct), and the cochlear aqueduct (which transmits the perilymphatic duct). The petrous apex is defined as the portion of the temporal bone lying anteromedial to the inner ear, between the sphenoid bone anteriorly and the occipital bone posteriorly. It is separated from the clivus by the petro-occipital fissure and the foramen lacerum. Meckel cave and the cavernous sinus are in close proximity to the petrous apex.

The *tympanic bone* has anterior, inferior, and posterior walls that form the majority of the adult bony external auditory canal.

The *styloid portion* of the temporal bone forms the styloid process.

The temporal bone contains three cavities: the external, middle, and inner ear (**Figs. 5.9 and 5.10**). The *external auditory canal* is composed of fibrocartilage laterally and bone medially (the tympanic bone and the vertical retromeatal portion of the squamous bone). The medial border of the external

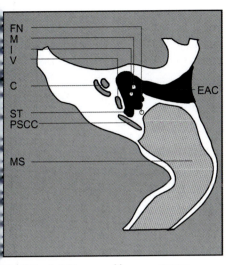

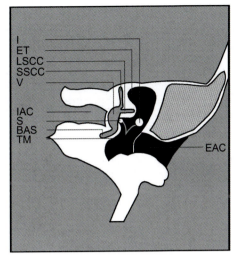

Fig. 5.9   Axial temporal bone anatomy.

C	cochlea
EAC	external auditory canal
FN	facial nerve canal (mastoid segment)
I	incus (long process)
M	malleus (neck)
MS	mastoid
PSCC	posterior semicircular canal
ST	sinus tympani
V	vestibulum

Fig. 5.10   Coronal temporal bone anatomy.

BAS	basal turn of the cochlea
EAC	external auditory canal
ET	epitympanum
I	incus
IAC	internal auditory canal
LSCC	lateral semicircular canal
S	stapes (footplate in oval window)
SSCC	superior semicircular canal
TM	tympanic membrane
V	vestibule

auditory canal is formed by the tympanic membrane. It attaches to the scutum superiorly and to the tympanic annulus inferiorly.

The *tympanic cavity* is a small cleftlike, air-containing space (~20 × 10 × 2 mm) within the petrous portion of the temporal bone bound by the anterior wall (carotid wall with the ostium tympanicum of the musculotubal canal in the hypotympanum), the posterior wall (with the aditus ad antrum in the upper part, the pyramidal eminence, the sinus tympani, and the facial nerve recess in the lower part), the tympanic membrane laterally, the labyrinthine wall with the cochlear promontory and the oval and round windows medially, the tegmen tympani superiorly, and the floor (jugular wall) inferiorly. The epitympanum (attic) is the tympanic cavity above the line drawn between the inferior tip of the scutum and the tympanic portion of the facial nerve. The aditus ad antrum connects the epitympanum to the mastoid antrum. Within the epitympanum are the malleus head and the body and short process of the incus. Prussak space, the most common site of pars flaccida cholesteatoma, is the area between the incus and the lateral sidewall of the epitympanum. The mesotympanum extends from the inferior tip of the scutum above to the line drawn parallel to the inferior aspect of the bony external auditory canal. The posterior inferior wall is comprised of the pyramidal eminence, the sinus tympani, and the facial nerve recess (contains the descending facial nerve). The mesotympanum contains the manubrium of the malleus, the long process of the incus, and the stapes, whose vibrations are modulated by the tensor tympani muscle (inserts on the malleus) and the stapedius muscle (attaches on the head of the stapes). The hypotympanum is a shallow trough in the floor of the middle ear and contains no vital structures. A vascular mass in the middle ear upon otoscopic inspection may represent a high-riding or dehiscent jugular bulb, aberrant carotid artery, persistent stapedial artery, vascular

granulation tissue, cholesterol granuloma, paraganglioma, or other tumor (e.g., hemangioma and meningioma).

The *inner ear* contains the membranous labyrinth set within the bony labyrinth (otic capsule), which forms the cochlea, vestibule, semicircular canals, and vestibular and cochlear aqueducts. The cochlea has approximately two and one half turns encircling a central bony axis, the modiolus. The basal first turn opens posteriorly into the round window niche. The vestibule, containing the utricle and saccule, is the central part of the labyrinth and is separated laterally from the middle ear by the oval window niche. The semicircular canals project off the superior, posterior, and lateral aspects of the vestibule. The upper bony margin of the superior semicircular canal forms a convexity on the petrous pyramid roof, called the arcuate eminence. The posterior semicircular canal points posteriorly along the line of the petrous ridge. The lateral semicircular canal juts into the epitympanum. The cochlear aqueduct, which contains the perilymphatic duct, is 6 to 10 mm in length and extends from the scala tympani of the basal turn of the cochlea (just anterior to the round window orifice) posteromedially to the lateral border of the jugular foramen and posteroinferiorly to the internal auditory canal. The vestibular aqueduct encompasses the endolymphatic duct. It extends from the vestibule, coursing posteroinferiorly to the posterior wall of the petrous pyramid, where it joins the endolymphatic sac.

The *internal auditory canal* enters the petrous pyramid from the posteromedial surface and functions as a conduit for the facial nerve, intramediate nerve, and vestibulocochlear nerves as they course from the brainstem to the inner ear. The medial opening of the internal auditory canal is known as the porus acusticus. The porus acusticus internus is shaped much like the beveled tip of a needle, with the maximum diameter in the same axis as the petrous pyramid. The posterior, superior, and inferior lips of the porus are prominent and made up of dense bone.

The anterior lip is usually poorly demarcated because it blends smoothly with the posteromedial surface of the petrous bone. Normally, the two internal auditory canals of the same patient are symmetric, but their shape varies considerably from one individual to the next. In 50% of cases, the canals are cylindrical, in 25% they have an oval shape, and in the remaining 25% the canals taper either medially or laterally. The canal's vertical diameter varies from 2 to 12 mm (mean 5 mm) and its length from 4 to 15 mm (mean 8 mm). In 95% of normal individuals, the difference between the two internal auditory canals does not exceed 1 mm in diameter and 2 mm in length. The lateral end of the internal auditory canal, known as the fundus, is separated from the inner ear by a vertical plate of bone that is perforated to allow passage of the nerves. The fundus is subdivided by a horizontal plate (falciform crest) and a vertical plate (Bill bar) into four compartments. The facial nerve lies anterosuperiorly with its nervus intermedius, the superior vestibular nerve posterosuperiorly, the cochlear nerve anteroinferiorly, and the inferior vestibular nerve posteroinferiorly.

The *facial nerve canal* originates at the foramen faciale of the fundus meatus acustici interni and terminates in the foramen stylomastoideum. The facial nerve canal has three segments and two genus. The labyrinthine segment courses with a gentle curve anterolaterally in the vestibulocochlear groove between the cochlea and vestibular labyrinth. At the geniculate fossa, the canal forms an acute angle (first genu), then courses posteriorly and laterally to become the tympanic segment. It runs along the superior portion of the internal wall of the tympanic cavity, above and medial to the cochleariform process, and beneath the plane of the horizontal semicircular canal above the oval window, faces the promontory that separates the round and oval windows, and extends to the posterior wall of the tympanum. The posterior extremity of the short process of the incus marks the point where the facial canal begins its second turn (posterior genu) into the styloid complex to become the mastoid segment. The stylomastoid foramen, the caudal opening of the mastoid portion of the intratemporal facial nerve canal located in the exocranial skull base surface anteromedial to the mastoid tip and posteromedial to the styloid process, transmits the facial nerve (CN VII) and extends directly into the parotid space. There may be congenital bony dehiscences in any portion of the facial canal (into the anterior epitympanic air cell, in the tympanic segment, or into the jugular fossa).

The *carotid canal,* located in the anterior part of the petrous pyramid, transmits the internal carotid artery and sympathetic plexus. Entering the skull base, the canal ascends vertically for ~1 cm, then proceeds horizontally in an anteromedial direction before ending above the foramen lacerum. The vertical portion is located inferior to the cochlea, anterior to the jugular fossa, and medial to the tympanic cavity. The horizontal portion is located anteromedial to the protympanum and posteromedial and parallel to both the eustachian tube and the semicanal for the tensor tympani muscle.

The *jugular foramen* is a bony channel that extends anteriorly, laterally, and inferiorly from the endocranium to the exocranium between the anterolaterally temporal and posteromedially occipital bones and transmits vessels and cranial nerves through the skull base into the carotid space. It can be divided into three compartments: a larger posterolateral venous compartment (sigmoid part), containing the sigmoid sinus and small meningeal arterial branches; a smaller anteromedial venous compartment (petrosal part), containing the inferior petrosal sinus; and a neural or intrajugular

compartment (pars nervosa), situated between the sigmoid and petrosal compartments, containing CN IX to XI. The sigmoid and the petrosal parts are separated by the intrajugular processes, which originate from the opposing surfaces of the temporal and occipital bones, as well as by a dural septum, which connects these two bony structures. The jugular foramen is separated from the hypotympanum by the bony lateral jugular plate, which may be normally dehiscent (dehiscent jugular bulb), and is medial to the descending facial canal and inferomedial to the posterior semicircular canal. The jugular foramen is separated from the anteromedial carotid canal by the caroticojugular spine and from the inferomedial hypoglossal canal by the jugular tubercle. Lesions can arise within the fossa or grow into the fossa from neighboring structures. The differential diagnosis of an erosive or destructive lesion in or about the jugular foramen includes paraganglioma, schwannoma (CN IX, X, XI, and XII), metastasis, meningioma, chordoma, chondrosarcoma, invasive squamous neoplasms (nasopharynx or external auditory canal), arteriovenous malformations (enlarging bulb), and cholesteatoma (primary or acquired).

The *musculotubal canal* proceeds from the inferior surface of the petrous bone, near the sphenopetrosal fissure, cranially in a dorsolateral direction to its orifice in the anterior wall of the tympanic cavity; it is divided by the cochleariform process into two semicanals: the lower for the bony part of the pharyngotympanic (auditor) tube, the upper for the tensor tympani muscle.

Imaging of the ear is requested for three main reasons: hearing loss (conductive or sensorineural), tinnitus, and dizziness. In other cases the main sign is external auditory meatus flow, facial palsy, or auricular malformation.

Conductive hearing loss may be congenital (congenital ossicular anomalies, which are isolated or associated with external auditory canal dysplasia, and congenital middle ear anomalies) or associated with cerumen, foreign body, exostosis, otitis, or tumor of the external ear; acute otitis media, serous otitis media, tympanic membrane perforation, tympanosclerosis, postinflammatory ossicular fixation, traumatic ossicular disruption, cholesteatoma, glomus tympanicum tumor, fenestral otosclerosis, and superior semicircular canal dehiscence syndrome; fibrous dysplasia; and Paget disease.

Neurosensory hearing loss may be caused by peripheral lesions (75%–80% of all cases of neurosensory hearing loss), such as congenital malformations of the labyrinth, transverse fractures of the petrous pyramid, labyrinthitis (serous, toxic, viral, or bacterial), ototoxicity (drugs such as streptomycin, gentamicin, and quinine), tumor destruction of the labyrinth, and otodystrophies (otosclerosis and Paget disease) or by retrocochlear processes (20%–25% of all cases of pure sensorineural hearing loss), such as cerebellopontine angle lesions (acoustic schwannoma, meningioma, and vascular loop), petrous apex lesions (congenital cholesteatoma, cholesterol granuloma, and glomus tumor), or central pathology involving the brainstem, cerebellum, and central auditory pathways (multiple sclerosis, tumors, ischemia, aneurysm, and intra-axial hemorrhage).

Tinnitus may be from intrinsic (vestibulocochlear) or extrinsic (muscular or vascular) causes. *Intrinsic tinnitus* is a common complaint, subjective and audible only to the patient (with Ménière disease, viropathies, drugs, allergy, noise, or systemic diseases). Often the cause is unclear, and treatment is lacking. *Extrinsic tinnitus* is far rarer, often objective, and potentially audible also to the examiner. Muscular tinnitus (with myoclonus of the palatal muscles or the tensor tympani) can be pulsatile but is not usually pulse synchronous. Vascular tinnitus is always pulse synchronous. Causes for vascular tinnitus may be arterial, arteriovenous, or venous. The arterial causes include the aberrant arteries (aberrant carotid artery, persistent stapedial artery, and laterally displaced artery), the stenotic arteries (fibromuscular dysplasia, atherosclerosis of the internal and external carotid, and styloid carotid compression), and petrous carotid aneurysm. Arteriovenous causes include paragangliomas, other vascular tumors, Paget disease of the bone, cerebral arteriovenous malformations, dural arteriovenous fistulas, and vertebral fistulas. Venous tinnitus may be caused by chronic anemia, pregnancy, thyrotoxicosis, intracranial hypertension, or a large or exposed jugular bulb, or it may be idiopathic.

Peripheral facial nerve paralysis may occur with *intracranial intra-axial lesions* (cavernoma, brainstem glioma, metastasis, multiple sclerosis, cerebrovascular accident, or hemorrhage), *intracranial extra-axial lesions* (cerebellopontine angle tumor: acoustic schwannoma, meningioma, or epidermoid; cerebellopontine angle inflammation: sarcoidosis or meningitis; and vascular: vertebrobasilar dolichoectasia, arteriovenous malformation, or aneurysm), *intratemporal processes* (fracture through the facial nerve canal, Bell palsy, otitis media, cholesteatoma, paraganglioma, hemangioma, facial nerve schwannoma, or metastasis), *extracranial lesions* (forceps delivery, penetrating facial trauma, malignant otitis externa, parotid surgery, or parotid malignancy) or *miscellaneous processes* (Möbius syndrome, diabetes mellitus, myasthenia gravis, or hyperparathyroidism).

Sixty percent of *congenital anomalies of the temporal bone* occur in the external auditory canal (range from mild stenosis to complete agenesis; pinna deformity [microtia] is often associated), middle ear (range from minor hypoplasia to agenesis; ossicular changes, e.g., rotation, fusion, or absence), or both. Inner ear abnormalities account for 30% of congenital defects and, because of a different embryogenesis of the inner ear, are not associated with external and middle ear deformities. Combined anomalies involving all three compartments make up to 10% and are limited to craniofacial dysplasias and trisomies (13, 18, and 21).

Computed tomography (CT) is ideal for outlining the bony architecture, whereas magnetic resonance imaging (MRI) provides soft tissue details. The causes of conductive hearing loss are best depicted by CT. MRI offers the best chance to find pathology in a clinical picture of vertigo, sensorineural hearing loss, or tinnitus. In cases such as congenital malformations, petrous apex lesions, and mixed hearing loss, CT and MRI are complementary and are often used together to demonstrate the full extent of disease.

The differential diagnosis list of diseased temporal bone is discussed in **Tables 5.3, 5.4, 5.5, 5.6,** and **5.7.**

Table 5.3   Temporal bone: diseases of the external auditory canal

Disease	CT Findings	Comments
Congenital/developmental lesions		
Atresia ▷ *Fig. 5.11*	In cases of stenosis, CT shows unilateral or bilateral narrowing of the external auditory canal from external opening of the canal to the tympanic membrane. **Membranous atresia** is characterized by cartilaginous plug in a bony external auditory canal. **Complete atresia** results in absence of the bony external auditory canal. The associated bony overgrowth about a deformed tympanic bone (atresia plate) may be thick, thin, complete, or incomplete. Middle ear findings depend on severity of atresia (hypoplastic middle ear and mastoid complex, ossicular chain deformities [rotation, fusion, or absence], hypoplasia or aplasia of the oval or round window, anterior displacement of the facial canal, and associated congenital cholesteatoma). Inner ear and internal auditory canal are usually normal.	Congenital bony, soft tissue, or mixed dysplasia of entire external auditory canal, including membranous and bony portions, usually unilateral by a 6:1 ratio, more commonly in right ear and in male patients. Patients usually present with a small deformity of the auricle, no visibly patent canal, or conductive hearing deficit. May be associated with inherited syndromes, including mandibulofacial dysostosis (Treacher Collins), acrofacial dysostosis (Nager), craniofacial dysostosis (Crouzon), oculoauriculovertebral dysplasia (Goldenhar), and Pierre Robin syndrome.
Low-lying dura	The low-lying dura may cover the roof of the external auditory canal, and when the canal is not developed, the middle cranial fossa deepens to form a groove lateral to the attic and labyrinth.	A depression of the tegmental plate is not unusual, particularly in patients with congenital atresia of the external auditory canal.
Inflammatory/infectious conditions		
Postinflammatory medial canal fibrosis	Homogeneous crescent soft tissue formation in the medial external auditory canal, unilateral or bilateral, abutting the tympanic membrane without underlying bone erosion or middle ear/mastoid involvement. May show slight enhancement of inflamed/edematous thickened external auditory canal walls in early stage.	Very rare. Distinct entity characterized by the formation of fibrous tissue in the medial bone external auditory meatus. Most cases occur in older patients (mean age 50 y; M:F = 1:2), with conductive hearing loss, tinnitus, otorrhea after chronic otitis externa and/or media, or as a complication of ear surgery.
Necrotizing (malignant) external otitis ▷ *Fig. 5.12*	Enhancing external auditory canal soft tissue mass with aggressive underlying bony changes (cortical bone erosions and associated osteomyelitis especially affect the inferior portion of the external auditory canal and mastoid), thickened auricle, extension to the temporomandibular joint, adjacent cellulitis or abscesses of the parotid, masticator and parapharyngeal spaces, and opacification of the middle ear and mastoid air cells. May progress to skull base osteomyelitis. Intracranial extension can lead to sigmoid sinus thrombosis, meningitis, intracranial empyema, and abscess.	Severe invasive infection of the external ear, usually caused by *Pseudomonas aeruginosa*. Occurs in elderly diabetic or otherwise immunocompromised patients (M:F = 2:1) with persistent otorrhea, otalgia, and cranial neuropathy (CN VII, IX to XII).
Keratosis obturans ▷ *Fig. 5.13*	Homogeneous soft tissue plug in the external auditory canal, often bilateral, without focal bone erosion of the canal. If the canal is diffusely widened, the bone walls appear smooth, without bone fragments. No enhancement of the tissue.	Rare abnormal accumulation and obstruction of the external auditory canal from desquamated keratin. Patients (< 40 y of age) present with acute, severe bilateral otalgia and a conductive hearing loss. Associated abnormalities are chronic sinusitis and bronchiectasis.
Cholesteatoma	Soft tissue mass within the external auditory canal with erosive osseous changes, usually seen as focal scalloping or irregular erosion of the inferior and/or posterior external auditory canal wall underneath the cholesteatoma mass. Foci of bony fragments (sequestrations of necrotic bone) may be present within the cholesteatoma matrix. The cholesteatoma may extend into the middle ear cavity or mastoid, or it may involve the facial nerve canal or tegmen tympani. May demonstrate rim enhancement.	Cholesteatoma of the external auditory canal is a rare entity. Most cases are spontaneous or occur after surgery, trauma, or with ear canal stenosis or obstruction. Occurs in older patients (age 40–75 y), usually as a unilateral process without other associated disease. Common symptoms are persistent otorrhea, chronic dull otalgia, and, less commonly, conductive hearing loss.

(continues on page 214)

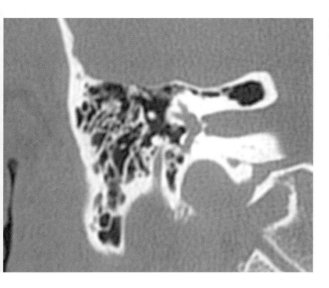

Fig. 5.11   Agenesis, external auditory canal. Coronal right T-bone CT image shows the absence of the bony external auditory canal. The mastoid and middle ear cavity are well developed and clear.

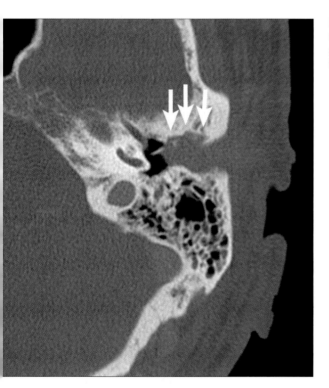

Fig. 5.12   Malignant necrotizing external otitis. Axial left T-bone CT image shows inflammatory changes in the region of the external auditory canal and auricle. The anterior bony external auditory canal is partially eroded (arrows).

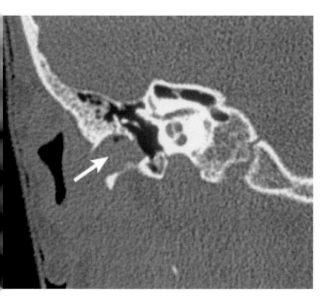

Fig. 5.13   Keratosis obturans. Coronal bone CT reconstruction reveals a homogeneous soft tissue filling (arrow) of the right external auditory canal without osseous changes. The middle ear is unaffected, and the overall size of the canal is slightly enlarged.

Table 5.3   (Cont.) Temporal bone: diseases of the external auditory canal

Disease	CT Findings	Comments
Benign neoplasms		
Exostoses ▷ *Fig. 5.14*	Broad-based bony expansion of the osseous external auditory canal wall with secondary stenosis. Bilaterality is the rule. The circumferential encroachment is usually located medial to the isthmus. Complete occlusion of external auditory canal is rare.	Benign bony overgrowth (not a true tumor) of bony external auditory canal in young adult male with chronic history of prolonged cold seawater exposure (surfer's ear, cold water ear). Conductive hearing loss may develop if the lesions are large. Other symptoms may be ear infection, pain, and tinnitus.
Osteoma	Solitary, unilateral, pedunculated, narrow-based, well-defined, osseous density mass, most commonly located lateral to the isthmus, near the osseous-cartilaginous junction of the external auditory canal. There are two varieties: the compact "ivory" type appears as a homogeneous dense bony mass, the "cancellous" type as a partially ossified mass.	Usually an incidental finding composed of mature bone. Much less common than exostoses. Occasionally identified at extracanalicular sites within the temporal bone, particularly in the mastoid. Secondary bacterial external otitis can occur medial to an obstructing osteoma. Cholesteatoma of the external auditory canal and/or middle ear may be an associated abnormality.
Benign ceruminous gland tumor	Polypoid soft tissue mass in the external auditory canal without bony destructive changes.	Benign tumors of ceruminous gland origin in the external auditory canal include ceruminous adenoma, chondroid syringoma, syringocystadenoma papilliferum, and ceruminous pleomorphic adenoma. They are very rare and are seen in adult patients (mean age 54 y; equal M:F distribution), which present with a painless mass of the outer half of the external auditory canal or with hearing changes. Occasionally symptoms of this tumor (pain, otorrhea) can result from an otitis externa secondary to meatus obstruction. The lesions have a tendency to recur after surgery and may degenerate into carcinoma.
Malignant neoplasms		Malignant tumors of the external auditory canal are relatively rare (squamous cell carcinoma > basal cell carcinoma > adenoid cystic carcinoma), mucoepidermoid carcinoma, adenocarcinoma; melanomas, and sarcomas are much less common.
Squamous cell carcinoma ▷ *Fig. 5.15*	Homogeneously or heterogeneously enhancing soft tissue mass filling the external auditory canal. Bone destruction may be quite extensive without bony flecks. Extension into the pinna, parotid gland, and soft tissues below temporal bone and mastoid tip is common. Involvement of the middle ear cavity and superior extension into middle cranial fossa are rare. Nodal drainage is to pre- and postauricular and parotid nodes.	Squamous cell carcinoma is the most common primary malignancy of the external auditory canal. Tumors may begin within the canal or in the middle ear. Patients (median age 65 y, more common in women) present with ulcerating external auditory canal mucosal lesion (may mimic otitis externa or external auditory canal cholesteatoma), otorrhea, otalgia, and conductive hearing loss. Late symptoms are facial nerve paresis, extensive bulky tumor, and nodal disease. **T staging:** T1: Tumor limited to external auditory canal without bony erosion or soft tissue involvement. T2: Tumor with limited osseous erosion or soft tissue involvement. T3: Tumor eroding osseous external auditory canal with limited soft tissue/middle ear/mastoid involvement. T4: Tumor eroding deeper inner ear structures/temporomandibular joint/extensive soft tissue extension, or facial nerve paresis.
Parotid malignancy (local invasion)	Enhancing inhomogeneous ill-defined soft tissue mass of the parotid gland with extraparenchymal extension and invasion of adjacent structures (skull base, deep spaces of the suprahyoid neck) filling the external auditory canal. There may be marked bony erosion.	When invasive parotid malignancy occurs in the cephalad aspect of the parotid gland, it may invade the external auditory canal and present as a mass in this area.
Metastases	Osteolytic and/or osteoblastic lesions in the bony external auditory canal, usually not associated with prominent soft tissue masses.	Originate most often from carcinomas of the lung, breast, prostate, and kidney or may present multiple myeloma and malignant lymphoma manifestations.

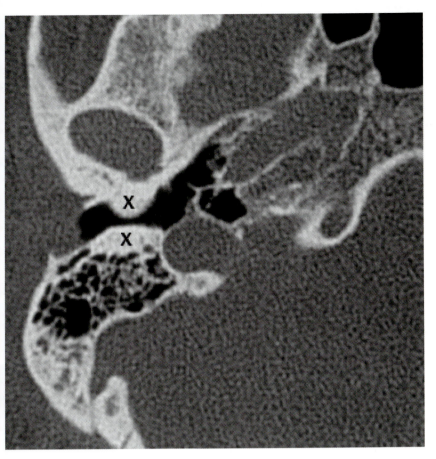

Fig. 5.14   External auditory canal exostosis. Axial right T-bone CT image demonstrates broad-based osseous external auditory canal encroachment on both anterior and posterior walls (x) medial to the isthmus with severe narrowing of the lumen.

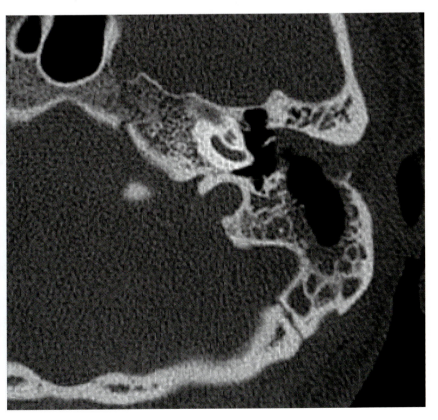

Fig. 5.15   External auditory canal squamous cell carcinoma. Axial left T-bone CT image shows a soft tissue density filling the external auditory canal with dorsal osseous destruction and invasion of the mastoid. The middle ear is unaffected.

Table 5.4 Temporal bone: diseases of the middle ear and mastoid

Disease	CT Findings	Comments
Congenital/developmental lesions		
Middle ear dysplasia	Malformations of the middle ear vary from minor hypoplasia with coarcted small and underdeveloped but aerated tympanic cavity to almost complete agenesis. Middle ear findings depend on severity of external auditory canal atresia and auricular dysplasia. Anomalies of the ossicular chain include rotation, fusion, or absence of the ossicles and abnormalities of the suspensory ligaments. Oval window atresia may be associated. An anomalous course of the intratemporal facial nerve is usual in middle ear dysplasia. The tympanic segment may be dehiscent, overlying oval, or round windows. The mastoid segment migrates anteriorly away from its normal position. A congenital cholesteatoma behind the atresia plate is identifiable in fewer than 10% of cases.	Middle and external ear dysplasia represents a spectrum of congenital anomalies resulting from abnormal embryogenesis of the first and second branchial arches and tympanic ring. The middle and external ear develop in concert from these structures, which explains the usual association of these anomalies. Abnormalities of the inner ear are less commonly associated, as these structures develop earlier in gestation. Dysplastic auricle, absent or stenotic external auditory canal, and conductive hearing loss are the most common symptoms. Occurs more commonly in male patients.
Mastoid dysplasia	CT reveals the development of the mastoid and the degree of pneumatization. Pneumatization can be completely absent, with absence of the corresponding mastoid process or with a solid block of bone. In case of a hypoplastic dense, sclerotic mastoid the pneumatization may be limited to a small mastoid antral cell. Possible associated findings are external auditory canal, middle ear and, less frequently, inner ear malformations. Hyperpneumatization of the temporal bone with extension into the occipital bone and even the parietal bone is a rare condition (associated complication: pneumatocele, pneumocephalus).	The development of the mastoid air cell system begins in utero. Unilateral or bilateral absence of the mastoid antrum is a rare clinical finding and it is usually systemic. Underdevelopment of mastoids may be isolated or in association with children with microtia, Treacher-Collins syndrome, Cornelia de Lange syndrome, trisomy 13, Down syndrome, and branchiooculofacial syndrome.
Primary cholesteatoma	Globular, well-marginated nonenhancing, hypodense, expansile mass, located in the posterior epitympanum (at tympanic isthmi) or near the stapes or the anterosuperior middle ear (adjacent to eustachian tube and anterior tympanic ring, medial to ossicles). Larger mass (late in disease) may erode ossicles, middle ear wall, and lateral semicircular canal or tegmen tympani and extend throughout cavity and mastoid complex.	Most common cause of mass in the middle ear cavity behind an intact tympanic membrane (other T-bone locations: petrous apex, mastoid, external auditory canal, squamous portion of the temporal bone). Histologically identical to epidermoid; congenital cholesteatomas consist of exfoliated keratin and solid cholesterin within a sac of stratified squamous epithelium, originating from ectodermal rests. Rarely associated with first branchial cleft remnant or middle and external ear dysplasia. Patients are usually between 4 and 20 y (M:F = 3:1) and present with unilateral progressive conductive hearing loss and no history of inflammatory ear disease. Late in disease large lesions can obstruct eustachian tube with resultant middle ear effusion and infection. Otoscopically, a white mass behind intact tympanic membrane may be seen.
Cephalocele ▷ *Fig. 5.16*	Well-defined middle ear mass with heterogeneous, mixed density (due to variable amounts of CSF and brain tissue) localized at the upper part of the attic with an apparent focal bone defect usually of the tegmen tympani. No contrast enhancement. Both ossicular chain and scutum are preserved. MRI is the best modality to clarify the temporal lobe herniation.	Protrusion of cranial contents into middle ear. Spontaneous in origin with congenital defect in the tegmen tympani or mastoideum, or as a result of previous temporal bone surgery or trauma. Can be associated with CSF leaks. Herniated brain is usually nonfunctional.

(continues on page 217)

Table 5.4 (Cont.) Temporal bone: diseases of the middle ear and mastoid

Disease	CT Findings	Comments
Aberrant internal carotid artery ▷ *Fig. 5.17*	Rounded tubular soft tissue density that enters the middle ear cavity posterolateral to the cochlea, crosses the mesotympanum along the cochlear promontory, and exits anteromedially to become the horizontal portion of the carotid canal. Carotid foramen and vertical segment of petrous internal carotid artery are absent. The inferior tympanic canaliculus, just anterolateral to the jugular bulb and posterior and lateral to where normal carotid foramen would be, is enlarged. Enhancement is equivalent to other arteries. CTA shows the aberrant nature of the enlarged collateral vessel traversing middle ear when internal carotid artery fails to develop.	Congenital vascular pseudomass: when the cervical portion and the first petrous portion of the internal carotid artery fail to develop, inferior tympanic artery, a branch of ascending pharyngeal artery, supplies petrous internal carotid artery via middle ear and caroticotympanic artery. Very rare disorder, with female and right side preference. May be an incidental finding or present with pulsatile tinnitus or conductive hearing loss. Otoscopically, a red retrotympanic pulsatile mass is seen.
Lateralized internal carotid artery	Dehiscent lateral wall of the petrous internal carotid artery as it borders the anterior middle ear cavity with protrusion of the enhancing internal carotid artery into middle ear. At the level of the cochlear promontory, CTA confirms the course of the laterally displaced petrous internal carotid artery (normal in size and contour) projecting into middle ear.	Vary rare vascular variant with failure of formation or ossification of the lateral wall of the petrous internal carotid artery. May be an incidental finding or present with pulsatile tinnitus. When prominent, a vascular retrotympanic mass may be seen otoscopically.
Persistent stapedial artery	CT scans will show absent ipsilateral foramen spinosum posterolateral to the normal foramen ovale (nonspecific; may be seen also when the middle meningeal artery takes its origin from the ophthalmic artery) and Y-shaped enlargement of the geniculate fossa with encroachment upon the adjacent anterior epitympanic recess. CTA may show the persistent stapedial artery arising from the genu of vertical and horizontal infracochlear petrous internal carotid artery and in the absence of a normal middle meningeal artery. It may occur with or without aberrant internal carotid artery.	The persistent stapedial artery is a very rare vascular congenital anomaly. If the embryological stapedial artery fails to involute (in the third fetal month), the artery courses from the infracochlear carotid through the stapedial obturator foramen, passes through the stapes footplate, crosses the medial wall of the middle ear cavity over the cochlear promontory, and passes superiorly into an enlarged anterior facial nerve tympanic segment. Intracranially, it becomes the middle meningeal artery. Most commonly asymptomatic finding on CT or during surgery.

(continues on page 218)

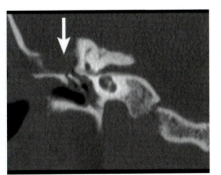

Fig. 5.16 Postoperative cephalocele, right middle ear. Right coronal T-bone CT image reveals a postmastoidectomy right ear with broad bone defect of the tegmen tympani (arrow) and soft tissue in the epitympanum.

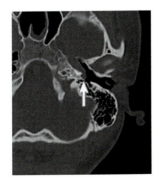

Fig. 5.17 Aberrant internal carotid artery. Left axial T-bone CT image shows the horizontal portion of the carotid canal extending too far posterolaterally into the middle ear (arrow). Note the absence of posterolateral margination. (Courtesy of Dr. B. Stinn, Zurich.)

II Head and Neck

Table 5.4   (Cont.) Temporal bone: diseases of the middle ear and mastoid

Disease	CT Findings	Comments
Dehiscent jugular bulb ▷ *Fig. 5.18*	Soft tissue mass low in the middle ear, contiguous with the internal jugular vein through a focal jugular (sigmoid) plate defect. The other margins of the adjacent jugular foramen are smooth and intact. Commonly seen with high-riding jugular bulb. The superolateral outpouching demonstrates similar enhancement characteristics to jugular bulb, sigmoid sinus, and internal jugular vein.	Congenital vascular pseudomass. Otoscopically, a retrotympanic vascular mass may be seen in the lower part of the middle ear behind the intact tympanic membrane. Does not grow with time. This is usually asymptomatic, but may cause pulsatile tinnitus or conductive hearing loss.
Prolapsing facial nerve	Soft tissue "mass" in the oval window niche along the undersurface of the lateral semicircular canal, best seen on coronal images. Concomitant anomalies of the stapes may be present.	Relatively rare congenital lesion. Facial nerve protrudes through a bony dehiscence as it courses along undersurface of the lateral semicircular canal. Usually it is an incidental finding.
Inflammatory/infectious conditions		
Otomastoiditis ▷ *Fig. 5.19*	In **acute uncomplicated otomastoiditis,** nonspecific fluid and enhancing inflammatory debris are apparent in the middle ear, and some or all of the mastoid and petrous apex air spaces are opacified by fluid or mucosal edema. The presence of air–fluid levels is pathognomonic for effusion. **Acute coalescent otomastoiditis** is characterized by erosion of bony walls, rarefaction of septa, and dehiscence into the inner ear and intracranial compartment. When there is associated abscess, a rim-enhancing fluid collection adjacent to eroded middle ear/mastoid cortex is present extracranially, either in the post- or preauricular soft tissues (subperiosteal abscess) or in and around the sternocleidomastoid muscle (Bezold abscess), or intracranially in the temporal lobe. The presence of pneumolabyrinth in the cochlea and vestibule indicates a fistula. Long-standing history of **chronic otitis media** may initiate ossicular erosions with absence of segment of ossicular chain. Tympanosclerosis appears as multifocal calcifications or ossifications within soft tissue debris in the middle ear cavity. Oval window involvement with a focus of calcification within occurs. An underdeveloped, poorly aerated sclerotic mastoid, granulation tissue in the middle ear, and retraction of thickened tympanic membrane also may be visible.	Acute otomastoiditis is a common infectious process that stems from upper respiratory infection and usually affects children. Bacterial etiology is the rule, with *Streptococcus pneumoniae* and *Haemophilus influenzae* accounting for the majority of cases. Common clinical symptoms are otalgia, fever, and postauricular swelling. Most aggressive cases are in young children. Tuberculous otitis and fungal disease are uncommon but occur more often in immunocompromised patients. Diagnostic imaging plays a key role in diagnosing complications, which may include subperiosteal abscess, labyrinthitis, meningitis, brain abscess, dural sinus thrombosis, and Bezold abscess. Manifestations of chronic otomastoiditis include cholesteatoma, granulation tissue, cholesterol granuloma, tympanosclerosis, postinflammatory ossicular erosions, and bony or fibrous tissue fixation.

(continues on page 220)

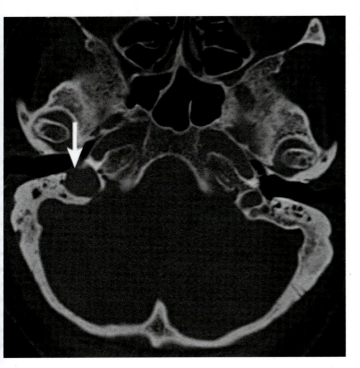

Fig. 5.18   Dehiscent jugular bulb. Axial bone CT image shows the sigmoid plate is dehiscent on the right side (arrow) with a soft tissue mass in the posteroinferior middle ear cavity contiguous with an enlarged jugular bulb.

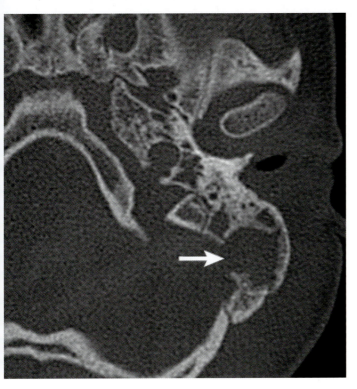

Fig. 5.19   Acute coalescent otomastoiditis. Left axial T-bone CT image demonstrates mastoid debris and confluence of mastoid air cells with trabecular and cortical erosions (arrow). Also seen is postauricular soft tissue swelling.

II   Head and Neck

Table 5.4 (Cont.) Temporal bone: diseases of the middle ear and mastoid

Disease	CT Findings	Comments
Acquired cholesteatoma ▷ *Fig. 5.20* ▷ *Fig. 5.21* ▷ *Fig. 5.22* ▷ *Fig. 5.23*	Nondependent, rounded, homogeneous hypodense mass (density less than that of the brain), associated with bone erosion or ossicular destruction. Cholesteatomas do not enhance with contrast. Tympanic membrane retraction may arise in the pars flaccida or pars tensa. **Pars flaccida cholesteatoma,** the most common form of acquired cholesteatoma (82%), develops primarily within Prussak space along the lateral attic wall, lateral to the ossicles, and may extend posteriorly into the posterolateral attic, then through the aditus ad antrum into the mastoid or inferiorly to the posterior middle ear recess. Erosion of the scutum is a classical finding in attic cholesteatoma and remodeling of the lateral attic wall. **Pars tensa cholesteatoma,** the far less common form of acquired cholesteatoma (18%), begins in the posterior mesotympanum medial to the ossicles and commonly involves the sinus tympani. Extension is toward the mastoid antrum medial to the incus. The **acquired mural cholesteatoma,** a particular type of lesion, does not present as a bulky mass, but appears to be quite invasive and has a propensity for developing numerous manifestations of bony erosion, including automastoidectomy, ossicular involvement, and fistula formation (at surgery, a fine non-CT-detectable membrane of cholesteatoma may be identified). Secondary findings relate to progressive bone erosion and may include destruction of the ossicles, facial nerve canal, labyrinth (particularly the lateral semicircular canal), mastoid (including Körner septum), tegmen tympani, or floor of the middle cranial fossa. Intracranial infections, sigmoid sinus thrombosis, and CSF leaks are rare complications.	Acquired cholesteatomas are usually a complication of chronic otomastoiditis, more common in men, and of any age. The accumulation of exfoliated keratin within a sac of stratified squamous epithelium (keratoma) within the middle ear produces a mass effect that erodes the bony walls and ossicles. It is believed to result from ingrowth of squamous epithelium through marginal tympanic membrane perforations, from retraction pockets, or from ingrowth into the middle ear of the basal layer of the tympanic membrane. Common symptoms are smelly aural discharge, conductive hearing loss, and otalgia. Late complications are vertigo, venous sinus thrombosis, and intracranial infections.
Cholesterol granuloma ▷ *Fig. 5.24*	Expansive, hypodense middle ear mass with smooth bony margins that does not enhance with contrast administration. When there is associated hemorrhage, a fluid level may be present. Although the mass fills the middle ear cavity, the ossicles are intact in most patients.	Cholesterol granuloma is a complication of chronic otomastoid inflammation that is characterized pathologically by specialized granulation tissue, blood breakdown products, and cholesterol crystals. Eustachian tube dysfunction is considered the most likely etiology, with secondary decreased intratympanic pressure, mucosal edema, and blood vessel rupture. In the temporal bone, cholesterol granuloma is seen within the middle ear cavity, mastoid, and petrous apex. When the lesion is in the middle ear, otoscopic examination reveals a "blue" tympanic membrane in the absence of pulsatile tinnitus.
Granulation tissue	On CT, granulation tissue causes contrast-enhancing, nondependent opacification of the middle ear without erosive bone changes; however, when there is associated hemorrhage, a fluid level may be present. Stranding soft tissue in middle ear is associated with inflammatory debris. (When the debris is globular, however, it cannot be differentiated from early cholesteatoma, where scalloping has not yet taken place.)	The development of granulation tissue in the middle ear is common both as an isolated phenomenon and in conjunction with other middle ear maladies, such as effusion and cholesteatoma. Granulation tissue is often vascular and has a distinct tendency to bleed, causing hemotympanum.

(continues on page 222)

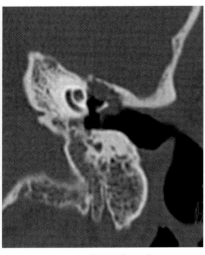

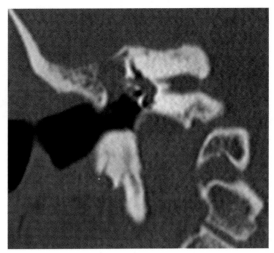

Fig. 5.20 Acquired pars flaccida cholesteatoma. Left coronal T-bone CT image shows an atticoantral nondependent, homogeneous soft tissue mass filling Prussak space. The scutum, lateral attic wall, and tegmen tympani are eroded. Also seen is the medially displaced malleus.

Fig. 5.21 Cholesteatoma with labyrinthine fistula. Right coronal T-bone CT image reveals opacification of the epitympanum with associated dehiscence of the lateral semicircular canal and tegmen tympani.

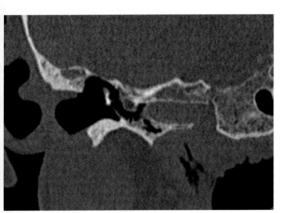

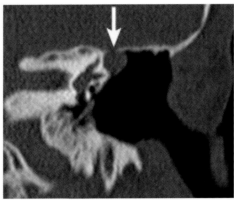

Fig. 5.22 Automastoidectomy (acquired mural cholesteatoma). Right coronal T-bone CT image demonstrates erosion of the scutum, lateral attic wall, tegmen tympani, and ossicles, as well as a ventilated common cavity connecting the enlarged middle ear and antrum.

Fig. 5.23 Recurrent cholesteatoma. Coronal T-bone CT image of the left postmastoidectomy ear reveals an abnormal soft tissue mass beneath a tegmen tympani defect (arrow).

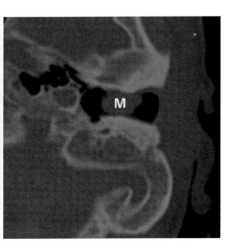

Fig. 5.24 Cholesterol granuloma, middle ear. Left axial T-bone CT image shows a smoothly expansile hypodense mass (M) of the middle ear, expanding into the external ear, without bone erosion or remodeling.

Table 5.4 (Cont.) Temporal bone: diseases of the middle ear and mastoid

Disease	CT Findings	Comments
Benign neoplasms		
Glomus tympanicum paraganglioma ▷ *Fig. 5.25*	Enhancing focal mass with flat base on the cochlear promontory, without connection to the jugular fossa. A large glomus tumor fills the middle ear cavity, creating attic block and resulting in fluid collection in mastoid, or extends into mastoid air cells or through tympanic membrane into the external auditory canal. The floor of the middle ear cavity is intact. The ossicles typically are spared. **Glasscock-Jackson classification** **Glomus tympanicum paraganglioma:** Type I: small mass limited to the promontory. Type II: mass completely fills the middle ear space. Type III: mass completely fills the middle ear space and extends into the mastoid. Type IV: mass fills the middle ear space and extends into the mastoid or through tympanic membrane to fill the external auricular canal; may extend anterior to carotid; may have intracranial extension.	Glomus tympanicum paraganglioma is a benign, neural crest tumor localized to the cochlear promontory of the middle ear cavity (along the course of the inferior tympanic nerve). The glomus tumor is the second most common cause of mass in the middle ear cavity behind an intact tympanic membrane. It is rarely associated with multicentric paragangliomas. Patients are usually female and between 40 and 60 y of age with pulsatile tinnitus and conductive hearing loss, rarely with facial nerve paralysis. Otoscopically, a red vascular mass is seen behind the anteroinferior quadrant of the eardrum.
Glomus jugulotympanicum paraganglioma ▷ *Fig. 5.26*	Homogeneous, intensely enhancing mass extending superolaterally from the jugular foramen into the middle ear cavity. Permeative-destructive bone changes along the superolateral margin of the jugular foramen mark extent of tumor. Bony floor of the middle ear cavity is invaded, and the jugular spine of the jugular foramen is eroded. The vertical segment of the petrous internal carotid artery is often dehiscent. Larger lesions may extend into the petrous bone, external auditory canal, and mastoid.	Glomus jugulare paraganglioma (GJP) is a benign tumor arising from paraganglia in and around the jugular foramen (jugular bulb, Jacobson nerve, and Arnold nerve). When middle ear extension occurs, such a tumor is called a glomus jugulotympanicum paraganglioma. GJP is the most common jugular foramen tumor and the second most common temporal bone tumor. In sporadic GJP, it is multicentric in 5% to 10% of patients. When familial (inherited as an autosomal dominant disease), multicentricity amounts to 25% to 50%. Patients are usually female and between 40 and 60 y of age with pulsatile tinnitus, conductive hearing loss, and cranial nerve involvement (CN IX, X, XI, and XII; VII and VIII less often). Otoscopically, a red vascular retrotympanic mass is seen.
Middle ear adenoma	Well-marginated, rounded enhancing soft tissue mass in the middle ear with minimal erosion. The ossicles may be encased. The mastoid is well pneumatized.	Very rare benign, indolent epithelial middle ear tumor, arising from modified respiratory mucosa. Mean age at presentation with conductive hearing loss is 45 y. No history of chronic otitis media. Otoscopically, a pink soft tissue mass is seen behind an intact tympanic membrane.
Middle ear schwannoma ▷ *Fig. 5.27*	Well-marginated, lobular, homogeneous, uniformly enhancing soft tissue mass in the middle ear cavity. Facial nerve schwannomas are most commonly centered on geniculate ganglion and emanating from facial canal. Jacobson nerve schwannoma reveals erosion of the cochlear promontory, possible enlargement of the inferior tympanic canaliculus, and absence of facial nerve involvement.	Schwannoma is one of the common benign middle ear space tumors. They may originate from the nerves of the tympanic cavity (facial nerve, Jacobson nerve, chorda tympani nerve, or Arnold nerve) or by expansion from outside the middle ear space (CN VIII, IX, X, and XI). Patients are adult and present with neural palsy and conductive hearing loss. Otoscopically, a fleshy white mass is seen behind an intact tympanic membrane.
Hemangioma	Poorly marginated, intensely enhancing mass with "honeycomb" bony matrix and/or spiculated appearance with intratumoral bone flecks. Most common sites of involvement are the labyrinthine segment of the facial nerve and the geniculate fossa area, but any segment of the facial nerve can be affected. Multisegmental involvement is also possible.	Intratemporal hemangiomas are rare extraneural vascular lesions arising from capillaries around the facial nerve, which can secondarily grow into the nerve. Often occurs with chronic, progressive, peripheral facial nerve paralysis. Pulsatile tinnitus may be present.

(continues on page 224)

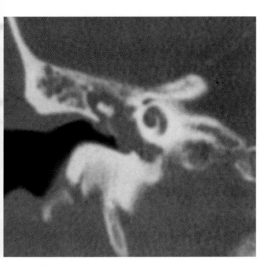

Fig. 5.25   Glomus tympanicum paraganglioma. Right coronal T-bone CT image shows complete opacification of the middle ear and mastoid air cells. The floor of the middle ear cavity is intact.

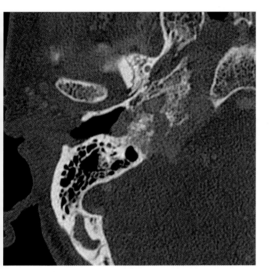

Fig. 5.26   Glomus jugulotympanicum paraganglioma. Right axial T-bone CT image demonstrates a large mass in the jugular foramen with adjacent permeative-destructive bone changes. The lesion extends through the bony floor into the middle ear. There is erosion of the posterior wall of the petrous carotid canal. (Courtesy of Dr. B. Stinn, Zurich.)

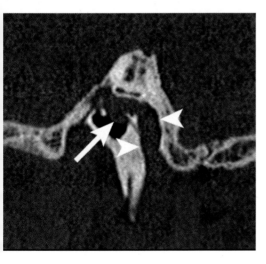

Fig. 5.27   Facial nerve schwannoma. Left sagittal T-bone CT image reveals a tubular soft tissue mass involving the mastoid and tympanic segments of the facial nerve. The tumor pedunculates into the middle ear cavity (arrow) and produces an expansion of the bony canal (arrowheads).

Table 5.4 (Cont.) Temporal bone: diseases of the middle ear and mastoid

Disease	CT Findings	Comments
Middle ear meningioma	Intensely uniform or heterogeneous enhancing, globular (most common) or en plaque soft tissue mass within the middle ear cavity with permeative-sclerotic bony changes in surrounding bones. Tegmen tympani and mastoid bones are affected in tegmen tympani meningioma; sigmoid plate and middle ear floor are affected in jugular foramen meningioma. Middle ear component may represent "tip of the iceberg" for larger jugular foramen or tegmen tympani meningioma.	Benign tumor arising from arachnoid cap cells. May extend up from jugular foramen into middle ear, extend down from dura overlying tegmen tympani, or arise within middle ear. Patients are usually middle-aged and female with conductive hearing loss (M:F = 1:3, average age at presentation 45 y). Otoscopically, a vascular (blue) retrotympanic mass may be seen.
Malignant neoplasms		
Squamous cell carcinoma ▷ *Fig. 5.28*	Holotympanic enhancing soft tissue mass. Bony destruction should be rather extensive. Destruction of the tegmen tympani or sinodural plate leads to intracranial involvement.	Primary malignant middle ear tumors in adults are rare and usually associated with a history of chronic otitis media. Squamous cell carcinoma can occur, as can various types of adenocarcinoma, particularly adenoid cystic carcinoma. Squamous cell carcinomas have a definite male predominance. The peak incidence is in the fifth to seventh decades. They are believed to originate in most patients from the tympanic mucosa. Adenocarcinomas of the middle ear have an equal gender incidence.
Middle ear rhabdomyosarcoma	Large, irregular, middle ear/mastoid mass with osteolytic, destructive bone and ossicle changes. The tumor enhances homogeneously. Possible areas of extension are the external auditory canal, internal auditory canal, middle and posterior cranial fossae, nasopharyngeal carotid space, masticator space, and parotid space.	Although rare, rhabdomyosarcoma is the most common primary middle ear tumor in the pediatric age group (bimodal: in children < 5 y and teens 15–19 y) with male predominance. Clinical symptomatology usually includes bloody otorrhea and ear pain; 30% of patients have neurologic deficits and nodal metastases at the time of diagnosis.
Metastases	Metastases involving the middle ear and mastoid usually extend from elsewhere, particularly the petrous apex, or disseminate hematogenously, and may be osteoblastic or osteolytic.	Primary sites include breast, lung, kidney, prostate, head and neck squamous neoplasms, and stomach.
Trauma		
		Damage to the temporal bone typically requires the application of great force and may cause fracture, hemorrhage, nerve trauma, vascular damage, or disruption of the middle or inner ear structures. Associated intracranial injuries, such as extra-axial hemorrhage, shear (or diffuse axonal injury), and brain contusion, are common. Twenty percent of patients with skull fracture have temporal bone fractures. Majority of fractures are actually oblique, transverse, longitudinal, or mixed. Potential complications of temporal bone fracture include infection (meningitis), hearing loss, facial (and other cranial) nerve injury, and CSF leak with otorrhea and/or rhinorrhea, and perilymphatic fistula.
Longitudinal fractures of the temporal bone ▷ *Fig. 5.29a, b*	Longitudinal fractures of the temporal bone course parallel to the long axis of the petrous pyramid, typically extralabyrinthine. It starts in the pars squamosa, mastoid, or external auditory canal, extends through the posterosuperior bony external auditory canal, continues across the roof of the middle ear space anterior to the labyrinth, and ends anteromedially in the middle cranial fossa in close proximity to the foramen lacerum and ovale. The most common course of the fracture is anterior and extralabyrinthine; however, although rare, intralabyrinthine extension is possible. Facial canal involvement is less common. Bilateral temporal bone fractures are present in 8% to 29% of all fractures. The **oblique fracture** crosses the external auditory canal in a horizontal plane and then extends upward obliquely toward the middle fossa. The fracture misses the otic capsule and may extend toward the petrous apex, where the fracture line may extend to the foramen lacerum. Conversely, the longitudinal fracture line is oriented in a more vertical plane.	Longitudinal fractures of the temporal bone are most common (70%–90% of all temporal fractures). They are usually secondary to blunt temporoparietal head trauma. Longitudinal fractures usually present with classic findings of laceration of the ear canal, tympanic membrane perforation, hematotympanum, ossicular injury (most commonly the incus), facial paralysis, and hearing loss. The hearing loss is predominantly conductive but may have a sensorineural component as well. Facial paralysis, often delayed and incomplete, occurs in ~10% to 20% of longitudinal fractures. Patients with longitudinal fractures usually develop CSF leaks from the tegmen, where the fracture line perforates the dura.

(continues on page 226)

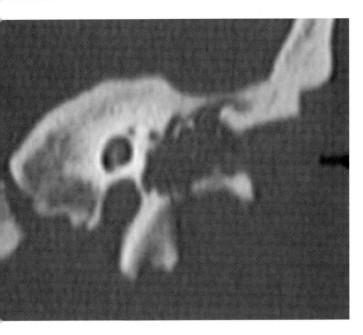

Fig. 5.28   Squamous cell carcinoma, middle ear. Left coronal T-bone CT image shows a large soft tissue mass filling the middle ear. There is marked bony erosion of the cavity walls and ossicular destruction.

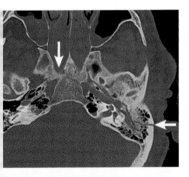
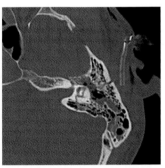
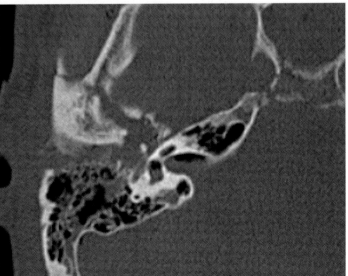

c

Fig. 5.29a–c   Temporal bone fractures. Left axial T-bone CT image (**a**) demonstrates an extralabyrinthine longitudinal fracture extending from the mastoid (arrow), crossing the middle ear cavity with associated ossicular derangement and hemotympanum, the carotid canal, and the greater wing of the sphenoid, reaching the clivus (arrow). Right axial T-bone CT image (**b**) reveals a mixed fracture with both longitudinal and oblique components. Also seen are associated ossicular derangement and hemotympanum, pneumolabyrinth, and air within the internal auditory canal. Left axial T-bone CT image (**c**) shows a transverse fracture extending through the bony labyrinth. Middle ear fluid is present, as well as an abnormal density filling of the mastoid cells.

Table 5.4   (Cont.) Temporal bone: diseases of the middle ear and mastoid

Disease	CT Findings	Comments
Transverse fractures of the temporal bone ▷ **Fig. 5.29c**	Transverse fractures of the temporal bone course perpendicular to the long axis of the petrous pyramid, usually medial or lateral to the arcuate eminence. Medially situated fractures involve the vestibule, cochlea, fundus of the internal auditory canal, and crus commune. A more unusual type of transverse fracture occurs medial to the vestibule and bisects the inner auditory canal. Laterally placed fractures involve the promontory, vestibule, and horizontal and posterior semicircular canals. Facial nerve canal involvement (geniculate fossa) is common.	Transverse fractures of the temporal bone are less common (10%–30% of all temporal fractures). They are usually secondary to blunt fronto-occipital head trauma. The fracture commonly begins in the vicinity of the jugular foramen or foramen magnum and extends to the middle cranial fossa. The tympanic membrane is usually spared. The ossicles are often spared. Clinical findings include persistent vertigo (due to transection of the vestibule, vestibular nerves, or vestibular aqueduct, perilymph fistula, labyrinthine concussion, or cupulolithiasis), often with spontaneous nystagmus, and permanent sensorineural hearing loss (due to damage to the cochlea or transection of the cochlear nerve). Facial paralysis is common (50%), often immediate and complete, due to edema, intraneuronal hematoma, impingement by fracture fragments, and complete transection. Patients with transverse fractures are more likely to develop CSF leaks from the vestibule defect. Also, because the tympanic membrane may be intact, they are more likely to present with CSF otorhinorrhea.
Ossicular injuries ▷ **Fig. 5.30**	**Incudomalleolar joint separation** appears as displacement of the head of the malleus (the "scoop of the ice cream" is usually displaced laterally) from the body and short process of the incus (the "cone" is usually displaced medially and anteriorly). **Incudostapedial joint separation** appears as abnormal enlargement of the dark cleft between the head of the stapes and the long process of the incus, as a fracture of the lenticular process of the incus, or as a fracture through the stapes superstructure. **Dislocation of the incus:** When incudomalleolar joint separation is associated with incudostapedial joint separation or a fracture of the stapes, the incus may remain in the epitympanic recess with rotation and superiorly, posteriorly, and laterally displace, prolapse into the lower part of the tympanic cavity or external auditory canal, or even disappear. **Dislocation of the malleoincudal complex** may be associated with an incudostapedial joint separation. The direction can be outward, inward, or downward. In cases of **stapediovestibular dislocation,** CT shows absence of the footplate from the oval window without labyrinthine fracture. The stapes is dislocated in the tympanic cavity or depressed into the vestibule. Pneumolabyrinth or perilymphatic fistula may be associated. **Fracture of the malleus** occurs at the neck or manubrium and is usually associated with other severe derangements. **Fractures of the incus** affect the long or lenticular process or the body of the incus. **Fractures of the stapes** may involve one crus or the arch and the footplate with or without displacement of fragments.	Trauma to the ossicular chain is a frequent complication of temporal bone injury after blows to the temporal, parietal, or occipital region, blasts, barotraumas, and lightning. Ossicular disruption can also occur following direct trauma to the ear by penetrating injury through the external auditory canal. Ossicular injury usually occurs as a dislocation. Incudostapedial and incudomalleolar disarticulation and dislocation of the incus and malleoincudal complex are common injuries, whereas stapediovestibular dislocation is rare. Fracture of the malleus, incus, or stapes is uncommon. Both axial and coronal images are needed for evaluation. Reformatted images may also be useful. There is a high incidence of conductive hearing loss secondary to ossicular injury.

(continues on page 227)

Table 5.4   (Cont.) Temporal bone: diseases of the middle ear and mastoid

Disease	CT Findings	Comments
Miscellaneous lesions		
Langerhans cell histiocytosis	CT can demonstrate a sharp-marginated, lytic temporal bone lesion with destruction of the middle and inner ear, with potential fistula formation toward the cochlea and all the semicircular canals. The soft tissue component enhances strongly. Fragments of bone within the soft tissue component are common.	Aggressive nonneoplastic lesion in the temporal bone, often bilateral or with other associated osseous lesions, causing extensive bone destruction with associated soft tissue mass; extracalvarial and/or intracranial extradural in young children with conductive hearing loss and otorrhea.
Mastoid pneumocele	Affect the mastoid air cells with surrounding extensive pneumatization of the skull base. All areas of pneumatization intercommunicate. There is focal or diffuse thinning of the surrounding bony structures and loss of the bony trabeculae. There may be dehiscence of the outer cortex of the temporal bone. Air may also be present within the atlanto-occipital joints and within adjacent extracranial soft tissues.	Uncommon symptomatic acquired lesion with abnormal pneumatization of the skull base extending from the temporal bone. Persistently increased intraluminal pressure has been proposed as a mechanism of pneumocele formation that causes the mastoid cells to expand throughout the skull base.

II Head and Neck

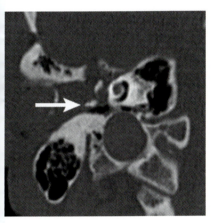

Fig. 5.30   Ossicular injuries. Right coronal T-bone CT image shows a comminuted mastoid fracture with ossicular disruption. The incus is rotated and displaced inferolaterally (arrow). Also present are a hemotympanum and blood in the external auditory canal.

Table 5.5 Temporal bone: diseases of the inner ear and internal auditory canal

Disease	CT Findings	Comments
Congenital/developmental lesions		
Labyrinthine aplasia (Michel deformity)	Petrous bone lacks cochlea, vestibule, and semicircular canals; amorphous bone instead of inner ear structures. Associated abnormalities: small or absent internal auditory canal, hypoplastic or absent petrous apex, flattened medial wall of middle ear (because neither the promontory nor the lateral semicircular canal bulges into the tympanic cavity), ossicle absence or fusion. Geniculate ganglion is posterior to normal location. Facial nerve bony canal is prominent.	Extremely rare congenital inner ear malformation characterized by complete lack of development of the inner ear. The developmental arrest occurs at the third gestational week. May be unilateral or bilateral. Seen in Klippel-Feil syndrome and thalidomide exposure. Sensorineural hearing loss from birth.
Cochlear aplasia	Complete absence of cochlea. Vestibule, semicircular canals, and internal auditory canal are variably affected: normal, hypoplastic, or dilated. Cochlear promontory is flat. Labyrinthine, geniculate ganglion, and anterior tympanic portions of facial nerve course occupy site where cochlea should be. External auditory canal, middle ear, ossicular chain, bony vestibular aqueduct, and endolymphatic duct are of normal size. **Cochlear hypoplasia:** The cochlea consists of a small 1- to 3-mm bud. The vestibule may be enlarged, and semicircular canals may be normal or deformed.	Extremely rare inner ear anomaly, usually bilateral. The developmental arrest occurs at the late third gestational week. Sensorineural hearing loss from birth.
Mondini malformation	The cochlea is small and consists of a normal base turn and a single ovoid cavity instead of the middle and apical turns with modiolar deficiency and interscalar septum absence. In the pseudo-Mondini malformation, the basal turn is enlarged too. Mondini malformation is associated in 20% of cases with anomalies of the vestibule, semicircular canals, and endolymphatic duct/sac.	Malformation of the bony inner ear with loss of the normal two and one half turns to the cochlea. May be unilateral or bilateral. Mondini malformation has been reported in campomelic dysplasia, CHARGE association, congenital CMV infection, hemifacial microsomia, trisomy 21, branchio-otorenal syndrome, Johanson-Blizzard syndrome, Klippel-Feil syndrome, Pendred syndrome, and Pierre Robin syndrome. Clinically the hearing loss is total. Because of an associated perilymph fistula, recurrent meningitis or recurrent CSF otorrhea that mimics otitis media with effusion may occur.
Cystic common cavity ▷ *Fig. 5.31*	Cochlea and vestibule are fused and seen as a common, featureless cavity without differentiation and of variable size (averaging 7–10 mm in diameter). The semicircular canals may be normal, deformed, or absent. Internal auditory canal, entering the anterior aspect of the common cavity, may be normal, small, or large. External auditory canal, middle ear structures, mastoid, and vestibular aqueduct are normal.	Rare congenital inner ear malformation, unilateral or bilateral, with congenital sensorineural hearing loss. Arrest of development occurs at the fourth gestational week.
Cystic cochleovestibular anomaly ▷ *Fig. 5.32*	"Snowman"-shaped bony inner ear with confluent cystic cochlea and vestibule with no internal structures visible. Semicircular canals are present but with variable shape and degree of dilation. The internal auditory canal may be dilated with defective fundus. External auditory canal, middle ear structures, mastoid, and vestibular aqueduct are normal.	Rare inner ear anomaly with congenital sensorineural hearing loss. Arrest of development occurs at the fifth gestational week. Sensorineural hearing loss from birth.
Semicircular canal dysplasia	**Sporadic semicircular canal dysplasia:** Dilated lateral semicircular canal forming single cavity with dilated vestibule. Posterior and superior semicircular canal may be normal, dilated, or hypoplastic. Cochlea can be normal or with incomplete apical and middle turn partition. Oval window atresia is commonly associated. **Syndromic semicircular canal dysplasia:** All semicircular canals are absent in both ears, the vestibule is small and dysmorphic, oval window atresia is always present, and cochlear anomalies (most common "isolated" cochlea with lack of cochlear aperture) are usually associated. **Semicircular canal dysplasia or aplasia** may be associated with labyrinthine aplasia, cochlear hypoplasia, or cystic common cavity deformity.	Rare inner ear anomaly with malformation, hypoplasia, or aplasia of one or all of semicircular canals. Arrest of development occurs at the sixth to eighth gestational week. May be part of genetic syndromes (CHARGE, Alagille, Kallmann, Noonan, Waardenburg, Crouzon, and Apert). Sensorineural hearing loss from birth. Conductive hearing loss often is present due to oval window atresia and ossicular chain anomalies.

(continues on page 230)

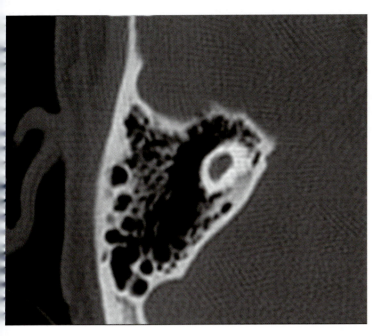

Fig. 5.31 **Cystic common cavity.** Right axial T-bone CT image shows the cochlea, vestibule, and semicircular canals as a common featureless small cavity without differentiation. (Courtesy of Dr. C. Ozdoba, Bern.)

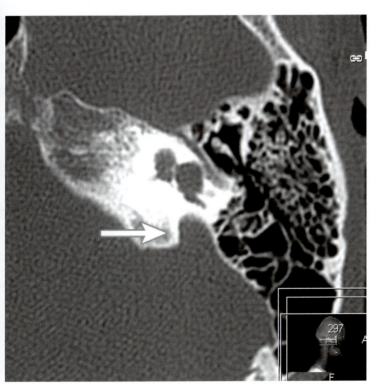

Fig. 5.32 **Cystic cochleovestibular anomaly.** Left axial T-bone CT image demonstrates a "snowman"-shaped inner ear with cystic featureless cochlea (absent modiolus) and dilated cystic vestibule. Also present is an enlarged bony vestibular aqueduct (arrow). (Courtesy of Dr. C. Ozdoba, Bern.)

Table 5.5   (Cont.) Temporal bone: diseases of the inner ear and internal auditory canal

Disease	CT Findings	Comments
Superior semicircular canal dehiscence ▷ *Fig. 5.33*	Uni- or bilateral small and complete defect in the bony wall of the one- to three-layer roof of the superior semicircular canal. Extreme thinning of tegmen tympani may be associated.	Treatable form of vestibular disturbance, most likely a developmental anomaly. Dehiscence of bone overlying the superior semicircular canal can result in a syndrome of slowly progressive dizziness and/or oscillopsia evoked by loud noises or by maneuvers that change middle ear or intracranial pressure, disabling disequilibrium, Tullio phenomenon (vertigo and/or nystagmus related to sound), conductive hearing loss in spite of normal middle ear function, and vertical-torsional eye movements in the plane of the superior semicircular canal evoked by sound and/or pressure stimuli. Mean age: 42 y (range 20–70 y).
Large vestibular aqueduct syndrome ▷ *Fig. 5.34a, b*	Describes the bony anomaly seen on temporal bone CT: V-shaped enlarged bony vestibular aqueduct with a midbony vestibular aqueduct diameter > than 1.5 mm, wider than the posterior semicircular canal diameter; 16% to 26% of ears with large vestibular aqueduct have a Mondini or pseudo-Mondini malformation. Associated vestibular (i.e., enlargement of the utricle area) and/or semicircular canal anomalies may be obvious. Complementary T2-weighted MRI can easily identify a corresponding enlarged endolymphatic duct and sac in foveal area and an associated cochlear dysplasia (CT does not give any information about the endolymphatic sac).	Most common congenital anomaly of the inner ear found by imaging. Arrested development of inner ear at seventh gestational week leaves large endolymphatic duct and sac associated with cochlear dysplasia. Bilateral anomaly in 90%. Most cases are sporadic, but it has been reported in brachio-otorenal syndrome, CHARGE association, congenital CMV infection, and Pendred syndrome. Sensorineural hearing loss develops with variable speed and may not be present until early adult life.
Internal auditory canal stenosis or atresia	The normal canal's vertical diameter varies from 2 to 12 mm (mean 5 mm) and its length from 4 to 15 mm (mean 8 mm). In 95% of normal individuals, the difference between the two internal auditory canals does not exceed 1 mm in diameter and 2 mm in length. A narrow internal auditory canal (IAC) can be diagnosed when the diameter of IAC is < 2 mm, and any acquired osseous condition predisposing to stenosis of the IAC is absent. A narrow internal auditory canal with duplication divided by bony septation is extremely rare. CT has a limited role in assessing the neural components of the internal auditory canal (MRI should be performed to look for the defect of neural structures in the IAC of patients with sensorineural hearing loss).	IAC anomalies, including atresia, stenosis, aplasia, and hypoplasia, are all rare congenital malformations of the temporal bone with or without congenital sensorineural hearing loss. It is theorized that this anomaly of the IAC results from altered cochleovestibular nerve development secondary to faulty chemotactic mechanisms or a lack of end-organ targets. Unilateral IAC anomalies are often seen in conjunction with other inner ear anomalies and occasionally with middle or external ear anomalies. Infrequently, it will occur as either an isolated or bilateral finding, associated with other systemic developmental anomalies, such as cardiac septal defects, polycystic kidney disease, skeletal deformities, and duodenal atresia. Acquired stenosis of the canal is caused by fibrous dysplasia, Paget disease, osteopetrosis, other more unusual bony dysplasias, osteomas, and meningiomas.
Epidermoid	Homogeneously hypodense, irregular, or lobulated nonenhancing cerebellopontine angle mass.	Epidermoid cyst usually occurs in the cerebellopontine cistern (4%–5% of cerebellopontine angle mass lesions), but is rarely seen within the internal auditory canal. Typical age: 20 to 50 y.
Inflammatory/infectious conditions		
Labyrinthine ossification	Diffuse or localized membranous labyrinthine fluid space ossification. Unilateral if tympanogenic, bilateral if meningogenic, or hematogenic. **Cochlear labyrinthine ossificans:** Fluid spaces of the cochlea itself are affected. **Noncochlear labyrinthine ossificans:** Fluid spaces of the semicircular canals or vestibule are affected. MRI can already show fibrous obliteration of membranous labyrinth in prelabyrinthine ossificans phase with labyrinthitis, whereas CT cannot.	Membranous labyrinth ossification is a healing response to infectious, inflammatory, traumatic, or surgical (i.e., previous labyrinthectomy) insult to inner ear. Labyrinthitis progresses to labyrinthine ossificans when suppurative. Infection may be tympanogenic (secondary to chronic otitis media or cholesteatoma), meningogenic (secondary to meningitis, usually bacterial in origin), or hematogenic (secondary to blood-borne infection, most often viral in origin, e.g., measles and mumps). Meningogenic labyrinthitis is the most common cause of acquired bilateral childhood deafness. Severe vertigo is an infrequent but devastating symptom.

(continues on page 232)

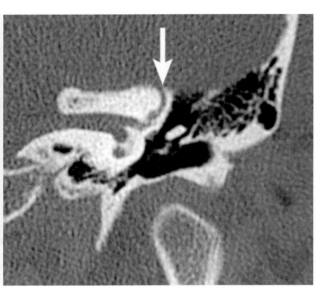

Fig. 5.33   Superior semicircular canal dehiscence. Left coronal T-bone CT image shows an unroofed superior semicircular canal (arrow) and associated thinning of the tegmen tympani. (Courtesy of Dr. A. von Hessling, Zurich.)

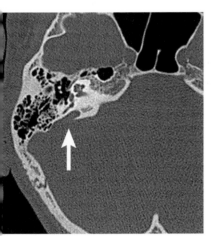

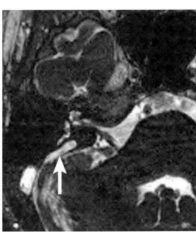

Fig. 5.34a, b   Large vestibular aqueduct syndrome. Right axial T-bone CT image (**a**) reveals an enlarged bony vestibular aqueduct on the posterior wall (arrow). (**b**) Right axial T2-weighted magnetic resonance imaging (MRI) demonstrates a conspicuous large endolymphatic sac (arrow) paralleling the posterior wall of the temporal bone.

b

Table 5.5 (Cont.) Temporal bone: diseases of the inner ear and internal auditory canal

Disease	CT Findings	Comments
Benign neoplasms		
Vestibulocochlear schwannoma	Well-delineated, enhancing mass centered near the porus acusticus with an elongated intracanalicular component and bulbous cisternal component in the cerebellopontine angle that result in an "ice cream cone" configuration. Pressure of the growing tumor results in erosion of the walls and consequent enlargement of the internal auditory canal. May bow the crista falciformis cephalad and flare the internal auricular canal when large. Usually solid but may show cystic or hemorrhagic change, particularly in large or rapidly growing tumors. Calcification is not present. Small ovoid lesions may be contained entirely within the internal acoustic meatus and may be missed with CT. (MRI is the preferred imaging modality for detecting and describing vestibulocochlear schwannomas. CT pneumocisternography is obsolete.)	Vestibulocochlear schwannoma is a common benign, slow-growing neoplasm that arises from Schwann cells of the vestibulocochlear nerve sheath (in particular at the glial-Schwann cell junction of the vestibular nerve), accounting for three fourths of all cerebellopontine angle masses and one tenth of all intracranial tumors. Schwannomas can affect other cranial nerves but have a predilection for the eighth nerve. Patients usually present in the fourth to six decades with slowly progressive unilateral sensorineural hearing loss and tinnitus, cerebellar dysfunction, or neuropathy of the lower cranial nerves. Vestibular symptoms (vertigo, dizziness) are less common. Bilateral vestibulocochlear schwannomas are the hallmark lesion of neurofibromatosis type 2, in a child or young adult. Other lesions found in NF2 are dural ectasia with no tumor mass within the dysplastic canal; meningiomas, sarcomas, and schwannomas of other cranial nerves; ependymomas; gliomas; and juvenile posterior subcapsular cataract.
Meningioma	Meningiomas limited to the internal auditory canal are rare and mimic a vestibulocochlear schwannoma both clinically and by imaging.	Meningiomas are the second most common tumor of the cerebellopontine angle and usually arise outside the internal auditory canal on the posterior surface of the petrous bone, although they may extend within the medial portion of the canal. They grow either as a solid mass with broad dural base and obtuse angle with the temporal bone or en plaque and may cause hyperostosis or erosion of the adjacent bony structures. Calcifications may occur.
Facial nerve schwannoma	Facial schwannomas may occur within the internal auditory canal but are usually recognizable because of the extension into the facial nerve canal as tubular or ovoid-shaped enhancing masses following the course of the intratemporal facial nerve with a smooth enlargement of the facial nerve canal and benign, sharply marginated remodeling of the geniculate fossa. A large tumor may extend into the middle ear cavity and protrude into the posterior cranial fossa.	Rare benign tumors of the Schwann cells that invest the peripheral facial nerve. Usually involve the geniculate ganglion but may involve any portion of the facial nerve (intratemporal > cerebellopontine angle/ internal acoustic canal > intraparotid). Patients present with facial nerve dysfunction or hearing loss.
Lipoma	Fat-density, nonenhancing lesion, usually located at the fundus of the internal auditory canal.	Lipomas are rare internal auditory canal lesions. They may also involve the cerebellopontine angle region and the labyrinth.
Facial nerve hemangioma ▷ *Fig. 5.35*	Poorly marginated enhancing soft tissue mass of the petrous pyramid, extending into the fundus of the internal auditory canal with distinctive amorphous "honeycomb" bone changes. Otic capsule is spared.	Rare intratemporal benign vascular tumor arising from capillaries around facial nerve, most commonly in the area of the geniculate fossa. Hemangioma limited to the lumen of the internal auditory canal is rare, usually located in the fundus. Larger hemangiomas involve the bone of the petrous pyramid and may extend within the internal auditory canal. Adult patients with internal auditory canal hemangioma present with relatively rapid onset of peripheral facial nerve paralysis and concomitant sensorineural hearing loss. Other vascular abnormalities within the internal auditory canal (e.g., varix malformation, aneurysm arising from the labyrinth artery) are extremely rare and may mimic the symptomatology of a schwannoma.
Endolymphatic papillary sac tumor	Inhomogeneously enhancing soft tissue mass with intratumoral bone spicules, centered in the fovea of the endolymphatic sac in the presigmoid, posterior surface of the petrous bone. The tumor erodes the posterior wall of temporal bone and infiltrates surrounding bone and connective tissue. Larger tumors spread to involve middle ear and inner ear, internal auditory canal, jugular foramen, and extend into the cerebellopontine angle cistern.	Rare, slow-growing, locally aggressive papillary adenomatous tumors that do not metastasize. Most endolymphatic sac tumors are sporadic. Seven percent of patients with von Hippel-Lindau disease will develop endolymphatic sac tumor. If the endolymphatic sac tumor is bilateral, von Hippel-Lindau disease is present. Patients usually present in the fourth decade with sensorineural hearing loss, facial nerve palsy, pulsatile tinnitus, or vertigo.

(continues on page 233)

Table 5.5   (Cont.) Temporal bone: diseases of the inner ear and internal auditory canal

Disease	CT Findings	Comments
Otosclerosis		
Fenestral otospongiosis/ otosclerosis ▷ *Fig. 5.36*	In active fenestral otosclerosis, the most frequent lesion is seen as a hypodensity in the labyrinthine capsule at the anterior margin of the oval window. It tends to extend posteriorly, fixing the stapes footplate and sometimes invading and thickening the footplate. Lucent lesions can also occur on the promontory or at the round window. Late, chronic bone CT findings are heaped upon new bone with dense, ossific plaques along oval and round window margins. It may obliterate the windows and bulge into the middle ear cavity.	In otosclerosis, the dense layer of ivory-like endochondral bone that surrounds the labyrinthine capsule is replaced by foci of spongy, vascular, irregular new bone. It is commonly a symmetrical disease. In fenestral otosclerosis (80%–90% of cases), the promontory, facial nerve canal, and oval and round windows are involved. Patients (M:F = 1:2) usually present in the second to third decades with bilateral progressive conductive hearing loss, tinnitus, and normal findings on otoscopic examination.
Cochlear otospongiosis/ otosclerosis ▷ *Fig. 5.37*	Focal radiolucencies in the otic capsules; when severe, the cochlea is completely surrounded by a ring of hypodense bone ("double-ring" sign). The demineralization may also be seen around the vestibule, semicircular canals, and internal auditory canal. Later, in the sclerotic phase, these foci may undergo remineralization and become indistinguishable from the normal otic capsule.	Retrofenestral otosclerosis is much less common and involves the bone around the cochlea or around the membranous labyrinth. It is invariably associated with fenestral otosclerosis. Becomes symptomatic in the second and third decades with bilateral, progressive, mixed hearing loss, tinnitus, and vertigo. May become worse during pregnancy or lactation.

II Head and Neck

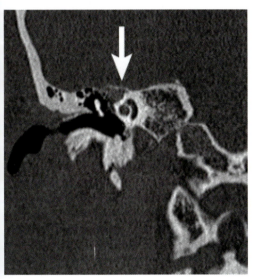

Fig. 5.35   Facial nerve hemangioma. Right coronal T-bone CT image reveals a mixed-density mass with irregular margins and "honeycomb" bony matrix centered in the region of the geniculate fossa (arrow). The otic capsule is spared.

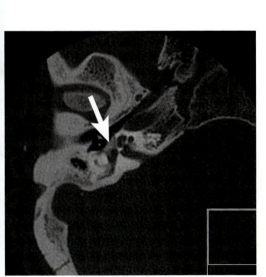

Fig. 5.36   Fenestral otosclerosis. Right axial T-bone CT image shows a radiolucent focus (arrow) on the anterior margin of the oval window (the location of the fissula ante fenestram). The otic capsule is otherwise spared. (Courtesy of Dr. C. Ozdoba, Bern.)

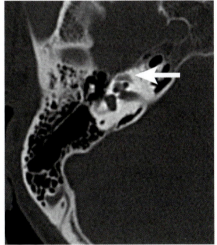

Fig. 5.37   Cochlear otospongiosis. Right axial T-bone CT image reveals a radiolucent focus in the pericochlear distribution (arrow).

Table 5.6   Temporal bone: lesions of the petrous apex

Disease	CT Findings	Comments
Congenital/developmental lesions		
Asymmetric fatty marrow ▷ *Fig. 5.38*	Nonpneumatized petrous apex with fatty marrow (petrous apex is considered pneumatized if it contains one or more air cells).	Approximately 33% of people have pneumatized petrous apices, of which 4% to 7% are asymmetrically pneumatized. Nonpneumatized petrous apex with fatty marrow is an incidental CT/MRI finding. Asymptomatic by definition.
Congenital cholesteatoma ▷ *Fig. 5.39a, b*	Smooth, sharply marginated, expansile lesion, centered within the petrous apex, hypodense with respect to brain, round or oval in shape, with lack of contrast enhancement. Large lesions may erode the horizontal petrous internal carotid artery canal, otic capsule, internal auditory canal, or jugular foramen.	Most petrous apex cholesteatomas are congenital. Absence of previous otologic disease and normal tympanic membrane are necessary to consider a cholesteatoma congenital. If congenital variant, may simultaneously affect mastoid area. Very rare petrous apex lesion usually associated with unilateral sensorineural hearing loss, headache, and aural fullness. Large lesions may cause dysfunction of CN X, XI, and XII if the lesion extends posterior or CN III, IV, and V if it extends anteromedially. Patients are 20 to 50 y old.
	Acquired cholesteatomas, which involve the petrous apex, are aggressive and may extensively erode the petrous bone.	Acquired cholesteatomas of the petrous apex are rare and usually occur by extension from the middle ear space along the supralabyrinthian air cell system along the anterior epitympanic space. Facial nerve dysfunction occurs in 20% to 50% of cases.
Subarcuate artery pseudolesion ▷ *Fig. 5.40*	Curvilinear vascular canal that passes through arch of superior semicircular canal from subarcuate fossa on posterior wall of petrous temporal bone in a lateral posterosuperior direction. The ease of visualization is dependent upon both the canal's size and the extent of adjacent pneumatization.	Normal temporal bone osseous canal through which passes the subarcuate artery (supplies otic capsule, semicircular canals, and posterior wall vestibule).
Benign obstructive processes		
Effusion (trapped fluid)	Nonexpansile fluid-attenuation opacification of the air cells. Cortical margin and air cell trabeculae are preserved. No contrast enhancement of petrous apex or adjacent meninges.	Most common radiographically identified lesion of the petrous apex. Presumed to represent sterile residual fluid collection in petrous apex air cells left behind after remote otomastoiditis with subsequent obstruction of the connection between the middle ear and apical air cells. Asymptomatic by definition. All ages affected. Incidental CT/MRI finding.
Mucocele	Smooth, expansile lesion, isodense to CSF, homogeneous, without contrast enhancement within the petrous apex. The presence of a large air cell on the opposite side can suggest a mucocele.	Mucocele of the petrous apex is very rare.
Cholesterol granuloma	Sharply and smoothly marginated ovoid lesion, isodense to brain, homogeneous and free of calcification without internal contrast enhancement, centered within and expanding the petrous apex especially posteriorly, where the overlying bone may be paper thin or absent. Large lesions may erode foramen magnum, hypoglossal canal, jugular foramen, and internal acoustic canal. (MRI: high signal on T1-, T2-, and diffusion-weighted images.)	Pneumatized petrous apex air cells are required. Inflammatory granulation tissue forms secondary to repeated hemorrhage leading to an expansile petrous apex lesion. Patients are young to middle-aged adults and present with sensorineural hearing loss and/or tinnitus, vertigo, and facial twitching. A previous history of chronic otomastoiditis is common.
Inflammatory/infectious conditions		
Apical petrositis	Middle ear and both mastoid and petrous air cells are usually involved simultaneously and opacified with peripheral contrast enhancement. As the infection progresses to osteomyelitis, trabecular breakdown and erosive cortical changes of the destroyed petrous apex become apparent. Advanced disease may cause possible complications of epidural empyema, abscess, or venous sinus thrombosis.	Apical petrositis is an acute infection of the pneumatized air cells of the petrous apex, usually caused by *Pseudomonas aeruginosa*. Patients are children or adolescents with acute otomastoiditis or adults with chronic suppurative ear or following mastoidectomy. They present with infectious symptoms and manifest some or all of the symptoms of Gradenigo syndrome: purulent otomastoiditis, otorrhea, abducens palsy, and deep facial and retro-orbital pain.

(continues on page 236)

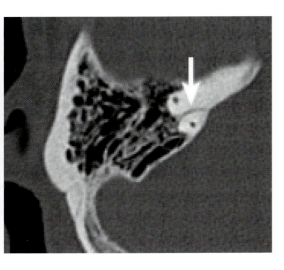

Fig. 5.38 Subarcuate artery pseudolesion. Right axial T-bone CT image in an adult reveals a normal curvilinear subarcuate artery canal (arrow) passing from the medial petrous ridge under the superior semicircular canal.

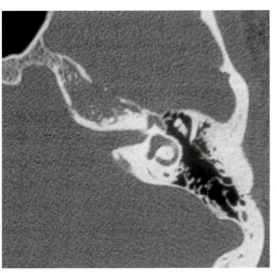

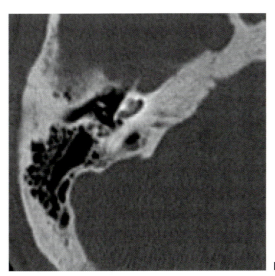

b

Fig. 5.39a, b Metastases. Left axial T-bone CT image (**a**) shows a permeative-destructive lesion of the petrous apex secondary to a breast malignancy. Right axial T-bone CT image (**b**) demonstrates diffuse blastic metastatic disease secondary to prostate carcinoma with involvement of the petrous apex.

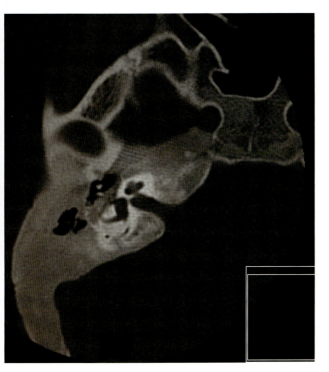

Fig. 5.40 Fibrous dysplasia. Right axial T-bone CT image reveals expansile "ground glass" appearance involving the posterior mastoid and petrous apex encroaching on the middle ear. (Courtesy of Dr. C. Ozdoba, Bern.)

Table 5.6   (Cont.) Temporal bone: lesions of the petrous apex

Disease	CT Findings	Comments
Benign neoplasms		
Meningioma	Extra-axial mass, either globose (spherical) or en plaque, attached to the petrous apex. May extend anteriorly under the temporal lobe and posteriorly along the edge of the tentorium. On CT scan, meningiomas typically are isodense to slightly hyperdense to brain. The density is generally homogeneous and sharply marginated. Typically, contrast produces a homogeneous, intense enhancement. Calcification may be present in a number of forms. Small punctate (psammomatous) calcifications are common. Occasionally, large nodular calcifications may be present. Dense calcification of the entire tumor that obscures contrast enhancement is not uncommon. Bony changes may be hyperostotic or osteolytic.	Although rarely originating from the petrous apex, meningiomas may infiltrate the region. Affect middle-aged women. Can remain clinically silent for many years.
Meckel cave trigeminal schwannoma	Dumbbell-shaped isodense or hypodense mass with smooth expansion of Meckel cave and petrous apex. May erode the superior petrous ridge. The marked contrast enhancement may be homogeneous, inhomogeneous, or even ring-shaped. Calcification is rare.	Meckel cave trigeminal schwannomas arising from the gasserian ganglion tend to enlarge superiorly into the middle cranial fossa and extend posteriorly into the posterior cranial fossa. Patients present in the third and fourth decades (mean age 44 y). Common symptoms include continuous facial pain and paresthesias.
Facial nerve hemangioma	Poorly marginated enhancing soft tissue mass of the petrous pyramid, emanating from geniculate fossa around intact otic capsule to the petrous apex with diffuse, mottled demineralization with multiple distinctive amorphous "honeycomb" bone changes.	Rare intratemporal benign vascular tumor arising from capillaries around facial nerve, most commonly in the area of the geniculate fossa. Patients are adults and present with relatively rapid onset of peripheral facial nerve paralysis.
Malignant neoplasms		
Chordoma	Expansile multilobulated inhomogeneous solid midline tumor centered in the clivus with lytic bone destruction, sharp margins of erosion, and at least some enhancement. Intralesional fragmented destroyed bone, hemorrhage, and mucoid areas may occur. Expanding tumor invades or displaces jugular foramen and petrous apex laterally.	Rare malignant bone tumors arising from notochordal remnants; 35% arise in the skull base as a destructive midline mass (clivus, sellar region, sphenoid sinus, nasopharynx, maxilla, and paranasal sinuses). Most commonly occur between the ages of 30 and 50 y (2:1 male predilection). Symptoms include ophthalmoplegia and headache.
Chondrosarcoma	Heterogeneously enhancing, relatively dense solid tumor located off the midline at the petro-occipital synchondrosis or near the spheno-occipital synchondrosis with arc or ringlike calcifications (50%). The infiltrating skull base mass shows usually a sharp, narrow, nonsclerotic transition zone to the adjacent normal bone.	Constitutes 6% of all skull base tumors. Typically centered in the petro-occipital and petrosphenoid synchondroses with frequent extension into the petrous apex or clivus. Most commonly occur between the ages of 10 and 80 y, with a mean age of 40 y (no gender predilection). Symptoms include insidious onset of headaches and cranial nerve palsies (usually CN VI; also III, V, VII, and VIII). May complicate Ollier disease and Maffucci syndrome. Osteosarcoma is rare in the temporal bone; may be seen secondarily in the setting of prior irradiation or Paget disease.
Plasmacytoma	Solitary intraosseous, usually homogeneous, mildly hyperdense expansile soft tissue mass with osteolytic destruction; scalloped, poorly marginated, nonsclerotic margins; and moderate, homogeneous or less commonly heterogeneous enhancement. Peripherally displaced osseous fragments may be seen.	Most common locations in head and neck are the sinonasal region, skull base (especially sphenoid and petrous temporal bones), and calvarial marrow space. Progression to multiple myeloma is common. Most present in the fifth to ninth decade, with male predilection. Symptoms include local pain and headache. Temporal bone lesions may present with sensorineural hearing loss and clival lesions with sixth cranial nerve palsy.
Metastases	Most petrous apex metastases appear lytic or permeative with bone cortex destruction and a varying amount of associated enhancing soft tissue mass. Breast cancer may be primarily lytic, blastic, or mixed. Metastatic prostate cancer is primarily osteoblastic but may be lytic. Other metastatic types that may be blastic are lung (carcinoid), stomach, bladder, and some CNS malignancies.	The petrous apex is the most common area in the temporal bone for hematogenous metastases to be found. In order of frequency, metastatic lesions of the following tumors have been found: breast, lung, kidney, prostate, and stomach. Metastasis to the temporal bone occurs late in the disease process, and there is usually either physical or radiologic evidence of other systemic lesions. Invasive extracranial lesions are most often primary nasopharyngeal tumors that extend into the cranial cavity by erosion of the skull base and petrous apex.

(continues on page 237)

Table 5.6   (Cont.) Temporal bone: lesions of the petrous apex

Disease	CT Findings	Comments
Metabolic/dysplastic lesions		
Paget disease	Paget disease of the temporal bone typically starts at the petrous apex and progresses inferolaterally. In the osteolytic stage, CT reveals decreased bone density due to demineralization. In the mixed phase, there can be a heterogeneous appearance of mixed lysis and sclerosis ("cotton wool" appearance). The sclerotic form of Paget disease is uncommon in the temporal bones. Bone thickening can be seen in the mixed and sclerotic phase. Involvement of the otic capsule with demineralization and encroachment upon the middle ear are late manifestations. Ossicular involvement may be limited to the stapes footplate.	Skull involvement alone or in association with changes elsewhere in the skeleton is quite common (28%–70%). The temporal bones may be involved by Paget disease, particularly the petrous apex, squamous portion, and mastoid area. Onset uncommon before age 40 (4:1 male predilection). Symptoms include hearing loss (sensorineural, conductive, or mixed), vertigo, and tinnitus. Malignant degeneration in ~1% of cases.
Fibrous dysplasia	All varieties of fibrous dysplasia are characterized by localized or diffuse increased bone volume of the affected temporal bone with thinning of the overlying cortical bone. Pagetoid fibrous dysplasia (50%) shows either classic "ground glass" or mixed sclerotic-cystic appearance. Sclerotic fibrous dysplasia (25%) shows homogeneous density approaching cortical bone. Cystic fibrous dysplasia (50%) shows a spherical or ovoid lucency surrounded by a dense bony shell. Lesion expansion may occasionally result in stenosis of the external and/or internal auditory canal, encroaching on the middle ear and ossicular chain, and obliteration of the otic capsule. In active phase, heterogeneous enhancement may be present.	The skull and facial bones are involved in 10% to 25% of cases of monostotic fibrous dysplasia and in 50% of polyostotic variety. Involvement of the temporal bone, however, is relatively rare. Most active in children and young adults; often ceases to grow by age 20 to 25 (3:1 female predilection). Symptoms include bulging, pain, and tenderness of the temporal area, stenosis of external auditory canal with recurrent otitis, and hearing loss (conductive, sensorineural, or mixed). May be associated with McCune-Albright syndrome. Malignant transformation is rare (< 0.5% of cases).
Osteopetrosis	The petrous bone shows a complete lack of pneumatization and a homogeneous diffuse, sclerotic appearance. Progression of the disease results in narrowing of the internal auditory canals.	Osteopetrosis is a rare bone disease characterized by formation of new bone while resorption of bone is diminished.
Miscellaneous lesions		
Langerhans cell histiocytosis	Destructive bone process with sharply defined "punched out" rather than expansile appearance. Fragments of bone within the heterogeneously enhancing soft tissue component are common.	Mastoid complex and temporal bone lesions are common. Bilateral disease occurs in 30%. Skull, skull base, mandible, maxilla, and vertebral body involvement also may occur. May be diffuse or multiple in more severe cases. Petrous apex disease is less common. Usually occurring in young patients (first decade, 2:1 male predilection). Symptoms include otalgia, otorrhea, hearing loss (conductive or sensorineural), facial nerve palsy, and vertigo.
Petrous carotid artery aneurysm	Fusiform or focal enlargement of the petrous internal carotid artery canal. Expansile mass with extension into adjacent structures. Curvilinear calcifications in the aneurysm wall. Enhancement is equivalent to other arteries. CTA shows aneurysmal dilation of petrous internal carotid artery.	Uncommon. Congenital aneurysm may be associated with additional intracranial aneurysms or anomalies, including neurofibromatosis and connective tissue disorders such as Marfan syndrome and fibromuscular dysplasia. Acquired aneurysms are posttraumatic or postinfectious. Presenting symptoms vary, depending on the adjacent structures and vessels involved: sensorineural hearing loss, headache, nasal congestion, and midface pressure and pain. A ruptured aneurysm may occur with otorrhagia, epistaxis, and neurologic deficit.
Petrous apex cephalocele	Hypodense, nonenhancing expansile lesion, centered outside petrous apex and extending from Meckel cave. The trigeminal notch and inferior border of the porus trigeminus are eroded, and the sharply marginated lesion extends a variable distance into the anterosuperior petrous apex. CT cisternogram may show contrast opacification of the defect in the petrous apex, proving communication with the subarachnoid space and Meckel cave.	Congenital or acquired, usually unilateral herniation of the posterolateral wall of Meckel cave into petrous apex. Rare lesion usually identified as an asymptomatic incidental nonoperative finding on MRI. In complicated cases, symptoms are trigeminal neuralgia, CSF otorrhea (with communication between cephalocele and middle ear), and recurrent meningitis.
Petrous apex arachnoid cyst	Hypodense, expansile lesion, without contrast enhancement at the petrous apex with smooth, noninvasive bony excavation.	Arachnoid cysts of the petrous apex are extremely rare lesions. Can be associated with petrous apex cephalocele. The cyst becomes symptomatic when the enlargement causes compression and dysfunction of neural structures (trigeminal neuralgia, midface paresthesia, and hearing loss) or alterations in CSF dynamics (CSF otorrhea or rhinorrhea).

Table 5.7 Temporal bone: jugular foramen lesions

Disease	CT Findings	Comments
Pseudomass		
Asymmetric jugular bulb	Temporal bone CT reveals normal, asymmetrically large jugular bulb, with intact cortical margins and jugular spine of jugular foramen. Normal, usually right-sided, asymmetrically large sigmoid sinus and jugular bulb demonstrate similar contrast enhancement characteristics as internal jugular vein.	Size of jugular foramen is greatly variable, even from side to side, and is associated with a corresponding large or small jugular bulb. Asymmetric jugular bulb is a normal variant, found incidentally on brain MRI during workup for unrelated symptoms. Large, asymmetric jugular bulb provides setting where MRI signal from slow, complex venous flow may mimic pathology (jugular bulb pseudolesion).
Congenital/developmental lesions		
High-riding jugular bulb	Jugular bulb reaching above the level of the inferior tympanic rim with a smoothly marginated bone defect behind the internal auditory canal. The bony plate separating the bulb from the middle ear cavity is preserved. The jugular bulb enhances to the same degree as the sigmoid sinus and internal jugular vein.	Normal variant, not to be confused with a mass lesion (present in 6% of temporal bones). More common on the right side. Does not change in size. Asymptomatic anatomical variation.
Dehiscent jugular bulb	Soft tissue mass low in the middle ear, contiguous with the internal jugular vein through a focal jugular (sigmoid) plate defect. The other margins of the adjacent jugular foramen are smooth and intact. Commonly seen with high-riding jugular bulb. The superolateral outpouching demonstrates similar enhancement characteristics to jugular bulb, sigmoid sinus, and internal jugular vein.	Congenital vascular pseudomass. Does not grow with time. This is usually asymptomatic, but it may cause pulsatile tinnitus or conductive hearing loss. Otoscopically, a retrotympanic vascular mass may be seen in the lower part of the middle ear behind the intact tympanic membrane.
Jugular bulb diverticulum ▷ *Fig. 5.41*	Well-corticated, focal polypoid mass extending from cephalad jugular bulb (usually superiorly and medially) into surrounding temporal bone just behind the internal auditory canal. The jugular bulb itself may be high. CTA shows fingerlike projection off jugular bulb.	Congenital vascular pseudomass; rare venous anomaly. More common on the left side. Does not change in size. Most common incidental finding, but may present with nonpulsatile tinnitus, sensorineural hearing loss, or symptoms mimicking Ménière disease. Otoscopic examination is negative.
Primary cholesteatoma (epidermoid)	Primary cholesteatoma originating in the immediate vicinity of the jugular foramen presents as smooth and rounded, homogeneous mass of low CT density (density less than that of brain), associated with expansion of the jugular fossa and erosion of the posteroinferior aspect of the petrous pyramid and adjacent occipital bone. Cholesteatomas do not enhance with contrast.	Primary cholesteatomas of the jugular fossa area are very rare. *Acquired cholesteatomas* of the temporal bone with infralabyrinthine extension inferior to the cochlea and internal auditory canal may break into the jugular fossa and cause Vernet syndrome with unilateral paresis of CN IX to XI.
Benign neoplasms		
Glomus jugulare paraganglioma ▷ *Fig. 5.42a, b*	Lobulated, homogeneous, intensive enhancing soft tissue mass (computer-generated density–time curve reveals a high, early, arterial peak), poorly marginated with cortical erosion, irregular enlargement of the jugular fossa, and permeative-destructive change of adjacent bone with no sclerosis. Jugular spine erosion is common. Routes of extension are superolateral through the floor of the middle ear, medial to the posteroinferior aspect of the petrous pyramid, and posterior with involvement of the occipital bone, hypoglossal canal, and foramen magnum. Inferior extension within and along the jugular vein occurs often. Up to 17% protrude extradurally into the middle and posterior cranial fossa. Glomus tumors frequently invade the jugular vein and obliterate the vessel partially or completely. **Glasscock-Jackson classification** **Glomus jugulare paraganglioma:** Type I: small tumor invading jugular bulb, middle ear, and mastoid process. Type II: tumor extending under internal auditory canal; may have intracranial extension. Type III: tumor extending to petrous apex; may have intracranial extension. Type IV: tumor extending beyond petrous apex into clivus or masticator space; may have intracranial extension.	Glomus jugulare paraganglioma (GJP) is a benign tumor arising from paraganglia surrounding the jugular bulb (in 85% of cases), Arnold nerve (branch of CN X), or Jacobson nerve (branch of CN IX). When middle ear extension occurs, such a tumor is called a glomus jugulotympanicum paraganglioma. GJP is the most common jugular foramen tumor and the second most common temporal bone tumor (after acoustic schwannoma). Multicentricity in sporadic forms is present in 10%. When familial (inherited as an autosomal dominant disease), multicentricity amounts to 25% to 50%. Increased risk of paragangliomas in MEN1 and NF1. Malignant transformation with regional lymph node metastases is seen in 4%. GJPs occur at any age but have a predilection for middle-aged women. Glomus jugulare tumors present with Horner syndrome and deficiencies of CN IX, X, XI, and XII. Cranial neuropathy of CN VII and VIII are seen less often. Glomus jugulotympanicum tumors present with pulsatile tinnitus, conductive hearing loss, and vascular retrotympanic mass. Endocrine syndrome may occur in 1% to 3% of cases.

(continues on page 240)

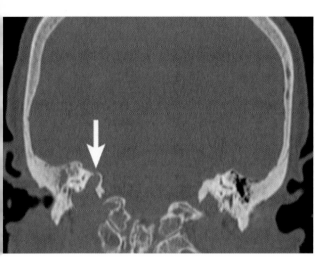

Fig. 5.41   Jugular bulb diverticulum. Coronal bone CT image shows an asymmetric large, high-riding right jugular bulb with a thumblike outpouching off the roof and projecting cephalad into the medial temporal bone (arrow).

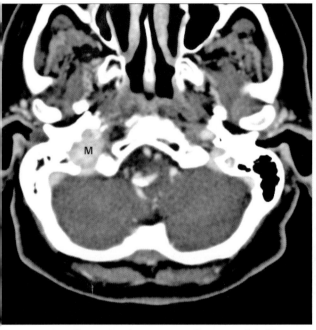

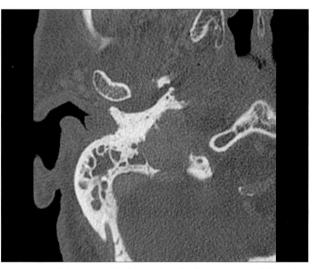

b

Fig. 5.42a, b   Glomus jugulare paraganglioma. Axial skull base contrast-enhanced CT image (**a**) shows a jugular foramen mass (M) on the right side with homogeneous intensive enhancement. Right axial T-bone CT image (**b**) demonstrates permeative-destructive bone changes along the lateral margin of the jugular foramen. (Courtesy of Dr. A. von Hessling, Zurich.)

Table 5.7 (Cont.) Temporal bone: jugular foramen lesions

Disease	CT Findings	Comments
Jugular foramen schwannoma ▷ *Fig. 5.43*	Schwannomas are fusiform or "dumbbell" tumors with well-defined margin, isodense or hypodense to brain, and dense contrast enhancement. Large tumors often show intramural cystic or fatty degeneration. Schwannomas cause smooth remodeled enlargement of the jugular foramen with well-defined, scalloped bone margins. Coronal bone CT plane may show amputation of lateral jugular tubercle ("bird's beak"). The vector of tumor growth follows a general craniocaudal course of CN IX to XI. The tumor may project superiorly into the posterior cranial fossa with extension into the cerebellopontine angle cistern and encroach on the brainstem. Some tumors grow inferiorly from jugular foramen into nasopharyngeal carotid space.	Second most common jugular foramen tumor (glomus jugulare paraganglioma first). Glossopharyngeal nerve most common nerve of origin. These tumors may become large before producing symptoms in middle-aged individuals. Sensorineural hearing loss may occur before clinical involvement of the nerves of the jugular foramen. Cranial nerve neurofibromas are extremely rare.
Hypoglossal schwannoma	Hypoglossal schwannomas are "dumbbell" tumors with well-defined margin, isodense or hypodense to brain, and dense contrast enhancement. Large tumors often show intramural cystic or fatty degeneration. They cause expansion and remodeling of the hypoglossal canal without osseous destruction. Hypoglossal schwannoma follows the course of CN XII with cephalad growth into anteroinferior basal cistern and cerebellopontine cistern and caudal growth into nasopharyngeal carotid space. Extension to involve the middle ear is not a feature of these tumors.	Schwannomas can also arise within the hypoglossal canal.
Jugular foramen meningioma	Poorly circumscribed, hyperdense jugular foramen mass (lobulated and en plaque morphotypes) with uniform, strong contrast enhancement. Meningiomas usually cause permeative-sclerotic bone changes at jugular foramen and of adjacent bone. Hyperostosis of adjacent jugular foramen cortex may be present. Dural-based tumor spread in basal cistern is most common. Meningiomas may also extend centrifugally in all directions from jugular foramen along dural surfaces and through surrounding bones. Less commonly, meningioma pedunculates up into basal cistern. Inferior spread dumbbells into nasopharyngeal carotid space.	Meningioma is the third most common jugular foramen mass. Meningiomas arise from arachnoid cap cells in meninges of skull base or CN IX to XI at the jugular foramen. They are typically large at presentation and more frequent in women, who are in the fourth to sixth decades of life, with complex cranial neuropathy involving CN IX to XI; less commonly, CN VII, VIII, and XII.
Malignant neoplasms		
Metastases	Metastases to the jugular foramen may be lytic, sclerotic, or mixed with variable enhancing, invasive jugular foramen mass.	Metastases to the jugular foramen occur most commonly with advanced metastatic disease and are usually part of other metastases in the skull base. Most common primary locations are breast, lung, kidney, and GI tract. Rapid symptom onset (often lower cranial nerve deficits). Retrograde perineural spread from malignancies of the face and oral cavity may give rise to jugular foramen metastases. Lymphoma, melanoma, and squamous cell carcinoma show this type of tumor extension. Enlargement and pathologic enhancement of the nerve root, as well as jugular foramen enlargement, are suggestive of perineural spread.
Plasmacytoma	Lytic bone destruction with scalloped, poorly margin-ated, nonsclerotic margins, along with enlargement of the jugular foramen due to a mildly hyperdense soft tissue mass with moderate homogeneous enhancement.	Plasmacytoma may manifest as a solitary lesion in the base of skull (especially sphenoid body and petrous temporal bone). Rarely, this tumor is located in the jugular fossa. Present in fifth to ninth decades. More common in male patients.

(continues on page 241)

Table 5.7   (Cont.) Temporal bone: jugular foramen lesions

Disease	CT Findings	Comments
Hemangiopericytoma	CT findings are similar to glomus tumors. There is lytic destruction with expansion of the jugular foramen. The soft tissue mass is irregular with marked contrast enhancement.	Hemangiopericytoma is a rare tumor in the jugular fossa. The tumor affects both genders equally and occurs in the fourth to sixth decades of life. At least 50% of hemangiopericytomas are malignant.
Chondrosarcoma	Chondrosarcoma of the jugular foramen reveals irregular bone destruction with enlargement of the foramen. The soft tissue component is relatively dense with variable contrast enhancement. Speckled, linear, or arclike calcifications may occur in tumor matrix.	Chondrosarcomas of the skull base characteristically arise from the petrosphenoidal or petro-occipital fissures. They may extend posterolaterally to involve the jugular foramen at its medial aspect. Chondrosarcomas confined to the jugular foramen are extremely rare tumors. Clinical profile: middle-aged patient with insidious onset of headaches and cranial nerve palsies. Expanding midline chordoma, centered in the clivus, may present an erosive and destructive lesion of the jugular fossa.
Nasopharyngeal squamous cell carcinoma	This tumor originates in the high posterolateral nasopharyngeal mucosal space, just below the skull base. CT shows an invasive soft tissue mass with simple skull base erosion, lytic destructive upward invasion of basisphenoid and basiocciput, and intracranial extension. Occasionally, sclerosis may be invoked in the skull base.	Nasopharyngeal squamous cell carcinoma can extend to involve the skull base, producing lower cranial nerve symptoms. Isolated extension to the jugular fossa is uncommon. Other secondary tumors with prominent extension (e.g., malignant parotid neoplasms and malignant tumors of the external auditory canal or middle ear cavity) may invade the base of the skull and temporal bone, including the jugular foramen.

II Head and Neck

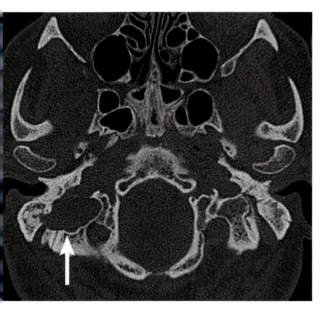

Fig. 5.43   Jugular foramen schwannoma (glossopharyngeal nerve). Axial skull base bone CT image reveals significant smooth enlargement of the right jugular foramen with thin, sclerotic margins (arrow).

6 Orbit and Globe

Wolfgang Zaunbauer and Francis A. Burgener

The paired orbits are pyramid-shaped cavities on either side of the ethmoid and sphenoid sinuses. The anterior cranial fossa lies above each orbit, the maxillary sinus below, the middle cranial fossa posterolaterally, and the temporal fossa anterolaterally.

Seven bones contribute to the bony orbit: the maxillary, frontal, lacrimal, and zygomatic bones, which are membranous in origin, and the sphenoid, palatine, and ethmoid bones, which are endochondral. The orbital plane of the frontal bone and the lesser wing of the sphenoid form the roof of the orbit. Portions of the frontal bone, the zygomatic bone, and the greater wing of the sphenoid bone form the lateral wall. The maxillary bone, zygoma, and orbital process of the palatine bone form the orbital floor. The medial wall is made up of the maxillary bone, lacrimal bone, ethmoid bone, lesser wing of the sphenoid bone, and frontal bone. The orbital apex is formed by the palatine bone and sphenoid bone.

The bony orbit is bordered by the periosteum (periorbita), which is loosely adherent to the surrounding bones except at the trochlear fossa, lacrimal crest, and margins of the fissures and canals, where it is more tightly bound. Anteriorly, at the margins of the orbit, the periorbita is continuous with the orbital septum, a membranous sheet forming the fibrous layer of the eyelids. It defines preseptal and postseptal compartments. The *preseptal space* consists of the lids and anterior soft tissues of the orbit. The *postseptal space* (orbit proper) contains the globe, extraocular muscles, optic nerve sheath complex, lacrimal system, and various neural and vascular structures surrounded by well-organized adipose tissue with fibrovascular septa. It can be divided into four major anatomical components: the globe, the optic nerve sheath complex, the conal–intraconal area, and the extraconal area (**Fig. 6.1**).

The globe, embedded in a fatty reticulum, has three coats and three fluid-filled intraocular chambers. It is roughly spherical in shape, measures about 2.5 cm long, is between 23 and 26 mm in equatorial diameter, and occupies approximately 20% of the total volume of the orbit.

The sclera, uvea, and retina compose the three layers of the globe. The sclera or outer layer is a fibrous capsule around the globe. It is contiguous with the transparent cornea anteriorly and the dural sleeve of the optic nerve posteriorly. The uvea or middle layer consists of the iris, ciliary body, and choroids. It is a vascular layer, which brings nutrients to the eye. It has an inner membrane (Bruch membrane) that separates the choroidal vessels from the retina. The retina consists of an outer pigmented layer and the sensorineural inner layer. The Tenon capsule envelops the eyeball from the margin of the cornea to the optic nerve and separates it from the central orbital fat. The episcleral space is a potential space between the Tenon capsule and the sclera that is filled with loose areolar tissue. Anteriorly, the conjunctiva covers the globe.

The lens apparatus divides the sphere of the globe into the anterior and posterior segments. The anterior segment, which is located between the cornea and lens and separated into the anterior and posterior chamber by the iris, is filled with an aqueous fluid, the aqueous humor. The posterior segment, located posterior to the lens and the ciliary muscle, is filled with vitreous humor. The thin hyaloid membrane envelops the vitreous body and is in contact with the posterior lens capsule, retina, and optic disk.

The *optic nerve* is not a true cranial nerve but rather an extension of the brain. The adult optic nerve is approximately 50 mm in length from the optic disk to the optic chiasm and 4 mm in diameter. The optic nerve can be divided into four different segments: the intraocular segment before the nerve penetrates the sclera, an intraorbital segment that traverses posteriorly in a slightly relaxed and undulating course through the orbital fat of the intraconal compartment, an intracanalicular segment within the optic canal, and an intracranial segment between the optic canal and the optic chiasm. The intraorbital portion is circumferentially invested by the pia–arachnoid, subarachnoid space, and dura mater, which blends with the sclera anteriorly and with the periosteum of the optic canal and the bony orbit posteriorly. The subarachnoid space that exists between the dura mater and the optic nerve pia is continuous with the intracranial subarachnoid space and reflects intracranial cerebrospinal fluid (CSF) pressure. The intracranial portion of the optic nerve is covered only by pia mater, as the dural sheath fuses with the periosteum of the optic canal.

The *orbital cone* consists of the extraocular muscles, which arise at the orbital apex from the annulus of Zinn and insert on the globe, and an envelope of fascia. This myofascial sling separates the retrobulbar space into the intraconal and extraconal compartments (**Fig. 6.2**). The *extraconal compartment* is the space outside the rectus muscle pyramid and contains the lacrimal gland and the lacrimal drainage apparatus, as well as cranial nerves (CNs) IV and V_1 (n. lacrimalis, n. frontalis), extraconal branches of the ophthalmic artery, and portions of the superior and inferior ophthalmic vein, embedded in peripheral orbital fat.

The *intraconal compartment* is the space inside the rectus muscle pyramid, filled with central orbital fat, and contains, in addition to the optic nerve and nerve–sheath complex, the intraconal branches of the ophthalmic artery, superior ophthalmic vein, and CN III, V_1, and VI.

Unlike the preseptal soft tissues, the retrobulbar space contains no lymphoid tissue or lymphatics.

The lacrimal system is composed of the lacrimal gland, the lacrimal drainage system (superior and inferior puncta, lacrimal canaliculi, common canaliculus, lacrimal sac, and nasolacrimal duct), and miscellaneous supporting structures. The orbital portion of the lacrimal gland lies in the bony lacrimal fossa, a postseptal extraconal space at the level of the zygomatic process of the frontal bone, just lateral to and superior of the globe adjacent to tendons of the levator palpebrae superioris and lateral rectus muscles. The smaller palpebral portion of the gland lies anterior to the orbital septum, where it projects onto the palpebral surface of the upper lid. These two portions of the lacrimal gland are connected by a small isthmus (its separation is not discernible on computed tomography [CT] scans). The nasolacrimal drainage apparatus is located within the bony lacrimal fossa in the preseptal portion of the inferomedial orbit at the suture of the frontal process of the maxilla and lacrimal bones, which, inferiorly, gives access to the nasolacrimal canal. It empties into the inferior nasal meatus.

The orbit communicates with multiple other compartments through various fissures and foramina. At the orbital apex, the optic canal forms a portal between the interior of the skull and the orbit and carries the optic nerve with its sheath, together with the ophthalmic artery and a complement of sympathetic nerves into the orbit. Sometimes the optic canal can project into

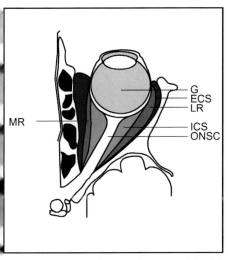

Fig. 6.1 Diagram of an axial section of the left orbit. ECS: extraconal space; G: orbital compartment globe; ICS: intraconal space; LR: lateral rectus muscle and sheath; MR: medial rectus muscle and sheath; ONSC: optic nerve–sheath complex.

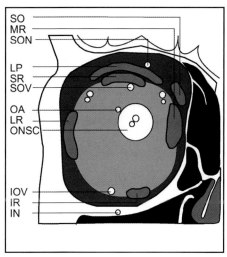

Fig. 6.2 Right coronal orbital anatomy. IN: infraorbital nerve; IOV: inferior ophthalmic vein; IR: inferior rectus muscle; LP: levator palpebrae muscle; LR: lateral rectus muscle; MR: medial rectus muscle; OA: ophthalmic artery; ONSC: optic nerve–sheath complex (with central retinal artery and vein); SO: superior oblique muscle; SOV: superior ophthalmic vein; SON: superior ophthalmic nerve; SR: superior rectus muscle.

the lumen of the sphenoid sinus or Onodi cells, and a bony dehiscence of its wall may be present.

The superior orbital fissure, formed from the greater and lesser wings of the sphenoid, connects the orbit with the middle cranial fossa, and the oculomotor (CN III), trochlear (CN IV), ophthalmic (CN V$_1$), and abducens (CN VI) nerves, sympathetic fibers, an orbital branch of the middle meningeal artery, and the superior ophthalmic vein pass through this fissure.

The inferior orbital fissure communicates with the pterygopalatine fossa and infratemporal fossa. Veins passing through the fissure connect the orbital venous system with the pterygoid plexus. Parts of CN V$_2$ (maxillary branch of the trigeminal nerve) and the infraorbital artery and vein also pass through this fissure.

The infraorbital groove and foramen transmit the infraorbital nerve and vasa infraorbitalis to the face.

The supraorbital foramen/incisure transmits the supraorbital artery and the superior ophthalmic vein (superior branch).

Near the suture between the frontal and ethmoid bones is the anterior and posterior ethmoid foramen. They transmit the anterior and posterior ethmoid nerves, arteries, and veins to the ethmoid sinus.

The nasolacrimal duct courses through the bony nasolacrimal canal and exits in the nasal cavity below the inferior turbinate.

CT demonstrates intrinsic contrast between bone, fat, and soft tissues. It is particularly useful in the evaluation of bony orbit, as well as pathology with potential calcification. The globe is well defined by CT. The higher density global wall is nicely contrasted by the very hypodense intraorbital fat posteriorly. The wall is uniform in width and density, except for a slight protuberance and change in density at the insertion of the optic nerve posteriorly (papilla). The various global layers cannot be differentiated on CT. The aqueous and vitreous chambers of the globe have a uniformly low density, whereas the lens stands out as a higher density structure in the anterior part of the globe. The CT density of the lens varies with the age, becoming progressively denser with age as it loses water content.

The extraocular muscles, lacrimal gland, Tenon capsule, intraorbital veins, ciliary muscle, optic sheath, and retinochoroidal layer significantly enhance with intravascular contrast media. The optic nerve normally does not enhance.

Proptosis is an abnormal protrusion of the globe beyond the orbital rim (> 21 mm anterior to the interzygomatic line on axial scans at the level of the lens). When associated with thyroid-associated orbitopathy, proptosis is sometimes called exophthalmos. Any space-occupying lesion within the orbit may cause proptosis. The

proptosis of thyroid-associated orbitopathy and idiopathic orbital inflammatory disease is typically axial, or projected away from the center of the orbit. This differs from proptosis associated with localized masses elsewhere in the orbit, which may cause nonaxial proptosis. Nonaxial proptosis is a frequent finding with dermoid cyst, subperiosteal abscess, subperiosteal hematoma, vascular malformations (e.g., encapsulated venous vascular malformation [cavernous hemangioma], venous lymphatic malformation, and orbital varix), arteriovenous malformation (AVM; high flow lesion), carotid-cavernous sinus fistula, and aneurysm, vascular tumors (capillary hemangioma, hemangiopericytoma, hemangioendothelioma, and angiofibroma), meningioma, schwannoma, neurofibroma, rhabdomyosarcoma, leukemia, lymphoproliferative lesions of the orbit, Langerhans cell histiocytosis, malignant fibrous histiocytoma, fibrosarcoma, metastatic neuroblastoma, and metastatic carcinoma. Proptosis is an uncommon finding in children, but the vast majority of space-occupying lesions in the orbit causing proptosis in children are benign. These include congenital/developmental lesions (dermoid, epidermoid, teratoma, and neurofibromatosis type 1), inflammatory/infectious conditions (cellulitis, abscess, and idiopathic orbital inflammatory disease), benign mesenchymal tumors (osteogenic, chondrogenic, histiocytomatous, lipomatous, myxomatous, and rhabdomyomatous), vascular malformations and tumors of vascular origin (encapsulated venous vascular malformation [cavernous hemangioma], venous lymphatic malformation, and capillary hemangioma), and neurogenic tumors (neurofibroma, plexiform neurofibromatosis, and glioma). The most common primary childhood orbital malignancy is rhabdomyosarcoma. Other orbital malignancies are malignant mesenchymal tumors, leukemia and lymphoproliferative lesions of the orbit, extension of retinoblastoma, secondary involvement by Ewing sarcoma, and metastases (neuroblastoma).

Enophthalmos refers to the relative depression of one globe back into the orbit. Any increase in size or volume of the orbit due to loss or defects of one or more walls of the orbit may cause enophthalmos. It is a finding with an orbita floor fracture and prolapse of fat and muscle into the maxillary sinus, or with a chronic sinusitis and the silent sinus syndrome. The absence of part of the sphenoid bone in neurofibromatosis type 1 may cause an enophthalmos. Breast carcinoma metastases may contract the orbital fat and cause enophthalmos. A phthisical, or end-stage contracted globe, may cause a pseudoenophthalmos. Cockayne syndrome may be associated with sunken eyes.

Leukokoria is an abnormal white, pink-white, or yellow-white pupillary light reflection that usually results from an intraocular abnormality and is seen most often in children. Common causes include retinoblastoma, medulloepithelioma, persistent hyperplastic primary vitreous (PHPV), retinopathy of prematurity (ROP), congenital cataract, choroidal colobomas, uveitis, toxocaral sclerosing endophthalmitis, congenital retinal folds, Coats disease, retina dysplasia, retinal astrocytic hamartoma (associated with tuberous sclerosis and von Recklinghausen disease), organized vitreous hemorrhage, and long-standing retinal detachment. CT demonstration of a calcified mass in a globe of normal size may be helpful for differentiating retinoblastoma from alternative diagnosis (PHPV, ROP, Coats disease, and a variety of other nonspecific causes of leukokoria). In toxocaral endophthalmitis, the eye is of normal size and has no calcifications. In Coats disease, true calcifications are rarely seen. PHPV is associated with unilateral microphthalmia, and ROP with bilateral microphthalmia; calcifications are often absent.

Microphthalmia is defined as an eye measuring less than two thirds of its normal size, or < 16 mm in axial dimension in adults and children. It may be divided into simple and complex types, and further subdivided into primary (congenital) and secondary (acquired) forms.

An anatomically correct but small eye characterizes simple primary microphthalmos, unilaterally or bilaterally, with no concurrent anomalies. The orbital cavity is small. The extraocular muscles are thin.

Simple secondary microphthalmos may be due to intrauterine infection (toxoplasmosis, rubella, and cytomegalovirus [CMV]) or vascular disorders (PHPV and ROP). The globe tends to be small but normally shaped. In adults, simple secondary microphthalmos may also result from trauma or infection (tuberculosis [TB] and acquired immunodeficiency syndrome [AIDS]-related CMV infection). These cause scarring and inward retraction of the globe, eventuating in phthisis bulbi. The bony orbits and retroocular structures have normal size and configuration. A small globe is also found in optic nerve atrophy.

Complex microphthalmia is congenital with intraocular malformations and may be divided into those eyes with and without colobomas and cysts. Complex microphthalmos may be associated with concurrent malformations, such as basal encephaloceles, dysgenesis of the corpus callosum, and the median cleft syndromes, as well as a wide variety of congenital syndromes and chromosomal abnormalities.

Congenital microphthalmia is seen on CT scans as a small globe associated with a small, underdeveloped bony orbit. In acquired microphthalmia, usually unilateral and found after trauma, surgery, inflammation with disorganization of the eye, or radiation therapy, CT scans show a shrunken, often calcified globe, termed phthisis bulbi, in a normal developed orbit. Bilateral microphthalmia and cataracts are seen with congenital rubella, PHPV, ROP, retinal folds, Lowe syndrome, Norrie disease, and Warburg syndrome. Nanophthalmos is a condition in which both eyes are abnormally small but otherwise normal.

Macrophthalmia (enlargement of the globe) is most commonly the result of juvenile glaucoma or myopia. Its most severe form, buphthalmos, is caused by juvenile-onset glaucoma. Macrophthalmia has to be differentiated from proptosis, indicating the anterior protrusion of a normal-sized globe.

Ocular calcification is commonly found in normal and abnormal tissues. Idiopathic scleral calcification (senile scleral plaque near the insertions of lateral and medial rectus muscles) is seen in many patients older than 70 y of age. Ciliary body calcification may be seen after trauma, inflammation, or in teratoid medulloepithelioma of the ciliary body. Choroidal calcification

often follows severe intraocular inflammation or trauma. Osteoma is an unusual but distinct cause of choroidal calcification peripapillary. Retinal astrocytic hamartoma (associated with tuberous sclerosis or neurofibromatosis), optic nerve head drusen (bilateral in 75%), and CMV retinitis may have retinal calcification. Tumor calcifications in the globe are characteristic of retinoblastoma. Meningioma of the optic nerve sheath infiltrating the posterior globe and hemangioblastoma (von Hippel–Lindau disease) may also produce intraglobal calcifications.

Extraglobal calcifications are most often of vascular origin (arteriosclerosis, phlebolith, encapsulated venous malformation, and AVM). Calcified hematoma, granuloma, and abscess also occur. The most common calcified tumor is a meningioma of the optic nerve sheath. Other calcified tumors are optic glioma, neurofibroma, neuroblastoma, lacrimal gland neoplasm, and dermoid. Lesions from the orbital wall and retinoblastoma with calcifications may occasionally extend into the extraglobal space.

Extraocular muscle enlargement (the maximum normal thickness in the belly of an extraocular muscle is 4.0 mm, measured in the axis perpendicular to the orbital wall) is a prominent feature of diseases such as thyroid-associated orbitopathy, myositis (idiopathic orbital pseudotumor, bacterial [from sinus extension], cysticercosis, trichinosis, and other, e.g., Lyme disease), vascular congestion (carotid-cavernous sinus fistula, dural AVM, superior ophthalmic vein or cavernous sinus thrombosis, and orbital apex mass), malignant neoplasm (metastases, adenoid cystic carcinoma, lymphoproliferative lesions of the orbit, and rhabdomyosarcoma), orbital lymphatic-venous malformation, trauma (edema and hemorrhage), acromegaly, and amyloidosis.

Optic nerve–sheath complex enlargement encompass a spectrum of disease entities, including primary and secondary neoplastic lesions (optic nerve glioma, optic nerve hemangioblastoma, optic nerve sheath meningioma, plexiform neurofibroma, leukemia, lymphoproliferative lesions, and metastases), inflammatory/infectious processes (idiopathic orbital pseudotumor, thyroid-associated orbitopathy, orbital sarcoidosis, TB, optic neuritis, and toxoplasmosis), trauma (perioptic hematoma), distended optic nerve sheath, and optic nerve sheath meningocele.

Enlargement of the superior ophthalmic vein can be associated with carotid-cavernous sinus fistula, dural AVM, superior ophthalmic vein or cavernous sinus thrombosis, orbital varix, orbital apex mass, thyroid-associated orbitopathy, idiopathic orbital pseudotumor, and normal variant.

Ocular detachment: there are basically three potential spaces in the eye that can accumulate fluid or blood, causing detachment of various layers of the globe: the posterior hyaloid space, the subretinal space, and the suprachoroidal space. Separation of the posterior hyaloid membrane from the sensory retina is referred to as *posterior hyaloid detachment*. It commonly occurs in the elderly with liquefaction of the vitreous, but it may also be present in children with PHPV.

Retinal detachment occurs when the sensory retina is separated from the retinal pigment epithelium. Retinal detachment may result from retraction associated with a mass, from a fibroproliferative disease in the vitreous, from endophthalmitis, or from retinal vascular leakage and hemorrhage.

Choroidal detachment is usually caused by ocular hypotony with accumulation of serous fluid or blood between the choroid and sclera, frequently after intraocular surgery or penetrating ocular trauma, and inflammatory choroidal disorders.

When considering orbital disease, it is helpful to localize the process to a compartment of the orbit, both for purposes of differential diagnosis and for therapeutic planning. The differential diagnosis of ocular lesions is discussed in **Table 6.1**, optic nerve–sheath complex lesions in **Table 6.2**, extraocular conal and intraconal lesions in **Table 6.3**, and extraocular extraconal lesions in **Table 6.4**.

Table 6.1   Ocular lesions

Disease	CT Findings	Comments
Congenital/developmental lesions		
Anophthalmos	Absence of a normal eye and optic nerve. In its place, there is a mass of amorphous soft tissue. The lens is absent. The extraocular muscles are thin; the muscle cone is narrowed and elongated. The bony orbit is small with thick walls. The optic chiasm may be hypoplastic or absent. The corpus callosum may be dysgenetic. The contralateral eye may be normal, small, or also absent.	Anophthalmos results from an insult to the developing globe during the first 4 weeks of gestation.
Microphthalmos ▷ *Fig. 6.3*	**Simple primary microphthalmos:** Small optic globe, anatomically correct, associated with small, underdeveloped orbit. Usually bilateral. Associated with cataracts, but with no concurrent anomalies. **Simple secondary microphthalmos:** The globe tends to be small but normally shaped; the lens is almost always identifiable; the posterior chamber of the eye tends to be hyperdense. There are no recognizable internal structures. The bony orbit and retroocular structures have normal size and configuration. **Phthisis bulbi** represents an end-stage atrophic globe that has undergone extensive degenerative changes: small, irregularly shaped globe with heavy subretinal calcification or ossification; the sclera becomes markedly thickened, irregular, and calcified. **Complex microphthalmos with coloboma:** All colobomatous eyes are small, enophthalmic, and malformed. The lenses are dysplastic. The size of the globe is inversely proportional to the size of the coloboma: the larger the outpouching, the smaller the globe. The bony orbit is also slightly small, the optic nerve and the extraocular muscles are thin. **Complex microphthalmos with cyst:** Small malformed globe associated with a large paraocular cyst (isodense to vitreous). The inner walls of the cyst may enhance. Proptosis may be present (depending on the size of the associated cyst). In most cases, only one eye is involved. **Cryptophthalmos** refers to severe microphthalmia. A rare congenital anomaly. Usually occurs bilateral.	Congenital causes: coloboma, congenital rubella, PHPV, ROP, retinal folds, Lowe syndrome, Norrie disease, and Warburg syndrome. Occurs as an isolated disorder or may be associated with other craniofacial anomalies (hemifacial microsomia, Goldenhar syndrome, hypomelanosis of Ito, Proteus syndrome, and Aicardi syndrome). Acquired causes: optic nerve atrophy, sequelae of trauma, infection, surgery, and radiation therapy.

(continues on page 246)

II   Head and Neck

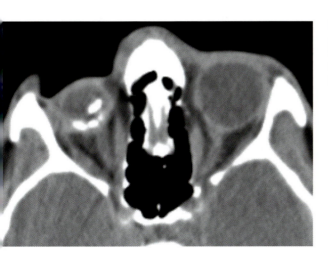

Fig. 6.3   Unilateral acquired microphthalmos and pseudoenophthalmos. Axial non-contrast-enhanced computed tomography (CT) image reveals a shrunken right bulb with heavy calcifications (phthisis bulbi) resulting in depression of the globe back into the normal-sized orbit.

Table 6.1   (Cont.) Ocular lesions

Disease	CT Findings	Comments
Congenital cystic eye	Solid and/or cystic mass that completely fills the orbit and protrudes anteriorly. Retroocular structures are not present or are extremely atrophic. The bony orbit is enlarged, and its walls are thin. The contralateral eye may be normal, small, or absent.	An extremely rare variant of anophthalmos in which the optic vesicle degenerates into a mass of disorganized, solid or cystic neuroectodermal, glial, and angiomatous elements. Orbital teratoma and microphthalmos with posterior cyst may exhibit similar imaging characteristics.
Coloboma	Colobomas appear as outpouchings of variable size and shape arising from the posterior globe. When bilateral, the colobomas are commonly asymmetric in size. All colobomatous eyes are small: the larger the outpouching, the smaller the globe.	Coloboma is a defect in closure of the fetal optic fissure. No gender predilection; may be associated with numerous other ocular, central nervous system (CNS), facial or systemic anomalies, including chromosomal syndromes. Differential diagnosis: buphthalmos, staphyloma, microphthalmic cyst, retrobulbar duplication cyst, retroocular dermoid, hydrops, and arachnoid cyst of the optic nerve sheath.
	Optic disk coloboma: Deformity of the posterior globe with focal small defect at optic nerve head insertion with crater- or funnel-shaped outpouching of vitreous, with fluid density; small unless associated with a retrobulbar microphthalmos cyst. Frequently bilateral. Associated findings: microcornea, microphthalmia, and optic tract and chiasm atrophy.	
	Choroidoretinal coloboma: Excavation separate from or extends beyond disk. Typically bilateral.	Rare. Female and right-side predilection. May present with leukocoria. Associated abnormalities: basal cephaloceles, moyamoya, and agenesis of corpus callosum.
	"Morning glory" disk anomaly: Usually unilateral congenital disk defect distinct from optic disk coloboma: funnel-shaped excavation, larger than simple optic disk coloboma, and central tuft of glial tissue within defect. Associated findings: aniridia, PHPV, and retinal detachment.	
Staphyloma ▷ **Fig. 6.4**	The eye shows a focal bulge posterior. Associated with axial myopia, staphylomas generally occur on the temporal side of the optic disk, but they are also seen anteriorly or along the equator of the eye. The sclera is thin at that level.	A staphyloma is a type of focal buphthalmia. Staphylomas may be seen with axial myopia, glaucoma, trauma, scleritis, and necrotizing infections. They have a high risk for chorioretinal degeneration, choroidal hemorrhage, posterior vitreous detachment, and retinal detachment. May present with visual loss in children and adults.
	Peripapillary staphyloma: Deep excavation of the posterior wall of the globe with connection to the vitreous cavity at optic nerve head. Usually unilateral.	Peripapillary staphyloma is an isolated congenital disk anomaly with extremely rare incidence. The disk is at the bottom of the excavated defect.
Coats disease	CT imaging characteristics are that of a retinal thickening with retinal detachment due to leakage of fluid with high cholesterol and lipoproteinaceous content, which presents as homogeneous hyperdensity involving part of or the entire vitreous in a normal-sized globe. The leaves of the detachment may mildly enhance. The lack of calcifications and lack of an enhancing mass in the globe are key findings to exclude retinoblastoma.	Coats disease is an idiopathic retinal disorder, characterized by telangiectatic, leaky retinal vessels that lead to exudative retinal detachment. It is usually a unilateral disorder that occurs in boys (peak age 6–8 y), rarely in adults (40–60 y). Leukocoria is a presenting symptom.
Norrie disease (retinal dysplasia)	Bilateral microphthalmia with hyperdense (hemorrhagic) vitreous, retinal detachment, optic nerve atrophy, small lens with retrolental pear-shaped bulge, and shallow anterior chamber.	Rare X-linked recessive syndrome associated with bilateral leukokoria and microphthalmia, retinal malformation, deafness, and mental retardation or deterioration. Developmental anomaly of the brain may also be present.
Warburg syndrome	Bilateral microphthalmia with retinal detachment, subretinal or vitreous hemorrhage, sometimes with layered blood levels. PHPV may be associated. The congenital nonattached retina exhibits a characteristic narrow, funnel-shaped or triangular intravitreal image adjacent to hyaloid (Cloquet) canal.	Rare autosomal recessive disorder consisting of bilateral leukokoria and microphthalmia, congenital unilateral or bilateral retinal nonattachment, profound mental retardation, lissencephaly, hydrocephaly, and with death in infancy.

(continues on page 247)

Table 6.1   (Cont.) Ocular lesions

Disease	CT Findings	Comments
Persistent hyperplastic primary vitreous (PHPV)	CT findings are unilateral (rarely bilateral) microphthalmos (can be absent), lens and anterior chamber hypoplasia, and increased density of the entire vitreous without calcification. A contrast-enhancing cone-shaped central retrolental intravitreal density is thought to represent the persistence of fetal tissue in Cloquet canal. Posterior hyaloid or retinal detachment with fluid levels may be associated.	Rare ocular malformation with persistence of various portions of the primary vitreous with hyperplasia and extensive proliferation of the associated embryonic connective tissue due to incomplete regression of embryonic ocular blood supply in Cloquet canal. It can reflect an isolated congenital defect or a manifestation of more extensive ocular or systemic involvement (e.g., trisomy 13, Norrie disease, Warburg syndrome, primary vitreoretinal dysplasia, and other congenital defects). Presents at birth or in infancy with leukocoria (it is the second most common cause of leukocoria), poor vision, and a small eye.
Retinopathy of prematurity (ROP)	Bilateral, often asymmetric microphthalmia with increased density of the vitreous chamber from previous hemorrhage or from neovascular ingrowth. Retinal detachment is frequently associated. A PHPV may be present. Lenticular and/or choroidal dystrophic calcifications are rare but may occur in the late stage of the disease.	Retrolental fibroplasia usually manifests in premature infants who received supplemental oxygen therapy after birth. It accounts for 3% to 5% of the cases of childhood leukokoria.
Inflammatory/infectious conditions		
Scleritis	Thickened, enhancing sclera. There may be associated thickening of Tenon capsule (sclerotenonitis), serous retinal detachment, disk swelling, or serous choroidal detachment. **Posterior nodular scleritis** is a focal, necrotizing, granulomatous inflammation. Unlike uveal melanoma or ocular lymphoma, no contrast enhancement is found.	Scleritis may be bacterial, fungal, or viral in origin, an idiopathic scleral inflammation, or associated with systemic disease (autoimmune disorders: rheumatoid arthritis, polyarteritis nodosa, relapsing polychondritis; other connective tissue diseases; metabolic conditions, e.g., gout; or Wegener granulomatosis, inflammatory bowel disease, Crohn disease, Cogan syndrome, and sarcoidosis). May be unilateral or bilateral, anterior or posterior, acute or chronic. Commonly affects women.
Endophthalmitis	Increased density of the vitreous without a mass. The uveoscleral coat may be thickened and demonstrate increased contrast enhancement (focal enhancement with abscess). Associated choroidal, retinal, and posterior vitreous detachment may be present. Variable degree of increased density in periocular soft tissue structures.	Refers to an intraocular infectious or noninfectious inflammatory process predominantly involving the vitreous cavity or anterior chamber. Exogenous endophthalmitis: due to surgical or nonsurgical penetrating trauma. Endogenous endophthalmitis: hematogenously from an infectious focus. Organisms: staphylococci, streptococci, meningococci, gram negatives, helminthic parasite, and cysticercosis.

(continues on page 248)

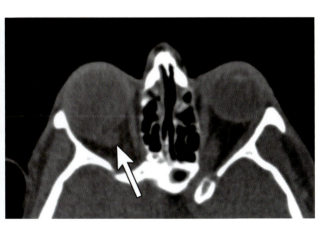

Fig. 6.4   Macrophthalmia and posterior staphyloma (due to progressive myopia). Axial non-contrast-enhanced CT image shows a posterior outpouching (arrow) of the posterolateral right eyeball. The anteroposterior diameter of the right globe is enlarged.

Table 6.1   (Cont.) Ocular lesions

Disease	CT Findings	Comments
Ocular toxocariasis (sclerosing endophthalmitis)	Spectrum of CT imaging characteristics: • Diffuse increased density of the eye by homogeneous intravitreal density, due to detached retina, organized vitreous, and inflammatory subretinal exudates. Absence of calcification. • Localized or diffuse ill-defined mass without enhancement. • Chronic abscess, seen as an irregularity of the uveoscleral coat with diffuse or local thickened, slightly enhanced uveosclera.	Uncommon, usually bilaterally ocular infection of children (average age 6 y) in close contact with dogs. The infection results from ingestion of eggs of the nematode *Toxocara canis*. The second-stage larva of *Toxocara* and the death of the larva result in a wide spectrum of intraocular inflammatory reactions (granuloma, abscess, and diffuse inflammatory infiltration of the choroids and sclera). Leukocoria is a presenting symptom. Imaging findings of toxocariasis may be similar to those seen in Coats disease and noncalcific retinoblastoma. Positive enzyme-linked immunosorbent assay (ELISA) is helpful in differential diagnosis.
Benign neoplasms		
Choroidal (cavernous) hemangioma	May present in two different forms: • As a circumscribed or solitary type, typically located posterior to the equator of the globe in the juxtapapillary or macular region of the fundus. The lenticular, solid soft tissue mass in the wall of the globe demonstrates intense contrast enhancement. May show peripheral calcification. • As a diffuse angiomatosis, often associated with facial nevus flammeus or variations of the Sturge–Weber syndrome. May involve as a flat, intensely enhancing mass the three components of the uvea and, occasionally, nonuveal tissues, such as the episclera, conjunctiva, and limbus. Unlike the melanomas, choroidal hemangiomas are not seen as an obvious lesion on noncontrast CT scans. Following contrast infusion, the hemangiomas exhibit bright enhancement. May be concealed by retinal detachment.	Congenital vascular hamartomas, typically seen in middle-aged to elderly individuals; isolated ocular finding or in association with neurocutaneous syndromes. Cavernous hemangiomas of the choroids are very uncommon, nonprogressive, benign lesions.
Choroidal osteoma	Choroidal osteoma (choriostoma) appears as a sharply demarcated, flat, platelike calcified thickening of the posterior choroids, typically in the juxtapapillary region. No soft tissue infiltration.	Rare benign choroidal tumor consisting of mature bone, found predominantly in otherwise healthy young women ages 10 to 30 y; 25% are bilateral, 15% multifocal. Can cause painless vision loss.
Uveal nevus	Small flat or minimally elevated lesion located most often in the posterior third of the choroid. Usually too little to be visualized.	Benign congenital lesion, usually diagnosed in the first decade of life. Most commonly misdiagnosed lesion to be enucleated under the presumption of malignant melanoma.
Ciliary body adenoma	May present as a well-defined tumor with moderate contrast enhancement arising from the ciliary body behind the iris, encroaching upon the lens.	Rare lesion. Although benign, adenoma of the nonpigmented ciliary epithelium can behave aggressively locally, causing cataract and vitreous hemorrhage. The most common presenting symptom is visual loss.
Uveal leiomyoma	Tends to occur in the ciliary body and peripheral choroidal region rather than in the posterior choroids. Appears as a protuberant, well-defined, elliptoid-ovoid mass that is isodense with respect to brain, with contrast enhancement.	Extremely rare benign tumor of the uveal tract, usually diagnosed in young adult women with decrease of visual acuity. Patients may develop cataract, secondary glaucoma, and retinal detachment.
Uveal schwannoma	Uveal schwannoma usually affects the ciliary body and peripheral choroids rather than the posterior choroids. The tumor appears as a solitary, well-defined, oval lesion, isodense with respect to the brain, with contrast enhancement. Displacement of the lens and bulge of the globe may be seen. Extraocular growth should not be seen.	Schwannoma of the uveal tract is a rarely encountered disease entity lesion that may be initially confused with malignant uveal melanoma. Most patients are women (second to sixth decades). Slowly progressive impairment of visual acuity can be explained by displacement of the lens and progression of an anterior subcapsular cataract. Rapid visual loss may be due to retinal detachment secondary to uveal schwannoma.

(continues on page 249)

Table 6.1 (Cont.) Ocular lesions

Disease	CT Findings	Comments
Choroidal cyst	Unilateral or, less commonly, bilateral cystic lesion that may cause retinal detachment.	Very rare lesion that may be mistaken for a solid choroidal tumor.
Retinal (capillary) hemangioma	This lesion, usually located in the midperipheral retina, is often small in size (1–2 mm) and can be inapparent on noncontrast scans, except the tumor is calcified or ossified. After contrast injection, it demonstrates significant enhancement. May be associated with exudates and retinal detachment.	Capillary hemangiomas of the retina, histologically similar to cerebellar hemangioblastomas, are extremely rare intraocular tumors, usually associated with von Hippel–Lindau disease (50% bilateral involvement, multiple in the affected eye in one third). These lesions can enlarge. Their propensity to bleed may cause exudative retinal detachment, glaucoma, cataract, and uveitis.
Retinal astrocytoma	Usually very small, thin, and translucent, or more dense, multilobulated, and minimally vascular nodule near the optic nerve. Single or multiple. Unlike retinoblastoma, it rarely grows. It may be associated with infiltration of the optic nerve, exudative retinal detachment, hemorrhage, and calcification.	Also called ocular (astrocytic) hamartoma. It is a rare, benign retinal tumor, occurring in children (8–15 y). May present as an isolated ocular pathologic finding (sporadic in one third of the cases) or in association with both tuberous sclerosis and neurofibromatosis type 1.
Malignant neoplasms		
Retinoblastoma ▷ *Fig. 6.5*	Calcified intraocular mass, hyperdense to vitreous in a normal-sized globe of a child younger than 3 y of age is highly suggestive of retinoblastoma. Punctuate, finely speckled, or diffuse, dense calcification is noted in 90%–95%. In contrast-enhanced CT scan, the tumor shows slight to moderate heterogeneous enhancement. Retinal detachment may occasionally be the only manifestation. **Endophytic growth pattern of retinoblastoma:** Irregular, solid, and heterogeneous peripheral intraocular mass, usually posterior to the equator, with inward protrusion into vitreous; associated with vitreous seeding. **Exophytic retinoblastoma:** Outward growth of the intraretinal tumor into the subretinal space; associated with a progressive retinal detachment. **Diffuse infiltrating form:** Rare; the tumor grows along the retina appearing as a placoid mass (which simulates inflammatory or hemorrhagic conditions), often without calcifications and usually outside the typical age group. Extension with optic nerve enlargement, abnormal soft tissue in orbit and intracranial extension may occur in 25% of cases, without calcifications.	Most common intraocular malignancy of infancy and childhood (average age at diagnosis 13 mo), congenital in origin, rarely occurs in adults, without gender or side predilection. Presents in 95% under the age of 5 y with leukocoria, severe vision loss, and eye pain. Unilateral in 70% to 75%, bilateral in 25% to 30%. *Trilateral retinoblastoma* refers to the association of bilateral retinoblastoma with a pinealoblastoma. *Tetralateral retinoblastoma:* bilateral disease plus pineal and suprasellar tumor. Sporadic: 60% of retinoblastomas. Inherited: 40% of retinoblastomas. Essentially all bilateral and multilateral disease. With risk of second malignancy (osteosarcoma, soft tissue sarcoma, and melanoma): 20% to 30% in nonirradiated patients, 50% to 60% radiation-induced.

(continues on page 250)

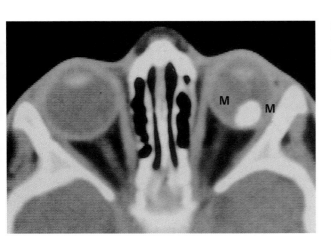

Fig. 6.5 Endophytic retinoblastoma. Axial non-contrast-enhanced CT image shows a large complex intraocular mass (M) of the posterior segment on the left side with ovoid tumor calcification.

II Head and Neck

Table 6.1   (Cont.) Ocular lesions

Disease	CT Findings	Comments
Ocular melanoma ▷ *Fig. 6.6* ▷ *Fig. 6.7*	Intraocular focal, well-defined, elevated dome, crescentic, flat, polypoid or mound shaped, solid, peripheral mass of the posterior segment, extending into the vitreous, with broad choroidal base, hyperdense to vitreous, with diffuse moderate enhancement. Mushroom shape implies penetration through Bruch membrane. Calcification is rare. Retinal detachment is frequently coexisting but often indistinguishable from the neoplasm without contrast enhancement. Transscleral penetration or optic nerve tumor invasion may be seen (5%).	Most common primary intraocular malignancy in adult Caucasian (peak incidence sixth and seventh decade), with slight male preference. The tumor is almost always unilateral, with 85% arising from the choroids, 10% from the ciliary body, and 5% from the iris. Congenital melanosis, ocular melanocytosis, ocudermal melanocytosis, and uveal nevi are conditions that may predispose to uveal melanoma. Presents with painless vision disturbance.
Ciliary body adenocarcinoma	May present as a well-defined, multilobulated mass with moderate contrast enhancement involving the ciliary body, the posterior and anterior chamber angle, and the iris. The invasive tumor can spread into choroid, corneoscleral, and episcleral tissues, as well as into the orbit and intracranially.	Ocular adenocarcinomas are extremely rare malignant lesions that may arise from the pigmented and nonpigmented epithelium of the ciliary body, iris, or retina. Associated uveitis, glaucoma, hemorrhage, and exudative retinal detachment are not uncommon. This intraocular neoplasm should be considered in middle-aged adults with a long-standing phthisical eye with an epibulbar mass and for proptosis of recent duration.
Medulloepithelioma	**Nonteratoid medulloepithelioma (diktymoma):** Appears as a dense, noncalcified mass in the region of the ciliary body, with moderate to marked enhancement. May be associated with cysts in the anterior part of the vitreous, lens coloboma, and lens subluxation. **Teratoid medulloepitheliomas (30%–50%):** with cartilaginous differentiation and associated calcification; appears as a dense, irregular, calcified mass in the region of ciliary body. In advanced medulloepithelioma involving the vitreous cavity and the retina, other causes of intraocular calcified lesions (retinoblastoma, CMV chorioretinitis, toxocara endophthalmitis, ROP, choroidal osteoma, and retinal astrocytoma) cannot be excluded. Retinal detachment is an associated finding seen in advanced cases.	Rare nonhereditary, unilateral embryonic neoplasm, malignant in most cases; usually diagnosed in the first decade of life (mean age 4 y); without racial, gender, or side predilection. It typically arises from the ciliary body epithelium but may also occur as a posterior mass in the retina or in the region of the optic nerve head and optic nerve. Presents with cataract, cyclitic membrane formation, and glaucoma. Ciliary body medulloepitheliomas may be associated with intracranial neoplasms (CNS medulloepithelioma and pinealoblastoma) and CNS malformations (agenesis of the corpus callosum, schizencephaly, and mass-like soft tissue prominence of the quadrigeminal plate). Extremely rare, these tumors can occur in adults and may mimic melanoma, adenoma or adenocarcinoma of the ciliary epithelium, mesoectodermal leiomyoma, neurilemoma, metastatic carcinoma, and intraocular inflammation, such as granulomatous uveitis or TB granuloma.
Ocular metastases ▷ *Fig. 6.8*	Metastatic tumor to the globe most commonly involves the posterior temporal portion of the uveal tract near the macula. The lesions are often multiple and bilateral (one third of cases) with small, flat, disk-like or lentiform shaped, thickened areas of increased density, and associated with exudative detachment. Less common presentations include circular uveal thickening. Contrast enhancement is variable, ranging from minimal to moderate.	Most patients with ocular metastases have a known primary malignancy with systemic metastases. The most common sources of secondary tumor within the eye are the lung and breast. In children, ocular metastases occur with neuroblastoma, Ewing sarcoma, Wilms tumor, and leukemia.
Leukemia	CT imaging of leukemic infiltration of the uvea, choroids, and retina reveals a localized or diffuse thickening of these structures, often bilateral. Intraocular hemorrhage due to hematologic alterations may be present.	Orbital involvement in leukemia is not common. It occurs in children with acute lymphatic leukemia and in adults with chronic lymphatic leukemia. Leukemia may involve every tissue of the eye; the choroids are the most consistently involved layer on histopathology. Intraocular findings include iritis and vitritis.
Ocular lymphoma	Orbital CT findings are usually normal and noncontributory but may include an ill-defined soft tissue density of the vitreous chamber, choroidal-scleral thickening, widening of the optic nerve, elevated chorioretinal lesions, and posterior vitreous and retinal detachment.	Primary intraocular lymphoma, considered part of primary CNS lymphoma, is a diffuse large B-cell lymphoma, a rare type of non–Hodgkin lymphoma. Involvement includes retina, subretinal space, vitreous, uvea, and optic nerve. Bilaterality occurs in about 90% of cases. Most patients diagnosed to have intraocular lymphoma are elderly (mean age 63 y) and have symptoms of vitritis with blurred vision and vitreous floaters, and a history of systemic lymphoma or CNS involvement.

(continues on page 252)

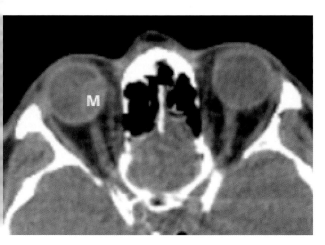

Fig. 6.6   Choroidal melanoma. Axial non-contrast-enhanced CT image reveals an intraocular focal, well-defined, dome-shaped peripheral mass (M) with a broad choroidal base at the nasal segment of the right globe.

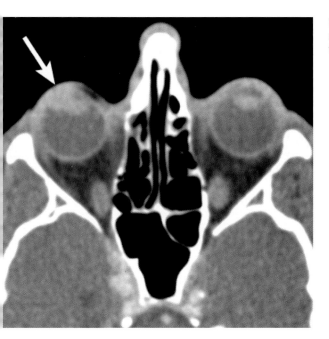

Fig. 6.7   Iris melanoma. Axial contrast-enhanced CT image demonstrates a polypoid solid mass with moderate enhancement involving the lateral iris and anterior chamber of the right globe (arrow).

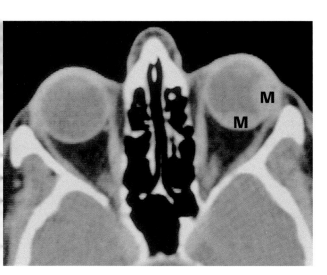

Fig. 6.8   Ocular metastases (from lung cancer). Axial non-contrast-enhanced CT image shows two intraocular peripheral, well-defined, lentiform-shaped solid masses (M) of the posterior temporal portion of the left globe.

Table 6.1 (Cont.) Ocular lesions

Disease	CT Findings	Comments
Trauma		
Eyeball injury ▷ *Fig. 6.9* ▷ *Fig. 6.10* ▷ *Fig. 6.11* ▷ *Fig. 6.12*	• **Ocular hemorrhage** Anterior chamber: distortion of the contours or increased density of the anterior chamber (anterior hyphema). Vitreous chamber hemorrhage: increased density of the vitreous without layering. Choroidal hematoma: hyperdense rounded or globular intraocular mass. Density of blood decreases with time. • **Ocular detachment** Retinal detachment. Choroidal detachment. • **Traumatic lens dislocation** Abnormal position of the lens. • **Eyeball rupture** Loss and flattening of the normal spherical contour of the eyeball ("pear" or "flat tire" sign). CT may show air within the globe and intraocular blood. • **Foreign body** CT may confirm the presence or absence of a foreign body and provide information with regard to its composition and location. It may also demonstrate other associated injuries and possible complications. • **Phthisis bulbi** In the chronic phase, the posttraumatic eyeball may appear small, deformed, retracted, calcified, and shrunken.	Intraocular hemorrhage may be spontaneous, posttraumatic, or associated with bleeding disorders and a variety of ocular disorders. The lens is more frequently subluxated than completely dislocated. Penetrating trauma or severe blunt trauma may cause laceration of the sclera with escape of the vitreous and decrease in the intraocular pressure. Foreign body can be classified as • Organic (wood, dirt, or other vegetable matter) • Inorganic (metallic ([steel, lead, iron, aluminum, and other metal alloys]) and nonmetallic (glass, plastic, stone, or other minerals). Phthisis bulbi is not unique to trauma. It is an end-stage appearance of an eyeball that has undergone degeneration and disorganization because of trauma, infection, inflammation, or tumor.
Miscellaneous lesions		
Macrophthalmia	Diffuse enlargement of the optic globe. **Pseudomacrophthalmia:** Apparent enlargement of one eye can occur with proptosis or when the contralateral eye is relatively small.	Macrophthalmia can result from glaucoma in children or may be seen as an isolated entity, secondary to massive intraocular tumor, or in association with neurofibromatosis. Axial myopia, characterized by elongation of the globe in the anteroposterior dimension, is the most common cause of eye enlargement with no intraocular masses. Retinoblastoma is the most common intraocular tumor to produce generalized eye enlargement. Buphthalmos ("ox eye"): diffuse extreme enlargement of the eye in children secondary to increased intraocular pressure, caused by congenital or infantile glaucoma.
Proptosis ▷ *Fig. 6.13*	Abnormal anterior protrusion of a normal-sized globe (extension > 21 mm anterior to the interzygomatic line on axial scans at level of lens). **Axial proptosis:** Globe projected away from the center of the orbit. **Nonaxial proptosis:** associated with localized masses elsewhere in the orbit.	Associated with thyroid ophthalmopathy, pseudotumor, infection (bacterial or fungal), sarcoidosis, Erdheim–Chester disease, Wegener granulomatosis, vasculitis and connective tissue diseases, lymphoproliferative disease, orbital mass lesions, including benign or malignant neoplasms, vascular lesions, abscesses, hematomas, fractures, mucoceles, Langerhans cell histiocytosis, fibrous dysplasia, and sphenoorbital dysplasia of neurofibromatosis type 1.
Enophthalmos ▷ *Fig. 6.14*	Relative depression of the globe back into the orbit.	May occur in orbital blow-out fracture, silent sinus syndrome, neurofibromatosis with absence of part of the sphenoid bone, breast carcinoma metastases, and Cockayne syndrome. Pseudoenophthalmos: end-stage-contracted globe.

(continues on page 254)

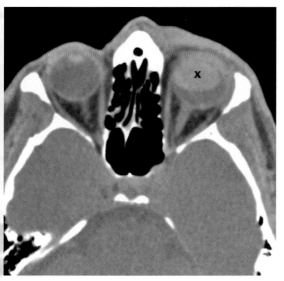

Fig. 6.9   Vitreous chamber hemorrhage. Axial non-contrast-enhanced CT image demonstrates increased density (x) of the left vitreous without layering.

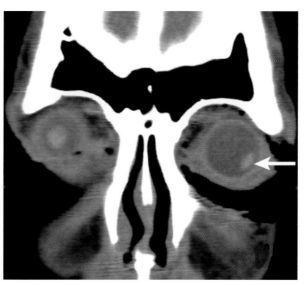

Fig. 6.10   Traumatic lens dislocation. Coronal reformatted section shows caudal-lateral luxation of the lens (arrow) into the vitreous body on the left side.

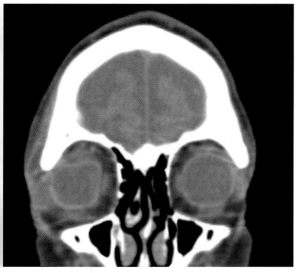

Fig. 6.11   Eyeball rupture. Coronal reformatted section reveals loss of the normal spherical contour of the right globe.

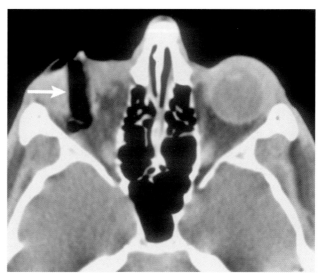

Fig. 6.12   Foreign body injury (wood). Axial non-contrast-enhanced CT image shows impalement injury (arrow) with double perforation of the right globe.

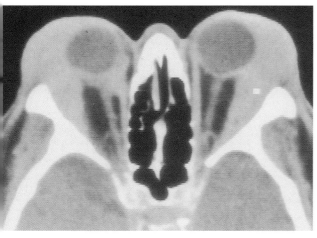

Fig. 6.13   Nonaxial proptosis. Axial non-contrast-enhanced CT image demonstrates bilateral abnormal protrusion of the globe with a lateral extraconal non-Hodgkin lymphoma mass involving the lacrimal gland and lateral rectus muscle (joystick point).

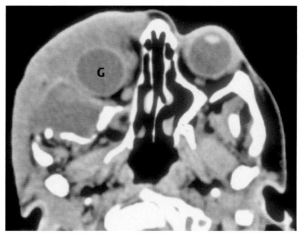

Fig. 6.14   Enophthalmos. Axial non-contrast-enhanced CT image in a patient with neurofibromatosis (NF1) reveals a broad sphenoid defect with relative depression of the right globe (G). Multiple plexiform neurofibromas are evident periorbitally.

Table 6.1 (Cont.) Ocular lesions

Disease	CT Findings	Comments
Posterior hyaloid detachment	Blood or other fluid accumulation occurs in the posterior hyaloid space between the detached posterior hyaloid membrane and sensory retina. On CT, the noncalcified mobile lesion tends to accumulate in the most dependent portion and may depict gravitational fluid–fluid levels. The detached posterior hyaloid membrane may be seen as an intravitreal curvilinear image extending toward the optic disk.	In adults older than 50 y, usually caused by accelerated vitreous liquefaction with myopia, surgical and nonsurgical trauma, and intraocular inflammation. In infants often associated with PHPV.
Retinal detachment ▷ *Fig. 6.15* ▷ *Fig. 6.16*	Blood or other fluid accumulation occurs in the subretinal space between the sensory retina and the retinal pigment epithelium. The leaves of the detached and folded sensory retina are limited at the ora serrata and at the optic disk and converge toward the optic disk, thereby producing a characteristic V-shaped configuration.	A rhegmatogenous retinal detachment occurs due to a hole, tear, or break in the retina that allows fluid to pass from the vitreous space into the subretinal space. Rhegmatogenous detachment is the most common. Risk factors include myopia, previous cataract surgery, and ocular trauma. A tractional retinal detachment occurs when fibrovascular tissue, caused by an injury, inflammation, or neovascularization, pulls the sensory retina from the retinal pigment epithelium. May occur in proliferative diabetic or sickle cell retinopathy. Secondary, serous, or exudative retinal detachment results in fluid accumulating underneath the retina without the presence of a hole, tear, or break. It occurs due to inflammation, injury, vascular abnormalities, and primary or metastatic choroidal tumors.
Choroidal detachment	Choroidal detachment is caused by the accumulation of fluid or blood in the potential suprachoroidal space. The choroid is firmly attached at the ciliary body and tethered at the vortex veins. This results in the typical appearance of choroidal detachment: it appears as a smooth, ring-shaped, crescentic, or dome-shaped, semilunar area of variable attenuation values. The detached leaves do not extent to the region of the optic nerve, form a U or, in a more advanced stage, the "kissing choroids" sign, and are restricted at the level of the scleral attachments of the vortex veins. The detached choroids can extend frontal to the ciliary body and result in ciliary detachment.	Ocular hypotony is the essential underlying cause of serous choroidal detachment and may be the result of ocular inflammatory disease (uveitis, scleritis, and Vogt–Koyanagi–Harada syndrome), accidental perforation of the eye, ocular surgery, or intensive glaucoma therapy. Other causes are myxedema, nanophthalmos, and idiopathic uveal effusion syndrome. Hemorrhagic choroidal detachment may occur spontaneously or as a complication of ocular surgery, ocular trauma, hemoglobinopathies, and anticoagulation therapy.
Macular degeneration	Irregular lesion of increased density, similar to uveal melanoma, related to hemorrhage in the retinal and subretinal space. Frequently complicated by scar formation or liquefaction of the vitreous with posterior hyaloid detachment. The lesion may show moderate to marked contrast enhancement.	Disciform degeneration of the macula in the elderly is a leading cause of legal blindness. The earliest changes at the macula are hyalinization and thickening of Bruch membrane, followed by ingrowth of choroidal neovascularization.
Optic nerve head drusen ▷ *Fig. 6.17*	Discrete, flat, round calcification of the optic nerve disk. Bilateral in 75% of cases.	Acellular accretions of hyalinelike material on or near the surface of the optic disk that become calcified. Most cases are idiopathic. Occasionally, drusen are associated with ocular diseases, such as retinitis pigmentosa. May be familial and asymptomatic or present with headache, visual field defects, and pseudopapilledema.

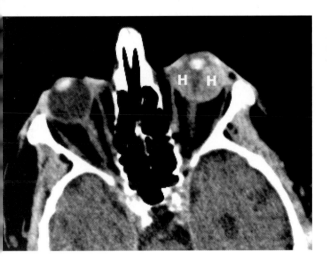

Fig. 6.15   Retinal detachment. Axial non-contrast-enhanced CT image shows subretinal hemorrhage (H) in the left globe with V-shaped configuration of the detached retinal layers. The apex is directed toward the optic disk.

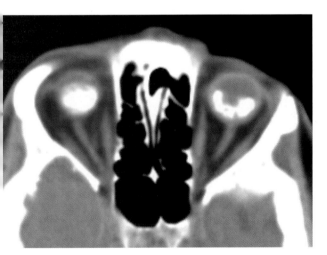

Fig. 6.16   Chronic retinal detachment. Axial non-contrast-enhanced CT image reveals heavy intraocular calcifications on both sides.

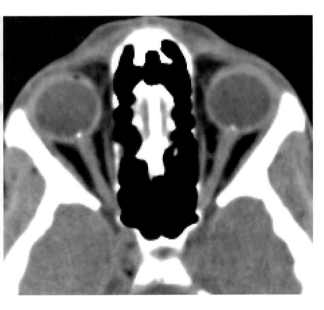

Fig. 6.17   Optic nerve head drusen. Axial non-contrast-enhanced CT image demonstrates the bilateral calcification of the optic nerve disc.

Table 6.2   Optic nerve-sheath complex lesions

Disease	CT Findings	Comments
Inflammatory/infectious conditions		
Optic perineuritis	Tubular thickening (uniform enlargement) or fusiform thickening (lens shaped, tapering at either end) of the optic nerve-sheath complex. May show perineural contrast enhancement, producing a form of "tram-track" sign.	Unusual localized form of orbital pseudotumor. In contrast to optic neuritis, pain is exacerbated with retrodisplacement of the globe, and patients are slightly older (mean age 39.5 y). Involvement of the optic nerve-sheath complex is rarely also found with viral, tuberculous, and syphilitic infections, radiation therapy, and sarcoidosis.
Optic neuritis	CT findings are usually normal but may include both mild swelling and enhancement of the optic nerve with irregular borders. Magnetic resonance imaging (MRI) is the best imaging modality to evaluate optic neuritis.	May be sporadic or a harbinger of multiple sclerosis. Patients (mean age 30 y) present with acute loss of visual acuity, evolving over hours to days, ipsilateral eye pain, and dyschromatopsia. Significant recovery of vision is typical. Approximately 50% of patients with idiopathic optic neuritis develop multiple sclerosis; 15% to 25% of patients with multiple sclerosis (MS) initially present with optic neuritis; 70% to 90% of patients with MS develop optic neuritis at some point. *Devic syndrome* (neuromyelitis optica): bilateral acute optic neuritis with transverse myelitis. Other, less common causes of optic neuritis include ischemia, pseudotumor, sarcoidosis, radiation therapy, systemic lupus erythematosus, viral infection (varicella, herpes, human immunodeficiency virus [HIV]-related optic neuropathy), toxoplasmosis, tuberculosis, syphilitic neuritis, and Sjögren syndrome.
Neoplasms		
Optic nerve glioma ▷ *Fig. 6.18*	Smooth, sharply marginated, tubular, fusiform, globular, or excrescent enlargement of the optic nerve, which is isodense to brain with slight to moderate contrast enhancement. Cystic degeneration, hemorrhage, necrosis, and calcification are uncommon. Kinking (buckling) and tortuosity can be noted. Intracranial extension along the optic pathway through the eroded optic canal is common with a dumbbell shape. Extension of glioma into the posterior optic pathway (chiasm, optic tracts, lateral geniculate bodies, or even optic radiations) may form a large mass growing into the adjacent brain. Bilateral involvement is more common in neurofibromatosis type 1.	Uncommon childhood disease (4% of all orbital tumors) but accounts for 80% of primary tumors of the optic nerve presenting with decreased vision and axial proptosis. The peak incidence is from 2 to 8 y of age, with slight female predominance. One third of patients have neurofibromatosis type 1; 15% of patients with neurofibromatosis type 1 have optic nerve or optic chiasm glioma. Histologically, childhood optic nerve glioma is commonly a pilocytic astrocytoma, whereas the much more rare adult optic nerve glioma (peak incidence 40–50 y of age, with male predominance) tends to be glioblastoma with much more aggressive behavior, bilateral, and predominantly involves the intracranial optic nerves and chiasm.
Ganglioglioma	The optic nerve shows diffuse enlargement unlike that observed in optic nerve glioma and optic nerve sheath meningioma.	Ganglioglioma is a rare tumor affecting the optic nerve.
Optic nerve hemangioblastoma	Well-enhanced, sharply demarcated, pear-shaped solid mass in the optic nerve. Apex tumors may grow unusually like a dumbbell, thereby widening the optic canal. In addition, optic nerve hemangioblastoma may be associated with optic nerve enlargement, chiasmal or optic tract edema, cysts, angiomatosis retinae, infratentorial hemangioblastomas, and cysts of the abdominal viscera.	Very rare tumor of optic nerve, seen in patients with von Hippel–Lindau disease or arises sporadically. More common in men. The age of diagnosis is between the third and fifth decades. Patients experience gradually progressive loss of vision either to blindness or surgical intervention, as well as proptosis with a dull eye pain.
Secondary optic nerve tumors	Metastasis of the optic nerve may appear as an irregular soft tissue mass with invasion of adjacent structures.	Secondary optic nerve tumors more frequent (82%) than primary optic nerve tumors (18%). These tumors include • Hematogenous metastases to the optic nerve–sheath complex (rare) • Direct extension from ocular tumors • Compression or invasion by tumor adjacent to the nerve in the orbital cavity • Extension of tumor from the sellar/parasellar area through the subarachnoid space • Seeding of tumor within the subarachnoid space from sources outside the neural axis, principally from carcinomas • CNS tumors extending to the chiasm and optic nerves, including primary neuroectodermal tumors, glioblastoma, and gliomatosis cerebri.

(continues on page 257)

Table 6.2 (Cont.) Optic nerve-sheath complex lesions

Disease	CT Findings	Comments
Optic nerve sheath meningioma ▷ *Fig. 6.19a, b*	Optic nerve sheath meningiomas are commonly seen as a diffuse tubular enlargement along the intraorbital portion of the optic nerve, but growth can be fusiform or as a localized, eccentric expansion of the optic nerve, often at the orbital apex, simulating a tumor within the orbit that has encroached on the optic nerve. They are infiltrative and may result in an irregular and serrated appearance. Meningiomas tend to be hyperdense on CT and frequently reveal globular, linear, plaquelike, or granular calcifications (calcification within the mass virtually excludes optic glioma). Meningiomas often show homogeneous and intense contrast enhancement surrounding the nonenhancing optic nerve embedded in the tumor ("tram-track" sign). Extension into the optic canal may cause enlargement and occasionally hyperostosis of the margin of the canal.	Optic nerve sheath meningiomas represent < 1% of all meningiomas and constitute 3% to 5% of orbital tumors. They may originate primarily from the meninges along the orbital segment of the optic nerve or may extend secondarily into the orbit from the intracranial meninges. Bilateral optic nerve sheath meningiomas are uncommon. They are the second most common primary neoplasm of the optic nerve-sheath complex and occur predominantly between the ages of 30 and 50 y but may occur at any age. Childhood optic nerve meningioma is often associated with neurofibromatosis type 2 and behaves aggressively. There is a female predominance (3–5:1). Patients present with optic nerve atrophy, progressive loss of vision over months, disk edema, or pallor and proptosis. Hemangiomas and hemangiopericytomas rarely originate in the perioptic nerve sheath.

(continues on page 258)

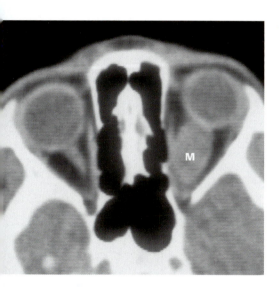

Fig. 6.18 Optic nerve glioma. Axial non-contrast-enhanced CT image shows a fusiform enlargement of the left intraorbital optic nerve (M).

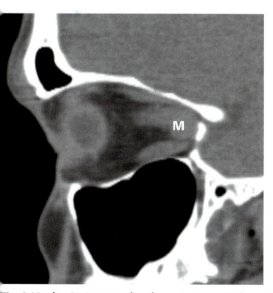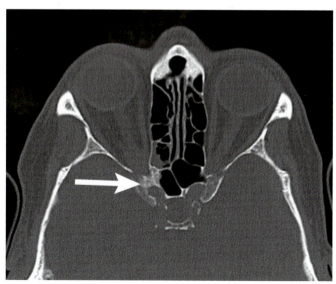

Fig. 6.19a, b Optic nerve sheath meningioma. Right sagittal orbit non-contrast-enhanced CT reconstruction (**a**) demonstrates a localized, eccentric expansion of the optic nerve sheath at the orbital apex (M). Axial bone CT image (**b**) reveals extension into the right optic canal with hyperostosis (arrow) of the margin of the canal.

Table 6.2   (Cont.) Optic nerve-sheath complex lesions

Disease	CT Findings	Comments
Lymphoproliferative disease	Lymphomatous optic neuropathy may produce a thickened, enlarged, and enhanced optic nerve sheath surrounding the nerve that does not enhance.	Lymphoma and leukemia may infiltrate the optic nerve–sheath complex as part of systemic disease. In leukemia, diffuse infiltration of the optic nerve can lead to rapid loss of vision. The spectrum of orbital disease in non–Hodgkin lymphoma includes well-defined mass lesions and diffusely infiltrative lesions in the extraconal and/or intraconal space, lacrimal gland masses, and conjunctival involvement.
Trauma		
Optic nerve injury ▷ *Fig. 6.20*	• Optic nerve injury from fracture fragments or foreign body that may impinge on the optic nerve. • Mass effect from edema and hemorrhage within the optic nerve sheath that may lead to ischemia. • Optic nerve avulsion.	Optic nerve injury is loss of vision or visual impairment secondary to direct or indirect damages of the optic nerve.
Miscellaneous lesions		
Distended optic nerve sheath	Bilateral or unilateral, tortuous, enlarged optic nerve–sheath complex with central density reflecting optic nerve.	Bilateral dilation of the perioptic nerve subarachnoid space may be idiopathic or result from increased intracranial pressure (intracranial mass lesions, hydrocephalus, malignant hypertension, diffuse cerebral edema, or increased venous pressure), elevated CSF protein level, and pseudotumor cerebri. Unilateral distention of the optic sheath may result from orbital apex obstruction by fracture or mass lesion of the optic nerve, inflammatory lesions, hydrops, optic atrophy, and arachnoid cyst.
Optic nerve sheath meningocele	Prominent focal or segmental enlargement of the dural arachnoid sheath around the optic nerve. The lumen is filled with CSF. May be associated with empty sella and enlarged subarachnoid cisterns, such as gasserian cisterns.	May occur primarily or secondarily in association with other orbital processes, such as meningioma, optic nerve pilocytic astrocytoma, and hemangioma. May present with changes in the visual acuity, visual field, and optic nerve appearance.

Table 6.3   Extraocular conal and intraconal lesions

Disease	CT Findings	Comments
Optic nerve–sheath complex lesions	See **Table 6.2**	
Inflammatory/infectious conditions		
Idiopathic orbital inflammatory disease (orbital pseudotumor) ▷ *Fig. 6.21*	CT is typically nonspecific and variable because the disease process, which is usually unilateral (75%) and multifocal, may present in many forms: • Enlargement of the extraocular muscles (myositic type) with involvement of any part of one or multiple extraocular muscles, including the tendinous insertion anteriorly, and with inward bowing of the medial contour of the muscle belly. Spillover of the inflammatory process into the orbital fat bordering the muscle makes the margin of the muscle indistinct or irregular rather than sharply marginated. • Diffuse oblong enlargement of lacrimal gland with moderate enhancement • Retrobulbar mass lesion (tumefactive type) with soft tissue density, irregular margins, and marked contrast enhancement, which may extend across multiple compartments, sometimes with extraorbital extension, but without bone destruction • Diffuse ill-defined infiltrations with obliteration of retrobulbar fat planes • Diffuse enlargement of the optic nerve–sheath complex (38%) with enhancement of the sheath contrasting against the central low density of the nerve • Uveal-scleral thickening (periscleritis) usually with extension along the most anterior portion of the optic nerve • Apical involvement with abnormal enhancement at the orbital apex extending into the enlarged cavernous sinus • Sclerosing pseudotumor with diffuse increase in density of the orbital fat with obliteration of the optic nerve, muscles, and circumferential involvement of the globe with complete fixation of the intraorbital structures.	Pseudotumor is the most common painful orbital mass in adults and the third most common ophthalmic disorder (5% of all orbital lesions). Orbital pseudotumor can involve retrobulbar fat (76%), extraocular muscles (57%), optic nerve–sheath complex (38%), uveal-scleral area (33%), and lacrimal gland (5%). Wegener granulomatosis, polyarteritis nodosa, lupus erythematosus, rheumatoid arthritis, sarcoidosis, fibrosing mediastinitis, retroperitoneal fibrosis, sclerosing cholangitis, primary orbital vasculitis, thyroiditis, or lymphoma can mimic this nongranulomatous acute, subacute, or chronic inflammatory process in the orbit. Presents with rapidly developing, painful ophthalmoplegia, proptosis, and chemosis. Optic nerve dysfunction results from inflammation of the perineural tissue or compression on the optic nerve from mass effect. Rapid and lasting response to steroid therapy is characteristic. No gender preference. Peak incidence: fifth decade. Pediatric pseudotumor encompasses 6% to 16% of orbital pseudotumors. A regional variant of pseudotumor is the Tolosa–Hunt syndrome, which is characterized by inflammatory infiltration on the orbital apex, including superior orbital fissure and cavernous sinus. It presents with a painful ophthalmoplegia (CN III, IV, and VI) and hypoesthesia of the periorbital skin.

(continues on page 260)

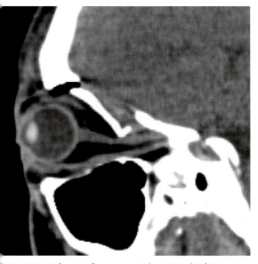

Fig. 6.20   Blow-in fracture. Right sagittal orbit non-contrast-enhanced CT reconstruction shows a fracture fragment of the orbital roof impinging on the right optic nerve.

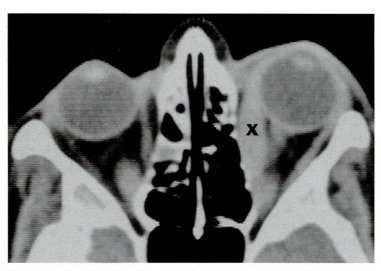

Fig. 6.21   Idiopathic orbital inflammatory disease (orbital pseudotumor, myositic type). Axial non-contrast-enhanced CT image shows left proptosis and enlargement of the medial rectus muscle (x), including the tendinous insertion anteriorly.

Table 6.3   (Cont.) Extraocular conal and intraconal lesions

Disease	CT Findings	Comments
Orbital cellulitis and abscess formation	Predisposing conditions such as sinusitis, foreign bodies, or fracture are usually evident. In preseptal inflammation, CT reveals a diffuse increase in density and thickening of the lid and conjunctiva. Low attenuation areas with or without rim enhancement reflect abscesses in the lid. In subperiosteal accumulation of inflammatory infiltrate or pus, usually originating from the ethmoid sinus, the medial rectus muscle is displaced laterally, often enhances slightly, and is thickened from the inflammatory edema. An enhancing rim indicates the displaced periosteum. A low-density area either localized or extending along the entire medial orbital wall reflects pus accumulation in the subperiosteal space. Demineralization, thinning, or loss of bone manifests inflammation or localized osteomyelitis of the lamina papyracea. Predisposing conditions such as sinusitis, foreign bodies, and fractures are usually evident. Extension of the infection into the intraconal space is manifested on CT by an ill-defined infiltrate with increased attenuation of the orbital fat (stranding and streaking giving rise to "dirty" appearance of the intraconal fat), and obliteration of the enhancing and swollen extraocular muscles and optic nerve–sheath complex. A low-density area with rim enhancement reflects an abscess. Air may be visible within the infiltrate caused either by anaerobic bacteria or leakage of air from the sinuses into the orbit. In diffuse extraconal and intraconal orbital infection, the least common type of orbital involvement, the entire orbital cavity, including the muscles and optic nerve, is obliterated by a diffuse increase in density with concomitant severe proptosis. In cases of severe inflammatory disease of the orbit, periorbital extension to the facial structures and the temporal and infratemporal fossae may occur. Posterior orbital extension may lead to superior orbital fissure syndrome, cavernous sinus thrombosis, and other intracranial complications.	Orbital cellulitis is a serious pyogenic infection of the orbit. It is most frequently the result of bacterial spread from contiguous paranasal sinus (particularly ethmoid) infection (84%). Other sources of infection are primary infections of the face, teeth, or pharynx, septicemia, retrograde thrombophlebitis, trauma, and penetrating foreign bodies. The patient is acutely ill with fever, ocular pain, lid edema, chemosis, proptosis, and limited ocular movements. Fungal infections (mucormycosis, aspergillosis) may occur as a complication of diabetic ketoacidosis and in immuncompromised and debilitated patients. They demonstrate a much more aggressive course with early bone destruction and invasion of arteries and veins.
Sarcoidosis ▷ *Fig. 6.22*	Ophthalmic manifestations of sarcoidosis may consist of • Unilateral or bilateral isodense enlargement or mass-like infiltration of the lacrimal glands and extraocular muscles, with contrast enhancement • Optic nerve–sheath complex thickening with abnormal enhancement of the optic nerve from the globe to the chiasm • Pseudotumor-like intraorbital enhancing masses Intracranial extension leads to leptomeningeal, dural, and parenchymal neurosarcoidosis with pathologic enhancement.	Systemic disease of unknown etiology characterized by noncaseating, granulomatous inflammation. It has a particular proclivity for adults younger than age 40 (slight female predominance) and for certain ethnic and racial groups (increased in African descent, Puerto Rican, Irish, and Scandinavian). Ophthalmic manifestations develop in ~25% of patients. In addition to the globe (uveitis, retinal vasculitis, and vitritis), the conjunctiva, extraocular muscles, retrobulbar space, lacrimal gland, optic nerve, chiasm, and optic radiation may be affected. The clinical signs consist of pain, proptosis, ophthalmoparesis, and visual loss.

(continues on page 261)

Table 6.3   (Cont.) Extraocular conal and intraconal lesions

Disease	CT Findings	Comments
Wegener granulomatosis	Characteristically, ocular and orbital involvement is bilateral. The CT appearance is similar to orbital pseudotumor with diffuse retrobulbar infiltration but with bony destruction. Wegener granulomatosis can affect the anterior optic pathways with infiltration of the optic chiasm and with enhancing lesions in the chiasmatic cistern, enhancement of the basal meninges, and thickening of the pituitary infundibulum. Enlargement of the lacrimal gland may be symmetric and extensive. Nasal and sinus involvement is usually also evident.	Systemic disease primarily affecting the upper respiratory tract, lungs, and kidneys. Orbital involvement is present in ~20% of cases. Ocular manifestations include scleritis, episcleritis, uveitis, and retinal vasculitis.
Erdheim–Chester disease ▷ **Fig. 6.23**	In Erdheim–Chester disease with orbital involvement, there may be infiltration of the anterior compartment (preseptal space) and/or posterior compartment of the orbit with intra- and extraconal enhancing lesions replacing the orbital fat and encasing the optic nerve and the extraocular muscles. Involvement of the ocular adnexa includes lacrimal gland enlargement.	Rare idiopathic systemic histiocytic disorder of adults characterized by xanthogranulomatous infiltrates with lipid-laden histiocytes and Touton giant cells in the long tubular bones, skin, soft tissue, heart, pericardium, blood vessels, lung, pleura, retroperitoneum, kidneys, hypothalamic/pituitary axis (diabetes insipidus), and dura. Orbital involvement is very rare and tends to be bilateral. These adult patients present with progressive proptosis, ophthalmoplegia, and visual loss.

(continues on page 262)

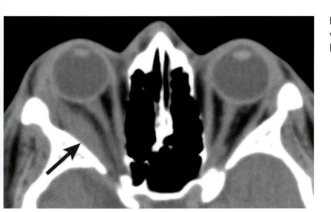

Fig. 6.22   Sarcoidosis. Axial non-contrast-enhanced CT image reveals enlargement of the right lateral rectus muscle (arrow) and right lacrimal gland. Increased orbital fat density is seen on the right side.

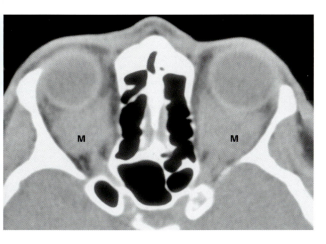

Fig. 6.23   Erdheim–Chester disease. Axial non-contrast-enhanced CT image demonstrates a bilateral intra- and extraconal soft tissue lesion (M), replacing the orbital fat and encasing the optic nerve and the extraocular muscles.

Table 6.3   (Cont.) Extraocular conal and intraconal lesions

Disease	CT Findings	Comments
Endocrine lesions		
Thyroid-associated orbitopathy (Graves disease) ▷ *Fig. 6.24a, b*	Characteristic CT findings are exophthalmos accompanied by enlargement of extraocular muscles with sparing of the tendinous attachments to the globe. The inferior recti, followed by medial and superior rectus muscles, are most often and most severely affected, but any muscle may be affected. About 90% of patients have bilateral muscle involvement, in 5% one isolated muscle belly is involved. There may be focal low-density areas within the muscle bellies, but the muscle margins remain sharp. The retroglobular fat is increased in volume, even in the absence of muscle enlargement, and cause anterior bulging of the orbital septum, prolapse of an enlarged lacrimal gland, and stretching and straightening of the optic nerve. Fatty replacement and a stringlike appearance of the extraocular muscles are findings of a later, chronic, noncongestive phase.	Autoimmune orbital inflammatory condition associated with thyroid dysfunction. However, 10% of patients have neither clinical nor laboratory evidence of hyperthyroidism (euthyroid ophthalmopathy). Most common cause of uni- or bilateral painless exophthalmos in young and middle-aged adults with female preference (M:F = 1:3–6). Visual loss from compressive and/or ischemic optic neuropathy results from increased extraocular muscle size and often massive increase in orbital fat.
Vascular lesions		
Orbital venous lymphatic malformation (lymphangioma)	Lobulated, poorly circumscribed, multicystic hypodense mass. The attenuation may change after infection or intralesional bleeding. Presence of blood products with fluid–fluid levels is highly suggestive. Bony remodeling may be present with large lesions. Punctuate calcification, or phleboliths, are uncommon. Usually exhibit cyst wall rim enhancement, but solid enhancement of venous components can also occur.	Orbital venous lymphatic malformation is a congenital hamartomatous lymphatic and venous vascular anomaly. Orbital venous lymphatic malformations tend to populate the extraconal space but may be located superficial (conjunctiva or lid), deep (retrobulbar), and often transspatial. They gradually and progressively enlarge during the growing years and do not involute (unlike capillary hemangioma). Occurs in children and young adults, with slight female predominance. The tendency toward spontaneous hemorrhage results in the sudden onset of proptosis, periorbital swelling, reduced eye mobility, and optic nerve compression.
Venous vascular malformation (cavernous hemangioma) ▷ *Fig. 6.25*	Unilateral, very rarely bilateral or multiple. Most commonly retrobulbar in the superior and lateral quadrants of the cone (80%). Appears as sharply circumscribed, rounded, ovoid, or lobulated homogeneous soft tissue mass of increased density. Calcified phleboliths are a nearly pathognomonic sign. Relatively uniform intense enhancement is the rule. The optic nerve is displaced by the tumor. Benign remodeling of bone in large lesions is not uncommon.	Cavernous hemangioma is a nonneoplastic, slow-growing hamartomatous vascular mass (low-flow lesion). It is the most common isolated orbital mass in adults 10 to 60 y of age (mean 40 y), with female predominance. Unilateral, slowly progressive, painless proptosis with diplopia and diminution of vision resulting from optic nerve compression is the usual presenting sign. Will not regress with age.
Orbital varix ▷ *Fig. 6.26a, b*	Uni- or bilateral dilation of one or more orbital veins seen as round or elongated, tubular, sharply marginated, intra- or extraconal structures, often superolateral, that enhances intensely with contrast. Phleboliths may be associated. Enlarges in a prone position and during a Valsalva maneuver. Proptosis may be present, which may also be enhanced during a Valsalva maneuver. Thrombosis in varicoid veins may show a primarily hyperdense, dilated vein. After intravenous administration of iodinated contrast medium the thickened vessel wall may enhance intensely, contrary to the nonenhancing luminal thrombus.	Orbital varix is an intraorbital mass composed of abnormally large veins. It may be a single vessel with saccular or segmental dilation or a tangled plexus of venous channels. The enormous dilation is either of congenital (low-flow venous malformation) or acquired origin. The lesion may also occur in association with intraorbital or intracranial AVM. May present at any age with intermittent proptosis, elicited by hanging head, jugular tourniquet, Valsalva maneuver, or coughing. A varix is a leading cause of spontaneous orbital hemorrhage. Thrombosis is common.

(continues on page 264)

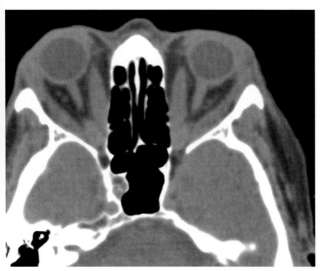
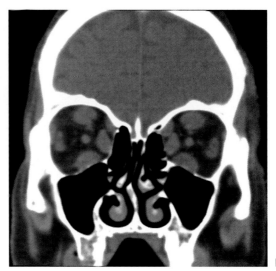

b

Fig. 6.24a, b   Thyroid-associated orbitopathy (Graves disease). Axial non-contrast-enhanced CT image (**a**) shows bilateral axial proptosis caused by the pouchlike, bilaterally symmetrical enlargement of the medial and (less marked) lateral rectus muscles, sparing the tendons. Coronal reformatted section (**b**) reveals bilaterally symmetrical thickening of all extraocular muscles, including both oblique and levator palpebrae muscles.

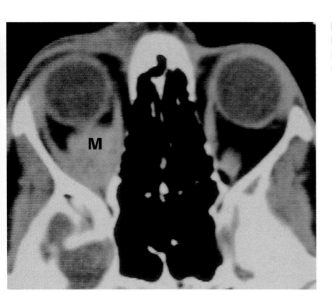

Fig. 6.25   Venous vascular malformation (cavernous hemangioma). Axial non-contrast-enhanced CT image shows an intraconal, sharply circumscribed, ovoid homogeneous soft tissue mass (M) of increased density on the right side.

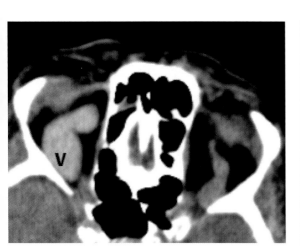
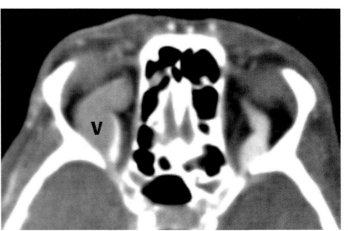

b

Fig. 6.26a, b   Bilateral orbital varix. Axial non-contrast-enhanced CT image (**a**) shows bilateral elongation and dilation of the superior ophthalmic vein, particularly on the right side. The hyperdense right varicoid vein (V) indicates thrombosis. Axial contrast-enhanced CT image (**b**) reveals only marginal luminal enhancement of the right superior ophthalmic vein (V) with nonenhancing luminal thrombus.

II Head and Neck

Table 6.3   (Cont.) Extraocular conal and intraconal lesions

Disease	CT Findings	Comments
Carotid-cavernous sinus fistula	On imaging, proptosis combined with ipsilateral widening of cavernous sinus, inferior petrosal sinus, pterygoid venous plexus, and superior ophthalmic vein and enlargement of extraocular muscles is indicative of carotid-cavernous fistula. Choroidal effusions can be associated. Occasionally, sellar erosion and enlargement of the superior orbital fissure are also evident. Associated findings may include partial venous thrombosis in the lumen of the superior ophthalmic vein or cavernous sinus. If trauma was the etiology, CT shows associated skull base fractures and intracranial complications.	Direct fast-flow carotid-cavernous sinus fistulas are spontaneous (primarily in diabetic older women and patients with osteogenesis imperfecta or Ehlers–Danlos syndrome) or posttraumatic arterio-venous communications between the cavernous carotid artery and cavernous sinus. Indirect lower-flow carotid-cavernous sinus fistulas, or dural AVMs, are multiple small shunts between the meningeal or dural branches of both the internal and external carotid artery and the dural veins around the cavernous sinus. Both types of carotid-cavernous sinus fistula may present with chemosis and pulsatile proptosis associated with an orbital bruit on auscultation. Palsies of CN III, IV, and VI may occur. Severe secondary glaucoma may lead to rapid monocular blindness.
Superior ophthalmic vein thrombosis	Enhancing walls and irregularity or absence of luminal enhancement of the dilated superior ophthalmic vein indicate partial or complete thrombosis.	Often associated with cavernous sinus thrombosis that is frequently a late complication of advanced paranasal sinus infection. Presents with ophthalmoplegia, proptosis, and chemosis.
Benign neoplasms		
Infantile hemangioma (capillary hemangioma)	The capillary hemangiomas may be primary to the orbit or primarily cutaneous involving the periocular tissues and lid with secondary orbital extension. The capillary hemangiomas in the subcutaneous space may form well-defined masses, but usually the lesions have a nodular, irregular margin. When there is no cutaneous component, and the lesion is deep in the orbit, it has a tendency to involve the superomedial portion of the orbit, but extensive ones infiltrate most of the orbit and may extend intracranially. CT usually shows a lobulated, irregularly marginated, infiltrative, heterogeneous, extra- and intraconal soft tissue mass, slightly hypodense, with intense, homogeneous enhancement.	Hemangiomas of infancy are high-flow neoplastic tumors. They grow rapidly during the first year of life and usually regress spontaneously by age 5 to 10. Although the tumor prefers the facial structures and the cutaneous portion of the eyelid, expansion may be seen in any orbital compartment. More common in girls. Presents with proptosis as well as eyelid and conjunctiva swelling.
Hemangiopericytoma	Spherical soft tissue mass with intense enhancement. In contrast to a cavernous hemangioma, the margins of the expansile mass are less well defined. Infiltration of muscles and erosion of the orbital bone may be present. Calcification is not a feature.	Uncommon vascular tumor that can arise wherever capillaries are present. Hemangiopericytomas may originate in the orbit or from the sinonasal cavities and then invade the orbit. They are aggressive lesions that can infiltrate the orbit in a multicompartmental fashion. About 50% of the cases are malignant. They become clinically manifest as progressing proptosis or lid swelling. There is no gender predominance. Mean age of presentation is the fourth decade. Hemangiopericytomas may be difficult to differentiate from other rare vasculogenic tumors, such as angio-leiomyoma, malignant hemangioendothelioma, and fibrous histiocytoma.

(continues on page 265)

Table 6.3   (Cont.) Extraocular conal and intraconal lesions

Disease	CT Findings	Comments
Neurofibroma ▷ *Fig. 6.27*	**Localized or circumscribed neurofibromas** present as a well-circumscribed, oval or fusiform, homogeneous tumor, more common in the superior quadrants, with density similar to brain, that enhances well with contrast. **Plexiform neurofibromas** present as elongated cords and nodules, poorly defined, irregular, and infiltrating, sometimes suggesting the image of a "bag of worms." **Diffuse neurofibromas** appear as a well-enhancing, ill-defined mass with extension into surrounding tissues (resulting in enlargement of extraocular muscles). The CT appearance of **malignant nerve sheath tumors** is similar to nonmalignant tumors with the exception of bone destruction.	Localized neurofibromas, unrelated to any syndrome, are seen in middle-aged patients and present as a painless mass leading to nonaxial proptosis. Plexiform neurofibromas are seen in the first decade of life. Involvement of the eyelid is considered to be virtually pathognomonic for von Recklinghausen disease. Neurofibromatosis type 1 can also be found in patients with multiple neurofibromas. Neurofibromas have a low but real malignant potential.
Schwannoma	Well-circumscribed, ovoid or fusiform, intraconal, heterogeneous mass with density similar to brain that enhances well with contrast. Low-density areas may represent cystic, necrotic, or hemorrhagic degeneration, regions of Antoni B cells or Antoni A cells intermixed with lipid-rich Schwann cells. The optic nerve may be compressed in lesions arising in the orbital apex, or it may be engulfed by the tumor.	Benign, slow-growing tumors of adults. Arise from the Schwann cells of the various nerve sheaths and constitute 1% to 8% of all orbital tumors. Branches of CN III, IV, V, and VI, sympathetic fibers, parasympathetic fibers, and the ciliary ganglion may be sources. The optic nerve is never the site of origin because it does not have Schwann cells. Usually an isolated lesion, 1% to 18% may be associated with neurofibromatosis type 2. Patients present with slowly progressive, painless proptosis, diplopia, and strabismus. Papilledema and optic atrophy with visual loss may be present with optic nerve compression.
Paraganglioma	Intraconal, retrobulbar, well-circumscribed, homogeneous, uniformly enhancing soft tissue mass lesion, is generally attached to an extraocular muscle and separate from the optic nerve. Prominent orbital veins may be present.	Paragangliomas of the orbit are extremely rare. The site of origin is thought to be the ciliary nerve, ciliary ganglion, or orbital neural tissue. Multiple paragangliomas can occur in 10% to 20% of patients. Paraganglioma may occur simultaneously in the orbit and carotid body. Present at any age, especially over age 50 y, without any gender bias, with progressive proptosis, eye motility restriction, conjunctival congestion, diplopia, papilledema, pain, and decreased vision. Five to 10% of all paragangliomas are malignant with local invasion and metastases.
Rosai–Dorfman disease	CT demonstrates large, heterogeneously enhancing, infiltrative soft tissue masses with striking proptosis. Fatty infiltration within the orbital mass is occasionally seen. Some cases have eyelid, lacrimal gland, and orbital involvement with extensive pre- and postseptal masses, but lesions can be purely retrobulbar with flattening of the globe. The optic nerve can be stretched and bowed by the abnormal orbital soft tissue. Sclerotic bone changes of the orbital wall are seen with sinonasal and intracranial extension.	Sinus histiocytosis with massive lymphadenopathy is a rare benign, idiopathic, proliferative disease of phagocytic histiocytes. Predominantly, it affects children and young adults, with slight male predominance. Most patients have painless bilateral cervical, axillary, and inguinal lymphadenopathy. Extranodal involvement includes the respiratory tract, skin, nasal cavity, intracranium, and skeletal system. Orbital involvement with proptosis, limited eye movement, eyelid edema, epiphora, and decreased visual acuity is usually unilateral.

(continues on page 266)

II Head and Neck

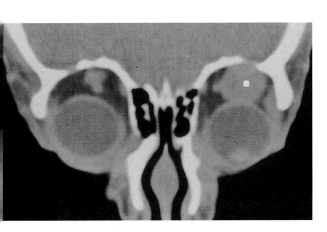

Fig. 6.27   Neurofibroma. Coronal reformatted section shows a well-circumscribed, oval homogeneous mass (joystick point) with density similar to brain in the superior quadrants causing nonaxial proptosis of the left globe.

Table 6.3   (Cont.) Extraocular conal and intraconal lesions

Disease	CT Findings	Comments
Malignant neoplasms		
Rhabdomyosarcoma	CT features include a well-defined intraconal and/or extraconal mass, isodense with the extraocular muscles, which becomes increasingly heterogeneous as it enlarges and with focal hemorrhage. The lesion demonstrates moderate to marked enhancement (dynamic CT reveals a low peak and slow washout on the density vs time curve). Invasion of the eyelid, sinuses, and base of the skull with associated bone destruction or remodeling is common.	Most common primary orbital malignancy in children and most common soft tissue malignancy of childhood, arising from pluripotential mesenchymal elements in the orbit or extraocular muscles. The peak incidence is in the first decade (average age 7–8 y). The characteristic clinical presentation is the rapid development of a painless unilateral proptosis in a child.
Lymphoproliferative lesions of the orbit ▷ *Fig. 6.28*	Bilateral orbital involvement is relatively common. In retrobulbar involvement the lymphoid tumor infiltrates and replaces the orbital fat by perineural and perivascular spread. The involvement may be diffuse and poorly defined but may produce an isolated, well-circumscribed and lobulated mass with irregular margins, isodense to extraocular muscles with moderate homogeneous enhancement that typically molds around existing orbital structures, such as the globe. There is no indentation of the globe. Infiltration and thickening of the extraocular muscles are not common. Lymphoma may encase the optic nerve, occasionally simulating meningioma or orbital pseudotumor.	Lymphoid tumors represent 10% to 15% of orbital masses. Usually non–Hodgkin lymphoma, they compromise a wide spectrum of proliferative disorders ranging from malignant lymphoma to the benign pseudolymphoma to the reactive hyperplasia. Orbital lymphoma typically occurs in the 45- to 60-y-old group. The presenting complaints are subacute development and progression of painless swelling, proptosis, and diplopia. It is not uncommon for orbital involvement to be the initial site of clinical presentation of lymphoma.
Orbital leukemia	CT findings are usually nonspecific. Diffuse thickening of the sclera or uvea, proptosis with infiltration of the retrobulbar fat, similar to orbital pseudotumor, Graves disease, or orbital cellulitis, or more circumscribed involvement of the optic nerve–sheath complex, and invasion of the extraocular muscles may be seen. Extraconal subperiosteal involvement is the result of direct infiltration of orbital bone or soft tissue by leukemic cells.	Orbital leukemia may be seen in adults with chronic lymphocytic leukemia. In children with acute myelogenous leukemia, the orbital infiltration may form a mass lesion, referred to as granulocytic sarcoma or chloroma.
Metastases ▷ *Fig. 6.29*	Intraconal metastatic lesions appear as a discrete infiltrating mass or diffuse lesion isodense to extraocular muscles and vascular structures. Mild to moderate contrast enhancement is noted. Metastatic scirrhous carcinoma of the breast may produce diffuse intraconal involvement with enophthalmos. Metastatic disease of the extraocular muscles may produce an asymmetric nodular configuration of the involved muscle or a diffuse muscle enlargement. When present, bony involvement may be osteolytic, osteoblastic, or both.	Metastases account for 10% of orbital neoplasmas. Nearly all systematic malignancies have been reported to metastasize to the orbit (the most common source is, in descending order of frequency, breast and lung cancer, unknown primary, prostate, and melanoma; childhood tumors reported to metastasize to the orbit include neuroblastoma, Ewing sarcoma, Wilms tumor, and medulloblastoma). Metastases to fat and bone occur twice as frequently as that of extraocular muscles. Sixty percent of lesions are extraconal, 20% intraconal. With time, most metastases produce diffuse orbital infiltration. Patients with orbital metastases frequently complain of diplopia, ptosis, proptosis, eyelid swelling, pain, and vision loss.

Table 6.4   Extraocular extraconal lesions

Disease	CT Findings	Comments
Congenital/developmental lesions		
Naso-orbital cephalocele	When present, there is a defect in the bony confines, and CSF, meninges, or brain may show mass effect on the orbital structures.	Cephaloceles are extracranial herniations of intracranial contents due to partial failure of rostral neural tube closure. In naso-orbital cephaloceles, the defect occurs between the ethmoid and frontal processes of the maxilla and may pass into the orbit, appearing as a medial orbital mass.
Dermoid ▷ **Fig. 6.30**	The superficial (simple, exophytic) subtype appears as a well-demarcated, ovoid mass, heterogeneous, cystic, with mixed fat and soft tissue density contents and mild, thin, rim enhancement, usually located extraconally in the superolateral aspect of the anterior orbit at the frontozygomatic suture, near the lacrimal gland, or in the superonasal aspect at the frontolacrimal suture. May contain fine or punctate calcifications in the cyst wall. Expansion or pressure erosions of the bony orbit may be associated. The deep (complicated, endophytic) subtype of adults may extend into sinuses, high deep masticator space, or intracranially, and cause a dumbbell-shaped dermoid. Ruptured orbital dermoid may be associated with irregular margins and reactive inflammatory changes indistinguishable from cellulitis.	The orbital ectodermal inclusion cysts are the most common congenital lesions of the orbit. Dermoids consist of epithelial elements plus dermal substructures including dermal appendages (e.g., hair or sweat glands in the wall). They most commonly present as superficial periorbital lesions in early childhood with proptosis. Most frequently presents in childhood and teenage years with painless subcutaneous mass, fixed to underlying bone, and slowly progressing, eccentric proptosis or progressive upper lid swelling. If ruptured, sudden growth, irregular margins, and inflammatory reactions may be present. Epidermoids are less common and can be differentiated from dermoids by features similar to fluid and more homogeneous appearance. Epidermoids contain epithelial elements only; do not contain fat.

(continues on page 268)

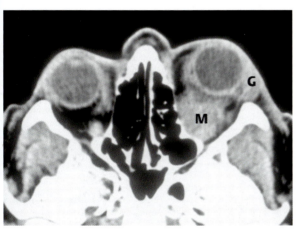

Fig. 6.28   Non–Hodgkin lymphoma. Axial non-contrast-enhanced CT image reveals an invasive mass (M) that occupies the left retrobulbar orbit filling the intraconal space and infiltrating the muscle cone. There is an additional lateral extraconal mass involving the left lacrimal gland (G).

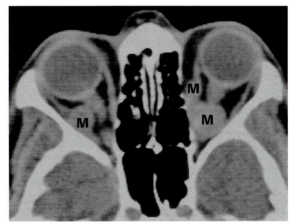

Fig. 6.29   Metastases. Axial non-contrast-enhanced CT image demonstrates bilateral conal masses (M) well-defined and isodense to extraocular muscles.

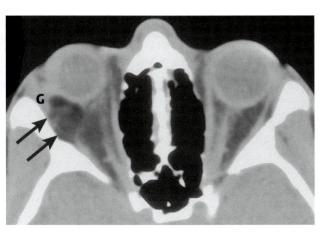

Fig. 6.30   Dermoid. Axial non-contrast-enhanced CT image shows a well-demarcated lobulated mass with mixed fat and soft tissue density, located extraconal in the superolateral aspect of the anterior right orbit (arrows) near the lacrimal gland (G).

II   Head and Neck

Table 6.4   (Cont.) Extraocular extraconal lesions

Disease	CT Findings	Comments
Orbital lymphatic-venous malformation ▷ *Fig. 6.31*	Lobulated, irregular, multicystic, hypodense mass with variable wall enhancement. Venous components may show a more diffuse enhancement. Layering hyperdense fluid-fluid levels correspond to blood products from spontaneous hemorrhage. Expansion or pressure erosions of the bony orbit may be associated. Calcifications or phleboliths are uncommon.	Congenital hamartomatous lymphatic and venous vascular malformation; orbital lymphangiomas tend to populate the extraconal space but are often trans-spatial. Lymphangiomas gradually and progresssively enlarge during the growing years (do not involute). The multilocular cystic lesions have a tendency to bleed. Orbital lymphatic-venous malformations occur in children and young adults, with slight female predominance. Most common clinical sign is progressive, painless proptosis with intermittent worsening. Optic nerve compromise is a late complication of large lesions.

Inflammatory/infectious conditions

Disease	CT Findings	Comments
Orbital subperiosteal abscess ▷ *Fig. 6.32*	Lentiform, low-density fluid collection running parallel to the wall of the orbit with adjacent sinus opacification and with central displacement of the extraocular muscle. Rarely, one may see a rim enhancement in this location or a small collection of gas. Demineralization, thinning, or loss of bone manifests inflammation or localized osteomyelitis of the adjacent bone. Cellulitic changes with stranding and streaking of the intraconal fat, enhancing and swollen extraocular muscles, or solid enhancing phlegmon retrobulbar may precede or follow abscess formation. Progression may lead to intraorbital abscess, superior ophthalmic vein thrombosis, cavernous sinus thrombosis, and intracranial extension.	Accumulation of pus between (usually medial) orbital wall and orbital periosteum, secondary to acute sinusitis and phlebitic transmission, or direct extension through dehiscence in the adjacent orbital bone (lamina papyracea). Uncommonly, due to trauma, bacteremia, or skin infection. Patients present with edema of the lids, painful proptosis, chemosis, eye muscle paralysis, visual disturbance, sinusitis, upper respiratory infection, and headache, fever, and chills.

Benign neoplasms

Disease	CT Findings	Comments
Meningioma	Sphenoid wing meningioma is the most common meningioma in the extraconal area. May involve the extraconal space from above or either side. A slightly hyperdense mass, with or without calcifications, and intense and uniform contrast enhancement is seen with sclerotic or lytic involvement of the adjacent orbital bone.	Extraconal meningiomas from the orbital wall periosteum or randomly located arachnoidal nests are infrequent. Meningiomas can involve the dura and contiguous bone of the orbital roof and greater wing of the sphenoid. Lesions can also involve the roof of the ethmoid or planum sphenoidale and can involve the sphenoid in the environs of the optic canal. Secondary extension into the orbit from intracranial meningiomas may also occur. Present most often in the fourth or fifth decade, occurring twice as often in females.
Ossifying fibroma	Well-circumscribed, expansile, mineralized mass, surrounded by a thick or thin radiodense rimming. There may be islands of bone formation within the lesion. Periosteal reaction is not a feature of benign fibro-osseous lesions. Enhancement is more pronounced in areas that are less mineralized.	Ossifying fibroma of the orbit and paraorbital region is often diagnosed incidentally, predilects to (black) women. Tends to occur in the third and fourth decades of life.
Psammomatoid active ossifying fibroma	Expansile mass with admixture of both soft tissue and bone density pattern. There may be areas of soft tissue–fluidlike level. The most characteristic feature is the presence of numerous round or oval calcified bodies of various sizes, representing the psammomatoid (cementicle) bodies. The lesion has an aggressive appearance with cortical break and extension into surrounding tissue.	Psammomatoid active ossifying fibroma typically occurs in the sinonasal tract (ethmoid sinus, supraorbital frontal region) and potentially may behave aggressively with locally invasive and destructive capabilities. Occurs in younger age groups (first and second decades), with no gender predilection.
Osteoma	Well-circumscribed, sharply delineated, round intrasinus mass, attached to the sinus wall broad-based or by a short pedicle, usually < 2 cm in size. Ivory osteomas are denser than adjacent bone; mature osteomas are isodense. Fibrous osteomas are lower and more variable in density. Most frequently seen in the frontal (80%) and ethmoid sinuses. Rarely, large osteoma in the frontal or ethmoid region may displace globe forward and cause proptosis. Obstruction of a sinus ostium may lead to infection or formation of a mucocele. Very rarely, an osteoma may erode through the dura, leading to rhinorrhea or intracranial infection.	Most common tumor of the paranasal sinuses. Osteomas are benign mature bone-forming hamartomatous lesions that are almost exclusively identified in the craniofacial skeleton (most common in the frontal and ethmoid sinuses). Symptoms associated with paraorbital osteomas include headaches, facial swelling or deformity, and proptosis and ocular disturbances. Paraorbital osteomas are more common in men, most often in the second to fourth decades of life. May be associated with Gardner syndrome.

(continues on page 269)

Table 6.4   (Cont.) Extraocular extraconal lesions

Disease	CT Findings	Comments
Osteoblastoma	Well-defined, round, expansile, mineralized lesion with prominent calcified rim (the central portion may have a similar appearance as ossifying fibroma).	Uncommon benign osteoblastic neoplasm. Head sites of involvement include the mandible, maxilla, temporal bone, paranasal sinuses, and orbit. Occurs more often in men younger than 30 y of age. Associated symptoms include pain, facial swelling, and asymmetry.
Giant cell tumor (osteoclastoma)	Lobulated, expansile, intraosseous, mildly hyperdense soft tissue mass with marked homogeneous or heterogeneous contrast enhancement. Overlying thinned cortical shell, focally interrupted, often sclerotic.	Giant cell tumors are benign but locally aggressive neoplasms. Giant cell tumors of the head and neck are uncommon (sites of occurrence include the sphenoid, temporal, and ethmoid bones). Symptoms of lesions of the paraorbital region include headache, diplopia, decreased vision, and proptosis.
Chondroma	Well-circumscribed lesion with endosteal scalloping composed of hyaline-type cartilage with varying degrees of calcification.	Chondromas of the paraorbital region, including the sinonasal tract (nasal cavity septum, ethmoid sinus) and nasopharynx are rare. There is equal gender predilection. Most patients are younger than 50 y of age. Symptomatic patients may present with nasal obstruction, enlarging, painless mass, proptosis, and headaches. Other, uncommon benign osseous neoplasms in the orbital region: chondroblastoma and chondromyxoid fibroma.
Malignant neoplasms		
Osteosarcoma	Destructive, poorly delineated osteolytic, osteosclerotic, or mixed mass lesion, with minimal or massive tumor bone formation within the tumor proper and invading surrounding tissue. Subperiosteal tumor bone formation and displaced periosteum are characteristic.	Craniofacial osteosarcomas occur in the jaws, paranasal sinuses, skull, and orbital region. They have an equal gender predilection and occur generally a decade or two later than those with extrafacial osteosarcomas. May be seen following radiation to the orbit for retinoblastoma.
Chondrosarcoma	May be seen as a nondestructive, fairly well delineated or destructive, and poorly delineated osteolytic or mixed lesion with coarse calcifications. There may be moderate to significant enhancement.	Craniofacial chondrosarcomas are slightly more common in men than in women and primarily occur in the fourth to seventh decades of life. An expanding mass may cause pain, proptosis, and visual disturbances.

(continues on page 270)

II Head and Neck

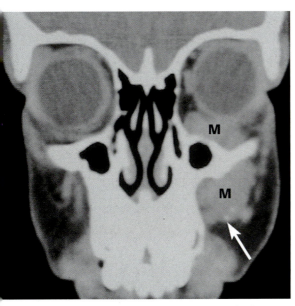

Fig. 6.31   Venous vascular malformation. Coronal reformatted non-contrast-enhanced CT image reveals a multilobulated soft tissue mass (M) in the left caudal extraconal space and buccal region containing phleboliths (arrow).

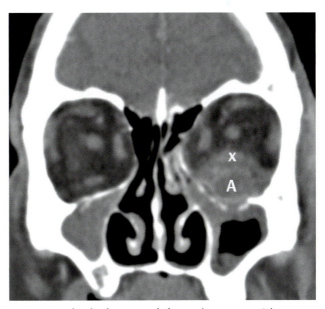

Fig. 6.32   Orbital subperiosteal abscess (posttraumatic). Coronal reformatted contrast-enhanced CT shows a rim-enhancing hypodense fluid collection (A) in the left caudal extraconal space with cranial displacement of the inferior rectus muscle (x). Also seen are outward displacement of dislocated fragments after an orbital floor fracture and mucosal thickening in the left and opacification of the right maxillary sinus.

Table 6.4   (Cont.) Extraocular extraconal lesions

Disease	CT Findings	Comments
Rhabdomyosarcoma	Extraconal and/or intraconal soft tissue mass commonly associated with bone destruction and possible extraorbital extension into the eyelid, adjacent sinus, and intracranial cavity. The tumor is isodense to muscle and may enhance moderately to markedly. Tumors with focal hemorrhage appear heterogeneous.	The most common primary malignant tumor of the orbit (excluding the globe) in children. About 90% occur before age 16. Patients present with rapidly progressive unilateral proptosis, ptosis, palpable mass, and ophthalmoplegia.
Metastases ▷ Fig. 6.33	Metastasis to the bony orbit presents on CT as bone destruction or hyperostosis. A soft tissue mass extending from the abnormal bone into the extraconal space or outside the orbit is often seen.	Metastatic disease to the bony orbit most commonly occurs in the greater sphenoid wing and may be limited to the bone or may have associated soft tissue components in the extraconal space or in the contiguous extraorbital location.
Secondary orbital tumors ▷ Fig. 6.34 ▷ Fig. 6.35	A low-density or soft tissue mass extending from outside the orbit into the extraconal space, sharply or poorly marginated, with or without contrast enhancement, with remodeling and bowing or with bony erosion and destruction of bony walls. The involvement of the orbit represents an advanced stage.	Malignant and benign tumors, including cysts, of the sinonasal cavities may invade the orbit. Tumors of the skin of the face can invade the orbit. Orbital invasion of intracranial tumors through the skull base may be present, either through natural foramina or by bone destruction. Malignant neoplasms of the oral cavity can extend along the perineural-perivascular pathway into the pterygopalatine fossa and then into the orbit.
Metabolic/dysplastic lesions		
Fibrous dysplasia	Involvement by fibrous dysplasia is usually unilateral, which leads to asymmetry. Expansion of involved bone with a homogeneous or heterogenous decreased ("ground glass") bone density, along with an intact thin cortex is typical, with an abrupt transition zone between the lesion and normal bone. May have cystic regions in the early, active phase of the disease, with centrally lucent lesions and thinned but sclerotic borders. The pagetoid (mixed) pattern of fibrous dysplasia shows mixed radiopacity and radiolucency. Obstructs osseous canals, foramina, pneumatic system, and sinuses. Contrast enhancement is often difficult to appreciate except in areas of lucent bone.	Fibrous dysplasia is a benign developmental skeletal disorder typically seen in adolescents and young adults younger than age 30. Can be monostotic or polyostotic. Orbital involvement may be focal or diffuse. Patients usually complain of diplopia and proptosis. Patients with orbitofacial neurofibromatosis type 1 may show sphenoid dysplasia with bony defects, middle fossa arachnoid cyst, optic nerve glioma, buphthalmos, and multiple plexiform neurofibromas. Often these patients present with pulsatile proptosis.
Paget disease	Thickened bone with both lytic and sclerotic areas. When involved, the roof and lateral orbital walls are the most frequently diseased areas.	Involvement of the bony orbit by Paget disease is infrequent, occurring only late in the disease process.
Trauma		
Orbital subperiosteal hematoma ▷ Fig. 6.36	The CT appearance of acute subperiosteal hematoma is a sharply defined, extraconal, homogeneous, high-density, nonenhancing, fusiform or biconvex mass. The muscles may be displaced inward by the extraconal collection. A swelling of the muscle and intraconal compartment may be associated. The CT appearance of chronic subperiosteal hematoma (hematic cyst) includes a well-defined extraconal, homogeneous or nonhomogeneous, nonenhancing mass, hyperdense (related to the protein-rich fluid and hemosiderin deposition) with osseous remodeling (erosion, expansion) in the majority of lesions.	Traumatic lesions of the orbital wall may form extraconal hematomas, usually along the roof or the floor and medial wall in association with a fracture. Nontraumatic acute and chronic subperiosteal hemorrhages of the orbit are rare and result from disruption of orbital vessels that penetrate the periosteum adjacent to the bone in association with sudden elevation of cranial venous pressure, bleeding diathesis, and paranasal sinusitis. They may present as orbital masses and may cause unilateral proptosis, limitation of eye mobility, and compressive optic neuropathy. The roof is the most common location; these hemorrhages occur almost exclusively in children and young adults (because the periosteal attachment to the roof tends to become stronger with age). Postoperative subperiosteal hematoma is a rare but severe complication after sinonasal operation.

(continues on page 272)

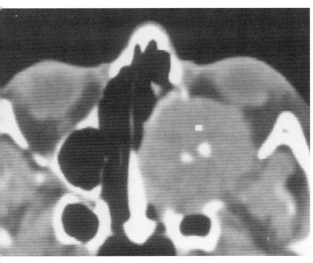

Fig. 6.33   Melanoma. Axial non-contrast-enhanced CT image demonstrates a soft tissue mass in the right maxillary sinus with destruction of bony walls and extension into the orbit, nasal cavity, and retromaxillary fat pad. There are a few remaining small bone fragments within the lesion.

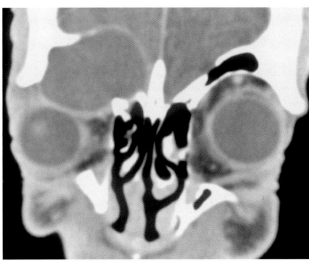

Fig. 6.34   Right frontal mucocele. Coronal reformatted non-contrast-enhanced CT image shows an opacified, expanded right frontal sinus with thinned cranial and caudal bony walls, and extra-axial dislocation of the right eye.

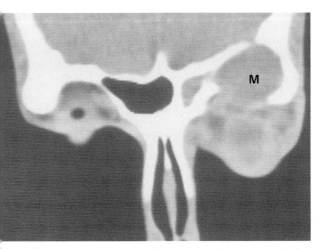

Fig. 6.35   Left orbitofrontal cholesterol granuloma. Coronal reformatted non-contrast-enhanced CT image demonstrates an eccentric, well-defined, hypodense, inhomogeneous mass (M) of the left lateral frontal sinus with dehiscence of the orbital roof and extra-axial dislocation of the left eye.

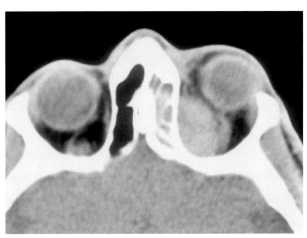

Fig. 6.36   Orbital subperiosteal hematoma. Axial non-contrast-enhanced CT image shows a sharply defined, biconvex, homogeneous, hyperdense, extraconal, and space-occupying lesion at the left orbital roof.

Table 6.4   (Cont.) Extraocular extraconal lesions

Disease	CT Findings	Comments
Orbital fractures ▷ *Fig. 6.37*	Direct fracture signs are alterations in skeletal contour and alignment, a linear lucency with irregular borders representing fracture line, traversing the orbital wall, with or without separation and displacement of the fragments, and changes in adjacent soft tissues. Indirect fracture signs, such as incorrectly located air (subcutaneous air inclusion, orbital emphysema, and pneumocephalus) or soft tissue densities (air-fluid levels in the sinus; the presence of a polypoid mass (teardrop) representing herniated and entrapped fibrofatty tissues and/or muscles between bone fragments; and a small local hematoma ("hanging drop" at the fracture site) can provide additional diagnostic assistance. **Orbital floor fractures** can occur as isolated injuries or in combination with zygomatic arch fractures, Le Fort type II or III midface fractures, and medial wall or orbital rim fractures. **Blow-out fractures** commonly represent isolated fractures of the orbital floor without involvement of the rim with outward displacement of the dislocated fragment, fat herniation into the maxillary sinus, and inferior rectus muscle herniation into the maxillary sinus, resulting in muscle entrapment. **Trapdoor fractures** are pure internal orbital fractures. The anteroposterior linear fracture is hinged medially by a greenstick fracture. It involves the orbital floor, medial to or within the infraorbital groove and canal or medial wall. Entrapment of orbital tissue commonly occurs; may incarcerate herniated tissue. **Medial blow-out fractures** may be isolated but are more common in conjunction with inferior blow-out fractures. Isolated orbital rim, orbital roof, and lateral orbital wall fractures are relatively uncommon. **Fracture of the zygomaticomaxillary complex** (the term *tripod fracture* is misleading) extends through the four articulations of the zygomatic bone: the zygomaticofrontal, the zygomaticosphenoidal, the zygomaticotemporal, and the zygomaticomaxillary sutures, with displacement and rotation of the zygoma. Additionally, this fracture may extend posteriorly to involve the pterygoid processes, greater sphenoid wing, and sphenotemporal buttress. **Le Fort II fracture** has a pyramidal shape and extends from the nasal bridge at or below the nasofrontal suture through the frontal processes of the maxilla, inferolaterally through the lacrimal bones and inferior orbital floor and rim through or near the infraorbital foramen, and inferiorly through the anterior wall of the maxillary sinus; it then travels under the zygoma, across the pterygomaxillary fissure, and through the pterygoid plates. **Le Fort III fractures** start at the nasofrontal and frontomaxillary sutures and extend posteriorly along the medial wall of the orbit through the nasolacrimal groove and ethmoid bones. The thicker sphenoid bone posteriorly usually prevents continuation of the fracture into the optic canal. Instead, the fracture continues along the floor of the orbit along the inferior orbital fissure and continues superolaterally through the lateral orbital wall, through the zygomaticofrontal junction and the zygomatic arch. Intranasally, a branch of the fracture extends through the base of the perpendicular plate of the ethmoid, through the vomer, and through the interface of the pterygoid plates to the base of the sphenoid.	Fractures of the orbital floor and medial wall occur with greater frequency than fractures of the roof, lateral wall, or complex orbital rim fractures. Isolated blow-in fractures of the four orbital walls are much less common than blow-up (superior blow-out) fractures or blow-out fractures of the orbital floor and the medial wall.

(continues on page 273)

Table 6.4   (Cont.) Extraocular extraconal lesions

Disease	CT Findings	Comments
	Orbital apex fractures are divided into (1) comminuted fractures, usually with fragment dislocation; (2) linear fractures, without dislocation of fragments; and (3) apex avulsion, with an intact optic canal; coexistent with orbital, facial, and skull base fractures.	
Miscellaneous lesions		
Langerhans cell histiocytosis	Osteolytic lesion, commonly in the superior or superotemporal orbit region with a fairly well-defined or diffuse soft tissue mass, with moderate to marked enhancement, encroaching lacrimal gland, lateral rectus, or even the globe. Multiple lesions may be present, resulting in multiple bony defects, on rare occasions in the orbital apex and superior orbital fissure. Similar lesions may be seen in facial bones, skull base, and calvarium.	Although Langerhans cell histiocytosis (LCH) is a rare disease, in patients with LCH, orbital involvement is not uncommon. Most of the patients are children 1 to 4 y old (age range birth-56 y). There is no gender predilection. Common symptoms of orbital LCH are unilateral or bilateral proptosis, edema, erythema of the eyelid, and periorbital pain, ptosis, optic nerve atrophy, and papilledema.
Giant cell reparative granuloma	These soft tissue lesions enhance with contrast and present in two forms: a peripheral form, involving soft tissues (e.g., paraorbital, sinonasal, or oral), and a central form, confined to intraosseous sites. The central lesion causes osteolysis and may have a bubble-like appearance; it is usually well delineated and may contain calcifications.	Giant cell reparative granuloma is a benign reactive osseous proliferation. In the head and neck area, the maxilla and mandible are the most common sites of occurrence; orbital, paraorbital, or nasopharyngeal involvement is less common. They are more common in women (most younger than 30 y). Paraorbital involvement is associated with pain and swelling.

(continues on page 274)

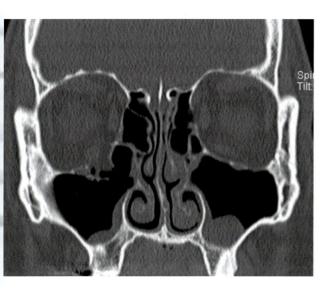

Fig. 6.37   Orbital floor fracture ("blowout" fracture). Coronal reformatted non-contrast-enhanced CT image demonstrates an isolated fracture of the right orbital floor with outward dislocated fragments and herniation of orbital fat into right maxillary sinus. Associated extraconal emphysema. Normal position of the enlarged inferior rectus muscle.

Table 6.4   (Cont.) Extraocular extraconal lesions

Disease	CT Findings	Comments
Lacrimal gland pathology		
Inflammatory lesions of the lacrimal gland		
Idiopathic orbital inflammatory disease ▷ **Fig. 6.38**	Inflammation tends to cause diffuse, at times massive, enlargement of a lacrimal gland (neoplasms usually spare the palpebral lobe), with moderate to marked contrast enhancement.	Most common nonneoplastic lacrimal mass; presents with tenderness in the upper outer quadrant of the orbit in the region of the lacrimal gland.
Dacryoadenitis	Contrast-enhanced CT typically demonstrates a massive contrast-enhancing lacrimal gland. Bilateral lacrimal masses are usually due to sarcoidosis (or lymphoproliferative lesions of the orbit). Abscess is diagnosed by identification of a characteristic low-density area with rim enhancement within an enlarged lacrimal gland.	Most acute, inflammatory enlargement of the lacrimal gland in younger patients results from postviral syndrome. Acute bacterial dacryoadenitis with suppuration and abscess formation is exceedingly rare and may develop secondary to an adjacent infection, from blood-borne spread or after trauma. Chronic dacryoadenitis, presenting with usually painless, slow lacrimal enlargement, may follow acute infection or is secondary to noninfectious inflammatory disorders such as sarcoidosis, Sjögren and Mikulicz syndrome, Kimura disease, and Wegener granulomatosis.
Lacrimal gland neoplasms		
Benign mixed tumor (pleomorphic adenoma)	Well-circumscribed, round or oval, predominantly solid, partly cystic, partly calcified extraconal tumor, with moderate contrast enhancement, and smooth, scalloped remodeling of lacrimal fossa. Irregularity at the edge of the tumor or infiltration of the adjacent orbital tissue may be seen in malignant transformation.	Tumors of the lacrimal gland may be epithelial, lymphoid, or metastatic. They comprise 40% to 50% of all lacrimal masses, one half of which are benign mixed tumors, with the other half constituting malignant tumors. Most common benign neoplasm of the lacrimal gland. Majority originates from the inner orbital lobe of the lacrimal gland. Clinical signs include a slow-growing, painless mass in the superolateral orbit of middle-aged patients (~40–50 y; without gender predilection), proptosis, and limited ocular motility. Other rare benign lacrimal gland tumors: oncocytoma, Whartin tumor.
Adenoid cystic carcinoma	Extraconal, irregular, isodense, solid, homogeneous, diffuse enhancing mass arising within the lacrimal gland, with invasion of the adjacent bony orbit. Regional intracranial extension in advanced tumors. Calcifications are not uncommon.	Although uncommon, adenoid cystic carcinoma is the most frequent malignant tumor of the lacrimal gland. High incidence of perineural tumor spread (best visualized with MRI). Occurs in young adults to old age (peak fourth decade), without gender predilection. Clinical profile: rapid onset of symptoms, painful mass, pain with paresthesia, proptosis, ptosis, and limited ocular motility. Other rare malignant epithelial lacrimal gland tumors: ex pleomorphic or other adenocarcinomas, mucoepidermoid carcinoma, squamous cell carcinoma, and undifferentiated carcinoma.
Lymphoproliferative lesions of the orbit ▷ **Fig. 6.39**	Homogeneous enhancing tumor, anywhere in orbit. Bilateral in 25%. Predilection for lacrimal gland (may be the only site): wedge-shaped enlargement of the lacrimal gland, isodense to slightly hyperdense, with moderate diffuse contrast enhancement. The extraconal mass may present with anterior and/or posterior extension and molds to and encases normal orbital structure. Malignant variants may have infiltrative appearance.	Lymphoproliferative lesions of the orbit include a wide spectrum, ranging from reactive hyperplasia, low-grade primary small B-cell lymphoma (especially mucosa-associated lymphoid tissue [MALT]), to diffuse large B-cell lymphoma, Burkitt lymphoma, and T-cell lymphoma. They comprise 5% to 10% of orbital masses. Although rare, primary lymphomas without systemic involvement appear to be the most common nonepithelial tumor of the lacrimal gland. Extramedullary plasmacytoma may also be seen in the lacrimal gland (extremely rare).
Metastases	Metastatic tumor in a lacrimal gland has a nonspecific CT appearance of diffuse enlargement of the gland. The lacrimal gland may be involved along with the adjacent periorbita and extraconal spaces.	Metastasis to the extraconal space may involve the lacrimal glands or the fat-containing spaces posterior to the orbital septa.

(continues on page 275)

Table 6.4 (Cont.) Extraocular extraconal lesions

Disease	CT Findings	Comments
Miscellaneous lesions of the lacrimal gland		
Focal amyloidosis	Amyloidoma of the lacrimal gland is associated with a unilateral lacrimal gland mass of soft tissue density, without contrast enhancement, frequently with punctate calcification, molding to surrounding orbital structures.	Focal amyloidosis is a very uncommon disorder. It may involve different orbital structures. Isolated involvement of the lacrimal gland may mimic inflammatory or even tumorous lesions. It typically affects middle-aged women with painless progressive proptosis but without visual morbidity. CT findings may mimic those seen in inflammatory or lymphoproliferative disorders of the lacrimal gland.
Lacrimal intraglandular cyst (dacryops) ▷ *Fig. 6.40*	Lacrimal gland enlargement due to cystic structures with fluid density and thin peripheral contrast enhancement that are contiguous with the palpebral lobe of the lacrimal gland. Calcifications are uncommon. No bone erosion.	Obstruction of the lacrimal gland ductules of the major and accessory lacrimal glands leads to the formation of dacryops, ductal cysts of the lacrimal glands. Dacryops is a rare clinical phenomenon, most commonly presenting unilaterally in the palpebral lobe. Patients frequently complain of painless swelling in the lateral portion of the upper eyelid. A history of trauma or inflammation of the conjunctiva or a congenital anomaly of the excretory duct can be the precipitating factor to cyst formation. Benign ductal cysts of the accessory lacrimal glands are uncommon lesions of the orbit arising from the glands of Krause and Wolfering.

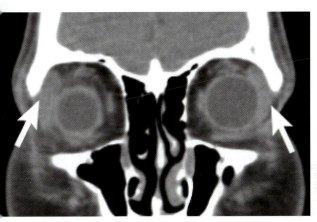

Fig. 6.38 Idiopathic orbital inflammatory disease. Coronal reformatted non-contrast-enhanced CT image shows bilateral enlargement of the lacrimal gland (arrows).

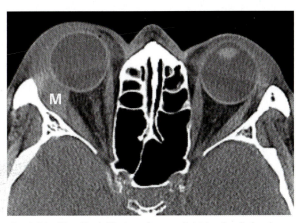

Fig. 6.39 Non-Hodgkin lymphoma, right lacrimal gland. Axial bone CT image reveals a mass of the right lacrimal gland (M), slightly flattening the circumference of the right globe.

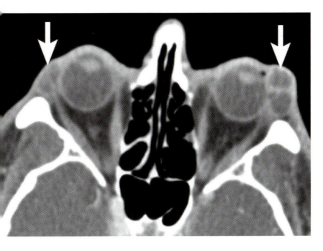

Fig. 6.40 Bilateral dacryops. Axial contrast-enhanced CT image demonstrates masses with fluid density and thin peripheral enhancement in the region of the diffuse enlarged lacrimal glands, lateral to the globes (arrows).

7 Nasal Cavity and Paranasal Sinuses

Wolfgang Zaunbauer and Francis A. Burgener

The triangular-shaped *nasal cavity* is divided in the midline by the nasal septum into two separate passages. Each passage has three bony projections along the lateral nasal wall that are formed by the superior, middle, and inferior turbinate bones, or conchae. The areas lateral and inferior to each turbinate represent the meatus of the nose. The superior margin of the nasal cavity is the cribriform plate; the inferior margin is the hard and soft palate. The nasal cavity is entered anteriorly through the nares. Posteriorly, it opens into the nasopharynx through the choanae.

The *paranasal sinuses* are named for the bones they occupy. Small aerated maxillary and ethmoid sinuses may be present at birth. Aeration of the sphenoid sinuses is generally apparent by 3 y of age, of the frontal sinuses by 6 y of age. Pneumatization may progress well into adult life. The *maxillary sinuses* are paired air cells within the maxilla. They drain via the maxillary ostium into the ethmoid infundibulum. The infundibulum opens into the middle nasal meatus through the semilunar hiatus. Accessory ostia are present in the medial wall in 15% to 40%. The *frontal sinuses* are paired, often asymmetric air cells within the frontal bone. Aplasia (5% of all adults) and hypoplasia are not uncommon. The frontal sinuses drain via the frontal ostium into the superior compartment of the frontal sinus drainage pathway (formed by frontoethmoidal air cells) and the inferior compartment of the frontal sinus drainage pathway, which is formed by either the ethmoid infundibulum or the middle nasal meatus. The *ethmoid sinuses* are paired groups of 3 to 18 air cells within ethmoid labyrinths, separated into anterior and posterior groups by the basal lamella of the middle turbinate. The anterior (or front) ethmoid cells empty into the middle nasal meatus, either via the ethmoid infundibulum and hiatus semilunaris or via the ethmoid bulla and the middle portion of the hiatus semilunaris. The posterior ethmoid cells empty into the superior nasal meatus and the sphenoethmoidal recess. The *sphenoid sinuses* occupy the medial sphenoid bone. They are asymmetrically divided by a septum that lies near the midline. The sphenoid sinus ostia lie in the anterosuperior wall. The sphenoid sinuses drain into the sphenoethmoidal recess, which is a recess of the nasal cavity, behind or near the superior turbinate.

The paranasal sinuses vary considerably in size from hypoplastic and even absent to very large. They tend to be symmetric in an individual, but occasionally considerable size differences occur. Hypoplastic or absent paranasal sinuses may be congenital (congenital hypoplasia or aplasia, cretinism, Down syndrome, and Kartagener syndrome) or associated with bony sinus wall overgrowth (fibrous dysplasia, Paget disease, thalassemia, and a variety of dysplasias). Pneumatization of the sphenoid sinus can be so extensive that it can surround the anterior clinoid process, optic nerve, foramen rotundum, vidian canal, pterygoid process, or maxilloethmoid process. Neural (maxillary and optic nerves) and vascular structures (internal carotid artery) can abut the sinus, protrude into its lumen, or even be exposed in the sinus.

The *ostiomeatal unit* is the crossroad of mucociliary drainage of the maxillary, anterior ethmoid, and frontal sinuses into the middle meatus of the nose (**Fig. 7.1**). Important components of the ostiomeatal unit include the maxillary sinus ostium and ethmoid infundibulum, uncinate process, ethmoid bulla, hiatus semilunaris, anterior and middle ethmoid air cells ostia, superior and inferior compartment of the frontal sinus drainage pathway, middle turbinate, and middle meatus contents, best visualized with coronal computed tomography (CT).

There is great variation in the intricate anatomy of sinonasal passages that may contribute to disease: nasal septal deviation (70% of nasal septa are deviated in patients older than age 14 y) nasal septal spur, and nasal septal pneumatization; paradoxically curved middle turbinate (reversal of curvature with a configuration that is convex laterally); concha bullosa (in 4%–15% of the population); pneumatized uncinate, medially deflected uncinate process, and atelectatic uncinate (usually associated with an ipsilateral silent sinus syndrome); Haller cells, which extend into the inferomedial floor of the orbit; giant ethmoid bulla; large agger nasi cells; Onodi cells with prominent superolateral pneumatization; asymmetric fovea ethmoidalis; dehiscence of lamina papyracea; and pneumatized crista galli.

Air–fluid levels in the paranasal sinuses are most often associated with acute sinusitis. Other causes are acute intrasinus hemorrhage or cerebrospinal fluid leak secondary to recent trauma, previous antral lavage, a recent surgical procedure, presence of a nasogastric tube, barotrauma, and spontaneous hemorrhages associated with bleeding disorders or anticoagulation. A large flabby retention cyst may mimic an air–fluid level when its upper surface flattens out.

The *sphenopalatine foramen,* located in the high posterolateral wall of the nasal cavity, connects the superior meatus of the nasal cavity with the pterygopalatine fossa. The *pterygopalatine fossa* is located between the posterior wall of the maxillary sinus, the pterygoid process of the sphenoid bone, and the vertical part of the palatine bone. It communicates through the pterygomaxillary fissure to the nasopharyngeal masticator space, through the inferior orbital fissure to the orbit, via the foramen rotundum and the vidian canal to the middle cranial fossa, and through the pterygopalatine canal with the oral cavity. Its contents are the maxillary nerve (cranial nerve [CN] V_2), parasympathetic pterygopalatine ganglion, distal internal maxillary artery and accompanying veins, and fat. Because of the complex connections of the pterygopalatine fossa, nasal cavity infections and tumors can access the orbit, nasopharyngeal masticator space, and intracranial space through this escape hatch.

The *nasolacrimal duct* drains inferiorly into the anterior part of the inferior nasal meatus.

With its multiplanar capability and exquisite characterization of tissue signal, magnetic resonance imaging (MRI) allows simultaneous evaluation of the sinonasal cavities, adjacent facial structures, and the brain. Despite the advantages of MRI, CT is more sensitive and accurate in assessing the osseous margins of the sinonasal cavity, the osseous floor of the anterior cranial fossa, and the walls of the orbit. CT remains the preferred imaging modality for evaluating sinonasal masses that contain calcifications or originate from bone or cartilage. It allows evaluation of fine bony details and osseous involvement.

The differential diagnosis of lesions in the nasal cavity and paranasal sinuses is discussed in **Table 7.1.**

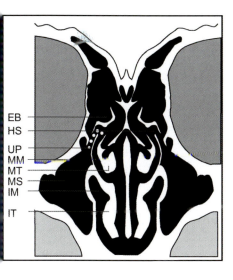

Fig. 7.1 Coronal graphic of osteomeatal unit. The maxillary sinus drains through the sinus ostium, infundibulum, and hiatus semilunaris into the middle nasal meatus. EB: ethmoid bulla; HS: hiatus semilunaris; IM: inferior nasal meatus; IT: inferior turbinate; MM: middle nasal meatus; MS: maxillary sinus; MT: middle turbinate; UP: uncinate process.

II Head and Neck

Table 7.1 Lesions in the nasal cavity and paranasal sinuses

Disease	CT Findings	Comments
Congenital/developmental lesions		
Choanal atresia ▷ *Fig. 7.2*	Narrowed choana occluded by a bony plate (90%) or membranous web (10%), unilateral or bilateral. There is medial bowing of the posterior maxilla, bony thickening of the posterolateral nasal wall and posterior vomer, with both curving toward the obstructed choana. Hypoplasia of the nasal cavity is frequently associated. **Choanal stenosis** with posterior nasal airway narrowed but not completely occluded is more common than true choanal atresia. Mucosal edema with choanal stenosis may imitate membranous atresia.	Most common congenital abnormality of nasal cavity. The nasal cavity on one or both sides does not communicate with the nasopharynx. Half of these lesions are isolated, and half are associated with other abnormalities (e.g., cleft palate, Treacher–Collins syndrome, and cardiovascular and abdominal malformations). Congenital nasal piriform aperture stenosis (< 11 mm) is an uncommon cause of nasal obstruction in the newborn caused by bony overgrowth and medialization of the nasal processes of the maxilla.

(continues on page 278)

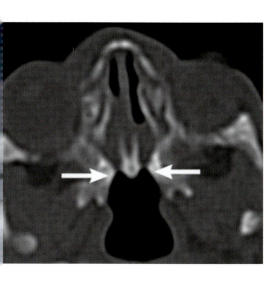

Fig. 7.2 Bilateral choanal atresia. Axial bone computed tomography (CT) image shows bowing of the posterior maxilla and bony thickening of the posterolateral nasal wall and posterior vomer, with both curving toward the obstructed choana on both sides (arrows).

Table 7.1 (Cont.) Lesions in the nasal cavity and paranasal sinuses

Disease	CT Findings	Comments
Nasopalatine cyst ▷ *Fig. 7.3*	A sharply demarcated cystic structure is seen arising in the nasopalatine canal in the midline of the maxillary alveolar bone. When enlarging, it may extend posteriorly into the hard palate (medial palatal cyst). Extensive nasopalatine cysts may also show remarkable nasolabial protrusion after penetration of the maxillary cortex.	Most common nonodontogenic cyst in the maxilla. Most common symptom is swelling of the anterior part of the palate (mean age 51.9 y, predilect to male).
Anterior cephalocele	Heterogeneous, mixed density mass due to variable amounts of cerebrospinal fluid (CSF) and brain tissue extending through a base of skull defect, contiguous with intracranial brain parenchyma. The apertura is smooth and defined by a rim of cortical bone. In case of herniation through the foramen cecum, the foramen cecum is enlarged and the crista galli hypoplastic or absent. The nasal septum may appear deformed or truncated anteriorly. (The instillation of a low dose of intrathecal contrast before CT may aid in distinguishing a simple meningocele from an encephalocele; although MRI is the best modality for confirming the presence of brain tissue in a cephalocele.) Frontoethmoidal cephaloceles are sincipital and subdivided into frontonasal, nasoethmoidal, and naso-orbital lesions. Transethmoidal, sphenoethmoidal, transsphenoidal, sphenoorbital, and sphenomaxillary cephaloceles are subtypes of basal cephaloceles.	A cephalocele is the protrusion of intracranial contents, including meninges and brain matter, through a defect in the skull base. Cephaloceles may be congenital or acquired secondary to surgery, trauma, or due to spontaneous causes. Anterior cephaloceles account for 25% of all congenital cephaloceles. They may be visible from the outside (sincipital) or not visible (basal). Rare congenital malformation. Affected patients typically present in the first year of life. Associated abnormalities are callosal hypogenesis, interhemispheric lipoma, dermoid, neuronal migration anomalies, colloid cyst, midline craniofacial dysraphisms, hypertelorism, microcephaly, microphthalmos, and hydrocephalus.
Nasal dermoid/epidermoid	**Dermoid:** Midline focal mass of fat density located anywhere from the glabella to the nasal columella. Findings that suggest intracranial extension include widened nasal septum, bifid septum, bifid perpendicular plate, bifid crista galli, interorbital widening, and defects in the cribriform plate. Dermal sinuses, complete or incomplete, are usually associated. **Epidermoid:** Mass with attenuation close to water located in the subcutaneous fat of the nose. Epidermoids are more common at the tip of the nose or slightly lateral to the nose.	Dermoid cysts are the most common midline congenital nasal masses. Nasal dermoids may be located anywhere from the glabella to the nasal tip and may extend intracranially. They may present with a nasal pit, dimple, or fistula containing a hair over the dorsum of the nose. Dermoids are slightly more common in male patients, whereas epidermoids have equal prevalence in both genders. They commonly become infected, may distort nasal growth, and are cosmetically unacceptable.
Nasal glioma	Well-circumscribed soft tissue mass, isodense to brain, located over nasal bones (extranasal glioma) or within nasal cavity (intranasal glioma). In patients with intranasal heterotopia, the foramen cecum may be deep and large, and the crista galli may be small or bifid. The anterior part of the nasal septum may be hypoplastic. With extranasal lesions, the nasal bones may be thinned.	Rare, developmental mass of dysplastic neurogenic tissue sequestered and isolated from the subarachnoid space ("encephalocele" that has lost its intracranial connection). Usually identified at birth as a congenital subcutaneous blue or red mass along the nasal dorsum. Nasal obstruction may be present with intranasal glioma due to firm, polypoid submucosal nasal cavity mass.
Protrusion of the internal carotid artery into the sphenoid sinus	Internal carotid artery is one of the neighboring structures of the sphenoid sinus. It courses through the area surrounded by bony structures such as the sphenoid sinus wall or clinoid processes and can be identified as a bulge in the sphenoethmoidal cell wall. The grade of protrusion increases as the sinus grows larger. In some instances, the bony plate separating the sphenoid sinus from the artery may be very thin or absent. When the sphenoid sinus is highly pneumatized, the internal carotid artery can course freely through the sphenoid sinus cavity.	One of the common anatomical variations of the sphenoid sinus, which can pose an endoscopic sinus surgical hazard if not recognized preoperatively. Protrusion of other neighboring structures (optic, maxillary, and vidian nerves) into the sphenoethmoid sinus lumen can also be seen.

(continues on page 279)

Table 7.1   (Cont.) Lesions in the nasal cavity and paranasal sinuses

Disease	CT Findings	Comments
Congenital dacryocystocele (dacryocele) ▷ *Fig. 7.4*	Well-circumscribed, rounded, hypodense, thin-walled lesion, anywhere from the lacrimal sac to the inferior aspect of the nasolacrimal duct at the inferior nasal meatus. There may be expansion of the nasolacrimal duct and erosion of adjacent bone. Unless infected, the density is homogeneous. If infected, there may be a rim of contrast enhancement around the cyst and enhancing inflammatory changes in surrounding soft tissues.	A dacryocele (lacrimal sac mucocele) is a cystic expansion of the nasolacrimal sac or a diverticulum of the sac caused by a distal block of the lacrimal drainage system combined with a one-way valve effect at the proximal end of the system. It is almost always associated with intranasal cysts. Dacryoceles are considered an uncommon congenital anomaly of the lacrimal drainage system and are usually present as a tense or fluctuant mass slightly nasal and inferior to the inner canthus in the first few days of life. Bilateral affectation is very rare. Most cases of congenital nasolacrimal duct cysts resolve spontaneously within 12 months. Secondary dacryocystitis, dacryopyocele, periorbital cellulites, and septicemia may ensue. Adult nasolacrimal sac mucocele is an uncommon mass arising in the medial canthal region of the orbit of middle-aged patients with a history of prior trauma, surgery, and postinflammatory or neoplastic stenosis. The cystic expansion is associated with distal nasolacrimal duct obstruction and proximal obstruction at the junction of the common canaliculus and sac. Canaliculocele is an extremely rare cause of a medial canthal mass. Nasolacrimal duct orifice cysts of the inferior nasal meatus are also rare acquired lesions.

(continues on page 280)

II Head and Neck

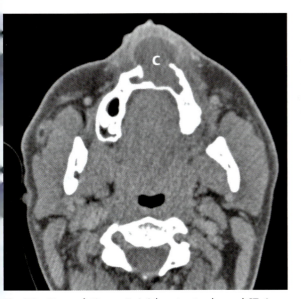

Fig. 7.3   Nasopalatine cyst. Axial contrast-enhanced CT. An extensive nasopalatine duct cyst (C) shows remarkable nasolabial protrusion after penetration of the maxillary cortex.

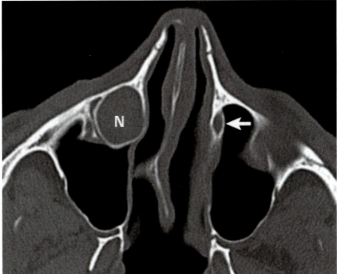

Fig. 7.4   Acquired dacryocystocele. Axial bone CT image demonstrates a smoothly enlarged right nasolacrimal duct (N). Note the normal nasolacrimal duct on the left (arrow).

Table 7.1   (Cont.) Lesions in the nasal cavity and paranasal sinuses

Disease	CT Findings	Comments
Maxillary sinus hypoplasia ▷ *Fig. 7.5*	Unilateral small maxillary sinus with orbital enlargement. The bones between the maxillary sinus and the floor of the orbit and the roof of the orbit and the floor of the frontal fossa are depressed. The floor of the orbit remains rounded. The wall between the nasal fossa and the hypoplastic sinus is displaced laterally. Sinus may be aerated without thickening of mucoperiosteal membranes. Maxillary sinus hypoplasia (MSH) shows three distinct patterns. Type I MSH characteristics are mild hypoplasia of the maxillary sinus, normal uncinate process, and a well-developed infundibular passage. Significant hypoplasia of the maxillary sinus, hypoplastic or absent uncinate process, and absent or pathologic infundibular passage are seen in type II MSH. Type III MSH is characterized by the absence of an uncinate process and cleftlike maxillary sinus hypoplasia.	The maxillary sinus develops in the fourth month of intrauterine life as a mucosal evagination in the center of the middle nasal meatus. If development is arrested at this stage, aplasia or hypoplasia occurs with incomplete pneumatization into the malar eminence and maxillary alveolar ridge. MSH occurs more frequently in syndromes of craniosynostosis, osteodysplasia (Melnick–Needles), as well as in cases of Down syndrome (hypoplasia of the frontal sinus). Conditions such as severe infection, trauma, tumor, irradiation, and congenital first arch syndrome arrest the growth of the maxilla, resulting in a small (hypoplastic) antrum.
Inflammatory/infectious conditions		
Acute rhinosinusitis	CT findings that correlate with acute sinusitis include air–fluid levels with bubbly or strandlike secretions, nodular or smooth mucosal thickening with contrast enhancement, and complete sinus opacification by fluid or soft tissue (mucosal edema). Imaging may reveal complications of sinusitis, such as secondary osteomyelitis, orbital complications, subcutaneous abscess (Pott puffy tumor), meningitis, epidural abscess, subdural empyema, and brain abscess.	Acute inflammatory process of sinonasal mucosa lasting for less than 4 weeks. Most cases follow viral upper respiratory infections. The bacteria most often involved are *Haemophilus influenzae* and *Streptococcus pneumoniae*. Predisposing factors include upper respiratory infections, systemic disease, nasal masses, trauma, anatomical variants, dental infections, and allergic mucosal edema. Manifests clinically as headache, local tenderness, facial pain, and purulent nasal drainage.
Chronic rhinosinusitis ▷ *Fig. 7.6*	In contrast with acute sinusitis, there is usually sclerosis and thickening of the affected sinus walls. Mucosal thickening may reflect inflammation or fibrosis. There is possibly dystrophic calcification of the mucosa. With coexistent acute disease, there may be enhancement of the inflamed mucosa. Signs of chronic rhinitis, including mucosal thickening, inflammatory polyps, and hyperplasia of the turbinates, may also be evident. Five different patterns of chronic rhinosinusitis may be described at CT: • **Infundibular pattern** is mainly due to the presence of mucosal thickenings or isolated polyps along the ethmoid infundibulum with blockage of maxillary sinus drainage alone. • **Ostiomeatal unit pattern** reflects obstruction of all drainage systems in the middle nasal meatus, leading to maxillary, frontal, and anterior ethmoid sinusitis. The most frequent causes are nonspecific mucosal thickenings and nasal polyps. This pattern may also be observed in the presence of benign or malignant neoplasms arising from the lateral nasal wall. • **Sphenoethmoidal recess pattern** is rather rare, consisting of sphenoid sinusitis and/or posterior ethmoiditis secondary to sphenoethmoid recess obstruction. • **Pattern of nasal polyposis** is characterized by bilateral involvement of the middle nasal meatus, as well as the ethmoid infundibular and paranasal cavities by inflammatory polyps. • **Sporadic pattern** includes a wide list of different conditions, such as isolated sinusitis, retention cyst, mucocele, and postsurgical changes.	Chronic sinusitis is an infection of the paranasal sinuses that persists beyond the acute stage (> 12 consecutive weeks' duration) or fails to respond to therapy. May be bacterial, allergic, or fungal in nature. All but one pattern of chronic rhinosinusitis (sporadic pattern) are based on the obstruction of different mucus-drainage pathways. Often associated conditions are underlying anatomical variations and primary ciliary dysmotility. All ages are affected. Common symptoms are facial pain and pressure, nasal obstruction, nasal discharge, hyposmia, and anosmia.

(continues on page 281)

Table 7.1   (Cont.) Lesions in the nasal cavity and paranasal sinuses

Disease	CT Findings	Comments
Fungal sinusitis ▷ *Fig. 7.7*	Localized *Aspergillus* sinusitis (mycetoma) usually affects a single sinus (maxillary > sphenoid > frontal > ethmoid sinuses). Presents with a focal polypoid mass within a partially or totally opacified sinus lumen with central areas of high density and/or fine, round to linear matrix calcifications. Thickened, inflamed mucosa at the periphery of the sinus may contrast enhance. The walls are thickened. **Chronic allergic hypersensitive aspergillus sinusitis** presents with usually asymmetrical pansinusitis, hypodense contrast-enhancing mucoperiosteal thickening, polyps, and hyperdense sinus contents, sinus expansion, and facial deformity. **Acute invasive fungal sinusitis** is most common in the maxillary and ethmoid sinuses, followed by the sphenoid sinus. The fulminant progressive disease presents with complete or partial soft tissue opacification of affected sinus, fungal colonization with increased density, absence of fluid levels, and multiple areas of focal bony destructions of sinus walls. Spread of sinus can extend into adjacent soft tissues and present with rhino-orbitocerebral disease. Vascular involvement can cause narrowing, dissection, and thrombosis.	*Aspergillus fumigatus* and Mucoraceae are the most common offending organisms. Acute invasive fungal sinusitis most often occurs in diabetic or immunocompromised patients with predisposing conditions (e.g., leukemia, bone marrow transplantation, severe malnutrition, or end-stage renal disease). Serious disease. Noninvasive continuous forms may occur in an otherwise healthy patient after change in local sinus microenvironment (sinus surgery, postradiation, marijuana smoking). Asymptomatic or mild sensation of a chronic rhinosinusitis.

(continues on page 282)

II Head and Neck

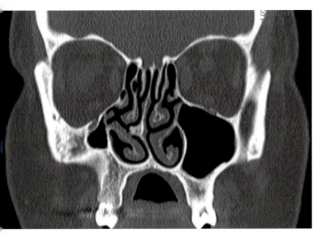

Fig. 7.5   Maxillary sinus hypoplasia (type II). Coronal reformatted bone CT image reveals a small aerated right maxillary sinus with orbital enlargement. No thickening of mucoperiosteal membranes is visible. The floor of the right orbit is depressed. The wall between the nasal fossa and the hypoplastic sinus is displaced laterally. Also seen is a hypoplastic right uncinate process.

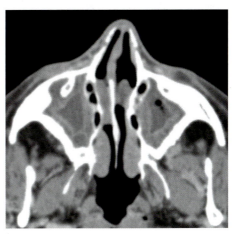

Fig. 7.6   Chronic rhinosinusitis. Axial contrast-enhanced CT image shows bilateral maxillary sinus mucosal thickening and enhancement of inflamed mucosa. Also noted are hypodensity of secretions and sclerosis and thickening of the affected maxillary sinus walls.

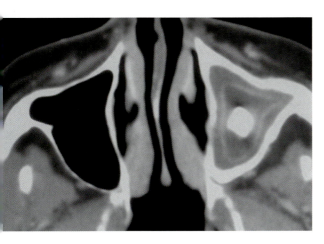

Fig. 7.7   Chronic noninvasive maxillary sinus aspergillosis. Axial contrast-enhanced CT image demonstrates left maxillary sinus mucosal thickening and enhancement of inflamed mucosa, associated with a central calcification. Also noted are hypodensity of secretions and sclerosis and thickening of the affected maxillary sinus walls.

Table 7.1   (Cont.) Lesions in the nasal cavity and paranasal sinuses

Disease	CT Findings	Comments
Infectious granulomatous sinonasal disease	Nodular or tumorlike masses in the nasal cavity and/or paranasal sinuses, commonly associated with bony destruction. External nasal involvement may also be present.	Bacterial infections with granulomatous lesions of the sinonasal cavities include actinomycosis, nocardiosis, tuberculosis, syphilis, leprosy, and glanders. Rhinoscleroma is a tumorlike expansion of the nose and upper lip, seen more commonly in Africa, Central and South America, and Eastern Europe. It is caused by *Klebsiella rhinoscleromatis*. It can also involve the nasopharynx, larynx, trachea, bronchi, middle ear, and orbit.
Cocaine nose	Granuloma of the nasal septum, which eventually may be eroded. Nonspecific mucosal inflammation of the nasal cavity and/or paranasal sinuses may be associated. The nasal septal destruction, loss of the structural integrity of the nasal cavity, and hard palate defect are recognized as a local complication.	Secondary to necrotizing vasculitis with prolonged cocaine abuse.
Wegener granulomatosis ▷*Fig. 7.8*	Favors nasal cavity (septum, turbinates) over sinuses. Presents with usually bilateral, irregular mucosal thickening and soft tissue nodules with contrast enhancement. Extensive bony destruction may occur without associated large soft tissue mass. Nasal septum perforation is common. May extend through hard palate. Orbital extension is the most common extrasinonasal site. As the disease becomes chronic, the walls of the residual paranasal sinuses (particularly the maxillary sinus) become markedly thickened, while the sinus volume is gradually reduced, and the nasal septum may completely disappear.	Systemic necrotizing granulomatous vasculitis that may also affect lungs and kidneys in addition to the sinonasal involvement. The antineutrophil cytoplasmic autoantibody assay is usually positive. Nasal manifestations of allergic granulomatosis and angiitis (Churg–Strauss syndrome) are similar to Wegener granulomatosis. Sarcoidosis may also present as granulomatous sinonasal disease with external nasal involvement and mucosal thickening of the septum and turbinates.
Retention cyst	Smooth, spherical mass of homogeneous water density adherent to the sinus wall. The mass does not enhance. Most arise in the floor of the maxillary antrum. A persistent rim of air and lack of sinus expansion distinguish the retention cyst from a mucocele. Retention cysts are usually not associated with mucosal thickening and edema.	Retention cyst, the most common mass of the maxillary sinus, results from the obstruction of ducts draining mucous glands; considered a complication of sinusitis. Retention cyst is most often asymptomatic. If large enough, it may become symptomatic by obstructing the sinus drainage.
Sinonasal polyposis	Multiple polypoid mucoid or soft tissue masses within the nasal fossa and paranasal sinuses. Polyps may be hyperdense with increased protein and decreased water content or colonization with fungal agent. Increased linear densities are due to trapped desiccated mucus. Curvilinear mucosal enhancement surrounding polyps is seen after intravenous (IV) contrast. Deossification of bony septa in ethmoid and nose, nasal cavity and sinus wall remodeling and expansion, enlargement of the infundibulum, lamina papyracea bulging into orbits, and even intracranial extensions are noted in severe cases (may have mucoceles associated).	The most common sinonasal masses develop from chronic nonneoplastic inflammatory swelling of the mucosa. Predisposing factors include chronic rhinosinusitis, allergy, cystic fibrosis, Kartagener syndrome, asthma, and aspirin sensitivity. Polyposis and allergic fungal sinusitis are frequently seen in association. Most commonly seen in adults; 60% are male. Patients present with nasal stuffiness and sometimes hypertelorism.
Antrochoanal polyp ▷*Fig. 7.9a, b*	A well-defined, homogeneous, low-density, mucuslike mass may be seen occupying the maxillary sinus, ipsilateral nasal cavity, and nasopharynx. Central increased density may be related to chronicity of polyp or fungal colonization. The maxillary ostium and infundibulum are considerably enlarged by passage of the dumbbell-shaped, nonenhancing polypoid lesion into the nose.	Inflammatory, solitary, peculiar variant of sinonasal polyp without significant allergic pathophysiology. Arises from the maxillary antrum; represents 3% to 6% of all sinonasal polyps. Most common in teenagers and young adults; predilection to male. Patients present with unilateral nasal obstruction, nasal drainage, cheek pain, and headaches. Bilateral obstructive maxillary sinusitis may be associated. Nasochoanal, sphenochoanal, and ethmochoanal polyps are less common variants.

(continues on page 284)

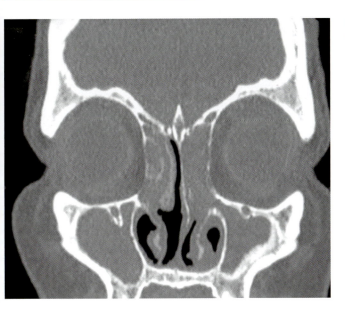

Fig. 7.8   Wegener granulomatosis. Coronal reformatted bone CT image shows bilateral obliteration of the nasal fossa and ethmoid and maxillary sinuses. There is erosion of the ethmoidal cell walls.

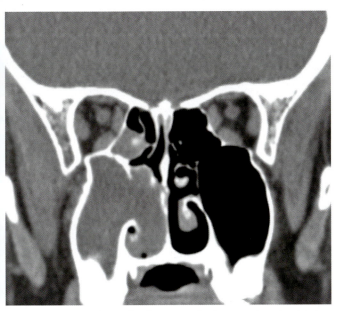

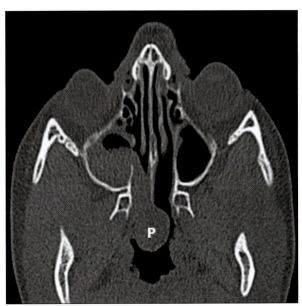

b

Fig. 7.9a, b   Antrochoanal polyp. Coronal reformatted section (**a**) shows a low-density, mucuslike mass filling the right maxillary sinus and the ipsilateral nasal cavity. Axial bone CT image (**b**) reveals the polyp extending from the right maxillary sinus through a wide ostium into the nasal cavity and nasopharynx (P).

Table 7.1 (Cont.) Lesions in the nasal cavity and paranasal sinuses

Disease	CT Findings	Comments
Mucocele ▷ *Fig. 7.10*	Airless, opacified, mucus-containing, nonenhancing enlarged and distorted sinus with smooth-walled expansion. High-density areas within the low-density or soft tissue density of the mucocele may be related to inspissated secretions or fungal colonization. Peripheral enhancement may suggest superinfection (mucopyocele). The sinus walls are remodeled and may even be thinned (thin peripheral rim of expanded bone) or focally absent due to pressure atrophy and erosion, but frank bone destruction and lytic changes are uncommon. Persistent expansion of the sinus is frequently associated with extension into the orbit or skull base and mass effect. In chronically infected mucoceles, a surrounding zone of sclerosis may be evident.	Most common expansile lesion of paranasal sinuses. Frontal sinuses are most frequently involved (65%), followed by the ethmoid sinus (25%), maxillary sinus (5%–10%), and sphenoid sinus (2%–5%). Results from chronic ostial obstruction of affected sinus from inflammation, trauma, surgery, or any space-occupying sinonasal mass lesion; may occur in septated sinuses and anatomical variants (concha bullosa, pneumatized crista galli, uncinate process, etc.). Most common in adults. Presenting symptoms depend on site of involvement, regional compression, and complications.
Silent sinus syndrome ▷ *Fig. 7.11*	Opacified, fully developed maxillary sinus with retraction and inward bowing of the orbital floor and the other sinus walls into sinus lumen. Uncinate process is apposed to inferomedial orbital wall, occluding maxillary sinus infundibulum. The adjacent middle nasal meatus is enlarged with varying degrees of lateral retraction of the middle turbinate. The decrease in sinus volume is associated with increased orbital volume and hypoglobus. The retroantral fat is widened.	Most cases are idiopathic, without a prior history of trauma or surgery. Characterized by painless enophthalmos associated with chronic maxillary sinus atelectasis after infundibular occlusion, seen in adults between the fourth and fifth decades. Symptoms related to sinusitis may or may not be present.
Cholesterol granuloma	CT features of the paranasal sinus cholesterol granuloma are of two types: a variety in which the changes are entirely nonspecific and cannot be differentiated from inflammatory or allergic sinus disease, and a more characteristic appearance of a cystlike lesion within the sinus cavity accompanied by expansion of the bony walls involved. CT of orbitofrontal cholesterol granuloma shows a lobular soft tissue expansile mass, isodense to brain, without contrast enhancement. Orbitofrontal cholesterol granulomas have a tendency to concentrate their expansion about the lateral margins of the frontal sinus affecting the superolateral orbital wall and adjacent soft tissues with a clear-cut area of osteolysis in the lateral part of the supraorbital ridge and frontal bone, characteristically extending into the zygomatic process as far as the frontomalar suture. Absent or minimal surrounding sclerosis.	Cholesterol granuloma is the result of a hemorrhagic foreign body response elicited by cholesterol crystals; usually occurs in the temporal bone (middle ear cavity, mastoid, and petrous apex). Cholesterol granuloma arising from the paranasal sinus is uncommon and occurs in the maxillary antrum, sphenoidal sinus, and frontal bone. It usually occurs in young or middle-aged men. Cholesterol granuloma of the maxillary sinus is usually an incidental finding. An expansive lesion of the sphenoid sinus may present with progressive visual deficit. The most common symptom of orbitofrontal lesions is gradual proptosis.
Benign neoplasms		
Osteoma	Sharply delineated round or lobulated mass of bone attenuation arising from and confined to bone or protruding into a sinus. Ivory osteomas are denser than adjacent bone. Non-ivory-type (fibrous) osteomas contain both dense calcifications and mildly calcific soft tissue. Larger frontal osteomas may invade the posterior wall of the sinus, leading to CSF leak, pneumocephalus, or subdural empyema and brain abscess. Osteomas also may occlude the sinus ostia, causing sinusitis or mucocele formation.	In the craniofacial skeleton, osteomas may be found in all sites but are most common in the frontal and ethmoid sinuses. Occur as a single lesion but may be associated with Gardner syndrome and multiple craniofacial osteomas. Osteomas are more common in men, reported in all ages (rare under age 10). Usually asymptomatic. Symptoms associated with sinus osteomas include headaches, facial swelling or deformity, and ocular disturbances.
Osteoblastoma	Osteoblastoma appears as a well-defined, round, expansile lesion with a prominent calcified rim. The central portion may appear similar to ossifying fibroma as a solitary cystlike or solid soft tissue lesion, with or without mineralized components. Osteoblastomas may show moderate to marked enhancement.	Uncommon osseous neoplasm. Head and neck sites of involvement include the mandible (most common site), maxilla, temporal bone, orbit, and paranasal sinuses. Osteoblastomas occur more often in men; most patients are younger than 30 y. Clinical symptoms include pain, facial swelling and asymmetry, and loosening of teeth.
Chondroma	Multilobulated, sharply demarcated soft tissue mass; can be hyperdense or hypodense relative to brain. Contrast enhancement is usually minimal. Calcifications within the tumor matrix are not often seen. These lesions tend to be expansile and can remodel bone. A distinction between a benign chondroma and a low-grade chondrosarcoma is not possible on sectional imaging.	Chondromas of the sinonasal tract are rare. Most frequent sites of occurrence include the nasal cavity (septum), the ethmoid sinus, and the nasopharynx. Most patients are younger than 50 y, and there is equal gender predilection. Patients may present with nasal obstruction, an enlarging, painless mass, proptosis, and headaches.

(continues on page 285)

Table 7.1   (Cont.) Lesions in the nasal cavity and paranasal sinuses

Disease	CT Findings	Comments
Ossifying fibroma ▷ *Fig. 7.12*	Unilocular, well-defined, expansile mixed soft tissue and bone density lesion. The low-attenuation fibrous center is surrounded either by a thick bony wall or a thin "eggshell" periphery of bone. Fibrous areas may show subtle contrast enhancement.	Monostotic lesion of osteogenic origin, occurring primarily in the mandibular premolar/molar region of women in the third and fourth decade, can occur in the craniofacial skeleton and involve the adjacent sinuses (maxillary, ethmoid, and frontal sinuses). May obstruct sinus drainage pathways, result in cosmetic deformity, and extend intracranially.
Schwannoma	Schwannomas appear as well-defined ovoid to fusiform, homogeneous soft tissue mass, hypodense relative to skeletal muscle, and reveal moderate to marked contrast enhancement. The larger lesions, however, may be inhomogeneous as well as cystic.	Neurogenic tumors are infrequent in the sinonasal cavities (nasal fossa, maxillary and ethmoid sinuses). They may arise from the first and second division of the trigeminal nerve and from the autonomic nerves (the olfactory nerve has no Schwann cells and therefore cannot be the site of these tumors).

(continues on page 286)

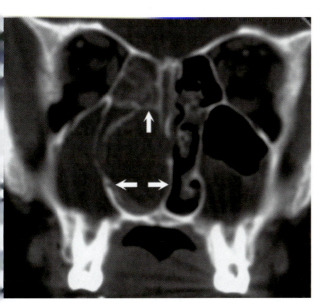

Fig. 7.10   Concha bullosa mucocele. Coronal bone CT image reveals a right intranasal mass expanding toward the medial wall of the right maxillary sinus, nasal septum, and right ethmoid cells (arrows). There is mucosal disease in both the maxillary and right ethmoid sinuses.

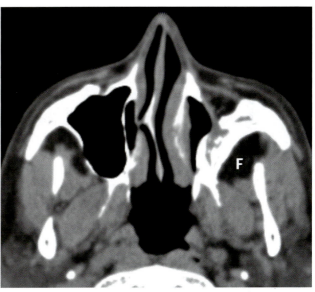

Fig. 7.11   Silent sinus syndrome (postsurgical). Axial non-contrast-enhanced CT image demonstrates retraction and inward bowing of the left maxillary sinus walls with diminished sinus volume. The retroantral fat pad is widened (F).

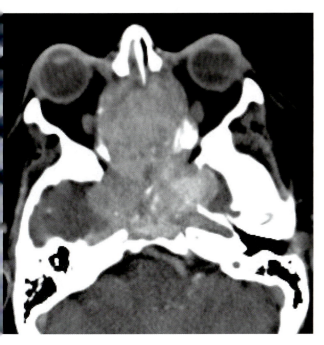

Fig. 7.12   Psammomatoid active ossifying fibroma. Axial contrast-enhanced CT image shows a large, well-circumscribed, expansile, midline located, inhomogeneous sinonasal mass with mixed calcific and enhancing soft tissue density components and a thin ossific outer margin.

Table 7.1   (Cont.) Lesions in the nasal cavity and paranasal sinuses

Disease	CT Findings	Comments
Hemangioma	Well-defined, lobular, diffusely enhancing soft tissue density mass. May cause bone remodeling and septal deviation. The CT appearance of intraosseous hemangiomas is variable and most commonly shows a characteristic sharply marginated expansile, rounded, well-defined bony lesion with intact, thinned, smooth inner and outer cortices and a sunburst or spoke-wheel-type pattern of radiating trabeculae. "Soap bubble" and "honeycomb" configuration may also occur. There is no associated periosteal reaction or soft tissue mass.	Nasal hemangiomas arise from the nasal septum or vestibule and are of the capillary type. Only a few arise from the lateral wall of the nose, and these are usually cavernous. In the paranasal sinuses, hemangiomas are even rarer. Patients (with a wide age range from infancy to late adulthood) present with epistaxis and nasal obstruction. Intraosseous hemangiomas of the facial bones are rare and most commonly arise in the maxilla, zygoma, mandible, and nasal bone. Patients usually present in the fourth decade of life, with a female predominance. Symptom: firm, nonpainful swelling.
Juvenile angiofibroma ▷ *Fig. 7.13*	Intensely enhancing lobular, well-circumscribed, soft tissue mass centered at the sphenopalatine foramen with multiple surrounding extensions into the nasal cavity, nasopharynx, paranasal sinuses, pterygopalatine fossa, masticator space, orbit (through the inferior orbital fissure), and intracranially (20%–36%; via superior orbital fissure, vidian canal, and foramen rotundum). Juvenile angiofibroma may cause adjacent compressive deossification or remodeling with enlarged ipsilateral nasal cavity and widening of the pterygopalatine fossa with anterior bowing of the posterior maxillary sinus wall (antral sign).	Rare, histologically benign, highly vascular, nonencapsulated, locally aggressive tumor arising from the fibrovascular stroma on the posterolateral nasal wall adjacent to the sphenopalatine foramen. Occurs almost exclusively in male adolescents with unilateral nasal obstruction and epistaxis, anosmia, serous otitis media, and pain.
Odontogenic neoplasms		Odontogenic tumors are neoplasms of the maxilla and mandible that originate from tooth-forming epithelial, mesenchymal tissue, or both. Clinically, they are generally asymptomatic but can cause bony swelling, tooth movement, tenderness, and pain when the bone is resolved.
	Ameloblastoma: Enhancing, expansile, uni- or multicystic, low-density mass with "bubbly" pattern, internal osseous septa, usually no calcifications in matrix, scalloped borders, and thinned cortical margins with focal areas of dehiscence. Extraosseous extension is rare. Unerupted molar tooth and resorption of adjacent tooth roots association is common. No evidence for perineural spread. Maxillary ameloblastomas occur most often in the molar-premolar region and can involve the adjacent maxillary sinus.	Most common odontogenic tumor (35%), mandible to maxilla ratio = 5:1. Twenty percent of ameloblastomas are thought to arise from dentigerous cysts. Most commonly presents at age 30 to 50 y with painless, slow-growing mandibular mass, loose teeth, bleeding, and trismus. Maxillary lesions may present with nasal obstruction. Malignant transformation is rare (1%).
	Odontogenic fibroma: Well-defined, expansile, unilocular, radiolucent lesion, mainly in the mandibular molar area or in the maxilla, associated with sharp resorption of the roots of adjacent teeth. Calcification is rare.	Rare disease, found in individuals age 20 y and younger.
	Odontogenic myxoma: Enhancing, expansile, multilocular lesion with straight and curved bony septa ("tennis racket" appearance), often accompanied by bulging of the bony cortex, which may be barely preserved, and inclination of adjacent teeth.	A locally aggressive tumor, occurring only in the jaws. This tumor develops in the third decade of life, with a slightly higher prevalence among women.
	Odontomas: Well-demarcated mass with amorphous areas of calcification (complex odontoma) and/or malformed teeth (compound odontoma) arranged in a disorderly pattern. A narrow radiolucent zone, along with a sharply defined bony rim representing the wall of the odontoma, frequently surrounds the tumor.	Hamartomatous malformation of odontogenic tissue. Compound odontoma is the more frequent variety and occurs most commonly in the maxillary incisor or canine region. Complex odontoma resembles a mature cementoma but is seen more often in the mandibular molar regions, develops in childhood and adolescence, and is more radiodense.

(continues on page 287)

Table 7.1 (Cont.) Lesions in the nasal cavity and paranasal sinuses

Disease	CT Findings	Comments
Schneiderian papilloma	Inverted papillomas usually originate from the lateral nasal wall in the vicinity of the middle turbinate. They show a unilateral bulky, polypoid soft tissue mass with variable enhancement pattern, from diffuse to heterogeneous, that involves the nasal vault and extends centrifugally into the adjacent sinuses, nasopharynx, and orbit. Rarely, they violate the meninges and intracranial structures. Foci of coarse calcification are occasionally present. They cause local bone remodeling and a unilateral ostiomeatal unit obstructive pattern of sinus opacification (obstructed sinus secretions do not enhance). Bilateral up to 13% due to transseptal extension.	Schneiderian papillomas are uncommon, representing 0.4% to 4.7% of all sinonasal tumors. Inverted papillomas account for 70% of sinonasal papillomas. This epithelial tumor of nasal mucosa is named for its characteristic endophytic rather than exophytic growth. Although histologically benign, they are locally aggressive tumors. An underlying or coexisting squamous cell carcinoma is present in 5.5% to 27% of cases. Peak incidence: 40 to 70 y, with male predominance. Patients present with nasal obstruction and discharge, epistaxis, anosmia, headache, and pain. Cylindric cell papillomas originate primarily from the lateral nasal wall. Fungiform papillomas arise on the nasal septum in young males and have a verrucous appearance.
Benign mixed tumor (pleomorphic adenoma)	Benign mixed tumors usually arise from the nasal septum, the lateral nasal cavity wall or turbinate, with secondary extension into the maxillary sinus. They appear as a broad-based or pedunculated, polypoid, well-demarcated, expanding intranasal soft tissue mass, generally associated with bone destruction.	Benign mixed tumors (pleomorphic adenomas) are the most common benign salivary-type neoplasms of the sinonasal tract. Patients (median age 20–60 y, equal gender distribution) usually complain of nasal obstruction, mass sensation, or epistaxis.

(continues on page 288)

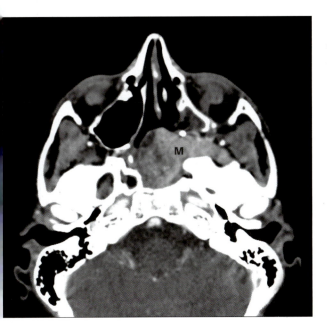

Fig. 7.13 Juvenile angiofibroma. Axial contrast-enhanced CT image reveals an intensely enhancing, lobular, well-circumscribed, soft tissue mass centered at the left sphenopalatine foramen (M) with extension into the nasopharynx, nasal cavity, left maxillary sinus, and pterygopalatine fossa. (Courtesy of Dr. A. von Hessling, Zurich.)

II Head and Neck

Table 7.1   (Cont.) Lesions in the nasal cavity and paranasal sinuses

Disease	CT Findings	Comments
Malignant neoplasms		
Squamous cell carcinoma ▷ *Fig. 7.14*	Large, poorly marginated, heterogeneous soft tissue density mass, with minimal to moderate contrast enhancement and extensive irregular destruction of adjacent bone. The tumor may show bone fragments or areas of punctate calcifications. Associated sinusitis or retained secretions are common due to ostial obstruction. Invasion of the retroantral fat pad and pterygopalatine fossa, maxillary alveolar ridge, buccal space, hard palate, and subcutaneous tissues of the cheek and nose occurs frequently. These tumors also have a propensity to grow insidiously toward the anterior and central skull base and orbits. Regional lymph nodes (retropharyngeal, submandibular, and/or jugulodigastric) are involved in 15% at presentation.	Malignant tumors of the nasal cavity and paranasal sinuses are relatively rare (3% of all head and neck tumors). Squamous cell carcinoma accounts for 80% of sinonasal malignancies. Twenty-five to 60% of these carcinomas involve the maxillary antrum; however, the maxillary sinus is secondarily involved by direct extension in 80% of patients. The nasal cavity is the site of origin in ~30% of cases, the ethmoid air cells in 10%, and the sphenoid and frontal sinus in < 2%. These are typically seen in patients who range in age from 60 to 70 y, more commonly in men. They are often clinically silent until advanced. First symptoms are usually from secondary obstructive sinusitis. **Staging:** T1: Tumor limited to antral mucosa. T2: Confined to suprastructure mucosa without bone destruction, or infrastructure with inferior or medial bony wall destruction. T3: Invades skin of cheek, posterior wall maxillary sinus, floor of medial wall orbit, masticator space, pterygoid plates, or ethmoid sinus. T4: Invades orbit or cribriform plate, posterior ethmoid or sphenoid sinuses, nasopharynx, soft palate, or skull base. Staging criteria are based on a theoretical plane joining the medial canthus of the eye with the angle of the mandible (Ohngren line). The area anteroinferior to this line is referred to as the infrastructure; the superoposterior is called the suprastructure of the maxillary antrum.
Glandular tumors of the sinonasal cavities ▷ *Fig. 7.15*	Well-circumscribed to poorly defined soft tissue density mass. Attenuation within the tumor is usually inhomogeneous due to cystic degeneration, necrosis, or serous and mucous collections; with diffuse, often heterogeneous contrast enhancement. Bone changes include bone remodeling, sclerotic reactions, erosion, and destruction. These tumors have a propensity to grow insidiously toward the anterior skull base and orbit. Perineural tumor spread may appear as obliteration and enlargement of the nerve sheath. Distant metastases are more common than lymph node involvement.	Tumors of minor salivary gland origin and other glandular neoplasms constitute 4% to 10% of malignant neoplasms of the sinonasal cavities. They can occur anywhere within the sinonasal cavities. However, they frequently arise from the minor salivary glands within the palate and then extend into the nasal cavity or paranasal sinuses. Adenoid cystic carcinoma is the most common malignant tumor of the minor salivary glands (47% maxillary, 32% nasal cavity, 7% ethmoid, 3% sphenoid, and 2% frontal). The others are adenocarcinoma, mucoepidermoid carcinoma, acinic cell carcinoma, and carcinoma ex pleomorphic adenoma. Adenocarcinomas more frequently arise in the ethmoid and are common in patients with occupational exposure to wood and leather dust. Age distribution shows a peak occurrence in the sixth and seventh decades, with a marked predominance of men. Low-grade tumors tend to present in younger patients. Patient often presents when the tumor is at an advanced stage with symptoms of obstruction, rhinorrhea, and epistaxis. Associated dull pain, paresthesia, or nerve paralysis due to perineural spread is highly suggestive of adenoid cystic carcinoma.

(continues on page 289)

Table 7.1 (Cont.) Lesions in the nasal cavity and paranasal sinuses

Disease	CT Findings	Comments
Merkel cell carcinoma	Hypervascular, homogeneously and massively enhancing mass expanding the nasal fossa with aggressive destruction of the nasal septum, intersinonasal wall, and orbital wall. No calcifications.	Highly aggressive neoplasm of neuroendocrine origin with poor prognosis. This rare tumor affects older patients (mean age 70 y), with a slight female predominance. The majority of the tumors are found on sun-exposed sites. Involvement of the nasal cavity and palatal mucosa is very uncommon.
Olfactory neuroblastoma (esthesioneuroblastoma)	Typically presents as a unilateral nasal homogeneous soft tissue mass with moderate to marked enhancement, often near the superolateral nasal wall near the frontoethmoidal complex. When large, the tumor may be inhomogeneous with areas of small or large cystic components. Punctate calcifications within the tumor matrix are unusual. Olfactory neuroblastomas have a marked propensity for crossing the cribriform plate and extending dumbbell-shaped intracranially. Other directions of tumor extension associated with bone remodeling mixed with destructive bone changes include ipsilateral ethmoid and maxillary sinuses. Orbital involvement is late.	Rare malignant nasal neoplasm of neuroectodermal origin that arises from the olfactory epithelium in the cribriform region, the upper third of the nasal septum, and along the superior and supreme nasal turbinates. They have a bimodal age distribution, presenting in boys and middle-aged adults (slight male predominance). Patients present with long-standing unilateral nasal obstruction and repeated episodes of epistaxis, anosmia, rhinorrhea, headache, pain, and ocular disturbances; 20% have malignant cervical nodes at presentation.

(continues on page 290)

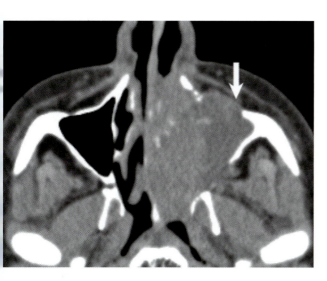

Fig. 7.14 Sinonasal squamous cell carcinoma. Axial non-contrast-enhanced CT image shows an aggressive soft tissue density mass of the left nasal cavity with extension into the left maxillary sinus. Also seen are multiple sites of sinus wall destruction with invasion of the left pterygopalatine fossa, retroantral fat pad, and cheek (arrow).

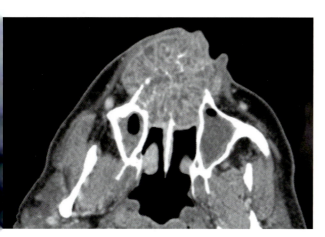

Fig. 7.15 Adenoid cystic carcinoma. Axial contrast-enhanced CT image reveals a large, relatively well-circumscribed, soft tissue density mass, inhomogeneous with heterogeneous contrast enhancement involving the nasal vault. Bone destruction of the maxilla (anterior nasal spine and palatine process) and nasal septum is visible, as well as extension into subcutaneous tissues.

II Head and Neck

Table 7.1 (Cont.) Lesions in the nasal cavity and paranasal sinuses

Disease	CT Findings	Comments
Osteosarcoma ▷*Fig. 7.16*	Poorly defined lesion with aggressive bone destruction, heterogeneous with ossified and nonossified soft tissue components, aggressive periosteal reaction with perpendicular spiculated pattern, and associated soft tissue extension; with enhancement of solid components after contrast.	Only about 7% of osteosarcomas arise in the head and neck. The mean age of these patients (35 y) is about 2 decades older than that of patients with osteosarcoma of the long bones. M:F = 1.5:1. Maxillary lesions arise from the sinus and alveolar ridge and usually produce no pain. Mandibular sarcomas occur in the body and ramus of the mandible and frequently cause a painful swelling. Ewing sarcoma of sinonasal cavities is extremely rare.
Chondrosarcoma	Typically large, multilobulated, sharply demarcated soft tissue mass with heterogeneous, predominantly peripheral enhancement, when first detected, with rings and crescents of calcium or amorphous tumor matrix calcification. Bone changes include erosion and destruction. Periosteal reaction, if present, is usually mild.	Sinonasal involvement is rare. These tumors occur in the wall of the maxillary sinus, at the junction of the nasal septum vomer with the sphenoid and ethmoid sinuses, and on the undersurface of the sphenoid bone. Most common in 30–45-y-old patients.
Rhabdomyosarcoma ▷*Fig. 7.17*	Large, poorly defined, inhomogeneous soft tissue mass, with intense contrast enhancement, destroying adjacent bone. Tumors of the ethmoid sinuses have a marked propensity for crossing the skull base and intracranial extension.	In adults, the ethmoid sinuses are the most common site of origin of head and neck rhabdomyosarcomas. Secondary sinonasal tumors may arise from adjacent orbital spread from orbital rhabdomyosarcoma or pharyngeal rhabdomyosarcoma.
Non–Hodgkin lymphoma	Lymphomas of the sinonasal cavities are often seen as relatively well-demarcated, polypoid, bulky masses of homogeneous soft tissue density; with moderate contrast enhancement, without calcification, with possible bone expansion. Lymphomas may also present as a poorly defined, sinus-obliterating soft tissue mass with bone erosion and destruction and surrounding infiltrations.	Lymphomas arising in the nose and paranasal sinuses are of the non-Hodgkin type and are frequently observed in patients who have disseminated lymphoma or acquired immunodeficiency syndrome (AIDS). Nasal fossa and maxillary sinuses are the most common locations. The disease is strongly associated with Epstein–Barr virus. It occurs mainly in Asian men, with a mean age of 50 y at the time of diagnosis. They can mimic the much more common entities of sinusitis, polyposis, granulomatous processes, and benign and malignant neoplasms.
Idiopathic midline granuloma	Destructive mass in the nasal septum leading to perforation. With progression, the disease spreads to the nose, face, hard and soft palates, adjacent sinuses, and orbits, with extensive bone destruction.	This entity is now clearly defined as a T-cell lymphoma.
Plasmacytoma	Fairly well-defined soft tissue density mass confined to the soft tissues with moderate to marked contrast enhancement. These lesions tend to be expansile and are associated with bone remodeling, as well as bone erosion. Multiple myeloma presents similarly to hematogenous metastases. It can have lytic lesions, which may also demonstrate diffuse osteopenia, and rarely sclerosis.	Extramedullary plasmacytoma accounts for 4% of all nonepithelial tumors of the sinonasal cavities. Nasal cavity, nasal septum, sphenoidal sinus, and nasopharynx are the most common locations.
Malignant melanoma	Well-defined, polypoid or sessile, lobular soft tissue mass in the nasal cavity, with diffuse contrast enhancement. Calcifications may be seen. Associated bone destruction often is present that involves the maxillary antrum, ethmoids, or cribriform plate area.	Less than 1% of all melanomas arise in the sinonasal cavities. Within the nasal cavity, the most common sites of melanomas are the anterior nasal septum, lateral nasal wall, and inferior turbinates. In the paranasal sinuses, the maxillary antrum is the site of origin in 80% of cases. Can be multicentric.
Metastases	The majority of metastases to the paranasal sinuses are to the bone. The tumor usually involves multiple sinuses, with bony wall destruction and extension into adjacent structures (e.g., intracranial and orbital).	A tumor metastatic to the nasal cavity and paranasal sinuses is rare. Renal cell carcinoma accounts for the majority. Other primary sites are lung, breast, colon, stomach, prostate, and thyroid. The sites of involvement are maxillary sinus > ethmoid sinus > frontal sinus > nasal cavity > sphenoid sinus. They occur in patients between 50 and 70 y of age. The clinical picture of metastatic lesions is similar to that of primary sinonasal malignancy.

(continues on page 292)

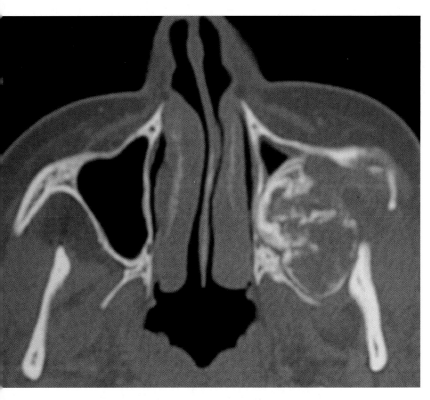

Fig. 7.16 Osteosarcoma. Axial bone CT image shows a large, relatively well-circumscribed, expansile mixed soft tissue and bone density mass of the lateral wall of the left maxillary sinus.

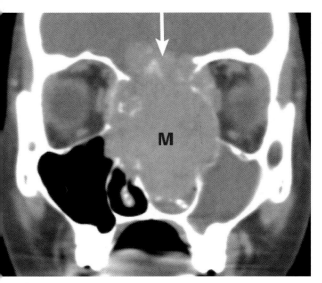

Fig. 7.17 Rhabdomyosarcoma. Coronal contrast-enhanced CT image shows extension of a large, markedly enhancing sinonasal cavity mass (M) into the orbits and intracranially (arrow).

Table 7.1   (Cont.) Lesions in the nasal cavity and paranasal sinuses

Disease	CT Findings	Comments
Craniofacial trauma		
Fracture ▷ *Fig. 7.18a, b* ▷ *Fig. 7.19* ▷ *Fig. 7.20*	Direct fracture signs on CT are fracture lines, discontinuity of bone, and displacement of bone. **Solitary strut (simple) fractures:** Include limited fractures (unilateral or midline) of the orbital floor, medial orbital wall, isolated orbital rim, zygomatic arch, nasal arch, and localized sinus wall (frontal, maxillary). **Complex strut fractures:** Limited fractures involving two adjacent anatomical areas: nasofrontal, naso-maxillary, nasoethmoidal, zygomaticomaxillary, and sphenotemporal. **Maxillary transfacial fractures:** Require pterygoid plate fractures; can be divided into Le Fort I fracture, Le Fort II fracture, Le Fort II with I fractures, Le Fort II with zygomaticomaxillary complex fractures, Le Fort III fractures, Le Fort III with I fractures, and Le Fort III with II fractures.	Maxillofacial fractures are common, often multiple, complex, and asymmetric. By approaching facial fractures in terms of the facial struts that are affected, these may be divided into three classes: limited, transfacial, and smash fractures. Traumatic midface injury often involves a combination of these fractures.

(continues on page 294)

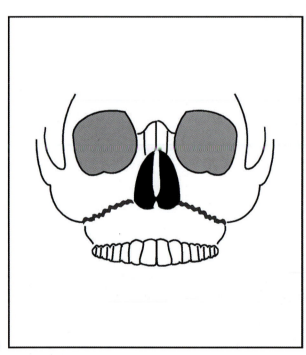
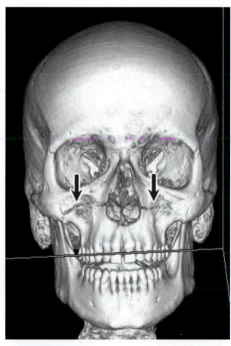

a   b

Fig. 7.18a, b   Le Fort I fracture. Drawing (**a**) of the Le Fort I fracture pattern involving fractures through the inferior portions of the medial and lateral maxillary buttresses ("floating palate"). Fractures include the nasal septum; the medial, anterior, lateral, and posterior wall of the maxillary sinus; and the pterygoid plates of the sphenoid. Three-dimensional reconstruction (**b**) shows detachment of the upper jaw from the remainder of the maxillofacial skeleton (arrows).

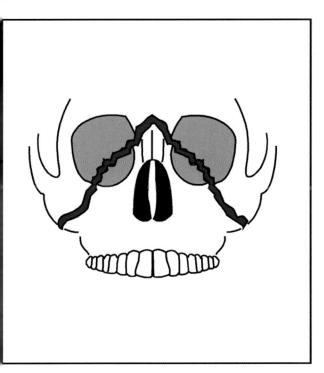

Fig. 7.19 Le Fort II fracture. Drawing of the Le Fort II fracture pattern involving fractures through the zygomaticomaxillary and frontomaxillary sutures ("floating maxilla"). Fractures include the nasal bone and septum, the frontal process of the maxilla, the medial orbital wall (ethmoid, lacrimal, and palatine) and floor of the orbit (inferior orbital fissure and canal), the infraorbital rim, the anterior and lateroposterior wall of the maxillary sinus, and the pterygoid plates of sphenoid.

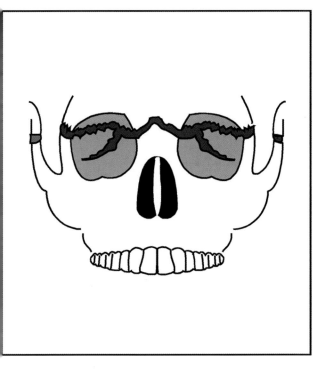

Fig. 7.20 Le Fort III fracture. Drawing of the Le Fort III fracture pattern involving complete craniofacial dissociation ("floating face"). Fractures include all from type II and pass through the lateral wall of the orbit, the zygomaticofrontal suture, and the zygomatic arch.

Table 7.1   (Cont.) Lesions in the nasal cavity and paranasal sinuses

Disease	CT Findings	Comments
▷ *Fig. 7.21a, b*	**Smash fractures:** Represent nasoethmoidal-orbital, central midface, and craniofacial fractures. Skull base fractures are present in a significant percentage of these patients. **Fracture of the zygomaticomaxillary complex:** Term *tripod* fracture is misleading; extends through the four articulations of the zygomatic bone: zygomaticofrontal, zygomaticosphenoidal, zygomaticotemporal, and zygomaticomaxillary sutures with displacement and rotation of the zygoma. Additionally, this fracture may extend posteriorly to involve the pterygoid processes, greater sphenoid wing, and sphenotemporal buttress. **Nasoethmoidal-orbital fracture:** Represents fractures of the lateral nasal bones, lower two thirds of the medial orbital rim, anterior ethmoidal structures, nasomaxillary buttress, and frontal process of the maxilla. Collapse of the nasoethmoidal complex and lateral displacement of the frontal process of the maxilla and medial orbital wall can result in a "blow-in" orbital fracture with traumatic telecanthus.	
Hemorrhage	Diffuse or polypoid mucosal thickening, air–blood level, or complete air replacement by blood are manifestations of sinus bleeding. The density varies with the age of the blood. Acute clot manifests as a hyperdense mass.	Occurs with trauma, surgery, neoplasm, vascular malformations, bleeding disorders, anticoagulation, and barotraumas (e.g., in divers and pilots of unpressurized aircraft).
CSF leak	A fracture through the inner table of the skull may be associated with a tear of the dura and arachnoid and a CSF leak. Frequently, the ethmoid, frontal, sphenoid, or petrous temporal bones may be involved. An air–fluid level in the adjacent paranasal sinuses might be due to blood or CSF. Pneumocephalus can occur in up to one third of all patients with posttraumatic or spontaneous CSF leak. CT cisternography or radionuclide cisternography may be useful if high-resolution, thin-section axial and coronal cranial and facial CT and MR cisternography do not show the CSF fistula.	Causes of CSF rhinorrhea include (1) blunt head trauma; (2) sequelae of skull base surgery; (3) destructive skull base lesions, including neoplasms (both benign and malignant) and empty sella; (4) developmental defects of the ethmoid, sphenoid, frontal, or petrous temporal bones with the formation of a meningocele or meningoencephalocele (with an intact tympanic membrane); and (5) fracture of the petrous temporal bone or other destructive processes in which CSF in the middle ear drains to the nose in the presence of an intact tympanic membrane. Head trauma accounts for 50% to 80% of all cases of CSF leak, and up to 16% are iatrogenic. Less than 5% of all cases of CSF rhinorrhea are spontaneous. Most cases of CSF rhinorrhea begin soon after a head injury and cease spontaneously within 7 to 180 days. Rhinorrhea may occur intermittently and can increase on bending forward, with Valsalva maneuver or jugular vein compression. CSF leak occurs often without nasal congestion, sneezing, lacrimation, or aural discharge

Miscellaneous		
Rhinolith and sinolith ▷ *Fig. 7.22*	Nasal or sinus mass. May be heavily calcified. The calcification appears as a cast surrounded by soft tissue related to inflammatory reactions.	Foreign body in sinonasal cavity acting as nidus may become encrusted with mineral salts when retained for a long period. Very rare. Rhinoliths may produce nasal obstruction, a malodorous nasal discharge with local pain, and epistaxis.
Pneumosinus dilatans	Focal or diffuse abnormal expansion and asymmetric dilation of a paranasal sinus with normal thickness of the displaced walls. The frontal sinus is most often affected, followed by the ethmoid and sphenoid sinuses.	Rare condition. Can occur separately or in association with meningioma, mucocele, fibrous dysplasia, acromegaly, arachnoid cyst, and cerebral hemiatrophy. A hypersinus is an enlarged paranasal sinus that does not expand the surrounding bone beyond its normal contours and has bony walls that are of normal thickness. Pneumoceles are hyperaerated paranasal sinuses or air cells associated with focal or generalized luminal enlargement and focal or diffuse thinning of adjacent bony wall. Pneumatoceles are extraosseous gas collections that usually form after trauma, infection, or surgery.

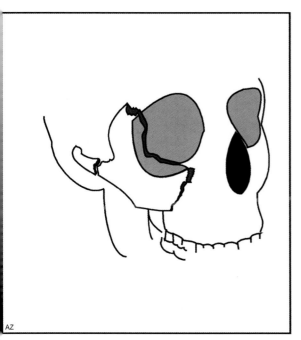

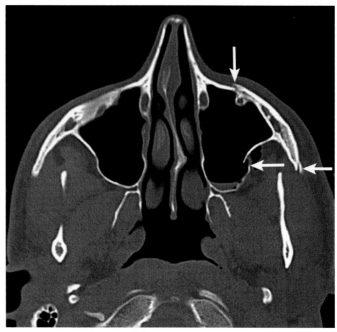

b

Fig. 7.21a, b   Zygomaticomaxillary complex fractures ("quadripod fracture"). Drawing (**a**). Fracture sites include the zygomaticofrontal suture, the zygomaticosphenoidal suture, the zygomaticomaxillary suture, and the zygomaticotemporal suture, with displacement and rotation of the zygoma. Axial bone CT image (**b**) shows an obvious detachment and displacement of the left zygoma (arrows).

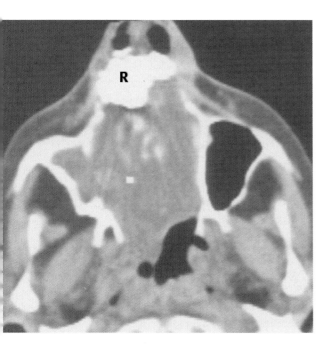

Fig. 7.22   Rhinolith. Axial non-contrast-enhanced CT reveals a heavily calcified mass lesion (R) anteriorly in the nasal cavity, associated with nasal obstruction, stagnation of nasal secretions, and acute and chronic sinonasal inflammation. Also visible is a large perforation of the nasal septum.

8 Suprahyoid Neck

Wolfgang Zaunbauer and Francis A. Burgener

The neck is the transitional area between the skull base superiorly and the thoracic inlet inferiorly that joins the head to the trunk and limbs. It serves as a major conduit for muscles, vessels, nerves, spinal cord, and spine. In addition, the cervical viscera with unique functions are located here: the larynx and trachea, the pharynx and esophagus, and the thyroid and parathyroid glands.

Structures in the neck are surrounded by a layer of subcutaneous tissue (superficial fascia) and are compartmentalized by three layers of the deep cervical fascia. The facial attachments to the hyoid bone functionally cleave the neck into the *suprahyoid neck*, extending longitudinally from the skull base to the hyoid bone, and the *infrahyoid neck*, extending from the hyoid bone to the thoracic inlet.

The suprahyoid neck represents the deep core tissues posterior to the sinonasal and oral cavity areas. It contains 12 distinct spaces defined by the layers of the deep cervical fascia (**Fig. 8.1**). The *pharyngeal mucosal, retropharyngeal, danger,* and *perivertebral* are midline nonpaired spaces. The *parapharyngeal, masticator, parotid,* and *carotid* are lateral paired spaces. The main characteristic of most of these spaces is their verticality. The carotid, retropharyngeal, danger, and perivertebral spaces extend across both the suprahyoid and the infrahyoid neck. The oral cavity is considered a unique region of the suprahyoid neck because the spaces of the oral cavity—the *sublingual* and *submandibular* spaces—do not display the same craniocaudal extent seen in the deep fascial spaces.

A main drawback of computed tomography (CT) imaging is its lack of specificity. By knowing the location and contents of each space, pathology (masses) may be identified and a differential diagnosis developed. Density helps to narrow the list of potential diagnosis of a given mass.

The *pharyngeal mucosal space* (PMS) is the area of the nasopharynx and oropharynx with the surface structures on the airway side of the middle layer of deep cervical fascia (buccopharyngeal fascia). Cranially, it butts a broad area of the sphenoid and occipital bones. The foramen lacerum is within the abutment area. The level of the glossoepiglottic and pharyngoepiglottic folds of the hypopharynx defines the caudal margin. Posterior to the pharyngeal mucosal space is the retropharyngeal space; bilateral to the pharyngeal mucosal space are the parapharyngeal spaces. The ventral airway side of the pharyngeal mucosal space has no fascial border. Critical contents of the pharyngeal mucosal space are the mucosa, lymphoid tissue of Waldeyer ring (adenoids and faucial and lingual tonsils), minor salivary glands, superior and middle constrictor muscles, salpingopharyngeus muscle, pharyngobasilar fascia (a tough aponeurosis that connects the superior constrictor muscle to the skull base), levator palatini muscle, and the cartilaginous end of the eustachian tube.

A generic pharyngeal mucosal space mass projects into the airway, disrupts the normal PMS mucosal and submucosal architecture, is centered medial to the laterally displaced parapharyngeal space, and invades the parapharyngeal space from medially to laterally. The most common lesion primary to the pharyngeal mucosal space is squamous cell carcinoma.

The *parapharyngeal space* (PPS) is the central space on each side of the core tissues of the deep face; it extends from the skull base to the level of the hyoid bone. It is symmetrical and situated between layers of the deep cervical fascia, with the pharyngeal mucosal space medial, the parotid space lateral, the masticator space anterior, and the carotid space and retropharyngeal space posterior. Inferiorly, at the pterygomandibular gap, the PPS is not separated from the posterior aspect of the submandibular space by fascia. The PPS contains mainly fat and connective tissue, small branches of the mandibular division of the trigeminal nerve (cranial nerve [CN] V$_3$), the external carotid artery branches (internal maxillary artery and ascending pharyngeal artery) and pharyngeal venous plexus, lymph nodes, and the rest of the minor salivary gland tissue.

A mass lesion of the PPS is centered within the fat of the space. It may displace the lateral wall of the pharyngeal mucosal space medially, the deep lobe of the parotid gland laterally, and the contents of the carotid space posteriorly. Masses of the surrounding spaces may displace the PPS in a characteristic fashion: a pharyngeal mucosal space mass pushes it from medial to lateral, a masticator space mass from anterior to posterior, a parotid space mass from lateral to medial, a carotid space mass from posterior to anterior, and a lateral retropharyngeal space mass from posteromedial to anterolateral. Usually the PPS serves as an "elevator shaft" through which infection and tumor originating from adjacent spaces may travel. Primary PPS masses (salivary gland tumors, neurogenic tumors, paragangliomas) are unusual.

The *posterior cervical space* (PCS) is a three-dimensional fascially defined space posteromedial to the sternocleidomastoid muscle and anteromedial to the trapezius muscle but superficial to the perivertebral space, largely corresponding to the posterior triangle of the neck seen on clinical examination. The PCS extends from a small superior component near the mastoid tip to a broader base at the level of the clavicle and is bordered superficially by the superficial layer of the deep cervical fascia, medially by the layer of the deep cervical fascia, and ventral by the carotid sheath. The majority of the posterior cervical space is below the hyoid bone. It contains fat, as well as the spinal accessory nerve, spinal accessory lymph node chain, preaxillary brachial plexus, dorsal scapular nerve, and sequestrations of primitive embryonic lymph sacs.

A mass lesion of the PCS is centered within the fat of the space. It may displace the carotid space anteromedially and the sternocleidomastoid muscle anterolaterally and flattens deeper prevertebral and paraspinal structures. The most common lesions of the PCS are reactive and suppurative lymph nodes, malignant nodal metastases, and lymphatic malformations.

The *retropharyngeal space* (RPS) is a midline space located just posterior to the pharynx. It is delimited anteriorly by the visceral fascia, laterally by the carotid sheath, and posteriorly by the prevertebral fascia. There is a very thin fascial layer of the prevertebral fascia (alar fascia) that divides the RPS into anterior and posterior compartments. The anterior compartment, the "true" RPS, extends from the skull base approximately to the third thoracic vertebral level in the mediastinum, where the alar fascia fuses with the visceral fascia. The posterior compartment, referred to as the danger space, extends from the skull

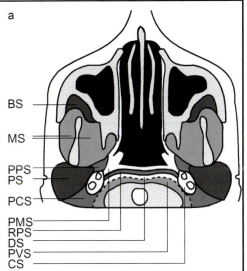
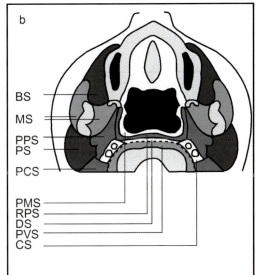
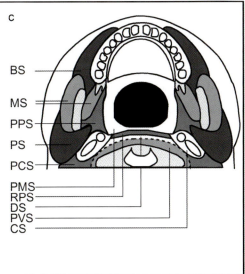
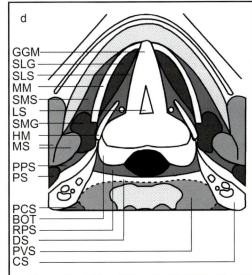

Fig. 8.1a–d   Anatomical drawing depicting the axial anatomy of the normal spaces of the suprahyoid neck. (a) At the level of the midnasopharynx. (**b**) At the level of the low nasopharynx. (**c**) At the level of the upper oral cavity. (**d**) At the level of the low oral cavity. BOT: base of tongue; BS: buccinator space; CS: carotid space; DS: danger space; GGM: genioglossus muscle; HM: hyoglossus muscle; LS: lingual septum; MM: mylohyoid muscle; MS: masticator space; PCS: posterior cervical space; PMS: pharyngeal mucosal space; PPS: parapharyngeal space; PS: parotid space; PVS: perivertebral space, prevertebral portion; RPS: retropharyngeal space; SLG: sublingual gland; SLS: sublingual space; SMG: submandibular gland; SMS: submandibular space.

base to the diaphragms and provides a direct pathway for head and neck infections to spread into the posterior mediastinum. In the suprahyoid neck, the RPS contains fat and retropharyngeal lymph nodes, which are divided into lateral (nodes of Rouviere) and medial groups. Both may extend from the skull base to C3. The danger space and the infrahyoid RPS contain only fat. Although separately defined fascial spaces, the RPS and danger space are considered together, because diseases affecting these spaces cannot be differentiated radiologically. A nodal mass of the suprahyoid RPS is centered posteromedial to the PPS, anterior to the prevertebral muscles, and directly medial to the carotid space. The nodal mass displaces the PPS fat anterolaterally and pushes the carotid space laterally (nodal pattern). An extranodal RPS mass, suprahyoidal or infrahyoidal, appears rectangular-shaped or oval, spans the RPS from side to side, and displaces the paired carotid spaces laterally and the pharyngeal mucosal space or visceral space anteriorly, while flattening the prevertebral space muscles posteriorly (nonnodal pattern).

The *perivertebral space* (PVS) is the cylindrical space surrounding the vertebral column, bordered by the tenacious deep layer of the deep cervical fascia. The attachment of the deep layer of the deep cervical fascia to the transverse process of the vertebral body divides the PVS into the anterior prevertebral portion and the posterior paraspinal portion. The PVS extends from the skull base across the neck to approximately the level of T4 in the posterior mediastinum. The prevertebral portion of the suprahyoid PVS sits directly behind the RPS. Anterolateral to the prevertebral portion of the PVS is the carotid space. The paired posterior cervical spaces are directly lateral to the prevertebral and paraspinal portions of the PVS. The prevertebral portion of the PVS contains the prevertebral muscles, scalene muscles, brachial plexus, phrenic nerve, vertebral artery and vein, vertebral body, and cervical disc. The paraspinal portion of the PVS contains paraspinal muscles, fat, and posterior elements of the vertebral body.

A mass lesion of the prevertebral portion of the PVS is centered within the prevertebral muscles or corpus of the vertebral body and elevates the prevertebral muscles, pushing the danger space/RPS anteriorly. A mass lesion of the paraspinal portion of the PVS is centered within the paraspinal musculature or the posterior elements of the vertebral body, pushing the PCS fat away from the posterior elements of the spine. The PVS is susceptible to inflammatory and infectious processes, as well as neoplasms.

The *carotid space* is a paired, tubular space encircled by the carotid sheath and composed by slips of all three layers of deep cervical fascia. The carotid space extends from the jugular foramen–carotid canal of the skull base to the aortic arch below. In the suprahyoid neck, the carotid space is bordered anteriorly by the PPS and the styloid process, laterally by the parotid space and the posterior belly of the digastric muscle, and medially by the RPS. Its suprahyoidal contents include the internal carotid artery, internal jugular vein, and CN IX to XII. The sympathetic plexus is embedded in the medial sheath walls (between the medial carotid space and the lateral RPS). The internal jugular nodal chain is closely associated but not in the carotid space.

A mass may be localized to the carotid space if it is centered within the area of the carotid artery and jugular vein, posterior to the PPS. A mass in the suprahyoid carotid space displaces PPS fat anteriorly and pushes the posterior belly of the digastric muscle and parotid space laterally. As a mass enlarges in the posterior suprahyoid carotid space, it pushes the internal carotid artery anteriorly. A carotid body paraganglioma may splay the external and internal carotid artery.

The *masticator space* is a large paired space anterolateral to the PPS, dorsal to the buccal space, anterior to the parotid space, deep to the zygomatic arch, and superficial to the pterygomaxillary fissure. It has a broad abutment with the skull base (sphenoid and temporal bones). Splitting of the superficial layer of the deep cervical fascia forms the masticator space. The lateral slip of the fascia with its origin from the inferior surface of the mandible runs up the lateral surface of the masseter muscle to attach to the zygomatic arch, then continues upward on the surface of the temporal muscle to attach high on the parietal calvarium (suprazygomatic masticator space). The medial slip of the fascia runs up the medial pterygoid muscle to insert on the skull base just medial to the foramen ovale (nasopharyngeal masticator space). The masticator space contains the medial and lateral pterygoid, temporalis, and masseter muscles, the mandibular nerve with two motor branches (the masticator and mylohyoid nerves) and sensory branches (lingual and inferior alveolar nerves), pterygoid venous plexus, inferior alveolar vein and artery, maxillary artery, temporomandibular joint, condylar and coronoid processes, ramus, and posterior body of the mandible.

A mass lesion of the masticator space is centered within the muscles of mastication or the mandible, displaces the parapharyngeal fat posteriorly, or invades the PPS from anterior to posterior. Malignant tumor of the masticator space and infection preferentially spread cephalad toward the skull base, within the muscles of the masticator space or perineurally, may pass through the skull base foramen, and can access the intracranial compartment (cavernous sinus).

The *buccal space* is bordered medially by the buccinator muscle and the outer cortex of the maxillary alveolar ridge, posteriorly by the masticator space, laterally by the parotid space, and anteriorly by the superficial muscles of facial expression (greater and lesser zygomaticus muscles and risorius) and the investing fascia. It does not have complete fascial coverings. Superiorly, the buccal fat blends imperceptibly into the fat of the temporal fossa. Inferiorly, there is no true boundary between the buccal space and the submandibular space. Posteriorly, there is often a direct communication between the medial buccal fat and the fat within the masticator space. The buccal space is composed primarily of adipose tissue. The other contents of the buccal space are the buccinator muscle, accessory parotid gland and minor salivary gland tissue, parotid duct, buccal lymph nodes, facial vein, facial and buccal artery, buccal branch of the facial nerve (CN VII), and buccal division of the mandibular nerve (CN V_3). The facial artery and vein lie just anterior to the buccal segment of the parotid duct, separating the buccal space into anterior and posterior compartments.

A mass lesion of the buccal space is centered within the fat of the space, adjacent to the outer surface of the buccinator muscle. It may displace the parotid duct posteriorly. Minor salivary gland tumors are the most common of primary buccal space masses, followed by venous malformations.

The *parotid space* is a paired lateral suprahyoid neck space, completely enclosed by the superficial layer of the deep cervical fascia. It is located posterolateral to the masticator space, posteriorly to the ramus of the mandible, extending from the external auditory canal above to the level of the mandibular angle below. The medial margin of the parotid space abuts the PPS. The posterior margin of the space relates to the carotid sheath vessels, the styloid process, and the posterior belly of the digastric muscle. The parotid space consists of the gland parenchyma, external carotid artery, retromandibular vein, extracranial facial nerve, intraparotid lymph nodes (~20), and parotid duct. The plane of the facial nerve, lateral to the retromandibular vein, divides the gland into a large superficial (about two thirds of the parotid space) and a deep lobe. The parotid tail is the most inferior aspect of the superficial lobe (inferior 2 cm of the gland). The parotid tail area is located deep and medial to the platysma, anterolateral to the sternocleidomastoid muscle, and posterolateral to the posterior belly of the digastric muscle, projecting into the posterior aspect of the submandibular space.

A mass is primary to the parotid space when the center of the lesion is within the parotid gland, lateral to the PPS. A larger, deep lobe parotid space mass displaces the PPS from lateral to medial with widening of the stylomandibular gap. A parotid space mass at the mandibular angle displaces the posterior belly of the digastric muscle medially. If perineural tumor is present, stylomastoid foramen fat will be replaced by tumor.

The oral cavity lies anterior to the oropharynx and below the sinonasal region. The oral cavity is separated from the oropharynx posteriorly by the circumvallate papillae, anterior tonsillar pillars, and soft palate. The oral mucosal space (OMS) lines the entire oral cavity, including the lips; buccal, gingival, and palatal surfaces; floor of the mouth (the semilunar mucosal surface overlying the mylohyoid and hyoglossus muscles); and the anterior two thirds of the oral tongue. No fascia exists to define the OMS. The retromolar trigone, a small region of mucosa behind the last molar on the mandibular ramus on both sides, is an anatomical crossroad of the oral cavity, oropharynx, soft palate, buccal space, masticator space, sublingual space, submandibular space, and PPS. The term *root of the tongue* is applied to the deep muscles (genioglossus and geniohyoid) of the oral tongue and the lingual septum. The mandible and maxilla are the defining bony margins of the oral cavity. Most masses in the oral cavity are amenable to direct clinical assessment. The vast majority of malignancies of OMS are squamous cell carcinomas, whereas minor salivary gland malignancies are relatively rare. Most infections of the oral cavity are dental in origin.

The *sublingual space* is a paired, nonfascial lined, fibrofatty space of the oral cavity within the oral tongue superomedial to the mylohyoid muscle, lateral to the genioglossus/geniohyoid muscles, and anterior to the lingual tonsil. It is a teacup-shaped space that is situated within the confines of the mylohyoid muscle below the tongue. Communication between sublingual spaces occurs in the midline superoranteriorly as a narrow isthmus beneath the frenulum. The sublingual space communicates freely with the submandibular space and the inferior PPS at the posterior margin of the mylohyoid muscle. The posterior aspect of the sublingual space is divided by the hypoglossal muscle into medial and lateral compartments. The lateral compartment contains the hypoglossal and lingual nerve, combined with the chorda tympani branch of the facial nerve, sublingual glands and ducts, deep portion of the submandibular gland, and submandibular duct. Normal occupants of the medial compartment are the glossopharyngeal nerve and lingual artery and vein.

A mass is confined to the sublingual space when the center of the lesion is superomedial to the mylohyoid muscle and lateral to the genioglossus muscle. Lesions may escape the sublingual space into the submandibular space at the posterior margin of the mylohyoid muscle or through a cleft of the mylohyoid muscle between its anterior one third and posterior two thirds. Larger lesions of the sublingual space may cross the anterior midline under the frenulum of the tongue and become bilobular. At times a lesion will be herniated from the posterior sublingual space into the adjacent cephalad submandibular space and low PPS. The most common lesions of the sublingual space include squamous cell carcinoma arising from the epithelial lining of the sublingual space, abscess formation from odontogenic infection, a variety of congenital/developmental lesions, ranula, and an obstructed submandibular duct.

The *submandibular space* is the most inferior space of the suprahyoid neck. It is a horseshoe-shaped, fascial-lined space located inferolaterally to the mylohyoid muscle sling and deep to the platysma muscle, below the mandible and superiorly to the hyoid bone. It continues inferiorly into the infrahyoid neck as anterior cervical space. The superficial layer of the deep cervical fascia splits to encircle the submandibular space, with the deeper slip of fascia running along the external surface of the mylohyoid muscle and a more shallow slip paralleling the deep margin of the platysma. There is no midline fascia separating the two sides of the submandibular space. No fascial separation

exists at the posterior margin of the mylohyoid muscle between the posterior submandibular and sublingual spaces and the inferior PPS. The principal contents of the submandibular space are the superficial portion of the submandibular gland, the submandibular and submental lymph nodes, the anterior belly of the digastric muscle, the facial vein and artery, and the inferior loop of the hypoglossal nerve and fat. The parotid gland tail may project into the posterior submandibular space.

A mass is primary to the submandibular space when its center is within the submandibular space inferolateral to the mylohyoid muscle. With rare exceptions, lesions of the submandibular space do not decompress into the sublingual space (in contrast to the tendency of large masses of the sublingual space to work their way into the submandibular space). Most lesions of the submandibular space are from either the submandibular gland or nodes. In children, the most common lesions are second branchial cleft cysts. In adults, the most common pathology of the submandibular space is metastatic lymph nodes from squamous cell carcinoma of the oral cavity.

There are few diseases that do not follow the spatial anatomical confinement or involve multiple spaces, either contiguously or noncontiguously. The term *transspatial* is applied to disease processes that involve multiple contiguous spaces of the neck (**Fig. 8.2**). Transspatial diseases can be divided into three broad categories: developmental lesions, infections, and tumors. Transspatial developmental lesions include thyroglossal duct cysts, branchial cleft cysts, infantile hemangioma, vascular malformations, and macrocystic lymphatic malformations. Transspatial infectious diseases include cellulitis and abscesses, as well as diving ranulas. Transspatial benign tumors include lipomas, schwannomas, neurofibromas, juvenile angiofibromas, and aggressive fibromatosis. Any malignant tumor of the neck (e.g., squamous cell carcinoma, both primary and metastatic, lymphoma, rhabdomyosarcoma, thyroid carcinoma, minor salivary gland malignancies, and melanoma), if large or aggressive enough, can be found in multiple contiguous spaces at presentation.

The term *multispatial* is applied to disease processes that involve multiple noncontiguous spaces of the neck. Multispatial diseases can be divided into nodal and nonnodal diseases

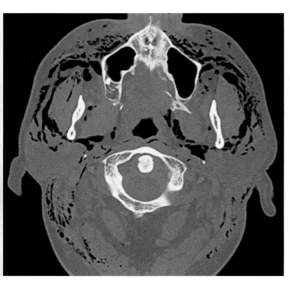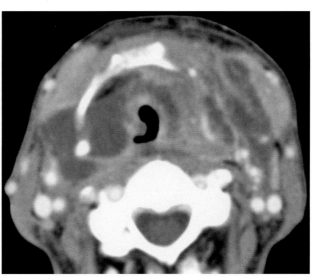

b

Fig. 8.2a, b   Transspatial disease. Axial bone computed tomography (CT) (**a**) reveals diffuse soft tissue emphysema with air in the subcutaneous layer of the skin and in every deep cervical space. Axial contrast-enhanced CT (**b**) shows necrotizing fasciitis of the neck with diffuse thickening of the skin, edema of the subcutaneous fat and platysma, and bilateral multiple fluid collections within the submandibular, visceral, retropharyngeal, and left carotid space.

(**Figs. 8.3, 8.4**). Multispatial nodal diseases include malignant adenopathy (lymph node metastases and lymphoma) and non-malignant inflammatory adenopathy (any upper respiratory infection, either viral or bacterial, with reactive adenopathy; less frequently, mononucleosis, tularemia, tuberculosis, cat scratch fever, sarcoidosis, human immunodeficiency virus, Castleman disease, and Kimura disease). Nonnodal multispatial diseases include neurofibromatosis and systemic metastases.

The *cervical lymph nodes* are arbitrarily grouped into levels I to VII (**Figs. 8.5, 8.6**). Level I includes all the nodes above the hyoid bone, below the mylohyoid muscles, and anterior to a transverse line drawn on each axial image through the posterior edge of the submandibular gland. Level IA represents the submental nodes that lie between the medial margins of the anterior bellies of the digastric muscles. Level IB represents the submandibular nodes that lie lateral and posterior to the medial edge of the anterior belly of the digastric muscle. Level II (upper jugular) nodes extend from the skull base to the lower body of the hyoid bone. They lie anterior to a transverse line drawn on each axial image through the posterior edge of the sternocleidomastoid muscle and posterior to a transverse line through the posterior edge of the submandibular gland. Level IIA nodes lie posterior to the internal jugular vein and are inseparable from the vein, or they lie anterior, medial, or lateral to the vein. Level IIB (upper spinal accessory) nodes lie posterior to the internal jugular vein with a fat plane separating the nodes and the vein. Retropharyngeal nodes, only present in suprahyoid neck, lie medial to the internal carotid artery. Level III (middle jugular) nodes lie between the level of the lower body of the hyoid bone and the lower margin of the cricoid cartilage. These nodes lie anterior to a transverse line drawn on each axial image through the posterior edge of the sternocleidomastoid muscle and lateral to the carotid arteries. Level IV (lower jugular) nodes lie between the level of the lower margin of the cricoid cartilage and the clavicle. These nodes lie anterior and medial to an oblique line drawn through the posterior edge of the sternocleidomastoid muscle and the posterolateral margin of the anterior scalene muscle

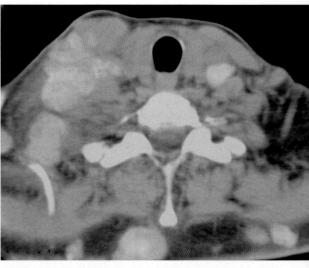

Fig. 8.4 Multispatial nonnodal disease. Axial non–contrast-enhanced CT shows bilateral, multiple nonnodal calcified hematogenous metastases (ovarian carcinoma) in noncontiguous spaces of the neck.

on each axial image. Level IV nodes lie lateral to the common carotid artery. Level V (posterior triangle) nodes extend from the skull base to the level of the clavicle. Level V nodes all lie anterior to a transverse line drawn through the anterior edge of the trapezius muscle. Above the bottom of the cricoid arch, level VA nodes lie posterior to a transverse line drawn on each axial image through the posterior edge of the sternocleidomastoid muscle. Below the bottom of the cricoid arch, level VB nodes lie posterior and lateral to an oblique line through the posterior edge of the sternocleidomastoid muscle and the lateral posterior edge of the anterior scalene muscle. Supraclavicular nodes are the low level IV or V nodes that are seen on the images that contain a portion of the clavicle. Level VI (anterior compartment or visceral) nodes lie inferior to the lower body of the hyoid

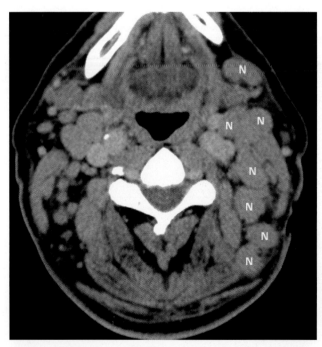

Fig. 8.3 Multispatial nodal disease. Axial contrast-enhanced CT demonstrates multiple nonnecrotic, well-circumscribed non–Hodgkin lymphoma nodes (N) in every level of the suprahyoid neck.

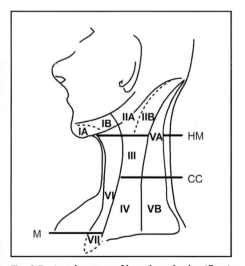

Fig. 8.5 Level system of lymph node classification. Level I nodes are submental (IA) and submandibular (IB) nodes, above the hyoid bone and below the mylohyoid muscle; level II nodes, upper deep cervical nodes; level III nodes, middle deep cervical nodes; level IV nodes, lower deep cervical nodes; level V nodes, spinal accessory and transverse cervical nodes; level VI nodes, prelaryngeal, pretracheal, and paratracheal nodes; level VII nodes, upper mediastinal nodes. CC: level of the lower margin of the cricoid cartilage arch; HM: level of the lower body of the hyoid bone; M: level of the top of the manubrium, separates levels VI and VII.

bone, superior to the top of the manubrium, and between the left and right carotid arteries. They include the juxtavisceral, anterior cervical, and external jugular nodes. Level VII (superior mediastinal) nodes lie caudal to the top of the manubrium in the superior mediastinum, between the left and right common carotid arteries. They extend caudally to the level of the innominate vein. Supraclavicular, retropharyngeal, parotid, facial, occipital, and postauricular nodal groups will still be referred to by their anatomical names.

A normal lymph node tends to be in the shape of a lima bean. The maximal diameter of a normal cervical lymph node varies from 3 to 11 mm; the greatest nodes are located in the submandibular and jugular digastric region. They are homogeneous, sharply delineated nodes, isodense to muscle with attenuation values from 40 to 50 Hounsfield units (HU), and enhancing slightly more than muscle on contrast-enhanced CT images. Fatty hilar metaplasia occurs almost exclusively at the periphery of the node as an area of low density. Cervical *nodal calcifications* are uncommon. In a child, metastatic neuroblastoma is the most common cause of calcified cervical lymph nodes. In adults, the most common cause of a calcified cervical lymph node is metastatic papillary thyroid carcinoma and scrofula. Other less

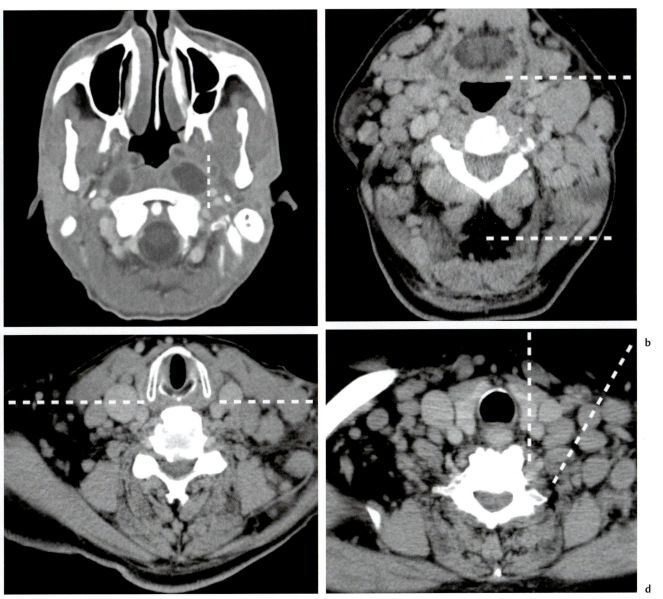

b

d

Fig. 8.6a–d The imaging-based nodal classification used on axial CT images. Axial contrast-enhanced CT (**a**) through the level of C1/C2 shows a sagittally oriented white line drawn along the medial edge of the internal carotid artery. Within 2 cm of the skull base, any node medial to this line is classified as a retropharyngeal node. A node lateral to this line is a level II node (tuberculous adenitis). Axial contrast-enhanced CT (**b**) just cranial to the hyoid bone shows a transverse white line through the posterior edge of each submandibular gland. The nodes anterior to this line are level I nodes. Nodes posterior to this line are level II nodes. Nodes posterior to the second transverse white line through the posterior edge of the sternocleidomastoid muscle are level V nodes (non–Hodgkin lymphoma). Axial contrast-enhanced CT (**c**) through the level of the glottis shows a transverse white line through the posterior edge of each sternocleidomastoid muscle. Nodes anterior to this line are level III, and nodes posterior to this line are level V nodes (non–Hodgkin lymphoma). Axial contrast-enhanced CT (**d**) through the thyroid gland reveals a vertical white line through the medial edge of the common carotid artery and an oblique white line through the posterior edge of the sternocleidomastoid muscle and the lateral posterior edge of the anterior scalene muscle. Nodes posterior to the oblique line are level V nodes, and nodes between the oblique and the vertical line are level IV nodes. Level VI nodes are medial to the vertical line between the common carotid arteries (non–Hodgkin lymphoma).

common causes of calcified lymph nodes are other nontubercular granulomatous infections, sarcoidosis, metastatic mucinous adenocarcinoma, and healed irradiated carcinomatous and lymphomatous nodes. Eggshell-type calcifications can occur in silicosis, sarcoidosis, tuberculosis, scleroderma, amyloidosis, sinus histiocytosis, and massive lymphadenopathy treated with interferon. *Cystic lymphadenopathy* is the term used to describe nodes completely replaced by material similar in density to water (0–20 HU) with a thin or imperceptible wall. Some cystic nodes have increased protein content resulting in higher attenuation on CT (> 20 HU). Cystic nodes are seen in metastatic

papillary thyroid carcinoma and in squamous cell cancer of the head and neck (base of the tongue and tonsil).

A space-specific differential diagnosis of pharyngeal mucosal space lesions as seen on CT is outlined in **Table 8.1**, of PPS lesions in **Table 8.2**, of masticator space lesions in **Table 8.3**, of parotid space lesions in **Table 8.4**, of suprahyoid carotid space lesions in **Table 8.5**, of suprahyoid RPS lesions in **Table 8.6**, of suprahyoid PVS lesions in **Table 8.7**, of lesions of the mucosal area of the oral cavity in **Table 8.8**, of submandibular space lesions in **Table 8.9**, of sublingual space lesions in **Table 8.10**, and of buccal space lesions in **Table 8.11**.

Table 8.1   Pharyngeal mucosal space lesions

Disease	CT Findings	Comments
Pseudomass		
Asymmetric lateral pharyngeal recess (fossa of Rosenmüller)	Unilaterally collapsed pharyngeal recess, inflammatory debris or fluid in the lateral pharyngeal recess, or asymmetric adenoid tissue may mimic a mass lesion. Maintenance of soft tissue planes in the adjacent parapharyngeal and retropharyngeal spaces strongly argues against a true mass lesion.	The lateral pharyngeal recess or fossa of Rosenmüller is the wide extent of the nasopharynx above the isthmus, located bilaterally just behind the opening of the auditory (eustachian) tube. A collapsed lateral pharyngeal recess can frequently be distended with the Valsalva maneuver, a modified Valsalva maneuver, or opening of the mouth widely.
Congenital/developmental lesions		
Tornwaldt cyst ▷ *Fig. 8.7*	Well-defined, round or ovoid, nonenhancing, fluid-filled, low-density mass with an imperceptible wall in the midline of the posterior nasopharyngeal wall between the longus capitis muscles without bone erosion. Size ranges from a few millimeters to 3 cm. Rare infected cyst may enhance peripherally.	Most common in young adults. Although usually asymptomatic, these cysts may become infected, giving rise to pain, halitosis, nasal discharge, and prevertebral muscle spasm. Differential diagnosis: Rathke pouch, a small epithelial cyst in the sphenoid body anterocephalad to Tornwaldt cyst. Uncommon and rare congenital cysts of the nasopharynx include transsphenoidal meningoencephalocele, neurenteric cyst, dermoid cyst, epidermoid cyst, cystic hamartoma, cystic teratoma, and extension of a second branchial cleft cyst or of a thymic cyst to the lateral pharyngeal wall.
Inflammatory/infectious conditions		
Adenoidal and tonsillar hyperplasia	Symmetric involvement of the lymphatic tissue in the nasopharynx and oropharynx with attenuation similar to that of muscle, usually associated with hypertrophic faucial tonsils and reactive retropharyngeal and cervical adenopathy. Lingual tonsillar hyperplasia may be very prominent.	Immunobiological overactivity results in hypertrophy of the lymphoepithelial tissue in the pharynx, most commonly the adenoid component, less commonly the faucial and lingual tonsils. Present in children and adolescents.
Tonsillitis, tonsillar (peritonsillar) abscess ▷ *Fig. 8.8*	*Tonsillitis* presents as nonspecific, uni- or bilaterally tonsillar enlargement, with heterogeneous contrast enhancement, consistent with early infection and edema, bulging into the airway. Inflammatory changes may extend into the soft palate, parapharyngeal space, and masticator space.	Acute tonsillitis may be caused by viral or bacterial infection. Beta-hemolytic *Streptococcus, Staphylococcus, Pneumococcus, Haemophilus,* and *Fusobacterium* are the most common organisms.

(continues on page 303)

Table 8.1 (Cont.) Pharyngeal mucosal space lesions

Disease	CT Findings	Comments
	Tonsillar abscess shows a swollen tonsil with central, uni- or multilocular low density and peripheral contrast-enhancing rim. When bilateral, tonsils may abut medially ("kissing tonsils"), obstructing the oropharyngeal airway. The abscess pocket is confined by the superior constrictor pharyngeal muscle to the pharyngeal mucosa space. No peritonsillar component is present. *Peritonsillar abscess* shows a pocket of fluid-like central areas of low attenuation within the enhancing cellulitic soft tissues of the peritonsillar area near the superior pole of the tonsil. When infection progresses, CT may show rupture of the abscess through the pharyngeal constrictor muscle into the parapharyngeal, masticator, and submandibular spaces. Most feared complication is extension of infection into the carotid space with septic thrombosis of the internal jugular vein or septic aneurysm of the carotid artery. Reactive bulky bilateral cervical adenopathy is common.	Usually occurs in children or young adults with sore throat and fever, followed by rapidly increasing painful swallowing, ear pain, and trismus. The disease is usually self-limited, but when it is severe, infection undergoes internal cavitations and suppuration, creating tonsillar or peritonsillar abscess. Peritonsillar abscess is the most common deep infection of the neck and chiefly involves patients between the ages of 10 and 40 y.
Tonsilloliths	Solitary or multiple calcifications in the tonsillar region, unilateral or bilateral, 1 to 7 mm in size or larger. Less commonly, calculi are seen in the adenoids or lingual tonsil.	Postinflammatory dystrophic calcifications within the tonsils exist in as much as 10% of the population (men < women, mean age 55 y). Phleboliths of a tonsillar venous malformation may simulate tonsillar calculi.
Postinflammatory mucus retention cyst	Well-defined, ovoid or pear-shaped, nonenhancing lesion of low (cystic) density in the nasopharynx, oropharynx, or vallecula, 1 to 2 cm, with no deep extension. Large cyst in the lateral pharyngeal recess may obstruct the eustachian tube, with resulting mastoid fluid.	Adult lesion. Usually an incidental finding. Rarely has any clinical significance. Nasopharyngeal pseudocysts have been postulated to be the result of a longus capitis perimyositis. Any of these cysts may become secondarily infected.

(continues on page 304)

II Head and Neck

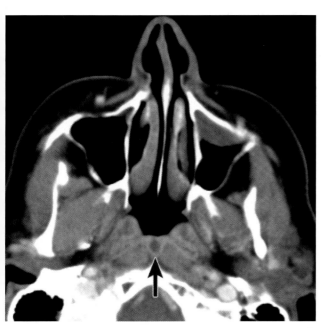

Fig. 8.7 Tornwaldt cyst. Axial contrast-enhanced CT shows a small midline cystic mass with ring enhancement in the posterior roof of the nasopharynx (arrow).

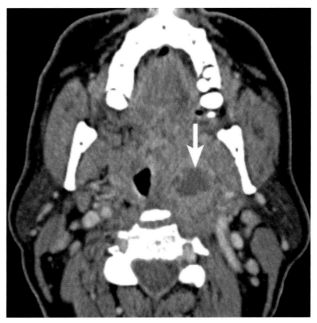

Fig. 8.8 Peritonsillar abscess. Axial contrast-enhanced CT demonstrates a swollen left tonsil and a peritonsillar fluid collection with central low density and a peripheral enhancing rim (arrow). Surrounding tissues are poorly defined. Oropharyngeal airway mass effect is present.

Table 8.1 (Cont.) Pharyngeal mucosal space lesions

Disease	CT Findings	Comments
Benign neoplasms		
Benign mixed tumor (pleomorphic adenoma)	Submucosal, exophytic or, when large, pedunculated, oval to round, well-circumscribed, moderate-enhancing soft tissue mass, isodense to surrounding mucosa and muscle, encroaching upon the nasopharyngeal, oropharyngeal, or oropalatal airway. It may appear inhomogeneous secondary to hemorrhage, calcification, and necrosis. If the tumor is adjacent to bone (e.g., hard palate), benign-appearing remodeling may be seen on CT.	Benign mixed tumors may arise in the minor salivary glands located in the submucosal layer of the pharyngeal mucosal space, palates (most common minor salivary gland site), or tongue base. Rarely multifocal. Symptoms are size and location dependent. Most common age of presentation: 30 to 60 (M:F = 1:2). Other benign growths in the pharynx are squamous papilloma, (vascular) polyps, vascular malformations, lymphatic malformations, ectopic pituitary adenoma, extension of pituitary adenoma, hamartoma, teratoma, developmental cysts, and pedunculated fibroma.
Malignant neoplasms		
Squamous cell carcinoma, nasopharynx ▷ *Fig. 8.9* ▷ *Fig. 8.10* ▷ *Fig. 8.11*	Usually large, polypoid or infiltrative, less-defined mass, isodense to muscle, with moderate contrast enhancement, most commonly arising from the lateral wall, including the fossa of Rosenmüller (82%), or from the midline (posterosuperior wall and inferior anterior wall of the nasopharynx) with asymmetrical thickening of the pharyngeal walls; tumor-caused deformity of the endopharyngeal contours, asymmetry of the fossa of Rosenmüller with blunting of the fossa, widening of the preoccipital soft tissue > 1.5 cm or nasopharyngeal soft tissue fullness. Nasopharyngeal carcinomas tend to grow via the mucosa or submucosa into the nasal cavity, oropharyngeal soft palate, and faucial tonsils. Because of its locally aggressive nature, nasopharyngeal cancer can penetrate the tough pharyngobasilar fascia and buccopharyngeal fascia with deep extension, loss of adjacent fat planes, and invasion into the parapharyngeal, masticator, carotid, and retropharyngeal space and prevertebral musculatures. Reactive increased sclerosis and destruction of the skull base usually occur directly over the tumor site, and extension through the skull base most often occurs via the foramen lacerum and the neural foramina of the middle cranial fossa floor. Perineural tumor spread primarily occurs after tumor has invaded the pterygopalatine fossa, foramen ovale, and hypoglossal canal. Further extension of tumor can involve the orbit, cavernous sinus, and even the brainstem. Nodal involvement may be extensive and bilateral. The nasopharyngeal carcinomas drain primarily into the lateral retropharyngeal lymph nodes and nodes of level II, followed by level V, level III, and the other cervical levels.	Malignant neoplasms of the nasopharynx include nasopharyngeal carcinomas (squamous cell carcinoma, low-grade papillary adenocarcinoma, other adenocarcinomas, and adenoid cystic carcinoma), non–Hodgkin lymphoma, Hodgkin lymphoma, Burkitt lymphoma, chloroma, extramedullary plasmocytoma, fibrosarcoma, carcinosarcoma, rhabdomyosarcoma, malignant schwannoma, liposarcoma, Kaposi sarcoma, mucosal melanoma, malignant fibrous histiocytoma, extraosseous chordoma, chondrosarcoma, and metastasis. Biopsy is the best way to establish diagnosis, as imaging cannot distinguish among malignancies of the nasopharynx. The overwhelming majority of nasopharyngeal malignancies are squamous cell carcinomas (80%) with varying degrees of cellular differentiation. Epstein–Barr virus, certain types of human leukocyte antigens (HLA), and salted fish and vegetables have a strong association. There is a demographic predilection among Chinese and North Africans. In the United States, it accounts for ~0.25% of all cancers, with a higher occurrence in men, usually over 40 y of age (there is an age peak among African Americans from 10 to 19 y old). A neck mass (due to jugular or spinal accessory lymphadenopathy) may be the first presenting symptom (at presentation, up to 90% of patients have regional nodal metastases, and at least 20% will have distant metastases). Tumor extension into the nasal cavity may present as epistaxis, nasal obstruction, or a nasal quality to the voice. Extension into the eustachian tube may present as hearing loss and serous otitis, whereas extension into the skull base with involvement of the cavernous sinuses may present as headache and cranial nerve palsies.

(continues on page 305)

Table 8.1 (Cont.) Pharyngeal mucosal space lesions

Disease	CT Findings	Comments
		Carcinoma of the nasopharynx: TNM classification **Primary tumor:** T1: Tumor confined to the nasopharynx or extends to soft tissue of oropharynx and/or nasal fossa T2: Tumor with parapharyngeal extension* T3: Tumor invades skull base and/or paranasal sinuses T4: Tumor with intracranial extension and/or involvement of cranial nerves, infratemporal fossa, masticator space, hypopharynx, or orbit **Regional lymph nodes:** N1: Unilateral cervical node(s): ≤ 6 cm in greatest dimension above supraclavicular fossa and/or retropharyngeal nodes N2: Bilateral node(s): ≤ 6 cm in greatest dimension above supraclavicular fossa N3a: Metastases in lymph node(s) > 6 cm in dimension N3b: Extension to the supraclavicular fossa **Distant metastasis:** M1: Distant metastasis *Parapharyngeal extension denotes posterolateral infiltration of tumor beyond the pharyngobasilar fascia.

(continues on page 306)

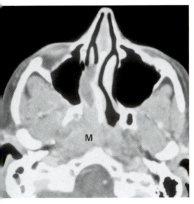

Fig. 8.9 Squamous cell carcinoma of the nasopharynx. Axial contrast-enhanced CT shows a large mass (M) filling the nasopharynx, intruding into the posterior nasal cavity, and invading the right parapharyngeal space.

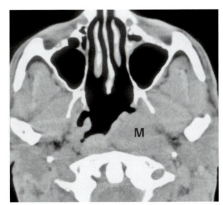

Fig. 8.10 Undifferentiated lymphoepithelial carcinoma (Schmincke–Regaud tumor). Axial non–contrast-enhanced CT reveals a mass (M) centered in the left lateral recess of the nasopharynx invading prevertebral muscles, the parapharyngeal space, and the masticator space.

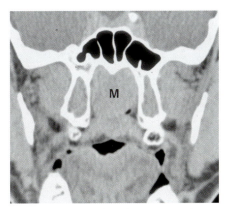

Fig. 8.11 Hodgkin lymphoma. Coronal reformatted, non–contrast-enhanced CT demonstrates a large, well-defined soft tissue mass (M) in the nasopharynx with no erosion of the skull base.

Table 8.1   (Cont.) Pharyngeal mucosal space lesions

Disease	CT Findings	Comments
Squamous cell carcinoma, oropharynx		**Clinical tumor stage of oropharyngeal carcinoma:** T1: Tumor $\leq$ 2 cm in its greatest dimension T2: Tumor $>$ 2 cm but $\leq$ 4 cm in its greatest dimension T3: Tumor $>$ 4 cm in its greatest dimension or extension to lingual surface of epiglottis T4a: Tumor invades the larynx, extrinsic muscles of the tongue, medial pterygoid, hard palate, or mandible T4b: Tumor invades lateral pterygoid muscle, pterygoid plates, lateral nasopharynx, or skull base, or encases carotid artery
	Squamous cell carcinoma of the base of the tongue Carcinoma of the base of the tongue is isodense to normal tongue muscle. Tumors are recognized as mucosal asymmetry, as mucosal-based exophytic lesion filling airway, by infiltration or obliteration of the normal fat planes of surrounding muscles, and by contrast enhancement of the tumor margins. Base of the tongue cancers may spread laterally into the mandible and medial pterygoid muscles; superiorly into the tonsillar fossa and soft palate; anteriorly into the mobile tongue and floor of the mouth; and inferiorly into the vallecula, pre-epiglottic space, and larynx or portions of the hypopharynx. The lingual tonsil carcinomas drain to nodes of level II, III, IV, and V.	Squamous cell carcinoma of the base of the tongue is an aggressive, deeply infiltrative tumor with a 75% incidence of lymph node metastases at presentation. Lesion is often asymptomatic until large in patients over 40 y of age (M > F) with a history of alcohol and tobacco use.
▷ *Fig. 8.12*	**Squamous cell carcinoma of the posterior pharyngeal wall** Carcinomas of the posterior pharyngeal wall commonly present as an enhancing flat, thick tumor of soft tissue density, spreading at the mucosal surface and often involving both the nasopharynx and the hypopharynx with irregular narrowing of the lumen. They spread submucosally, invading the pharyngeal constrictors and the retropharyngeal space. Deep invasion of the prevertebral muscles is unusual at initial presentation.	Carcinomas of the posterior pharyngeal wall have the worst prognosis of all oral cavity and oropharyngeal squamous cell carcinomas. Lesion is often asymptomatic until large in patients over 40 y of age (M > F) with a history of alcohol and tobacco use.

(continues on page 307)

Table 8.1 (Cont.) Pharyngeal mucosal space lesions

Disease	CT Findings	Comments
▷ *Fig. 8.13*	**Squamous cell carcinoma of the faucial tonsil** Cancers of the tonsillar fossa usually arise near the upper pole of the tonsil as an enhancing mass with invasive deep margins. They may extend posterolaterally to the lateral pharyngeal wall, parapharyngeal space, and pterygoid muscles; inferiorly to the glossotonsillar sulcus, base of the tongue, and floor of the mouth; superiorly to the soft palate and nasopharynx; and anteriorly and posteriorly to the tonsillar pillars. Cancers of the anterior tonsillar pillar tend to spread superiorly into the soft and hard palate, nasopharynx, pterygoid muscles, and skull base; anteriorly into the buccinator muscle; and inferiorly along the palatoglossus muscle into the base of the tongue. Cancers of the posterior tonsillar pillar tend to spread superiorly into the soft palate, posteriorly into the posterior pharyngeal wall, and inferiorly into the pharyngoepiglottic fold. Bone erosion and carotid artery encasement are present in advanced stages. Lymph node metastases occur primarily in the upper jugular or retropharyngeal nodes, but the spinal accessory and submandibular nodes are also at risk. Carcinomas of the tonsil tend to produce cystic metastases.	Carcinomas of the tonsil account for 1.5% to 3% of all cancers. They have an overall 70% chance of having clinically positive nodal metastases at initial presentation. Lesion is often asymptomatic until large in patients over 40 y of age (M > F) with a history of alcohol and tobacco use.

(continues on page 308)

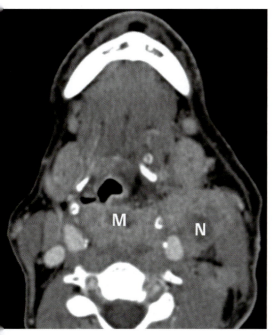

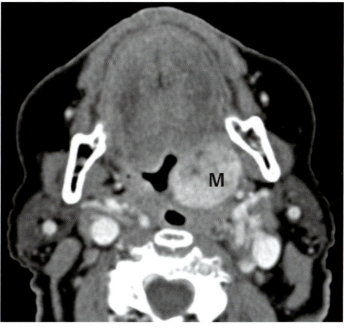

Fig. 8.12 Squamous cell carcinoma of the posterior pharyngeal wall. Axial contrast-enhanced CT shows a large, enhancing mass with central necrosis (M), arising from the posterior pharyngeal wall, filling the oropharynx, reaching the carotid sheath on both sides, without deep invasion. Also visible is an associated large, left level IIA necrotic metastatic node (N) with circumferential disease.

Fig. 8.13 Squamous cell carcinoma of the faucial tonsil. Axial contrast-enhanced CT reveals a large, intensely enhancing left tonsillar mass (M) with invasion of the adjacent lingual tonsil and parapharyngeal space.

II Head and Neck

Table 8.1   (Cont.) Pharyngeal mucosal space lesions

Disease	CT Findings	Comments
Non–Hodgkin lymphoma	Involvement of the lymphatic tissue in the nasopharynx and oropharynx with smoothly marginated, exophytic, bulky submucosal mass, with attenuation similar to that of muscle. Deep invasion and bone destruction are uncommon. Associated adenopathy may be nonnecrotic, often bulky, and may be in atypical locations. Rarely associated extra-nodal sites are sinonasal cavity, orbit, parotid gland, larynx, and thyroid gland.	Second most common pharyngeal mucosal space malignancy in the adult. Patients are usually older than 40 y and may present with an adenoidal or tonsillar mass, associated systemic symptoms (fever, malaise, and hepatospleno-megaly), and distant adenopathy (present in 50% of cases).
Minor salivary gland malignancy ▷ *Fig. 8.14*	Enhancing, well-circumscribed, smooth exophytic or irregular infiltrating pharyngeal mucosal space mass, often with deep exten-sion into adjacent deep facial spaces. Rarely, minor salivary gland malignancies have metastatic adenopathy at presentation.	Rare, aggressive tumors arising from minor salivary glands in the pharyngeal mucosal space (soft palate > sinonasal cavity > tongue > lin-gual tonsil). Histologically, these tumors include adenoid cystic carcinoma, adenocarcinoma, mucoepidermoid carcinoma, malignant mixed tumors, and acinic cell adenocarcinoma. More common in adult women, with submucosal, pain-ful pharyngeal wall mass. More invasive lesions can have cranial neuropathy (cranial nerve [CN] V_2, CN V_3).
Rhabdomyosarcoma	Bulky, heterogeneous, poorly marginated nasopharyngeal mass with variable, typically heterogeneous enhancement pattern. Associ-ated osseous destructive changes to the skull base or remodeling of bone can be present.	In children, rhabdomyosarcoma is the third most common malignancy in the head and neck, following brain tumors and retinoblastoma. Rhabdomyosarcomas comprise 4% to 8% of all malignant tumors in children younger than 15 y. Forty percent of rhabdomyosarcomas arise in the head and neck, with the orbit and nasopharynx most commonly involved, followed by the para-nasal sinuses and middle ear. In the oropharynx, the base of the tongue is the predilection site.

Table 8.2   Parapharyngeal space lesions

Disease	CT Findings	Comments
Pseudomass		
Asymmetric pterygoid venous plexus ▷ *Fig. 8.15*	Unilateral pterygoid venous plexus enlarge-ment with curvilinear contrast enhancement medial to pterygoid muscles and in the parapharyngeal space. Often seen on side of larger internal jugular vein. May be seen secondary to carotid-cavernous fistula.	Normal variant with unilateral prominence of an extensive network of small vascular channels in the medial masticator space and parapharyngeal space, draining the cavernous sinus and other in-tracranial venous channels (through the foramina ovale, spinale, lacerum, and foramen of Vesalius) and the deep facial vein to the maxillary vein. Usually asymptomatic; incidental CT or MRI find-ing may be mistaken for a focal vascular tumor.
Congenital/developmental lesions		
Atypical second branchial cleft cyst	Nonenhancing, thin, smooth-walled, round or ovoid mass of fluid attenuation values ex-tending from the deep margin of the faucial tonsil into the parapharyngeal fat toward the skull base and causing lateral pharyngeal wall displacement. When infected, the cyst wall may become thickened and irregular, the cyst content develops higher attenuation, and the sur-rounding fat planes may become obscured.	Although the most common location for a second branchial cleft cyst is the submandibular space, they can atypically present in the parapha-ryngeal space. Although congenital, the cysts most commonly present in young adults with parotid gland bulge, dysphagia, and vague neck discomfort, often after an upper respiratory tract infection.

(continues on page 310)

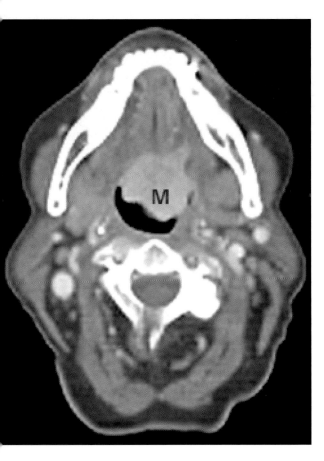

Fig. 8.14   Mucoepidermoid carcinoma of the base of the tongue. Axial contrast-enhanced CT demonstrates a midline large, enhancing mass (M) at the tongue base–lingual tonsil extending anteriorly to involve the left sublingual space and laterally to involve the glossotonsillar sulcus.

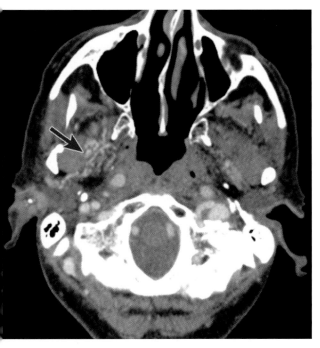

Fig. 8.15   Asymmetric pterygoid venous plexus. Axial contrast-enhanced CT demonstrates a unilateral prominent venous plexus in and around pterygoid muscles in the right masticator and parapharyngeal spaces (arrow).

Table 8.2   (Cont.) Parapharyngeal space lesions

Disease	CT Findings	Comments
Inflammatory/infectious conditions		
Parapharyngeal space infection ▷ *Fig. 8.16*	CT may show an inflammatory mass or abscess of the parapharyngeal space with expansion and medial displacement of the tonsil and lateral pharyngeal wall. **Cellulitis/phlegmon** may appear as a soft tissue mass, often ill defined and enhancing, with obliteration of the parapharyngeal fat and obscuration of the adjacent enlarged muscles and pharyngeal mucosal space structures. **Abscesses** may present as uniloculated or multiloculated masses with air or fluid attenuation centers. Thick, irregular enhancing wall suggests mature abscess. Potential complications constitute internal jugular vein thrombosis, cavernous sinus thrombosis, and arterial rupture and pseudo-aneurysm formation of the carotid arteries.	In the absence of penetrating trauma, a primary infectious process located in the pharynx, tonsils, adenoids, teeth, parotid gland, and paranasal sinuses may cause parapharyngeal space infection. Patients with parapharyngeal space infection are very sick, presenting with sudden onset of fever and chills. Trismus and CN IX to XII palsy and Horner syndrome may also be present.
Benign neoplasms		
Benign mixed tumor (pleomorphic adenoma) ▷ *Fig. 8.17*	Small tumors appear as sharply marginated, round or ovoid, isodense or hyperdense with parotid gland tissue, homogeneously mild to moderate enhancing mass centered within the parapharyngeal fat. Large tumors (> 2 cm) present as lobulated, well-circumscribed, inhomogeneously enhancing mass (in two-phase CT, these tumors present with an increase in attenuation during the second phase), with areas of low attenuation representing foci of necrosis, old hemorrhage, cysts, or fat. Focal areas of high-attenuation values represent dystrophic calcifications or ossifications in the tumor matrix. To diagnose an extraparotid origin, an intact fat plane between the tumor and the deep portion of the parotid gland must be clearly demonstrated.	Salivary gland tumors represent ~40% to 50% of parapharyngeal space masses (neurogenic tumors 17%–25%, paraganglioma ~10%). Benign mixed tumor is the most common salivary gland tumor. Benign mixed tumors in the parapharyngeal space commonly arise from the deep lobe of the parotid gland and extend into the parapharyngeal space through the stylomandibular tunnel. However, they can also arise from minor salivary glands of the pharyngeal mucosa or primarily within the parapharyngeal space from congenital rests of salivary gland tissue. Benign mixed tumors are typically seen in middle-aged women and present as a slowly growing painless mass, pushing a tonsil into the pharyngeal airway.
Lipoma	Well-defined, nonenhancing fat density mass (−65 to −125 HU), homogeneous without any internal soft tissue stranding. Liposarcoma may also be a concern if there is prominent internal stranding, enhancing nodularity, or inhomogeneity.	Uncommon lesions in the parapharyngeal space. Peak age of occurrence is 40 y and older (M:F = 2.5:1).
Malignant neoplasms		
Malignancies of salivary gland origin	Moderate enhancing soft tissue mass with irregular, ill-defined margins or infiltration of surrounding tissues. Differentiation from benign tumors may be difficult, as two thirds of salivary gland malignancies have smooth, well-defined margins.	Malignant tumors of the parapharyngeal space are much less common than benign lesions and include malignant lesions of salivary gland origin (especially mucoepidermoid carcinoma, adenoid cystic carcinoma, and acinic cell carcinoma), along with direct invasion of malignancies of the adjacent spaces.

(continues on page 311)

Table 8.2   (Cont.) Parapharyngeal space lesions

Disease	CT Findings	Comments
Contiguous tumor extension	Obliteration of the parapharyngeal fat due to an infiltrating soft tissue mass with its center in the pharyngeal mucosal space (squamous cell carcinoma, non–Hodgkin lymphoma, and minor salivary gland malignancy); in the masticator space (e.g., sarcoma of the mandible or surrounding soft tissues and malignant neurogenic lesion); in the parotid space (e.g., mucoepidermoid carcinoma and adenoid cystic carcinoma); and in the submandibular space (squamous cell carcinoma of the oral cavity) or the skull base (metastatic disease).	Direct spread of malignant tumor from adjacent deep facial space: these malignant tumors break out of their space of origin and invade the parapharyngeal space.

II Head and Neck

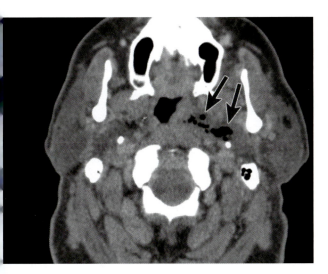

Fig. 8.16   Parapharyngeal abscess. Axial contrast-enhanced CT shows an inhomogeneous, multilocular gas collection (arrows) within the left parapharyngeal space with perifocal edema. Nasopharyngeal airway mass effect is present.

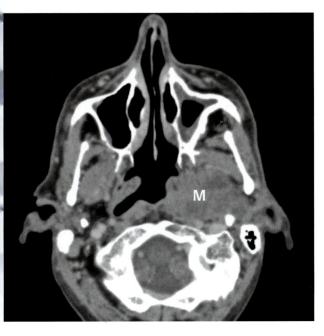

Fig. 8.17   Benign mixed tumor. Axial contrast-enhanced CT reveals a large, lobulated, inhomogeneously enhancing mass (M) centered within the left parapharyngeal space, pushing the pharyngeal mucosal space medially, the left medial pterygoid muscle superolaterally, and the carotid artery posteriorly. The left stylomandibular notch is widened. No intact fat plane can be demonstrated between the tumor and the deep lobe of the parotid gland (the left parotid gland was compressed and displaced with no connection to the mass at surgery).

Table 8.3   Masticator space lesions

Disease	CT Findings	Comments
Pseudomass		
Asymmetric pterygoid venous plexus	Unilateral pterygoid venous plexus enlargement with curvilinear contrast enhancement medial to pterygoid muscles and in the parapharyngeal space. Often seen on side of larger internal jugular vein. May be seen secondary to carotid-cavernous fistula.	Normal variant with unilateral prominence of an extensive network of small vascular channels in the medial masticator space and parapharyngeal space, draining above the cavernous sinus and other intracranial venous channels (through the foramina ovale, spinale, lacerum, and foramen of Vesalius) and the deep facial vein to the maxillary vein. Usually asymptomatic; incidental CT or MRI finding may be mistaken for a focal vascular tumor.
Benign masticator muscle hypertrophy	Unilateral or bilateral diffuse, homogeneous enlargement of masticator muscles. The masseter muscle is most obviously affected. Enlarged muscles are isodense to normal skeletal muscles and enhance normally. Cortical thickening affecting mandible and zygomatic arch may be observed, or a rough bony projection of cortical bone along the anterior surface of the mandible at the site of the masseter insertion; also, normally preserved fascial and soft tissue planes.	Presents as nontender lateral facial mass; may be familial. Acquired form is usually secondary to nocturnal teeth clenching. Temporomandibular joint (TMJ) dysfunction or malocclusion may also contribute.
CN V₃ denervation atrophy	Most frequently unilateral. CT is relatively insensitive to acute and subacute denervation changes. Long-standing chronic denervation is manifested by marked loss of volume and extensive fatty replacement of the affected muscles of mastication. Ipsilateral asymmetry of the torus tubarius and fluid in the mastoid cells due to tensor veli palatini denervation and eustachian tube dysfunction are additional findings. Contralateral masticator muscle atrophy makes normal masticator space appear hypertrophic.	Damage to the mandibular nerve may be seen with malignant or benign tumors involving the third division of the trigeminal nerve, after surgery and trauma, and with infection; more common in adults due to prevalence of head and neck tumors and surgery. If all muscles innervated by mandibular nerve are involved (medial and lateral pterygoid, masseter, temporalis, tensor veli palatini, mylohyoid, and anterior belly of digastric muscle), then lesion is between root exit zone of lateral pons and foramen ovale. If only mylohyoid and anterior belly digastric muscle are involved, lesion is between the skull base and mandibular foramen.
Congenital/developmental lesions		
Infantile hemangioma (capillary hemangioma)	Solitary, multifocal, or transspatial, lobular cervicofacial soft tissue mass, homogeneous and isodense with muscle. Contrast enhancement is uniform and intense. No calcifications. Can be very large, occupying, filling, and expanding the masticator space. Commonly involves the masseter muscle. Bony deformity or skeletal hypertrophy may be associated with infantile hemangioma, but intraosseous invasion is extremely uncommon. Size, enhancement, and vascularity of tumor regress in involutional phase with internal, low-density fat.	Most common infant tumors; typically present in early infancy with rapid growth and ultimately involute via fatty replacement by adolescence. Infantile hemangiomas are high-flow lesions during their proliferative phase, low-flow lesions in their involutional phase. Sixty percent of infantile hemangiomas occur in head and neck, with superficial strawberry-colored lesions and facial swelling and/or deep lesions, often in parotid, masticator, and buccal spaces. Retropharyngeal, sublingual, and submandibular spaces, along with oral mucosa, are other common locations.
Venous vascular malformation (cavernous hemangioma)	Extraparotid, lobulated or poorly marginated soft tissue mass, isodense to muscle, with rounded calcifications (phleboliths). May be superficial or deep, localized or diffuse, solitary or multifocal, circumscribed or transspatial, with or without satellite lesions. Contrast enhancement is patchy or homogeneous and intense. Bony deformity of the adjacent mandible or posterolateral wall of the maxillary antrum may occur, as well as fat hypertrophy in adjacent soft tissues.	Venous vascular malformations are congenital low-flow, nontumorous vascular malformations, have an equal gender incidence, may not become clinically apparent until late infancy or childhood, virtually always grow in size with the patient during childhood, and do not involute spontaneously. Most are found in the buccal region. Masticator space, sublingual space, tongue, orbit, and dorsal neck are other common locations. Frequently, venous malformations do not respect fascial boundaries and commonly involve more than one deep fascial space. They are soft and compressible. Lesion may increase in size with Valsalva maneuver, bending over, or crying. Swelling and enlargement can occur following trauma or hormonal changes (e.g., pregnancy). Pain is common and often caused by thrombosis.

(continues on page 313)

Table 8.3   (Cont.) Masticator space lesions

Disease	CT Findings	Comments
Lymphatic malformation (lymphangioma, cystic hygroma)	Uni- or multiloculated, nonenhancing, fluid-filled low-density mass with imperceptible wall, which tends to invaginate between normal structures. Often found in multiple contiguous cervical spaces (transspatial). Rapid enlargement of the lesion, areas of high attenuation values and fluid–fluid levels suggest prior hemorrhage. Lymphatic and venous malformation may coexist.	Lymphatic malformations represent a spectrum of congenital low-flow vascular malformations, differentiated by size of dilated lymphatic channels. Macrocystic lymphatic malformation is the most common subtype. Sixty-five percent are present at birth; 90% are clinically apparent by 3 y of age. The remaining 10% present in young adults. In the suprahyoid neck, the masticator and submandibular spaces are the most common locations. May be sporadic or part of congenital syndromes (e.g., Turner, Noonan, and fetal alcohol syndromes).
Inflammatory/infectious conditions		
Masticator space infection ▷ *Fig. 8.18* ▷ *Fig. 8.19*	**Cellulitis/phlegmon** of the masticator space may appear as a soft tissue mass, often ill-defined, with swollen enhancing masticator muscles and obliteration of fat planes. The parapharyngeal space may be compressed posteromedially by edematous medial pterygoid muscle. Overlying subcutaneous tissues often demonstrate linear stranding or mottled increased attenuation beneath thickened skin. **Abscesses** may present as uniloculated or multiloculated, ovoid to round mass with air or fluid attenuation centers. A thick, irregular enhancing wall suggests mature abscess. Surrounding tissues are edematous. Masticator space infection may be accompanied by mandibular osteomyelitis and airway encroachment. Infection may spread into the suprazygomatic and nasopharyngeal masticator spaces, causing osteomyelitis of the skull base, or extend inferiorly into the floor of the mouth and upper neck.	Masticator space infection originates most commonly from second or third molar tooth infection (parodontal or periapical abscess in the mandible that may demonstrate signs of osteomyelitis) or following dental procedure. Masticator space cellulitis and abscess formation may also occur as a complication of mandibular or zygomatic arch fractures, especially when treated with internal fixation. Infection may also extend to the masticator space from adjacent areas in the neck. Odontogenic abscess is the most common lesion of the masticator space. Painful jaw swelling, fever, trismus, induration over the angle and ramus of the mandible, and elevated white blood cell count (WBC) are often present.

(continues on page 314)

II Head and Neck

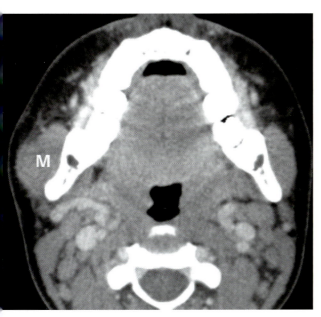

Fig. 8.18   Masseteric myositis. Axial contrast-enhanced CT shows an enlarged right masseter muscle (M) with subtle, homogeneous enhancement. Linear markings are visible in the adjacent subcutaneous and buccal fat.

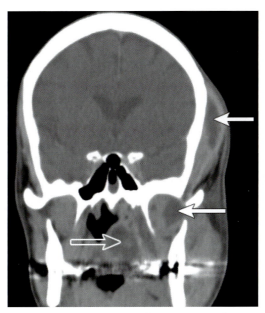

Fig. 8.19   Masticator space abscesses. Coronal reformatted, contrast-enhanced CT depicts focal fluid densities with an enhancing rim within the masticator muscles of the left supra- and infrazygomatic space (arrows) arising from a parapharyngeal space abscess (open arrow). (Courtesy of Dr. N. Stahr, Winterthur.)

Table 8.3   (Cont.) Masticator space lesions

Disease	CT Findings	Comments
Mandibular osteomyelitis ▷ *Fig. 8.20*	CT findings include periosteal new bone formation, localized cortical breakdown associated with increased attenuation within the medullary cavity and poorly defined lucencies within the bone, often accompanied by extension of infection into the adjacent spaces with sinus tracts, myositis, fasciitis, cellulitis, and abscess formation. In long-standing infection, bony sequestra and sclerosis may be seen.	Acute osteomyelitis of the mandible most often results from tooth infection, less often from adjacent deep space infection, from dental manipulation, following surgical procedures or penetrating trauma.

Benign neoplasms

Disease	CT Findings	Comments
Ameloblastoma ▷ *Fig. 8.21* ▷ *Fig. 8.22*	Expansile, unilocular or "bubbly," multilocular, mixed cystic-solid mass emanating from the molar/ramous area of the mandible or from the premolar/first molar region of the maxilla with scalloped borders. May have a honeycombed appearance with bony septa. A matrix calcification is rare with the exception of desmoplastic ameloblastoma. An unerupted molar tooth association and resorption of adjacent teeth are common. The lesion often demonstrates marked expansion with thinned or imperceptible cortical shell. Larger lesions with extraosseous extension show extensive soft tissue enhancement mixed with cystic low-density areas.	Most common odontogenic and benign mandibular tumor. Mandible:maxilla ratio = 5:1. Most commonly manifests from age 30 to 50 y (M = F) with a slow-growing painless mass of the affected area. High recurrence rate (33%); malignant transformation is rare (1%). Other benign expansile mandibular masses include odontogenic keratocyst, dentigerous cyst, giant cell reparative granuloma, brown tumor, giant cell tumor, aneurysmal bone cyst, hemangioma, cystic fibrous dysplasia, and ossifying fibroma.
Schwannoma	Sharply and smoothly marginated, ovoid to fusiform, homogeneous soft tissue mass along the course of the mandibular division of the trigeminal nerve, isodense to hypodense relative to muscle, with variable, often intense contrast enhancement. Large tumors may undergo cystic degeneration and present with central unenhancing and peripheral enhancing areas. Calcifications are exceptional. Smooth, corticated enlargement of the bony foramen and canal involved are typical of change from V_3 schwannoma.	Schwannomas of the masticator space are usually of mandibular nerve origin (CN V_3) and may be located anywhere along its extracranial course. However, involvement of the mandibular nerve is rare. Schwannomas more rarely affect CN V_3 branches, including inferior alveolar and mental nerves. Can be multifocal in patients with neurofibromatosis type 2; occurs in patients in their 30s to 40s. Even large lesions may be asymptomatic. Long-standing chronic denervation is manifested by marked loss of volume and extensive fatty replacement of the affected muscles of mastication.
Neurofibroma	**Solitary neurofibroma:** Fusiform, ovoid or tubular sharply circumscribed mass, isodense to hypodense relative to cervical cord, smooth and surrounded by fat planes. Differs from schwannoma by an overall lower density that may approach water and conspicuous absence of contrast enhancement. Rarely undergoes cystic degeneration. **Plexiform neurofibroma:** Usually large, diffuse, ill-defined, lobulated, multinodular, low-density mass involving multiple cervical compartments (transspatial), including the masticator space. A typical sign is the target sign with central punctate enhancement surrounded by peripheral low attenuation within multiple tumor nodules. Neurofibromas observed in von Recklinghausen disease characteristically occur at multiple sites and are often confluent, multiple, or plexiform.	About 50% of all neurofibroma cases are sporadic, ~50% are associated with neurofibromatosis type 1. Neurofibromas of the masticator space arise from the inferior alveolar nerve, mylohyoid branch, or masticator nerve branch of the mandibular division of the trigeminal nerve (CN V_3). Can occur at any age, with average 35 y (female predominance). These neoplasms grow slowly and are painless. Two to 6% of lesions in neurofibromatosis type 1 may undergo malignant transformation.
Aggressive fibromatosis (extra-abdominal desmoid fibromatosis, juvenile fibromatosis)	"Malignant-appearing," poorly marginated inhomogeneously enhancing transspatial soft tissue mass with local invasion of muscle, vessels, nerves, and bone. Most common locations are perivertebral space, supraclavicular area, and masticator space.	Benign soft tissue tumor of fibroblastic origin arising from aponeurotic neck structures. Associated abnormality: Gardner syndrome. Seen at all ages (70% younger than 35 y). Significantly more women affected. Patients present with firm, painless neck mass. Paresis depends on site. Postoperative recurrence rate may reach 25%.

(continues on page 316)

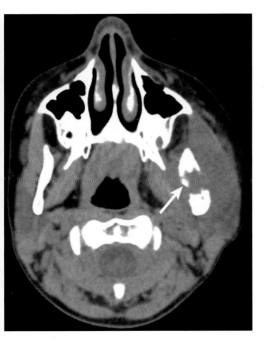

Fig. 8.20   Mandibular osteomyelitis. Axial non–contrast-enhanced CT demonstrates a lytic lesion of the left mandibular ramus with sequestrum (arrow), marked swelling of the left masseter and medial pterygoid muscle, involvement of the left parotid space, and perifocal edema.

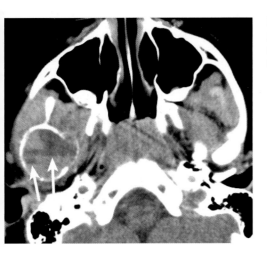

Fig. 8.21   Aneurysmal bone cyst. Axial non–contrast-enhanced CT reveals a markedly expansile osteolytic lesion of the right condylar process with well-defined scalloped margins and fluid–fluid levels (arrows). The muscles of the masticator space are displaced away.

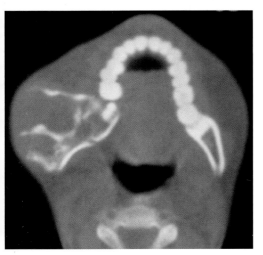

Fig. 8.22   Hemangioma. Axial non–contrast-enhanced CT shows an extensive expansile multicystic, septated, osteolytic lesion in the ramus of the right mandible. The cortex is thinned, expanded, and disrupted.

Table 8.3   (Cont.) Masticator space lesions

Disease	CT Findings	Comments
Malignant neoplasms		
Contiguous tumor extension	Invasive masticator space mass, often demonstrating cortical erosion or destruction of the adjacent mandible.	Invasion of the masticator space is usually a late manifestation of carcinoma of the oral cavity, oropharynx, paranasal sinuses, nasopharynx, external auditory canal, or salivary gland. Squamous cell carcinoma and adenoid cystic carcinoma may enter the masticator space by direct extension from the faucial tonsil or retromolar trigone, by way of direct mandibular invasion from the floor of the mouth, or via perineural tumor spread along the mandibular and lingual nerves, which originate from the mandibular division of the trigeminal nerve.
Sarcomas	Sarcomas of the masticator space present as often large, poorly marginated, heterogeneous masses with intermediate attenuation values and variable, heterogeneous contrast enhancement. Bone production or calcifications are most commonly seen in osteosarcoma, chondrosarcoma, synovial sarcoma, and Ewing sarcoma. Bone fragments within tumors can be present in any masticator space sarcoma with extensive bone destruction of the mandibular, zygomatic arch, or pterygoid plate. There may be invasion of adjacent fascial planes and spaces. Masticator space sarcomas can spread by direct extension into the middle cranial fossa or into the pterygopalatine fossa. Perineural tumor spread on CN V_3 can occur anywhere along its course with enhancement of the enlarged nerve, obscuration of the fat planes around the nerve, and enlargement of its foramen or canal.	Primary malignant tumors of the masticator space are uncommon. They include sarcomas of the mandible or surrounding soft tissues and malignant neurogenic lesions. Chondrosarcoma arises from the TMJ and jaws. Soft tissue extension of osteosarcomas involves the masticator space when the angle, ramus, or condyle is the primary site of involvement. The most common masticator space sarcoma in the pediatric population is a rhabdomyosarcoma (first and second decades, rare in adults).
Malignant schwannoma	Tubular mass along the course of the mandibular division of the trigeminal nerve and its primary branches within the masticator space. Extension through the enlarged foramen ovale to involve the gasserian ganglion is not uncommon with this lesion.	Malignant nerve sheath tumors arising from the mandibular division of the trigeminal nerve are rare.
Non–Hodgkin lymphoma	Ill-defined and infiltrative masticator space mass, isolated or associated with nodal disease, extranodal lymphatic disease (Waldeyer ring), and/or involvement of other extranodal, extralymphatic sites (e.g., sinus, nose, and orbit).	Patients may have CN V_3 symptoms and masticator space mass as part of systemic non–Hodgkin lymphoma or as the first manifestation of limited head and neck disease.
Mandibular metastases ▷ *Fig. 8.23*	Metastases typically manifest as ill-defined mandibular destructive soft tissue attenuating masses, often with extension into surrounding tissues. The posterior body and angle are most commonly affected. Some blastic lesions, such as prostate metastasis, may occur.	Metastases to the mandible are four times more common than to the maxilla. However, metastasis to the mandible is uncommon. Usually occurs as a multifocal disease in the setting of known primary tumor (breast, lung, renal, or prostate cancer). Metastases may be asymptomatic or may cause pain and CN V_3 numbness.
Metabolic disorder		
Calcium pyrophosphate dihydrate deposition disease ▷ *Fig. 8.24*	CT usually demonstrates fine irregular and linear periarticular and intra-articular calcifications (chondrocalcinosis) with degenerative changes of the joint (metabolic arthritis). Tumorous calcified collections with mass effect or destruction of the temporal bone and mandibular condyle are occasionally observed in the TMJ.	Metabolic arthritis, which can accompany calcium pyrophosphate dihydrate deposition disease ("pseudogout"), is rare in the TMJ. Men and women older than 50 y are equally affected. Symptoms related to TMJ involvement are sudden attacks with pain, joint swelling, trismus, abnormal occlusion, and conductive hearing loss. Other crystal-associated arthropathies are gout, calcium hydroxyapatite crystal deposition disease, and chronic renal failure.

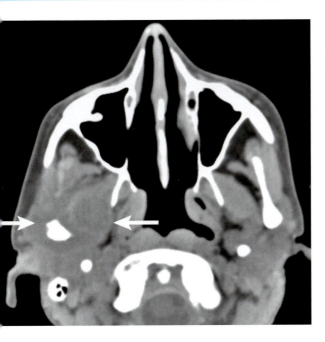

Fig. 8.23 Metastatic disease (rectal carcinoma). Axial non–contrast-enhanced CT demonstrates a lytic lesion of the right condylar process with widespread soft tissue mass extension (arrows), hypodense to normal muscle, into the masticator space.

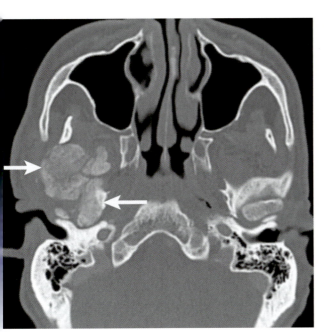

Fig. 8.24 Calcium pyrophosphate dihydrate deposition disease. Axial bone CT shows large calcified masses (arrows) centered within the right glenoid fossa bulging into the masticator space. Note the absence of the destructed right mandibular condyle.

II **Head and Neck**

Table 8.4 Parotid space lesions

Disease	CT Findings	Comments
Congenital/developmental lesions		
First branchial cleft cyst ▷ *Fig. 8.25*	Well-defined, unilocular, ovoid to round, nonenhancing or rim-enhancing fluid attenuation mass located periauricular (anterior, below, or posterior to pinna [type I]) or immediate periparotid (superficial, parotid, and parapharyngeal spaces [type II]); may have a direct connection with the external auditory canal. If infected, the wall may thicken and enhance, and the cyst content develops higher attenuation.	First branchial cleft cysts are very rare (only 8% of all branchial cleft remnants). Both children and adults may be affected. Most commonly seen in middle-aged women with recurrent abscesses around the ear or at the angle of the mandible; unresponsive to treatment. May be associated with branchial cleft fistula or sinus. Otorrhea commonly occurs if the cyst drains into the external auditory canal.
Infantile hemangioma (capillary hemangioma)	Solitary, multifocal or transspatial, lobular soft tissue mass, homogeneous and isodense with muscle. No calcifications. Infantile hemangiomas can be well circumscribed, replacing the parotid gland, or can be infiltrative and might involve periparotid structures. Contrast enhancement is uniform and intense. Size, enhancement, and vascularity of tumor regress in involutional phase with internal, low-density fat.	By far the most common parotid gland lesion in the first year of life. A cutaneous hemangioma may also be found overlying the parotid region as an associated finding. True capillary hemangiomas are neoplastic conditions; typically display a rapid proliferation phase during the first year of life followed by an involution phase with fatty replacement. Occur predominantly in girls. Infantile hemangiomas are high-flow lesions during their proliferative phase, low-flow lesions in their involutional phase. Hemangiomas may enlarge rapidly due to bleeding within.
Lymphatic malformation (lymphangioma, cystic hygroma) ▷ *Fig. 8.26*	Lymphatic malformations can involve the parotid gland directly or by local extension. Tend to appear as cystic masses filled with homogeneous low-attenuation material and without contrast enhancement. Cysts usually have thin walls, and most commonly there are multiple intercommunicating cystic components. Infected lesions show higher attenuation, an enhanced thickening of the cyst wall, and infiltration of the adjacent soft tissues. In the case of hemorrhage, fluid–fluid levels may be observed.	Lymphatic malformations represent a spectrum of congenital low-flow vascular malformations, differentiated by size of dilated lymphatic channels. May be sporadic or part of congenital syndromes (Turner, Noonan, and fetal alcohol syndrome). Macrocystic lymphatic malformation is the most common subtype. Sixty-five percent are present at birth; 90% are clinically apparent by 3 y of age, with the remaining 10% present in young adults. In children, the most common location is the posterior cervical space, followed by the oral cavity. In adults, lymphatic malformations are rare, may be posttraumatic, and are more commonly seen in the sublingual, submandibular, and parotid spaces. Often found in multiple contiguous spaces (transspatial). Other cystic lesions of the parotid gland are sialoceles and dermoid, epidermoid, mucus retention and sebaceous cysts.
Polycystic disease of the parotid glands	Bilateral, markedly enlarged parotid glands with small areas of decreased density producing a mildly inhomogeneous appearance.	Rare inherited familial disorder, affecting predominantly women (gender linked?) with bilateral, enlarged, nontender parotid swelling, due to multiple cystic areas replacing the parenchyma, present for months or years. Hormonal changes (e.g., during pregnancy) may cause expression or exacerbation.
Inflammatory/infectious conditions		
		Acute viral, bacterial, and calculus-induced parotitis are the most common salivary gland abnormalities.
Acute viral parotitis	Usually bilateral. The involved parotid glands are somewhat enlarged, dense, and enhance slightly. Submandibular and sublingual glands may also be involved.	Mumps is the most frequent acute viral infection of the parotid glands. Other viral etiologies are *Coxsackie viruses, parainfluenza viruses, influenza virus type A, herpes virus, echovirus,* and *choriomeningitis virus.* Viral infection is associated with systemic infection.
Acute suppurative parotitis and abscess	Usually unilateral. Diffuse swollen, enhancing parotid gland with focal area of rim-enhancing fluid attenuation. The parotid duct may be dilated with or without calculus. There are secondary inflammatory changes in the overlying subcutaneous fat and skin. Intraparotid and periparotid lymph nodes may be involved in the inflammatory reaction. The abscess may extend into the masticator and parapharyngeal spaces or upper neck.	Bacterial infection with unilateral cheek swelling associated with fever, chills, and elevated WBC. Most common bacterial organisms are *Staphylococcus aureus* (50%–90%), *Streptococcus viridans, Haemophilus influenzae, Escherichia coli, anerobes,* and *Streptococcus pneumoniae.*

(continues on page 319)

Table 8.4   (Cont.) Parotid space lesions

Disease	CT Findings	Comments
Benign lymphoepithelial lesions (BLLs) of human immunodeficiency virus	Usually bilateral parotid gland enlargement with multiple, predominantly superficial intraglandular masses with a homogeneous cystic appearance, hypodense (10–25 HU) with thin rims of enhancement, varying in size from a few millimeters to several centimeters (rare). Intraparotid lymph nodes may also be enlarged. Often with coexistent diffuse homogeneous cervical lymphadenopathy and adenoidal, faucial, and lingual tonsillar hypertrophy. No calculi are identified in the glands or ducts.	Lymphoepithelial cysts in the parotid gland may be secondary to incomplete ductal obstruction by periductal lymphocytic infiltration or arise within the intraparotid lymph nodes. Occurs with painless facial swelling in HIV-positive patients (CD4 level usually below 500/mL) and may be the first manifestation of the infection.
Chronic recurrent parotitis	Unilateral, diffusely enlarged parotid gland, often slightly denser than normal, with or without dystrophic calcifications. Cystic changes in the gland and dilated Stensen duct with or without calculi may be evident. Irregular intraglandular sialectasis can only be appreciated on CT sialogram. Chronic inflammatory disease of the salivary glands can result in loss of parenchymal as well as fatty matrix and consequent shrinkage of the gland.	Strictures, calculi, or both within the main salivary gland duct may result in chronic sialodochitis and sialadenitis. Chronic recurrent sialadenitis is clinically characterized by recurrent diffuse or localized painful swelling of the salivary gland.
Granulomatous parotitis ▷ **Fig. 8.27**	Unilateral or, less commonly, bilateral diffuse enlargement of the parotid gland, with multiple small nodular "foamy" densities distributed throughout the gland or a solitary mass. There is often an associated cervical lymphadenopathy.	The granulomatous diseases that may involve the major salivary glands include sarcoidosis, tuberculosis, atypical mycobacterial infection, syphilis, cat scratch fever, toxoplasmosis, and actinomycosis. These diseases may affect the intraparotid or juxtaglandular lymph nodes or the gland parenchyma directly. Presents usually as a nontender, painless, chronic enlargement of the gland.

(continues on page 320)

II   Head and Neck

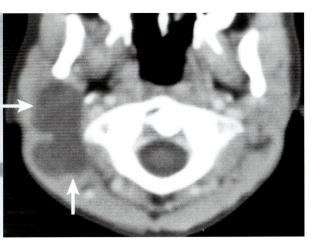

Fig. 8.25   First branchial cleft cyst (type II). Axial contrast-enhanced CT shows a well-defined, bilobed, nonenhancing, fluid attenuation mass (arrows) in the right parotid space.

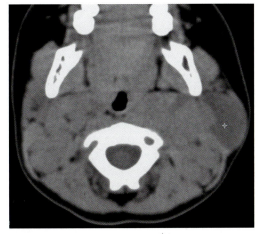

Fig. 8.26   Lymphatic malformation. Axial non–contrast-enhanced CT reveals a cystic mass with thin walls filled with homogeneous low-attenuation material in the left parotid space (joystick point).

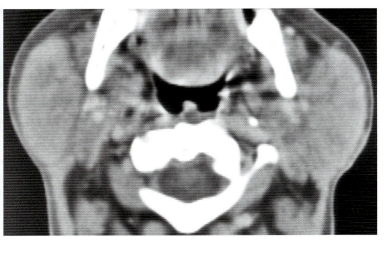

Fig. 8.27   Granulomatous parotitis (sarcoidosis). Axial contrast-enhanced CT reveals bilateral diffuse parotid enlargement and slight heterogeneity with multiple small nodular densities.

Table 8.4 (Cont.) Parotid space lesions

Disease	CT Findings	Comments
Sjögren syndrome	In the early stage of disease, CT demonstrates nonspecific enlargement of the parotid glands. In later stages, CT may demonstrate an increased density of the glands, a tiny honeycomb glandular appearance, or an inhomogeneous pattern with cysts, solid nodules, and premature fat depositions with heterogeneous enhancement and punctate calcifications. There is no diffuse cervical lympadenopathy. Parotid sialogram reveals a normal central duct system and numerous globular collections of contrast material, 1 to 3 mm in diameter, uniformly scattered throughout the gland.	Sjögren syndrome is an autoimmune disease with chronic inflammation of the exocrine glands that occurs either alone (primary Sjögren syndrome) or with any of several connective tissue diseases (secondary Sjögren syndrome). The adult form predominantly affects women over 40 y of age with keratoconjunctivitis sicca, xerostomia, and xerorhinia. Associated with clearly increased risk of developing non–Hodgkin lymphoma in intra- or extraparotid sites.
Benign neoplasms		
Benign mixed tumor (pleomorphic adenoma) ▷ Fig. 8.28	Small tumors appear as sharply marginated, intraparotid, round or ovoid, isodense or hyperdense with parotid gland tissue, homogeneously mild to moderate enhancing mass. Large tumors (> 2 cm) present as lobulated, well-circumscribed, inhomogeneously enhancing mass (in two-phase CT, these tumors present with an increase in attenuation during the second phase), with areas of lower attenuation representing foci of necrosis, old hemorrhage, cysts, or fat. Benign mixed tumors are the most common salivary tumors to have calcifications or ossifications in the tumor matrix. A large, deep, pear-shaped mass may widen the stylomandibular notch and displace the parapharyngeal space anteromedially.	Benign mixed tumor follows the rule of 80s: 80% of parotid tumors are benign; 80% of benign parotid tumors are benign mixed tumors; 80% of parotid benign mixed tumors are in the superficial lobe; 80% of salivary gland benign mixed tumors are parotid; 80% of untreated benign mixed tumors remain benign. Most common parotid tumor; slow-growing, painless benign neoplasm in the cheek. Most common in Caucasians, rare in African Americans (M:F = 1:2; age range 30–60 y).
Warthin tumor (papillary cystadenoma lymphomatosum) ▷ Fig. 8.29	Usually located in the posterior aspect of the tail of the parotid gland; appear as round to ovoid, smoothly marginated, strong and homogeneously enhancing soft tissue masses, measuring 2 to 4 cm, that contain no calcification. Cyst formations with mural nodule are common. In two-phase CT, these tumors present with a decrease in attenuation during the second phase. There is no evidence of cervical lymphadenopathy.	Nearly exclusive to the parotid and the most common parotid neoplasm to become manifest, either multiple in one gland, bilaterally, or as cystic lesions. Most commonly occurs in men. Smoking predisposes to parotid adenolymphoma. There is a peak incidence in the fifth to seventh decades. Clinical symptoms can be attributed to enlargement of the lesion. Malignancy developing is extremely rare.
Oncocytoma	Similar in appearance to benign mixed tumor and solid Warthin tumor.	Rare tumor that occurs in the major salivary glands, exclusively in adults older than 50 y.
Lipoma	Well-circumscribed, homogeneous mass, isodense to fat (−65 to −120 HU), without contrast enhancement. Angiolipoma is similar to ordinary lipomas except for associated angiomatous proliferation. CT demonstrates marked enhancement around the fatty components.	Lipomas represent ~1% of all parotid tumors, invade deeply into the intraglandular septa, and occur in all age groups.
Facial schwannoma	Tend to occur along the facial nerve as well-defined, fusiform soft tissue mass with varying degrees of contrast enhancement. Some of the parotid facial nerve tumors may be extensive, multilobulated, with areas of cystic formation and inhomogeneous enhancement.	Facial schwannomas are usually solitary and manifest as a slowly enlarging, painless mass. These tumors can occur at any age, most commonly between 20 and 50 y, with a female predominance.
Neurofibroma	Intraparotid, most often ovoid, well-demarcated, heterogeneous, low-density mass, solitary or multiple. Absence of contrast enhancement is conspicuous. Plexiform neurofibroma shows a usually large, ill-defined, more infiltrative, heterogeneous mass with a mixed density pattern. A typical finding is the target sign with a punctate high attenuation centrally surrounded by peripheral low attenuation within multiple small tumor nodules.	Neurofibroma may arise from the facial nerve trunk or its branches and may therefore lie within the parotid gland. May be localized, solitary or multiple, or plexiform. Multiple or plexiform neurofibromas are seen in patients with von Recklinghausen disease.

(continues on page 322)

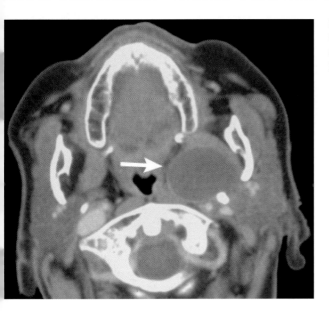

Fig. 8.28 Parotid benign mixed tumor. Axial contrast-enhanced CT demonstrates a large, deep parotid lobe tumor on the left side, sharply marginated, ovoid, hypodense to surrounding parotid, pushing the parapharyngeal space medially (arrow).

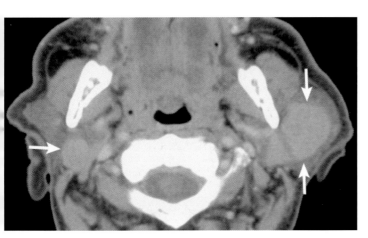

Fig. 8.29 Warthin tumor. Axial contrast-enhanced CT shows bilateral superficial parotid lobe tumors (arrows), ovoid, smoothly marginated, homogeneously dense, solid, and mildly enhancing.

Table 8.4 (Cont.) Parotid space lesions

Disease	CT Findings	Comments
Malignant neoplasms		
Mucoepidermoid carcinoma ▷ *Fig. 8.30*	Low-grade carcinomas may be benign in appearance with well-circumscribed, smooth borders. The ovoid mass is isodense to muscle. Cystic areas are occasional and focal calcifications rarely present. High-grade carcinomas demonstrate infiltrating margins, particularly when associated with adjacent soft tissue or muscle invasion and an inhomogeneous aspect. Malignant adenopathy is often present (levels 2 and 5; intra- and periparotid nodes).	Parotid tumors are uncommon neoplasms; 15% to 20% are malignant. Mucoepidermoid carcinoma is the most common malignant tumor of the parotid gland. It represents 10% of all salivary gland tumors and 30% of all salivary gland malignancies. There is a male predominance between the ages of 35 and 65 y (may also be seen in the pediatric population). Presents with a rock-hard parotid mass and associated pain or itching in the facial nerve distribution. Facial nerve paralysis is an ominous sign. **Major salivary gland carcinoma: TNM classification Primary tumor:** T1: Tumor < 2 cm without extraparenchymal extension T2: Tumor 2 to 4 cm without extraparenchymal extension T3: Tumor > 4 cm with or without extraparenchymal extension T4a: Tumor invades skin, mandible, ear canal, and/or facial nerve T4b: Tumor invades skull base and/or pterygoid plates and/or encases carotid artery **Regional lymph nodes:** N1: Single ipsilateral node < 3 cm N2a: Single ipsilateral node 3 to 6 cm N2b: Multiple ipsilateral nodes ≤ 6 cm N2c: Bilateral or contralateral nodes ≤ 6 cm N3: Node(s) > 6 cm **Distant metastasis:** M1: Distant metastasis
Adenoid cystic carcinoma ▷ *Fig. 8.31*	Parotid mass, isodense to muscle with homogeneous enhancement. May be well defined or poorly defined, depending on grade. Prone to perineural spread on CN V and VII.	Second most common parotid malignancy (and the most common in submandibular, sublingual, and minor salivary glands), with slight female preponderance between the ages of 50 and 70 y. Squamous cell carcinoma, adenocarcinoma, acinic cell carcinoma (most common multifocal parotid malignancy), undifferentiated carcinoma, epithelial-myoepithelial carcinoma, and atypical carcinoid are much less common and cannot be distinguished on CT because margins, architecture, and CT density overlap.
Non–Hodgkin lymphoma ▷ *Fig. 8.32*	CT may demonstrate unilateral or bilateral, solitary or multiple well-circumscribed, homogeneous, non-necrotic, enlarged intraparotid lymph nodes with mild to moderate homogeneous enhancement, or a diffuse parotid infiltration with moderate to high density, with or without extension into adjacent spaces. Periparotid and cervical lymphadenopathy is often present. Leukemic infiltration of the parotid gland is indistinguishable from infiltrative lymphoma.	Primary malignant lymphoma arising from the parotid gland is rare, whereas secondary involvement is common. An increased incidence is noted in Sjögren syndrome.
Intraglandular metastases	Single or multiple, unilateral or bilateral intra- and periparotid soft tissue masses, round or with infiltrating or invasive margins, often inhomogeneous with central necrosis.	Metastatic disease from a primary malignancy outside the parotid gland is a rare condition (4% of all salivary neoplasms, M:F = 2:1, seventh decade). Malignant melanoma and cutaneous squamous cell carcinoma (face, auricle, and scalp) account for the majority of lymphatic metastases to the parotid gland. Primary disease of the breast, lung, kidney, prostate, and gastrointestinal (GI) tract account for the majority of systemic metastases to the parotid gland.
Miscellaneous lesions		
Sialosis or sialadenosis	Parotid disease is usually bilateral and symmetric, but it can be unilateral or asymmetric. The parotid glands are enlarged but may appear either dense or fatty, depending on the dominant pathologic change.	Metabolic or endocrine related salivary gland disorders with nonneoplastic, noninflammatory, nontender, chronic or recurrent enlargement of the major or minor salivary glands. May be associated with diabetes, cirrhosis, alcoholism, malnutrition, hormonal imbalance, and drugs.

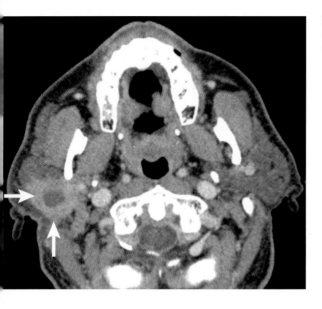

Fig. 8.30   Mucoepidermoid carcinoma. Axial contrast-enhanced CT shows an enhancing, solid-cystic mass with poorly defined margins (arrows) in the superficial lobe of the right parotid gland.

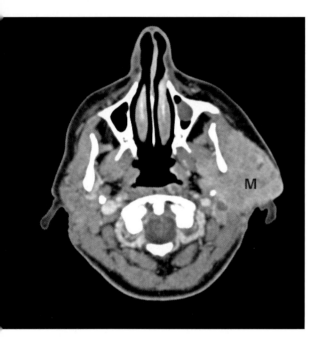

Fig. 8.31   Adenoid cystic carcinoma. Axial contrast-enhanced CT reveals a holoparotid, inhomogeneous, enhancing mass (M) with poorly defined margins and adjacent soft tissue invasion.

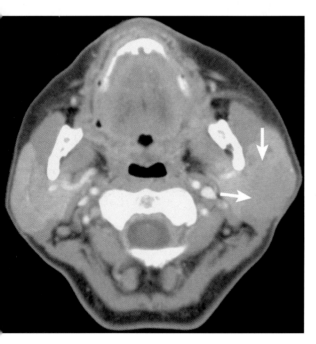

Fig. 8.32   Sjögren syndrome with parenchymal parotid non–Hodgkin lymphoma. Axial contrast-enhanced CT demonstrates findings of later-stage Sjögren syndrome with bilateral enlargement, heterogeneity, and increased CT density of the parotid glands. Also seen is an associated left parotid mass with invasive margins and less enhancement compared with parotid gland tissue (arrows).

II   Head and Neck

Table 8.5 Suprahyoid carotid space lesions

Disease	CT Findings	Comments
Pseudomass		
Ectatic carotid artery ▷ *Fig. 8.33*	One or both internal carotid arteries may have a retropharyngeal course and are imposing as round enhancing structure in the widened retropharyngeal space. Bilateral tortuous internal carotid arteries migrating medially to touch in the midline of the retropharyngeal space are called "kissing carotids." If the carotid artery folds sharply on itself, the appearance of an enhancing carotid space mass may be suggested. Sectional imaging, reconstructions, and CT angiography (CTA) easily define the vascular nature of the tubular, tortuous, elongated, sometimes dilated carotid artery.	A tortuous internal carotid artery can manifest as a pulsatile mass in the carotid triangle at physical examination. It can also present as a submucosal mass displacing the pharyngeal posterior wall. Increasing incidence of medial loop is seen with increasing age.
Asymmetric internal jugular vein	The size of the internal jugular veins can be variable and asymmetric due to their reciprocal size relationship to the external jugular veins and positional and anatomical factors. The right internal jugular vein is usually larger than the left.	A wide range of normal variation exists in symmetry of the internal jugular veins, from complete absence of one vein to perfect bilateral symmetry.
Congenital/developmental lesions		
Congenital absence of the internal carotid artery ▷ *Fig. 8.34a, b*	Demonstrating an absence of the bony carotid canal with skull base CT will confirm the diagnosis of agenesis. Similarly, demonstrating the presence of a diminutive carotid canal with CT will permit one to differentiate hypoplasia of the internal carotid artery from acquired conditions resulting in a small-caliber internal carotid artery (e.g., chronic dissection, fibromuscular dysplasia, and severe atherosclerosis).	Agenesis, aplasia, and hypoplasia of the internal carotid artery are rare congenital anomalies (in < 0.01% of the population). Congenital absence may be unilateral (with left-sided predominance) or bilateral. Collateral blood flow may allow these patients to remain asymptomatic.
Inflammatory/infectious conditions		
Reactive lymphadenopathy	In reactive adenopathy, the suprahyoid deep cervical lymph nodes (level II) may by definition enlarge to a maximum diameter of 1.5 cm but maintain their normal oval shape, isodensity to muscle, and their homogeneous internal architecture with variable, usually mild enhancement. Enhancing linear markings within node may be seen. Postinflammatory fatty infiltration of nodes appears as low-density nodal hilus, mimicking necrosis, in a node with pronounced lima-bean shape.	The internal jugular nodal chain is closely associated, but not in the carotid space. Reactive hyperplasia is a nonspecific lymph node reaction, current or prior to any inflammation in its draining area. Can occur at any age, but most common in the pediatric age group.
Viral lymphadenitis	Viral adenitis may present as bilateral diffuse lymph node enlargement without necrosis, similar in appearance to lymphoma and sarcoidosis.	Nonspecific imaging finding that may be observed in a variety of viral infections, such as *adenovirus, rhinovirus, enterovirus, measles, mumps, rubella, varicella zoster, herpes simplex virus, Epstein–Barr virus,* and *cytomegalovirus.* However, in the presence of parotid lymphoepithelial cysts and hyperplastic adenoids, HIV infection should be strongly suggested.
Suppurative lymphadenitis ▷ *Fig. 8.35*	In suppurative adenopathy, the involved nodes are enlarged, ovoid to round, with poorly defined margins and surrounding inflammatory changes. Contrast-enhanced CT images show thick enhancing nodal walls with central hypodensity, similar to metastatic adenopathy with necrotic center. Extracapsular spread of infection from the suppurative lymph nodes may result in abscess formation.	Common in pediatric age group with acute onset of tender neck mass and fever. Organisms have predilection for specific ages (infants: *Staphyloccoccus aureus,* group B, *Streptococcus,* Kawasaki disease; children 1–4 y: *S. aureus,* group A, *Streptococcus,* atypical mycobacteria; children 5–15 y: anaerobic bacteria, toxoplasmosis, cat scratch disease, tularemia; immunocompromised adults: histoplasmosis, coccidioidomycosis, *Cryptococcus, Pneumocystis carinii,* and toxoplasmosis).
Carotid space infection	*Cellulitis* may present as a soft tissue mass with obliteration of adjacent fat planes. It is often ill defined, enhancing, and extending along fascial planes and into subcutaneous tissues beneath thickened skin. *Abscesses* often appear as a poorly marginated soft tissue mass in the expanded carotid space with single or multiloculated low-density center, with or without gas collections, and usually thick abscess wall. Contrast-enhanced CT images show a thick, irregular peripheral rim enhancement and enhancement of the inflamed adjacent soft tissues.	Infection of the carotid space often evolves from a suppurative adenitis of internal jugular chain lymph nodes draining areas of submandibular, tonsillar, or pharyngeal infection. It may also result from extension of cellulitis or abscess from adjacent spaces or after direct penetrating trauma. Carotid space infection may result in a septic thrombophlebitis of the internal jugular vein or in an internal carotid artery erosion, thrombosis, or pseudoaneurysm formation.

(continues on page 326)

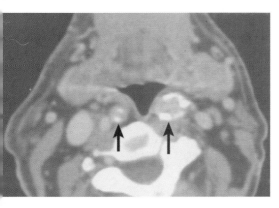

Fig. 8.33 Ectatic carotid artery. Axial contrast-enhanced CT reveals a retropharyngeal course of both internal carotid arteries. They are imposing as round, wall-calcified, enhancing structures (arrows) in the widened retropharyngeal space.

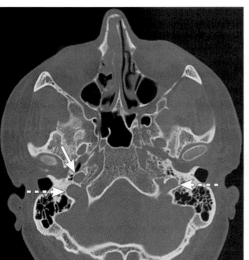 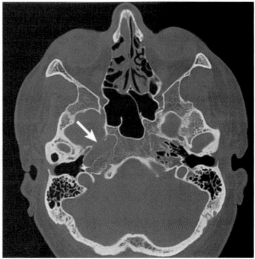

b

Fig. 8.34a, b Isolated agenesis of the left internal carotid artery. Axial bone CT (**a**) shows the absent vertical segment of the bony carotid canal on the left side (arrow: right carotid canal; bilateral dashed arrow: jugular foramen). Axial bone CT (**b**) demonstrates the absent horizontal portion of the bony carotid canal on the left side (arrow: right carotid canal). (Courtesy of Dr. B. Stinn, Zurich.)

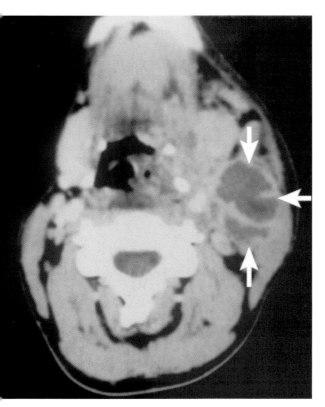

Fig. 8.35 Toxoplasma lymphadenitis. Axial contrast-enhanced CT demonstrates a left confluent suppurative nodal mass (level II) with rim enhancement and surrounding inflammatory changes (arrows). (Courtesy of Dr. R. Schôpf, Landeck.)

II Head and Neck

Table 8.5   (Cont.) Suprahyoid carotid space lesions

Disease	CT Findings	Comments
Vascular lesions		
Jugular vein thrombophlebitis or thrombosis	**Jugular vein thrombophlebitis:** Characterized by enlargement of the internal jugular vein by intraluminal hyperdense acute thrombus; also, increased density in fat and loss of soft tissue planes surrounding the thrombus-filled vein from edema/cellulitis. After intravenous (IV) administration of contrast material, the thickened vessel wall may enhance intensely, contrary to the nonenhancing luminal thrombus. Edema fluid may be present in the retropharyngeal space. **Jugular vein thrombosis:** The vein is dilated, with low-attenuation intraluminal content and enhancement of the wall, without adjacent inflammation. Collateral veins bypassing the thrombosed jugular vein may be seen.	In the acute-subacute thrombophlebitis phase (< 10 d after acute event), the clinical findings are most commonly those of a swollen, hot, tender, ill-defined, nonspecific neck mass with fever. In the chronic jugular vein thrombosis phase (> 10 d after acute event), patients present with a tender, vague, deep, and nonspecific neck mass, in comparison with a palpable cord encountered when the external vein is thrombosed. A history of central venous catheter placement, pacemaker insertion, previous neck surgery, local malignancy, infective cervical adenopathy, deep space infection, polycythemia, or drug abuse is often available. The hallmarks of the Lemierre syndrome are (1) septic jugular vein thrombosis after a primary oropharyngeal infection and (2) metastatic infection.
Venous aneurysm ▷ **Fig. 8.36**	Fusiform or saccular dilation of a cervical vein with attenuation values similar to the brachiocephalic vein before and after contrast administration that enlarges on Valsalva maneuver.	Aneurysmal dilations in cervical veins are rare due to low pressure in the venous system. They are observed in any cervical vein, most frequently in the internal and external jugular veins. Congenitally elastic layers and muscle cells are insufficient or even absent in the wall of venous aneurysms. May appear as a soft, compressible mass in the neck.
Internal carotid artery aneurysm ▷ **Fig. 8.37**	Fusiform, eccentric, or saccular dilation of the internal carotid artery with attenuation values similar to the aorta before and after contrast administration, often associated with parietal thrombus. Curvilinear calcification of the dilated vascular wall is common.	Extracranial carotid aneurysms are uncommon. Atherosclerosis, fibromuscular dysplasia, trauma, spontaneous dissection, and infection are causes of extracranial aneurysms. Most arise from the bifurcation or proximal internal carotid artery and can rupture, thrombose, or cause distal emboli. Ischemic symptoms and mass effect are the typical clinical presentation.
Carotid artery dissection ▷ **Fig. 8.38**	Internal carotid artery dissection typically spares the carotid bulb and terminates near the skull base. In the case of a subintimally located dissection, the mural hematoma will protrude the intima into the vessel lumen and produce a variable degree of stenosis up to occlusion. Dissections that occlude the internal carotid artery may terminate in a rat tail–shaped tapered occlusion. However, if the dissection occurs in the subadventitial layer, vessel wall thickening and considerable wall expansion into the carotid space may occur without causing relevant vessel narrowing. Focal outpouchings of the enhancing arterial lumen (pseudoaneurysms), without associated thrombus, may be seen on CT or CTA. A discrete intimal flap and patent double lumens are rarely seen findings.	Carotid artery dissections result from intimal injury, laceration of the arterial wall, or spontaneous hemorrhage of the vasa vasorum, causing subintimal or intramural hematoma. Nontraumatic dissection can be in association with an underlying vasculopathy (e.g., fibromuscular dysplasia), hypertension, migraine headaches, vigorous physical activity, pharyngeal infections, sympathomimetic drugs, and oral contraceptives. Dissections may cause headache, neck or suboccipital pain, cerebral ischemia, and infarction (from either flow reduction or thromboembolic complications). Symptom onset may be delayed. Some patients develop postganglionic Horner syndrome or lower cranial nerve palsies.
Carotid artery pseudoaneurysm	Pseudoaneurysm is seen as a carotid space mass. Axial contrast-enhanced CT scans demonstrate focal outpouchings of the enhancing arterial lumen, often in an orientation parallel to the vessel with a double lumen sign. The false lumen of a large pseudoaneurysm may compress the true lumen of the displaced parent carotid artery. Enhancement may be irregular with associated intraluminal thrombus. Wall calcification occurs if chronic.	Rupture of all three arterial layers accompanied by an organized hematoma that then cavitates and communicates with the true vessel lumen results in a pseudoaneurysm. Pseudoaneurysms do not contain normal arterial wall components. The development of a pseudoaneurysm of the extracranial carotid arteries is rare. Patients with advanced neck cancer, radiation therapy, and iatrogenic injury during surgery, after blunt or penetrating trauma, are at risk. Symptoms vary from an asymptomatic neck mass to sudden rupture with devastating hemorrhage and death.

(continues on page 328)

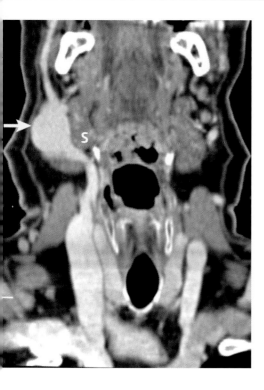

Fig. 8.36 Venous aneurysm. Coronal reformatted contrast-enhanced CT reveals fusiform dilation of the right anterior facial vein (arrow), coursing along the supero-lateral aspect of the submandibular gland (S). (Courtesy of Dr. T. Hertle, Dresden.)

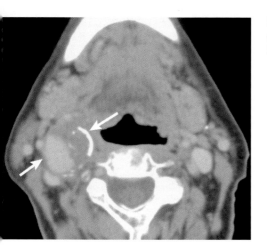

Fig. 8.37 Internal carotid artery aneurysm. Axial contrast-enhanced CT shows eccentric dilation of the right internal carotid artery (arrows) with irregular enhancing lumen associated with thick wall thrombus. Also visible is wall calcification.

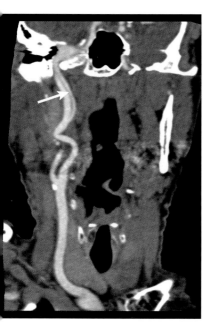

Fig. 8.38 Internal carotid artery dissection. Coronal reformatted, contrast-enhanced CT demonstrates dilation, dissection flap (arrow), and double lumen in the distal subcranial segment of the right internal carotid artery. Dissection stops at the skull base.

Table 8.5   (Cont.) Suprahyoid carotid space lesions

Disease	CT Findings	Comments
Carotid artery rupture	The soft tissue hematoma appears as a well to poorly defined, often inhomogeneous mass lesion that may displace the adjacent structures. CT densities range from 80 HU (acute) to 20 HU (chronic). Rarely, a fluid–fluid level is evident, caused by the setting of cellular elements within the hematoma. Contrast-enhanced CT images may show active extravasation of contrast material. CTA can be very effective in identifying the site or source of bleeding.	Rupture of the extracranial carotid artery or its branches is a rare but serious complication accompanied by life-threatening bleeding, pseudoaneurysm, or arteriovenous fistula. This "carotid blowout" syndrome is usually a result of radiation therapy for head and neck cancer, more extensive surgery, wound breakdown, infection, and tumor recurrence; may occur in patients with retropharyngeal abscess, parapharyngeal abscess, and necrotic fasciitis; is secondary to a pseudoaneurysm or as a result of trauma. The site of the hemorrhage is the internal carotid artery in 62% of cases, followed by the external carotid artery (25%) and common carotid artery (13%). Patients with an impending carotid rupture present with a sentinel hemorrhage with profuse but self-limited bleeding. Acute carotid blowout refers to acute uncontrolled hemorrhage.
Benign neoplasms		
Glomus vagale paraganglioma	Sharply defined, ovoid mass, isodense to adjacent muscles, and surrounded by fat planes. The tumor is intensely and homogeneously enhancing after IV bolus injection of contrast material. On dynamic CT scanning, glomus tumors have a vascular curve. At suprahyoid levels, the carotid space paraganglioma typically displaces the internal carotid artery anteromedially (without widening of the carotid bifurcation), the internal jugular vein posterolaterally, the parapharyngeal space and the styloid muscles anteriorly, the styloid process anterolaterally, and the posterior belly of the digastric muscle laterally. Upper cervical paraganglioma may show vertebral destruction. When the tumor extends to the level of the jugular foramen, permeative bone changes may be noted.	Glomus vagale paragangliomas (2.5% of all paragangliomas) are usually centered in the nasopharyngeal carotid space, 2 cm below the skull base (nodose ganglion of the vagus nerve) but can arise from anywhere along the course of the vagus nerve. Occurs in sporadic and familial forms. Five percent are multicentric in the nonfamilial group and may be multiple in 30% of patients with a positive family history of paraganglioma. They can be associated with medullary carcinoma of the thyroid, other visceral neoplasms, in familial multiple endocrine neoplasia syndromes (especially multiple endocrine neoplasia [MEN] type 1), neurofibromatosis, and multiple mucocutaneous neuromas. The majority of patients are younger than 40 y (slight female predominance). Glomus vagale tumors may present as an asymptomatic, slowly enlarging, nontender, pulsatile neck mass or posterolateral pharyngeal mass but more commonly present with symptoms of vagus nerve dysfunction (vocal cord paralysis) or with symptoms from involvement of the hypoglossal or glossopharyngeal nerves. Glomus vagale tumor is rarely hormonally active. Malignant paragangliomas are very rare.
Schwannoma	Usually well-circumscribed, ovoid to fusiform, homogeneous soft tissue mass, isodense or, rarely, hypodense to adjacent muscles with variable, often intense contrast enhancement. On dynamic CT scanning, schwannomas show either a rapid or a gradual enhancement pattern. Large tumors may undergo cystic degeneration and therefore present with central unenhancing and peripheral enhancing areas (target appearance). Calcifications are exceptional. In suprahyoid neck, carotid space schwannomas, surrounded by fat planes, typically grow in a craniocaudal direction posterior to the internal carotid artery and the internal jugular vein, tend to separate the vessels, and displace the internal carotid artery anteromedially, the internal jugular vein posterolaterally, the parapharyngeal space and styloid muscles anteriorly, the styloid process anterolaterally, and the posterior belly of the digastric muscle laterally. If the jugular foramen is involved, an expanded jugular foramen with sharp, sclerotic margins is characteristic.	Schwannomas are rare (5% of all benign soft tissue tumors). Schwannomas of the suprahyoid carotid space arise from CN IX to XII, the cervical nerve roots, or the sympathetic chain. Mean age at onset is 18 to 63 y (male predominance). Schwannomas are usually solitary and present as a slowly enlarging, painless anterolateral neck mass and/or posterolateral pharyngeal wall mass. Ipsilateral vocal cord paralysis represents the most common symptom of a vagus nerve schwannoma. May be multiple with neurofibromatosis type 2. Malignant transformation is exceedingly rare.

(continues on page 329)

Table 8.5   (Cont.) Suprahyoid carotid space lesions

Disease	CT Findings	Comments
Neurofibroma ▷ *Fig. 8.39*	**Solitary neurofibroma:** Fusiform, ovoid or tubular, sharply circumscribed mass, isodense to cervical cord, smooth and surrounded by fat planes. Differs from schwannoma by an overall lower density that may approach water and absence of contrast enhancement. In suprahyoid neck, carotid space solitary neurofibromas grow posterior to the internal carotid artery and the internal jugular vein, tend to separate the vessels, and displace the internal and external carotid artery anteromedially, the internal jugular vein posterolaterally, the parapharyngeal space and styloid muscles anteriorly, the styloid process anterolaterally, and the posterior belly of the digastric muscle laterally. **Plexiform neurofibroma:** Usually large, diffuse, ill-defined, lobulated, multinodular, low-density mass involving multiple cervical compartments (transspatial), including the carotid space. A typical sign is the target sign with central punctate enhancement surrounded by peripheral low attenuation within multiple tumor nodules. Neurofibromas observed in von Recklinghausen disease characteristically occur at multiple sites and are often confluent, multiple, or plexiform.	About 50% of all neurofibroma cases are sporadic, ~50% are associated with neurofibromatosis type 1. Neurofibromas of the suprahyoid carotid space arise from the sympathetic chain, vagus nerve, or hypoglossal nerve. They can occur at any age, with the average 35 y (female predominance). These neoplasms grow slowly and are painless. Large masses can result in complex lower cranial nerve palsies. Two to 6% of lesions in neurofibromatosis type 1 may undergo malignant transformation.
Meningioma	The jugular foramen meningioma is a dural-based, well-circumscribed mass, isodense or hyperdense, or even calcified. Compared with schwannoma it enhances strongly and may demonstrate dural origin. The adjacent cortex shows sclerosis, remodeling, or erosion. As the tumor extends out of the foramen, it may cause smooth enlargement of the foramen and assume a dumbbell shape with intra- and larger extracranial components. The internal carotid artery is pushed anteriorly by the emerging carotid space meningioma.	Extracranial extension of a dumbbell-type jugular foramen meningioma, though rare, may descend into the carotid space and present as a slow-growing carotid space mass with gradual symptom progression of complex lower cranial neuropathy (female predominance; age 40–60 y).

(continues on page 330)

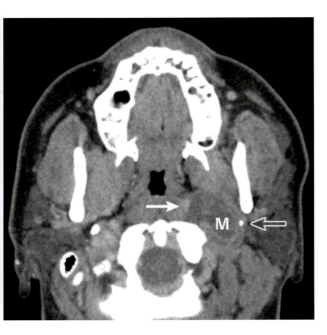

Fig. 8.39   Nasopharyngeal carotid space neurofibroma. Axial contrast-enhanced CT demonstrates on the left side an ovoid, well-circumscribed, low-density, nonenhancing mass (M). Internal carotid artery is seen on the anteromedial surface (arrow). Also noted is displacement of the parapharyngeal space anteriorly and the styloid process (open arrow) laterally.

II Head and Neck

Table 8.5 (Cont.) Suprahyoid carotid space lesions

Disease	CT Findings	Comments
Malignant neoplasms		
Nodal metastases ▷ *Fig. 8.40* ▷ *Fig. 8.41*	Lymph nodes in the upper internal jugular chain are considered abnormal when > 1.5 cm in diameter or when there is evidence of central hypodensity suggesting necrosis.	The lymphatics of the nasopharynx, oral cavity, oropharynx, supraglottic larynx, and pyriform sinus may drain to the upper internal jugular nodes. Level II nodes are the most commonly metastatic involved with regard to all head and neck squamous cell carcinoma.
Lymphoma	Hodgkin and non–Hodgkin lymphomas can present with multiple or single nodal enlargement as isolated symptom or as part of a more advanced stage. In general, there is a homogeneous enhancement, although rim enhancement or spotty or dentritic enhancement on CT is sometimes seen.	The upper internal jugular lymph node chain may also be involved by malignant lymphoma.
Contiguous tumor extension	Soft tissue mass within the carotid space, obliterating the normal fat planes and enhancing vessels.	Squamous cell carcinoma may extend outside the pharyngeal mucosal space. The most common malignant processes involving the suprahyoid carotid space are direct invasion by nasopharyngeal or tonsillar carcinoma.

Table 8.6 Suprahyoid retropharyngeal space lesions

Disease	CT Findings	Comments
Pseudomass		
Tortuous carotid artery	One or both internal carotid arteries may have a retropharyngeal course and are imposing as round enhancing structure in the widened retropharyngeal space (in fact, the artery is not contained within the retropharyngeal space; instead, it bows the alar fascia medially and projects into the retropharyngeal space). Bilateral ectatic internal carotid arteries migrating medially to touch in the midline of the retropharyngeal space are called "kissing carotids." If the carotid artery folds sharply on itself, the appearance of an enhancing carotid space mass may be suggested. Sectional imaging, reconstructions, and CTA easily define the vascular nature of the tubular, tortuous, sometimes dilated carotid artery.	A tortuous internal carotid artery can manifest as a pulsatile mass in the carotid triangle at physical examination. It can also present as a submucosal pulsatile mass displacing the pharyngeal posterior wall. Increasing incidence of medial loop, coiling, and kinking are seen with increasing age.
Retropharyngeal edema ▷ *Fig. 8.42a, b*	Uniform low-density fluid collection in the retropharyngeal space without significant mass effect, without wall enhancement, or surrounding cellulitis. Sharp demarcation from pharynx and prevertebral muscles.	Accumulation of noninfected fluid in the retropharyngeal space, seen with superior vena cava syndrome, internal jugular vein thrombosis, lymphatic obstruction secondary to lower neck or mediastinal tumor, trauma, neck surgery, or radiation. It is also seen in patients with acute calcific prevertebral tendinitis (longus colli tendinitis) or as a result of infections of the pharynx or vertebral column. Retropharyngeal fluid itself is asymptomatic.

(continues on page 332)

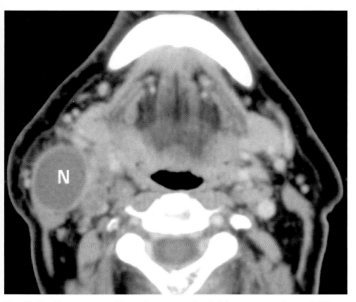

Fig. 8.40 Squamous cell carcinoma node. Axial contrast-enhanced CT shows a large right jugulodigastric (level II) node (N) with a necrotic, cystic center and mild peripheral rim enhancement (cystic lymphadenopathy).

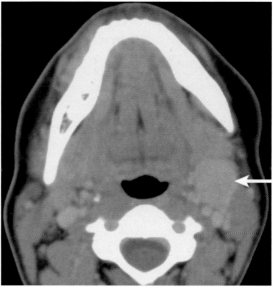

Fig. 8.41 Neoplastic node from thyroid cancer. Axial contrast-enhanced CT demonstrates an enlarged, round left jugulodigastric node with uniform intense enhancement (arrow).

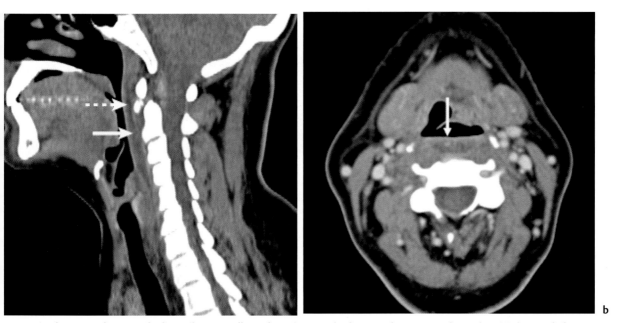

b

Fig. 8.42a, b Retropharyngeal edema (longus colli tendinitis). Sagittal reformatted, contrast-enhanced CT (**a**) shows calcification at the longus colli muscle insertion (dashed arrow at C1–C2 level) and uniform low-density fluid collection in the retropharyngeal space (arrow). Axial contrast-enhanced CT (**b**) demonstrates low-density fluid collection in the retropharyngeal space (arrow) without significant mass effect or rim enhancement. (Courtesy of Dr. S. Leschka, Zurich.)

Table 8.6   (Cont.) Suprahyoid retropharyngeal space lesions

Disease	CT Findings	Comments
Congenital/developmental lesions		
Infantile hemangioma (capillary hemangioma)	Solitary or multifocal, lobular soft tissue mass, homogeneous and isodense with muscle. Contrast enhancement is uniform and intense. No calcifications. Infantile hemangiomas are usually infiltrative lesions that do not respect the fascial boundaries and may extend into the retropharyngeal space as part of multiple space involvement (transspatial diseases). Size, enhancement, and vascularity of tumor regress in involutional phase with internal, low-density fat.	True capillary hemangiomas are neoplastic conditions; they typically display a rapid proliferation phase during the first year of life followed by an involution phase with fatty replacement. They have a female predilection. Infantile hemangiomas are high-flow lesions during their proliferative phase, low-flow lesions in their involutional phase. Sixty percent of infantile hemangiomas occur in the head and neck, with superficial strawberry-colored lesions and facial swelling and/or deep lesions, often in parotid, masticator, and buccal spaces. Retropharyngeal, sublingual, and submandibular spaces and oral mucosa are other common locations.
Venous vascular malformation (cavernous hemangioma)	Lobulated or poorly marginated soft tissue mass, isodense to muscle, with rounded calcifications (phleboliths). May be superficial or deep, localized or diffuse, solitary or multifocal, circumscribed or transspatial, with or without satellite lesions. Contrast enhancement is patchy or homogeneous and intense. Bony deformity of the adjacent mandible and fat hypertrophy in adjacent soft tissues may occur.	As opposed to infantile hemangiomas, vascular malformations are not tumors but true congenital low-flow vascular anomalies, have an equal gender incidence, may not become clinically apparent until late infancy or childhood, virtually always grow in size with the patient during childhood, and do not involute spontaneously. Vascular malformations are further subdivided into capillary, venous, arterial, lymphatic, and combined malformations. Venous vascular malformations, usually present in children and young adults, are the most common vascular malformations of the head and neck. The buccal region and dorsal neck are the most common locations. Masticator space, sublingual space, tongue, lips, and orbit are other common locations. Frequently, venous malformations do not respect fascial boundaries and involve more than one deep fascial space (transspatial disease). They are soft and compressible. Lesion may increase in size with Valsalva maneuver, bending over, or crying. Swelling and enlargement can occur following trauma or hormonal changes (e.g., pregnancy). Pain is common and often caused by thrombosis.
Lymphatic malformation (lymphangioma, cystic hygroma)	Uni- or multiloculated, nonenhancing, fluid-filled mass with imperceptible wall, which tends to invaginate between normal structures. Often found in multiple contiguous cervical spaces (transspatial) with secondary extension into the retropharyngeal space. Large retropharyngeal lymphangioma may cause mass effect on pediatric airway. Rapid enlargement of the lesion, areas of high attenuation values, and fluid–fluid levels suggest prior hemorrhage. Lymphatic and venous malformation may coexist.	Lymphatic malformations represent a spectrum of congenital low-flow vascular malformations, differentiated by size of dilated lymphatic channels. May be sporadic or part of congenital syndromes (Turner, Noonan, and fetal alcohol syndromes). Macrocystic lymphatic malformation is the most common subtype. Sixty-five percent are present at birth. Ninety percent are clinically apparent by 3 y of age; the remaining 10% present in young adults. In the suprahyoid neck, the masticator and submandibular spaces are the most common locations. In the oral cavity, lymphatic malformations can occur in the tongue, floor of the mouth, cheek, and lips. The anterior tongue is the most common location for oral cavity lymphangiomas, commonly presenting as an enlarged tongue.
Inflammatory/infectious conditions		
		Infection of the retropharyngeal space is most common in children age 6 y or younger in whom pharyngitis or infection of the faucial tonsils of the oropharyngeal mucosal space or the adenoids of the nasopharyngeal mucosal space, most often with streptococci or staphylococci, spread to the retropharyngeal lymph node chains. Infection of the retropharyngeal space is uncommon in adults, in whom it is most often due to accidental (foreign body, fish bones, or gunshots) or iatrogenic (endoscopy, intubation, or assisted ventilation) pharyngeal perforation. Typically, retropharyngeal space infections progress in four successive phases and can be stopped at any stage by appropriate treatment:
Reactive lymphadenopathy	In reactive lymphadenopathy, the suprahyoid retropharyngeal lymph nodes are enlarged (> 8 mm) but maintain their normal oval shape, isodensity to muscle, and homogeneous internal architecture with variable, usually mild enhancement. Enhancing linear markings within the node may be seen.	1. Phase: Reactive hyperplasia is a nonspecific lymph node reaction current or prior to any inflammation in its draining area. Reactive lymphadenopathy also represents the first response of the retropharyngeal lymph nodes to the spread of infection.

(continues on page 333)

Table 8.6   (Cont.) Suprahyoid retropharyngeal space lesions

Disease	CT Findings	Comments
Suppurative lymphadenitis	In suppurative lymphadenitis, the involved retropharyngeal nodes are enlarged, ovoid to round, with poorly defined margins and surrounding inflammatory changes. Contrast-enhanced CT images show thick, enhancing nodal walls with central hypodensity, similar to metastatic adenopathy with necrotic center.	2. Phase: The infected nodes suppurate with consequent development of an intranodal abscess.
Cellulitis	Cellulitis is seen as horizontal, rectangle, or oval widening in the posterior midline of the retropharyngeal space (nonnodal pattern of retropharyngeal space involvement: mass displaces carotid spaces laterally, pharyngeal mucosal space anteriorly, while flattening prevertebral muscles posteriorly) with poorly defined areas of low density and an amorphous enhancement following contrast media injection. The process may extend into the adjacent spaces and inferiorly into the mediastinum.	3. Phase: Early spread of the organism outside an infected suppurative lymph node may result in retropharyngeal cellulitis, causing the tissues to swell without focal fluid collections.
Abscess ▷ *Fig. 8.43*	Tense fluid collection (the attenuation value of the liquefied content usually exceeds 25 HU), distending the retropharyngeal space in a nonnodal pattern of retropharyngeal space involvement and producing pharyngeal airway narrowing. Presence of gas within is virtually diagnostic. Thick, irregular enhancing wall suggests mature abscess. Adjacent cellulitis/phlegmon may obscure the prevertebral muscles and pharyngeal mucosal space structures. Complications may result from spread to adjacent spaces (mediastinitis with 50% mortality, jugular vein thrombosis or thrombophlebitis, narrowing of the internal carotid artery [ICA] caliber, and ICA pseudoaneurysm and rupture).	4. Phase: Extracapsular spread of infection from a suppurative lymph node rupture results in abscess formation. Can also result from ventral spread of diskitis/osteomyelitis and prevertebral infection or from accidental or iatrogenic pharyngeal perforation. Most patients are children (< 6 y). Increasing frequency in adult population because of diabetes, HIV, alcoholism, and malignancy. Common signs: septic male patient with neck pain and sore throat.
Benign neoplasms		
Lipoma	Retropharyngeal, well-defined, nonenhancing fat density mass (−65 to −125 HU), homogeneous without any internal soft tissue stranding. Benign infiltrating lipoma may involve multiple contiguous neck spaces.	Lipomas of the retropharyngeal space are rare and do not cause symptoms until they reach a large size and have a significant mass effect on the pharynx (obstructive sleep apnea). Such fatty tumors also carry the rare possibility of being liposarcomas (inhomogeneous mass with soft tissue and fatty components and contrast enhancement), which further warrants their excision.

(continues on page 334)

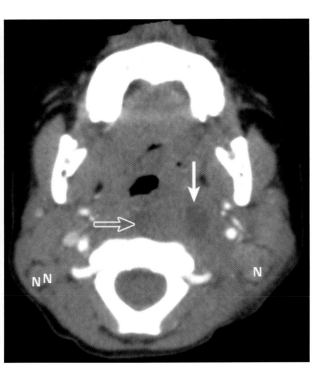

Fig. 8.43   Suppurative lymphadenitis and abscess. Axial contrast-enhanced CT reveals enlargement of a left lateral retropharyngeal lymph node with central hypodensity and a thick, slightly enhancing nodal wall (arrow). Also seen is an irregular, ill-defined, low-density fluid collection (open arrow) after medial rupture into the retropharyngeal space, as well as additional bilateral reactive nodes (N).

II Head and Neck

Table 8.6 (Cont.) Suprahyoid retropharyngeal space lesions

Disease	CT Findings	Comments
Malignant neoplasms		
Nodal metastases ▷ *Fig. 8.44*	Uni- or bilateral round retropharyngeal mass with a nodal pattern of suprahyoid retropharyngeal space involvement; the center of the lesion is anterior to the prevertebral musculature, posteromedial to the parapharyngeal space, and medial to the carotid space. Displacement of the parapharyngeal space is anterolateral. The mass flattens and remains anterior to the prevertebral musculature. Necrosis appears as central low density with a variably thick, irregular enhancing wall. Ill-defined margins and stranding of surrounding fat are features of extracapsular spread. May have significant mass effect on pharynx.	Metastatic involvement of lateral and medial retropharyngeal lymph nodes is most commonly seen with a nasopharyngeal primary squamous cell carcinoma, but also with an oropharyngeal, nasal cavity, and hypopharynx carcinoma. In addition, the retropharyngeal lymph nodes may be involved by thyroid carcinoma, malignant melanoma, and breast carcinoma.
Lymphoma ▷ *Fig. 8.45*	Involved nodes initially appear enlarged, homogeneous, and mildly enhancing. Central hypodense necrosis is uncommon. Later extranodal progression may cause the lymphomatous tissue to fill the entire retropharyngeal space.	The retropharyngeal lymph node chain may be involved by non–Hodgkin lymphoma, Hodgkin disease, and chronic lymphocytic leukemia, either as an initial site or as part of a multiple chain and/or extranodal lymphatic or extranodal extralymphatic involvement.
Contiguous tumor extension	At the level of the nasopharynx, an ill-defined soft tissue mass of the posterior wall may be seen with extrapharyngeal tumor spread into the soft tissues of the retropharyngeal space in a nonnodal pattern of retropharyngeal space involvement. Once inside, the retropharyngeal tumor can move in a cephalocaudal direction. Associated malignant lymphadenopathy in the suprahyoid retropharyngeal space may be present.	Squamous cell carcinoma may extend outside the pharyngeal mucosal space. The most common malignant processes involving the suprahyoid retropharyngeal space are direct contiguous extension from nasopharyngeal, posterior oropharyngeal wall, or tonsillar carcinoma. Nasopharyngeal lymphoma, rhabdomyosarcomas, or minor salivary gland malignancies may also involve the retropharyngeal space by direct extension from the nasopharynx (visceral space) or involvement of the retropharyngeal lymph nodes.
Trauma		
Emphysema	Interstitial radiolucent gaseous collections in the retropharyngeal space and in several other spaces, including subcutaneous tissues. Extensive soft tissue emphysema may extend downward, giving rise to pneumomediastinum.	Gas in the retropharyngeal space secondary to laryngeal trauma and accidental (foreign body, fish bones, and gunshots) or iatrogenic pharyngeal perforation (endoscopy, intubation, and assisted ventilation) is well known.
Hematoma ▷ *Fig. 8.46*	Tense fluid collection distending the retropharyngeal space in a nonnodal pattern of retropharyngeal space involvement producing pharyngeal airway narrowing. In the acute stage, the hematoma may be hyperdense and homogeneous. In the subacute stage, the hematoma may be either isodense or slightly hypodense, with patchy or inhomogeneous appearance. When completely liquefied, the hematoma again has a homogeneous density that is lower than muscle and may be surrounded by a pseudocapsule, which enhances after contrast administration.	Hematomas in the retropharyngeal space are unusual and are most often related to blunt head and neck trauma. Nontraumatic causes of retropharyngeal hematoma include anticoagulant therapy and complications of aneurysms, tumors, and infection. Life-threatening airway obstruction can result from retropharyngeal hematomas.

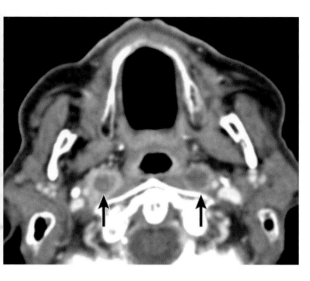

Fig. 8.44   Nodal squamous cell carcinoma. Axial contrast-enhanced CT reveals an enlarged spherical lateral retropharyngeal lymph node bilaterally with a central area of low density and peripheral rim enhancement (arrows).

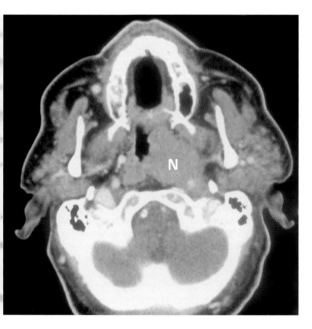

Fig. 8.45   Nodal non–Hodgkin lymphoma. Axial contrast-enhanced CT demonstrates an enlarged, ovoid, left lateral retropharyngeal lymph node (N) with homogeneous minor enhancement.

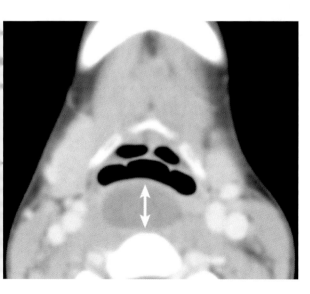

Fig. 8.46   Retropharyngeal hematoma. Axial contrast-enhanced CT demonstrates widening of the retropharyngeal space by a hypoattenuating ovoid mass (double arrow) without rim enhancement that displaces the mesopharynx anteriorly.

Table 8.7   Suprahyoid perivertebral space lesions

Disease	CT Findings	Comment
Pseudomass		
Levator scapulae muscle hypertrophy	Altered contour of the neck with homogeneous enlargement of levator scapulae muscle and denervated atrophic trapezius muscle. Absent ipsilateral internal jugular vein and sternocleidomastoid muscle from radical neck dissection, or an ipsilateral jugular foramen mass are findings of underlying cause.	Asymmetry of the levator scapulae muscles is an unusual cause of a palpable posterior triangle mass. Damage to the spinal accessory nerve secondary to radical neck dissection or, less commonly, an ipsilateral jugular foramen mass (paraganglioma, schwannoma, meningioma, or metastasis) leads to denervation atrophy of the trapezius muscle with compensatory hypertrophy of the levator scapulae muscle. In case of levator scapulae muscle atrophy secondary to cervical spondylosis with spinal nerve compression of the C3, C4, and C5 roots, the normal-sized contralateral levator scapulae muscle may present as a palpable mass.
Levator claviculae muscle	Uni- or bilaterally, the levator claviculae muscles arise from the anterior portion of the transverse processes of the upper cervical vertebrae (most likely above the C3 level), then head inferiorly and laterally, coursing lateral to the scalene muscles, anterior to the levator scapulae muscle, and medial to the sternocleidomastoid muscle, and insert in the lateral third of the clavicle, blending with the trapezius.	A normal variant not to be mistaken for an abnormality (lymphadenopathy or unenhanced vessel).
Vertebral body osteophyte	The classic sign of spondylosis is osteophytosis. Osteophytes are bony spurs that originate on the anterolateral aspect of the vertebral bodies a few millimeters from the discovertebral junction (at the site of attachment of the peripheral fibers of the annulus fibrosus). At the beginning, they extend in a horizontal direction; in the more advanced phase, they become hooked and grow vertically. Sometimes osteophytes develop on both sites of a disc space and grow until they fuse together to form a "bridge" osteophyte.	Spondylosis deformans of the cervical spine is the most typical consequence of age- or load-related degeneration of the vertebral body. It is found in 60% of women and 80% of men after the age of 50. C5–C6 is the most common level, followed by C6–C7, then C4–C5. Only when degenerative alterations are severe and symptomatic (e.g., cervical osteophytic dysphagia) should they be considered pathologic. Osteophytes can be distinguished from syndesmophytes of ankylosing spondylitis, paravertebral ossification of psoriasis and reactive arthritis, and bulky anterior-flowing ossification of the anterior longitudinal ligament of diffuse idiopathic skeletal hyperostosis.
Facet degenerative arthropathy	Osseous facet overgrowth ("mushroom cap" facet appearance) and bone excrescences impinging on neural foramina and the spinal canal in conjunction with articular joint space narrowing with sclerosis and intra-articular gas (vacuum phenomenon). Enhancing inflammatory soft tissue changes surrounding the facet joint are common. Frequently seen in conjunction with spondylosis deformans.	Hypertrophic degenerative facet may be perceived as a cervical mass on physical examination. Arthropathy most common in middle/lower cervical spine. Frequently seen in the elderly population. No gender preference.
Congenital/developmental lesions		
Venous vascular malformation (cavernous hemangioma)	Lobulated soft tissue mass, isodense to muscle, containing rounded calcifications (phleboliths). Contrast enhancement may be patchy and delayed or homogeneous and intense. Fat hypertrophy in adjacent soft tissues may be present.	Most common vascular malformation of head and neck, commonly in buccal region. Dorsal neck is another common location. These are usually infiltrative transspatial lesions and may extend into the perivertebral space as part of multiple space involvement. Present clinically in children, adolescents, or young adults.

(continues on page 337)

Table 8.7 (Cont.) Suprahyoid perivertebral space lesions

Disease	CT Findings	Comment
Lymphatic malformation (lymphangioma, cystic hygroma)	Uni- or multiloculated, nonenhancing, fluid-filled mass with imperceptible wall, which tends to invaginate between normal structures. Often found in multiple contiguous cervical spaces (transspatial). Rapid enlargement of the lesion, areas of high attenuation values, and fluid–fluid levels suggest prior hemorrhage. Lymphatic and venous malformation may coexist.	Lymphatic malformations represent a spectrum of congenital low-flow vascular malformations, differentiated by size of dilated lymphatic channels. May be sporadic or part of congenital syndromes (Turner, Noonan, and fetal alcohol syndrome). Macrocystic lymphatic malformation is the most common subtype; 65% are present at birth. Ninety percent are clinically apparent by 3 y of age; the remaining 10% present in young adults. In the suprahyoid neck, the masticator and submandibular spaces are the most common locations. In the oral cavity, lymphatic malformations can occur in the tongue, floor of the mouth, cheek, and lips. The anterior tongue is the most common location for oral cavity lymphangiomas, commonly presenting as an enlarged tongue.

Inflammatory/infectious conditions

Disease	CT Findings	Comment
Vertebral body osteomyelitis	Infectious spondylitis of the cervical spine is discocentric and extends from one vertebral body to adjacent vertebra across a disc; may reveal involvement at a single level or at two contiguous levels. The typical CT findings of pyogenic vertebral osteomyelitis include irregularity and loss of vertebral end plate cortex of two adjacent vertebrae; Swiss cheese–like, diffuse lytic vertebral body destruction with extensive bone sequestration (particularly in the subchondral bone region); and destruction of the intervertebral disc with loss of the adjoining disc space height. The paraspinal soft tissue component with soft tissue swelling, cellulitis with diffusely enhancing soft tissue edema, and abscess formation tend to involve the entire prevertebral space. Gas within both bone and adjacent soft tissue is a reliable indicator of infection. Spinal cord compression may occur because of intraspinal extension. The prevertebral space infection may secondarily involve the retropharyngeal space and carotid space. Osteomyelitis involving the posterior elements of the spine with an inflammatory mass in the paraspinal portion of the perivertebral space is rare. The classic CT findings of tuberculous spondylitis are large, frequently calcified paraspinal soft tissue masses with thick, irregular rim enhancement and focal lytic anterior vertebral body destruction, associated with marginal sclerosis. Isolated posterior element involvement is possible.	The cervical spine is an uncommon site for osteomyelitis. C5 and C6 levels are most frequently affected (6.5% of all spinal segments involved). *Mycobacterium tuberculosis* is the most common causative agent worldwide. *S. aureus* is the most common pathogen in the United States. *Brucella, Pseudomonas, Serratia,* and *Candida* are common organisms in long-standing IV drug addicts and immunocompromised patients. Vertebral osteomyelitis is usually caused by hematogenous spread to the vertebral body, whereas infection of the intervertebral disc is due to osteomyelitis of the adjacent vertebral body that secondarily invades the disc or to direct contamination of the disc during surgical spine procedures or penetrating trauma. Adults are more often affected. Diabetics, pediatric and elderly patients, IV drug addicts, and patients with urinary tract infection, pneumonia, or skin infection are at risk.
Soft tissue infection	Phlegmon of the perivertebral space may present as focal or diffuse muscle enlargement and obliteration of soft tissues, fascial planes and skin, due to diffuse soft tissue edema, with enhancement. Often associated with abscess formation: peripherally enhancing, low-density liquefied collection, with or without gas.	Soft tissue infection of the prevertebral and/or paraspinal portion of the perivertebral space from direct extension from adjacent infection (spondylodiscitis and septic facet arthritis), hematogenous spread from distant sites, or transcutaneous direct inoculation of deep tissue. Most common causative agents are *S. aureus, Mycobacterium tuberculosis,* and *E. coli.* Fungal infections are rare, more common in immunocompromised host. Predisposing factors are diabetes mellitus, alcoholism, cirrhosis, chronic renal failure, IV drug abuse, and immunocompromised state.
Longus colli tendinitis	Focal soft tissue thickening with calcification in the prevertebral area anterior to C1 and C2. It is associated with a retropharyngeal space edema, extending as a uniform low-density fluid collection in the retropharyngeal space down to C5, without significant mass effect, without wall enhancement, or surrounding cellulitis. Sharp demarcation is seen from the pharynx and prevertebral muscles. Calcifications may resolve on imaging follow-up.	Calcific tendinitis of the longus colli muscle is characterized by the deposition of calcium hydroxyapatite into the longus colli tendon. Patients (third to sixth decade) often complain of odynophagy, neck pain, paraspinal muscle spasm, and mild fever for 2 to 7 days.

(continues on page 338)

II Head and Neck

Table 8.7　(Cont.) Suprahyoid perivertebral space lesions

Disease	CT Findings	Comment
Vascular lesions		
Vertebral artery dissection	Extracranial vertebral artery dissections are usually located in the extradural segment between the skull base and C2 (V_3), less commonly in the foraminal segment (V_2). In the case of a subintimal dissection, the mural hematoma will protrude the intima into the vessel lumen and produce a variable degree of stenosis, irregular stenosis, long segment stenosis ("string" sign), multiple focal stenosis ("string of pearls" sign), up to a rat tail–shaped tapered or abrupt vascular occlusion. However, if the dissection occurs in the subadventitial layer, considerable wall expansion may occur without causing relevant vessel narrowing. Although rare, an intimal flap, a double lumen (dissecting aneurysm), or a focal aneurysmal dilation (pseudoaneurysm) may be seen on CT or CTA. A thin rim of contrast enhancement can sometimes be seen surrounding the mural hematoma (possibly resulting from enhancement of the vasa vasorum). Multivessel involvement may occur in up to two thirds of cases.	Dissection of the vertebral artery is an often overlooked cause of stroke in young adults (< 45 y). Vertebral artery dissections are caused by a primary intramural hematoma (due to ruptured vasa vasorum) or by penetration of blood into the arterial wall through a primary intimal tear. Vertebral artery dissections can be traumatic or nontraumatic. Nontraumatic dissection can be either spontaneous or in association with an underlying vasculopathy (e.g., fibromuscular dysplasia or cystic media necrosis), a predisposing connective tissue disorder (Marfan syndrome, Ehlers–Danlos syndrome, osteogenesis imperfecta, or autosomal dominant polycystic kidney disease), hyperhomocysteinemia, hypertension, migraine, vigorous physical activity, pharyngeal infections, sympathomimetic drugs, and oral contraceptives. Dissections may cause headache or neck/suboccipital pain, accompanied or followed by ischemic symptoms, originating in the vertebrobasilary territory (either from flow reduction or thromboembolic complications). Subarachnoid hemorrhage from intracranial extension may occur in 10%. Rarer clinical manifestations include cervical spine cord ischemia and cervical root impairment.
Benign neoplasms		
Schwannoma ▷ *Fig. 8.47*	Although some may emanate from the neural canal, thereby widening the spinal neural foramen ("dumbbell" lesion), still others may derive from the branches beyond the foramen and present as a well-circumscribed ovoid to fusiform homogeneous soft tissue mass, isodense to cord, with variable, often intense contrast enhancement. Large tumors may undergo cystic degeneration and therefore present with central unenhancing and peripheral enhancing areas. Calcifications are exceptional.	Tumors of neurogenic origin are some of the more frequently seen benign neoplasms of the perivertebral space. They can produce a mass effect in the paraspinal space. This consists mainly of anterior displacement and effacement of the longus muscle at suprahyoid levels and of the anterior scalene muscle at infrahyoid levels. The occurrence of multiple peripheral nerve schwannomas in patients with neurofibromatosis type 2 is characteristic.
Neurofibroma	Sporadic neurofibromas may present as solitary or multiple ovoid or fusiform heterogeneous low-density masses with well-circumscribed margins. Absence of contrast enhancement is conspicuous. In neurofibromatosis type 1 (NF1), localized neurofibromas have similar imaging characteristics to solitary neurofibromas, but they are often bilateral, multilevel, diffuse, or plexiform and follow the cervical nerve roots with intraforaminal extension, the brachial plexus, the vagus nerves, and peripheral subcutaneous nerve branches.	Ninety percent of neurofibromas occur as sporadic, solitary tumors. Sixteen to 65% of patients with NF1 have neurofibromas (57% single lesions), most commonly in patients between the ages of 20 and 40 y. Sudden painful enlargement of a neurofibroma in NF1 should suggest malignant transformation (3%–5% of patients with NF1 develop malignant peripheral nerve sheath tumors).
Aggressive fibromatosis (extra-abdominal desmoid fibromatosis, juvenile fibromatosis)	"Malignant-appearing," poorly marginated inhomogeneously enhancing soft tissue mass with local invasion of muscle, vessels, nerves, and bone. Most common locations are perivertebral space, supraclavicular area, and masticator space.	Benign soft tissue tumor of fibroblastic origin arising from aponeurotic neck structures. Associated abnormality: Gardner syndrome. Seen at all ages (70% younger than 35 y). Significantly more women are affected. Patients present with a firm, painless neck mass. Paresis depends on the site. Postoperative recurrence rate may reach 25%.
Other benign mesenchymal tumors	Well-defined homogeneous soft tissue mass with usually moderate, uniform contrast enhancement.	Other benign mesenchymal tumors of the perivertebral space are relatively rare and include (myo)fibroblastic tumors, fibrohistiocytic tumors, rhabdomyoma, mesenchymoma, or myxoma. Clinically, these present as a mass of increasing size, associated with discomfort or pain.

(continues on page 339)▶

Table 8.7   (Cont.) Suprahyoid perivertebral space lesions

Disease	CT Findings	Comment
Osteochondroma	Sessile or pedunculated osseous "cauliflower" lesion with marrow and cortical continuity with parent vertebra, usually in the posterior elements of the cervical spine. May compress the spinal cord or nerve roots.	Only 2% to 3% of osteochondromas (sporadic, hereditary multiple exostosis) occur in the spine: cervical (50%, C2 predilection) > thoracic > lumbar > sacrum. Peak age 10 to 30 y; M:F = 3:1. Many spinal osteochondromas are asymptomatic. Complications include deformity, fracture, vascular compromise, neurologic sequelae, mechanical impingement symptoms, and malignant transformation (< 1% solitary lesions; 3%–5% familial osteochondromatosis).
Aneurysmal bone cyst	Aneurysmal bone cysts arise in the posterior elements of the vertebra as a markedly expansile ("ballooning") multicystic osteolytic lesion with well-defined scalloped margins and displacement of the paraspinal musculature away from the spine. Fluid–fluid levels (due to hemorrhage and blood product sedimentation) are characteristic. Enhancement is confined to the periphery and septations interposed between the blood-filled spaces. Spinal cord compression may occur because of intraspinal extension. Occasionally, the expansile lesion may affect two or more contiguous vertebrae. Solid aneurysmal bone cyst is a rare variant. The solid component predominates and enhances diffusely.	Primary lesions are usually observed in the first, second, and third decades of life, with slight female predominance; 20% occur in the spine. Can coexist with osteoblastoma, giant cell tumor, or enchondroma.
Giant cell tumor	Lytic, expansile lesion centered in the vertebral body, with heterogeneous contrast enhancement; may contain fluid attenuation regions due to necrosis or focal aneurysmal bone cyst component. Zone of transition is narrow, margin usually not sclerotic. May have cortical breakthrough with apparent soft tissue extension.	In spine, peak incidence in second and third decades of life, with female preponderance. Can undergo sarcomatous transformation (spontaneously or in response to radiation therapy). Primary malignant giant cell tumors are rare. May be associated with aneurysmal bone cyst.
Osteoblastoma	Involvement of posterior elements of the vertebra is typical. The expansile, lytic lesion with thin, sclerotic margins may contain partially calcified matrix.	Histologically identical to osteoid osteoma but larger and occurs typically in the spine. May be associated with aneurysmal bone cyst.
Malignant neoplasms		
Vertebral body metastases	Focal, multifocal, or diffuse involvement of the cervical spine with osteolytic, osteoblastic, or mixed-type lesions. The vertebral body is involved before the neural arch. Associated cortical bone destruction and contiguous enhancing soft tissue extension into the perivertebral space are common. Multiple vertebral involvement is seen with intervertebral disc sparing. Bone expansion is virtually limited to lytic metastases from carcinomas of the kidney, thyroid, and lung and osteoblastic metastases from prostatic carcinoma that may mimic Paget disease. Pathologic fracture is common. Spinal cord compression may occur because of intraspinal extension.	Metastatic disease to the vertebral body with extraosseous tumor extension through cortical perforations is the most common malignant lesion of the perivertebral space. Present in 10% to 40% of patients with systemic cancer (primary tumor in adults: lung, breast, prostate, kidney, GI, or unknown primary [15%–25%]; primary tumor in children: hematologic malignancies, neuroblastoma, and Ewing sarcoma). Most common symptoms are spine pain, focal tenderness, soft tissue mass, and neurologic compromise from cord compression.

(continues on page 340)

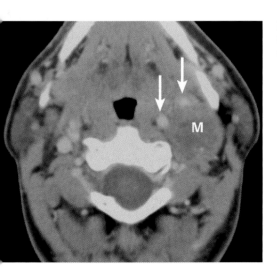

Fig. 8.47   Paraspinal schwannoma. Axial contrast-enhanced CT reveals a centrally lucent soft tissue mass (M) in the left paraspinal space with anterior/medial displacement of the carotid space vessels (arrows).

Table 8.7 (Cont.) Suprahyoid perivertebral space lesions

Disease	CT Findings	Comment
Chordoma	Chordoma appears as a destructive vertebral body mass with osseous erosion and expansion, sparing posterior elements. May extend into the disc space and involve adjacent vertebrae. A large associated soft tissue mass of low attenuation with extension into the perivertebral space may be the dominant finding. Mild/moderate contrast enhancement with inhomogeneous necrotic areas is characteristic. Extension along nerve roots and enlargement of neural foramina mimics peripheral nerve sheath tumors. Spinal cord compression may occur because of intraspinal extension. Up to 50% of these tumors may show coarse, amorphous calcified matrix. Anteroinferiorly expanding tumor of the clivus may invade or displace the nasopharyngeal perivertebral space and nasopharynx.	Rare primary malignant tumor of notochord origin. Originates from the sacrum and coccyx region (50%), sphenooccipital region (35%), and spine (15%), especially C2–C5 and lumbar. Cervical spine chordomas occur in 40- to 60-y-old patients (M:F = 2:1) and present with gradual onset of neck pain, numbness, and motor weakness.
Lymphoma	Involves vertebral body more than neural arch. Multiple vertebrae involvement is common; may cross disc space. Lytic, permeative bone destruction with enhancing poorly defined soft tissue mass involving adjacent structures (epidural, paraspinal muscles) is characteristic. "Ivory" vertebral body is rare. Epidural extension from adjacent vertebral or paraspinous disease is common.	Both in Hodgkin disease and non–Hodgkin lymphoma, bone involvement is usually secondary (hematogenous or invasion from adjacent soft tissues and lymph nodes). Most common presenting symptom is pain, most often in patients between the ages of 40 and 70 y. Slight male predominance.
Plasmocytoma	Solitary, large, expansile, osteolytic lesion with scalloped, poorly marginated, nonsclerotic margins, associated with soft tissue masses, with mild/moderate homogeneous contrast enhancement. The vertebral body is more frequently involved by plasmocytoma, but the disease may also affect the posterior elements. No tumoral calcifications, but peripherally displaced osseous fragments may be seen. Primary sclerotic form is extremely rare, but sclerosis may occur after proper treatment. May involve intervertebral disc and adjacent vertebrae. Epidural extension and/or variable degrees of pathologic fractures (vertebra plana) may cause spinal cord compression.	Solitary intra- or extramedullary tumor of plasma cells, with no evidence of multiple myeloma elsewhere. Represent only 3% of plasma cell neoplasms. Spine is the most common site. Cervical spine plasmocytomas occur in patients older than 40 y, with male predominance; can be asymptomatic or present with local neck pain, low levels of serum/urine monoclonal proteins, and neurologic compromise from cord compression. Progression to multiple myeloma is common.
Multiple myeloma	Polyostotic. Common spine presentations are multiple or diffuse lytic lesions, sometimes associated with irregular dense hypertrophy of the remaining vertical trabeculae or diffuse osteopenia. Vertebral destruction and pathologic fractures with variable spinal canal narrowing are common.	Most common primary tumor of bone with multifocal malignant proliferation of monoclonal plasma cells within bone marrow. Occur in 40- to 80-y-old patients (M:F = 3:2), more common in African Americans than Caucasians or Asians. Patients present with bone pain, anemia, hypercalcemia, proteinuria (including Bence–Jones proteins), renal failure, and monoclonal gammopathy (high erythrocyte sedimentation rate, abnormal electrophoresis).
Malignant mesenchymal tumors ▷ *Fig. 8.48* ▷ *Fig. 8.49*	Fairly well to poorly defined, inhomogeneous soft tissue mass with necrotic and hemorrhagic components and considerable contrast enhancement. The center of a mass in the paraspinal portion is within the paraspinal musculature or posterior vertebral body elements, and the mass displaces the paraspinal musculature and posterior cervical space fat away from the spine. Erosion/destruction of adjacent cervical spine is common.	Several different primary neoplasms can arise in the soft tissues of the perivertebral space: malignant fibrous histiocytoma, fibrosarcoma, neurofibrosarcoma, hemangiopericytoma, synovial sarcoma, and rhabdomyosarcoma. The clinical presentation is commonly a painless, slowly growing mass. Acute painful presentations are associated with tumor necrosis or hemorrhage. Metastatic disease within the muscles of the perivertebral space is rare and is seen most frequently with advanced disease.

(continues on page 341)

Table 8.7   (Cont.) Suprahyoid perivertebral space lesions

Disease	CT Findings	Comment
Contiguous tumor extension	Imaging findings of obliteration of the retropharyngeal fat stripe, irregular muscle contour, and postcontrast muscle enhancement are suggestive of direct extension from pharyngeal or tonsillar carcinoma with actual prevertebral muscle invasion, but nonspecific (because these findings may also be due to peritumoral edema without actual muscle invasion).	Late cases of pharyngeal squamous cell carcinoma, particularly those arising in the posterior pharyngeal wall, may rarely invade the perivertebral space.
Trauma		
Hematoma ▷ *Fig. 8.50*	Soft tissue hematoma appears as prevertebral soft tissue swelling or as a non-neoplastic heterogeneous mass in the paraspinal portion of the perivertebral space, nonenhancing, with adjacent parenchymal hemorrhage and surrounding edema. Unlike hematoma, muscle hemorrhage has little mass effect, with preservation of fascial planes.	Soft tissue hemorrhage can collect as hematoma. Hematomas are a common finding after sport and other injuries associated with cervical spine and muscle injury. Hematomas can be seen in the muscle, in the intermuscular fat planes, or within the subcutaneous tissues.

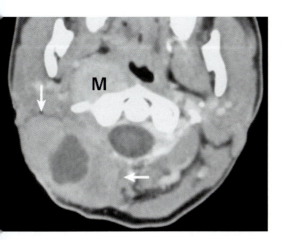

Fig. 8.48   Malignant fibrous histiocytoma. Axial contrast-enhanced CT shows masses in the prevertebral (M) and paraspinal (arrows) portion of the perivertebral space on the right involving prevertebral and paraspinal muscles with variable enhancement and a central region of decreased attenuation.

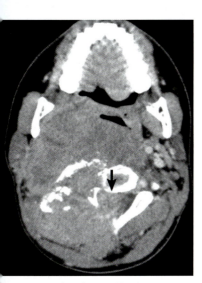

Fig. 8.49   Infantile myofibromatosis. Axial contrast-enhanced CT shows a very large solid soft tissue mass in the prevertebral and paraspinal portion of the perivertebral space on the right involving prevertebral and paraspinal muscles with inhomogeneous enhancement. There is lytic destruction of the vertebral body (C1–C3), pedicle, and lamina with bony debris. Extension into epidural space is present (arrow).

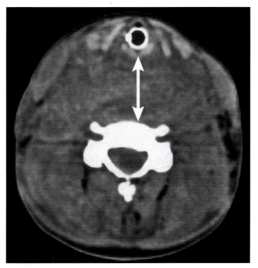

Fig. 8.50   Hematoma and edema. Axial non–contrast-enhanced CT reveals massive swelling of the perivertebral space with extreme anterior displacement of the pharyngeal mucosal space/visceral space (double arrow) after pediatric cervical spine (C2–C3) craniocaudal distraction injury.

Table 8.8 Lesions of the mucosal area of the oral cavity

Disease	CT Findings	Comment
Congenital/developmental lesions		
Infantile hemangioma (capillary hemangioma)	Solitary, multifocal or transspatial, lobular soft tissue mass, homogeneous and isodense with muscle. Contrast enhancement is uniform and intense. No calcifications. Size, enhancement, and vascularity of tumor regress in involutional phase with internal, low-density fat.	True capillary hemangiomas are neoplastic conditions; they typically display a rapid proliferation phase during the first year of life, followed by an involution phase with fatty replacement. They have a female predilection. Infantile hemangiomas are high-flow lesions during their proliferative phase, low-flow lesions in their involutional phase. Sixty percent of infantile hemangiomas occur in the head and neck, with superficial strawberry-colored lesions and facial swelling and/or deep lesions, often in the parotid, masticator, and buccal spaces. Retropharyngeal, sublingual, and submandibular spaces and oral mucosa are other common locations.
Venous vascular malformation (cavernous hemangioma)	Lobulated or poorly marginated soft tissue mass, isodense to muscle, with rounded calcifications (phleboliths). May be superficial or deep, localized or diffuse, solitary or multifocal, circumscribed or transspatial, with or without satellite lesions. Contrast enhancement is patchy or homogeneous and intense. Bony deformity of the adjacent mandible and fat hypertrophy in adjacent soft tissues may occur.	As opposed to infantile hemangiomas, vascular malformations are not tumors but true congenital low-flow vascular anomalies, have an equal gender incidence, may not become clinically apparent until late infancy or childhood, virtually always grow in size with the patient during childhood, and do not involute spontaneously. Vascular malformations are further subdivided into capillary, venous, arterial, lymphatic, and combined malformations. Venous vascular malformations, usually present in children and young adults, are the most common vascular malformation of the head and neck. The buccal region and dorsal neck are the most common locations. Masticator space, sublingual space, tongue, lips, and orbit are other common locations. Frequently, venous malformations do not respect fascial boundaries and involve more than one deep fascial space (transspatial disease). They are soft and compressible. Lesion may increase in size with Valsalva maneuver, bending over, or crying. Swelling and enlargement can occur following trauma or hormonal changes (e.g., pregnancy). Pain is common and often caused by thrombosis.
Lymphatic malformation (lymphangioma, cystic hygroma)	Uni- or multiloculated, nonenhancing, fluid-filled mass with imperceptible wall, which tends to invaginate between normal structures. Often found in multiple contiguous cervical spaces (transspatial). Rapid enlargement of the lesion, areas of high attenuation values, and fluid–fluid levels suggest prior hemorrhage. Lymphatic and venous malformation may coexist.	Lymphatic malformations represent a spectrum of congenital low-flow vascular malformations, differentiated by size of dilated lymphatic channels. May be sporadic or part of congenital syndromes (Turner, Noonan, and fetal alcohol syndrome). Macrocystic lymphatic malformation is the most common subtype; 65% are present at birth. Ninety percent are clinically apparent by 3 y of age; the remaining 10% present in young adults. In the suprahyoid neck, the masticator and submandibular spaces are the most common locations. In the oral cavity, lymphatic malformations can occur in the tongue, floor of the mouth, cheek, and lips. The anterior tongue is the most common location for oral cavity lymphangiomas, commonly presenting as an enlarged tongue.
Lingual (ectopic) thyroid gland	Well-circumscribed midline or paramedian lobulated tongue mass along the course of the thyroglossal duct (foramen cecum area), less commonly in the sublingual space or tongue root. Due to its high iodine content and metabolic activity, the thyroid tissue will appear dense with strong enhancement. Goitrous calcifications and low-density areas may be present. The thyroid gland can be absent from its usual cervical location (complete arrest).	Thyroid tissue in abnormal location in tongue base or floor of mouth. May undergo goitrous or carcinomatous transformation.

(continues on page 343)

Table 8.8   (Cont.) Lesions of the mucosal area of the oral cavity

Disease	CT Findings	Comment
Torus palatinus ▷ *Fig. 8.51*	Torus palatinus is seen as a flat, spindle-shaped, nodular, or lobular exostosis, which arises in the midportion of the hard palate. Exostoses that are composed of compact bone are of uniform increased bone density. Those that contain a marrow space have trabeculations. Torus mandibularis is an exostosis involving the lingual surface of the mandible just above the mylohyoid line and opposite the premolars; less common than torus palatinus; bilateral in 90% of cases.	Exostoses are localized outgrowths of bone on the surface of the maxilla or mandible (torus mandibularis) that are variable in size, shape, and number (single, multiple exostosis). They are more common in Asian and Inuit populations and twice as common in women. They are more common in early adulthood and can increase in size.
Inflammatory/infectious conditions		
Ludwig angina	CT demonstrates massive edema and an enhancing diffuse, ill-defined infiltration of the superficial and deep tissues of the floor of the mouth, submandibular and sublingual spaces, with low-attenuation areas reflecting abscesses or localized areas of phlegmon. Air in the soft tissues can be the result of gas-producing anaerobic infection. Elevation and backward displacement of the tongue, secondary to marked diffuse swelling, may lead to severe acute airway compromise.	Ludwig angina refers to a potentially lethal acute bilateral cellulitis of the floor of the mouth and submandibular and sublingual spaces that produces gangrene or serosanguineous phlegmon but little or no frank pus. Further spread occurs into the parapharyngeal, retropharyngeal, and carotid spaces, or even into the mediastinum. The source of infection is usually odontogenic, but sublingual or submandibular sialadenitis, trauma, and surgical procedures of the floor of the mouth are also causes of infection. Patients between the ages of 20 and 60 y (rarely seen in children) often present with rapidly progressive facial swelling and induration, oral pain, fever, trismus, dysphagia, dysphonia, and dyspnea. Ludwig angina represents a clinical emergency!
Odontogenic infection ▷ *Fig. 8.52*	Abscesses appear as single or multiloculated, low-density areas, with or without gas collections, and demonstrate peripheral rim enhancement. Common associated findings are extensive adjacent tongue and soft tissue cellulitis, edematous subcutaneous skin changes with stranding and dermal thickening, increased density of fatty tissue with streaky, irregular enhancement (edematous, "dirty" fat), thickening and enhancement of fasciae, muscular enlargement with enhancement (myositis), and reactive or suppurative adenopathy of submandibular lymph nodes.	Odontogenic infection is most often caused by periapical or periodontal disease related to poor oral hygiene or by extraction of a carious tooth. Odontogenic infection may result in cellulitis, myositis, fasciitis, osteomyelitis, and abscess formation. Odontogenic infections of the maxillary molars may extend into the buccal and masticator spaces. Further spread occurs into the retromolar trigone, parapharyngeal, and submandibular spaces and the floor of the mouth. Infections arising from the mandibular first molar and premolar teeth (the roots of which do not reach below the attachment of the mylohyoid muscle) tend to involve the sublingual space. Infections arising from the lower second and third molar teeth (the roots of which reach below the attachment of the mylohyoid muscle) spread into the submandibular space.

(continues on page 344)

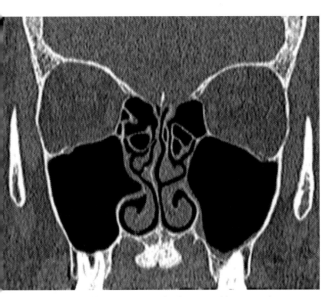

Fig. 8.51   Torus palatinus. Coronal reformatted bone CT shows a lobular exostosis that arises in the middle of the hard palate.

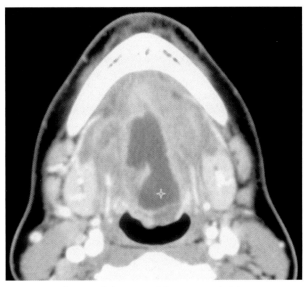

Fig. 8.52   Abscess of the root of the tongue. Axial contrast-enhanced CT demonstrates a central midline rim-enhancing fluid collection (joystick point) between the genioglossus muscles in the lingual septum, along with edema of the base of the tongue.

Table 8.8   (Cont.) Lesions of the mucosal area of the oral cavity

Disease	CT Findings	Comment
Benign neoplasms		
Benign mixed tumor (pleomorphic adenoma) of the minor salivary glands	Solitary, exophytic, broad-based or pedunculated, sharply marginated, oral submucosal mass, oval to round, isodense to muscle, minimally enhancing, projecting into the oral cavity. May be inhomogeneous with calcifications or cystic components. No deep extension. If the tumor is adjacent to bone (e.g., hard palate), benign-appearing remodeling of bone may be seen.	Benign mixed tumor is the most common benign salivary gland tumor (60%–80%). Eighty percent occur in parotid glands, 8% in submandibular glands, 0.5% in sublingual glands. Seven percent of these benign, heterogeneous tumors arise spontaneously from minor salivary glands that normally line all surfaces of the upper aerodigestive tract. The hard and soft palates are the most common locations. May be found at any age (most common: 50–60 y; M = F). The patient typically presents with a slowly enlarging, painless submucosal tumor. Malignancy may develop in 2% to 10% of lesions (carcinoma ex pleomorphic adenoma).
Malignant neoplasms		
Squamous cell carcinoma of the oral cavity		Squamous cell carcinoma accounts for 95% of all neoplasms of the oral cavity. It represents 5% of malignant neoplasms in the United States. **Clinical tumor stage of oral cavity carcinoma:** T1: Tumor is ≤ 2 cm in its greatest dimension. T2: Tumor is > 2 cm but not > 4 cm in its greatest dimension. T3: Tumor is > 4 cm in its greatest dimension. T4a (oral cavity): Tumor invades through cortical bone, into deep/extrinsic muscle of tongue, maxillary sinus, or skin of face. T4a (lip): Tumor invades through cortical bone, inferior alveolar nerve, floor of mouth, or skin (chin or nose). T4b: Tumor invades the masticator space, pterygoid plates, and skull base or encases the internal carotid artery. Thirty to 70% of oral cavity squamous cell carcinomas have malignant lymph nodes at presentation. Distant metastases are not frequent.
▷ Fig. 8.53	**Squamous cell carcinoma of the lip:** On CT, the primary tumor may appear as a variably enhancing, invasive soft tissue mass with or without areas of ulceration. Bone erosion usually occurs along the buccal surface of the mandibular or maxillary alveolar ridge. Large tumors may extend directly into the mandible or involve the mental nerve without cortical bone destruction. Metastases to lymph nodes are late and infrequent (< 10% in lower lip cancers). Lower lip lesions metastasize to the submental and submandibular lymph nodes, upper lip lesions to the preauricular, submental, and submandibular lymph nodes.	Most common malignant neoplasm of the oral cavity. 95% of all lip carcinomas originate in the lower lip (0.6% of all cancers in men). Carcinomas of the lips have an indolent and often protracted clinical course. Most common in white men. Peak: fifth to seventh decade. When patients are younger than 40 y, oral cavity malignancy is associated with acquired immunodeficiency syndrome (AIDS) or marijuana use.
	Squamous cell carcinoma of the oral tongue: Variably enhancing, infiltrative, ulcerative, and/or exophytic mucosal mass lesion, usually originating along the lateral border or ventral surface of the anterior two thirds of the tongue (lingual tonsil is part of the oropharynx). Advanced tumors tend to grow into the glossotonsillar sulcus, base of the tongue, tonsillar fossa, floor of the mouth, and submandibular space, to cross lingual septum to the opposite half of the tongue, or may invade the mandible. Forty to 70% of patients have regional adenopathy (submandibular nodes, high and midjugular nodes, or lower jugular nodes) at presentation, half of these bilaterally.	Carcinoma of the oral tongue is the second most common site of oral cavity cancer (20% of all oral carcinomas). It is a disease of men. Peak: seventh to eighth decade, but may also be seen in the young. Predisposing factors are poor oral hygiene, tobacco and alcohol use, preexisting Plummer–Vinson syndrome (Scandinavian women), and the coincidence of syphilis. Involvement of the lingual nerve is responsible for the pain in the ipsilateral ear.

(continues on page 345)

II Head and Neck

Table 8.8 (Cont.) Lesions of the mucosal area of the oral cavity

Disease	CT Findings	Comment
Squamous cell carcinoma of the oral cavity (continued)	**Squamous cell carcinoma of the floor of the mouth:** Poorly circumscribed mass with evidence of invasion on deep margins. Most tumors originate in the anterior portion of the floor of the mouth slightly off the midline. Inferior spread occurs into the sublingual space and may result in obstruction of the submandibular duct and chronic inflammation or infection of the submandibular gland. Infiltration into the mylohyoid muscle signifies involvement of the submandibular space. Superiorly and posteriorly, the tumors tend to involve the ventral surface of the tongue, the adjacent lingual neurovascular bundle, and the base of the tongue. Anteriorly and laterally, the tumor may advance into the adjacent gingival mucosa and may then destroy the cortex of the mandible. The prevalence of lymph node metastasis (submandibular nodes, high jugulodigastric chain) is between 30% and 70%. Bilateral involvement is common.	Squamous cell carcinoma of the floor of the mouth is the third most common tumor of the oral cavity (10%–15% of all oral carcinomas). Occurs predominantly in men in their 60s. It is the most common intraoral site in Africans.
	Squamous cell carcinoma of the buccal mucosa: The growth pattern of buccal carcinomas is usually exophytic, ulcerative, and verrucous. These variably enhancing mass lesions tend to invade the masticator space, the buccinator muscle with subsequent involvement of the skin, the anterior tonsillar pillar, and the soft palate. Pathways of lymphatic spread are variable and include the submandibular, facial, intraparotid, and preauricular nodes. Lymph node metastases are seen early and are present in 50% of cases.	Most buccal carcinomas are encountered in men in their seventh decade with a history of tobacco use or betel nut chewing. Infiltration of the medial pterygoid muscle causes trismus; this may be the first presenting symptom.
	Squamous cell carcinoma of the gingiva: Frequently occurs in the molar and premolar regions along the gingival margin of a tooth. Destruction of the underlying bone is a frequent finding. Fifty percent of patients have submandibular lymph node metastases at presentation.	The lower jaw is more often affected than the upper jaw. Tumors may present as ulcerating, plaquelike, or nodular lesion.
	Squamous cell carcinoma of the retromolar trigone: Can spread to any of the adjacent structures, including the buccal region, tonsils, base of the tongue, skull base, nasopharynx, and floor of the mouth. Osseous invasion of the mandible is common.	

(continues on page 346)

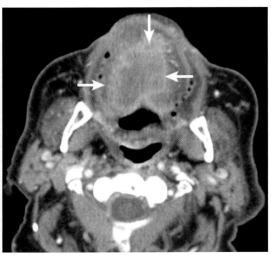

Fig. 8.53 Squamous cell carcinoma of the oral tongue. Axial contrast-enhanced CT demonstrates an extensive, invasive, irregularly defined, heterogeneous right oral tongue mass with rim enhancement that crosses the lingual septum to the contralateral side.

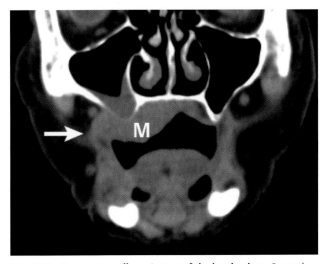

Fig. 8.54 Squamous cell carcinoma of the hard palate. Coronal reformatted, non–contrast-enhanced CT reveals a soft tissue mass (M) arising to the right side of the hard palate, crossing the midline, and causing an extrinsic defect in the oral cavity. There is erosion of the right alveolar process of the maxilla with invasion of the sinus and lateral tumor extension into the right buccal space (arrow).

Table 8.8   (Cont.) Lesions of the mucosal area of the oral cavity

Disease	CT Findings	Comment
Squamous cell carcinoma of the oral cavity (continued) ▷ *Fig. 8.54*	**Squamous cell carcinoma of the hard palate:** Often confined to its site of origin at the time of diagnosis. Advanced tumors may invade the maxilla, nasal cavity, buccal mucosa, tongue, or retromolar trigone. Perineural extension via the palatine nerves into the pterygopalatine fossa is common. Pathways of lymphatic spread include the facial and retropharyngeal lymph nodes and the upper jugular chain. Thirty percent of patients present with lymph node metastases.	Malignant tumors arising from the hard palate are of squamous cell origin in 50% of cases and of minor salivary gland origin in the remaining 50%. Squamous cell carcinoma of the hard palate predominantly affects elderly men and is strongly related to smoking.
Minor salivary gland malignancy	Enhancing, poorly circumscribed, diffusely infiltrating, submucosal soft tissue mass, extending into adjacent structures (hard palate, maxilla, sinuses, and buccal mucosa), and adjacent spaces, and invading muscles. Very coarse calcifications may be seen in adenocarcinoma. Associated malignant adenopathy is rare.	Histologically, these tumors include adenoid cystic carcinoma, mucoepidermoid carcinoma, adenocarcinoma, acinic carcinoma, and pleomorphic adenocarcinoma. Adenoid cystic carcinoma is the most frequent malignant tumor of minor salivary gland origin (25%). Unlike squamous cell carcinoma, tumors of minor salivary gland origin occur in younger patients (third to sixth decade), have an equal male to female ratio, and grow slowly. The patient typically presents with a slowly enlarging, painless submucosal oral cavity mass. Most common locations in the oral cavity are the hard palate–soft palate junction and buccal, labial, and lingual regions.

Table 8.9   Submandibular space lesions

Disease	CT Findings	Comments
Pseudomass		
Mandibular nerve motor atrophy	Chronic CN V_3 denervation atrophy demonstrates severe atrophy and fatty replacement of the tensor tympani and tensor veli palatini muscles, the muscles of mastication (medial and lateral pterygoid, temporalis, and masseter muscles), and the mylohyoid and anterior belly of the digastric muscles.	Damage to the mandibular nerve anywhere along its course may produce denervation atrophy. Loss of CN V_3–innervated muscle volume produces a "hollow concavity" of the cheek (masseter muscle atrophy) or the temporal fossa (temporalis muscle atrophy). The jaw deviates toward the affected side. Denervation of the tensor veli palatini muscle results in a diminutive torus tubarius and eustachian tube function, with accumulation of mastoid fluid. Denervation of the tensor tympani muscle may result in loss of acoustic dampening. May present as pseudotumors because of the relative prominence of the contralateral normal side.
Accessory salivary tissue	Ovoid to lobulated, homogeneous or heterogeneous submandibular mass, commonly anterior to submandibular gland, with density and contrast enhancement following normal submandibular gland.	Normal salivary tissue in abnormal position within the submandibular space. Usually found incidentally. May present as mass. Accessory salivary gland tissue is susceptible to pathology of normal salivary glands.
Congenital/developmental lesions		
Typical second branchial cleft cyst ▷ *Fig. 8.55*	Ovoid or rounded, unilocular, low-density cyst (isodense to cerebrospinal fluid), nonenhancing with no discernible wall. Typically occur at the level of the mandibular angle in the posterior submandibular space, anteromedial to the sternocleidomastoid muscle, lateral to carotid space, and posterolateral to the submandibular gland. A beak on the cyst pointing medially between the internal and external carotid arteries is pathognomonic if visualized. If infected, peripheral wall is thicker and enhances, and the density of content increases. "Dirty" fat lateral to the cyst indicates surrounding cellulitis.	Second branchial cleft anomalies represent 95% of all branchial disorders, and cysts are far more common than sinuses and fistulas. Twenty percent are diagnosed in infants and young children and 75% in patients between 20 and 40 y old. Patients present with a painless, compressible lateral neck mass. May get larger with upper respiratory tract infection. If infected, mass becomes painful. If associated fistulous tract is present, cutaneous opening is typically at anterior border of the sternocleidomastoid muscle near middle or lower portion.

(continues on page 347)

Table 8.9   (Cont.) Submandibular space lesions

Disease	CT Findings	Comments
Suprahyoid thyroglossal duct cyst	Well-circumscribed, thin-walled mass of fluid density, unilocular or multilocular, with characteristic anterior midline location entirely within the tongue muscles or in the region of the mylohyoid muscle between the anterior bellies of the digastric muscles, clearly separated from the hyoid bone. Inflammation can alter the density of the cyst, with peripheral rim enhancement and inflammatory changes in the adjacent tissues. A solid mass within the cyst may indicate either associated ectopic thyroid tissue or carcinoma. Calcifications within the soft tissue component may be an indicator of papillary adenocarcinoma.	Thyroglossal duct cysts are the result of incomplete obliteration of the embryonic thyroglossal duct anywhere along its course. Only 20% of these lesions are suprahyoid and may be found from the level of the hyoid bone to the foramen cecum at the tongue base. Presents as a midline mass in the suprahyoid region with fullness in the floor of the mouth, usually detected before the age of 20, frequently following infection.
Developmental cyst ▷ *Fig. 8.56*	**Dermoid:** Unilocular, thin-walled, well-demarcated ovoid mass, with fatty, fluid, or mixed contents. Globules of fat floating within the lesion may produce a characteristic "sack of marbles" appearance. Alternatively, fat–fluid levels may be present. Calcification (< 50%) and a subtle rim enhancement of wall are sometimes seen. **Epidermoid:** Low-density, unilocular, well-demarcated mass, with fluid contents only, a thin enhancing wall, and no significant surrounding inflammatory changes. **Teratoma:** Multilocular, heterogeneous, mixed-density mass containing solid, fatty, and cystic components, and calcifications.	Developmental cysts are a rare cause of head and neck masses. They are usually located in the midline or slightly off the midline within the floor of the mouth, the submandibular or sublingual space, submandibular gland, and root of the tongue. The teratomatous lesions are categorized by their germ cell tissue composition. Epidermoids seem to involve the sublingual space more commonly; dermoids, the submandibular space. They typically become manifest at 5 to 50 y (M:F = 3:1) as a painless subcutaneous or submucosal mass in the suprahyoid region with fullness in the floor of the mouth. The identification of the cyst location in relationship to the mylohyoid muscle on CT or MRI is extremely helpful in surgical planning.
Infantile hemangioma (capillary hemangioma)	Solitary, multifocal, or transspatial, lobular soft tissue mass, homogeneous and isodense with muscle. Contrast enhancement is uniform and intense. No calcifications. Can be very large, occupying, filling, and expanding the spaces. Size, enhancement, and vascularity of tumor regress in involutional phase with internal, low-density fat.	Congenital capillary hemangioma is the most common infant tumor. Typically presents in early infancy with rapid growth and ultimately involutes via fatty replacement by adolescence. Infantile hemangiomas are high-flow lesions during their proliferative phase, low-flow lesions in their involutional phase. Sixty percent of infantile hemangiomas occur in the head and neck, with superficial strawberry-colored lesions and facial swelling and/or deep lesions, often in the parotid, masticator, and buccal spaces. Retropharyngeal, sublingual, and submandibular spaces and oral mucosa are other common locations.

(continues on page 348)

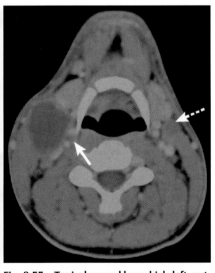

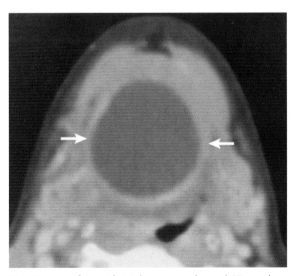

Fig. 8.55   Typical second branchial cleft cyst. Axial contrast-enhanced CT shows an ovoid, well-circumscribed, thin-walled mass of fluid density in the right posterior submandibular space. A beak on the cyst pointing medially between the internal and external carotid arteries is present (arrow). A smaller second branchial cleft cyst is seen on the left side (dashed arrow).

Fig. 8.56   Epidermoid. Axial contrast-enhanced CT reveals a midline, low-density, unilocular, well-circumscribed ovoid mass (arrows) between the anterior bellies of the digastric muscles in the submandibular space, with a thin wall and no surrounding inflammatory changes.

Table 8.9 (Cont.) Submandibular space lesions

Disease	CT Findings	Comments
Venous vascular malformation (cavernous hemangioma)	Lobulated or poorly marginated soft tissue mass, isodense to muscle, with rounded calcifications (phleboliths). May be localized or diffuse, solitary or multifocal, circumscribed or transspatial, with or without satellite lesions. Contrast enhancement is patchy or homogeneous and intense. Bony deformity of the adjacent mandible and fat hypertrophy in adjacent soft tissues may occur.	As opposed to infantile hemangiomas, vascular malformations are not tumors but true congenital low-flow vascular anomalies, have an equal gender incidence, may not become clinically apparent until late infancy or childhood, virtually always grow in size with the patient during childhood, and do not involute spontaneously. Vascular malformations are further subdivided into capillary, venous, arterial, lymphatic, and combined malformations. Venous vascular malformations, usually present in children and young adults, are the most common vascular malformation of head and neck. The buccal region and dorsal neck are the most common locations. Masticator space, sublingual space, tongue, lips, and orbit are other common locations. Frequently, venous malformations do not respect fascial boundaries and involve more than one deep fascial space (transspatial disease). They are soft and compressible. Lesion may increase in size with Valsalva maneuver, bending over, or crying. Swelling and enlargement can occur following trauma or hormonal changes (e.g., pregnancy). Pain is common and often caused by thrombosis.
Lymphatic malformation (lymphangioma, cystic hygroma)	Uni- or multiloculated, nonenhancing fluid-filled mass with imperceptible wall, more commonly in the submandibular than sublingual space. Tends to invaginate posteriorly from the submandibular into the sublingual space or anteriorly into the contralateral submandibular space. Rapid enlargement of the lesion, areas of high attenuation values, and fluid–fluid levels suggest prior hemorrhage. Cyst walls and septa may enhance after contrast material injection. Lymphangiomas may involve the salivary glands directly or by extension. Lymphatic and venous malformation may coexist.	Lymphatic malformations represent a spectrum of congenital low-flow vascular malformations, differentiated by size of dilated lymphatic channels. Macrocystic lymphatic malformation is the most common subtype; 65% are present at birth. Ninety percent are clinically apparent by 3 y of age; the remaining 10% present in adults. They may occur sporadically or with congenital syndrome (e.g., Turner, Noonan, and fetal alcohol syndrome). In the suprahyoid neck, the parotid, masticator, submandibular, sublingual, and parapharyngeal spaces are the most common locations. Compressive symptoms may result from sudden rapid enlargement or following infection or posttraumatic hemorrhage.
Inflammatory/infectious conditions		
Reactive lymphadenopathy	In reactive lymphadenopathy, the submental and submandibular lymph nodes are enlarged (> 10 mm) but maintain their normal oval shape, isodensity to muscle, and homogeneous internal architecture with variable, usually mild enhancement. Enhancing linear markings within the node may be seen. Associated enlargement of lymph nodes in other node-bearing regions of the neck is common. The lingual, faucial, and adenoidal tonsils are often enlarged.	Reactive hyperplasia is a nonspecific lymph node reaction, current or prior to any inflammation in its draining area. Reactive lymphadenopathy also represents the first response of the submandibular lymph nodes to the spread of infection.
Suppurative lymphadenitis	In suppurative lymphadenitis, the involved nodes are enlarged, ovoid to round, with poorly defined margins and surrounding inflammatory changes. Contrast-enhanced CT images show thick, enhancing nodal walls with central hypodensity, similar to metastatic adenopathy with necrotic center. Extracapsular spread of infection from the suppurative lymph nodes may result in abscess formation.	Infections of the nodal level I lymph nodes commonly occur from dental, floor of the mouth, or buccal infections. Reactive nodes transform into suppurative nodes with intranodal abscess. Common in young patients. Acute/subacute onset of tender mass and fever is seen.

(continues on page 349)

Table 8.9 (Cont.) Submandibular space lesions

Disease	CT Findings	Comments
Submandibular sialadenitis ▷ *Fig. 8.57* ▷ *Fig. 8.58* ▷ *Fig. 8.59*	In acute submandibular sialadenitis and sialodochitis secondary to calculus, the submandibular gland duct is dilated, enlarged, and enhancing with surrounding inflammatory changes. Frank abscess formation is rare. In chronic-obstructive submandibular sialadenitis, the submandibular gland is shrunken, fatty infiltrated, with little or no enhancement, and usually associated with duct dilation and calculi. If associated with ductal obstruction from the anterior floor of the mouth squamous cell carcinoma, CT may show an enlarged duct emerging from invasive, enhancing mass and leading to an enlarged, enhancing submandibular gland. If no stone is seen and no tumor is present, sialography will reveal radiolucent stones or a ductal stenosis with a transition in the ductal caliber.	Inflammation of the submandibular gland results from ductal obstruction due to sialolithiasis, fibrous strictures, or a neoplasm obliterating the orifice of Wharton duct. Primary glandular inflammation in Sjögren disease, AIDS, or bacterial or viral infection is rare. Acute submandibular sialadenitis represents with unilateral, painful submandibular gland swelling and colicky pain on eating. **Sialolithiasis:** Calculi are more common in submandibular gland duct (85%–90%) than parotid gland duct (10%). Sublingual and minor salivary glands are rarely affected. Most calculi (80%–90%) are radiopaque; 25% of patients may have multiple calculi. Submandibular gland duct calculi form at the hilum of the gland or are found in the ductal system. The sialolith may be palpable in the floor of the mouth.

(continues on page 350)

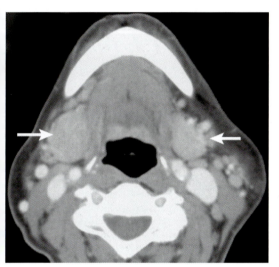

Fig. 8.57   Sjögren syndrome. Axial contrast-enhanced CT demonstrates bilateral enlargement and increased density of the submandibular glands (arrows).

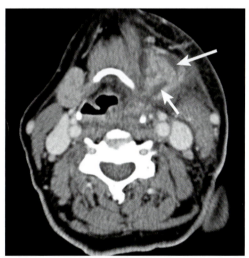

Fig. 8.58   Acute suppurative sialadenitis with abscess formation. Axial contrast-enhanced CT reveals a diffuse, enlarged and inhomogeneous, enhanced left submandibular gland with multilocular collections of fluid (arrows). Associated cellulitis with obliteration of adjacent fat planes, thickening of the platysma, and infiltration of the subcutaneous fat are present.

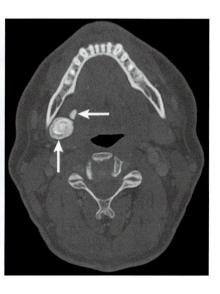

Fig. 8.59   Sialolithiasis. Axial bone CT demonstrates two radiopaque calculi (arrows) at the hilum of the right submandibular gland and proximal Wharton duct. (Courtesy of Dr. A. von Hessling, Zurich.)

Table 8.9   (Cont.) Submandibular space lesions

Disease	CT Findings	Comments
Diving ranula ▷ *Fig. 8.60*	Unilocular or multilobular, well-circumscribed, low-density mass emanating from sublingual space and extending into adjacent submandibular space (and inferior parapharyngeal space). Diving ranula may be characteristically comet-shaped with collapsed cyst in the sublingual space ("tail" sign) and large pseudocystic component (its "head") in the posterior submandibular space. Large, horseshoe-shaped ranula may extend across the midline through the anterior isthmus of the sublingual space.	Simple ranula is a mucus retention cyst, acquired secondarily (after trauma to the neck or oral cavity or inflammation) to obstructed sublingual or minor salivary glands, and arises within the sublingual space. The term *diving* or *plunging ranula* is used when a simple ranula becomes large and ruptures out of the posterior sublingual space into the submandibular space, creating a pseudocyst lacking epithelial lining. Median age at presentation with painless sublingual and submandibular mass is 30 y.
Submandibular gland retention cyst (mucocele)	Well-circumscribed, nonenhancing mass lesion of low attenuation values in place of the submandibular gland, conforming to the fascial boundaries of the posterior submandibular space. No sublingual space extension.	Mucus retention cyst of the submandibular gland can be differentiated from a diving ranula by the submandibular gland involvement.
Cellulitis	Cellulitis of the submandibular space may present as a soft tissue mass with obliteration of adjacent fat planes. It is often ill-defined, enhancing, without focal rim-enhancing fluid collection extending along fascial planes and into subcutaneous tissues beneath thickened skin. Infection of the submandibular space readily extends posteriorly into the parapharyngeal space.	Infection of the submandibular and sublingual spaces is common and can easily pass from one space to the other. Infection of the submandibular space most commonly occurs from suppurative adenopathy associated with dental, floor of the mouth, or buccal infections. Submandibular space infections are often precipitated by submandibular gland inflammation secondary to ductal stenosis or calculus, or it may result directly from odontogenic infection.
Abscess	Abscesses often appear as a poorly marginated soft tissue mass in the expanded submandibular space with single or multiloculated low-density center, with or without gas collections, and usually thick abscess wall. Contrast-enhanced CT images show a thick, irregular peripheral rim enhancement. May be part of a transspatial abscess. Tooth with periapical abscess and focal mandibular cortex dehiscence or mandibular osteomyelitis with permeative bone changes, focal bone destruction, and periosteal reaction may refer to the source of the infection. Edematous subcutaneous skin changes with stranding and dermal thickening, increased density of fatty tissue with streaky, irregular enhancement (edematous, "dirty" fat), muscular enlargement with enhancement (myositis), and reactive or suppurative adenopathy of submandibular lymph nodes are common associated findings.	Focal collection of pus within oral cavity spaces: sublingual space, submandibular space, root of the tongue, or transspatial. The source of infection is usually odontogenic (tooth root abscess/mandibular osteomyelitis). Infections arising from the lower second and third molar teeth (the roots of which reach below the attachment of the mylohyoid muscle) spread into the submandibular space. Submental space infection may complicate apical and periodontal disease of the incisor teeth. Submandibular duct calculus, sublingual or submandibular sialadenitis, and penetrating trauma are other causes of infection. Further spread occurs into the parapharyngeal and retropharyngeal space. Present in elderly patients with sublingual or submandibular swelling, painful tongue, dysphagia, and dysphonia. Elevation and backward displacement of the tongue may compromise airway.
Benign neoplasms		
Lipoma	Thin-walled, encapsulated, nonenhancing fat-density mass (−65 to −125 HU), homogeneous without any internal soft tissue stranding. Can be transspatial.	Most common sites of origin in the neck are the posterior cervical and submandibular spaces. More common in men (fifth to sixth decade, sometimes in children).
Benign mixed tumor (pleomorphic adenoma) of submandibular gland	Single, homogeneous ovoid soft tissue mass, with fairly well-defined margins within an enlarged submandibular gland. When large, the intraglandular tumor may pedunculate off the margin of the gland into the submandibular space. Sometimes foci of fat, necrosis, hemorrhage, or focal calcifications may be seen. The contrast enhancement, mild to moderate, may be uniformly homogeneous or heterogeneous.	Fifty-five percent of submandibular gland tumors are benign, 45% malignant. Benign mixed tumor is the most common tumor of the submandibular gland; 8% of all head and neck benign mixed tumors arise in the submandibular gland. Presents as slow-growing, painless submandibular space mass. Peak age of occurrence is 40 y and older; (M:F = 1:2). If left untreated, 10% to 25% of benign mixed tumors will undergo malignant transformation.
Pedunculated parotid tail mass	Solid or cystic mass at the level of the mandibular angle, located anterolateral to sternocleidomastoid muscle and lateral to posterior belly of digastric muscle, medial and deep to the platysma muscle. May mimic a posterior submandibular space lesion.	A pedunculated parotid tail tumor can easily be mistaken for a nonparotid mass on axial images. Benign mixed tumor and Warthin tumor are the most common solitary mass lesions of the most inferior aspect of the superficial parotid gland lobe.

(continues on page 351)

Table 8.9   (Cont.) Submandibular space lesions

Disease	CT Findings	Comments
Ameloblastoma ▷ *Fig. 8.61* ▷ *Fig. 8.62*	Usually centered in third molar, mandibular ramus region. Enhancing, expansile, uni- or multicystic, low-density mass with "bubbly pattern," internal osseous septa, usually no calcifications in matrix, scalloped borders, and thinned cortical margins with focal areas of dehiscence. Unerupted molar tooth and resorption of adjacent tooth roots association are common. No evidence of perineural spread. Extraosseous extension into the major areas of the oral cavity or masticator space is rare.	Most common benign mandibular tumor. Most common odontogenic tumor (35%), mandible:maxilla = 5:1. Twenty percent of ameloblastomas are thought to arise from dentigerous cysts. Most commonly presents in 30- to 50-y-olds with painless, slow-growing mandibular mass, loose teeth, bleeding, and trismus. Malignant transformation is rare (1%). Other benign odontogenic tumors are calcifying epithelial odontogenic tumor, ameloblastic fibroma, adenomatoid odontogenic tumor, dentinoma, calcifying odontogenic cyst, odontogenic ameloblastoma, odontomas, and cementomas. Benign nonodontogenic tumors and cysts are found not only in the jaw bone but also in other areas of the skeleton.

(continues on page 352)

II **Head and Neck**

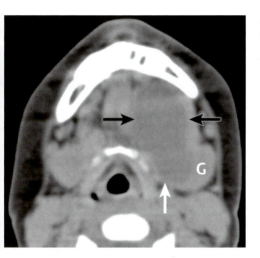

Fig. 8.60   Diving ranula. Axial non–contrast-enhanced CT reveals a large, well-defined, unilocular sublingual space mass of fluid density (black arrows) herniating into the adjacent posterior submandibular space (white arrow) with mass effect on the left submandibular gland (G).

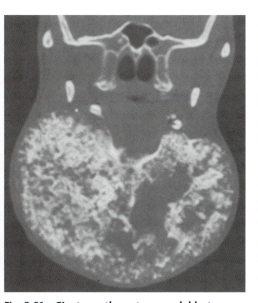

Fig. 8.61   Giant acanthomatous ameloblastoma. Coronal reformatted bone CT shows a facial deformity due to extensive and grotesque deformity of the expanded mandibular body. There are coarse internal calcifications, exhibiting a trabecular appearance, and surrounding cortical destructions. Marked mass effect on oral cavity areas is obvious.

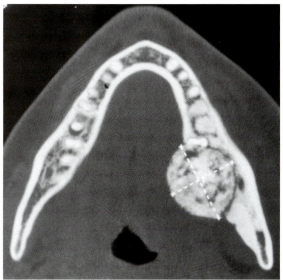

Fig. 8.62   Benign cementoblastoma. Axial bone CT demonstrates a circular, heterogeneous radiopaque mass with a radiolucent halo associated with the root of the second mandibular molar, extending into the left submandibular space.

Table 8.9   (Cont.) Submandibular space lesions

Disease	CT Findings	Comments
Malignant neoplasms		
Nodal metastases	Single or grouped lymph nodes centered within the fat of the submandibular space outside the submandibular gland, round (with a longitudinal-to-transverse diameter ratio < 2), variable in size (maximal longitudinal diameter > 15 mm), with heterogeneous enhancement. Nodal tumor necrosis appears as a central nonenhancing low-density mass with variably thick, irregular, moderately enhancing wall. Metastatic nodes may be completely cavitated by cystic degeneration, mimicking a benign cyst (e.g., squamous cell carcinoma of the area of Waldeyer ring and papillary thyroid carcinoma). Ill-defined margins and stranding of surrounding fat are features of extracapsular spread.	Malignant tumor of the submandibular space is nodal tumor in the vast majority of cases. Metastatic involvement of submental (level IA) and submandibular (level IB) lymph nodes typically occurs in association with primary head and neck squamous cell carcinomas of the skin of face, oral cavity structures, nose, and anterior sinus regions. A painless, firm submandibular space mass may be the presenting symptom, most commonly in patients with known primary (M > F, > 40 y).
Nodal non–Hodgkin lymphoma	Bilateral, multiple, well-demarcated, homogeneous, nonnecrotic enlarged nodes throughout submandibular space, isodense to muscle, with variable diffuse enhancement and generally no extracapsular extension. Dominant node may reach 5 to 10 cm in size. Extranodal tumor extension, nodal necrosis, calcification, and hemorrhage are rare prior to treatment (high-grade non–Hodgkin lymphoma may show central node necrosis, mimicking metastasis from squamous cell carcinomas).	Nodal non–Hodgkin lymphoma of the submandibular space usually occurs in association with manifestations in various deep lymphatic chains of the neck. Clinical: painless, multiple, rubbery submandibular space masses. Systemic symptoms include night sweats, recurrent fevers, unexplained weight loss, and fatigue (median age of occurrence 50–55 y; M:F = 1.5:1).
Adenoid cystic carcinoma of the submandibular gland ▷ *Fig. 8.63*	Smaller tumors may present as a well-circumscribed, relatively homogeneous mass with mild enhancement arising within or from the enlarged submandibular gland. When large, the inhomogeneous enhancing mass may show irregular calcifications and emanate from the submandibular gland into the submandibular space with invasive margins. Adenoid cystic carcinoma has a propensity to infiltrate and spread along perineural planes.	Malignancy of the submandibular gland is rare. Adenoid cystic carcinoma is the most common submandibular gland carcinoma. It accounts for 4% to 8% of total salivary gland tumors, 30% of minor salivary gland tumors, 15% of sublingual gland tumors, 12% of submandibular gland tumors, and 2% to 6% of parotid gland tumors. Most patients with a submandibular gland carcinoma are women in their fourth to sixth decades who present with a painless submandibular swelling.
Mucoepidermoid carcinoma of the submandibular gland	Low-grade lesions are generally better circumscribed, contain more cysts, may be hemorrhagic, and may appear benign with well-defined margins. Higher-grade lesions are more solid, isodense, and aggressive and may show infiltration, necrosis, and calcification. Contrast enhancement is usually mild to moderate.	Mucoepidermoid carcinoma accounts for < 10% of salivary gland tumors and 30% of salivary gland malignancies. Fifty-four percent are present in the major salivary glands, 46% in the intraoral minor salivary glands. Exposure risk: radiation. It usually occurs in patients younger than age 50, but it is the most common malignant salivary gland tumor in children.
Metastases to the submandibular gland ▷ *Fig. 8.64*	May be a fairly well-circumscribed mass or less defined and infiltrative, replacing portions of the enlarged submandibular gland.	Metastatic deposits in the submandibular gland are extremely rare and due to direct extension from a primary oral cavity lesion or as a result of hematogenous spread (melanoma, breast cancer, papillary thyroid cancer, and uterine leiomyosarcoma).
Contiguous tumor extension	Carcinoma of the tongue and floor of the mouth has CT density similar to normal tongue muscle. Direct invasion of the sublingual and submandibular spaces is recognized by obliteration of the normal fat planes and by contrast enhancement of the tumor margins.	Advanced carcinomas of the tonsil, tongue, and floor of the mouth may spread into the sublingual spaces, tongue muscles, and submandibular spaces.
Malignant mandibular tumors	In advanced cases, cortical breakthrough with tumor outside of the jaw is a common finding. When the body or symphysis is the principal site of tumor, soft tissue extension involves the submandibular space or sublingual space, depending on from which side of the mylohyoid muscles the mass originates.	Malignant mandibular neoplasms are rare and often occur in younger people. They include osteogenic sarcoma, chondrosarcoma, fibrosarcoma, Ewing sarcoma, malignant lymphoma, multiple myeloma, Burkitt lymphoma, leukemia, and metastases.

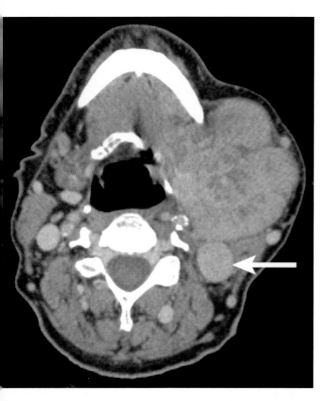

Fig. 8.63 Adenoid cystic carcinoma of the submandibular gland. Axial contrast-enhanced CT reveals a very large, inhomogeneously enhancing mass emanating from the left submandibular gland. An associated left spinal accessory nodal metastasis is present (arrow).

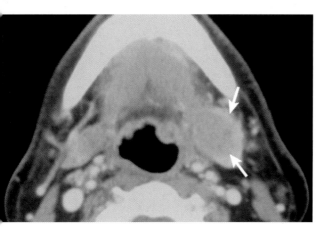

Fig. 8.64 Metastatic malignant melanoma. Axial contrast-enhanced CT shows a poorly defined mass involving the left enlarged submandibular gland, with less enhancement compared with submandibular gland tissue (arrows).

Table 8.10   Sublingual space lesions

Disease	CT Findings	Comments
Pseudomass		
Hypoglossal nerve motor atrophy ▷ *Fig. 8.65*	In CN XII injury, the intrinsic and extrinsic tongue muscles are affected. Long-standing chronic denervation is manifested by marked loss of hemitongue volume, extensive fatty replacement, absence of contrast enhancement, and ipsilateral deviation of the midline fatty septum. A characteristic finding in chronic hypoglossal denervation is the prolapse of the affected hemitongue posteriorly into the oropharynx.	Damage to the hypoglossal nerve anywhere along its course may produce denervation atrophy. Patients who have denervation atrophy of muscles innervated by the hypoglossal nerve demonstrate loss of hemitongue volume, loss of normal papillae, and deviation of the tongue toward the side of pathologic change on protrusion.
Congenital/developmental lesions		
Infantile hemangioma (capillary hemangioma)	Solitary, multifocal, or transspatial, lobular soft tissue mass, homogeneous and isodense with muscle. Contrast enhancement is uniform and intense. No calcifications. Size, enhancement, and vascularity of tumor regress in involutional phase with internal, low-density fat.	True capillary hemangiomas are neoplastic conditions; they typically display a rapid proliferation phase during the first year of life, followed by an involution phase with fatty replacement. They have a female predilection. Infantile hemangiomas are high-flow lesions during their proliferative phase, low-flow lesions in their involutional phase. Sixty percent of infantile hemangiomas occur in the head and neck, with superficial strawberry-colored lesions and facial swelling and/or deep lesions, often in the parotid, masticator, and buccal spaces. Retropharyngeal, sublingual, and submandibular spaces and oral mucosa are other common locations.
Venous vascular malformation (cavernous hemangioma)	Lobulated, well-defined, or poorly marginated soft tissue mass, isodense to muscle, with rounded calcifications (phleboliths). May be localized or diffuse, solitary or multifocal, circumscribed or transspatial, with or without satellite lesions. Contrast enhancement is patchy or homogeneous and intense. Fat hypertrophy in adjacent soft tissues may be present.	As opposed to hemangiomas, vascular malformations are not tumors but true congenital low-flow vascular anomalies, have an equal gender incidence, may not become clinically apparent until late infancy or childhood, virtually always grow in size with the patient during childhood, and do not involute spontaneously. Vascular malformations are further subdivided into capillary, venous, arterial, lymphatic, and combined malformations. Venous vascular malformations, usually present in children and young adults, are the most common vascular malformation of the head and neck. The buccal region and dorsal neck are the most common locations. Sublingual space, masticator space, tongue, lips, and orbit are other common locations. Frequently, venous malformations do not respect fascial boundaries and involve more than one deep fascial space. They are soft and compressible. Lesion may increase in size with Valsalva maneuver, bending over, or crying. Rapid swelling and enlargement can occur following trauma or hormonal changes (e.g., pregnancy). Pain is common and often caused by thrombosis.
Lymphatic malformation (lymphangioma, cystic hygroma)	Uni- or multilocular, often poorly circumscribed and transspatial, insinuating nonenhancing, fluid-density mass. Fluid–fluid levels may be seen. If uninfected, the wall may be very thin.	Lymphatic malformations represent a spectrum of congenital low-flow vascular malformations, differentiated by size of dilated lymphatic channels. May be sporadic or part of congenital syndromes (Turner, Noonan, and fetal alcohol syndromes). Macrocystic lymphatic malformation is the most common subtype; 65% are present at birth. Ninety percent are clinically apparent by 3 y of age; the remaining 10% present in young adults. In the suprahyoid neck, involvement of the masticator, submandibular, parotid, and parapharyngeal spaces is more common than involvement of the sublingual space. Lymphatic malformations may involve the salivary glands directly or by extension. Large lesions can present with airway obstruction.

(continues on page 355)▶

Table 8.10 (Cont.) Sublingual space lesions

Disease	CT Findings	Comments
Developmental cyst	**Dermoid:** Unilocular, thin-walled, well-demarcated ovoid mass with fatty, fluid, or mixed contents. Globules of fat floating within the lesion may produce a characteristic "sack of marbles" appearance. Alternatively, fat–fluid levels may be present. Calcification (< 50%) and subtle rim enhancement of the wall are sometimes seen. **Epidermoid:** Low-density, unilocular, well-demarcated mass with fluid contents only, a thin enhancing wall, and no significant surrounding inflammatory changes. **Teratoma:** Multilocular, heterogeneous, mixed-density mass containing solid, fatty, and cystic components and calcifications.	Developmental cysts are a rare cause of head and neck masses. They are usually located in the midline or slightly off the midline within the floor of the mouth, the anterior submandibular or sublingual space, the submandibular gland, and the root of the tongue. The teratomatous lesions are categorized by their germ cell tissue composition. Epidermoids seem to involve the sublingual space more commonly; dermoids, more commonly the submandibular space. Present from birth, oral cavity space cysts typically become manifest at age 5 to 50 y (M:F = 3:1) as a painless subcutaneous or submucosal mass in the suprahyoid region with fullness in the floor of the mouth. The identification of the cyst location in relationship to the mylohyoid muscle on CT or MRI is extremely helpful in surgical planning.
Lingual thyroid tissue	High-density mass secondary to iodine accumulation, sharply margined, with avid homogeneous enhancement, usually at the midline of the base of the tongue along the expected tract of the thyroglossal duct. Less commonly found in the sublingual space or tongue root.	Aberrant thyroid can be found in many locations in the neck and mediastinum. A lingual (base of the tongue) location of the thyroid may represent the only undescended thyroid tissue in the body. Ectopic thyroid tissue has a high female-to-male preponderance. There are two presentation age peaks: around puberty and in the elderly. Symptoms may arise from local mass effect; hyperthyroidism is rare. Lesions that occur in a cervical thyroid gland can also be found in ectopic glandular tissue, including goiter and different types of carcinoma, but most commonly papillary carcinoma.

(continues on page 356)

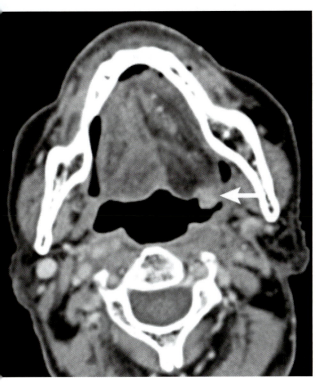

Fig. 8.65 Left hypoglossal nerve motor atrophy. Axial contrast-enhanced CT demonstrates fatty atrophy of the left intrinsic tongue muscles and decrease in size of the extrinsic genioglossus and hyoglossus muscles. Also noted is deviation of the midline septum to the left, as well as slight prolapse of the tongue on the left side posteriorly (arrow: left oropharyngeal carcinoma).

II Head and Neck

Table 8.10 (Cont.) Sublingual space lesions

Disease	CT Findings	Comments
Inflammatory/infectious conditions		
Ludwig angina	CT demonstrates massive edema and an enhancing diffuse, ill-defined infiltration of the superficial and deep tissues of the floor of the mouth, submandibular and sublingual spaces, with low-attenuation areas reflecting abscesses or localized areas of phlegmon. **Cellulitis** appears as thickening of the cutis and subcutis and increased density of fatty tissue with streaky, irregular enhancement (edematous, "dirty" fat). **Myositis** appears as thickening and enhancement of muscles. **Fasciitis** appears as thickening and enhancement of fasciae. Air in the soft tissues can be the result of gas-producing anaerobic infection. Elevation and backward displacement of the tongue, secondary to marked swelling, may lead to severe acute airway compromise.	Ludwig angina refers to a potentially lethal acute bilateral cellulitis of the floor of the mouth and submandibular and sublingual spaces that produces gangrene or serosanguineous phlegmon but little or no frank pus. Further spread occurs into the parapharyngeal, retropharyngeal, and carotid spaces, or even into the mediastinum. The source of infection is usually odontogenic, but sublingual or submandibular sialadenitis, trauma, or surgical procedures of the floor of the mouth are also causes of infection. Patients between the ages 20 and 60 y (rarely in children) often present with rapidly progressive facial swelling, oral pain, fever, dysphagia, dysphonia, and dyspnea. Ludwig angina represents a clinical emergency.
Abscess ▷ *Fig. 8.66*	Abscesses appear as single or multiloculated, low-density areas, with or without gas collections, and demonstrate peripheral rim enhancement. Central root of the tongue abscesses begin in the midline septum area between the genioglossus muscles. Sublingual space abscesses may be unilateral, with fluid collection superomedial to the mylohyoid muscle, or bilateral, with a horseshoe-shaped fluid collection connected by anterior isthmus. Tooth with periapical abscess and focal mandibular cortex dehiscence or mandibular osteomyelitis with permeative bone changes, focal bone destruction, and periosteal reaction may refer to the source of the infection. Edematous subcutaneous skin changes with stranding and dermal thickening, increased density of fatty tissue with streaky, irregular enhancement (edematous, "dirty" fat), muscular enlargement with enhancement (myositis), and reactive or suppurative adenopathy of submandibular lymph nodes are common associated findings.	Focal collection of pus within oral cavity spaces (sublingual space, submandibular space, root of the tongue, or transspatial). The source of infection is usually odontogenic (tooth root abscess/mandibular osteomyelitis). Infections arising from the mandibular first molar and premolar teeth (the roots of which do not reach below the attachment of the mylohyoid muscle) tend to involve the sublingual space. Infections arising from the lower second and third molar teeth (the roots of which reach below the attachment of the mylohyoid muscle) spread into the submandibular space. Submandibular duct calculus, sublingual or submandibular sialadenitis, and penetrating trauma are other causes of infection. Further spread occurs into the parapharyngeal and retropharyngeal space.
Necrotizing fasciitis	The CT findings consist of thickening of the cutis and subcutis, thickening and enhancement of the cervical fascia and muscles (fasciitis and myositis), and fluid collections in multiple neck spaces (including oral cavity, carotid, parapharyngeal, retropharyngeal, perivertebral, and masticator spaces), air collections with fluid collections, and reactive lymphadenopathy. Vascular complications include erosion and rupture of the carotid artery and thrombosis of the internal jugular vein.	Necrotizing fasciitis is a severe, acute, and potentially life-threatening streptococcal or mixed bacterial soft tissue infection with a very rapid clinical evolution. It can follow any infection in the neck and is usually characterized in the early stages by neck swelling, erythema, and fever. The infection spreads rapidly throughout the tissue planes of the neck. Failure to treat may lead to sepsis and mediastinitis. It occurs predominantly in immunocompromised and elderly patients.
Dilated submandibular gland duct	CT demonstrates a dilated submandibular gland duct in the sublingual space that can be followed back into the gland (confirming that this is not a ranula). Complete obstruction of the duct leads to atrophy of the gland.	Partial obstruction of the submandibular gland duct can be congenital or caused by calculus or stricture secondary to calculus, trauma, infection, or neoplasm. Thirty percent of salivary glands with sialolithiasis have associated single or multiple stenoses. Symptoms include intermittent swelling, pain with eating, and superimposed infection secondary to stasis.
Sialocele	**True sialocele:** Sublingual space mass, smoothly bordered, ovoid to lenticular with fluid density in the course of the dilated submandibular duct. If associated with sialolithiasis, CT may show duct enlargement with enhancing enlarged submandibular gland and enhancing adjacent inflammatory soft tissues. With **false sialocele,** fluid collection is distinct from the submandibular duct.	Partial obstruction of the distal end of the submandibular duct, usually caused by sialolithiasis, inflammation, or a tumor, will produce dilation of the duct with focal distention representing an epithelial-lined salivary mucocele or salivary retention cyst. Disruption of the duct, usually caused by trauma or surgery, will cause extrusion of saliva into the adjacent tissue, resulting in a pseudocyst, contained within a fibrous pseudocapsule (false sialocele).

(continues on page 357)

Table 8.10   (Cont.) Sublingual space lesions

Disease	CT Findings	Comments
Ranula, simple or diving	**Simple ranula:** Sharply marginated, unilateral, oval to lenticular, unilocular, homogeneous, low-density (0–20 HU) mass confined to the sublingual space with thin, nonenhancing wall. Wall thickening and minimal internal septa formation can be noted after infection or surgery. **Diving ranula:** Unilocular or multilobular, well-circumscribed, low-density mass emanating from the sublingual space and extending into the adjacent submandibular space and inferior parapharyngeal space. Diving ranula may be characteristically comet-shaped with collapsed cyst in the sublingual space ("tail" sign) and large pseudocystic component (its "head") in the posterior submandibular space. Large, horseshoe-shaped ranula may extend across the midline through the anterior isthmus of the sublingual space.	Ranulas are rare lesions. Simple ranula is a mucus retention cyst, acquired secondarily (after trauma or inflammation) to obstructed sublingual or minor salivary glands, that arises within the sublingual space. The term *diving* or *plunging ranula* is used when a simple ranula becomes large and ruptures out of the posterior sublingual space into the submandibular and inferior parapharyngeal spaces, creating a pseudocyst lacking epithelial lining. Simple ranulas are seen as intraoral mass lesions. Diving ranulas are seen as submandibular or neck masses with no clinically apparent oral connection.
Benign neoplasms		
Benign mixed tumor (pleomorphic adenoma) of sublingual gland origin ▷ *Fig. 8.67*	Single, homogeneous, ovoid soft tissue mass with fairly well-defined margins in the sublingual space. Sometimes foci of necrosis, hemorrhage, or focal calcifications may be seen. The contrast enhancement, mild to moderate, may be uniformly homogeneous or heterogeneous.	Only 0.5% to 1% of all head and neck benign mixed tumors arise in the sublingual gland. Presents as slow-growing, painless sublingual space mass. Peak age of occurrence 40 y and older; M:F = 1:2.

(continues on page 358)

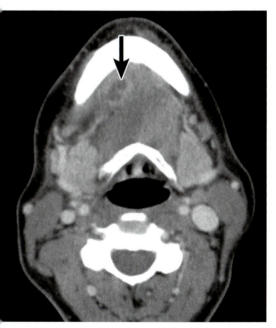

Fig. 8.66   Sublingual space abscess (odontogenic infection after dental decay). Axial contrast-enhanced CT shows infection spread into the sublingual space with rim-enhancing fluid collection superomedial to the right mylohyoid muscle.

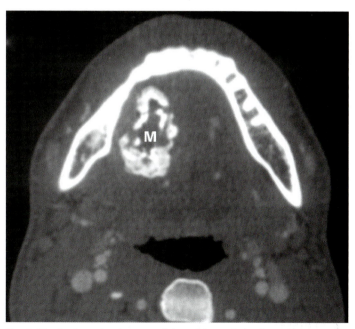

Fig. 8.67   Benign mixed tumor of the sublingual gland. Axial bone contrast-enhanced CT shows a large, sharply defined, irregular, heterogeneous mass (M) with extensive calcification in the right sublingual space.

II   Head and Neck

Table 8.10   (Cont.) Sublingual space lesions

Disease	CT Findings	Comments
Malignant neoplasms		
Contiguous tumor extension ▷ *Fig. 8.68*	Aggressive, fairly enhancing mixed-density mass lesion violating the sublingual space. Tongue base carcinoma invades the sublingual space from posterior to anterior, oral tongue carcinoma invades it from superior to inferior.	The most common malignant lesion of the sublingual space is a squamous cell carcinoma arising from the epithelial covering of the sublingual space or related to direct extension of oropharyngeal carcinoma.
Malignant sublingual gland or minor salivary gland tumor	Small well defined or larger poorly, irregular defined soft tissue mass in the sublingual space with heterogeneous enhancement. Mucoepidermoid carcinomas have a strong tendency to spread into local lymph nodes. Distant adenoid cystic carcinoma metastases occur most often in lungs.	Eighty percent of all sublingual gland masses are malignant. Malignant tumors of the sublingual gland, and minor salivary gland origin include adenoid cystic carcinoma, mucoepidermoid carcinoma, malignant mixed tumor (carcinoma ex pleomorphic adenoma), metastasizing benign mixed tumor, and carcinosarcoma. Patients (30–60 y, M = F) present with painless sublingual space swelling.

Table 8.11   Lesions of the buccal space

Disease	CT Findings	Comments
Pseudomass		
Accessory parotid gland ▷ *Fig. 8.69*	Accessory parotid tissue may be unilateral or bilateral, overlying the anterior margin of the masseter muscle outside the masticator space, and has the same attenuation as the tissue in the main parotid gland.	In 20% to 35% of healthy patients, accessory parotid tissue is present in the buccal space, separate from and anterior to the parotid gland, immediately to the parotid duct. May mimic a buccal mass on clinical examination.
Congenital/developmental lesions		
Developmental cyst	**Dermoid:** Cystic, well-demarcated mass, localized in the buccal space, adjacent to the skin and distinct from the buccinator muscle, with fatty, fluid, or mixed contents. Globules of fat floating within the lesion may produce a characteristic "sack of marbles" appearance. Alternatively, fat–fluid levels may be present. Calcifications (< 50%) and a subtle rim enhancement of wall are sometimes seen. **Epidermoid:** Low-density, unilocular, well-demarcated mass localized in the buccal space, with fluid contents only, a thin wall, and no significant surrounding inflammatory changes. **Teratoma:** Multilocular, heterogeneous, mixed-density mass, containing solid, fatty, and cystic components and calcifications.	Developmental cysts are a rare cause of head and neck masses. They typically become manifest during the second or third decade of life.
Infantile hemangioma (capillary hemangioma)	Solitary, multifocal or transspatial, lobular soft tissue mass, homogeneous and isodense with muscle. Contrast enhancement is uniform and intense. No calcifications. Size, enhancement and vascularity of tumor regress in involution phase with internal, low-density fat.	True capillary hemangiomas are neoplastic lesions. They tend to be small or absent at birth, typically enter a rapid proliferation phase during the first year of life, followed by a stationary period and, finally, an involution phase with fatty replacement. They have a female predilection. Infantile hemangiomas are high-flow lesions during their proliferative phase, low-flow lesions in their involutional phase. Sixty percent of infantile hemangiomas occur in the head and neck, with superficial strawberry-colored lesions and facial swelling and/or deep lesions, often in the parotid, masticator, and buccal spaces. Retropharyngeal, sublingual, and submandibular spaces and oral mucosa are other common locations.

(continues on page 360)

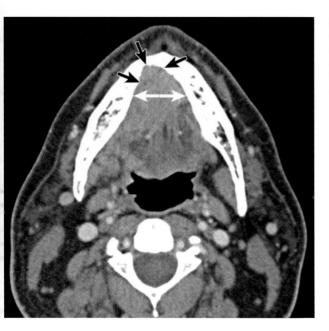

Fig. 8.68 Squamous cell carcinoma of the tongue. Axial contrast-enhanced CT reveals that the large enhancing tumor crosses the midline (double arrow) and involves both genioglossus muscles, the right sublingual space, and the right mylohyoid muscle. There is a large area of bone destruction of the medial mandibular cortical wall underlying the tumor (arrows).

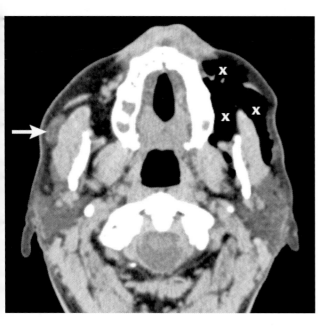

Fig. 8.69 Accessory parotid gland. Axial non–contrast-enhanced CT reveals ovoid tissue overlying the right masseter (arrow) that has the same attenuation as the parotid gland. Large emphysema in the left buccal space (x) is coincident.

Table 8.11 (Cont.) Lesions of the buccal space

Disease	CT Findings	Comment
Venous vascular malformation (cavernous hemangioma)	Multilobulated, well-defined, or poorly marginated soft tissue mass, isodense to muscle. May be located superficially or involve deep structures, localized or diffuse, solitary or multifocal, circumscribed or transspatial, with or without satellite lesions. Contrast enhancement is patchy or homogeneous and intense. The presence of characteristic phleboliths will strongly suggest the diagnosis.	Unlike infantile hemangiomas, vascular malformations are true congenital low-flow vascular anomalies, have an equal gender incidence, are always present at birth, and enlarge proportional to growth. They never involute and remain present throughout life. Vascular malformations are further subdivided into capillary, venous, arterial, lymphatic, and combined malformations. Venous vascular malformations, usually present in children and young adults, are the most common vascular malformation of the head and neck. The buccal region and dorsal neck are the most common locations. Masticator space, sublingual space, tongue, lips, and orbit are other common locations. Frequently, venous malformations do not respect fascial boundaries and involve more than one deep fascial space (transspatial disease). They are soft and compressible. Lesions may increase in size with Valsalva maneuver, bending over, or crying. Rapid swelling and enlargement can occur following trauma or hormonal changes (e.g., pregnancy). Pain is common and often caused by thrombosis.

Inflammatory/infectious conditions

Disease	CT Findings	Comment
Cellulitis	Cellulitis may present as a soft tissue mass with edematous obliteration of adjacent fat planes but without a definite low-density collection of pus. It is often ill defined, enhancing, and extending along fascial planes and into subcutaneous tissues beneath thickened skin.	Buccal space cellulitis may arise from an infection of the masticator space or oral cavity. Commonly occurs in children younger than 3 y (F = M) in fall/winter with fever, buccal swelling, and blue-red skin color; 17% are associated with ipsilateral serous otitis media.
Abscess	Abscesses often appear as a poorly marginated soft tissue mass in the expanded buccal space with single or multiloculated low-density center, with or without gas collections, and usually thick abscess wall. Contrast-enhanced CT images show a thick, irregular peripheral rim enhancement and enhancement of the inflamed adjacent soft tissues. From the buccal and masticator space, the abscesses may spread into the retromolar trigone, parapharyngeal space, submandibular space, and floor of the mouth.	Odontogenic infections of the maxillary molars may produce bacterial abscesses in the buccal space and masticator space. Less commonly, they may result from infections of buccal lymph nodes or minor salivary glands. They may occur in all age groups with an acute onset (risk factors: history of diabetes mellitus and Crohn disease). Patients may be toxic, febrile, dehydrated, and present with a tender, swollen cheek and a fluctuating mass.

Benign neoplasms

Disease	CT Findings	Comment
Benign epithelial tumors of salivary gland origin	Well-circumscribed, rounded, isoattenuating mass with moderate contrast enhancement. Central areas of low attenuation and rim enhancement, calcifications, and cysts are possible in larger tumors.	The most common primary masses in the buccal space are salivary gland tumors. Benign mixed tumor (pleomorphic adenoma) is the most common benign tumor of the salivary glands. It is 9 times as common in the accessory parotid gland as in minor salivary glands. Presents as slow-growing, nontender buccal space mass. Peak age of occurrence 40 y and older; M:F = 1:2. Other benign salivary gland lesions (e.g., monomorphic adenomas and ductal papillomas) may have similar clinical and imaging characteristics.
Lipoma	Well-defined, nonenhancing fat-density mass (−65 to −125 HU), homogeneous without any internal soft tissue stranding.	Lipomas of the buccal space are uncommon. Present as slowly enlarging palpable mass. Peak age of occurrence 40 y and older; M:F = 2.5:1.

(continues on page 361

Table 8.11 (Cont.) Lesions of the buccal space

Disease	CT Findings	Comment
Neurofibroma	May present as solitary or multiple, rounded or ovoid, well-demarcated, heterogeneous, low-density mass. Absence of contrast enhancement is conspicuous. Plexiform neurofibroma shows a usually large, ill-defined, more infiltrative, heterogeneous mass with a mixed-density pattern. A typical finding is the target sign with a punctate high attenuation centrally surrounded by peripheral low attenuation within multiple small tumor nodules.	Neurofibromas involving the buccal space are usually associated with neurofibromatosis type 1. They may be localized, solitary or multiple, or plexiform.
Schwannoma	Schwannomas tend to occur as a well-defined, fusiform soft tissue mass with varying degrees of contrast enhancement. Some of the nerve tumors may be extensive, multilobulated, with areas of cystic formation and inhomogeneous enhancement.	Schwannomas of the buccal space are very rare. They are usually solitary and manifest as a slowly enlarging, painless mass along the branches of the facial or mandibular nerves. These tumors can occur at any age, most commonly between the age of 20 and 50 y, with a female predominance.
Solitary fibrous tumor	Well-defined, solid mass, isodense to muscle, with heterogeneously or homogeneously strong enhancement and occasional calcification or necrosis.	The buccal space is an uncommon location for this ubiquitous neoplasm.
Nodular fasciitis	Well-circumscribed, round, solid soft tissue mass in the buccal space, isodense to muscle, with heterogeneously or homogeneously strong contrast enhancement and occasional calcification or necrosis.	Nodular fasciitis is a rare benign proliferation of fibroblasts and myofibroblasts. A history of trauma may precede these mesenchymal tumors. The lesions are generally small and solitary, slowly progressive, commonly seen in the head and neck region of infants and children, and seen in the upper extremities in young adults.
Malignant neoplasms		
Squamous cell carcinoma	Tumors originating in adjacent spaces may extend or secondarily involve the buccal space as aggressive, diffusely infiltrating, fairly enhancing mixed-density mass lesion, with obliteration of the normal fat planes and contrast enhancement of the tumor margins.	Squamous cell carcinoma is the most common malignant tumor involving the buccal space. The tumor may project or extend into the buccal space from deep extension of carcinomas originating in the skin, subcutaneous tissues, buccal mucosa, masticator space, alveolar ridge of the maxilla, retromolar trigone, mandible, base of the tongue, and nasal vestibule.
Nodal metastases	Metastatic buccal lymphadenopathy typically manifests as a single node > 10 mm in maximum diameter or as a grouping of nodes. Suggestive of nodal metastasis is a round, mildly enhancing soft tissue mass, centered within fat of the anterior or posterior buccal space. Most reliable imaging finding of metastatic disease is the presence of central nodal necrosis. Necrosis appears as central nonenhancing low density with a variably thick, irregular enhancing wall. Ill-defined margins and stranding of surrounding fat are features of extracapsular spread.	Metastatic buccal lymphadenopathy typically occurs in association with clinically evident, deeply infiltrating facial neoplasms, or in recurrent squamous cell carcinoma of the sinuses and gingivobuccal sulcus. Patients (> 40 y) present with smooth, nontender, mobile buccal masses.

(continues on page 362

Table 8.11   (Cont.) Lesions of the buccal space

Disease	CT Findings	Comment
Lymphoma ▷ *Fig. 8.70*	**Intranodal lymphoma:** Hodgkin and non–Hodgkin lymphomas of buccal nodes can present with multiple or single nodal enlargement as isolated symptom or as part of a systemic disease. Lymph node masses commonly demonstrate homogeneous soft tissue attenuation. In general, there is homogeneous enhancement, although rim enhancement and spotty or dentritic enhancement on CT are sometimes seen. **Extranodal lymphoma:** Ill-defined and infiltrative buccal space mass along the course of the parotid duct, isolated or associated with nodal disease, extranodal lymphatic disease (Waldeyer ring), and/or involvement of other extranodal extralymphatic sites (e.g., sinus, nose, and orbit).	Buccal space lymphoma may either arise within the buccal lymph nodes or be extranodal. The latter is more common in non–Hodgkin lymphoma and has a poor prognosis. Patients (> 50 y) may have CN V_3 symptoms and a buccal space mass as part of systemic non–Hodgkin lymphoma or as the first manifestation of limited head and neck disease.
Rhabdomyosarcoma	Bulky, heterogeneous, locally invasive, ill-defined soft tissue mass, isodense with muscle, with moderate to marked contrast enhancement. May be heterogeneous due to focal hemorrhage or necrotic areas. Contiguous soft tissues and osseous structures are often involved by direct invasion.	Rhabdomyosarcomas are rare malignant mesenchymal tumors; 40% of these will involve the head and neck. Involvement of the buccal space is uncommon. They tend to occur in children (< 5 y). The most characteristic presenting features are a rapid onset and progression.
Liposarcoma	Well-differentiated liposarcomas present as a lobulated, fatty mass with some enhancing internal septations or nodules. Calcifications may occur. Less well-differentiated liposarcomas display as heterogeneous, enhancing soft tissue mass with or without amorphous fatty foci, often with unsharp, infiltrating borders.	Only 3 to 6% of liposarcomas occur in the head and neck region. Within the oral cavity, they may be located in the cheek, palate, floor of the mouth, and submental regions. They may occur in all age groups (30–60 y) and show no gender predilection.
Mucoepidermoid carcinoma	Single mass with hyperattenuating, well-defined or infiltrative margins, central iso- or hypoattenuating area (necrotic), and prominent enhancement. Adjacent malignant adenopathy may be present.	Usually occurs in the accessory parotid gland (exceptionally within Stensen duct). Patients (40–50 y, F ≥ M) present with a nontender, mobile palpable buccal mass that has been present for 1 to 5 y.
Adenoid cystic carcinoma	Moderate enhancing soft tissue mass with irregular, ill-defined margin or infiltration of surrounding tissues. Differentiation from benign tumors may be difficult, as two thirds of salivary gland malignancies have smooth, well-defined margins.	Adenoid cystic carcinoma is the most frequent malignant tumor of the minor salivary glands (25%). Commonly occurs in women of early middle age. Pain is common.
Acinic cell carcinoma	Moderate enhancing soft tissue mass with irregular, ill-defined margin or infiltration of surrounding tissues. Differentiation from benign tumors may be difficult, as two thirds of salivary gland malignancies have smooth, well-defined margins.	Twice as common in the accessory parotid gland as in salivary rests. Has a varying biological behavior. Tumor affects women more than men (40–60 y).
Parotid duct		
Sialectasia of Stensen duct ▷ *Fig. 8.71*	Parotid duct ectasia may present as • Beadlike or rosary-like dilations and stenoses of Stensen duct over the full length • Cystic dilation of the parotid duct. The width of the duct is moderately distended proximal and distal to the cystic area. • Sialectasis with fusiform dilation of the parotid duct	Most commonly due to an obstructed calculus located at the orifice of Stensen duct. With idiopathic parotid duct ectasia, results of the workup for a cause of the duct dilation such as a tumor, inflammation, stricture, or stones are negative. Congenital cystic dilation of the parotid duct with formation of multilocular cystic areas is very rare, may be unilateral or bilateral, and may manifest in infancy or appear later. Painless recurrent tubular swelling over the lateral aspect of the face with an associated intraoral submucosal distention. It sometimes results in recurrent parotitis.

(continues on page 363)

Table 8.11 (Cont.) Lesions of the buccal space

Disease	CT Findings	Comment
Trauma		
Emphysema	Interstitial radiolucent gaseous collections in the buccal space and in other spaces, including subcutaneous tissues.	Buccal emphysema may occur spontaneously, following trauma or surgery, with pneumoparotitis, or as part of a cervicofacial emphysema.
Hematoma ▷ *Fig. 8.72*	Buccal hematoma may appear as soft tissue swelling or as a nonenhancing mass, with hemorrhage and edema of adjacent subcutaneous tissue. In the acute stage, the hematoma may be hyperdense. In the subacute stage, the hematoma might be poorly defined and is either isodense or slightly hypodense. When completely liquefied, the hematoma has a homogeneous density that is lower than muscle and may be surrounded by an enhancing pseudocapsule.	Soft tissue hemorrhage can collect as hematoma. Hematomas of the buccal space are a common finding after sports injuries and other blunt head and neck traumas.

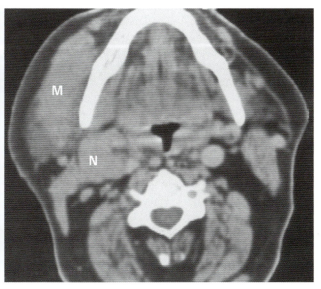

Fig. 8.70 **Non–Hodgkin lymphoma.** Axial contrast-enhanced CT demonstrates a homogeneous, poorly enhancing, multilobulated right buccomasseteric mass (M). Right level II nodal involvement is present (N).

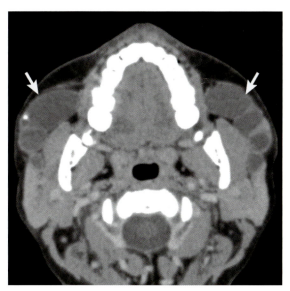

Fig. 8.71 **Sialectasia of the Stensen duct.** Axial non–contrast-enhanced CT reveals bilateral "rosary-like" dilations and stenosis of the Stensen duct (arrows). A small calculus is present on the right side.

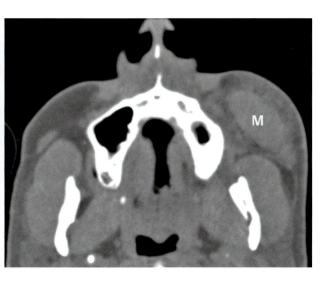

Fig. 8.72 **Buccal hematoma.** Axial non–contrast-enhanced CT shows a well-circumscribed, ovoid soft tissue mass (M) in the left buccal space. Also seen is fat stranding of subcutaneous fat, with thickened overlying skin.

9 Infrahyoid Neck

Wolfgang Zaunbauer and Francis A. Burgener

As in the suprahyoid neck, the structures of the infrahyoid neck are surrounded by a layer of subcutaneous tissue (superficial cervical fascia) and are compartmentalized by three layers of the deep cervical fascia: superficial (investing), middle (visceral), and deep (prevertebral). The infrahyoid neck contains 10 distinct spaces defined by the layers of the deep cervical fascia (**Fig. 9.1**). The visceral space, retropharyngeal space, danger space, and perivertebral space are midline, nonpaired spaces. The anterior cervical space, carotid space, and posterior cervical space are lateral, paired spaces. Of these spaces, only the visceral space and the paired anterior cervical space are unique to the infrahyoid neck. The carotid, retropharyngeal, danger, and perivertebral spaces all traverse both the suprahyoid and infrahyoid neck.

The *visceral space* is a cylindrical space in the anterior midline of the infrahyoid neck, completely enclosed by the middle layer (visceral fascia) of the deep cervical fascia. It is the largest space of the infrahyoid neck, extending from the hyoid bone to the upper mediastinum. It is bordered posteriorly by the retropharyngeal space and posterolaterally by the carotid space bilaterally. Paired anterior cervical spaces are lateral to the visceral space and are continuous with the submandibular spaces superiorly. The contents of the visceral space include the larynx, cervical trachea, hypopharynx, cervical esophagus, thyroid gland, parathyroid glands, recurrent laryngeal nerves, and lymph nodes (level VI group).

A visceral space mass presentation depends on the structures involved. The center of a *thyroid mass* is within the thyroid gland, with thyroid tissue seen surrounding the lesion. The ipsilateral carotid space is displaced laterally, and the trachea and esophagus are displaced to the side opposite the lesion. The center of a *parathyroid mass* is between the thyroid gland anteriorly and the longus colli muscle posteriorly (tracheoesophageal groove). When large, parathyroid lesions displace the thyroid lobe anteriorly and the adjacent carotid space anterolaterally. The best indicator of a *hypopharyngeal malignancy* is a bulky mass with invasion and destruction of submucosal and deep structures, as well as associated necrotic lymph nodes. *Cervical esophageal mass lesions* are centered in the middle of the posterior visceral space, immediately posterior to the trachea, abutting or surrounding the esophagus, and displace the trachea and thyroid gland anteriorly. The esophagus can pouch out from its normal, retrotracheal location into the tracheoesophageal groove and mimic a paraesophageal nodal mass. *Laryngeal lesions* are centered within the cartilaginous edifice of the larynx. A *cervical tracheal mass lesion* is centered in the tracheal wall and may displace the thyroid gland laterally and the esophagus posteriorly.

The *retropharyngeal space* (RPS), a midline space just posterior to the aerodigestive tract, continues into the infrahyoid neck from the suprahyoid neck above and extends inferiorly to the level of the upper thoracic spine. Unlike the suprahyoid RPS, which contains both fat and lymph nodes, the infrahyoid RPS contains only fat, defined by the visceral fascia anteriorly and the alar fascia posteriorly. The *danger space* lies between the RPS and perivertebral space in the midline. It continues into the infrahyoid neck from the suprahyoid neck above and extends inferiorly to the diaphragm. It is a potential space, normally containing only fat, and is formed between two parallel slips of the deep layer of the deep cervical fascia, the alar fascia anteriorly and laterally and the prevertebral fascia posteriorly. Although separately defined fascial spaces, the "true" RPS and the danger space are considered together, because they cannot be differentiated from one another by means of sectional imaging.

A mass of the infrahyoid RPS appears rectangular shaped or oval and is centered anterior to the prevertebral muscles and posterior to the visceral space. A mass remains anterior to and flattens prevertebral muscles, as it enlarges and may displace the carotid space laterally. The infrahyoid RPS may be involved by processes arising from tissues within this space, but more commonly it is affected by external invasion from adjacent spaces.

The *perivertebral space* (PVS), a large cylindrical space surrounding the vertebral column, continues into the infrahyoid neck from the suprahyoid neck above and extends inferiorly to the upper mediastinum. The PVS is completely bordered by the tenacious deep layer of the deep cervical fascia. The attachment of the fascia to the transverse processes of the vertebral body divides the PVS into the anterior prevertebral portion and the posterior paraspinal portion. The contents of the prevertebral portion include the prevertebral muscles, scalene muscles, brachial plexus roots, phrenic nerve, vertebral artery and vein, and vertebral body. The paraspinal portion contains the paraspinal muscles, fat, and posterior elements of the vertebral body. In the infrahyoid neck, the PVS is bordered anteriorly by the RPS, anterolaterally by the carotid space, and posteriorly and laterally by the posterior cervical space.

A mass lesion of the prevertebral portion is centered within the prevertebral muscles or corpus of the vertebral body and elevates the prevertebral muscles, pushing the retropharyngeal space anteriorly. A mass lesion of the paraspinal portion is centered within the paraspinal musculature or the posterior elements of the spine, pushing the fat of the posterior cervical space away. This space is susceptible to the same inflammatory, infectious, and neoplastic processes as the suprahyoid component.

The *carotid space* is a paired tubular space, encircled by the carotid sheath, composed by slips of all three layers of the deep cervical fascia. The infrahyoid carotid space contains the common carotid artery, internal jugular vein, and vagus nerve. The sympathetic plexus is embedded in the medial sheath walls (between the medial carotid space and the lateral RPS). The internal jugular nodal chain (nodal levels III and IV) is found along the length of the internal jugular vein within the outer layers of the carotid sheath. In the infrahyoid neck, the carotid space is bordered anteriorly by the anterior cervical space, laterally by the sternocleidomastoid muscle, posteriorly by the posterior cervical space and prevertebral space, and medially by the visceral space and RPS.

The center of a carotid space mass in the infrahyoid neck is typically in close association with the carotid artery and the jugular vein. As a carotid space mass enlarges, it may engulf the vessels or push them apart.

The *posterior cervical space* (PCS) represents the paired posterolateral compartment of the neck confined anteriorly by the carotid space, medially by the deep layer of the deep cervical fascia enveloping the perivertebral space, and laterally and posteriorly by the superficial layer of the deep cervical fascia,

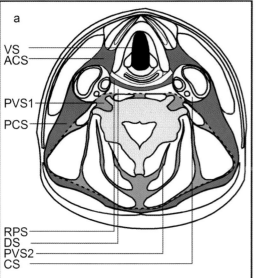 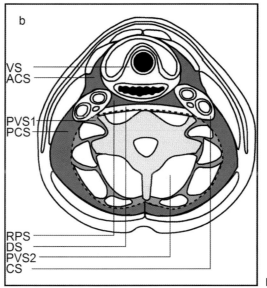

Fig. 9.1a, b   Anatomical drawing depicting the axial anatomy of the normal spaces of the infrahyoid neck. (a) At the level of the glottis. **(b)** At the level of the thyroid gland. ACS: anterior cervical space; CS: carotid space; DS: danger space; PCS: posterior cervical space; PVS1: prevertebral portion, periverterbral space; PVS2: paraspinal portion, periverterbral space; RPS: retropharyngeal space; VS: visceral space; Dashed line: deep layer of deep cervical fascia, with the prevertebral fascia anteriorly.

just deep to the sternocleidomastoid muscle and the trapezius muscle. Most of the PCS is below the hyoid bone, although the very top of this space extends well into the suprahyoid neck. The contents of the PCS include fat, the spinal accessory nerve, the spinal accessory lymph node chain (node level V), and the preaxillary brachial plexus.

A PCS mass is centered in the fat of the PVS. A strip of fat must separate the mass from the carotid space. Large tumors displace the carotid space anteromedially, elevate the sternocleidomastoid muscle, and compress deeper prevertebral and paraspinal structures.

The *anterior cervical space* (ACS) is a small, paired space of the ventral infrahyoid neck, encircled by layers of the deep cervical fascia. It is lateral of the visceral space, medial of the sternocleidomastoid muscle, and ventral of the carotid space. The ACS is the inferior extension of the submandibular space into the infrahyoid neck and contains only fat.

An ACS mass is centered in the fat of the ACS. Large masses elevate the sternocleidomastoid muscle, displace the carotid space vessels posteromedially, and may compress the thyroid gland lobe. The ACS may be important for mediastinal extension of cervical abscesses.

The *larynx* has a framework consisting of a cartilaginous skeleton connected by membranes and ligaments and moved by muscles. The laryngeal skeleton consists of the hyoid bone, cricoid, thyroid, epiglottis, and paired arytenoid cartilages. This framework supports the mucosa-covered surfaces of the larynx. The endolarynx can be subdivided into the supraglottis, glottis, and subglottis. The *supraglottis* extends from the tip of the epiglottis above to the laryngeal ventricle below. The *glottis* includes the true vocal cords and both the anterior and posterior commissures. The *subglottis* extends from the inferior border of the glottic region to the inferior edge of the cricoid cartilage. There are three intralaryngeal compartments: the paired lateral paraglottic space and the midline preepiglottic space. The *paraglottic space* lies between the mucosa and the laryngeal framework and is paired and symmetric. The *preepiglottic space* is a triangular, C-shaped, fat-filled space set between the hyoid bone anteriorly and the epiglottis posteriorly. All structures that predominantly

contain fat (preepiglottic space, paraglottic spaces, aryepiglottic folds, and false cords) are hypoattenuating on computed tomography (CT) images. Ossified cartilage shows a high-attenuating outer and inner cortex and a central low-attenuating medullary space due to fatty tissue. Nonossified hyaline cartilage and nonossified fibroelastic cartilage have the attenuation values of soft tissue. On contrast-enhanced CT, neither the mucosal surface nor the submucosal structures of the larynx show enhancement. The abducted position of the true vocal cords during quiet breathing facilitates evaluation of the anterior and posterior commissures. Additional scans obtained with phonation or modified Valsalva maneuvers facilitate evaluation of the aryepiglottic fold, laryngeal ventricle, and hypopharynx.

The primary sign of tumor spread to the deep paralaryngeal spaces on CT is replacement of fatty tissue with fat density by tumor tissue with intermediate density. Neoplastic cartilage invasion occurs preferentially where the attachments of Sharpey fibers interrupt the perichondrium, thus acting as direct pathways for tumor spread into the cartilaginous tissue. These areas typically include the anterior commissure, the junction of the anterior one fourth and posterior three fourths of the lower thyroid lamina, the posterior border of the thyroid lamina, the cricoarytenoid joint, and the area of attachment of the cricothyroid membrane. The diagnosis of neoplastic cartilage invasion on CT is mainly based on the presence of tumor on both sides of a laryngeal cartilage (extralaryngeal tumor spread), combined with erosion or lysis in the thyroid, cricoid, and arytenoid cartilage and sclerosis in the cricoid and arytenoid (but not the thyroid) cartilage.

The *hypopharynx* is the most caudal portion of the pharynx and extends from the level of the hyoid bone and valleculae to the upper esophageal sphincter. It is formed for the most part by the inferior pharyngeal constrictor muscles. The hypopharynx includes the piriform sinuses, the postcricoid region, and the posterior hypopharyngeal wall. The piriform sinus is situated bilaterally between the thyroid cartilage and the aryepiglottic fold, and is adjacent to the paraglottic space and the cricoid cartilage. The postcricoid region extends from the cricoarytenoid joints to the lower edge of the cricoid cartilage (cricopharyngeus muscle). The posterior wall of the hypopharynx is the inferior continuation of the posterior oropharynx wall. The mucosal surface of the hypopharynx frequently displays a distinct contrast enhancement; the muscular tissue is not enhancing. The hypopharynx may be filled with air or may be collapsed during quiet respiration (a modified Valsalva maneuver may distend this region and rule out the presence of a tumor).

Thyroid lesions are primarily evaluated with radionuclide scanning and ultrasonography. Because of its iodide content, the normal thyroid gland has a density of 80 to 100 HU on CT. After injection of contrast material, the thyroid gland enhances tremendously (drawback: because of iodine uptake from the contrast agent, thyroid localization with nuclear scintigraphy and radioactive iodine treatment must be delayed 4 to 8 weeks after administration of iodinated contrast agents). *Thyroid nodules* are common and comprise adenomas, cysts, focal thyroiditis, multinodular goiter, and malignant tumors. A multiplicity of nodules in an enlarged thyroid gland usually suggests a benign process or metastases. *Calcification* occurs in 13% of all thyroid lesions, including 17% of all malignancies and 11% of all benign processes. Punctate, linear, nodular, amorphous, and peripheral eggshell-like calcifications occur in benign and malignant thyroid tumors, whereas fine punctate calcification is more indicative of malignancy. *Cystic areas* occur in many thyroid masses; 38% of malignancies have cystic components, and 62% of benign masses may be entirely or partly cystic. *Hemorrhage* may be found in papillary carcinomas or goiters.

Once a lesion is identified as in an infrahyoid neck space, the differential diagnosis should be reviewed. The differential diagnosis of the visceral space lesions as seen on CT is discussed in **Table 9.1**, of laryngeal lesions in **Table 9.2**, of thyroid gland lesions in **Table 9.3**, of infrahyoid carotid space lesions in **Table 9.4**, of posterior cervical space lesions in **Table 9.5**, of infrahyoid retropharyngeal space lesions in **Table 9.6**, of infrahyoid perivertebral space lesions in **Table 9.7**, and of anterior cervical space lesions in **Table 9.8**.

Table 9.1   Visceral space lesions

Disease	CT Findings	Comments
Laryngeal lesions	See **Table 9.2**	See **Table 9.2**
Thyroid gland lesions	See **Table 9.3**	See **Table 9.3**
Congenital/developmental lesions		
Infrahyoid thyroglossal duct cyst ▷ *Fig. 9.2* ▷ *Fig. 9.3*	Nonenhancing, smooth, thin-walled low-density (cystic), round or ovoid midline neck mass, usually between 2 and 4 cm, occasionally septated, located at the level of the hyoid bone (~50% of cases) or below it (~25% of cases), deep to or embedded in the infrahyoid strap muscles ("claw" sign). The more inferior the cyst, the more likely it is to be off the midline. The wall may thicken and enhance, and the cyst content may develop higher attenuation, if infected. Any associated nodularity or chunky calcification within the cyst suggests associated thyroid carcinoma. Persistent thyroid tissue may occur anywhere along the thyroglossal duct and typically enhances markedly on postcontrast CT.	The thyroglossal duct cyst, found along the course of the embryonic thyroglossal duct, is the most common midline neck mass. Ninety percent of the lesions are diagnosed before the age of 10 y (M < F). Associated abnormalities are thyroid agenesis, ectopia, and pyramidal lobe.
Cervical thymic cyst ▷ *Fig. 9.4*	Nonenhancing, smooth, thin-walled, low-density (cystic) mass in the lateral infrahyoid neck, lateral visceral space, or adjacent to the carotid space. The lateral left infrahyoid neck, at the level of thyroid gland, is the most common location. May be unilocular or multilocular. Cyst wall may be nodular (aberrant thymic tissue, lymphoid aggregates, or parathyroid tissue). Larger cyst may present as a dumbbell cervicothoracic mass.	Rare remnant of the thymopharyngeal duct, found from the pyriform sinus to the mediastinum. Most present between 2 and 15 y of age (only 33% present after first decade). Slightly more common in male patients. Often asymptomatic. When large, may be associated with respiratory distress or vocal cord paralysis.
Fourth branchial anomaly	Nonenhancing, rounded or ovoid, sharply marginated, thin-walled lesion with central fluid density, attached to the thyroid cartilage or with involvement of the left thyroid lobe. When **fourth branchial sinus** connection with pyriform sinus is maintained, air may be seen in the sinus tract, cyst, and/or left thyroid lobe area, and infection of the cyst and left thyroid lobe is likely. Thyroiditis and thyroid abscess may obscure the cyst itself. **Fourth branchial fistula** denotes two openings, one in the low anterior neck and the other in the pyriform sinus apex.	Remnants of the fourth branchial apparatus. Most cases occur anywhere from the left pyriform sinus apex to the thyroid lobe. Rarest of all forms of branchial cleft anomalies (1%–2%). Present as recurrent suppurative thyroiditis or perithyroid abscess in pediatric patients. More common in female patients.

(continues on page 368)

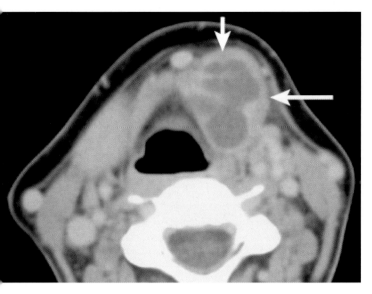

Fig. 9.2   Infrahyoid thyroglossal duct cyst. Axial contrast-enhanced computed tomography (CT) shows a septated, hypodense, paramedian left neck mass embedded in the infrahyoid strap muscles (arrows). A thick enhancing rim suggests prior infection.

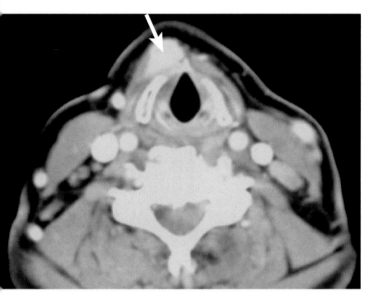

Fig. 9.3   Persistent thyroid tissue. Axial contrast-enhanced CT reveals a strongly enhancing solid nodule of ectopic thyroid tissue (arrow) embedded in the right strap muscles.

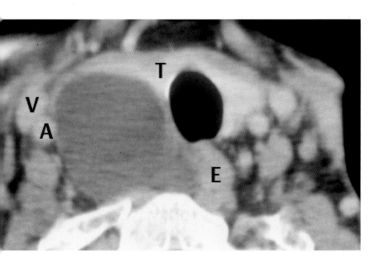

Fig. 9.4   Cervical thymic cyst. Axial contrast-enhanced CT shows a nonenhancing, unilocular, well-circumscribed visceral space mass with fluid density, displacing the carotid space laterally (V, A) and impinging on the right thyroid lobe (T), trachea, and esophagus (E).

Table 9.1 (Cont.) Visceral space lesions

Disease	CT Findings	Comments
Inflammatory/infectious conditions		
Abscess	Poorly marginated soft tissue mass in the expanded visceral space with single or multiloculated low-density center (the attenuation value of the liquefied content usually exceeds 25 HU), with or without gas collections, and usually thick abscess wall. Contrast-enhanced CT images show a thick, irregular peripheral rim enhancement and enhancement of the inflamed adjacent soft tissues.	Abscess originating in the visceral space is rare and usually secondary to penetrating trauma or superinfection of a hematoma.
Parathyroid lesions		
Parathyroid adenoma ▷ *Fig. 9.5*	Moderately contrast enhancing, round or oval, well-circumscribed, usually homogeneous soft tissue mass, hypodense to thyroid gland, typically 1 to 3 cm in size, either in the thyroid bed or in an ectopic location. Cystic degeneration and hemorrhage may occur. In a small percentage of cases (2%–5%), multiple adenomas are present.	Normal parathyroid glands (5 × 3 × 1 mm) are usually not seen on CT. Most people (83%) have four parathyroid glands located behind the upper and lower poles of the thyroid gland. Ectopic glands may be located within the thyroid gland (8%) or along the thymopharyngeal duct tract, extending from the angle of the mandible to the lower anterior mediastinum (15%–20%). Primary hyperparathyroidism and hypercalcemia are caused by a solitary adenoma (in 75%–85%, more common in women), multiple adenomas (in 2%–3%), parathyroid hyperplasia (in 10%–15%), or parathyroid carcinoma (in < 1%).
Parathyroid carcinoma	Parathyroid carcinoma is usually indistinguishable from benign adenoma on sectional imaging. Only the presence of local invasion into the thyroid gland, muscles, or vessels or nodal metastases (in one third of cases) and hematogenous metastases (in 21%–28%) would suggest this diagnosis.	Parathyroid carcinoma causes hyperparathyroidism in 85% to 90% of patients. Men and women are affected equally.
Parathyroid cyst	Nonenhancing, well-defined, ovoid, usually large (2–12 cm), low-density mass, thin-walled, unilocular, homogeneous, typically found in the tracheoesophageal groove, near the lower pole of the thyroid gland, more common on the left side. The cervicothoracic type may be dumbbell shaped.	Rare entity. Classified as nonfunctioning parathyroid cyst (congenital colloidal cyst, diagnosed in the fourth or fifth decade of life, slightly more common in women) or functioning parathyroid cyst, producing primary hyperparathyroidism (10%; these are pseudocysts with cystic necrosis or degeneration of a parathyroid adenoma, more common in men). Large cysts may compress the adjacent trachea, esophagus, and recurrent laryngeal nerve, causing recurrent laryngeal nerve palsy.
Hypopharyngeal lesions		
Hypopharyngeal carcinoma ▷ *Fig. 9.6* ▷ *Fig. 9.7* ▷ *Fig. 9.8*	Invasive mucosal mass, isodense to muscle, with moderate contrast enhancement, arising from the pyriform sinus (60%), postcricoid region (25%), or posterior hypopharyngeal wall (15%) with asymmetrical thickening of the pharyngeal walls, tumor-caused deformity of the endopharyngeal contours, and restrictive extensibility with phonation or modified Valsalva maneuver.	More than 90% of tumors of the hypopharynx are squamous cell carcinomas occurring usually in men older than 50 y with a history of tobacco and alcohol abuse. Tumors associated with Plummer–Vinson syndrome typically occur in women. Up to 15% of patients with hypopharyngeal squamous cell carcinoma have second primary tumors. Because of a prolonged asymptomatic preclinical interval, hypopharyngeal cancers are usually in an advanced stage at presentation. Up to 75% of patients have nodal metastases, and 20% to 40% of patients have distant metastases at the time of diagnosis.

(continues on page 370)

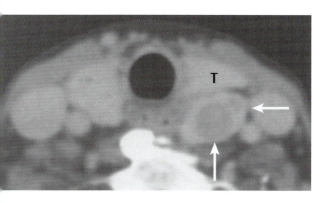

Fig. 9.5 Parathyroid adenoma. Axial contrast-enhanced CT demonstrates an ovoid, well-circumscribed, heterogeneously enhancing, soft tissue mass (arrows) in the left tracheoesophageal groove posterior to the left lobe of the thyroid gland (T).

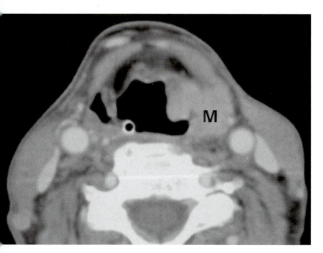

Fig. 9.6 Pyriform sinus carcinoma. Axial contrast-enhanced CT demonstrates a left pyriform sinus tumor (M) with involvement of the aryepiglottic fold and endolaryngeal paraglottic fat.

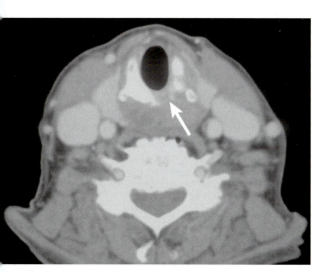

Fig. 9.7 Postcricoid carcinoma of the hypopharynx. Axial contrast-enhanced CT reveals a bulky postcricoid hypopharyngeal tumor eroding cricoid cartilage (arrow).

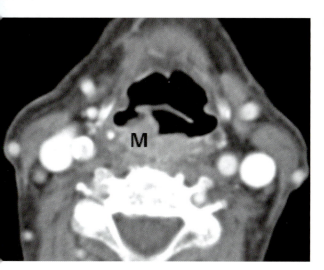

Fig. 9.8 Posterior hypopharyngeal wall carcinoma. Axial contrast-enhanced CT shows a moderately enhancing, asymmetrical thickening of the posterior pharyngeal wall (M).

Table 9.1   (Cont.) Visceral space lesions

Disease	CT Findings	Comments
Hypopharyngeal carcinoma (continued)	Tumors arising from the **lateral wall of the pyriform sinus** tend to spread through the thyrohyoid membrane into the soft tissues of the neck (carotid artery) very early. Tumors originating from the medial wall of the pyriform sinus may infiltrate the larynx by growing anteriorly into the paraglottic space with cord fixation, or they may spread to the postcricoid region and cervical esophagus. Once an advanced pyriform sinus tumor has reached the apex, it may spread into the larynx, invading the arytenoid cartilage, cricoarytenoid joint, and subglottis. Pyriform sinus carcinoma frequently invades the laryngeal framework. Pyriform sinus tumors primarily drain into group II, III, and V lymph nodes. **Postcricoid area** tumors tend to spread submucosally, either circumferentially or toward the cervical esophagus, with thickening of the postcricoid region and anterior displacement of the arytenoid and cricoid cartilages. Invasion of the cricoid cartilage is common. Growth beyond the posterior cricoarytenoid muscle into the thyroid gland and cervical trachea and perineural infiltration along the branches of the recurrent laryngeal nerve with fixation of the vocal cord are other common features. Postcricoid area tumors tend to metastasize to group III, IV, and VI lymph nodes. **Posterior hypopharyngeal wall** cancers commonly involve both the hypopharynx and oropharynx with asymmetrical thickening of the posterior pharyngeal wall. Invasion of the retropharyngeal space is common. Rarely, these tumors cause invasion of the prevertebral muscles at presentation. Posterior hypopharyngeal wall cancers have a tendency to involve primarily the retropharyngeal lymph nodes and secondarily the internal jugular chain lymph nodes.	Two to 7% of all hypopharyngeal tumors are atypical forms of squamous cell carcinoma (verrucous carcinoma, spindle cell carcinoma, basaloid cell carcinoma, and undifferentiated carcinoma of the nasopharyngeal type). **Carcinoma of the hypopharynx: TNM classification** **Primary tumor** T1: Tumor limited to one subsite* of the hypopharynx and ≤ 2 cm in greatest dimension T2: Tumor invades more than one subsite* of hypopharynx or an adjacent site or measures > 2 cm but < 4 cm in greatest dimension without fixation of hemilarynx T3: Tumor measures > 4 cm in greatest dimension, or with fixation of hemilarynx or extension to esophagus T4a: Tumor invades any of the following: thyroid or cricoid cartilage, hyoid bone, thyroid gland, esophagus, central compartment soft tissue (prelaryngeal strap muscles and subcutaneous fat) T4b: Tumor invades prevertebral fascia, encases carotid artery, or invades mediastinal structures **Regional lymph nodes** N1: Metastasis in a single ipsilateral lymph node, < 3 cm N2a: Metastasis in a single ipsilateral lymph node between 3 and 6 cm N2b: Metastasis in multiple ipsilateral lymph nodes, none > 6 cm in greatest dimension N2c: Metastasis in bilateral or contralateral lymph nodes, none > 6 cm in greatest dimension N3: Metastasis in a lymph node > 6 cm **Distant metastasis** M1: Distant metastasis * Hypopharyngeal subsites include the paired pyriform sinuses, the postcricoid area, and the posterior pharyngeal wall. Less than 5% of tumors of the hypopharynx are of nonsquamous cell origin and unrelated to tobacco and alcohol. These include benign tumors (e.g., lipomas, retention cysts of minor salivary glands, leiomyomas, papillomas, adenomas, and angiomatous tumors) and nonsquamous cell malignancies, such as various sarcomas, malignant lymphoma, and malignant minor salivary gland tumors.
Pharyngocele	Air-filled saccular formation arising either from the lateral side of the pyriform sinus (ostium of junction located between the middle and inferior constrictor muscles) or from the vallecula (ostium of junction located between the superior and middle pharyngeal constrictor muscles). More frequently seen unilateral. Increase in volume with Valsalva maneuver and phonation.	Acquired lateral pharyngeal wall herniation. Presumably, pharyngoceles arise from increased intrapharyngeal pressure, as in chronic coughers, wind instrumentalists, or glass blowers. More common in men (fifth and sixth decade).

(continues on page 371)

Table 9.1   (Cont.) Visceral space lesions

Disease	CT Findings	Comments
Zenker diverticulum ▷*Fig. 9.9*	May appear as a nonenhancing, thin-walled, unilocular oval expansion of the hypopharynx, off the midline in the posterior visceral space, filled with food, debris, and air, often with an air–fluid level.	Outpouching of mucosa and submucosa at the pharyngoesophageal junction through a weaker area in the posterior pharyngeal wall (Kilian dehiscence). Presenting sometimes with dysphagia or chronic aspiration.
Esophageal lesions		
Esophageal duplication cyst	Cystic-appearing, homogeneous, well-circumscribed, nonenhancing esophageal mass in the visceral space, off the midline, with mass effect on the trachea and adjacent structures. May extend inferiorly into the upper mediastinum.	Esophageal duplication cysts—a type of gastro-intestinal duplication—are rare; 20% occur in the upper third of the esophagus. The cyst lining can be squamous, respiratory, intestinal, or mixed. Gradual enlargement occurs with secretory endothelium. Cysts rarely communicate with the esophagus lumen. Most present in early childhood with dysphagia or respiratory distress.
Cervical esophageal carcinoma ▷*Fig. 9.10*	Often eccentric, poorly marginated, infiltrating, enhancing soft tissue esophageal mass centered in the posterior midline visceral space behind the trachea. Cervical esophageal carcinomas tend to spread in a submucosal fashion to the hypopharynx. Larger lesions are transspatial (retropharyngeal, periverterbral, and carotid space) and may show invasion of thyroid and cricoid cartilage, trachea, and recurrent laryngeal nerve. CT cannot reliably delineate the individual layers of the esophageal wall and therefore cannot distinguish between T1 and T2 lesions. Infiltration of the tumor into the periesophageal fat on CT denotes a T3 tumor. Tumor involving adjacent structures denotes a T4 lesion. Cervical esophageal cancers tend to metastasize to group VI, low level IV or V nodes, and mediastinal lymph nodes. The group VI lymph nodes are involved usually (71%) at the time of diagnosis.	Twenty percent of esophageal squamous cell carcinomas arise in the cervical esophagus (M:F = 4:1; peak range 55–65 y; history of tobacco and alcohol abuse, Plummer–Vinson syndrome, caustic stricture, achalasia, or prior radiation). Frequently detected late with poor prognosis. Diagnosis is established with barium swallow, endoscopy, and biopsy. Cross-sectional imaging is considered complementary and may be performed for staging. **Esophageal carcinoma: TNM classification** **Primary tumor** T1: Tumor invades lamina propria, muscularis mucosa T2: Tumor invades muscularis propria T3: Tumor invades adventitia T4: Tumor invades adjacent structures **Regional lymph nodes** N1: Regional lymph node metastasis **Distant metastasis** M1a: Cervical nodal metastasis M1b: Distant metastasis Fifteen percent of patients have synchronous or metachronous tumors.

(continues on page 372)

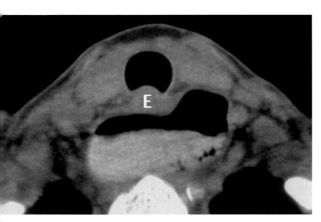

Fig. 9.9   Zenker diverticulum. Axial non–contrast-enhanced CT demonstrates an ovoid sac posterior and left of the collapsed esophagus (E) with air–fluid level after contrast medium swallow.

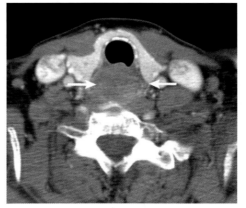

Fig. 9.10   Cervical esophageal carcinoma. Axial contrast-enhanced CT shows an ill-defined enhancing circumferential mass centered on the cervical esophagus (arrows) with obscured esophageal lumen and invasion of trachea.

Table 9.1   (Cont.) Visceral space lesions

Disease	CT Findings	Comments
Juxtavisceral nodal lesions		
Nodal metastases from thyroid carcinoma	Lymph node metastases from thyroid carcinoma are round or spherical in shape and may have, irrespective of size, a variable aspect, including homogeneously enhancing nodes, hemorrhagic nodes with high density, central necrotic nodes with peripheral nodal enhancement, or completely cystic nodes (can be filled with high concentration of thyroglobulin that gives low density on CT). Malignant nodal calcification may be seen in metastatic papillary, follicular, and medullary thyroid cancer (42% of cases). An enhancing nodal rim, which is irregular and thick with infiltration to the adjacent fat planes, reflects extracapsular tumor spread.	Juxtavisceral lymph nodes include prelaryngeal, paratracheal, and paraesophageal lymph nodes (level VI nodes). Thyroid carcinoma is the most common neck tumor to involve these nodes exclusively. Papillary carcinoma has the highest incidence of thyroid malignancies for cervical lymph node metastases (50%).
Lymphoma	In cases of Hodgkin and non–Hodgkin lymphoma, either a single dominant node with scattered surrounding smaller nodes or a multiple nodal disease may be present. Involved lymph nodes range in size from 1 to 10 cm, are round or oval, well circumscribed, often with a thin nodal capsule. Nodal density is equal or less than muscle. In general, there is a homogeneous contrast enhancement, although a thin peripheral rim enhancement or spotty or dendritic enhancement on CT is sometimes seen. Nodal necrosis can occur, albeit less frequently than with metastatic squamous cell carcinoma. Intranodal calcification may be seen after radiation or chemotherapy. Rarely, it may be seen prior to therapy in aggressive high-grade lymphoma.	Both Hodgkin and non–Hodgkin lymphomas involve juxtavisceral lymph nodes, either as an isolated symptom or as part of a more advanced stage.
Tracheal lesions		
Cervical tracheal carcinoma ▷ *Fig. 9.11*	Soft tissue mass within the outline of the tracheal wall (tracheal cartilage), with narrowing of the tracheal lumen and often with large extratracheal components of tumor (30%–40%). Paratracheal lymph nodes are involved in 30% at presentation.	Primary tracheal malignancy is exceedingly uncommon (0.1%–0.4% of all diagnosed malignancies). Most prevalent histology worldwide is squamous cell carcinoma (60%–90%; men are more often afflicted than women, the usual presenting age in the sixth decade of life, with cough, dyspnea, stridor, hemoptysis, and dysphonia). Other histologies are adenoid cystic carcinoma, carcinoid, mucoepidermoid carcinoma, carcinosarcoma, and chondrosarcoma. **Tracheal carcinoma: TNM classification** **Primary tumor** T1: Primary tumor confined to trachea, < 2 cm T2: Primary tumor confined to trachea, > 2 cm T3: Spread outside the trachea but not to adjacent organs or structures T4: Spread to adjacent organs or structures **Regional lymph nodes** N1: Positive regional nodal disease **Distant metastasis** M1: Distant metastasis The incidence of multiple primary carcinomas in tracheal carcinoma is 28%. Carcinomas of the larynx, thyroid gland, esophagus, and lung are most commonly responsible for secondary invasion of the trachea. Neoplasms may also involve the trachea by metastasizing from distant sites.

(continues on page 373)

Table 9.1   (Cont.) Visceral space lesions

Disease	CT Findings	Comments
Benign tracheal tumors	Eccentric, broad-based or pedunculated, well-defined, polypoid mass confined within the tracheal lumen without evidence of adjacent invasion. The lipomas manifest as fat density; the other benign tumors are enhancing soft tissue–density masses.	Benign tumors of the trachea are quite rare (~10% of primary tumors): juvenile laryngotracheal papillomatosis, solitary papilloma, leiomyoma, lipoma, pleomorphic adenoma, granular cell tumor, hemangioma, neurogenic tumor, glomus tumor, fibroma, chondroma, and amyloidoma. These neoplasms may present with symptoms of airway obstruction.
Paratracheal air cyst ▷ *Fig. 9.12*	Air cyst, unilocular or multilocular, with rounded margins, 1 to 15 mm in size, in the right posterior paratracheal region at the thoracic inlet, with one or more narrow communicating necks with the trachea.	Relatively common tracheal diverticula (3.7% of the population). Should not be confused with pneumomediastinum in patients who have sustained a traumatic injury, or an apical lung herniation on the right.

(continues on page 374)

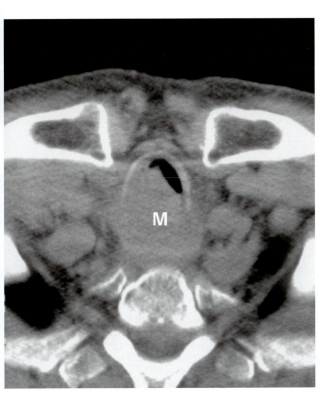

Fig. 9.11   Cervical tracheal carcinoma. Axial contrast-enhanced CT reveals a large lobulated, intraluminal mass (M) with severe luminal narrowing of the trachea and large extratracheal spread.

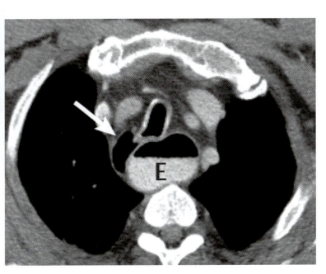

Fig. 9.12   Paratracheal air cyst. Axial contrast-enhanced CT shows a unilocular, air-filled tracheocele (arrow) in the right paratracheal region originating from the posterolateral aspect of the trachea at the level of the thoracic inlet. Accidental megaesophagus (E) with air–fluid level is visible after contrast medium swallow.

Table 9.1 (Cont.) Visceral space lesions

Disease	CT Findings	Comments
Acquired tracheal stenosis ▷ *Fig. 9.13*	**Acute postintubation stenosis** results from mucosal edema or granulation tissue, seen as focal narrowing of tracheal lumen by eccentric or concentric soft tissue thickening internal to normal-appearing tracheal cartilage. Outer tracheal wall has normal configuration, and trachea has normal oval shape. In patients with **chronic stricture,** the tracheal lumen is narrowed primarily because of collapse and inward displacement of calcified tracheal cartilage. Mucosa and submucosa may be normal or thickened by fibrosis. CT findings of **tracheobronchopathia osteochondroplastica** include thickened tracheal cartilage with small 3- to 8-mm calcific nodules along its inner aspect, protruding into the tracheal lumen with irregular narrowing. Diffuse **amyloidosis** leads to concentric, smooth, or nodular thickening of the submucosal tracheal wall. Cartilage is normal, but concentric submucosal calcification or ossification may occur. **Respiratory relapsing polychondritis** is characterized by wall thickening limited to the anterior and lateral tracheal walls, sparing of the posterior membrane, collapse of the cartilage, and narrowing of the lumen. If cartilage calcification is present, the cartilage may appear thicker than normal. The inner and outer borders of the thickened tracheal wall are smooth.	Symptomatic tracheal stenoses are usually caused by prolonged intubation or tracheostomy. Other rare causes of acquired cervical tracheal stenosis are tracheobronchopathia osteochondroplastica, amyloidosis, and relapsing polychondritis. Wall thickening and narrowing of the tracheal lumen may also be seen in Wegener granulomatosis, miscellaneous inflammatory lesions (sarcoidosis, ulcerative colitis) and various infectious processes (healing stage of tuberculous tracheitis).

Table 9.2 Laryngeal lesions

Disease	CT Findings	Comments
Congenital/developmental lesions		
Thyroglossal duct cyst	The infrahyoid thyroglossal duct cyst is typically seen anterior to the larynx as a nonenhancing, smooth, well-circumscribed hypoattenuated mass within or beneath the strap muscles. Occasionally, a thyroglossal duct cyst can protrude into the preepiglottic space through the incisura of the thyroid cartilage. The paraglottic space is spared (as opposed to laryngoceles).	Thyroglossal duct cysts arise from the thyroglossal duct remnant. Other congenital nonneoplastic lesions of the larynx are hamartoma, ectopic thyroid, and thymus.
Venous vascular malformation (cavernous hemangioma)	Venous vascular malformations appear as well-circumscribed soft tissue masses that display uniform intense contrast enhancement. Phleboliths within the lesion are pathognomonic for venous vascular malformations.	Venous vascular malformations of the larynx typically occur in the subglottis arising from the posterior wall (infantile type) or originate from the true vocal cords or, less common, from the supraglottis (adult type). Hemangiomas in adults may be isolated lesions or associated with cervicofacial angiodysplasia.
Degenerative/acquired lesions		
Laryngocele ▷ *Fig. 9.14* ▷ *Fig. 9.15* ▷ *Fig. 9.16*	Laryngoceles are usually unilateral (75%). An **internal (simple) laryngocele** is an air–filled, well-defined, thin-walled cystic mass, identified deep to the false cord in the paraglottic space, which can be followed down to the level of the laryngeal ventricle. Less common **external laryngoceles** protrude through the thyrohyoid membrane into the anterior cervical space with dilation of only the external portion of the lesion. **Mixed laryngoceles** pass through the thyrohyoid membrane, with dilation of both the interior and exterior segments. A fluid-filled laryngocele is called a **laryngeal mucocele:** CT density can vary depending on the presence of proteinaceous secretions and other debris. An infected, pus-filled laryngocele with wall thickening and a peripheral rim enhancement is termed a **pyolaryngocele.** Laryngeal neoplasms may present indirectly with a secondary laryngocele.	Laryngoceles are commonly an acquired expansion of the saccule of the anterior laryngeal ventricle into the paraglottic space of the supraglottic larynx, with gradual enlargement over time, and with or without extension laterally through the thyrohyoid membrane into the anterior cervical space. Presumably they arise from increased intralaryngeal pressure, as in chronic coughers, wind instrumentalists, and glass blowers. A congenital predisposition is considered a likely possibility. Obstruction of the sacculus by tumor, postinflammatory stenosis, trauma, or amyloid is a less common cause of laryngocele (15%). Laryngoceles present commonly in adulthood; more common in men. Many are asymptomatic. When symptomatic, they may be associated with airway obstruction, hoarseness, and dysphagia and present endoscopically as a submucosal supraglottic mass or cause a compressible swelling of the neck.

(continues on page 376)

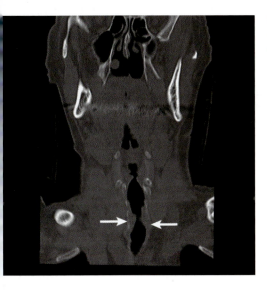

Fig. 9.13 Postintubation tracheal stenosis. Axial contrast-enhanced CT demonstrates an asymmetrical soft tissue wall thickening with associated luminal narrowing, producing an "hourglass" configuration (arrows).

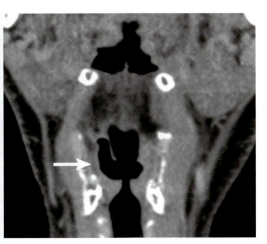

Fig. 9.14 Internal simple laryngocele. Coronal reformatted non–contrast-enhanced CT shows an air-filled expansion of the right saccule of the anterior laryngeal ventricle into the paraglottic space (arrow).

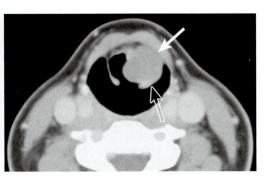

Fig. 9.15 Internal laryngeal mucocele. Axial contrast-enhanced CT during "E" phonation shows a fluid-filled dilated laryngeal saccule extending superiorly in the left paraglottic space (arrow) and aryepiglottic fold (open arrow).

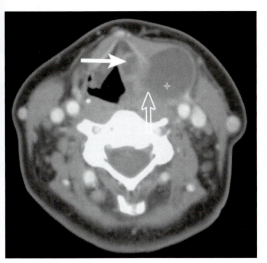

Fig. 9.16 Mixed laryngomucocele. Axial contrast-enhanced CT reveals a fluid-filled dilated laryngeal saccule with slight enhancement of the wall (arrow) extending through the thyrohyoid membrane (open arrow) into the soft tissues of the neck (joystick point).

Table 9.2 (Cont.) Laryngeal lesions

Disease	CT Findings	Comments
Retention cyst	Fluid-filled cystic mass measuring up to several centimeters in diameter with submucosal deformity. Often protrudes into the airway.	Mucosal cysts can arise from obstruction of mucous gland ducts. With the exception of the free margin of the vocal cord, they can occur anywhere in the larynx. A vallecular cyst (oropharyngeal lesion, more common in children) bulges between the base of the tongue and the free anterior margin of the epiglottis, unilateral or bilateral. Congenital laryngeal cysts originate in the aryepiglottic fold and may bulge into the laryngeal vestibule, preepiglottic space, or lateral neck.
Fibrous and fibroangiomatous polyp	Nodular isodense lesion on the free margin of the true vocal cord, commonly located at the junction of the anterior and middle thirds. Frequently bilateral and occasionally with multiple lesions.	Nonneoplastic stromal reaction in patients with a history of vocal abuse (e.g., singers and professional speakers).
Gout	May manifest as acute gouty cricoarytenoiditis with vocal fold immobility and asymmetrical soft tissue swelling around the arytenoid cartilages, with airway obstruction, or as chronic tophaceous involvement of the thyroid lamina.	Gouty involvement of the larynx must be considered in any patient with a history of gout who presents with hoarseness, odynophagia, dysphagia, stridor, or neck lump.
Amyloid ▷ *Fig. 9.17*	Focal or diffuse laryngeal thickening with nodules, plaques, and calcifications, commonly in the epiglottis, ventricles, and true and false cords. Laryngeal amyloidoma sometimes mimics a laryngocele filled by high-density fluid.	Submucosal amyloid deposition from larynx to distal airways; incidental finding or associated with systemic disease. Usually occurs in the fifth decade of life. Common symptom is hoarseness.
Inflammatory/infectious conditions		
Laryngotracheobronchitis (croup)	Edematous mucosal swelling, most significant in the subglottic area, with steeple-shaped airway narrowing.	Parainfluenza or respiratory syncytial virus infection in young children (3 m–3 y) and, rarely, in adults. The onset is gradual, with several days of upper and lower respiratory tract symptoms followed by the development of a classic barking cough and stridor.
Acute epiglottitis	Symmetric edematous swelling of the larynx, including the epiglottis, arytenoids, and aryepiglottic folds, with airway obstruction and ballooning of the pharynx.	Caused by *Haemophilus influenzae, Pneumococcus,* or *Streptococcus,* usually in children between 1 and 5 y of age. Can cause acute severe respiratory compromise. The term *supraglottitis* refers to a disease in adults with inflammation of the supraglottis, valleculae, base of the tongue, uvula, soft palate, platysma muscle, and prevertebral soft tissues. *Angioneurotic edema* has identical presentation on CT. Associated thickening of the retropharynx may be present with angioneurotic edema but not with epiglottitis.
Tuberculosis (TB)	Laryngeal TB manifests as diffuse bilateral laryngeal thickening with or without a focal mass. Inadequate treatment of TB can lead to laryngeal stenosis or cricoarytenoid fixation.	Results from pooling of infected secretions in the posterior larynx or from hematogenous dissemination to the anterior larynx. A variety of other granulomatous diseases, such as syphilis, fungal infections, sarcoidosis, plasma cell granuloma, Wegener granulomatosis, and Langerhans cell histiocytosis, may affect the larynx with diffuse or focal laryngeal thickening and ulceration; cannot be differentiated radiologically from neoplasia.
Rheumatoid arthritis	Cricoarytenoid subluxation, cricoarytenoid and subglottic swelling, sometimes with polypoid rheumatoid nodules.	Laryngeal abnormalities are seen in up to 50% of patients with advanced rheumatoid disease.
Relapsing polychondritis	Laryngotracheal involvement can be localized or diffuse. Initially, a soft tissue swelling around the laryngeal and tracheal cartilages is present with airway narrowing. Later, the weakened cartilages collapse or are destroyed. Calcification may be seen in the abnormal soft tissues.	Rare connective tissue disease that causes inflammation that may affect cartilage throughout the body. The clinical features include auricular chondritis, arthritis, laryngotracheal symptoms, nasal chondritis, ocular inflammation, and audiovestibular and cardiovascular symptoms. The peak onset is in the fourth and fifth decades; average age is 47 y, with a female predominance of 3:1.
Benign neoplasms		
Papilloma	Solitary or multiple small nodular lesions, frequently located in the anterior half of the larynx at the level of the vocal cords. Subglottic extension with spread to the trachea and bronchi may be associated.	Squamous cell papilloma caused by human papillomavirus infection is the most common benign laryngeal tumor. It typically occurs in children younger than 10 y with juvenile papillomatosis; solitary in adults.

(continues on page 377)

Table 9.2   (Cont.) Laryngeal lesions

Disease	CT Findings	Comments
Chondroma ▷ Fig. 9.18	Chondromas of the larynx primarily affect the cricoid and thyroid cartilages. The relatively circumscribed, lobulated, hypoattenuating tumor expands the involved site and has stippled or coarse intratumoral calcifications, characteristic of a chondrogenic tumor. However, there are no reliable CT criteria that enable differentiation between chondrosarcoma and benign chondroma.	True chondromas of the larynx are extremely unusual and are greatly outnumbered by laryngeal chondrosarcoma. They may be an incidental finding or cause minor symptoms, such as hoarseness. A clinically significant cartilaginous neoplasm > 2 cm in dimension more likely represents laryngeal chondrosarcoma. Other benign tumors of the cartilaginous skeleton occur but are even more unusual, including aneurysmal bone cyst, giant cell tumor, aggressive osteoblastoma, and brown tumor.
Lipoma	Laryngeal lipoma commonly arises in the supraglottic region and typically manifests as a homogeneous, nonenhancing lesion with attenuation values from −65 to −125 HU. Internal architecture is minimal.	Laryngeal lipomas comprise < 0.5% of benign neoplasms at these sites, occur in all ages, and affect both genders equally. The symptoms are nonspecific but often include airway obstruction. At endoscopy, the tumor may manifest as a solitary, sessile, or pedunculated polypoid submucosal mass.
Paraganglioma	Occurs in the supraglottic larynx and presents as a submucosal mass in the region of the aryepiglottic fold–false vocal cord. The right side of the larynx is more often involved. On CT, the highly vascularized neoplasm shows homogeneous intense enhancement.	Laryngeal paragangliomas are very rare. These neuroendocrine tumors are three times more common in women and have been described in patients from 5 to 83 y of age (median age 44 y). Patients present with hoarseness, dysphagia, dyspnea, stridor, hemoptysis, and foreign body sensation in the throat. Functioning laryngeal paragangliomas are exceptional.
Nerve sheath tumors (schwannoma, neurofibroma) ▷ Fig. 9.19	Present as round, well-defined supraglottic masses hypoattenuated on unenhanced CT images and slightly enhanced with intravenous (IV) administration of contrast material. A target appearance with central nonenhancing and peripheral enhancing areas may be seen.	Laryngeal nerve sheath tumors are very unusual. These smooth-surfaced submucosal tumors arise from the superior laryngeal nerve, single or multiple, unilateral or bilateral. They occur as isolated cases or in patients with von Recklinghausen disease and neurofibromatosis 2. Dysphonia and hoarseness may be the presenting symptoms. Other submucosal benign neoplasms of the larynx (e.g., leiomyoma, rhabdomyoma, ganglioneuroma, and granular cell tumor) occur but are even more unusual.

(continues on page 378)

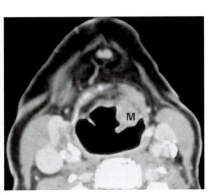

Fig. 9.17   Localized amyloidosis. Axial contrast-enhanced CT shows an expansile submucosal mass (M) with slightly high absorption and small calcifications arising within the left aryepiglottic fold and paraglottic space.

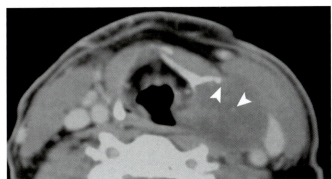

Fig. 9.18   Chondroma. Axial contrast-enhanced CT demonstrates a hypoattenuating tumor arising from the left thyroid cartilage with stippled intratumoral calcifications (arrowheads).

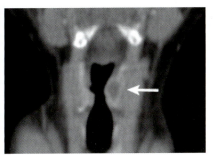

Fig. 9.19   Schwannoma. Coronal reformatted non–contrast-enhanced CT reveals a hypodense mass (arrow) beneath an intact mucosa at the level of the left false and true vocal cord passing the ventricle in a vertical direction.

Table 9.2   (Cont.) Laryngeal lesions

Disease	CT Findings	Comments
Malignant neoplasms		
Squamous cell carcinoma ▷ **Fig. 9.20** ▷ **Fig. 9.21** ▷ **Fig. 9.22** ▷ **Fig. 9.23** ▷ **Fig. 9.24** ▷ **Fig. 9.25**	The imaging criteria used to define the site and the extent of tumor consist of the detection of a solid mass projecting into the lumen, thickening of soft tissues, abnormal enhancement, and fat tissue effacement. The imaging that correlates to tumoral fixation of the cord includes cricoarytenoid joint involvement, interarytenoid disease, and paraglottic spread. Extralaryngeal tumor and eroded edges or lysis of thyroid cartilage and sclerosis or lysis of cricoid and arytenoid cartilage should raise suspicion for cartilage invasion. **Supraglottic carcinomas** originating from the epiglottis primarily invade the preepiglottic space. Tumors that originate from the petiole often invade the low preepiglottic space and, via anterior commissure, the glottis or subglottis. Tumors originating from the aryepiglottic fold, false cord, and laryngeal ventricle primarily infiltrate the paraglottic space. Tumors arising in the arytenoid and interarytenoid region usually infiltrate submucosally toward the hypopharynx. Supraglottic carcinoma tends to spread into the pyriform sinus or toward the base of the tongue, but it rarely invades the glottis and thyroid cartilage. Deep cervical lymph node metastases occur early and are often bilateral. **Glottic carcinoma** typically arises from the anterior half of the vocal cord and primarily spreads into the anterior commissure, which should not exceed 1 mm in thickness. From the anterior commissure, glottic tumors may grow into the infra- or supraglottic regions or into the contralateral vocal cord, or they gain access via the thyroid cartilage and cricothyroid membrane to the prelaryngeal soft tissues of the neck. Alternatively, tumor may grow posteriorly to the posterior commissure, arytenoids, cricoarytenoid joints, subglottic space, or postcricoid region. Lymphatic metastases from localized glottic carcinoma are uncommon. **Subglottic carcinoma** is diagnosed by demonstrating any soft tissue inside the cricoid cartilage, as there is no normal tissue between the mucosal surface and cricoid cartilage. The tumor may spread to the vocal cord and supraglottis, thyroid gland, hypopharynx, cervical esophagus, and tracheal wall. Subglottic carcinoma is very often accompanied by lymph node metastases, both paratracheal and pretracheal.	Over 95% of laryngeal tumors are squamous cell carcinomas. They occur mainly in men who abuse tobacco and alcohol. Glottic carcinomas (60%) are diagnosed early due to hoarseness. Supraglottic (30%) and subglottic (5%) carcinomas are symptomatic late in the course of the disease and therefore usually present in the advanced stage. Their submucosal extension cannot be evaluated by endoscopic examination alone. **Carcinoma of the larynx: TNM classification** **Primary tumor** *Supraglottis* T1: Tumor confined to one subsite* T2: Tumor invades mucosa of more than one subsite* or glottis or region outside the supraglottis with normal cord mobility T3: Tumor limited to the larynx with fixation of vocal cord and/or extension into the postcricoid area, medial wall of pyriformis sinus, or preepiglottic space or slight erosion of thyroid cartilage T4a: Tumor invades through thyroid cartilage and/or extends beyond the larynx: trachea, soft tissues of the neck, extrinsic tongue muscles, thyroid gland, esophagus, strap muscles T4b: Tumor invades prevertebral space, mediastinum, or encases carotid artery * Subsites include epiglottis, aryepiglottic folds, and false cords, including the laryngeal ventricles. *Glottis* T1: Tumor confined to one (T1a) or both vocal cords (T1b), including anterior or posterior commissures with normal cord mobility T2: Tumor extends to supraglottis and/or subglottis and/or associated with impaired vocal cord mobility T3: Tumor limited to the larynx with vocal cord fixation, and/or invades paraglottic space, and/or inner cortex of thyroid cartilage T4a: Tumor invades through thyroid cartilage and/or extends beyond the larynx: trachea, soft tissues of the neck, extrinsic tongue muscles, thyroid gland, esophagus, strap muscles T4b: Tumor invades prevertebral space, mediastinum, or encases carotid artery *Subglottis* T1: Tumor confined to subglottis T2: Tumor invades vocal cord(s) with normal or impaired mobility T3: Tumor confined to larynx with vocal cord fixation T4a: Tumor invades through cricoid or thyroid cartilage and/or extends beyond the larynx: trachea, soft tissues of the neck, extrinsic tongue muscles, thyroid gland, esophagus, strap muscles T4b: Tumor invades prevertebral space, mediastinum, or encases carotid artery **Regional lymph nodes** N1: Single ipsilateral node < 3 cm N2a: Single ipsilateral node 3 to 6 cm N2b: Multiple ipsilateral nodes < 6 cm N2c: Bilateral or contralateral nodes < 6 cm N3: Node(s) > 6 cm **Distant metastasis** M1: Distant metastasis

(continues on page 380)

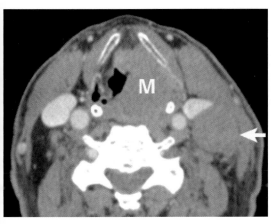

Fig. 9.20   Supraglottic squamous cell carcinoma. Axial contrast-enhanced CT demonstrates a large, moderately enhancing, exophytic and invasive mass (M) with involvement of the left paraglottic and preepiglottic fat. Also visible is associated left level III adenopathy (arrow).

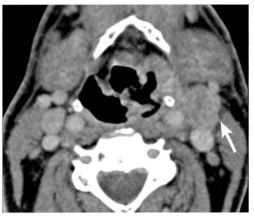

Fig. 9.21   Supraglottic squamous cell carcinoma. Axial contrast-enhanced CT reveals a left, large, ulcerating, aryepiglottic fold tumor. Also seen is associated left level II adenopathy (arrow).

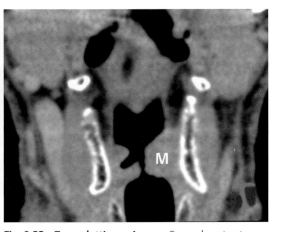

Fig. 9.22   Transglottic carcinoma. Coronal contrast-enhanced CT reconstruction shows a glottic and supraglottic tumor (M) with invasion of the left paraglottic space passing the left ventricle in a vertical direction. No cartilage invasion is apparent.

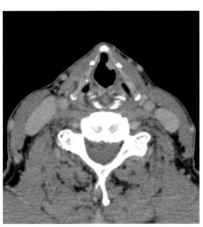

Fig. 9.23   Glottic squamous cell carcinoma. Axial contrast-enhanced CT shows a small exophytic left true vocal cord mass with homogeneous enhancement.

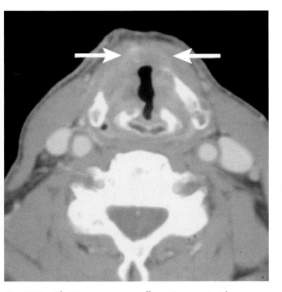

Fig. 9.24   Glottic squamous cell carcinoma. Axial contrast-enhanced CT demonstrates a large mass involving both vocal cords and the anterior commissure. Bilateral destruction of the anterior thyroid lamina and invasion of the prelaryngeal muscles (arrows) are obvious. The left arytenoid cartilage shows major sclerosis, indicating cartilage invasion.

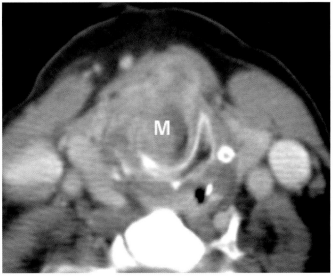

Fig. 9.25   Subglottic squamous cell carcinoma. Axial contrast-enhanced CT demonstrates a large inhomogeneous mass (M) filling the airway at the level of the cricoid cartilage, aggressively extending through the right cricoid ring to involve the right thyroid lobe, and anterior through the cricothyroid membrane into the strap musculature.

Table 9.2 (Cont.) Laryngeal lesions

Disease	CT Findings	Comments
Laryngeal chondrosarcoma ▷ *Fig. 9.26* ▷ *Fig. 9.27*	Laryngeal chondrosarcomas arise predominantly in the ossified hyaline cartilages. The posterior and posterolateral aspect of the cricoid is most frequently involved, followed by the thyroid cartilage (inferolateral); the arytenoid cartilage, epiglottis, and hyoid bone are rare locations. CT shows an expansile solid hypodense (to muscle), moderately enhancing mass with intrinsic arc and ringlike, stippled, coarse or "popcorn" calcifications and cortical destruction. The tumor may remain endolaryngeal and lead to significant airway narrowing or more commonly extend into the immediate exolaryngeal soft tissues.	Sarcomas of the larynx are extremely rare neoplasms that account for ~1% of all tumors of this organ. Chondrosarcoma is the most common sarcoma of the larynx and predominantly affects men in their sixth or seventh decade of life. Patients present with progressive hoarseness, dyspnea, stridor, or dysphagia. An indolent external neck mass may be palpable. At endoscopy, the tumor may manifest as a solitary, lobulated submucosal mass with intact mucosal surfaces. Other malignant tumors of the cartilaginous skeleton occur, including osteosarcoma and multiple myeloma, but they are even more unusual.
Malignant minor salivary gland tumor	None of these unusual types of submucosal carcinomas have any imaging characteristics to distinguish them from squamous cell carcinoma.	Malignant minor salivary gland tumors may arise from the minor salivary glands in the supraglottic and subglottic regions. **Adenoid cystic carcinoma** most commonly arises in the subglottis, invades the entire larynx submucosally, and infiltrates the thyroid gland and the esophagus. Common symptoms include pain and paralysis of the recurrent laryngeal nerve. No gender predilection. **Mucoepidermoid carcinoma:** Men are affected six times more often than women; the epiglottis is the most commonly affected site. **Adenocarcinoma:** Most commonly found in the fifth to seventh decade with a male predominance. Presents with extensive submucosal tumor spread and invasion of the laryngeal skeleton.
Non–Hodgkin lymphoma	Laryngeal non–Hodgkin lymphoma is typically a submucosal homogeneously enhancing soft tissue mass centered in the supraglottis and may spread to involve the glottis and subglottis. Deep tumor invasion into cartilage or strap muscles may occur, as well as cervical lymphadenopathy. Involvement of the hypopharynx and superior extension to the oropharynx or even nasopharynx should raise the possibility of non–Hodgkin lymphoma.	Non–Hodgkin lymphoma of the larynx is rare. Patients with laryngeal lymphoma (M:F = 1:3, mean age 58 y) commonly present with progressive hoarseness, cough, dysphagia, or, less frequently, systemic symptoms.
Metastases to the larynx	Melanoma and renal adenocarcinoma usually metastasize to the soft tissues, mainly the vestibular and aryepiglottic folds. Lung and breast carcinomas may metastasize to the marrow spaces of the ossified thyroid, cricoid, and arytenoid cartilages with destruction of the laryngeal skeleton.	Metastases to the larynx are rare, most often found in men. The primary sources of metastatic tumor are skin, kidney, breast, lung, prostate, colon, stomach, and ovary. Common sites of involvement are the supraglottic and subglottic regions.
Trauma		
Dislocation of joints	Dislocation of the cricoarytenoid joint is straightforward to diagnose due to the abnormal position of the arytenoid relative to the cricoid cartilage (the arytenoid cartilage is tipped forward and rotated medially), edema of the aryepiglottic fold, and bowed hypomobile vocal cord. Cricothyroid dislocation appears as a rotation of the cricoid ring relative to the thyroid with widening of the space between the lower thyroid and the cricoid. It is most commonly associated with thyroid or cricoid fracture.	The mechanism of external laryngeal injury can be divided into blunt trauma, in which the larynx and upper trachea are crushed against the spine, and penetration trauma. Blunt trauma tends to be associated with motor vehicle accidents, sports injuries, falls, and strangulation, whereas penetrating trauma is related to assaults. Internal laryngeal injury is related to intubation, instrumentation, ingestion from foreign bodies and caustic substances, and radiation.

(continues on page 382)

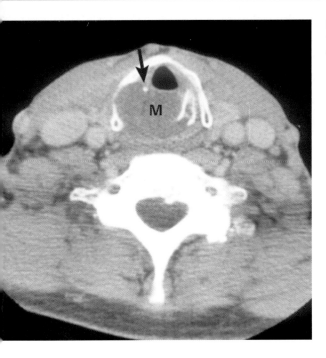

Fig. 9.26   Chondrosarcoma, larynx. Axial contrast-enhanced CT reveals a predominantly hypodense expansile mass (M), containing stippled peripheral calcification (arrow), arising from the destroyed posterior lamina of the cricoid cartilage. Also noted is marked airway narrowing.

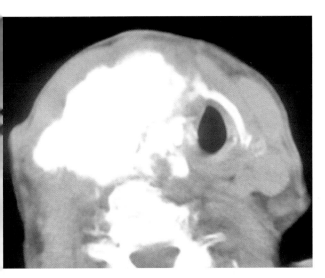

Fig. 9.27   Osteosarcoma, larynx. Axial bone CT demonstrates a huge expansile lesion with increased bone density, arising from the destroyed right thyroid cartilage lamina.

Table 9.2   (Cont.) Laryngeal lesions

Disease	CT Findings	Comments
Cartilage fracture ▷ *Fig. 9.28a, b*	Fractures of the thyroid cartilage may be vertical or horizontal, or the entire thyroid cartilage may be shattered with dislocation of fragments of cartilage. Fractures of the cricoid cartilage tend to occur bilaterally and lead to the collapse of the cricoid ring. Fractures are invariably associated with soft tissue abnormalities (subcutaneous emphysema, mucosal tears, edema, and hematoma with loss of internal laryngeal landmarks).	A hyoid fracture is often associated with avulsion of the posteriorly displaced epiglottis. Laryngotracheal separation shows malalignment between the larynx and trachea
Submucosal hematoma	Distention and increased soft tissue densities in the preepiglottic and paraglottic spaces, swelling of the aryepiglottic folds, true and false vocal cords, and increased soft tissue densities within and around the cricoid cartilage.	Endolaryngeal soft tissue hemorrhages are usually associated with trauma, with or without cartilage damage. Spontaneous hemorrhage occurs with bleeding disorders and anticoagulation.
Vocal cord paralysis ▷ *Fig. 9.29a, b*	CT imaging features are explained by atrophy of the thyroarytenoid muscle and include an enlarged ventricle, ipsilateral enlargement of the pyriform sinus, thickening and anteromedial displacement of the aryepiglottic fold, and paramedian position, decreased size, and fatty infiltration of the true vocal cord. Left is more common than right.	Immobilization of true vocal cord by denervation. Many cases are idiopathic, toxic, or inflammatory/infectious etiologies. Lesions compressing or injuring vagus or recurrent laryngeal nerves are surgery, trauma, and masses, both cancerous and noncancerous. In a patient with vocal cord paralysis of unknown origin, CT should be extended to the skull base and the mediastinum to include the entire pathway of the vagus and recurrent laryngeal nerve.
Subglottic stenosis	Eccentric or circumferential subglottic or tracheal luminal narrowing with wall thickening due to submucosal edema, granulation tissue, or collapsed cartilage.	Congenital or acquired (e.g., complication of prolonged intubation or tracheostomy, or sequelae of cricoid cartilage fracture).

Table 9.3   Thyroid gland lesions

Disease	CT Findings	Comments
Pseudomass		
Pyramidal lobe of the thyroid gland	An accessory lobe usually arises from the isthmus and extends superiorly, superficial to the thyroid cartilage, along the course of the distal thyroglossal duct. It may be attached to the hyoid bone. Uncommonly, the pyramidal lobe may arise from the medial right or left thyroid lobe.	Normal variant. May be present in 10% to 40% of the population. A pyramidal lobe is most commonly recognized in patients with Graves disease.
Prominent thyroid isthmus	Infrequently, the thyroid isthmus may reside anterior to the cricoid cartilage.	The thyroid isthmus (1.25–2 cm in width and height, < 0.6 cm thick) is a midline structure, anterior to the trachea (usually overlying the first through third tracheal rings).
Congenital/developmental lesions		
Ectopic thyroid	Ectopic thyroid tissue is dense (80–100 HU) because of its iodine content and typically enhances markedly on postcontrast CT.	Any disruption of thyroid descent may lead to either lingual thyroid, seen with complete failure of descent, or ectopic thyroid, with thyroid tissue anywhere along the course of the thyroglossal duct. Overdescent of the thyroid may result in ectopic thyroid in the mediastinum, on rare occasions in the trachea or heart. Ectopic thyroid is subject to the same diseases as the anatomically correctly positioned thyroid. Development of a mass lesion is often the reason why these ectopic thyroids become symptomatic.

(continues on page 384)

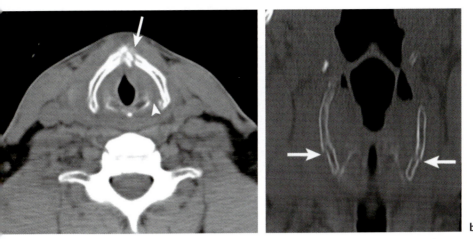

Fig. 9.28a, b   Laryngeal trauma. Axial non–contrast-enhanced CT (**a**) shows a shattered thyroid cartilage with posterior displacement of a fragment (arrow). There is left cricothyroid dislocation (arrowhead). Coronal reformatted bone CT (**b**) reveals bilateral horizontal thyroid lamina fractures.

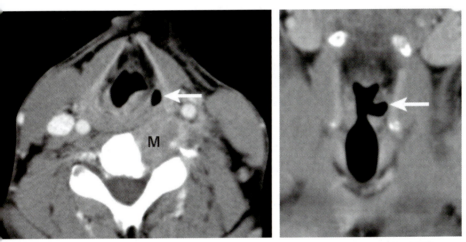

Fig. 9.29a, b   Left recurrent laryngeal nerve paralysis. Axial contrast-enhanced CT (**a**) during quiet respiration shows thickening and anteromedial displacement of the left aryepiglottic fold and dilated left piriform sinus (arrow). There is a malignant peripheral nerve sheath tumor in the left paraspinal space (M) with infiltration of the left longus muscle and carotid space. Coronal contrast-enhanced CT (**b**) reconstruction during quiet respiration demonstrates a paramedian position and "pointing" of the paralytic thinned left true vocal cord and distention of the ipsilateral laryngeal ventricle (arrow).

Table 9.3 (Cont.) Thyroid gland lesions

Disease	CT Findings	Comments
Thyroglossal duct cyst	Nonenhancing, smooth, thin-walled, low-density (cystic) round or ovoid midline neck mass (usually 2–4 cm), occasionally septated, located either at or below the level of the hyoid bone (80%), or suprahyoidal at the base of the tongue or within the posterior floor of the mouth (20%). The more inferior the cyst, the more likely it is to be off the midline, deep to or embedded in the infrahyoid strap muscles ("claw" sign). The wall may thicken and enhance and the cyst content develop higher attenuation, if infected. Any associated nodularity or chunky calcification within the cyst suggests associated thyroid carcinoma. Occasionally associated with thyroid agenesis, ectopia, and pyramidal lobe.	Failure of the hollow thyroglossal duct to involute may result in a persistent fistulous tract or cyst along the path of migration between the foramen cecum and thyroid bed in the infrahyoid neck. Thyroglossal duct cysts are the most common embryologic remnant in the neck, usually detected before the age of 20 y, frequently following infection. There is no gender predilection.
Thyroid hemiagenesis	Absence of a thyroid lobe and enlargement of the contralateral lobe.	Thyroid agenesis is uncommon. Hemi-agenesis is also rare; however, when it does occur it often involves the left lobe. Occasionally the isthmus may be absent.
Inflammatory/infectious conditions		
Hashimoto thyroiditis	Diffuse moderately enlarged, lobular, generally hypodense thyroid gland with mild heterogeneity and less well-defined margins. No calcifications or areas of necrosis or adenopathy are evident. In 12%, there may be atrophy and fibrosis of the gland.	Chronic, autoimmune-mediated lymphocytic inflammation of thyroid gland, leading to gland destruction and hypothyroidism; associated with an elevated risk of thyroid gland lymphoma and papillary carcinoma. It occurs most often in women over the age of 40 y. Familial predisposition.
De Quervain thyroiditis	Usually mild unilateral or bilateral and symmetric thyroid enlargement with diffusely decreased attenuation (isodense/hypodense to muscle) and only moderate contrast enhancement. There may be atrophy of the thyroid gland over time.	Uncommon, subacute, presumably viral thyroiditis presenting with painful gland enlargement, fever, and fatigue after an upper respiratory tract infection. Most commonly affects middle-aged women. Hyperthyroidism is present in half of all patients, sometimes followed by transient hypothyroidism. It is a self-limited disease; complete recovery in weeks to months is characteristic.
Riedel thyroiditis	Unilateral or bilateral, often asymmetric and irregular enlargement of a diffusely hypodense thyroid gland. Decreased contrast enhancement increases the contrast between the residual normal thyroid tissue and the fibrotic parenchyma. Compression of the trachea, esophagus, and vessels and/or obliteration of the adjacent soft tissue planes may simulate an infiltrative mass.	Extremely rare form of chronic thyroiditis (immune-mediated?), characterized by replacement of the normal thyroid parenchyma by a dense fibrosis that extends beyond the thyroid capsule and invades adjacent structures of the neck. Multifocal fibrosclerosis (retroperitoneal and mediastinal fibrosis, sclerosing cholangitis, and orbital pseudotumor) may be associated. Occurs preferentially in women around 50 y of age. Patients present with an enlarging mass causing compression of the trachea, hoarseness, difficulty in swallowing, and hypothyroidism.
Suppurative thyroiditis	Neck and glandular swelling secondary to edema with hazy lobe margins and a low-density parenchymal mass, usually unilateral, with left-sided predominance. In the presence of an abscess, a single or multiloculated area of fluid density with or without air and air–fluid levels may be identified in the thyroid or in the perithyroid soft tissues of the neck with peripheral rim enhancement.	Acute suppurative thyroiditis is uncommon, mainly caused by *Streptococcus haemolyticus, Staphylococcus,* and *Pneumococcus.* Can occur in immunosuppressed persons, but also in otherwise healthy patients after trauma or irradiation. Preexisting thyroid disease, particularly nodular goiter, is present in 50% of adult patients. A special form is recurrent infection caused by a pyriform fossa sinus tract, as found in third or fourth branchial cleft anomalies, or by a thyroglossal duct fistula. Patients present with acute anterior neck pain, fever, and dysphagia. These patients usually have euthyroidism.

(continues on page 385)

Table 9.3   (Cont.) Thyroid gland lesions

Disease	CT Findings	Comments
Degenerative lesions		
Thyroid cyst ▷ *Fig. 9.30*	Unilateral, large cystic mass within normal thyroid tissue. Cysts are usually hypodense but become isodense when the protein content, including thyroglobulin, is elevated. The wall is thin and smooth. Bleeding may occasionally occur into a cyst, resulting in a sudden increase of the cyst.	Thyroid cysts account for 15% to 25% of all thyroid nodules. True thyroid cysts lined with epithelium are rare. Most cysts are the result of degeneration of thyroid adenomas, with the accumulation of serous fluid, colloid substance, or blood. A cervical thymic cyst in contiguity with the lower pole of the thyroid may mimic a thyroid cyst.
Amyloid deposition	Diffuse glandular enlargement. The enlarged cervical lymph nodes may be homogeneously enhanced. Involvement of the airways shows subglottic and tracheal narrowing.	Amyloidosis involving the thyroid gland is very rare and may be seen both in patients with Hashimoto thyroiditis and in patients with systemic amyloidosis. Amyloid deposition in systemic amyloidosis may also be seen in the cervical lymph nodes, larynx, and trachea.
Metabolic disorders		
Multinodular goiter ▷ *Fig. 9.31*	Well-marginated, diffuse, asymmetric enlargement of the thyroid gland with heterogeneous appearance. Degenerative and colloidal cysts appear as multiple hypodense areas; solid adenomatous nodules and fibrosis contribute to variably sized, intermediate-attenuation masses; and hemorrhage has a high density. Focal amorphous, ringlike, and curvilinear calcifications are present in 90%. Substernal and mediastinal extension occurs in 37% of patients. Secondary manifestations of goiter include compression and displacement of the trachea, esophagus, and adjacent vessels. No associated lymphadenopathy.	*Goiter* refers to any enlargement of the thyroid gland, related to genetic and environmental factors. Endemic goiters are prevalent in iodine-deficient areas. Most simple diffuse goiters progress to multinodular goiter. There is a 2 to 4:1 female predominance, and the incidence grows with age. Patients usually present with local compression symptoms and cosmetic disfigurement. Multinodular goiters may or may not be associated with functional thyroid abnormalities. In toxic nodular goiter (Plummer disease), hyperthyroidism is caused by the autonomous function of one or more adenomas. Anaplastic thyroid carcinoma may arise from multinodular goiter in 5% (risk factors: radiation exposure, family history of thyroid carcinoma, and rapid growth).

(continues on page 386)

II Head and Neck

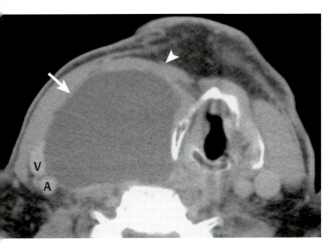

Fig. 9.30   Colloid cyst. Axial contrast-enhanced CT reveals a large cystic mass within the visceral space originating from the right thyroid lobe with mass effect on the larynx, right strap muscles (arrowhead), sternocleidomastoid muscle (arrow), and carotid space (A, V).

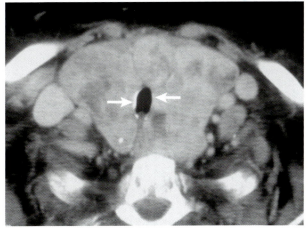

Fig. 9.31   Multinodular goiter. Axial contrast-enhanced CT demonstrates enlargement of the thyroid gland and multiple thyroid nodules with central low-attenuation areas and a few calcifications. There is mass effect on the trachea with narrowing and displacement (arrows).

Table 9.3 (Cont.) Thyroid gland lesions

Disease	CT Findings	Comments
Benign neoplasms		
Thyroid adenoma ▷ *Fig. 9.32*	Inhomogeneous hypodense mass, 1 to 4 cm in diameter, within the focal enlarged thyroid gland. Margins are well circumscribed. Large adenomas enhance more heterogeneously because of hemorrhage, cyst formation, fibrosis, and multiple amorphous calcifications within it. Absence of invasive features and lymphadenopathy suggests thyroid adenoma (biopsy is always required to rule out malignancy). Thyroid nodules with calcifications in males, thyroid nodules with blurred calcifications, and calcifications in the margin of the lesion may suggest malignant disease.	True benign neoplasm of differing histopathologic types, usually solitary and nonfunctioning, often incidentally detected in young and middle-aged adults (M:F = 1:4). Most thyroid cysts represent spontaneous degeneration of adenomas. Sudden enlargement of an adenoma is usually related to spontaneous hemorrhage within the lesion. A toxic adenoma is an autonomous functioning adenoma that usually exceeds 3 cm in diameter before it produces clinically apparent hyperthyroidism. The colloid or adenomatous nodule is composed of focal hyperplastic epithelium and is not a true neoplasm. Rarely, a parathyroid adenoma has an ectopic intrathyroid location. Thyroid nodules are common and comprise adenomas, cysts, focal thyroiditis, multinodular goiter, and malignant tumors. The incidence of malignancy in a single nodule is 10% to 15%, in a multinodular goiter 4% to 7.5%. Most thyroid cancers present as cold nodules on radionuclide scans.
Malignant neoplasms		
Papillary carcinoma ▷ *Fig. 9.33*	The primary tumor appearance is highly variable. The tumor is isodense with muscle interspersed with low-attenuation areas representing cystic or necrotic areas. Psammomatous or amorphous calcifications are present in up to 35% of patients. The size of the tumor ranges from small to large. The neoplasm may be multifocal. Less commonly, the tumor may be diffuse and invasive with extrathyroidal extension. Aggressive forms may invade the larynx and trachea or esophagus. Metastases to lymph nodes may be solid and hypervascular, solid and cystic, or cystic and display calcifications. In some cystic metastases, the wall may be smooth and thin, simulating a cystic lesion.	Papillary carcinoma is the most common thyroid cancer (60%–80%, peak incidence in the third and fourth decades, with a female predominance [3:1]). As many as 20% are multifocal. In up to 50% lymph node metastases may precede the clinical recognition of a tumor in the thyroid gland and may occur in the paratracheal and supraclavicular areas (levels IV–VI), midjugular and upper jugular nodes (levels III and II), as well as in retropharyngeal and superior mediastinal nodes. Distant metastases (lung, bone) occur in 5% to 7%.
Follicular carcinoma ▷ *Fig. 9.34*	The tumor appearance is a reflection of the pathologic changes ranging from a well-delimited nodule to an ill-defined invasive tumor with necrosis and calcification. They rarely become cystic. A small percentage invades the larynx, trachea, and esophagus. Nodal spread is rare (10%); distal spread is more common (20%).	Follicular carcinoma constitutes ~20% to 25% of thyroid carcinomas, has a female predominance, and occurs a decade later than papillary carcinoma, with a peak incidence in the fifth decade. The majority of follicular carcinomas are slow growing, solitary, and encapsulated, resembling an adenoma. The widely invasive form extends outside the gland and penetrates the surrounding tissue.
Anaplastic carcinoma	Usually large, irregular, heterogeneously dense-hyperdense thyroid mass with central low-attenuation areas, reflecting hemorrhage and necrosis (75%), and dense amorphous, globular calcifications (58%). Extrathyroidal extension with invasion of neighboring soft tissue structures, aerodigestive system, carotid artery, and jugular vein is common (26%–53%). Mediastinal extension is encountered in 25%. Lymph node metastases (40%), often necrotic, and distant hematogenous metastases (50%) are common.	Anaplastic (undifferentiated) carcinoma accounts for < 5% of thyroid malignancies. It is the most aggressive neoplasm in the thyroid and has a female predominance, with a peak incidence in the sixth or seventh decade. In almost 50% of cases, the anaplastic carcinoma develops within a goiter or may arise from differentiated thyroid cancer.

(continues on page 388)

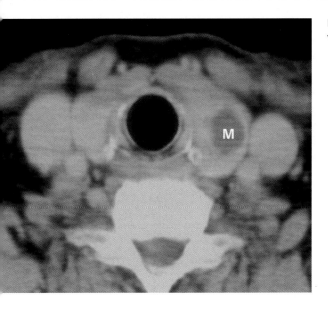

Fig. 9.32 Thyroid adenoma. Axial contrast-enhanced CT shows a well-defined, hypodense mass (M) with an enlarging left thyroid lobe.

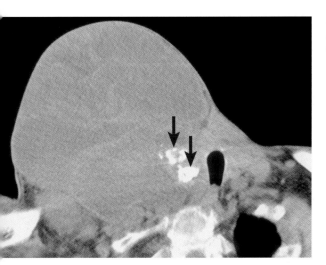

Fig. 9.33 Papillary carcinoma. Axial non–contrast-enhanced CT shows a large, solid, well-circumscribed, heterogeneous mass with coarse focal calcification (arrows).

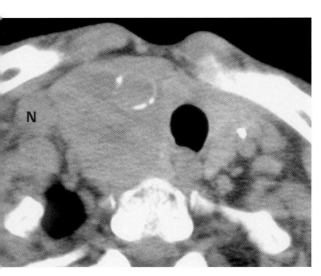

Fig. 9.34 Follicular carcinoma. Axial non–contrast-enhanced CT reveals a large heterogeneous tumor with focal calcification originating from the right thyroid lobe. Also visible is a right level V lymph node metastasis (N).

Table 9.3   (Cont.) Thyroid gland lesions

Disease	CT Findings	Comments
Medullary thyroid carcinoma	Solid nonenhancing, low-density, well-circumscribed mass in the thyroid gland, frequently multifocal and bilateral. Fine, punctate, or coarse calcifications may be found in the tumor and in nodal metastases.	Rare neuroendocrine malignancy arising from thyroid parafollicular cells (4%–5% of all thyroid gland malignancies). Although medullary cancer is associated with multiple endocrine neoplasia type 2 (MEN 2) syndromes and hereditary, familial forms, 80% occur sporadically. Patients who have sporadic medullary carcinoma typically present with a painless palpable nodule in the fifth or sixth decade of life, with bilateral tumors in 20%, but up to 75% have lymphadenopathy at presentation. There is a slight female preponderance (1.5:1). MEN 2 syndromes occur in children and younger adults (mean age 35 y), with multifocal and bilateral manifestation in 80%. Distant metastases may settle in the lungs, liver, and bone.
Lymphoma ▷ *Fig. 9.35*	The CT aspect is variable and includes an isolated nodule (80%), bilateral nodules (20%), or bulky mass involving the entire gland. The tumor is often homogeneous, solid, and hypodense and shows only minor enhancement. Necrosis and calcifications are uncommon. A diffusely infiltrated gland results in a hypodense thyromegaly with extraglandular extension. When present, enlarged cervical lymph nodes are usually multiple, bilateral, nonenhancing, hypodense, and solid.	Thyroid non–Hodgkin lymphoma (2%–5% of all thyroid malignancies; M:F = 1:4; peak incidence sixth decade) is either primary (defined as an extranodal, extralymphatic lymphoma that arises from the thyroid gland) or secondary as part of systemic lymphoma. Most thyroid lymphomas are non-Hodgkin B-cell lymphomas. Less common are mucosa-associated lymphoid tissue (MALT) lymphomas, rarely Hodgkin lymphoma, Burkitt cell lymphoma, and T-cell lymphoma. Patients with Hashimoto thyroiditis are predisposed to thyroid gland lymphoma. Patients usually present with a rapidly enlarging thyroid mass and obstructive symptoms related to compression of the aerodigestive tract.
Metastases to the thyroid gland	Single or multiple thyroid masses of variable size demonstrating low density. In advanced forms, the entire thyroid gland may be invaded, indistinguishable from a primary thyroid tumor.	Metastatic disease to the thyroid gland usually is clinically occult, although 2% to 4% of patients dying of malignant disease (skin [metastatic melanoma], breast, lung, kidney, or colon) may present metastases at autopsy. A separate category includes malignant tumors that invade the thyroid from adjacent structures, such as carcinomas of the larynx, pharynx, trachea, and esophagus.

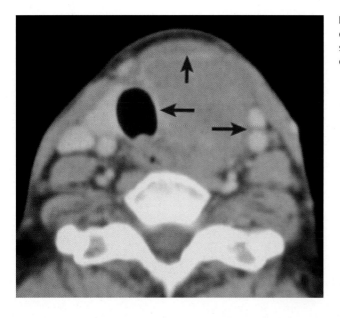

Fig. 9.35   Primary thyroid non–Hodgkin lymphoma. Axial contrast-enhanced CT reveals a large, nonenhancing, homogeneous, solid, hypodense left thyroid lobe mass. The tumor compresses but does not invade surrounding structures (arrows).

Table 9.4   Infrahyoid carotid space lesions

Disease	CT Findings	Comments
Pseudomass		
Carotid bulb asymmetry	Unilateral or asymmetric prominent carotid artery bifurcation without thrombus in older patients with atherosclerosis.	The carotid bulb is the most proximal aspect of the cervical internal carotid artery. The bulb may form a significant focal dilation where the internal carotid artery originates from the common carotid artery at a slight angle.
Carotid artery ectasia	Round, enhancing structure in the widened retropharyngeal space. Sectional imaging, reconstructions, and computed tomography angiography (CTA) easily define the nature of the retropharyngeal structure as a tubular, tortuous, sometimes dilated carotid artery.	One or both distal common carotid arteries may have a retropharyngeal course. Increasing incidence of medial loop with increasing age. This normal variant may present clinically as a pulsatile retropharyngeal mass.
Cervical aortic arch	Abnormal, enhancing, tubular structure, continuous with the ascending and descending aorta. Its apex lies well above the medial ends of the clavicles, on the right or on the left side of the vertebral column. In both instances, branching of the arch vessels is variable and may be aberrant. Frequently, the descending aorta is contralateral to the aortic arch.	In this very uncommon congenital anomaly, the aortic arch lies above the manubrium and may present as a pulsatile neck mass; > 80% are right-sided. Patients often have a benign or asymptomatic course, but it may occur with other cardiovascular congenital abnormalities. Only women with cervical aortic arch may develop aneurysms.
Jugular vein asymmetry ▷ *Fig. 9.36*	The size of the internal jugular veins can be variable and asymmetric due to their reciprocal size relationship to the external jugular veins and positional and anatomical factors. The right internal jugular vein is usually larger than the left.	Incidental finding on CT without any pathologic significance. Sometimes a large vein can be felt in the neck as a soft mass. Phlebectasia of the internal jugular vein is a rare benign focal fusiform dilation of the inferior aspect of the internal jugular vein with enlargement during Valsalva maneuver and decrease at rest, usually seen in children and young adults. Phlebectasia should be differentiated from true venous aneurysms.

(continues on page 390)

II Head and Neck

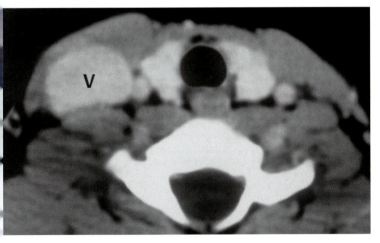

Fig. 9.36   Jugular vein asymmetry. Axial contrast-enhanced CT reveals phlebectasia of the right internal jugular vein (V). Note the absent left internal jugular vein.

Table 9.4 (Cont.) Infrahyoid carotid space lesions

Disease	CT Findings	Comments
Congenital/developmental lesions		
Atypical second branchial cleft cyst	Rarely, a second branchial cleft cyst can extend into the infrahyoid neck but still maintain close proximity to the carotid artery and internal jugular vein. CT reveals a well-circumscribed, ovoid or rounded, homogeneously hypoattenuated, unilocular mass, surrounded by a uniform thin and regular wall. The mural thickness may increase after infection. A focal projection of cyst extending between the carotid bifurcation, termed a "notch" sign, is considered pathognomonic for a second branchial cleft cyst.	Second branchial cleft cysts can occur anywhere along the line from the tonsillar fossa to the supraclavicular region. They may manifest as an often chronic, recurrent, painless, compressible neck mass in a child or young adult, increasing in size with upper respiratory tract infections.
Inflammatory/infectious conditions		
Reactive lymphadenopathy	In reactive adenopathy, the infrahyoid deep cervical lymph nodes (levels III and IV) may by definition enlarge to a maximum diameter of 1 cm but maintain their normal oval shape, isodensity to muscle, and their homogeneous internal architecture with variable, usually mild enhancement. Enhancing linear markings within the node may be seen. Postinflammatory fatty infiltration appears as low-density nodal hilus, mimicking necrosis, in a node with pronounced lima bean shape.	The internal jugular nodal chain is closely associated but not in the carotid space. Reactive hyperplasia is a nonspecific lymph node reaction, current or prior to any inflammation in its draining area. Can occur at any age but most common in the pediatric age group.
Viral lymphadenitis	Viral adenitis may present as bilateral diffuse lymph node enlargement without necrosis, similar in appearance to lymphoma and sarcoidosis.	Nonspecific imaging finding that may be observed in a variety of viral infections, such as *adenovirus, rhinovirus, enterovirus, measles, mumps, rubella, varicella zoster, herpes simplex virus, Epstein–Barr virus,* and *cytomegalovirus.* However, in the presence of parotid lymphoepithelial cysts and hyperplastic adenoids, human immunodeficiency virus (HIV) infection should be strongly suggested.
Suppurative lymphadenitis	In suppurative adenopathy, the involved nodes are enlarged, ovoid to round, with poorly defined margins and surrounding inflammatory changes. Contrast-enhanced CT images show thick enhancing nodal walls with central hypodensity, similar to metastatic adenopathy with necrotic center. Extracapsular spread of infection from the suppurative lymph nodes may result in abscess formation.	Common in pediatric age group with acute onset of tender neck mass and fever. Organisms have predilection for specific ages (infants: *Staphylococcus aureus,* group B, *Streptococcus,* Kawasaki disease; children 1–4 y: *S. aureus,* group A, *Streptococcus,* atypical mycobacteria; children 5–15 y: anaerobic bacteria, toxoplasmosis, cat scratch disease, tularemia; immunocompromised adults: histoplasmosis, coccidioidomycosis, *Cryptococcus, Pneumocystis carinii,* and toxoplasmosis).
Tuberculous lymphadenitis	Tuberculous nodes are multiple in presentation, most often bilateral, and may have a variable appearance, ranging from mild reactive hyperplasia to frank caseation and necrosis. Some enlarged nodes may enhance, some may be isoattenuated with muscle, and some may be of a lower attenuation than muscle. Although there may be effacement of the fat planes in the immediate region of the involved nodes, there usually is little infiltration of the adjacent neck. The presence of a multichambered, low-density nodal mass with ringlike areas of enhancement both within and around the mass and a large, low-density mass with a thick, sometimes corrugated rim of enhancement about the periphery ("cold abscess") are highly suggestive of tuberculous lymphadenitis. Fibrocalcific changes occur in the chronic phase or after treatment.	Tuberculous lymphadenitis occurs when mycobacteria involve the nodes of the infrahyoid neck chains. Nontuberculous mycobacterial infection is the most common cause of granulomatous disease in children, caused by *Mycobacterium avium intracellulare, M. bovis, M. scrofulaceum,* and *M. kansasii.* Atypical mycobacterial diseases have a propensity to be unilateral or asymmetric. The imaging findings are similar to those of TB.

(continues on page 391)

Table 9.4   (Cont.) Infrahyoid carotid space lesions

Disease	CT Findings	Comments
Cat scratch disease	Contrast-enhanced CT may demonstrate enlarged lymph nodes with surrounding edema and areas of central hypodensity, due to necrosis.	Cat scratch disease is a self-limiting infectious disease, caused by *Bartonella henselae* that may follow the scratch or bite of a cat or other animal. Following inoculation, an erythematous papule forms; several weeks later, a painful regional lymphadenopathy develops in up to 30% of cases.
Kimura disease	Marked contrast enhancement of enlarged round cervical lymph nodes.	Unusual inflammatory disease with cervical lymphadenopathy, involvement of parotid and submandibular regions, peripheral eosinophilia, and elevated serum immunoglobulin E (IgE) that occurs predominantly in Asian men in their second and third decades.
Kawasaki syndrome	Unilateral or bilateral cervical lymphadenopathy with enlarged oval reactive nodes.	Kawasaki disease is an acute systemic inflammatory condition that occurs in children younger than 10 y with high fever, oral cavity mucositis, rash, nonpurulent conjunctivitis, cardiac manifestations, and cervical lymphadenopathy (may be seen in 50%–70%).
Histiocytic necrotizing lymphadenitis (Kikuchi–Fujimoto disease)	Generally unilateral cervical lymphadenopathy with multiple enlarged oval nodes, with or without necrosis.	Kikuchi–Fujimoto disease is a rare inflammatory disease, typically seen in women in their third decade of life with tender cervical lymphadenopathy, fever, flulike symptoms, leukopenia, generalized lymphadenopathy, and hepatosplenomegaly.
Posttransplantation lymphoproliferative disorder	Presents in the neck either with diffuse bilateral nodal enlargement or a large nodal mass with central low attenuation.	In 1% to 10% of patients following organ transplantation, lymphadenopathy may be seen, but disease in the neck is uncommon. Can be associated with a mass lesion in Waldeyer ring.
Abscess	Poorly marginated soft tissue mass in the expanded carotid space with single or multiloculated, low-density center, with or without gas collections, and usually thick abscess wall. Contrast-enhanced CT images show a thick, irregular peripheral rim enhancement and enhancement of the inflamed adjacent soft tissues.	Carotid space abscesses commonly arise from extracapsular spread of suppurative lymphadenitis of the internal jugular chain or are due to penetrating trauma, vascular surgery, and intravenous (IV) drug abuse.
Nodal sarcoidosis	Multiple, most often bilateral, enlarged, homogeneously enhancing nodes, with sharp margins and a "foamy" aspect. Eggshell calcification is less frequently in the neck. Positive mediastinal nodes are common.	Sarcoidosis is a chronic multisystem granulomatous disease. The most common manifestations in the head and neck include parotid gland, ocular, and lacrimal gland involvement, as well as facial nerve and cervical lymph nodes.
Giant lymph node hyperplasia (Castleman disease)	Large, single or multiple conglomerate, nonnecrotic nodes; often show massive contrast enhancement. Calcifications may be seen occasionally.	Castleman disease is a rare nodal disease with benign lymphoid tissue hyperplasia, most commonly in the mediastinum (70%); 14% occur in the head and neck, mainly in the cervical nodes, parotid and submandibular regions, and Waldeyer ring. Castleman disease may also occur as a soft tissue mass in extranodal neck sites. It typically affects men younger than 30 y.
Sinus histiocytosis (Rosai–Dorfman disease)	Very large, round, nonnecrotic cervical nodes bilateral with homogeneous contrast enhancement.	Rosai–Dorfman disease is a rare benign histiocytic proliferation occurring most commonly in the first two decades of life with massive painless cervical lymphadenopathy. Extranodal disease is common in the upper respiratory tract, orbit, and salivary glands.

(continues on page 392)

Table 9.4   (Cont.) Infrahyoid carotid space lesions

Disease	CT Findings	Comments
Vascular lesions		
Jugular vein thrombosis ▷ *Fig. 9.37* ▷ *Fig. 9.38*	**Jugular vein thrombophlebitis:** Enlargement of the internal jugular vein by intraluminal hyperdense acute thrombus, increased density in fat, and loss of soft tissue planes surrounding the thrombus-filled vein from edema/cellulitis. After IV administration of contrast material, the thickened vessel wall may enhance intensely, contrary to the nonenhancing luminal thrombus. Edema fluid may be present in the retropharyngeal space. **Jugular vein thrombosis:** The vein is dilated, with low-attenuation intraluminal content and contrast-enhancement of the wall without adjacent inflammation. Collateral veins bypassing the thrombosed jugular vein may be seen.	In the acute-subacute thrombophlebitis phase (< 10 d after acute event), the clinical findings are most commonly those of a swollen, hot, tender, ill-defined, nonspecific neck mass with fever. In the chronic jugular vein thrombosis phase (> 10 d after acute event), patients present with a tender, vague, deep, nonspecific neck mass, in comparison to a palpable cord encountered when the external vein is thrombosed. A history of central venous catheter placement, pacemaker insertion, previous neck surgery, local malignancy, infective cervical lymphadenopathy, deep space infection, polycythemia, or drug abuse is often available. The hallmarks of Lemierre syndrome are septic jugular vein thrombosis after a primary oropharyngeal infection and metastatic infection.
Carotid artery aneurysm	Fusiform or saccular dilation of the carotid artery with attenuation values similar to the aorta before and after contrast administration. Curvilinear calcification of the dilated vascular wall is common. A thrombus may be seen. An intimal flap indicates dissecting aneurysm.	Common conditions associated with aneurysms of the extracranial carotid artery include atherosclerosis, congenital defects (Ehlers–Danlos, Marfan, Kawasaki, and Maffucci syndromes), trauma, and infection (mycotic aneurysm).
Hemorrhage and hematoma ▷ *Fig. 9.39*	Well to poorly defined, often inhomogeneous mass lesion that may displace the adjacent structures. CT densities range from 80 HU (acute) to 20 HU (chronic). Rarely, a fluid–fluid level is evident, caused by the setting of cellular elements within the hematoma and in anticoagulated patients.	Nontraumatic (spontaneous) and traumatic etiologies.
Benign neoplasms		
Carotid body paraganglioma ▷ *Fig. 9.40*	Sharply defined, ovoid mass, isodense to adjacent muscles, with mass center in the crotch of the common carotid bifurcation and superior extension. The tumor is intensely and homogeneously enhancing after IV bolus injection of contrast material and shows incorporation of carotid branches into the tumor density and characteristically splaying internal and external carotid artery, unlike other hypervascular lesions, such as metastases from renal cell carcinoma, thyroid cancer, and melanoma, or amyloid deposition.	In the infrahyoid neck, paragangliomas most commonly arise from paraganglia in carotid body, which is situated in the carotid bifurcation (60%–67% of all paragangliomas). Carotid body paragangliomas may affect all age groups but typically present as slow-growing, pulsatile, painless mass below the angle of the mandible, in women, in the fourth decade of life, and may be multiple in as many as 30% of patients with a positive family history of paraganglioma. Twenty percent have vagal and/or hypoglossal neuropathy. Most display no functional activity (paroxysmal hypertension, palpitations, and flushing from catecholamine secretion). Living in areas of high altitude predisposes to the formation of carotid body tumors. Paragangliomas have a tendency to occur multifocally. They can be associated with medullary carcinoma of the thyroid, in familial MEN syndromes, neurofibromatosis, and multiple mucocutaneous neuromas. As many as 10% of all carotid body paragangliomas are malignant.
Schwannoma ▷ *Fig. 9.41*	Usually well-circumscribed, ovoid to fusiform homogeneous soft tissue mass, isodense or, rarely, hypodense to adjacent muscles with variable, often intense contrast enhancement. Large tumors may undergo cystic degeneration and therefore present with central nonenhancing and peripheral enhancing areas. Calcifications are exceptional. In infrahyoid neck, carotid space schwannomas typically grow between the common carotid artery and the internal vein, tend to separate the vessels, and displace the common carotid artery anteromedially, the internal jugular vein posterolaterally, the anterior scalene muscle posteriorly, the sternocleidomastoid muscle anteriorly, the visceral space to the contralateral neck, and the posterior cervical space posterolaterally.	Only 13% of schwannomas occur in the extracranial head and neck along the sympathetic chain, brachial plexus, vagus nerve, and cervical nerve roots. In infrahyoid carotid space schwannoma, patients present with an asymptomatic palpable infrahyoid anterolateral neck mass. There is a male predominance, age range from 18 to 63 y. May be multiple in neurofibromatosis type 2.

(continues on page 393)

Table 9.4   (Cont.) Infrahyoid carotid space lesions

Disease	CT Findings	Comments
Neurofibroma	Sporadic neurofibromas may present as solitary or multiple, ovoid or fusiform, heterogeneous, low-density masses with well-circumscribed margins. Absence of contrast enhancement is conspicuous. Large lesions can encase the carotid artery. Plexiform neurofibromas may appear as more infiltrative, poorly circumscribed and marginated fluid-density lesions that often surround the carotid artery.	Infrahyoid carotid space neurofibromas arise from the cervical sympathetic chain or vagus nerve. Women in the third decade of life are most commonly affected. About 50% of all neurofibroma cases are associated with neurofibromatosis type 1. Five to 10% of lesions may undergo malignant transformation.
Primitive neuroectodermal tumor (PNET)	The CT findings are variable and include homogeneous tumors with or without calcifications or heterogeneous lesions with cystic, necrotic areas and solid portions. After injection of contrast material, intense enhancement may be seen.	Primitive neural tumors include neuroblastoma, ganglioneuroblastoma, and ganglioneuroma. Primary or metastatic neuroblastoma in the neck typically occurs in children younger than 5 y and presents with large masses that encroach on the pharynx and larynx and that may involve cranial nerves (CN) IX to XII or the sympathetic ganglia, producing dysphagia, dyspnea, and Horner syndrome.

(continues on page 394)

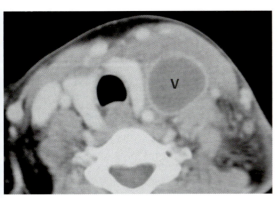

Fig. 9.37   Internal jugular vein thrombophlebitis. Axial contrast-enhanced CT demonstrates enlargement of the left internal jugular vein (V) with vessel wall enhancement and low-density nonenhancing intraluminal filling defect. Note increased density in fat and loss of soft tissue planes surrounding the thrombus-filled vein from edema/cellulites.

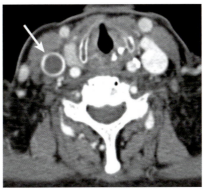

Fig. 9.38   Internal jugular vein thrombosis. Axial contrast-enhanced CT shows a low-density intraluminal filling defect and a rim of high density surrounding the nonenhancing thrombus in the right internal jugular vein (arrow). Note the absence of adjacent soft tissue inflammatory changes.

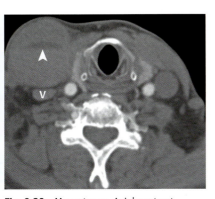

Fig. 9.39   Hematoma. Axial contrast-enhanced CT demonstrates a large right infrahyoid nonenhancing carotid space mass with fluid–fluid level (arrowhead) and mass effect on the internal jugular vein (V), visceral space, and sternocleidomastoid muscle.

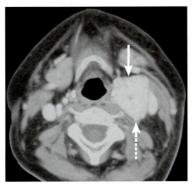

Fig. 9.40   Carotid body paraganglioma. Axial contrast-enhanced CT reveals a large avidly enhancing mass splaying external (arrow) and internal (dashed arrow) carotid arteries at the carotid bifurcation.

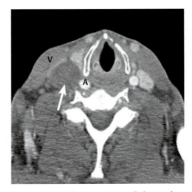

Fig. 9.41   Schwannoma of the right vagus nerve. Axial contrast-enhanced CT shows a large infrahyoid carotid space tumor with inhomogeneous and minor enhancement displacing the right common carotid artery (A) medially and the internal jugular vein (V) laterally and anteriorly (arrow).

Table 9.4   (Cont.) Infrahyoid carotid space lesions

Disease	CT Findings	Comments
Malignant neoplasms		
Nodal metastases from squamous cell carcinoma ▷ *Fig. 9.42*	Metastasis is probable if the minimal axial diameter of a lymph node of the internal jugular chain (level III and IV) is > 10 mm, the nodal shape is spherical, the ratio of the maximal longitudinal nodal length to the nodal width has a value < 2, or if a grouping of three or more lymph nodes with a minimal axial diameter of 8 to 9 mm in the drainage chains of the primary tumor is present. Nodal calcification from untreated metastatic squamous cancer is uncommon. More reliable imaging findings of metastatic disease are the presence of a central area of low density with a peripheral rim or an inhomogeneous nodal texture on contrast-enhanced CT images, due to tumor cells, interstitial fluid, necrosis, or cystic cavitation. Indistinct nodal margins, an enhancing irregular and thick nodal rim with infiltration of the adjacent fat planes and invasion of adjacent structures are straightforward CT findings for extranodal tumor extension. Obliteration of a cervical lymph node region with nodal conglomerates is an imaging feature of extensive extracapsular infiltration.	The most common neoplasms involving cervical lymph node groups are metastases from head and neck squamous cell carcinoma. The incidence of metastatic adenopathy at initial presentation varies from < 10% in glottic cancer to 90% in nasopharyngeal cancer. CT criteria for assessing nodal metastases are based on nodal size and shape, the presence of central necrosis, the presence of a localized group of nodes in an expected node-draining area for a specific primary tumor, and extranodal tumor extension. However, CT is insensitive to the presence of nonnecrotic tumor within normal-sized lymph nodes.
Nodal metastases from systemic primary	Most metastatic neck nodes from distant sites occur in the supraclavicular area (low-level IV and V). The CT appearance may be variable, including solid nodes, necrotic nodes, hypervascular nodes with areas of hemorrhage (renal cell carcinoma, malignant melanoma), and calcified nodes (colon cancer).	Systemic malignancy sites that more commonly create cervical neck metastatic nodes are melanoma, esophagus, breast, lung, and abdomen carcinoma or unknown primary with metastases to cervical nodes.
Nodal metastases from papillary thyroid carcinoma	The involved nodes may be homogeneous, may enhance, have small scattered calcifications, have hemorrhage within the node, appear indistinguishable from reactive adenopathy, or be completely cavitated with a low density on CT (secondary to a high intranodal concentration of thyroglobulin), mimicking the appearance of a benign cyst.	Metastatic papillary thyroid carcinoma may have a variety of appearances at imaging. Papillary thyroid carcinoma is a relatively common cause of intranodal calcification, which may also be seen in metastatic follicular and medullary thyroid cancer.
Nodal non–Hodgkin lymphoma ▷ *Fig. 9.43*	In cases of non–Hodgkin lymphoma, a single dominant node with scattered surrounding smaller nodes, nodal chain, or bilateral diffuse nodal disease may be present. Involved lymph nodes range in size from 1 to 10 cm, round or oval, well-circumscribed, often with a thin nodal capsule. Nodal density is equal or less than muscle, with homogeneous minor enhancement or a thin peripheral rim enhancement. Nodal necrosis can occur, albeit less frequently than with metastatic squamous cell carcinoma. Intranodal calcification may be seen after radiation or chemotherapy. Rarely, it may be seen prior to therapy in aggressive high-grade lymphoma.	Non–Hodgkin lymphoma is the second most common neoplasm of the head and neck region (behind squamous cell carcinoma) and presents with • Enlarging or persistent painless noncontiguous lymphadenopathy (levels II–V, superficial nodes; also in nodal sites atypical of the usual drainage routes for squamous cell carcinoma: retropharyngeal, submandibular, parotid, occipital nodes) • Frequent involvement (23%–30%) of extranodal lymphatic (Waldeyer ring) and extranodal extralymphatic sites (orbit, sinonasal cavities, deep facial spaces, mandible, thyroid gland, salivary gland, skin, and larynx) • With or without associated constitutional symptoms (night sweats, recurrent fevers, unexplained weight loss, fatigue, and pruritic skin rash) Incidence increases with age. Risk factors for non–Hodgkin lymphoma include congenital or acquired immunodeficiency, autoimmune disorders, immunosuppressive regimens, Sjögren syndrome, and Epstein–Barr virus infection.

(continues on page 396)

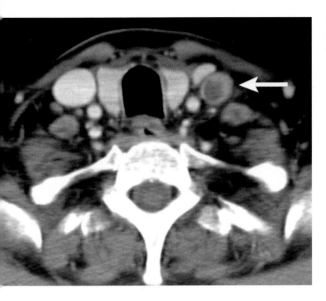

Fig. 9.42   Squamous cell carcinoma nodes. Axial contrast-enhanced CT shows an enlarged necrotic left level IV node with thick rim enhancement (arrow).

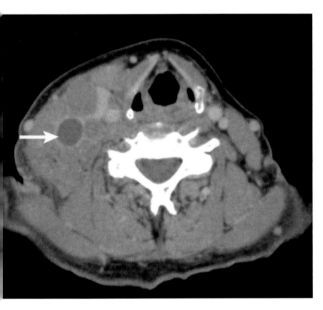

Fig. 9.43   Non–Hodgkin lymphoma. Axial contrast-enhanced CT reveals bulky right internal jugular chain adenopathy (level III) with necrosis, seen as low-density center (arrow), mass effect, and infiltration of adjacent structures (sternocleidomastoid muscle).

Table 9.4   (Cont.) Infrahyoid carotid space lesions

Disease	CT Findings	Comments
Nodal Hodgkin lymphoma ▷ *Fig. 9.44*	Classically, Hodgkin lymphoma involves a single node or nodal cluster of the internal jugular chain, uni- or bilateral, and spreads contiguously. The neck adenopathies in Hodgkin lymphoma are large (2–10 cm) and homogeneous. Nodal density is either normal or decreased, with variable, usually mild homogeneous nodal enhancement. Necrosis, seen as low-density center, is uncommon prior to treatment. Intranodal calcification may be seen after radiation or chemotherapy. Rarely, it may be seen prior to therapy.	Imaging cannot reliably distinguish Hodgkin lymphoma and non–Hodgkin lymphoma. Hodgkin lymphoma is less common than non–Hodgkin lymphoma. Hodgkin lymphoma most commonly involves upper anterior mediastinal and cervical lymph nodes (internal jugular, spinal accessory, and transverse cervical nodal chains). Associated mediastinal adenopathy is more common with Hodgkin lymphoma and abdominal adenopathy with non–Hodgkin lymphoma. In distinction to non–Hodgkin lymphoma, Hodgkin lymphoma primarily affects lymph nodes (> 90%) and only rarely presents in extranodal sites. Hodgkin lymphoma has a bimodal age distribution, with an early peak at 20 to 24 y and a later peak at 80 to 84 y. The median age at diagnosis for patients with Hodgkin lymphoma is ~28 y as compared with 67.2 y for patients with non–Hodgkin lymphoma. Forty percent of patients have category B symptoms (fever, weight loss, and night sweats).
Contiguous tumor extension	Because of its locally aggressive nature, nasopharyngeal cancer can penetrate the tough pharyngobasilar fascia and buccopharyngeal fascia with deep extension, loss of adjacent fat planes, and invasion into the carotid space. Carotid artery encasement may be present in advanced stages of squamous cell carcinoma of the faucial tonsil. Tumors arising from the lateral wall of the pyriform sinus tend to spread through the thyrohyoid membrane into the soft tissues of the neck and carotid space very early.	The carotid space may be invaded by a pharyngeal squamous cell carcinoma, which may spread further craniocaudally along the neurovascular structures. Extrathyroidal extension of anaplastic carcinomas with invasion of neighboring soft tissue structures and extension into the carotid space is common (26%–53%).

Table 9.5   Posterior cervical space lesions

Disease	CT Findings	Comments
Pseudomass		
Levator claviculae muscle	This muscle has its origin in the upper cervical spine and inserts into the middle or lateral third of the clavicle and appears as nodular soft tissue structure in the posterior cervical space.	Normal anatomical variant, occurring in 2% to 3% of the population. Rarely, the muscle itself causes the impression of a posterior neck mass lesion.
Congenital/developmental lesions		
Third branchial cleft cyst	Rounded or ovoid, sharply marginated lesion in the posterior cervical space with central fluid density. The cyst wall is nearly imperceptible. The sternocleidomastoid muscle is usually laterally displaced. May contain air if the cyst communicates with the pyriform sinus via patent tract. When infected, the cyst wall may become thickened and irregular, the cyst content develops higher attenuation, and the surrounding fat planes may become obscured.	Rare lesion (accounts for only 3% of all branchial anomalies). May occur anywhere along the course of the third branchial cleft or pouch. Presents in adulthood as painless fluctuant mass in the posterior triangle of the neck. May be associated with third branchial cleft sinus or fistula.

(continues on page 397)

Table 9.5   (Cont.) Posterior cervical space lesions

Disease	CT Findings	Comments
Venous vascular malformation (cavernous hemangioma)	Lobulated soft tissue mass, isodense to muscle, containing rounded calcifications (phleboliths). Contrast enhancement may be patchy and delayed or homogeneous and intense. Fat hypertrophy in adjacent soft tissues may be present.	Vascular malformations are not tumors but true congenital low-flow vascular anomalies, have an equal gender incidence, may not become clinically apparent until late infancy or childhood, virtually always grow in size with the patient during childhood, and do not involute spontaneously. Vascular malformations are further subdivided into capillary, venous, arterial, lymphatic, and combined malformations. Venous vascular malformations, usually present in children and young adults, are the most common vascular malformations of the head and neck. The buccal region and dorsal neck are the most common locations. Frequently, venous malformations do not respect fascial boundaries and involve more than one deep fascial space (transspatial disease). They are soft and compressible. Lesion may increase in size with Valsalva maneuver, bending over, or crying. Swelling and enlargement can occur following trauma or hormonal changes (e.g., pregnancy). Pain is common and often caused by thrombosis.
Lymphatic malformation (cystic hygroma, lymphangioma) ▷ *Fig. 9.45*	Thin-walled, multiseptated or unilocular, nonenhancing cystic mass that may insinuate in and around normal structures. Fluid–fluid levels may be present due to hemorrhage.	Lymphatic malformations represent a spectrum of congenital low-flow vascular malformations, differentiated by size of dilated lymphatic channels. Macrocystic lymphatic malformation is the most common subtype. Ninety percent of lymphatic malformations become clinically apparent by 3 y of age, whereas the remaining 10% present as neck mass in the young adult. May be sporadic or part of congenital syndromes (Turner, Noonan, and fetal alcohol syndromes). Most lymphatic malformations arise in the posterior cervical space and supraclavicular region. Up to 10% of all cervical cystic hygromas extend into the mediastinum. Rapid enlargement of a lymphangioma is usually due to hemorrhage into the cystic spaces of the mass.

(continues on page 398)

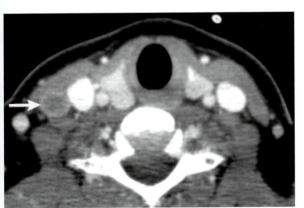

Fig. 9.44   Hodgkin lymphoma. Axial contrast-enhanced CT demonstrates unilateral enlarged right low jugular chain nodal mass (arrow) with necrotic low-density center and mild peripheral enhancement.

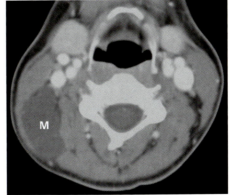

Fig. 9.45   Lymphatic malformation. Axial contrast-enhanced CT shows a well-circumscribed, nonenhancing, septated low-density right posterior cervical space mass (M).

II Head and Neck

Table 9.5   (Cont.) Posterior cervical space lesions

Disease	CT Findings	Comments
Inflammatory/infectious conditions		
Reactive lymphadenopathy	In reactive adenopathy, cervical lymph nodes may by definition enlarge to a maximum diameter of 1.5 cm but maintain their normal oval shape, isodense to muscle, and their homogeneous internal architecture with variable, usually mild enhancement. Enhancing linear markings within the node may be seen. Multiple nodal locations are typically present. Postinflammatory fatty infiltration appears as low-density nodal hilus (which is peripheral rather than central), mimicking necrosis in a node with pronounced lima bean shape (fat usually has a lower attenuation than tumor necrosis).	Reactive hyperplasia is a nonspecific lymph node reaction, current or prior to any inflammation in its draining area. Can occur at any age but is most common in the pediatric age group.
Suppurative lymphadenitis	Enlarged node with internal low attenuation (intra-nodal abscess) and ringlike contrast enhancement of the peripheral portion. The node has ill-defined margin and increased density in the adjacent fatty tissue, reflecting inflammation/edema.	Patients are usually septic with tender neck mass. Suppurative lymphadenopathy tends to occur with unusual pathogens (e.g., tularemia, atypical myco-bacteria, and cat scratch fever).
Tuberculous lymphadenitis	Several CT patterns of nodal disease can be seen in the course of disease, ranging from mild reactive hyperplasia to frank caseation and necrosis. Some enlarged nodes may enhance, some may be isoat-tenuated with muscle, and some may be of a lower attenuation than muscle. Although there may be effacement of the fat planes in the immediate region of the involved nodes, there usually is little infiltration of the adjacent neck. The presence of a multicham-bered, low-density nodal mass with ringlike areas of enhancement both within and around the mass and a large, low-density mass with a thick, sometimes corrugated rim of enhancement about the periphery ("tuberculous abscess") are highly suggestive of tuberculous adenitis. Fibrocalcified nodes occur in the chronic phase or after treatment.	Cervical tuberculous adenitis is a manifestation of a systemic disease process. Bilateral posterior cervical space nodes are commonly involved. Coexisting disease in the anterior triangle may be present. The vast majority of cases are found in patients who have emigrated from endemic areas. It is most prevalent in the 20- to 30-y age group but can occur at any age. Patients often present with an asymptomatic neck mass and few if any constitutional symptoms (fever, night sweats, or weight loss).
Abscess	Poorly marginated soft tissue mass in the expanded posterior cervical space with single or multiloculated low-density center, with or without gas collections, and usually thick abscess wall. Contrast-enhanced CT images show a thick, irregular peripheral rim enhancement and enhancement of the inflamed adjacent soft tissues.	Abscesses within the posterior cervical space com-monly arise from extracapsular spread of suppurative lymphadenitis of the nodal chain along the spinal accessory nerve.
Nodal sarcoidosis	Produces multiple, most often bilateral diffusely en-larged, homogeneously enhancing nodes, with sharp margins and a "foamy" aspect. Eggshell calcification is less frequently seen in the neck. Positive mediasti-nal nodes are common.	Sarcoidosis is a chronic multisystem granulomatous disease. The most common manifestations in the head and neck include parotid gland, ocular, and lacrimal gland involvement, as well as facial nerve and cervical lymph nodes.
Benign neoplasms		
Lipoma ▷ *Fig. 9.46*	Homogeneous, well-defined, nonenhancing mass with fat density (–65 to –125 HU) in the posterior cer-vical space with a thin capsule having smooth convex margins. Internal architecture is minimal.	Most head and neck lipomas are located subcutaneously and in the posterior cervical space. Other common locations are the submandibular, anterior cervical, and parotid spaces. Can be multiple, transspatial, and intramuscular. Associated syndromes: Madelung disease, Dercum disease, familial multiple lipomatosis, and Gardner syndrome. More common in men (fifth to sixth decade).
Intramuscular myxoma	Usually solitary, intramuscular, well-defined, lobu-lated, homogeneous mass with tissue attenuation intermediate between that of water and muscle. CT values approaching those of fat may also occur.	Myxoma is commonly located in the large muscles of the thigh, shoulder, buttocks, and upper arm. It is rare in the head and neck and can arise from the paraspinal muscles, scalene muscles, geniohyoid muscle, and sternocleidomastoid muscle. The tumor usually occurs between age 40 and 70 y and is slightly more common in women.

(continues on page 399)

Table 9.5   (Cont.) Posterior cervical space lesions

Disease	CT Findings	Comments
Schwannoma	Up to 5 cm, well-circumscribed ovoid to fusiform, homogeneous soft tissue mass, isodense or hypodense to adjacent muscles with variable, often intense contrast enhancement. Large tumors may undergo cystic or necrotic degeneration and therefore present with central nonenhancing and peripheral enhancing areas. Calcifications are exceptional. Displaces jugular vein anteriorly and medially.	Schwannoma in the posterior cervical space arises from a distal brachial plexus root, cervical sensory nerve, or CN XI. Most commonly sporadic and isolated. May be multiple in neurofibromatosis type 2.
Neurofibroma	Sporadic neurofibromas may present as solitary or multiple, ovoid or fusiform, heterogeneous, low-density masses with well-circumscribed margins. Absence of contrast enhancement is conspicuous. In von Recklinghausen disease (neurofibromatosis type 1 [NF1]), localized neurofibromas have similar imaging characteristics to solitary neurofibromas, but they are often bilateral and follow the cervical nerve roots with intraforaminal extension, as well as the brachial plexus, vagus nerve, and peripheral subcutaneous nerve branches. Plexiform neurofibromas may appear as more infiltrative, poorly circumscribed and marginated, fluid-density lesions.	Cervical neurofibromas may be solitary lesions (although rare), or they may be seen in patients with NF1, most commonly in patients between the ages of 20 and 40 y. Sudden painful enlargement of a neurofibroma in NF1 should suggest malignant transformation.
Malignant neoplasms		
Liposarcoma	Well-differentiated liposarcomas present as a lobulated, fatty mass with some enhancing internal septations or nodules. Calcifications may occur. Less well-differentiated liposarcomas display as a heterogeneous, enhancing soft tissue mass with or without amorphous fatty foci, often with unsharp, infiltrating borders.	Liposarcoma is the second most common soft tissue sarcoma after malignant fibrous histiocytoma. Only 3% to 6% of liposarcomas occur in the head and neck region (posterior cervical space, larynx, and cheek). They show no gender predilection (age peak third to sixth decade). Other soft tissue malignant neoplasms are uncommon.
Nodal metastases from squamous cell carcinoma	Single or multiple, oval to round, mildly enhancing soft tissue masses centered within fat of the posterior cervical space, variable in size from < 1 cm to very large. Necrosis appears as central nonenhancing, low density with a variably thick, irregular enhancing wall (central nodal tumor may show a slight enhancement of the low-attenuation node). Ill-defined margins and stranding of surrounding fat are features of extracapsular spread.	The most common disease of the posterior cervical space is metastatic squamous cell carcinoma. Nodes of the spinal accessory lymph node chain (classified as level V) containing metastatic squamous cell carcinoma should prompt examination of the pharyngeal mucosal space, larynx, and base of the tongue.

(continues on page 400)

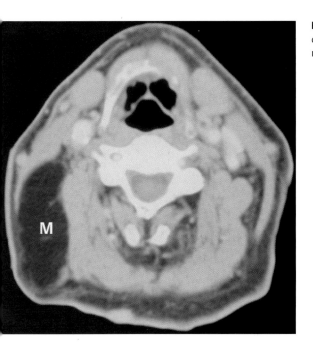

Fig. 9.46   Lipoma. Axial contrast-enhanced CT demonstrates a well-defined, homogeneous, nonenhancing, fat-density mass (M) within the right posterior cervical space.

II Head and Neck

Table 9.5   (Cont.) Posterior cervical space lesions

Disease	CT Findings	Comments
Nodal metastases from systemic primary	Most metastatic neck nodes from distant sites occur in the supraclavicular area (low-level IV [Virchow node] and V). The CT appearance may be variable, including solid nodes, necrotic nodes, hypervascular nodes with areas of hemorrhage (renal cell carcinoma, malignant melanoma), and calcified nodes (colon cancer).	Systemic malignancy sites that more commonly create cervical neck metastatic nodes are esophagus, breast, lung, and abdominal carcinoma, melanoma, or unknown primary with metastases to cervical nodes. In patients with predominantly low posterior cervical space lymphadenopathy, the primary tumor should be sought in the thyroid, thorax, or abdomen.
Nodal metastases from differentiated thyroid carcinoma	The involved lymph nodes may enhance, have small scattered calcifications, have hemorrhage within the node, appear indistinguishable from reactive adenopathy, or be completely cavitated, mimicking the appearance of a benign cyst.	Differentiated thyroid carcinoma may present with posterior cervical space lymphadenopathy.
Nodal non–Hodgkin lymphoma	Nodes invaded by non–Hodgkin lymphoma are typically multiple, large, solid, homogeneous, slightly enhancing, round masses. Extracapsular spread is uncommon. Nodal necrosis can occur in high-grade non–Hodgkin lymphoma. Intranodal calcification may be seen after radiation or chemotherapy. Rarely, it may be seen prior to therapy in aggressive high-grade lymphoma.	Non–Hodgkin lymphoma in the posterior triangle of the neck presents with enlarging or persistent painless lymphadenopathy along the spinal accessory and transverse cervical chain. Lymphadenopathy in other lymph node chains in the adjacent neck is typically present. Associated involvement of extranodal lymphatic (Waldeyer ring) and extranodal extralymphatic sites (orbit, sinonasal cavities, deep facial spaces, mandible, thyroid gland, salivary gland, skin, and larynx) are frequent.
Nodal Hodgkin lymphoma	The neck adenopathies in Hodgkin lymphoma are large (2–10 cm) and homogeneous. Nodal density is either normal or decreased, with variable, usually mild homogeneous nodal enhancement. Necrosis, seen as low-density center, is uncommon prior to treatment. Intranodal calcification may be seen after radiation or chemotherapy. Rarely, it may be seen prior to therapy.	Hodgkin lymphoma is less common than non–Hodgkin lymphoma. Hodgkin lymphoma most commonly involves upper anterior mediastinal and cervical lymph nodes (internal jugular, spinal accessory, and transverse cervical nodal chains). Associated mediastinal adenopathy is common with cervical Hodgkin lymphoma. In distinction to non–Hodgkin lymphoma, Hodgkin lymphoma primarily affects lymph nodes (> 90%) and only rarely presents in extranodal sites. Hodgkin lymphoma has a bimodal age distribution, with an early peak at 20 to 24 y and a later peak at 80 to 84 y. The median age at diagnosis for patients with Hodgkin lymphoma is around 28 y. Forty percent of patients have category B symptoms (fever, weight loss, and night sweats).
Trauma		
Seroma ▷ *Fig. 9.47* 	Uniloculated, nonenhancing, cystic mass at the surgery site.	A seroma is a pocket of clear serous fluid that sometimes develops after surgery (e.g., neck dissection). Seromas are different from hematomas, which contain red blood cells, and from abscesses, which contain pus and result from an infection.

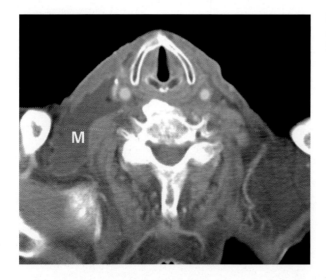

Fig. 9.47   Seroma (after cervical diskectomy). Axial contrast-enhanced CT demonstrates a well-defined, homogeneous, nonenhancing low-attenuation mass (M) within the right posterior cervical space.

Table 9.6 Infrahyoid retropharyngeal space lesions

Disease	CT Findings	Comments
Pseudomass		
Edema/lymph fluid	Uniform low-density fluid collection in the retropharyngeal space without significant mass effect, wall enhancement, or surrounding cellulitis. Sharp demarcation from pharynx and prevertebral muscles.	Nonabscess fluid in the retropharyngeal space, seen with superior vena cava syndrome, internal jugular vein thrombosis, lymphatic obstruction secondary to lower neck or mediastinal tumor, trauma, neck surgery, or radiation. It is also seen in patients with longus colli tendinitis (acute calcific prevertebral tendinitis). Retropharyngeal fluid itself is asymptomatic.
Congenital/developmental lesions		
Third branchial cleft cyst	Rounded or ovoid, sharply marginated lesion in the retropharyngeal space with central fluid density. The cyst wall is nearly imperceptible. May contain air if the cyst communicates with the pyriform sinus via the patent tract. When infected, the cyst wall may become thickened and irregular, the cyst content develops higher attenuation, and the surrounding fat planes may become obscured.	Rarely, a third branchial cleft cyst may be seen in the retropharyngeal space, simulating a retropharyngeal abscess. Cyst presents in adulthood. Patients with retropharyngeal third branchial cleft cyst will often present with recurrent retropharyngeal infection. May be associated with third branchial cleft sinus or fistula.
Venous vascular malformation (cavernous hemangioma)	Lobulated or poorly marginated soft tissue mass, isodense to muscle. The presence of phleboliths is highly suggestive of the diagnosis. May be superficial or deep, localized or diffuse, solitary or multifocal, circumscribed or transspatial, with or without satellite lesions. Contrast enhancement is patchy or homogeneous and intense. Fat hypertrophy in adjacent soft tissues may occur.	As opposed to infantile hemangiomas, vascular malformations are not tumors but true congenital low-flow vascular anomalies, have an equal gender incidence, may not become clinically apparent until late infancy or childhood, virtually always grow in size with the patient during childhood, and do not involute spontaneously. Vascular malformations are further subdivided into capillary, venous, arterial, lymphatic, and combined malformations. Venous vascular malformations, usually present in children and young adults, are the most common vascular malformations of the head and neck. The buccal region and dorsal neck are the most common locations. Masticator space, sublingual space, tongue, lips, and orbit are other common locations. Frequently, venous malformations do not respect fascial boundaries and involve more than one deep fascial space (transspatial disease). They are soft and compressible. Lesion may increase in size with Valsalva maneuver, bending over, or crying. Swelling and enlargement can occur following trauma or hormonal changes (e.g., pregnancy). Pain is common and often caused by thrombosis.
Lymphatic malformation (lymphangioma, cystic hygroma)	Uni- or multiloculated, nonenhancing fluid-filled mass with imperceptible wall, which tends to invaginate between normal structures. Often found in multiple contiguous cervical spaces (transspatial) with secondary extension into the retropharyngeal space. Rapid enlargement of the lesion, areas of high attenuation values, and fluid–fluid levels suggest prior hemorrhage. Lymphatic and venous malformation may coexist.	Lymphatic malformations represent a spectrum of congenital low-flow vascular malformations, differentiated by size of dilated lymphatic channels. May be sporadic or part of congenital syndromes (Turner, Noonan, and fetal alcohol syndromes). Macrocystic lymphatic malformation is the most common subtype; 65% are present at birth. Ninety percent are clinically apparent by 3 y of age; the remaining 10% present in young adults. Most lymphatic malformations arise in the posterior cervical space and supraclavicular region. Large retropharyngeal lymphangioma may cause mass effect on pediatric airway.

(continues on page 402)

Table 9.6   (Cont.) Infrahyoid retropharyngeal space lesions

Disease	CT Findings	Comments
Inflammatory/infectious conditions		
Cellulitis	Cellulitis is seen as widening of the retropharyngeal space with poorly defined areas of low density and an amorphous enhancement following contrast media injection. The process may extend into the adjacent spaces and inferiorly into the mediastinum.	Retropharyngeal space infection occurs most commonly in children (< 6 y), but also in adult patients. It is usually caused by infection of the pharynx, paranasal sinuses, and nose. Patients present with high fever and other clinical signs of infection.
Abscess ▷ *Fig. 9.48*	Tense fluid collection distending the retropharyngeal space and producing pharyngeal airway narrowing. Thick, irregular enhancing wall suggests mature abscess. Adjacent cellulitis/phlegmon may obscure the prevertebral muscles and pharyngeal mucosal space structures. Complications may result from spread to adjacent spaces (mediastinitis with 50% mortality, jugular vein thrombosis or thrombophlebitis, narrowing of internal carotid artery [ICA] caliber, ICA pseudoaneurysm, and rupture).	Can result from suprahyoid suppurative retropharyngeal node rupture, ventral spread of diskitis/osteomyelitis and prevertebral infection, or from pharyngeal penetrating foreign body. Most patients are children (< 6 y). Increasing frequency in adult population because of diabetes, HIV, alcoholism, and malignancy. Common signs: septic male patient, neck pain, sore throat.
Benign neoplasms		
Lipoma	Well-defined, nonenhancing fat-density mass (–65 to –125 HU), homogeneous without any internal soft tissue stranding. Hibernomas (fetal lipomas) are benign encapsulated tumors consisting of brown fat, with slightly higher and subtly inhomogeneous attenuation than lipoma.	More common in men (fifth to sixth decade). Can be seen in contiguous spaces (transspatial). Multiple in 5% of cases. Usually asymptomatic. May have significant mass effect on pharynx. Lipoma variants include fibrolipoma, angiolipoma, spindle cell lipoma, pleomorphic lipoma, and myolipoma with imaging features usually not distinguishable from liposarcoma.
Malignant neoplasms		
Contiguous tumor extension	Retropharyngeal solid enhancing soft tissue mass due to an infiltrating tumor with its center in the adjacent infrahyoidal cervical spaces. Once inside, the retropharyngeal tumor can move in a cephalocaudal direction.	Squamous cell carcinoma frequently involves the retropharyngeal space by direct invasion. The level of involvement depends on the location of the primary tumor. Malignant extension into the infrahyoid retropharyngeal space is most common from the hypopharynx.
Synovial sarcoma	This rare malignant neoplasm is usually a circumscribed mass posterior to the pharynx with soft tissue attenuation or a heterogeneous mass of mixed fluid and soft tissue attenuation. Most of these tumors enhance. Hemorrhage and calcification may occur.	In the neck, synovial sarcomas are most commonly found in or about the retropharyngeal space. They are often painful and present with hoarseness, dysphagia, or dyspnea.

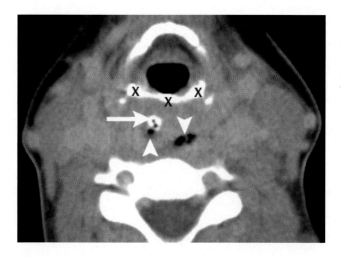

Fig. 9.48   Infrahyoid retropharyngeal abscess. Axial contrast-enhanced CT demonstrates a radiopaque foreign body (arrow) after toothpick ingestion and retropharyngeal perforation. Tense fluid and gas collection (arrowheads) is widening the retropharyngeal space and is causing mass effect on the hypopharynx (x = contrast medium within the hypopharynx).

Table 9.7   Infrahyoid perivertebral space lesions

Disease	CT Findings	Comments
Pseudomass		
Cervical rib	CT scans show a prominent cervical transverse process or a cervical rib as bony projection in the absence of any other abnormality.	A cervical rib is a supernumerary rib above the normal first rib that arises from the seventh cervical vertebra. A prominent cervical transverse process is probably a form of supernumerary cervical rib developing at a level above the lowest cervical vertebra. May present clinically as a palpable supraclavicular mass.
Vertebral body osteophyte	The classic sign of spondylosis is osteophytosis. Osteophytes are bony spurs that originate on the anterolateral aspect of the vertebral bodies a few millimeters from the discovertebral junction (at the site of attachment of the peripheral fibers of the annulus fibrosus). At the beginning, they extend in a horizontal direction; in the more advanced phase, they become hooked and grow vertically. Sometimes osteophytes develop on both sites of a disk space and grow until they fuse together to form a "bridge osteophyte."	Spondylosis deformans of the cervical spine is the most typical consequence of age- or load-related degeneration of the vertebral body. It is found in 60% of women and 80% of men after the age of 50. C5–C6 is the most common level, followed by C6–C7, then C4–C5. Only when degenerative alterations are severe and symptomatic (e.g., cervical osteophytic dysphagia) should they be considered pathologic. Osteophytes can be distinguished from the syndesmophytes of ankylosing spondylitis, paravertebral ossification of psoriasis and reactive arthritis, and flowing ossification of diffuse idiopathic skeletal hyperostosis.
Hypertrophic facet joint	Osseous facet overgrowth ("mushroom cap" facet appearance) and bone excrescences impinging on neural foramina and the spinal canal in conjunction with articular joint space narrowing with sclerosis and intra-articular gas (vacuum phenomenon). Enhancing inflammatory soft tissue changes surrounding facet joint are common. Frequently seen in conjunction with degenerative disk disease.	Hypertrophic degenerative facet may be perceived as a cervical "mass" on physical examination. Degenerative facet joint disease is most common in middle/lower cervical spine. Frequently seen in the elderly population. No gender preference.
Levator claviculae muscle	Uni- or bilaterally, the levator claviculae muscles arise from the anterior portion of the transverse processes of the upper cervical vertebrae (most likely above the C3 level), then head inferiorly and laterally, coursing lateral to the scalene muscles, anterior to the levator scapulae muscle, and medial to the sternocleidomastoid muscle, and insert in the lateral third of the clavicle, blending with the trapezius.	A normal variant, not to be mistaken for an abnormality (lymphadenopathy, unenhanced vessel).
Levator scapulae muscle hypertrophy	Altered contour of the neck with homogeneous enlargement of the levator scapulae muscle and denervated atrophic trapezius muscle. Absent ipsilateral internal jugular vein and sternocleidomastoid muscle from radical neck dissection and an ipsilateral jugular foramen mass are findings of underlying cause.	Asymmetry of the levator scapulae muscles is an unusual cause of a palpable posterior triangle mass. Damage to spinal accessory nerve secondary to radical neck dissection and, less commonly, ipsilateral jugular foramen mass (paraganglioma, schwannoma, meningioma, and metastasis) lead to denervation atrophy of trapezius muscle with compensatory hypertrophy of the levator scapulae muscle. In case of a levator scapulae muscle atrophy secondary to cervical spondylosis with spinal nerve compression of the C4 and C5 roots, the normal-sized contralateral levator scapulae muscle may present as a palpable mass.

(continues on page 404)

Table 9.7 (Cont.) Infrahyoid perivertebral space lesions

Disease	CT Findings	Comments
Congenital/developmental lesions		
Omovertebral bone ▷ *Fig. 9.49*	High position of the scapula (Sprengel anomaly) and a relative large triangular bone that extends from the medial border of the scapula to the spinous process, lamina, or transverse process of C5 to C7.	Sprengel anomaly is caused by the failure of scapular descent. The condition is usually sporadic and unilateral. Other skeletal anomalies, mainly Klippel–Feil syndrome, may be present. An omovertebral bone is seen in only one third of children affected by Sprengel anomaly.
Inflammatory/infectious conditions		
Calcific tendinitis of the longus colli muscle	Soft tissue thickening with calcification, seen in the prevertebral area at the level of C1 and C2, associated with retropharyngeal space edema, extending from C2 to C5.	Acute longus colli tendinitis secondary to calcium hydroxyapatite deposition, self-limiting, with neck pain, mild fever, and odynophagia (for 2–7 d, third through sixth decade).
Vertebral osteomyelitis	Signs of spondylodiskitis with disk space narrowing, irregular end-plate destruction, and soft tissue involvement of the prevertebral and epidural space with soft tissue swelling, cellulitis with diffusely enhancing soft tissue edema, and abscess formation. Osteomyelitis involving the posterior elements of the spine with an inflammatory mass in the paraspinal portion of the perivertebral space is rare.	Infection involving cervical vertebral body, disk space, epidural space, and associated perivertebral space. C5 and C6 levels are most frequently affected in cervical spine. Most common causative agents are *Staphylococcus aureus, Streptococcus, Mycobacterium tuberculosis, Escherichia coli, Proteus, Brucella, Pseudomonas, Serratia,* and *Candida.* May be caused by hematogenous spread, direct inoculation, or contiguous spread. Adults are more often affected. Diabetics, elderly, IV drug addicts, and patients with urinary tract infection, pneumonia, and skin infection are at risk.
Perivertebral space abscess	Poorly marginated soft tissue mass in the expanded prevertebral or paraspinal portion of the perivertebral space with single or multiloculated low-density center, with or without gas collections, and usually thick abscess wall. Contrast-enhanced CT images show a thick, irregular peripheral rim enhancement and enhancement of the inflamed adjacent soft tissues.	Soft tissue infection of the prevertebral and/or paraspinal portion of the perivertebral space from direct extension from adjacent infection, hematogenous dissemination from distant sites, or transcutaneous infection of deep tissue. Most common pathogens are *S. aureus, M. tuberculosis,* and *E. coli.* Fungal infections are rare, more common in immunocompromised host. Predisposing factors are diabetes mellitus, alcoholism, cirrhosis, chronic renal failure, IV drug abuse, and immunocompromised state.
Benign neoplasms		
Schwannoma	Although some ("dumbbell" lesion) may emanate from the neural canal, thereby widening the spinal neural foramen, still others may derive from the branches beyond the foramen and present as well-circumscribed, ovoid to fusiform, homogeneous soft tissue mass, isodense to cord, with variable, often intense contrast enhancement. Large tumors may undergo cystic degeneration and therefore present with central nonenhancing and peripheral enhancing areas. Calcifications are exceptional.	Tumors of neurogenic origin are some of the more frequently seen benign neoplasms of the perivertebral space. They can produce a mass effect in the paraspinal space. This consists mainly of anterior displacement and effacement of the longus muscle at suprahyoid levels and of the anterior scalene muscle at infrahyoid levels. The occurrence of multiple peripheral nerve schwannomas in patients with neurofibromatosis type 2 is characteristic.
Neurofibroma ▷ *Fig. 9.50*	Sporadic neurofibromas may present as solitary or multiple, ovoid or fusiform, heterogeneous, low-density masses with well-circumscribed margins. Absence of contrast enhancement is conspicuous. In neurofibromatosis type 1 (NF1), localized neurofibromas have similar imaging characteristics to solitary neurofibromas, but they are often bilateral, multilevel, diffuse, or plexiform and follow the cervical nerve roots with intraforaminal extension, the brachial plexus, the vagus nerve, and peripheral subcutaneous nerve branches.	Ninety percent of neurofibromas occur as sporadic, solitary tumors; 16% to 65% of patients with NF1 have neurofibromas (57% single lesions), most commonly in patients between the ages of 20 and 40 y. Sudden painful enlargement of a neurofibroma in NF1 should suggest malignant transformation (3%–5% of patients develop malignant peripheral nerve sheath tumors).
Aggressive fibromatosis (extra-abdominal desmoid fibromatosis, juvenile fibromatosis) ▷ *Fig. 9.51*	"Malignant-appearing," poorly marginated, inhomogeneously enhancing soft tissue mass with local invasion of muscle, vessels, nerves, and bone. Most common locations are perivertebral space, supraclavicular area, and masticator space.	Benign soft tissue tumor of fibroblastic origin arising from aponeurotic neck structures. Associated abnormality: Gardner syndrome. Seen at all ages (70% < 35 y). Significantly more women affected. Present with firm, painless neck mass. Paresis depends on site. Postoperative recurrence rate may reach 25%.

(continues on page 405)

Table 9.7 (Cont.) Infrahyoid perivertebral space lesions

Disease	CT Findings	Comments
Other benign soft tissue tumors	Well-defined, homogeneous soft tissue masses with usually moderate, uniform contrast enhancement.	They include (myo)fibroblastic tumors, fibrohistiocytic tumors, rhabdomyoma, mesenchymoma, and myxoma. Clinically, these present as a mass of increasing size, associated with discomfort or pain.
Osteochondroma	Sessile or pedunculated osseous "cauliflower" lesion with marrow and cortical continuity with parent vertebra, usually in the posterior elements of the cervical spine. May compress the spinal cord or nerve roots.	Only 2% to 3% of osteochondromas (sporadic, hereditary multiple exostosis) occur in the spine: cervical (50%, C2 predilection) > thoracic > lumbar > sacrum. Peak age 10 to 30 y; M:F = 3:1. Many spinal osteochondromas are asymptomatic. Complications include deformity, fracture, vascular compromise, neurologic sequelae, mechanical impingement symptoms, and malignant transformation (< 1% solitary lesions; 3%–5% familial osteochondromatosis).
Aneurysmal bone cyst	Aneurysmal bone cysts arise in the posterior elements of the vertebra as a markedly expansile ("ballooning") multicystic osteolytic lesion with well-defined scalloped margins, and displacement of the paraspinal musculature away from the spine. Fluid–fluid levels (due to hemorrhage and blood product sedimentation) are characteristic. Enhancement is confined to the periphery and septations interposed between the blood-filled spaces. Spinal cord compression may occur because of intraspinal extension. Occasionally, the expansile lesion may affect two or more contiguous vertebrae. Solid aneurysmal bone cyst is a rare variant. The solid component predominates and enhances diffusely.	Primary lesions are usually observed in the first, second, and third decades of life with slight female predominance; 20% occur in the spine. Can coexist with osteoblastoma, giant cell tumor, or enchondroma.
Giant cell tumor	Centered in the vertebral body. Lytic, expansile lesion with heterogeneous contrast enhancement. May contain fluid attenuation regions due to necrosis or focal aneurysmal bone cyst component. Zone of transition is narrow, margin usually not sclerotic. May have cortical breakthrough with apparent soft tissue extension.	In spine, peak incidence are second and third decades of life, with female preponderance. May be associated with aneurysmal bone cyst. Can undergo sarcomatous transformation (spontaneously or in response to radiation therapy). Primary malignant giant cell tumors are rare.
Osteoblastoma	Involvement of posterior elements of the vertebra is typical. Expansile, lytic lesion with thin sclerotic margins; may contain partially calcified matrix.	Histologically identical to osteoid osteoma but larger. Occurs typically in the spine. May be associated with aneurysmal bone cyst.

(continues on page 406)

II Head and Neck

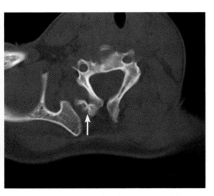

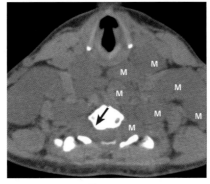

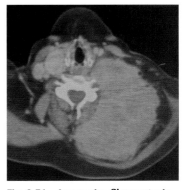

Fig. 9.49 Omovertebral bone. Axial bone CT shows a high position of the right scapula (Sprengel anomaly) and a small transverse/oblique bone (arrow) extending from the right lamina of C6 to the medial border of the right scapula.

Fig. 9.50 Neurofibromatosis type 1. Axial non–contrast-enhanced CT demonstrates bilateral multiple hypodense neurofibromas (M) involving cervical nerve roots, the brachial plexus, vagus nerves, and peripheral subcutaneous nerve branches. Note also intraforaminal extension (arrow).

Fig. 9.51 Aggressive fibromatosis. Axial contrast-enhanced CT reveals a huge, inhomogeneously, intense enhancing soft tissue mass centered in the left perivertebral space.

Table 9.7   (Cont.) Infrahyoid perivertebral space lesions

Disease	CT Findings	Comments
Malignant neoplasms		
Malignant mesenchymal tumors	Fairly well to poorly defined, inhomogeneous soft tissue mass with necrotic (hypodense) areas and considerable contrast enhancement. Erosion/destruction of adjacent cervical spine is common.	They include malignant fibrous histiocytoma, fibrosarcoma, synovial sarcoma, and rhabdomyosarcoma. The clinical presentation is commonly a painless, slow-growing mass. Acute painful presentations are associated with tumor necrosis or hemorrhage.
Chordoma ▷ *Fig. 9.52*	Chordoma appears as a destructive vertebral body mass with osseous erosion and expansion, sparing posterior elements. May extend into the disk space and involve adjacent vertebrae. A large associated soft tissue mass of low attenuation with extension into the perivertebral space may be the dominant finding. Extension along nerve roots and enlargement of neural foramina mimics peripheral nerve sheath tumors. Spinal cord compression may occur because of intraspinal extension. Up to 50% of these tumors may show coarse, amorphous calcified matrix.	Rare primary malignant tumor of notochord origin. Originates from the sacrum and coccyx region (50%), sphenooccipital region (35%), and spine (15%), especially C2–C5 and lumbar. Cervical spine chordomas occur in 40- to 60-y-old patients (M:F = 2:1) and present with gradual onset of neck pain, numbness, and motor weakness. Ewing sarcoma, chondrosarcoma, and osteosarcoma originate infrequently in the cervical spine.
Vertebral body metastases	Involves vertebral body, often with extension into the neural arch. Destructive lesion, more permeative, less expansile with associated soft tissue mass. When the tumor breaks out of the vertebral body in an anterior direction, the prevertebral portion of the perivertebral space is involved early with epidural extension occurring late. Early epidural involvement with moderate perivertebral space tumor is seen when the metastatic disease breaks out of the vertebral body in a posterior, epidural direction.	Over 95% of tumors of the spine are metastases.
Lymphoma	Involves vertebral body more than neural arch. Multiple vertebrae involvement is common. May cross disk space. Lytic, permeative bone destruction with enhancing, poorly defined soft tissue mass, involving adjacent structures (epidural, paraspinal muscles). "Ivory" vertebral body is rare. Epidural extension from adjacent vertebral or paraspinous disease is common.	Both in Hodgkin disease and non–Hodgkin lymphoma, bone involvement is usually secondary (hematogenous spread, or invasion from adjacent soft tissues and lymph nodes). Most common presenting symptom is pain, most commonly in patients between the ages of 40 and 70 y. Slight male predominance.

Table 9.8   Anterior cervical space lesions

Disease	CT Findings	Comments
Pseudomass		
Enlarged anterior jugular vein ▷ *Fig. 9.53*	The size of the anterior jugular veins can be variable and asymmetric.	Incidental finding on CT without any pathologic significance.
Congenital/developmental lesions		
Branchial cleft cyst	Ovoid or rounded, unilocular, low-density cyst (isodense to cerebrospinal fluid), nonenhancing with no discernible wall. If infected, peripheral wall is thicker and enhances, and the density of content increases. "Dirty" fat lateral to the cyst indicates surrounding cellulitis.	Second branchial cleft cysts can occur anywhere along the line from the tonsillar fossa to the supraclavicular region. The anterior cervical space is an unusual location.
Lymphatic malformation (cystic hygroma, lymphangioma)	Uni- or multiloculated, nonenhancing fluid-filled mass with imperceptible wall, which tends to invaginate between normal structures. Rapid enlargement of the lesion, areas of high attenuation values, and fluid–fluid levels suggest prior hemorrhage.	Lymphatic malformations represent a spectrum of congenital low-flow vascular malformations, differentiated by size of dilated lymphatic channels. Macrocystic lymphatic malformation is the most common subtype. May be sporadic or part of congenital syndromes (Turner, Noonan, and fetal alcohol syndromes). Sixty-five percent are present at birth; 90% are clinically apparent by 3 y of age. The remaining 10% present in young adults. Often found in multiple contiguous cervical spaces (transspatial). A secondary extension into the anterior cervical space is rare.

(continues on page 407)

Table 9.8 (Cont.) Anterior cervical space lesions

Disease	CT Findings	Comments
Degenerative/acquired lesions		
Laryngocele	Thin-walled air- or fluid-filled cystic mass within the anterior cervical space and with or without a paraglottic space component.	External or mixed laryngocele extending from laryngeal ventricle with lateral extensions through thyrohyoid membrane.
Inflammatory/infectious conditions		
Anterior cervical space infection ▷ *Fig. 9.54*	**Cellulitis** may present as a soft tissue mass with obliteration of adjacent fat planes. It is often ill defined, enhancing, and extending along fascial planes and into subcutaneous tissues beneath thickened skin. **Abscesses** may appear as a poorly marginated soft tissue mass in the expanded anterior cervical space with single or multiloculated low-density center, with or without gas collections, and usually thick abscess wall. Contrast-enhanced CT images show a thick, irregular peripheral rim enhancement and enhancement of the inflamed adjacent soft tissues.	It may result from extension of cellulitis or abscess from adjacent spaces or after direct penetrating trauma.
Benign neoplasms		
Lipoma	Well-defined, nonenhancing, fat-density mass (−65 to −125 HU), homogeneous without any internal soft tissue stranding. Benign infiltrating lipoma may involve multiple contiguous neck spaces. Liposarcoma may also be a concern if there is prominent internal stranding, enhancing nodularity, or inhomogeneity.	Lipomas of the anterior cervical space are rare and do not cause symptoms until they reach a large size and have a significant mass effect.
Malignant neoplasms		
Contiguous tumor extension	Obliteration of the fat of the anterior cervical space due to an infiltrating mass with its center in the adjacent infrahyoidal cervical spaces.	These malignant tumors break out of their space of origin and invade the anterior cervical space.

II Head and Neck

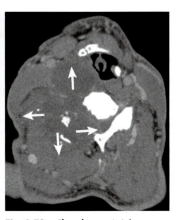

Fig. 9.52 Chordoma. Axial contrast-enhanced CT shows lytic destruction of the right posterior C5 vertebral body, pedicle, and lamina, associated with a large contiguous low-attenuation soft tissue mass (arrows) extending into the anterior prevertebral portion and posterior paraspinal portion of the right perivertebral space and epidural space. Note bony debris and small tumor calcifications.

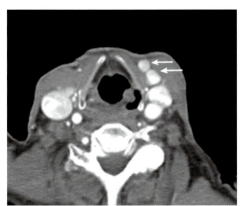

Fig. 9.53 Double anterior jugular vein. Axial contrast-enhanced CT shows the left anterior jugular vein separated into enlarged anterior and posterior branches (arrows).

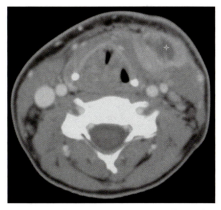

Fig. 9.54 Abscess. Axial contrast-enhanced CT reveals a rim-enhancing focal fluid collection (joystick point) in the left anterior cervical space. Also seen are associated cellulitis with obliteration of adjacent fat planes, thickening of the left sternocleidomastoid muscle and platysma, and infiltration of the subcutaneous fat.

III Spine

10 Computed Tomography of Spinal Abnormalities

Steven P. Meyers

Computed tomography (CT) is a useful imaging modality for evaluating normal spinal anatomy and pathologic conditions involving the vertebrae and sacrum. Because of its high spatial resolution, CT can be utilized to evaluate pathologic disorders of vertebrae (neoplasms, inflammatory diseases, etc.), epidural soft tissues, disks, thecal sac, facet joints, and paravertebral structures.

The normal spine is comprised of 7 cervical, 12 thoracic, and 5 lumbar vertebrae. The upper two cervical vertebrae have different configurations than the other vertebrae. The atlas (C1) has a horizontal ringlike configuration with lateral masses that articulate with the occipital condyles superiorly and the superior facets of C2 inferiorly. The dorsal margin of the upper dens is secured in position in relation to the anterior arch of C1 by the transverse ligament. Various anomalies occur in this region, such as atlanto-occipital assimilation, segmentation (e.g., block vertebrae), basiocciput hypoplasia, condylus tertius, and os odontoideum. The lower five cervical vertebral bodies have rectangular shapes with progressive enlargement inferiorly. Superior and lateral projections from the C3 to C7 cervical vertebral bodies form the uncovertebral joints. The transverse processes are located anterolateral to the vertebral bodies and contain the foramina transversaria within which the vertebral arteries and veins are located. The posterior elements consist of paired pedicles, articular pillars, laminae, and spinous processes. The cervical spine has a normal lordosis.

The 12 thoracic vertebral bodies and 5 lumbar vertebral bodies progressively increase in size caudally. The posterior elements include the pedicles, transverse processes, laminae, and spinous processes. The transverse processes of the thoracic vertebrae also have articulation sites for ribs. The thoracic spine has a normal kyphosis and the lumbar spine a normal lordosis. Anterior and posterior longitudinal ligaments connect the cervical vertebrae, and interspinous ligaments and ligamenta flava provide stability for the posterior elements.

The cortical margins of the vertebral bodies have dense compact bone structure. The medullary compartments of the vertebrae are comprised of bone marrow and trabecular bone. Pathologic processes such as tumor, inflammation, and infection result in bone lysis with or without extension of the intramedullary lesions through destroyed cortical bone. Contrast enhancement may also be seen at the pathologic sites. Because of direct visualization of these pathologic processes in the marrow, magnetic resonance imaging (MRI) can often detect these abnormalities sooner than CT, which relies on later indirect signs of trabecular destruction for confirmation of disease.

The intervertebral disks enable flexibility of the spine. The two major components of normal disks, the nucleus pulposus and anulus fibrosus, are seen as structures with intermediate attenuation. The outer anulus fibrosus is made of dense fibrocartilage. The central nucleus pulposus is made of gelatinous material. The combination of various factors, such as decreased turgor of the nucleus pulposus and loss of elasticity of the anulus with or without tears, results in degenerative changes in the disks. CT features of disk degeneration include decreased disk heights, vacuum disk phenomena, disk bulging, and associated vertebral body osteophytes. Radial tears of the anulus fibrosus are often clinically significant and are associated with disk herniations. The term *disk herniation* usually refers to extension of the nucleus pulposus through an annular tear beyond the margins of the adjacent vertebral body end plates. Disk herniations can be further subdivided as protrusions (when the head of the herniation equals the neck in size), extrusions (when the head of the herniation is larger than the neck), or extruded fragments (when there is separation of the herniated disk fragment from the disk of origin). Disk herniations can occur in any portion of the disk. Posterior and posterolateral herniations can cause compression of the thecal sac and contents, as well as compression of epidural nerve roots in the lateral recesses or within the intervertebral foramina. Lateral and anterior disk herniations are less common but can cause hematomas in adjacent structures. Disk herniations that occur superiorly or inferiorly result in focal depressions of the vertebral cortical end plates (i.e., Schmorl nodes). On CT, recurrent disk herniations may be difficult to delineate from scar or granulation tissue. MRI, however, can be used in these situations because herniated disks do not typically enhance after gadolinium contrast administration, whereas scar tissue typically shows contrast enhancement.

The thecal sac is a meningeal covered compartment containing cerebrospinal fluid (CSF), which is contiguous with the basal subarachnoid cisterns and extends from the upper cervical level to the level of the sacrum. The thecal sac contains the spinal cord and exiting nerve roots. The distal end of the conus medullaris is normally located at the T12–L1 level in adults. Lesions within the thecal sac are categorized as intradural intra- or extramedullary. Intramedullary lesions directly involve the spinal cord, whereas extramedullary lesions do not primarily involve the spinal cord. Extra- or epidural lesions refer to spinal lesions outside the thecal sac.

Evaluation of the spinal cord, intradural nerves, and spinal subarachnoid space can be done with CT using myelography by placement of iodinated contrast into the thecal sac by percutaneous needle injection. Diffuse or focal abnormal expansion of the spinal cord, intradural extramedullary lesions, and nerve root compression can be evaluated with CT myelography. MRI with high soft tissue contrast resolution, however, is typically superior to CT in the evaluation of the spinal cord and various intramedullary pathologic conditions, such as congenital malformations, neoplasms, benign mass lesions (dermoid, arachnoid cyst, etc.), inflammatory/infectious processes, traumatic injuries (contusions and hematomas), and ischemia/infarction, as well as the adjacent CSF and nerve roots. MRI after the intravenous administration of gadolinium contrast agents is also useful for evaluating lesions within the spinal cord, as well as neoplastic or inflammatory diseases within the thecal sac.

The normal blood supply to the spinal cord consists of seven or eight radicular arteries that enter the spinal canal through the intervertebral foramina to supply the three main vascular territories of the spinal cord (cervicothoracic: cervical and upper three thoracic levels, midthoracic: T4 level to C7 level, and thoracolumbar: T8 level to lumbosacral plexus). The cervicothoracic vascular distribution is supplied by radicular branches arising from the vertebral arteries and costocervical trunk. The midthoracic territory is often supplied by a radicular branch at the C7 level. The thoracolumbar territory is supplied by a single artery arising from the ninth, tenth, eleventh, or twelfth intercostal arteries (75%); the fifth, sixth, seventh, or eighth intercostal arteries (15%); or the first or second lumbar arteries (10%). The radicular arteries supply the longitudinally oriented anterior spinal artery, which is located in the midline anteriorly adjacent to the spinal cord and supplies the gray matter and central white matter of the spinal cord. The radicular arteries also supply the two major longitudinally oriented posterior spinal arteries that course along the posterolateral sulci of the spinal cord, as well as one third to one half of the outer rim of the spinal cord via a peripheral anastomotic plexus. Ischemia or infarcts involving the spinal cord represent rare disorders associated with atherosclerosis, diabetes, hypertension, abdominal aortic aneurysms, and abdominal aortic surgery. Vascular malformations can be seen within the thecal sac, with or without involvement of the spinal cord.

Epidural structures of clinical importance include the (1) lateral recesses (anterolateral portions of the spinal canal located between the thecal sac and pedicles that contains nerve roots, vessels and fat), (2) dorsal epidural fat pad, (3) posterior elements and facet joints, and (4) posterior longitudinal ligament and ligamentum flavum. The intervertebral foramina represent the bony channels between the pedicles through which the nerves traverse.

Narrowing of the thecal sac, lateral recesses, and intervertebral foramina can result in clinical signs and symptoms. The narrowing can result from disk herniations, posterior vertebral body osteophytes, hypertrophy of the ligamentum flavum and facet joints, synovial cysts, excessive epidural fat, epidural neoplasms, abscesses, hematomas, spinal fractures, spondylolisthesis, or spondylolysis. CT is useful for evaluating these disorders and for categorizing the degree of narrowing of the thecal sac, as well as compression of nerve roots in the lateral recesses and intervertebral foramina.

CT plays a major role in the evaluation of traumatic injuries to the spine. The high definition and detail of bone anatomy displayed with CT using reformatted images in coronal and sagittal planes enable detection of complex and/or subtle vertebral fractures, retropulsed fracture fragments into the spinal canal and/or intervertebral foramina, and disruption of the foramina transversaria with associated injuries of the vertebral arteries. Stability of fractures can be related to findings on CT using the Denis three-column model. The *anterior column* consists of the anterior half of the vertebral body and disk, along with the anterior longitudinal ligament. The *middle column* consists of the posterior half of the vertebral body and disk, along with the posterior longitudinal ligament. The *posterior column* consists of the posterior bony vertebral arch, inter- and supraspinous ligament complex, ligamentum flavum, and facet joints and capsule. Minor injuries involve only part of one column and typically do not lead to instability. *Compression fractures* involving only the anterior column with disruption of the anterior end plate (often between T6–T8 and T12–L3) with an intact spinal canal are considered stable. *Burst fractures* that result from an axial loading injury with disruption of the anterior and middle columns (often at the thoracolumbar junction and T10–L5) can be seen with CT as buckling of the anterior, superior, and posterior end plates with or without retropulsed bone fragments into the spinal canal and are often unstable. *Seat belt fractures (Chance fractures)* are flexion-compression fractures involving the anterior, middle, and posterior columns and are typically unstable. *Fracture-dislocation* fractures represent unstable fractures involving all three columns from combinations of compression, tension, and rotation/shear forces.

Table 10.1 Spine: Congenital and developmental abnormalities

Lesions	CT Findings	Comments
Congenital		
Chiari I malformation ▷ *Fig. 10.1*	Cerebellar tonsils extend > 5 mm below the foramen magnum in adults, 6 mm in children younger than 10 y. Syringohydromyelia in 20% to 40%; hydrocephalus in 25%; basilar impression in 25%. Less common association: Klippel–Feil syndrome, atlanto-occipital assimilation.	Cerebellar tonsillar ectopia. Most common anomaly of central nervous system (CNS). Not associated with myelomeningocele.
Chiari II malformation (Arnold–Chiari malformation) ▷ *Fig. 10.2*	Small posterior cranial fossa with gaping foramen magnum through which there is an inferiorly positioned vermis associated with a cervicomedullary kink; beaked dorsal margin of the tectal plate. Myeloceles or myelomeningoceles seen in nearly all patients. Hydrocephalus and syringohydromyelia are common. Dilated lateral ventricles are seen posteriorly (colpocephaly).	Complex anomaly involving the cerebrum, cerebellum, brainstem, spinal cord, ventricles, skull, and dura. Failure of fetal neural tube to develop properly results in altered development affecting multiple sites of the CNS.
Chiari III malformation	Features of Chiari II plus lower occipital or high cervical encephalocele.	Rare anomaly associated with high mortality.
Myelomeningocele/myelocele	Posterior protrusion of spinal contents and unfolded neural tube (neural placode) through defects in the bony dorsal elements of the involved vertebrae or sacral elements. The neural placode is usually located at the lower lumbar-sacral region with resultant tethering of the spinal cord. If the neural placode is flush with the adjacent skin surface, the anomaly is labeled a myelocele. If the neural placode extends above the adjacent skin surface, the anomaly is labeled a myelomeningocele; with or without syringohydromyelia.	Failure of developmental closure of the caudal neural tube results in an unfolded neural tube (neural placode) exposed to the dorsal surface in the midline without overlying skin. Other features associated with myelomeningoceles and myeloceles include dorsal bony dysraphism, deficient dura posteriorly at the site of the neural placode, and Chiari II malformations. By definition, the spinal cords are tethered. Usually repaired surgically soon after birth.
Terminal myelocystocele	Posterior lower spina bifida through which the distal portion of a tethered spinal cord (containing a localized cystic dilation), cerebrospinal fluid (CSF), and meninges extends beneath the dorsal subcutaneous fat.	Represent 1% to 5% of skin-covered masses at dorsal lumbosacral region. Anomalous development of the lower spinal cord, vertebral column, sacrum, and meninges, with or without association with anomalies of genitourinary tract (epispadias, caudal regression syndrome, and anomalies of the genitourinary system and hindgut).
Lipomyelocele/ lipomyelomeningocele	Unfolded caudal neural tube (neural placode) covered by a lipoma that is contiguous with the dorsal subcutaneous fat through defects (spina bifida) involving the bony dorsal vertebral elements. The neural placode is usually located at the lower lumbar-sacral region with resultant tethering of the spinal cord, with or without syringohydromyelia. With lipomyelomeningocele, the dorsal lipoma that extends into the spinal canal is asymmetric, resulting in rotation of the placode and meningocele.	Failure of developmental closure of the caudal neural tube results in an unfolded neural tube (neural placode) covered by a lipoma that is contiguous with the subcutaneous fat. The overlying skin is intact, although the lipoma usually protrudes dorsally. The nerve roots arise from the placode. Features associated with lipomyelomeningoceles and lipomyeloceles include tethered spinal cords, dorsal bony dysraphism, and deficient dura posteriorly at the site of the neural placode. Not associated with Chiari II malformations. Diagnosis often in children, occasionally in adults.
Intradural lipoma	Focal dorsal dysraphic spinal cord attached to a lipoma with low attenuation that often extends from the central canal of the spinal cord to the pial surface; intact dorsal dural margins and posterior vertebral elements.	Intradural lipomas are usually in the cervical or thoracic region.
Diastematomyelia	Division of spinal cord into two hemicords usually from T9 to S1, with or without fibrous or bony septum partially or completely separating the two hemicords. Hemicords located either within a common dural tube (50%, type I) or within separate dural tubes (50%, type II), with or without syringohydromyelia at, above, or below the zone of diastematomyelia. Often associated with tethering of the conus medullaris, osseous anomalies (spina bifida with laminar fusion, butterfly vertebrae, hemivertebrae, and block vertebrae). Diastematomyelia seen in 15% of patients with Chiari II malformations.	Developmental anomalies related to abnormal splitting of the embryonic notochord with abnormal adhesions between the ectoderm and endoderm. Can present in children with clubfeet or adults and children with neurogenic bladder, lower extremity weakness, and chronic pain; with or without association with nevi, lipomas.

(continues on page 413)

Table 10.1   (Cont.) Spine: Congenital and developmental abnormalities

Lesions	CT Findings	Comments
Os odontoideum ▷ *Fig. 10.3a, b*	Separate corticated bony structure positioned superior to the C2 body at site of normally expected dens, often associated with enlargement of the anterior arch of C1 (may sometimes be larger than os odontoideum).	Independent bony structure positioned superior to the C2 body at site of normally expected dens, often associated with hypertrophy of the anterior arch of C1, with or without cruciate ligament incompetence/instability (with or without zone of high signal on T2-weighted images in spinal cord). Os odontoideum associated with Klippel–Feil anomaly, spondyloepiphyseal dysplasia, Down syndrome, and Morquio syndrome. Etiology suggested to be normal variant or childhood injury (before age 5–7 y) with fracture/separation of the cartilaginous plate between the dens and body of axis.

(continues on page 414)

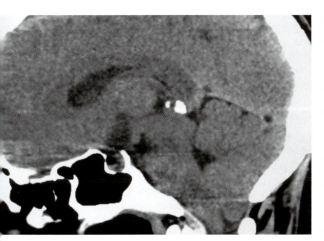

Fig. 10.1   Chiari I malformation. Sagittal image shows extension of the cerebellar tonsils below the foramen magnum to the level of the posterior arch of C1, as well as a normal-shaped fourth ventricle.

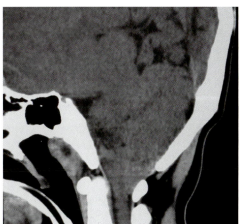

Fig. 10.2   Chiari II malformation. Sagittal image shows a small posterior cranial fossa, inferior extension of the cerebellum through a widened foramen magnum, and an abnormal-shaped fourth ventricle.

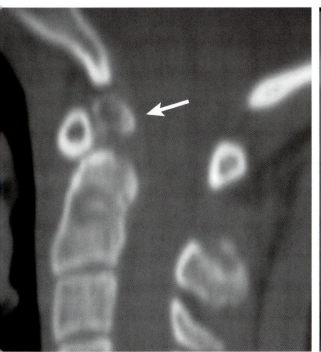

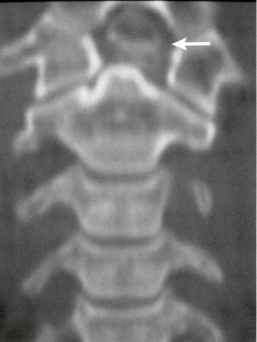

b

Fig. 10.3a, b   Os odontoideum. Sagittal (**a**) and coronal (**b**) images show a corticated bony structure positioned superior to the C2 body at the site of a normally expected dens (arrows).

Table 10.1 (Cont.) Spine: Congenital and developmental abnormalities

Lesions	CT Findings	Comments
Ossiculum terminale ▷ *Fig. 10.4a, b*	Small corticated bone located cranial to the dens and superior to the level of the transverse ligament.	Congenital nonunion of the upper margin of the dens with a terminal ossicle located superior to the transverse ligament. No associated spinal instability.
Short pedicles: congenital/developmental spinal stenosis	Narrowing of the anteroposterior dimension of the thecal sac to < 10 mm resulting predominantly from developmentally short pedicles. May occur at one or multiple levels.	Developmental variation with potential predisposition to spinal cord injury from traumatic injuries or disk herniations, as well as early symptomatic spinal stenosis from degenerative changes.
Achondroplasia ▷ *Fig. 10.5*	**Anomalies of vertebrae:** Shortening and flattening of vertebral bodies, with or without anterior wedging of one or multiple vertebral bodies, shortened pedicles with spinal stenosis. **Anomalies at the craniovertebral junction:** Small foramen magnum, basioccipital hypoplasia, odontoid hypoplasia, basilar invagination, hypertrophy of posterior arch of C1, platybasia, and atlanto-occipital dislocation.	Achondroplasia represents a congenital type of osteochondrodysplasia that results in short-limbed dwarfism (decreased rate of endochondral bone formation). Usually autosomal dominant/sporadic mutations.
Klippel–Feil anomaly ▷ *Fig. 10.6*	Fusion of vertebral bodies that have either a narrow tall configuration or wide/flattened configuration, absent or small intervening disk, with or without fusion of posterior elements, occipitalization of atlas, congenital scoliosis, and kyphosis.	Represents congenital fusion of two or more adjacent vertebrae resulting from failure of segmentation of somites (third to eighth weeks of gestation). Can be associated with Chiari I malformations, syringohydromyelia, diastematomyelia, anterior meningocele, and neurenteric cyst.
Hemivertebrae ▷ *Fig. 10.7*	Wedge-shaped vertebral body, with or without molding of adjacent vertebral bodies toward shortened side of hemivertebra.	Disordered embryogenesis in which the paramedian centers of chondrification fail to merge, resulting in failure of formation of the ossification center on one side of the vertebral body; with scoliosis.
Butterfly vertebra	Paired hemivertebrae with constriction of height in midsagittal portion of vertebral body, with or without molding of adjacent vertebral bodies toward midsagittal constriction.	Disordered embryogenesis in which there is persistence of separate ossification centers in each side of the vertebral body (failure of fusion).
Tripediculate vertebra ▷ *Fig. 10.8a, b*	Wedge-shaped vertebral body containing two pedicles on enlarged side and one pedicle on the shortened side; may be multiple levels of involvement, with or without adjacent hemivertebrae, with or without molding of adjacent vertebral bodies toward shortened side of involved segments; with scoliosis.	Disordered embryogenesis at more than one level with asymmetric malsegmentation, with scoliosis.
Spina bifida occulta	Minimal defect near midline where laminae do not fuse; no extension of spinal contents through defect. Most commonly seen at the S1 level; other sites include C1, C7, T1, and L5.	Mild anomaly with failure of fusion of dorsal vertebral arches (laminae) in midline; usually benign normal variation.

(continues on page 416)

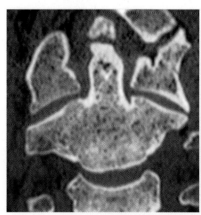
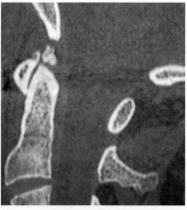

a   b

Fig. 10.4a, b Ossiculum terminale. Coronal (**a**) and sagittal (**b**) images show a small corticated bone located cranial to the dens and superior to the level of the transverse ligament.

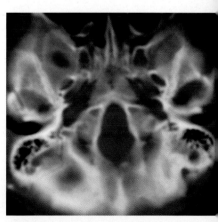

Fig. 10.5 Achondroplasia. Axial image shows a narrow foramen magnum.

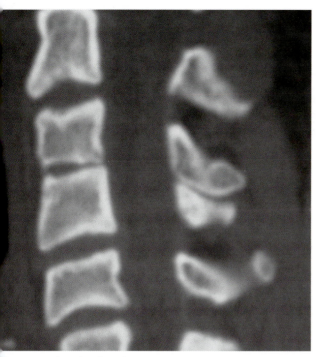

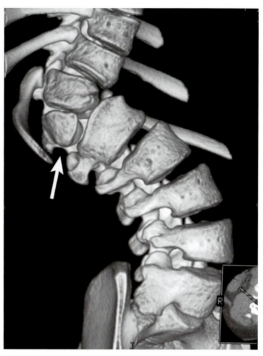

Fig. 10.6 Klippel-Feil syndrome. Sagittal image shows a segmentation anomaly involving the C3 and C4 vertebral bodies, which have narrowed anteroposterior dimensions with a small intervening disk. Partial fusion of the posterior elements is also seen involving these vertebrae.

Fig. 10.7 Hemivertebra. Volume-rendered image shows a hemivertebra causing scoliosis (arrow).

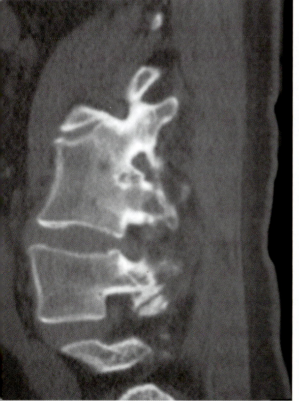

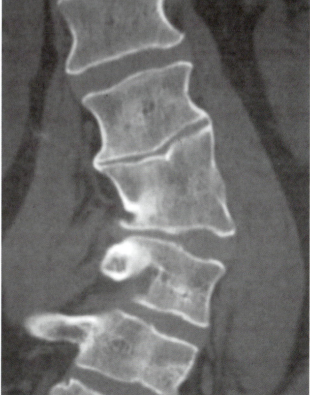

b

Fig. 10.8a, b Tripediculate vertebra. Sagittal (**a**) and coronal (**b**) images show a vertebra with two pedicles on the left side and one pedicle on the right.

Table 10.1   (Cont.) Spine: Congenital and developmental abnormalities

Lesions	CT Findings	Comments
Spina bifida aperta (spina bifida cystica) ▷ *Fig. 10.9a, b*	Wide defect where lamina are unfused, and through which spinal contents extend dorsally (myelocele, myelomeningocele, meningocele, lipomyelocele, lipomyelomeningocele, myelocystocele).	Usually associated with significant clinical findings related to the severity and type of neural tube defect.
Meningoceles	Vertebral defect either from surgical laminectomies or congenital anomaly. Sacral meningoceles can alternatively extend anteriorly through a defect in the sacrum.	Meningoceles resulting from congenital dorsal bony dysraphism. Anterior sacral meningoceles can result from trauma or be associated with mesenchymal dysplasias (neurofibromatosis 1 [NF1], Marfan syndrome, and syndrome of caudal regression).
Syndrome of caudal regression ▷ *Fig. 10.10a–c*	Partial or complete agenesis of sacrum/coccyx, with or without involvement of lower thoracolumbar spine. Symmetric sacral agenesis > lumbar agenesis > lumbar agenesis with fused ilia > unilateral sacral agenesis. Prominent narrowing of thecal sac and spinal canal below lowermost normal vertebral level; with or without myelomeningocele, diastematomyelia, tethered spinal cord, thickened filum, and lipoma.	Congenital anomalies related to failure of canalization and retrogressive differentiation resulting in partial sacral agenesis and/or distal thoracolumbar agenesis; with or without association with other anomalies, such as imperforate anus, anorectal atresia/stenosis, malformed genitalia, and renal dysplasia. May not have clinical correlates in mild forms; with or without distal muscle weakness, paralysis, hypoplasia of lower extremities, sensory deficits, lax sphincters, and neurogenic bladder.

Table 10.2   Solitary osseous lesions involving the spine

Lesions	CT Findings	Comments
Neoplasms (malignant)		
Metastatic tumor	Single or multiple well-circumscribed or poorly defined infiltrative lesions involving the vertebral marrow, dura, and/or leptomeninges; low to intermediate attenuation; may show contrast enhancement, with or without medullary and cortical bone destruction (radiolucent), with or without bone sclerosis, with or without pathologic vertebral fracture, with or without epidural tumor extension causing compression of neural tissue or vessels. Leptomeningeal tumor often best seen on postcontrast images.	May have variable destructive or infiltrative changes involving single or multiple sites of involvement.
Myeloma/plasmacytoma ▷ *Fig. 10.11a, b*	Multiple (myeloma) or single (plasmacytoma), well-circumscribed or poorly defined, diffuse infiltrative radiolucent lesions involving the vertebra(e), and dura; involvement of vertebral body lesions typically radiolucent/bone lysis, rarely involves posterior elements until late stages, low to intermediate attenuation; may show contrast enhancement. Pathologic vertebral fracture, with or without epidural tumor extension causing compression of neural tissue or vessels.	May have variable destructive or infiltrative changes involving the axial and/or appendicular skeleton.

(continues on page 418)

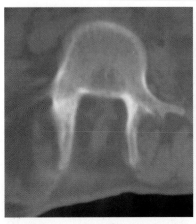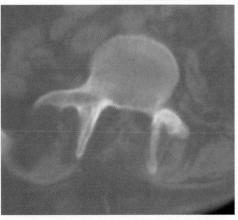

a   b

Fig. 10.9a, b   Spina bifida aperta. Axial image show widely separated laminae in a patient who had postnatal surgery for a myelocele (Chiari II malformation).

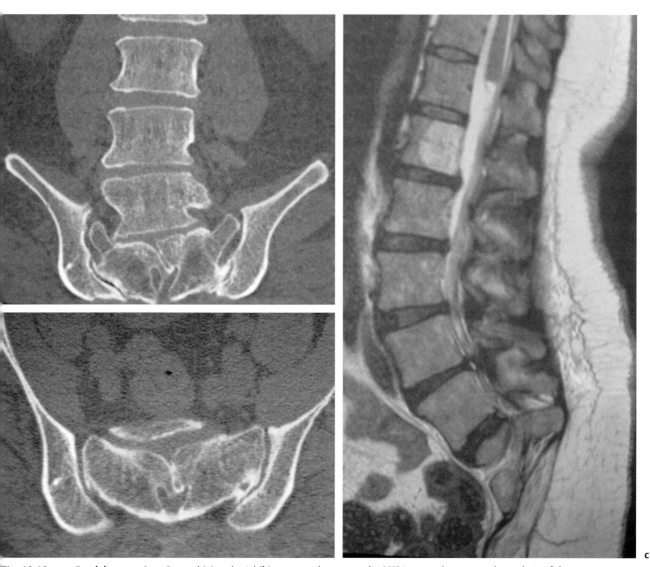

c

Fig. 10.10a–c   Caudal regression. Coronal (**a**) and axial (**b**) computed tomography (CT) images show severe hypoplasia of the sacrum as seen on a sagittal T2-weighted magnetic resonance imaging (MRI) (**c**).

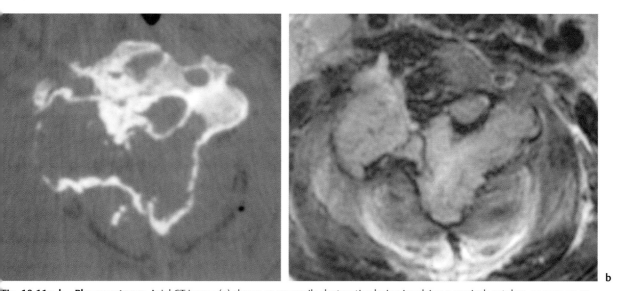

b

Fig. 10.11a, b   Plasmacytoma. Axial CT image (**a**) shows an expansile destructive lesion involving a cervical vertebra, as seen on an axial T2-weighted image (**b**). The tumor causes spinal cord compression.

III Spine

Table 10.2   (Cont.) Solitary osseous lesions involving the spine

Lesions	CT Findings	Comments
Lymphoma and leukemia	Single or multiple, well-circumscribed or poorly defined, infiltrative radiolucent lesions involving the marrow of the vertebrae, dura, and/or leptomeninges; low to intermediate attenuation, pathologic vertebral fracture, with or without epidural tumor extension causing compression of neural tissue or vessels. May show contrast enhancement, with or without bone destruction. Diffuse involvement of vertebra with Hodgkin lymphoma can produce bone sclerosis, as well as an "ivory vertebra" pattern that has diffuse high attenuation. Leptomeningeal tumor often best seen on postcontrast images.	May have variable destructive or infiltrative marrow/bony changes involving single or multiple vertebral sites. Lymphoma may extend from paraspinal lymphadenopathy into the spinal bone and adjacent soft tissues within or outside the spinal canal or initially involve only the epidural soft tissues or only the subarachnoid compartment. Can occur at any age (peak incidence third to fifth decades).
Chordoma ▷ *Fig. 10.12a–d*	Well-circumscribed, lobulated radiolucent lesions, low to intermediate attenuation, usually shows contrast enhancement (usually heterogeneous); locally invasive associated with bone erosion/destruction; usually involves the dorsal portion of the vertebral body with extension toward the spinal canal. Also occurs in sacrum.	Rare, slow-growing tumors (~3% of bone tumors); usually occur in adults 30 to 70 y old; M > F (2:1); sacrum (50%) > skull base (35%) > vertebrae (15%).
Chondrosarcoma ▷ *Fig. 10.13a–c*	Lobulated radiolucent lesions, low to intermediate attenuation, with or without matrix mineralization; may show contrast enhancement (usually heterogeneous); locally invasive associated with bone erosion/destruction, encasement of vessels and nerves; can involve any portion of the vertebra.	Rare, slow-growing malignant cartilaginous tumors (~16% of bone tumors), usually occur in adults (peak in fifth to sixth decades), M > F; sporadic (75%), malignant degeneration/transformation of other cartilaginous lesion, enchondroma, osteochondroma, etc. (25%).
Osteogenic sarcoma ▷ *Fig. 10.14a, b*	Destructive malignant lesions, low to high attenuation, usually with matrix mineralization/ossification within lesion or within extraosseous tumor extension; can show contrast enhancement (usually heterogeneous). Cortical bone destruction and epidural extension of tumor can compress the spinal canal and spinal cord.	Malignant bone lesions rarely occur as primary tumor involving the vertebral column; locally invasive, high metastatic potential. Occurs in children as primary tumors and adults associated with Paget disease, irradiated bone, chronic osteomyelitis, osteoblastoma, giant cell tumor, and fibrous dysplasia.

(continues on page 420)

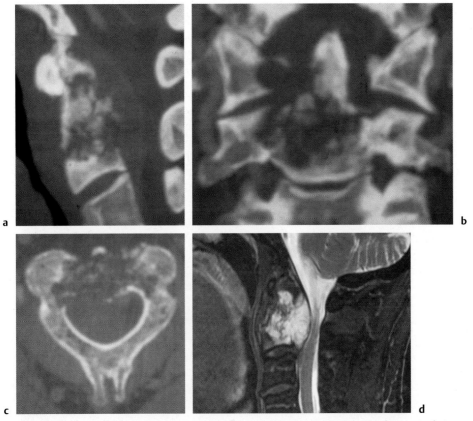

a   b   c   d

Fig. 10.12a–d   Chordoma. Sagittal (**a**), coronal (**b**), and axial (**c**) CT images show a destructive lesion involving the C2 vertebra that has high signal on a fat-suppressed, T2-weighted sagittal image (**d**).

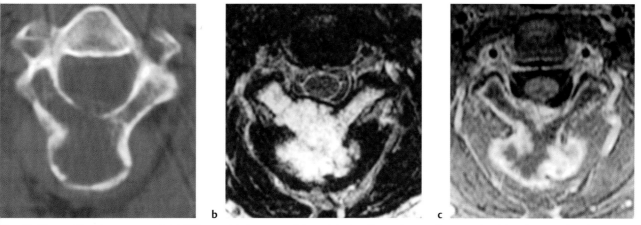

Fig. 10.13a–c   Chondrosarcoma. Axial CT image (**a**) shows a radiolucent destructive and expansile tumor involving the posterior elements that has high signal on axial T2-weighted MRI (**b**) and shows contrast enhancement on axial fat-suppressed, T1-weighted MRI (**c**).

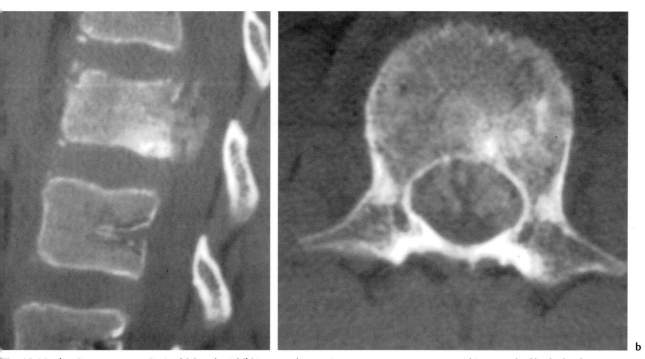

Fig. 10.14a, b   Osteosarcoma. Sagittal (**a**) and axial (**b**) images show an intraosseous osteosarcoma within a vertebral body that has malignant ossified mineralization with extension into the spinal canal.

III Spine

Table 10.2 (Cont.) Solitary osseous lesions involving the spine

Lesions	CT Findings	Comments
Ewing sarcoma	Destructive malignant lesions involving the vertebral column, radiolucent with low to intermediate attenuation; typically lack matrix mineralization; can show contrast enhancement (usually heterogeneous). Cortical bone destruction and epidural extension of tumor can compress the spinal canal and spinal cord.	Usually occurs between the ages of 5 and 30, M > F; rarely occurs as primary tumor involving the spinal column; locally invasive, high metastatic potential.
Malignant fibrous histiocytoma (MFH)	Tumors are often associated with zones of cortical destruction and extraosseous soft tissue masses. Tumors have low to intermediate attenuation, can show contrast enhancement. Cortical bone destruction and epidural extension of tumor can compress the spinal canal and spinal cord.	Malignant tumors involving soft tissue and rarely bone that are presumed to derive from undifferentiated mesenchymal cells. The World Health Organization (WHO) now uses the term *undifferentiated pleomorphic sarcoma* for pleomorphic MFH.
Hemangioendothelioma	Lesions usually have sharp margins that may be slightly lobulated and often have low to intermediate attenuation; can be intraosseous radiolucent lesions or extradural soft tissue lesions. Can be multifocal. Extraosseous extension of tumor through zones of cortical destruction can be seen. Lesions can show contrast enhancement.	Vasoformative/endothelial low-grade malignant neoplasms that are locally aggressive and rarely metastasize compared with high-grade angiosarcoma.
Hemangiopericytoma	Tumors often have well-defined margins; intraosseous lesions can be radiolucent with or without lobulated margins; extraosseous lesions can have low to intermediate attenuation. Lesions may contain slightly prominent vessels centrally or peripherally, with or without hemorrhagic zones. Can show contrast enhancement.	Rare malignant tumors of pericytic origin that occur in soft tissues and less frequently in bone.

Neoplasms (benign)

Lesions	CT Findings	Comments
Enchondroma	Lobulated radiolucent lesions, low to intermediate attenuation, with or without matrix mineralization; can show contrast enhancement (usually heterogeneous). Locally invasive associated with bone erosion/destruction; usually involves posterior elements.	Rare, slow-growing tumors (~12% of bone tumors); usually occur in children and young adults (10–30 y), M = F.
Chondroblastoma	Tumors are typically radiolucent with lobular margins and typically have low to intermediate attenuation. Up to 50% have chondroid matrix mineralization. May show contrast enhancement. Cortical destruction is uncommon. Bone expansion secondary to the lesion can result in spinal cord compression.	Benign cartilaginous tumors with chondroblast-like cells and areas of chondroid matrix formation that rarely occur in the spine. Spinal tumors most often involve the thoracic vertebrae and usually involve both the body and pedicles.
Osteoid osteoma ▷ Fig. 10.15	Intraosseous circumscribed radiolucent lesion often < 1.5 cm in diameter located in posterior elements, central zone with low to intermediate attenuation that can show contrast enhancement, surrounded by a peripheral zone of high attenuation (reactive bone sclerosis).	Benign osseous lesion containing a nidus of vascularized osteoid trabeculae surrounded by osteoblastic sclerosis; 14% of osteoid osteomas are located in the spine; usually occurs between the ages of 5 and 25 y, M > F. Focal pain and tenderness associated with lesion are often worse at night, relieved with aspirin.
Osteoblastoma ▷ Fig. 10.16	Expansile radiolucent vertebral lesion often > 1.5 cm in diameter located in posterior elements (90%) with or without extension into vertebral body (30%), with or without epidural extension (40%), low to intermediate attenuation, often surrounded by a zone of bone sclerosis; can show contrast enhancement, with or without spinal cord/spinal canal compression.	Rare benign bone neoplasm (2% of bone tumors) usually occurs between age 6 and 30 y. One third of osteoblastomas involve the spine.
Giant cell tumor ▷ Fig. 10.17a, b	Circumscribed radiolucent vertebral lesion with low to intermediate attenuation; can show contrast enhancement. Location: vertebral body > vertebral body and vertebral arch > vertebral arch alone. With or without spinal cord/spinal canal compression, with or without pathologic fracture.	Locally aggressive lesions that rarely metastasize. Account for 5% of primary bone tumors. Usually involve lone bones; only 4% involve vertebrae. Occur in adolescents and adults (age 20–40 y).
Aneurysmal bone cyst ▷ Fig. 10.18a–c	Circumscribed vertebral lesion usually involving the posterior elements with or without involvement of the vertebral body; variable low, intermediate, high, and/or mixed attenuation, with or without surrounding thin shell of bone, with or without lobulations, with or without one or multiple fluid/fluid levels, with or without pathologic fracture.	Expansile blood/debris-filled lesions that may be primary or occur secondary to other bone lesions, such as giant cell tumor, fibrous dysplasia, and chondroblastoma. Most occur in patients younger than 30 y. Locations: lumbar > cervical > thoracic. Clinical findings can include neurologic deficits and pain.

(continues on page 422)

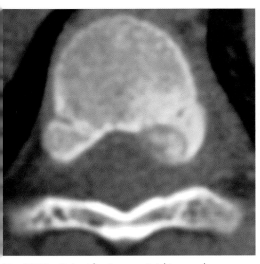

Fig. 10.15   Osteoid osteoma. Axial image shows a small, circumscribed radiolucent lesion in the posterior left portion of the vertebral body that has a central zone with low to intermediate attenuation containing calcifications surrounded by a peripheral zone of high attenuation (reactive bone sclerosis).

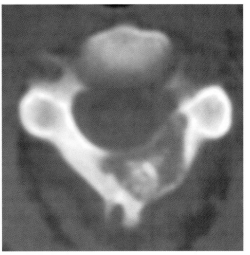

Fig. 10.16   Osteoblastoma. Axial image shows an expansile radiolucent lesion involving the left lamina with low to intermediate attenuation containing calcifications and surrounded by a zone of bone sclerosis.

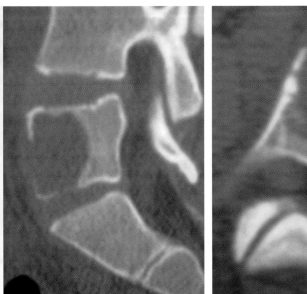

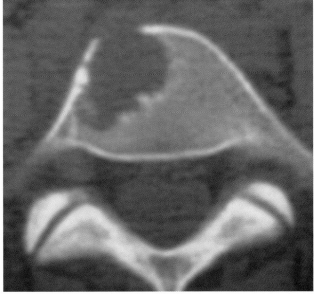

b

Fig. 10.17a, b   Giant cell tumor. Sagittal (**a**) and axial (**b**) images show a circumscribed radiolucent lesion in the L5 vertebral body associated with focal destruction of the anterior cortical margin.

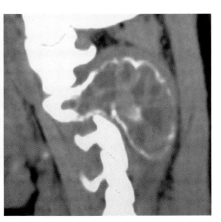

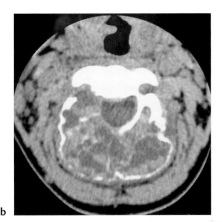

b

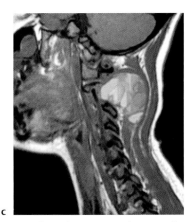

c

Fig. 10.18a–c   Aneurysmal bone cyst. Sagittal (**a**) and axial (**b**) CT images show a large expansile lesion involving the posterior elements of C2 with a thinned surrounding shell of bone and containing multiple fluid–fluid levels, as seen on sagittal T1-weighted MRI (**c**).

Table 10.2 (Cont.) Solitary osseous lesions involving the spine

Lesions	CT Findings	Comments
Osteochondroma ▷ *Fig. 10.19a, b*	Circumscribed sessile or protuberant osseous lesion typically arising from posterior elements of vertebrae, central zone contiguous with medullary space of bone, with or without cartilaginous cap. Increased malignant potential when cartilaginous cap is > 2 cm thick.	Benign cartilaginous tumors arising from defect at periphery of growth plate during bone formation with resultant bone outgrowth covered by a cartilaginous cap. Usually benign unless associated with pain and increasing size of cartilaginous cap. Can occur as multiple lesions (hereditary exostoses) with increased malignant potential.
Hemangioma ▷ *Fig. 10.20*	Circumscribed or diffuse vertebral lesion usually radiolucent without destruction of bone trabeculae, located in the vertebral body with or without extension into pedicle or isolated within pedicle; typically low to intermediate attenuation with thickened vertical trabeculae; can show contrast enhancement; multiple in 30%. Location: thoracic (60%) > lumbar (30%) > cervical (10%).	Most common benign lesions involving vertebral column, F > M, composed of endothelial-lined capillary and cavernous spaces within marrow associated with thickened vertical trabeculae and decreased secondary trabeculae; seen in 11% of autopsies. Usually asymptomatic; rarely cause bone expansion and epidural extension resulting in neural compression (usually in thoracic region); increased potential for fracture with epidural hematoma.
Other tumorlike lesions		
Paget disease ▷ *Fig. 10.21a–c*	Expansile sclerotic/lytic process involving a single or multiple vertebrae with mixed intermediate to high attenuation. Irregular/indistinct borders between marrow cortical bone; can also result in diffuse sclerosis, "ivory" vertebral pattern.	Chronic disease with disordered bone resorption and woven bone formation. Usually seen in older adults; polyostotic in 66%; can result in narrowing of neuroforamina and spinal canal.
Fibrous dysplasia ▷ *Fig. 10.22*	Expansile process involving one or more vertebrae with mixed intermediate and high attenuation, often a "ground glass" appearance.	Benign medullary fibro-osseous lesion of bone usually seen in adolescents and young adults; can result in narrowing of the spinal canal and neuroforamina; mono- and polyostotic forms (with or without endocrine abnormalities such as with McCune-Albright syndrome/precocious puberty).
Arachnoid cyst	Well-circumscribed, extra-axial lesions with low attenuation similar to CSF. No contrast enhancement. Usually cause mass effect on the adjacent spinal cord. Chronic erosive changes can be seen at the vertebrae adjacent to the cyst.	Nonneoplastic acquired, developmental, or congenital extra-axial cysts filled with CSF. Cysts can be small or large, asymptomatic or symptomatic.

(continues on page 424)

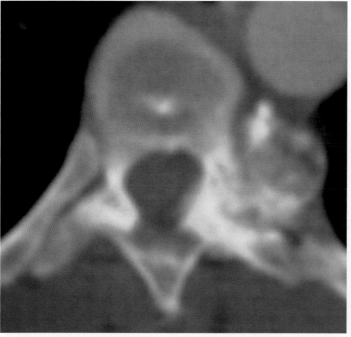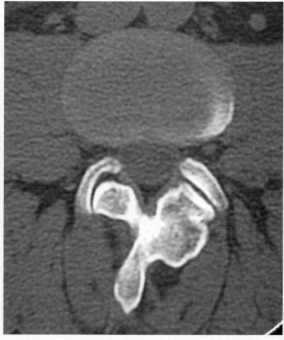

a

Fig. 10.19a, b   Osteochondroma. Axial images in two patients show protuberant osseous lesions arising from posterior elements with central zones contiguous with medullary spaces of adjacent bone.

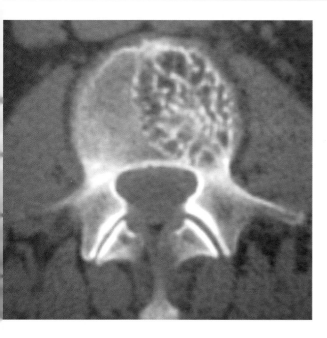

Fig. 10.20   Hemangioma. Axial image shows a circumscribed vertebral lesion with low to intermediate attenuation and thickened vertical trabeculae.

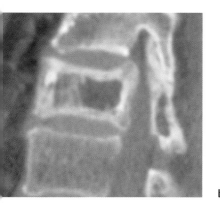
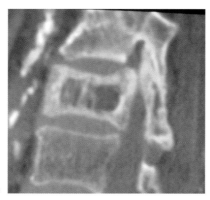
b
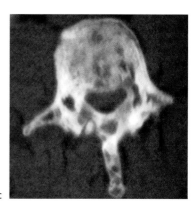
c

Fig. 10.21a–c   Paget disease. Sagittal (**a,b**) and axial (**c**) images show enlargement of a vertebral body with thickened cortical margins, indistinct borders between marrow and cortical bone, and mixed osteosclerotic and radiolucent zones.

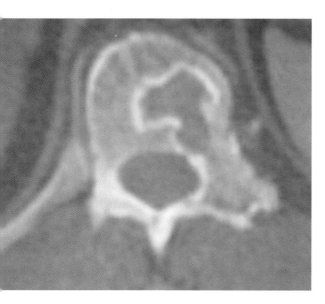

Fig. 10.22   Fibrous dysplasia. Axial image shows a circumscribed lesion involving the left side of the vertebral body that extends into a widened left pedicle. The lesion has mixed intermediate and high attenuation.

Table 10.2 (Cont.) Solitary osseous lesions involving the spine

Lesions	CT Findings	Comments
Tarlov cyst (perineural cyst) ▷ *Fig. 10.23a, b*	Well-circumscribed cysts with CSF attenuation involving nerve root sleeves associated with chronic erosive changes involving adjacent bony structures. Sacral (with or without widening of sacral foramina) > lumbar nerve root sleeves. Usually range from 15 to 20 mm in diameter but can be larger.	Typically represent incidental asymptomatic anatomical variants associated with prior dural injury.
Dermoid	Well-circumscribed, spheroid or multilobulated, intradural extramedullary or intramedullary lesions that can contain zones with low, intermediate, and/or high attenuation and calcifications; usually show no contrast enhancement, with or without fluid–fluid or fluid–debris levels. Lumbar region most common location in spine. Can cause chemical meningitis if dermoid cyst ruptures into the subarachnoid space. Commonly located at or near midline.	Nonneoplastic congenital or acquired ectodermal inclusion cystic lesions filled with lipid material, cholesterol, desquamated cells, and keratinaceous debris; usually mild mass effect on adjacent spinal cord or nerve roots. Adults: M slightly > F; with or without related clinical symptoms.
Epidermoid	Well-circumscribed, spheroid or multilobulated, intradural extramedullary lesion with low to intermediate attenuation; typically shows no contrast enhancement.	Nonneoplastic extramedullary epithelial-inclusion lesions filled with desquamated cells and keratinaceous debris; usually mild mass effect on adjacent spinal cord and/or nerve roots. May be congenital (with or without associated with dorsal dermal sinus, spina bifida, hemivertebrae) or acquired (late complication of lumbar puncture).
Neurenteric (endodermal) cyst	Well-circumscribed, spheroid, intradural extramedullary lesions with low to intermediate attenuation; usually show no contrast enhancement. Lesions may extend into the spinal cord in 10%.	Developmental failure of separation of notochord and foregut resulting in sinus tract or cysts between ventrally located endoderm and dorsally located ectoderm. Distal long tract symptoms and progressive spinal cord compression.
Synovial cyst ▷ *Fig. 10.24a, b*	Circumscribed lesion located adjacent to the facet joint. A thin rim of intermediate attenuation surrounds a central zone that may have low to intermediate attenuation. No contrast enhancement is usually seen, but a thin rim of peripheral enhancement may be observed.	Represents protrusion of synovium with fluid from degenerated facet joint into the spinal canal medially or dorsally into the posterior paraspinal soft tissues. Variable CT attenuation and MRI signal is related to the contents, which may include serous or mucinous fluid, blood, hemosiderin, and/or gas.
Bone island	Usually appears as a circumscribed radiodense ovoid or spheroid focus in medullary bone that may or may not contact the endosteal surface of cortical bone.	Bone islands (enostoses) are nonneoplastic intramedullary zones of mature compact bone composed of lamellar bone that are considered to be developmental anomalies resulting from localized failure of bone resorption during skeletal maturation.
Trauma		
Fracture ▷ *Fig. 10.25* ▷ *Fig. 10.26*	**Traumatic and osteopenic vertebral fracture:** Acute/subacute fractures have sharply angulated cortical margins, no destructive changes at cortical margins of fractured end plates, with or without convex outward angulated configuration of compressed vertebral bodies, with or without spinal cord and/or spinal canal compression related to fracture deformity, with or without retropulsed bone fragments into spinal canal, with or without subluxation, with or without kyphosis, with or without epidural hematoma. **Malignancy-related vertebral fracture:** Fractures related to radiolucent and/or sclerotic lesions, with or without destructive changes at cortical margins of vertebrae, with or without convex outward-bowed configuration of compressed vertebral bodies, with or without paravertebral mass lesions, with or without spheroid or poorly defined lesions in other noncompressed vertebral bodies.	Vertebral fractures can result from trauma, primary bone tumors/lesions, metastatic disease, bone infarcts (steroids, chemotherapy, and radiation treatment), osteoporosis, osteomalacia, metabolic (calcium/phosphate) disorders, vitamin deficiencies, Paget disease, and genetic disorders (osteogenesis imperfecta, etc.).

(continues on page 426)

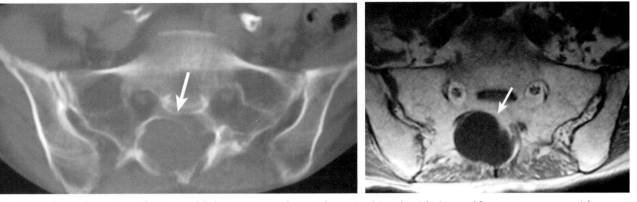

Fig. 10.23a, b   Tarlov cyst. Axial CT image (**a**) shows an expansile cystic lesion involving the right S1 sacral foramen, as seen on axial T1-weighted MRI (**b**) (arrows).

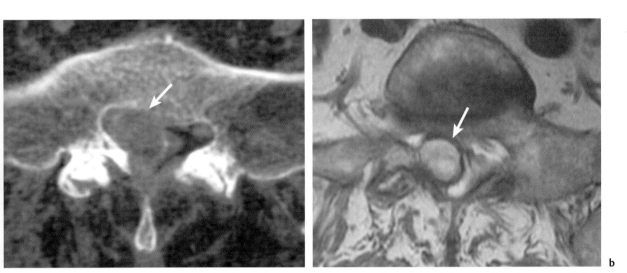

Fig. 10.24a, b   Synovial cyst. Axial CT image (**a**) shows a large synovial cyst arising from the medial aspect of the degenerated left facet joint, as seen on axial T2-weighted MRI (**b**). The synovial cyst compresses and displaces the thecal sac (arrows).

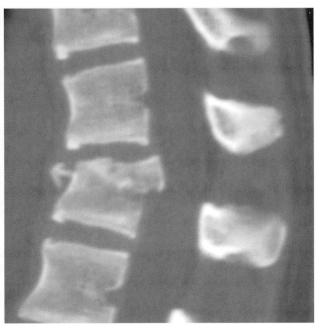

Fig. 10.25   Traumatic fracture. Sagittal image shows compression fractures involving the anterior, superior, and posterior cortical margins of a vertebral body.

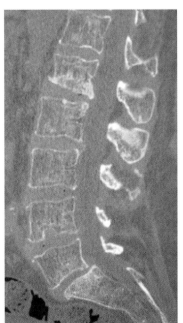

Fig. 10.26   Osteopenia-related fracture. Sagittal image shows diffuse osteopenia in an elderly patient, as well as a compression fracture deformity involving the inferior end plate of the L1 vertebral body.

Table 10.2   (Cont.) Solitary osseous lesions involving the spine

Lesions	CT Findings	Comments
Inflammation/infection		
Rheumatoid arthritis ▷ *Fig. 10.27a–c*	Erosions of vertebral end plates, spinous processes, and uncovertebral and apophyseal joints. Irregular enlarged enhancing synovium (pannus: low to intermediate attenuation) at atlantodens articulation results in erosions of dens and transverse ligament, with or without destruction of transverse ligament with C1 on C2 subluxation and neural compromise; with or without basilar impression.	Most common type of inflammatory arthropathy that results in synovitis, causing destructive/erosive changes of cartilage, ligaments, and bone. Cervical spine involvement in two thirds of patients, juvenile and adult types.
Eosinophilic granuloma ▷ *Fig. 10.28a, b*	Single or multiple circumscribed radiolucent lesions in the vertebral body marrow associated with focal bony destruction/erosion with extension into the adjacent soft tissues. Lesions usually have low to intermediate attenuation and involve the vertebral body and not the posterior elements; can show contrast enhancement, with or without enhancement of the adjacent dura. Progression of the lesion can lead to vertebra plana (a collapsed flattened vertebral body), with minimal or no kyphosis and relatively normal-sized adjacent disks.	Single lesion: Commonly seen in male patients younger than 20 y; proliferation of histiocytes in medullary cavity with localized destruction of bone with extension into adjacent soft tissues. Multiple lesions: Associated with syndromes such as Letterer–Siwe disease (lymphadenopathy, hepatosplenomegaly), children younger than 2 y; Hand–Schüller–Christian disease (lymphadenopathy, exophthalmos, and diabetes insipidus), children between 5 and 10 y.
Hematopoietic		
Amyloidoma	Amyloid lesions in bone can occur as zones of osteopenia, permeative radiolucent destruction or uni- or multifocal radiolucency. Lesions can have low to intermediate attenuation and can show contrast enhancement.	Uncommon disease in which various tissues (including bone, muscle, tendons, tendon sheaths, ligaments, and synovium) are infiltrated with extracellular eosinophilic material composed of insoluble proteins with beta-pleated sheet configurations (amyloid protein). Amyloidomas are single sites of involvement. Amyloidosis can be a primary disorder associated with an immunologic dyscrasia or secondary to a chronic inflammatory disease.
Bone infarcts	Focal ringlike lesion or poorly defined zone with increased attenuation in medullary bone; usually no contrast enhancement, with or without associated fracture.	Bone infarcts can occur after radiation treatment, surgery, corticosterioid medications, chemotherapy, or trauma.
Congenital		
Myelomeningocele/myelocele	Imaging is usually performed after surgical repair of myeloceles or myelomeningoceles. Posterior protrusion of spinal contents is seen with unfolded neural tube (neural placode) through defects in the bony dorsal elements of the involved vertebrae or sacral elements. The neural placode is usually located at the lower lumbar-sacral region with resultant tethering of the spinal cord. If the neural placode is flush with the adjacent skin surface, the anomaly is labeled a myelocele. If the neural placode extends above the adjacent skin surface, the anomaly is labeled a myelomeningocele, with or without syringohydromyelia.	Failure of developmental closure of the caudal neural tube results in an unfolded neural tube (neural placode) exposed to the dorsal surface in the midline without overlying skin. Other features associated with myelomeningoceles and myeloceles are dorsal bony dysraphism, deficient dura posteriorly at the site of the neural placode, and Chiari II malformations. By definition, the spinal cords are tethered. Usually repaired surgically soon after birth.
Meningoceles	Protrusion of CSF and meninges through a dorsal vertebral defect either from surgical laminectomies or congenital anomaly. Sacral meningoceles can alternatively extend anteriorly through a defect in the sacrum.	Acquired meningoceles are more common than meningoceles resulting from congenital dorsal bony dysraphism. Anterior sacral meningoceles can result from trauma or be associated with mesenchymal dysplasias (NF1, Marfan syndrome, and syndrome of caudal regression).

(continues on page 427)

Table 10.2   (Cont.) Solitary osseous lesions involving the spine

Lesions	CT Findings	Comments
Lipomyelomeningocele	Unfolded caudal neural tube (neural placode) covered by a lipoma that is often contiguous with the dorsal subcutaneous fat through defects (spina bifida) involving the bony dorsal vertebral elements. The neural placode is usually located at the lower lumbar-sacral region with resultant tethering of the spinal cord, with or without syringohydromyelia.	Failure of developmental closure of the caudal neural tube results in an unfolded neural tube (neural placode) covered by a lipoma that is contiguous with the subcutaneous fat. The overlying skin is intact, although the lipoma usually protrudes dorsally. The nerve roots arise from the placode. Features associated with lipomyelomeningoceles and lipomyeloceles include tethered spinal cords, dorsal bony dysraphism, and deficient dura posteriorly at the site of the neural placode. Not associated with Chiari II malformations. Diagnosis often in children, occasionally in adults.

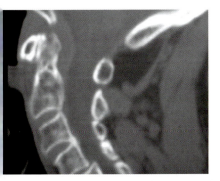 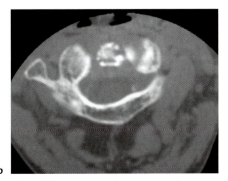 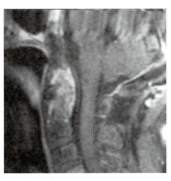

Fig. 10.27a–c   Rheumatoid arthritis. Sagittal (**a**) and axial (**b**) CT images show erosive changes involving the dens from a contrast-enhancing pannus, as seen on sagittal fat-suppressed T1-weighted MRI (**c**).

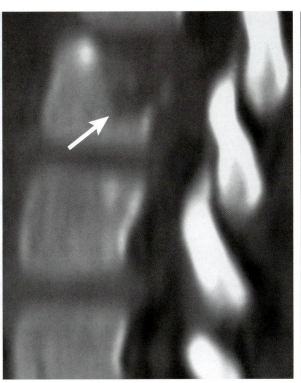 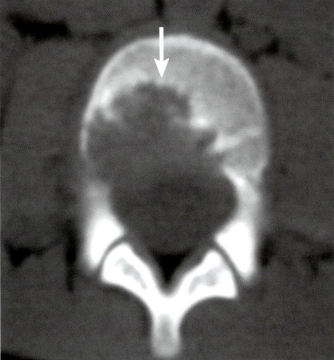

Fig. 10.28a, b   Eosinophilic granuloma, 6-year-old boy. Sagittal (**a**) and axial (**b**) images show a destructive osteolytic lesion involving the upper dorsal portion of a vertebral body (arrows).

Table 10.3   Multifocal lesions involving the spine

Lesions	CT Findings	Comments
Neoplasms (malignant)		
Metastatic tumor ▷ *Fig. 10.29a–c*	Single or multiple well-circumscribed or poorly defined infiltrative lesions involving the vertebral marrow, dura, and/or leptomeninges; low to intermediate attenuation; may show contrast enhancement, with or without medullary and cortical bone destruction (radiolucent), with or without bone sclerosis, with or without pathologic vertebral fracture, with or without epidural tumor extension causing compression of neural tissue or vessels. Leptomeningeal tumor often best seen on postcontrast images.	May have variable destructive or infiltrative changes involving single or multiple sites of involvement.
Myeloma/plasmacytoma ▷ *Fig. 10.30a, b*	Multiple (myeloma) or single (plasmacytoma), well-circumscribed or poorly defined, diffuse infiltrative radiolucent lesions involving the vertebra(e) and dura; involvement of vertebral body lesions typically radiolucent/bone lysis, rarely involves posterior elements until late stages; low to intermediate attenuation; may show contrast enhancement. Pathologic vertebral fracture, with or without epidural tumor extension causing compression of neural tissue or vessels.	Malignant monoclonal plasma cell tumors, may have variable destructive or infiltrative changes involving the axial and/or appendicular skeleton.
Lymphoma and leukemia ▷ *Fig. 10.31a, b*	Single or multiple, well-circumscribed or poorly defined infiltrative radiolucent lesions involving the marrow of the vertebrae, dura, and/or leptomeninges; low to intermediate attenuation, pathologic vertebral fracture, with or without epidural tumor extension causing compression of neural tissue or vessels. May show contrast enhancement, with or without bone destruction. Diffuse involvement of vertebra with Hodgkin lymphoma can produce bone sclerosis, as well as an "ivory" vertebra pattern, which has diffuse high attenuation. Leptomeningeal tumor often best seen on postcontrast images.	Tumors of malignant lymphocytes, may have variable destructive or infiltrative marrow/bony changes involving single or multiple vertebral sites. Lymphoma may extend from paraspinal lymphadenopathy into the vertebrae, adjacent soft tissues within or outside the spinal canal, initially involve only the epidural soft tissues or only the subarachnoid compartment. Can occur at any age (peak incidence third to fifth decades).
Neoplasms (benign)		
Hemangioma	Circumscribed or diffuse vertebral lesion, usually radiolucent–deficiency of bone trabeculae, located in the vertebral body with or without extension into pedicle or isolated within pedicle; typically have low to intermediate attenuation with thickened vertical trabeculae; can show contrast enhancement; multiple in 30%. Location: thoracic (60%) > lumbar (30%) > cervical (10%).	Most common benign lesions involving vertebral column, women > men, composed of endothelial-lined capillary and cavernous spaces within marrow associated with thickened vertical trabeculae and decreased secondary trabeculae; seen in 11% of autopsies. Usually asymptomatic, rarely cause bone expansion and epidural extension resulting in neural compression (usually in thoracic region); increased potential for fracture with epidural hematoma.

(continues on page 430)

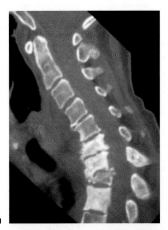 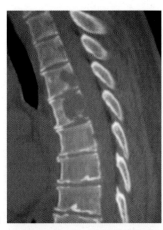 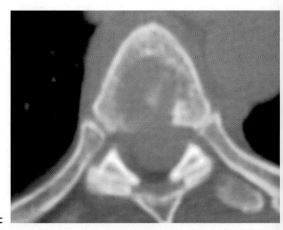

a   b   c

Fig. 10.29a–c   Metastatic disease. Sagittal image (**a**) shows osteosclerotic and osteolytic metastatic lesions involving multiple vertebrae, as well as a compression fracture of the T1 vertebral body. Sagittal (**b**) and axial (**c**) images in another patient show osteolytic tumors.

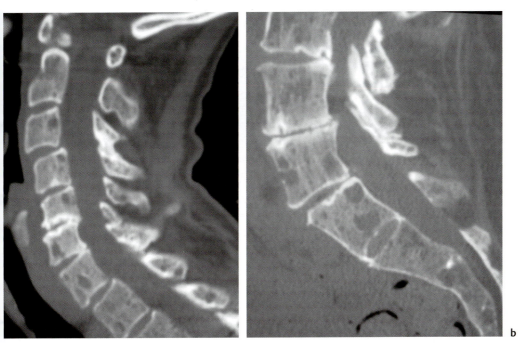

Fig. 10.30a, b **Multiple myeloma.** Sagittal images (**a,b**) show multiple osteolytic lesions in multiple vertebrae.

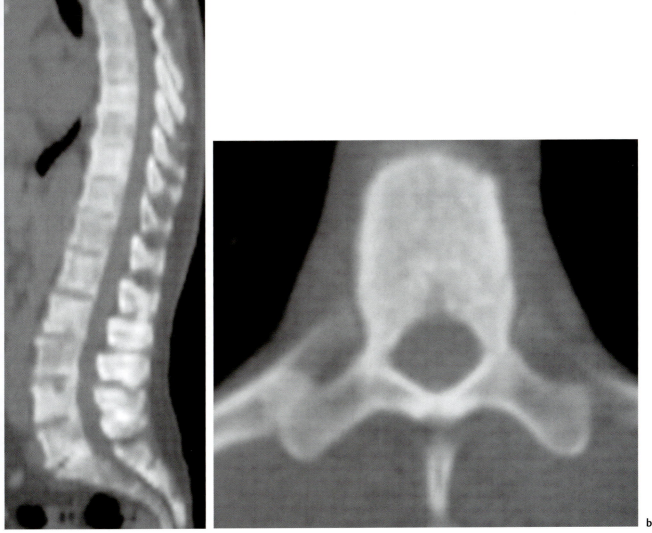

Fig. 10.31a, b **Hodgkin lymphoma.** Sagittal (**a**) and axial (**b**) images show multiple osteosclerotic lesions.

Table 10.3 (Cont.) Multifocal lesions involving the spine

Lesions	CT Findings	Comments
Other tumorlike lesions		
Tarlov cyst (perineural cyst)	Well-circumscribed cysts with CSF attenuation involving nerve root sleeves associated with chronic erosive changes involving adjacent bony structures. Sacral (with or without widening of sacral foramina) > lumbar nerve root sleeves. Usually range from 15 to 20 mm in diameter but can be larger.	Typically represent incidental asymptomatic anatomical variants associated with prior dural injury.
Bone island	Usually appear as a circumscribed, radiodense, ovoid or spheroid focus in medullary bone that may or may not contact the endosteal surface of cortical bone.	Nonneoplastic intramedullary zones of mature compact bone composed of lamellar bone which are considered to be developmental anomalies resulting from localized failure of bone resorption during skeletal maturation.
Melorheostosis ▷ *Fig. 10.32*	Attenuation of these lesions is based on the relative proportions of chondroid, mineralized osteoid, and soft tissue components. Mineralized zones typically have high attenuation along sites of thickened cortical bone; typically no contrast enhancement is seen in bone lesions. Nonmineralized portions can have low to intermediate attenuation and can show contrast enhancement. **Osteopoikilosis** typically appears as multiple circumscribed, radiodense, ovoid or spheroid foci in medullary bone that usually measure 3 to 5 mm. The long axis of the foci are often parallel to the adjacent bone trabeculae. Some foci may contact the endosteal surface of cortical bone.	Rare bone dysplasia with cortical thickening that has a "flowing candle wax" configuration. Associated soft tissue masses occur in ~25%. The soft tissue lesions often contain mixtures of chondroid material, mineralized osteoid, and fibrovascular tissue. Surgery is usually performed only for lesions causing symptoms. Osteopoikilosis (osteopathia condensans disseminate or spotted bone disease) is a sclerosing bone dysplasia in which numerous small round or oval radiodense foci are seen in medullary bone, giving the appearance of multiple bone islands. Can occur at any age, usually asymptomatic. In 25%, bone lesions may be associated with subcutaneous nodules, keloid formation, and scleroderma-like lesions (Buschke–Ollendorff syndrome). Osteopoikilosis may also occur as an overlap syndrome with other sclerosing bone dysplasias, such as melorheostosis and osteopathia striata.
Paget disease ▷ *Fig. 10.33a, b*	Expansile sclerotic/lytic process involving a single or multiple vertebrae with mixed intermediate to high attenuation. Irregular/indistinct borders between marrow cortical bone; can also result in diffuse sclerosis, "ivory" vertebral pattern.	Chronic disease with disordered bone resorption and woven bone formation. Usually seen in older adults, polyostotic in 66%; can result in narrowing of neuroforamina and spinal canal.
Trauma		
Fracture ▷ *Fig. 10.34a, b* ▷ *Fig. 10.35*	**Traumatic and osteopenic vertebral fracture:** Acute/subacute fractures have sharply angulated cortical margins, no destructive changes at cortical margins of fractured end plates. With or without convex outward angulated configuration of compressed vertebral bodies, with or without spinal cord and/or spinal canal compression related to fracture deformity, with or without retropulsed bone fragments into spinal canal, with or without subluxation, with or without kyphosis, with or without epidural hematoma. **Malignancy-related vertebral fracture:** Fractures related to radiolucent and/or sclerotic lesions, with or without destructive changes at cortical margins of vertebrae, with or without convex outward-bowed configuration of compressed vertebral bodies, with or without paravertebral mass lesions, with or without spheroid or poorly defined lesions in other noncompressed vertebral bodies.	Vertebral fractures can result from trauma, primary bone tumors/lesions, metastatic disease, bone infarcts (steroids, chemotherapy, and radiation treatment), osteoporosis, osteomalacia, metabolic (calcium/phosphate) disorders, vitamin deficiencies, Paget disease, and genetic disorders (osteogenesis imperfecta, etc.).

(continues on page 432)

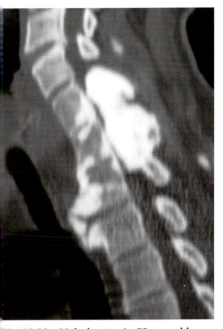

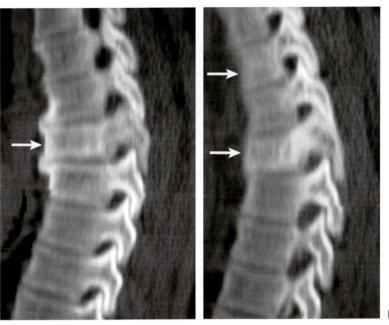

Fig. 10.32   Melorheostosis, 53-year-old man. Sagittal image shows heavily ossified zones and thickened cortical bone involving multiple cervical vertebrae.

Fig. 10.33a, b   Paget disease. Sagittal images show expansile osteosclerotic changes involving a thoracic vertebra with mixed intermediate and high attenuation. Irregular/indistinct borders between marrow and cortical bone are seen. Similar but less pronounced findings are seen in another vertebra two levels above (arrows).

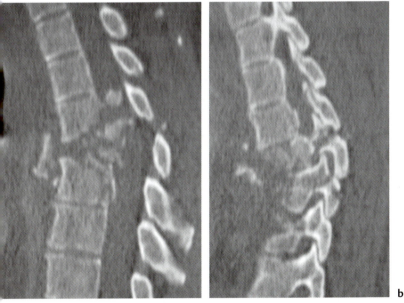

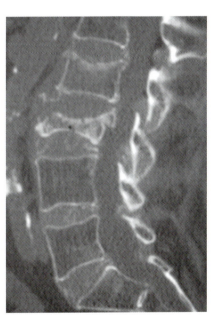

Fig. 10.34a, b   Fracture, traumatic. Sagittal images show severe unstable compression fractures of adjacent thoracic vertebrae with displaced fragments within the spinal canal.

Fig. 10.35   Fracture, osteoporotic. Sagittal image shows diffuse osteopenia and compression fracture deformities involving the L3 and L2 vertebral bodies.

III Spine

Table 10.3   (Cont.) Multifocal lesions involving the spine

Lesions	CT Findings	Comments
Inflammation/infection		
Pyogenic vertebral osteomyelitis/diskitis ▷ *Fig. 10.36a, b*	Poorly defined radiolucent zones involving the end plates and subchondral bone of two or more adjacent vertebral bodies, with or without fluid collections in the adjacent paraspinal soft tissues; may show contrast enhancement in marrow and paravertebral soft tissues; variable enhancement of disk (patchy zones within disk) and/or thin or thick peripheral enhancement; with or without epidural abscess/paravertebral abscess; with or without vertebral compression deformity; with or without spinal cord or spinal canal compression.	Vertebral osteomyelitis represents 3% of osseous infections, results from hematogenous source (most common) from distant infection or intravenous (IV) drug abuse; complication of surgery, trauma, diabetes; spread from contiguous soft tissue infection. Initially involves end arterioles in marrow adjacent to end plates with eventual destruction and spread to the adjacent vertebrae through the disk. Seen in children and adults older than 50 y. Gram-positive organisms (*Staphylococcus aureus, Staphylococcus epidermidis, Streptococcus*, etc.) account for 70% of pyogenic osteomyelitis, and gram-negative organisms (*Pseudomonas aeruginosa, Escherichia coli, Proteus*, etc.) represent 30%. Fungal osteomyelitis can appear similar to pyogenic infection of spine.
Vertebral osteomyelitis tuberculosis ▷ *Fig. 10.37a–c*	Poorly defined radiolucent zones involving the end plates and subchondral bone of two or more adjacent vertebral bodies, with or without fluid collections in the adjacent paraspinal soft tissues; may show contrast enhancement in marrow and paravertebral soft tissues; variable enhancement of disk (patchy zones within disk) and/or thin or thick peripheral enhancement; with or without epidural abscess/paravertebral abscess; with or without vertebral compression deformity; with or without spinal cord or spinal canal compression. Can show limited disk involvement early in disease process.	Initially involves marrow in the anterior portion of the vertebral body with spread to the adjacent vertebrae along the anterior longitudinal ligament, often sparing the disk until later in disease process; usually associated with paravertebral abscesses that may be more prominent than the vertebral abnormalities.
Rheumatoid arthritis	Erosions of vertebral end plates, spinous processes, and uncovertebral and apophyseal joints. Irregular enlarged enhancing synovium (pannus: low to intermediate attenuation) at atlantodens articulation results in erosions of dens and transverse ligament, with or without destruction of transverse ligament with C1 on C2 subluxation and neural compromise; with or without basilar impression.	Most common type of inflammatory arthropathy that results in synovitis, causing destructive/erosive changes of cartilage, ligaments, and bone. Cervical spine involvement seen in two thirds of patients, juvenile and adult types.
Ankylosing spondylitis ▷ *Fig. 10.38a, b*	Inflammation occurs at entheses (sites of attachment of ligaments, tendons, and joint capsules to bone). Squaring of vertebral bodies with mineralized syndesmophytes across many disks, osteopenia, erosions at sacroiliac joints with eventual fusion across these joints and facets. The spine in these cases is referred to as "bamboo spine."	Chronic progressive autoimmune inflammatory disease involving the spine and sacroiliac joints. Associated with human leukocyte antigens (HLA) B27 in 90%, onset in patients 20 to 30 y old, M:F 3:1. Fractures can occur in the horizontal plane through the osteopenic and fused "bamboo spine" at the level of the disks and/or vertebral bodies, as well as involving the posterior elements.

(continues on page 434)

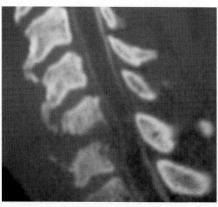 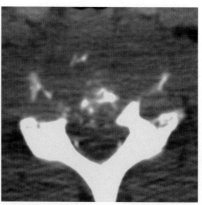

Fig. 10.36a, b   Osteomyelitis. Sagittal (**a**) and axial (**b**) postmyelographic CT images show destructive changes involving the end plates of two adjacent vertebral bodies from pyogenic osteomyelitis/diskitis.

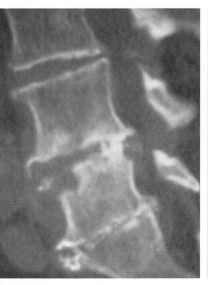
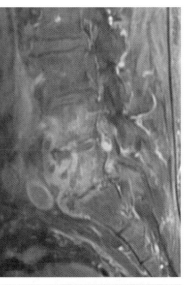

Fig. 10.37a–c   Osteomyelitis, tuberculosis.
Sagittal (**a**) and coronal (**b**) images show destructive changes involving the end plates of two adjacent vertebral bodies, as well as paraspinal collections representing old abscesses (arrows). Abnormal contrast enhancement is seen at the site of infection on a sagittal fat-suppressed, T1-weighted image (**c**).

c

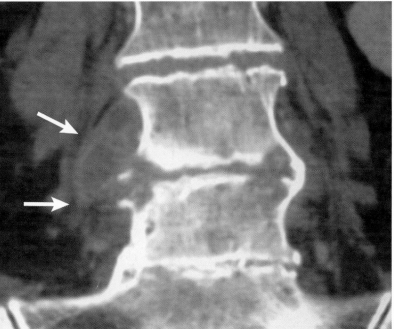
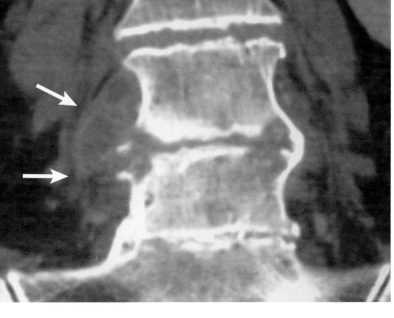

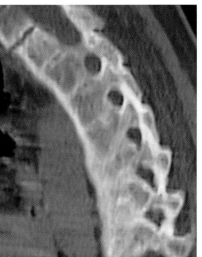
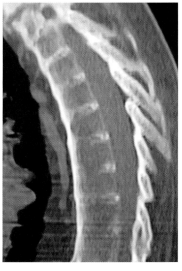

Fig. 10.38a, b   Ankylosing spondylitis. Sagittal images show squaring of vertebral bodies with mineralized syndesmophytes across the disks, osteopenia, and fusion across the facet joints ("bamboo spine"). Also seen is a horizontally oriented fracture through the upper thoracic spine.

b

Table 10.3   (Cont.) Multifocal lesions involving the spine

Lesions	CT Findings	Comments
Eosinophilic granuloma	Single or multiple, circumscribed radiolucent lesions in the vertebral body marrow associated with focal bony destruction/erosion with extension into the adjacent soft tissues. Lesions usually have low to intermediate attenuation and involve the vertebral body and not the posterior elements; can show contrast enhancement, with or without enhancement of the adjacent dura. Progression of lesion can lead to vertebra plana (collapsed flattened vertebral body) with minimal or no kyphosis and relatively normal-sized adjacent disks.	**Single lesion:** Commonly seen in male patients younger than 20 y; proliferation of histiocytes in medullary cavity with localized destruction of bone with extension into adjacent soft tissues. **Multiple lesions:** Associated with syndromes such as Letterer–Siwe disease (lymphadenopathy, hepatosplenomegaly), children younger than 2 y; Hand–Schüller–Christian disease (lymphadenopathy, exophthalmos, diabetes insipidus), children 5 to 10 y old.
Sarcoidosis	Sarcoid lesions can be multiple with variable sizes or solitary within marrow. Lesions can have circumscribed and/or indistinct margins within marrow and usually are radiolucent with low to intermediate attenuation; rarely are sclerotic; can show contrast enhancement.	Chronic systemic granulomatous disease of unknown etiology in which noncaseating granulomas occur in various tissues and organs, including bone.
Mastocytosis ▷ *Fig. 10.39a–c*	Radiographs and CT can show indistinctly marginated sclerotic lesions, radiolucent zones, or mixed sclerotic and radiolucent lesions in medullary bone.	Heterogeneous uncommon disorders with pathologic accumulation of mast cells in various tissues (age ranges from first to seventh decades, mean in fourth decade) and can be classified into four clinical categories. Category 1 is the most common and includes 1A, which involves the skin (cutaneous mastocytosis or urticaria pigmentosa), and 1B or systemic mastocytosis, with mast cells occurring in various tissues (bone marrow, spleen, gastrointestinal [GI] tract, and lymph nodes). Category 1 usually has a favorable prognosis. Category 2 includes mastocytosis associated with a myeloproliferative or myelodysplastic disorder. Prognosis depends on the associated degree of myelodysplasia. Category 3 (lymphadenopathic mastocytosis with eosinophilia or aggressive mastocytosis) is associated with a poor prognosis related to large mast cell burdens. Category 4 results from mast cell leukemia and has a very poor prognosis.
Hematopoietic		
Hematopoietic disorders	Red marrow hyperplasia can be seen as diffuse expansion of the diploic space of the skull with or without thinning of cortical bone.	Red marrow reconversion from erythroid hyperplasia can result from anemia secondary to sickle cell disease, thalassemia major, hereditary spherocytosis. Similar findings of red marrow expansion can be seen with polycythemia rubra. Medications (such as exogenous erythropoietin and granulocyte macrophage colony-stimulating factor in patients with anemia and neutropenia, respectively) can also cause red marrow reconversion in adults and children.

(continues on page 435)

Table 10.3   (Cont.) Multifocal lesions involving the spine

Lesions	CT Findings	Comments
Extramedullary hematopoiesis	Lesions can have low or intermediate attenuation depending on the proportions and distribution of fat and red marrow.	Represents proliferation of erythroid precursors outside medullary bone secondary to physiologic compensation for abnormal medullary hematopoiesis from congenital disorders such as hemoglobinopathies (sickle cell, thalassemia, etc.), as well as acquired disorders, such as myelofibrosis, leukemia, lymphoma, myeloma, or metastatic carcinoma.
Bone infarcts	Focal ringlike lesion or poorly defined zone with increased attenuation in medullary bone; usually no contrast enhancement, with or without associated fracture.	Bone infarcts can occur after radiation treatment, surgery, corticosterioid medications, chemotherapy, or trauma.
Congenital		
Dural ectasia	Scalloping of the dorsal aspects of vertebral bodies, dilation of optic nerve sheaths, dilation of intervertebral and sacral foraminal nerve sheaths, lateral meningoceles.	Dural dysplasia associated with NF1. Dural ectasia can also result from Marfan syndrome.

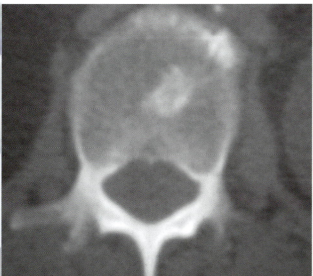
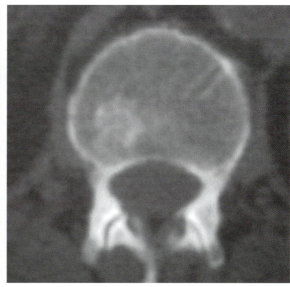

b

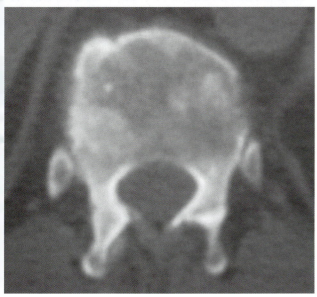

Fig. 10.39a–c   Mastocytosis. Axial images show multiple sclerotic foci within multiple vertebrae.

III Spine

Table 10.4 Spine: Extradural lesions

Lesions	CT Findings	Comments
Neoplasms		
Metastatic tumor ▷ *Fig. 10.40*	Single or multiple, well-circumscribed or poorly defined lesions involving the vertebral marrow, dura, and/or leptomeninges; low to intermediate attenuation; usually with contrast enhancement, with or without bone destruction, with or without pathologic vertebral fracture, with or without compression of neural tissue or vessels. Leptomeningeal tumor often best seen on postcontrast images.	Metastatic tumor may have variable destructive or infiltrative changes involving single or multiple sites of involvement.
Lymphoma ▷ *Fig. 10.41a–c*	Single or multiple well-circumscribed or poorly defined infiltrative lesions involving the vertebrae, epidural soft tissues, dura, and/or leptomeninges; low to intermediate attenuation; usually with contrast enhancement, with or without bone destruction. Diffuse involvement of vertebra with Hodgkin lymphoma can produce an "ivory" vertebra. Leptomeningeal tumor often best seen on postcontrast images.	Lymphoma may have variable destructive or infiltrative marrow/bony changes involving single or multiple vertebral sites. Lymphoma may extend from bone into adjacent soft tissues within or outside the spinal canal or initially involve only the epidural soft tissues or only the subarachnoid compartment. Can occur at any age (peak incidence third to fifth decades).
Myeloma/plasmacytoma ▷ *Fig. 10.42a, b*	Multiple (myeloma) or single (plasmacytoma), well-circumscribed or poorly defined diffuse infiltrative lesions involving the vertebra(e), and dura; involvement of vertebral body typical; rarely involves posterior elements until late stages, low to intermediate attenuation, usually with contrast enhancement, with bone destruction.	Myeloma may have variable destructive or infiltrative changes involving the axial and/or appendicular skeleton.
Osteosarcoma ▷ *Fig. 10.43a, b*	Destructive malignant lesions, usually with matrix mineralization/ossification within lesion or within extraosseous tumor extension; can show contrast enhancement (usually heterogeneous). Cortical bone destruction and epidural extension of tumor can compress the spinal canal and spinal cord.	Malignant bone lesions rarely occur as primary tumor involving the vertebral column, locally invasive, high metastatic potential. Occurs in children as primary tumors and adults (associated with Paget disease, irradiated bone, chronic osteomyelitis, osteoblastoma, giant cell tumor, and fibrous dysplasia).

(continues on page 438)

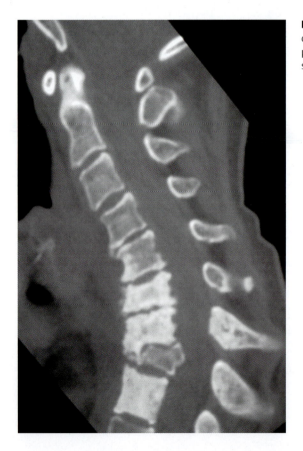

Fig. 10.40 Metastatic disease. Sagittal image shows osteosclerotic and osteolytic metastatic lesions involving multiple vertebrae, as well as a compression fracture of the T1 vertebral body that extends dorsally toward the spinal canal.

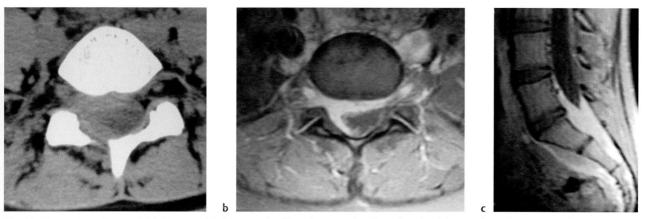

Fig. 10.41a–c   Lymphoma. Axial CT image (**a**) shows epidural lymphoma within the right side of the spinal canal, as seen as abnormal epidural contrast enhancement on axial (**b**) and sagittal (**c**) fat-suppressed, T1-weighted MRI.

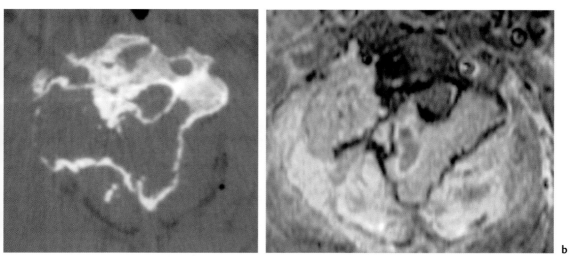

Fig. 10.42a, b   Myeloma/plasmacytoma. Axial CT image (**a**) shows an expansile destructive lesion involving a cervical vertebra, as seen on axial postcontrast, fat-suppresed T1-weighted MRI (**b**). The tumor causes spinal cord compression.

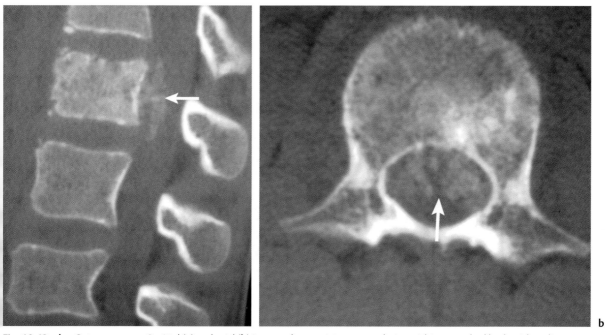

Fig. 10.43a, b   Osteosarcoma. Sagittal (**a**) and axial (**b**) images show an intraosseous lesion within a vertebral body with malignant ossified mineralization. The tumor extends into the spinal canal, causing spinal canal compression (arrows).

III Spine

Table 10.4   (Cont.) Spine: Extradural lesions

Lesions	CT Findings	Comments
Chordoma ▷ *Fig. 10.44a–d*	Well-circumscribed, lobulated radiolucent lesions, low to intermediate attenuation; usually shows contrast enhancement (usually heterogeneous); locally invasive associated with bone erosion/destruction; usually involves the dorsal portion of the vertebral body with extension toward the spinal canal. Also occurs in sacrum.	Rare, slow-growing, destructive notochordal tumors (~3% of bone tumors); usually occur in adults 30 to 70 y; M > F (2:1); sacrum (50%) > skull base (35%) > vertebrae (15%).
Chondrosarcoma ▷ *Fig. 10.45a–c*	Lobulated radiolucent lesions, low to intermediate attenuation, with or without matrix mineralization; may show contrast enhancement (usually heterogeneous); locally invasive associated with bone erosion/destruction, encasement of vessels and nerves; can involve any portion of the vertebra.	Rare, slow-growing, malignant cartilaginous tumors (~16% of bone tumors), usually occur in adults (peak in fifth to sixth decades), M > F; sporadic (75%), malignant degeneration/transformation of other cartilaginous lesion enchondroma, osteochondroma, etc. (25%).
Aneurysmal bone cyst ▷ *Fig. 10.46a, b*	Circumscribed vertebral lesion usually involving the posterior elements with or without involvement of the vertebral body; with variable low, intermediate, high, and/or mixed attenuation, with or without surrounding thin shell of bone, with or without lobulations, with or without one or multiple fluid–fluid levels, with or without pathologic fracture.	Expansile blood/debris filled lesions that may be primary or occur secondary to other bone lesions, such as giant cell tumor, fibrous dysplasia, and chondroblastoma. Most occur in patients younger than 30 y. Locations: lumbar > cervical > thoracic. Clinical findings can include neurologic deficits and pain.

(continues on page 440)

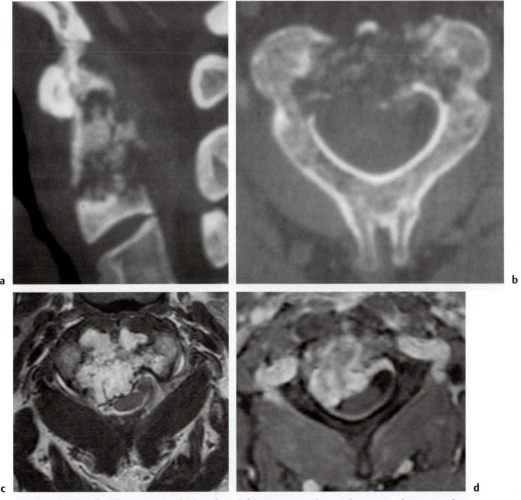

Fig. 10.44a–d   Chordoma. Sagittal (**a**) and axial (**b**) CT images show a destructive lesion involving the C2 vertebra that has high signal on axial T2-weighted MRI (**c**) and shows contrast enhancement on axial fat-suppressed, T1-weighted MRI (**d**). The tumor extends into the spinal canal, compressing the spinal cord.

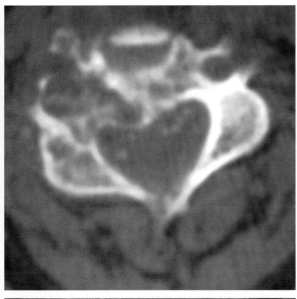

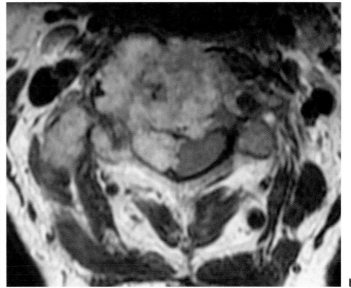

b

Fig. 10.45a–c Chondrosarcoma. Axial CT image (**a**) show a destructive lesion involving the C3 vertebra that has high signal on axial T2-weighted MRI (**b**) and shows contrast enhancement on axial fat-suppressed, T1-weighted MRI (**c**). The tumor extends into the spinal canal, compressing the spinal cord.

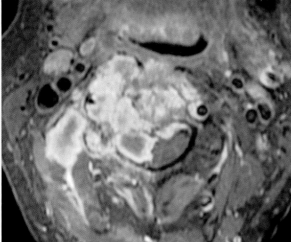

III Spine

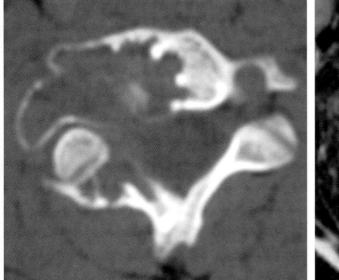

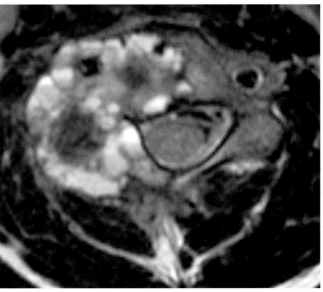

b

Fig. 10.46a, b Aneurysmal bone cyst. Axial CT image (**a**) shows an expansile radiolucent lesion that has mixed low, intermediate, and high signal on axial T2-weighted MRI (**b**).

Table 10.4   (Cont.) Spine: Extradural lesions

Lesions	CT Findings	Comments
Hemangioma ▷ *Fig. 10.47a–d*	Circumscribed or diffuse vertebral lesion, usually radiolucent–destruction of bone trabeculae, located in the vertebral body with or without extension into pedicle or isolated within pedicle; typically low to intermediate attenuation with thickened vertical trabeculae; can show contrast enhancement; multiple in 30%. Location: thoracic (60%) > lumbar (30%) > cervical (10%). Occasionally, lesions extend from bone into the epidural soft tissues.	Most common benign lesions involving vertebral column, F > M; composed of endothelial-lined capillary and cavernous spaces within marrow associated with thickened vertical trabeculae and decreased secondary trabeculae; seen in 11% of autopsies. Usually asymptomatic; rarely cause bone expansion and epidural extension resulting in neural compression (usually in thoracic region); increased potential for fracture with epidural hematoma.
Osteochondroma ▷ *Fig. 10.48*	Circumscribed sessile or protuberant osseous lesion typically arising from posterior elements of vertebrae, central zone contiguous with medullary space of bone, with or without cartilaginous cap. Increased malignant potential when cartilaginous cap is > 2 cm thick.	Benign cartilaginous tumors arising from defect at periphery of growth plate during bone formation with resultant bone outgrowth covered by a cartilaginous cap. Usually benign lesions unless associated with pain and increasing size of cartilaginous cap. Can occur as multiple lesions (hereditary exostoses) with increased malignant potential.
Paget disease ▷ *Fig. 10.49a, b*	Expansile sclerotic/lytic process involving a single or multiple vertebrae with mixed intermediate to high attenuation. Irregular/indistinct borders between marrow cortical bone; can also result in diffuse sclerosis, "ivory" vertebral pattern.	Chronic disease with disordered bone resorption and woven bone formation. Usually seen in older adults, polyostotic in 66%; can result in narrowing of neuroforamina and spinal canal.
Melorheostosis ▷ *Fig. 10.50a, b*	Attenuation of these lesions is based on the relative proportions of chondroid, mineralized osteoid, and soft tissue components. Mineralized zones typically have high attenuation along sites of thickened cortical bone; typically no contrast enhancement is seen in bone lesions. Nonmineralized portions can have low to intermediate attenuation and can show contrast enhancement.	Rare bone dysplasia with cortical thickening that has a "flowing candle wax" configuration. Associated soft tissue masses occur in ~25%. The soft tissue lesions often contain mixtures of chondroid material, mineralized osteoid, and fibrovascular tissue. Surgery is usually performed only for lesions causing symptoms.

(continues on page 442)

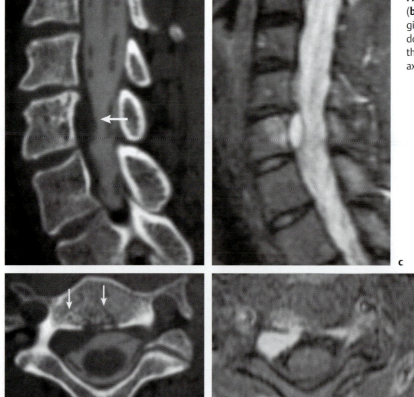

Fig. 10.47a–d   Hemangioma. Sagittal (**a**) and axial (**b**) postmyelographic CT images show a hemangioma in the vertebral body with epidural extension dorsally indenting the right anterior margin of the thecal sac, as seen on postcontrast sagittal (**c**) and axial (**d**) fat-suppressed T1-weighted MRI (arrows).

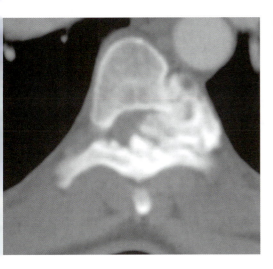

Fig. 10.48   Osteochondroma. Axial image shows an osteochondroma involving the left pedicle that extends into the spinal canal, displacing the thecal sac and spinal cord to the right.

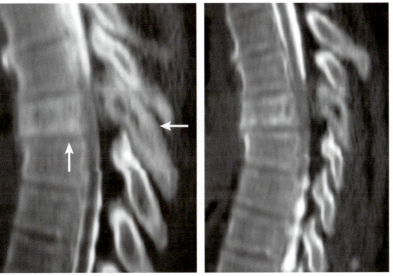

b

Fig. 10.49a, b   Paget disease. Sagittal postmyelographic images show expansion of a thoracic vertebral body and posterior elements from Paget disease, causing narrowing of the spinal canal (arrows).

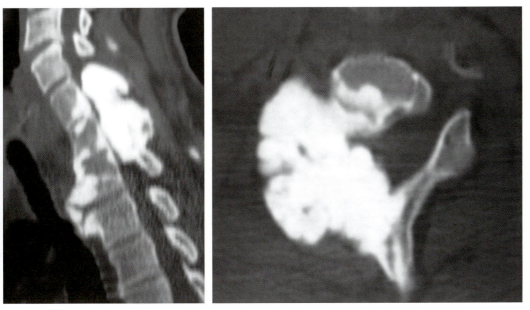

b

Fig. 10.50a, b   Melorheostosis. Sagittal (**a**) and axial (**b**) images show extensive proliferative osseous changes involving the right sides of multiple cervical vertebrae with resultant narrowing of the spinal canal.

Table 10.4   (Cont.) Spine: Extradural lesions

Lesions	CT Findings	Comments
Neoplasms and other masses		
Schwannoma (neurinoma)	Circumscribed or lobulated extramedullary lesions, intermediate attenuation, with contrast enhancement. Contrast enhancement can be heterogeneous in large lesions due to cystic degeneration and/or hemorrhage.	Encapsulated neoplasms arising asymmetrically from nerve sheath; most common type of intradural extramedullary neoplasm; usual presentation in adults with pain and radiculopathy, paresthesias, and lower extremity weakness. Multiple schwannomas seen with NF2.
Neurofibroma	Lobulated extramedullary lesions with or without irregular margins, with or without extradural extension of lesion with dumbbell shape, intermediate attenuation, with contrast enhancement. Contrast enhancement can be heterogeneous in large lesions; with or without erosion of foramina, with or without scalloping of dorsal margin of vertebral body (chronic erosion or dural ectasia/NF1).	Unencapsulated neoplasms involving nerve and nerve sheath; common type of intradural extramedullary neoplasm often with extradural extension; usual presentation in adults with pain and radiculopathy, paresthesias, and lower extremity weakness. Multiple neurofibromas seen with NF1.
Hemangiopericytoma	Extra- or intradural extramedullary lesions; can involve vertebral marrow, often well circumscribed, intermediate attenuation, with contrast enhancement (may resemble meningiomas), with or without associated erosive bone changes.	Rare neoplasms in young adults (M > F) sometimes referred to as angioblastic meningioma or meningeal hemangiopericytoma; arise from vascular cells/pericytes; frequency of metastases > meningiomas.
Arachnoid cyst	Well-circumscribed intradural extramedullary lesions with low attenuation similar to CSF, no contrast enhancement; with or without associated erosive bone changes.	Nonneoplastic congenital, developmental, or acquired extra-axial lesions filled with CSF; usually mild mass effect on adjacent spinal cord or nerve roots.
Teratoma	Circumscribed lesions with variable low, intermediate, and/or high attenuation; with or without contrast enhancement. May contain calcifications and cysts, as well as fatty components that can cause chemical meningitis if ruptured.	Second most common type of germ cell tumors; occurs in children, M > F; benign or malignant types; composed of derivatives of ectoderm, mesoderm, and/or endoderm.
Disk herniation		
Preoperative ▷ *Fig. 10.51* ▷ *Fig. 10.52a, b* ▷ *Fig. 10.53a, b* ▷ *Fig. 10.54a, b*	**Disk herniation/protrusion:** Disk herniation in which the head of the protruding disk is equal in size to the neck on sagittal reconstructed images; disk herniation usually similar in attenuation to disk of origin. Can be midline in position, off-midline in lateral recess, posterolateral within intervertebral foramen, lateral or anterior; with or without compression or displacement of thecal sac and/or nerve roots in lateral recess and/or foramen. **Disk herniation/extrusion:** Disk herniation in which the head of the disk herniation is larger than the neck on sagittal reconstructed images; attenuation of disk herniation usually similar to disk of origin. Can be midline, off-midline in lateral recess, posterolateral within intervertebral foramen, lateral, or anterior. Can extend superiorly, inferiorly, or both directions; with or without associated epidural hematoma; with or without compression or displacement of thecal sac and/or nerve roots in lateral recess and/or foramen. Can be calcified or contain gas if originating from a disk with vacuum phenomenon. **Disk herniation/extruded disk fragment:** Disk herniation that is not in contiguity with disk of origin, attenuation of disk herniation usually similar to disk of origin. Can be midline, off-midline in lateral recess, posterolateral within intervertebral foramen, lateral, or anterior. Can extend superiorly, inferiorly, or both directions. Rarely extend into dorsal portion of spinal canal or into thecal sac; with or without associated epidural hematoma; with or without compression or displacement of thecal sac and/or nerve roots in lateral recess and/or foramen.	Type of disk herniation (focal > broad-based) that results from inner annular disruption or subtotal annular disruption with extension of nucleus pulposus toward annular weakening/disruption with expansive deformation. Type of disk herniation (focal > broad-based) with extension of nucleus pulposus through zone of annular disruption with expansive deformation. Herniated fragment of nucleus pulposus without connection to disk of origin.

(continues on page 444)

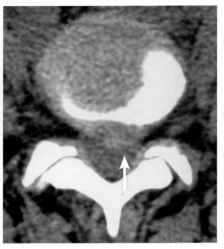

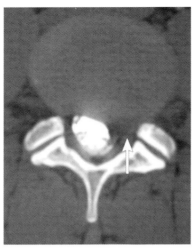

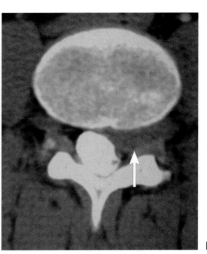

Fig. 10.51 Disk herniation/protrusion. Axial image shows a posterior disk herniation centrally and eccentric to the left (arrow).

Fig. 10.52a, b Disk herniation/extrusion. Axial postmyelographic images show a posterior disk herniation/extrusion on the left that extends superiorly into the left foramen, compressing the nerve in this location (arrows).

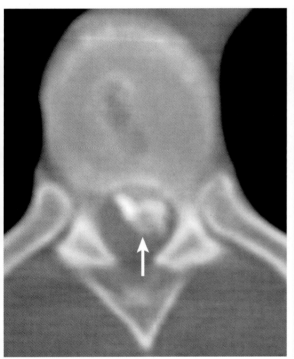

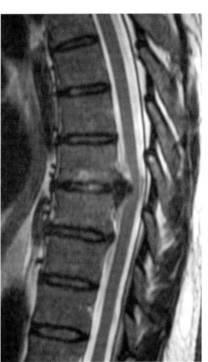

Fig. 10.53a, b Calcified disk herniation. Axial CT image (**a**) shows a calcified posterior thoracic disk herniation that has low signal on sagittal T1-weighted MRI (**b**) (arrow).

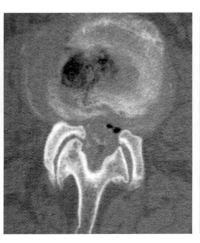

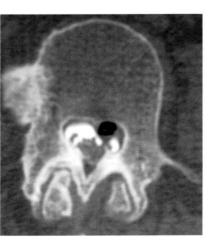

Fig. 10.54a, b Disk herniation with vacuum phenomenon. Axial postmyelographic images show a posterior disk herniation on the left with vacuum phenomenon.

Table 10.4   (Cont.) Spine: Extradural lesions

Lesions	CT Findings	Comments
Postoperative edema, scar/granulation tissue	**Postdiskectomy changes:** Soft tissue material located in anterior epidural space with intermediate attenuation; with or without mass effect on thecal sac resulting from edema and tissue injury from surgery; with or without contrast enhancement; changes progressively involute after 2 months.	Changes from diskectomy evolve from localized edema with or without hematoma with mass effect on the thecal sac during the immediate postoperative period to granulation tissue and scar (peridural fibrosis), which may show contrast enhancement usually without associated mass effect, with or without retraction of adjacent structures.
Degenerative changes		
Posterior disk bulge/osteophyte complex ▷ *Fig. 10.55a–c*	Diffuse broad-based bulge of disk usually with accompanying osteophytes from the adjacent vertebral bodies. Disks usually have decreased heights, low to intermediate attenuation related to disk degeneration and desiccation of the nucleus pulposus; with or without vacuum disk phenomenon.	With aging, altered disk metabolism, trauma, or biomechanical overload; the proteoglycan content in a disk can decrease resulting in disk desiccation, loss of turgor pressure in the disk, decreased disk height, bulging of the anulus fibrosus, with or without spinal canal stenosis, with or without narrowing of the intervertebral foramina, with or without thickening of spinal ligaments.
Degenerative facet hypertrophy ▷ *Fig. 10.56a, b*	Hypertrophic degenerative facets indent the dorsal lateral margins of the thecal sac and can result in spinal canal stenosis.	Degenerative arthritic changes involving the facet joints often lead to facet hypertrophy, which can result in spinal canal stenosis, usually in association with posterior disk bulge/osteophyte complexes.
Ossification of the posterior longitudinal ligament (PLL) ▷ *Fig. 10.57a, b*	Occurs as midline ossification at the dorsal aspects of the disks and vertebral bodies over several levels. A thin radiolucent line may be seen between the PLL and dorsal vertebral body margin secondary to connective tissue between the nonossified inner layer and ossified outer layers of the PLL.	The PLL extends from the C2 level to the sacrum and is attached to the anulus fibrosus of the disks and dorsal margins of the vertebral bodies. Ossification of the outer fibers of the PLL consists of lamellar bone and calcified cartilage, involves the cervical spine in 70%, thoracic in 15%, and lumbar region in 15%. Can result in spinal canal stenosis.
Synovial cyst ▷ *Fig. 10.58a, b*	Circumscribed structure located adjacent to the medial aspect of a degenerated facet joint, thin rim of intermediate attenuation surrounding a central zone that can have low or intermediate attenuation. Typically no contrast enhancement centrally.	Represents protrusion of synovium with fluid (ganglion cyst) from degenerated facet joint into spinal canal; variable MRI signal related to contents that may include mucinous or serous fluid, blood, hemosiderin, or air.

(continues on page 446)

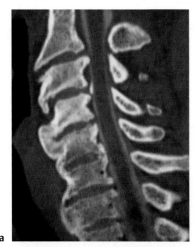
a
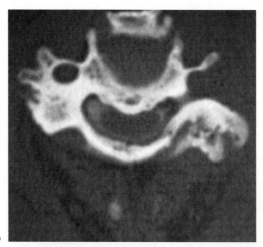
b
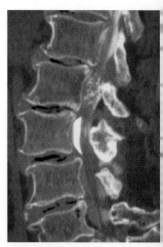
c

Fig. 10.55a–c   Disk bulge/osteophyte and spinal canal stenosis. Sagittal (**a,c**) and axial (**b**) postmyelographic CT images show posterior disk bulge/osteophyte complexes causing multilevel spinal canal stenosis.

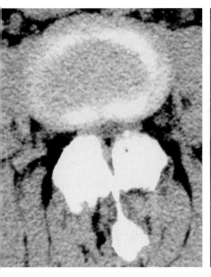 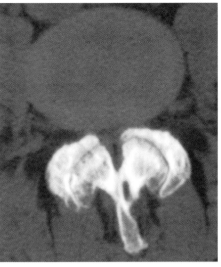

Fig. 10.56a, b   Facet hypertrophy causing spinal canal stenosis. Axial images show prominent degenerative facet arthropathy indenting the thecal sac and causing spinal canal stenosis.

III Spine

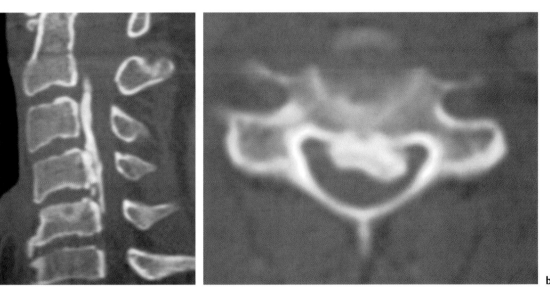

Fig. 10.57a, b   Ossification of the posterior longitudinal ligament (PLL). Sagittal (**a**) and axial (**b**) images show ossification of the PLL causing spinal canal stenosis.

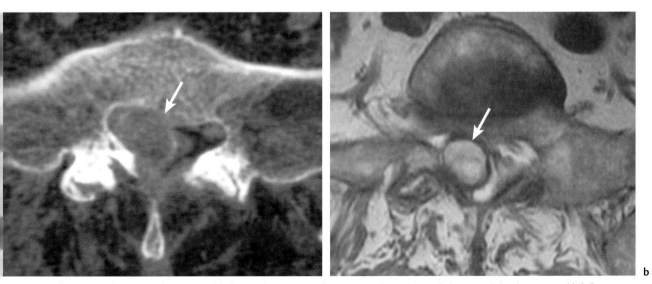

Fig. 10.58a, b   Synovial cyst. Axial CT image (**a**) shows a large synovial cyst arising from the medial aspect of the degenerated left facet joint, as seen on axial T2-weighted MRI (**b**). The synovial cyst compresses and displaces the thecal sac (arrows).

Table 10.4 (Cont.) Spine: Extradural lesions

Lesions	CT Findings	Comments
Fracture fragments ▷ *Fig. 10.59a, b*	Acute/subacute fractures have sharply angulated cortical margins, no destructive changes at cortical margins of fractured end plates; with or without convex outward angulated configuration of compressed vertebral bodies, with or without spinal cord and/or spinal canal compression related to fracture deformity, with or without retropulsed bone fragments into spinal canal, with or without subluxation, with or without kyphosis, with or without epidural hematoma.	Vertebral fractures can result from trauma, primary bone tumors/lesions, metastatic disease, bone infarcts (steroids, chemotherapy, and radiation treatment), osteoporosis, osteomalacia, metabolic (calcium/phosphate) disorders, vitamin deficiencies, Paget disease, and genetic disorders (osteogenesis imperfecta, etc.).
Epidural hematoma	Epidural collection with variable low, intermediate, and/or slightly high attenuation, with or without spinal cord compression.	Attenuation of epidural hematomas can vary secondary to stage of blood clotting and hematocrit. Older epidural hematomas can have mixed attenuation related to the various states of hemoglobin and breakdown products. Can be spontaneous or result from trauma or complication from coagulopathy, lumbar puncture, myelography, or surgery.
Spondylolysis ▷ *Fig. 10.60a, b*	Spondylolisthesis associated with cortical discontinuity of one or both pars interarticularis regions.	Fractures of the pars interarticularis regions from traumatic or stress injuries can lead to spondylolisthesis with narrowing of the spinal canal and/or neural foramina.
Epidural abscess ▷ *Fig. 10.61a, b*	Epidural collection with low signal attenuation surrounded by a peripheral rim (thin or thick) of contrast enhancement, with or without associated vertebral osteomyelitis/diskitis, with or without air collections, often extend over two to four vertebral segments; can result in compression of spinal cord and spinal canal contents.	Epidural abscess can evolve from an inflammatory phlegmonous epidural mass, extension from paravertebral inflammatory process or vertebral osteomyelitis/diskitis. May be associated with complications from surgery, epidural anesthesia, diabetes, distant source of infection, immunocompromised status. Organisms commonly involved include *S. aureus*, gram-negative bacteria, tuberculosis, coccidioidomycosis, candidiasis, aspergillosis, and blastomycosis. Clinical findings include back and radicular pain, with or without paresthesias and paralysis of lower extremities.
Epidural lipomatosis ▷ *Fig. 10.62*	Increased extradural fat is seen within the spinal canal with resultant narrowing of the thecal sac.	Epidural lipomatosis is a condition in which there is prominent deposition of unencapsulated mature adipose tissue in the epidural space. May be related to obesity, chronic use of steroid medication, or endogenous hypercortisolemia. Thoracic 60%, lumbar 40%.

(continues on page 448)

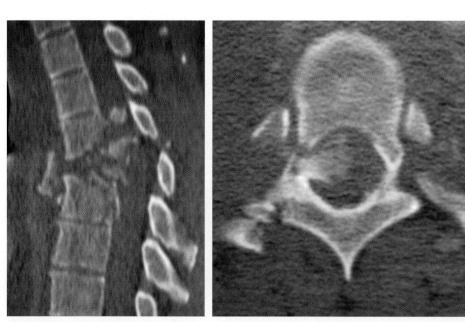

a　　　　　　　　　　　　　　　　　　　　　　　　　　b

Fig. 10.59a, b   Displaced fracture fragments. Sagittal images show comminuted vertebral fractures with fragments displaced into the spinal canal.

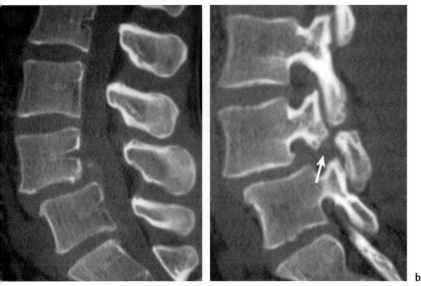

Fig. 10.60a, b   Spondylolysis. Sagittal images show spondylolisthesis (**a**), as well as fragmentation of the pars interarticularis region (**b**) (arrow).

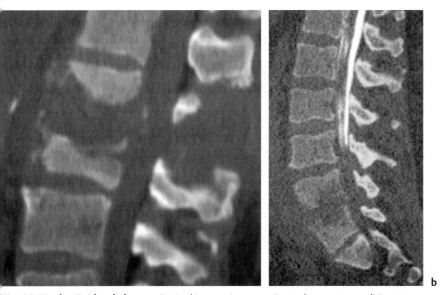

Fig. 10.61a, b   Epidural abscess. Sagittal images in two patients show osteomyelitis at two adjacent vertebral bodies with destructive end plate changes and dorsal epidural abscesses compressing the thecal sac.

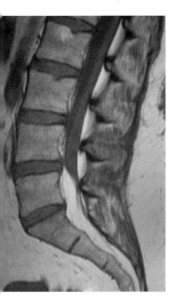

Fig. 10.62   Epidural lipomatosis. Narrowing of the thecal sac is seen from prominent epidural fat extending from the L4–L5 level inferiorly on sagittal T1-weighted MRI.

III Spine

Table 10.4   (Cont.) Spine: Extradural lesions

Lesions	CT Findings	Comments
Inflammation/infection		
Rheumatoid arthritis ▷ *Fig. 10.63a, b*	Erosions of vertebral end plates, spinous processes, and uncovertebral and apophyseal joints. Irregular enlarged synovium (pannus: intermediate attenuation) at atlantodens articulation results in erosions of dens and transverse ligament, with or without destruction of transverse ligament with C1 on C2 subluxation and neural compromise, with or without basilar impression.	Most common type of inflammatory arthropathy that results in synovitis, causing destructive/erosive changes of cartilage, ligaments, and bone. Cervical spine involvement seen in two thirds of patients, juvenile and adult types.
Eosinophilic granuloma ▷ *Fig. 10.64a, b*	Single or multiple, circumscribed soft tissue lesions in the vertebral body marrow associated with focal bony destruction/erosion with extension into the adjacent soft tissues. Lesions usually involve the vertebral body and not the posterior elements, with low to intermediate attenuation, with or without contrast enhancement, with or without enhancement of the adjacent dura. Progression of lesion can lead to vertebra plana (a collapsed flattened vertebral body), with minimal or no kyphosis and relatively normal-sized adjacent disks.	**Single lesion:** Commonly seen in male patients younger than 20 y; proliferation of histiocytes in medullary cavity with localized destruction of bone with extension into adjacent soft tissues. **Multiple lesions:** Associated with syndromes such as Letterer–Siwe disease (lymphadenopathy, hepatosplenomegaly), children younger than 2 y; Hand–Schüller–Christian disease (lymphadenopathy, exophthalmos, diabetes insipidus), children 5 to 10 y old.
Gout	Radiographic features may include erosions at the diskovertebral junctions or facet joints, osteophytes, spinal deformities with subluxations and pathologic fractures. Soft tissue swelling with or without calcifications can be seen with tophi that occur in the late phases of gout. Tophi often have 160 HU, which may be used for narrowing the differential diagnosis with respect to other joint diseases.	Inflammatory disease involving synovium resulting from deposition of monosodium urate crystals. Occurs when the serum urate level exceeds its solubility in various tissues and body fluid (> serum urate level of 7 mg/dL in men and 6 mg/dL in women). Can be a primary disorder of hyperuricemia resulting from inherited metabolic defects in purine metabolism or inherited abnormalities involving renal tubular secretion of urate. Primary gout accounts for up to 90% of cases in men. Secondary gout results from acquired metabolic alterations caused by medications (thiazide diuretics, alcohol, salicylates, and cyclosporine) that diminish renal excretion of uric acid salts.
Calcium pyrophosphate deposition disease (CPDD) ▷ *Fig. 10.65a, b*	Radiographs and CT show chondrocalcinosis, which can be seen at the C1–odontoid articulation. At C1–C2, hypertrophy of synovium may occur, which can have low to intermediate attenuation containing calcifications seen with CT.	CPDD is a common disorder usually seen in older adults in which there is deposition of calcium pyrophosphate crystals resulting in calcifications of hyaline and fibrocartilage; associated with cartilage degeneration, subchondral cysts, and osteophyte formation. Symptomatic CPDD is referred to as pseudogout because of overlapping clinical features with gout. Usually occurs in the knee, hip, shoulder, elbow, and wrist, rarely at the odontoid–C1 articulation.

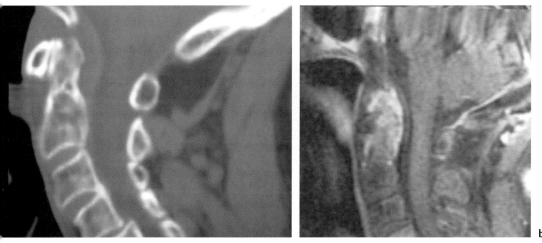

Fig. 10.63a, b   Rheumatoid arthritis. Sagittal CT image (**a**) shows erosive changes at the dens from a contrast-enhancing pannus, as seen on a postcontrast fat-suppressed, T1-weighted sagittal image (**b**).

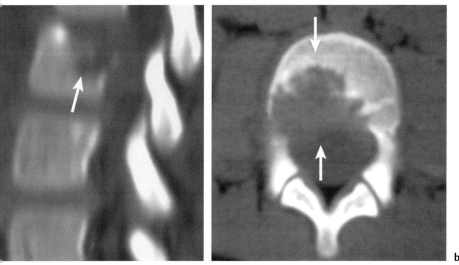

Fig. 10.64a, b   Eosinophilic granuloma. Sagittal (**a**) and axial (**b**) images show destructive changes at the upper dorsal portion of a vertebral body with epidural extension (arrows).

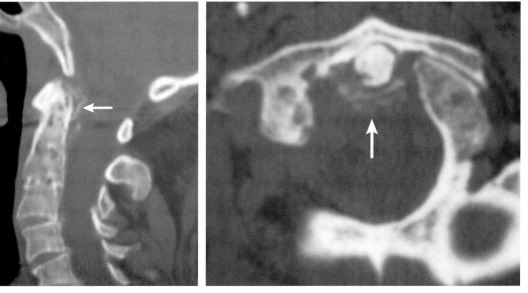

Fig. 10.65a, b   Calcium pyrophosphate deposition disease (CPDD). Sagittal (**a**) and axial (**b**) images show soft tissue/synovial thickening at the atlantodens articulation containing amorphous small calcifications (arrows).

Table 10.5   Spine: Traumatic lesions

Lesions	CT Findings	Comments
Fracture (traumatic/osteopenic) ▷ *Fig. 10.66* ▷ *Fig. 10.67*	**Traumatic vertebral fracture:** Acute/subacute fractures have sharply angulated cortical margins, no destructive changes at cortical margins of fractured end plates; with or without convex outward angulated configuration of compressed vertebral bodies, with or without spinal cord and/or spinal canal compression related to fracture deformity, with or without retropulsed bone fragments into spinal canal, with or without subluxation, with or without kyphosis, with or without epidural hematoma. **Osteopenic vertebral fracture:** Acute/subacute fractures usually have sharply angulated cortical margins, no destructive changes at cortical margins of fractured vertebral bodies; with or without compression deformities involving other vertebral bodies, with or without convex outward angulated configuration of compressed vertebral bodies, with or without spinal cord and/or spinal canal compression related to fracture deformity, with or without retropulsed bone fragments into spinal canal, with or without subluxation, with or without kyphosis, with or without epidural hematoma. **Chronic healed fractures** usually have normal or near normal signal in compressed vertebral body. Occasionally, persistence of signal abnormalities in vertebral marrow results from instability and abnormal axial loading.	Vertebral fractures can result from trauma in normal bone or as pathologic fractures in abnormal bone associated with primary bone tumors/lesions, metastatic disease, bone infarcts (steroids, chemotherapy, and radiation treatment), osteoporosis, osteomalacia, metabolic (calcium/phosphate) disorders, vitamin deficiencies, Paget disease, and genetic disorders (osteogenesis imperfecta, etc.).
Occipital condyle fractures ▷ *Fig. 10.68a–c*	Rough edge fragments of one or both occipital condyles. Fractures may extend to involve the hypoglossal canals and jugular foramina.	**Type 1:** Traumatic fracture of condyle with minimal displacement from axial loading mechanism from high-energy blunt trauma (often stable if only unilateral). **Type 2:** Fracture of occipital condyle from shear mechanism extending into skull base (can be stable if unilateral or unstable). **Type 3:** Transverse fracture of condyle from rotation/bending with injury to alar ligaments that extend from upper lateral portions of the dens to the medial aspects of the occipital condyles. Injury to the alar ligaments results in instability at the occipitocervical junction.
Atlanto-occipital dislocation	Abnormal increased distance from the basion of the clivus to the tip of the odontoid using the basion-axial interval (BAI) and/or basion-dental interval (BDI). The BAI is the distance from the basion to a line drawn along the dorsal surface of the C2 body (normal BAI for adults ranges from −4 to 12 mm, children 0 to 12 mm). The BDI is only used in patients older than 13 y and is the distance from the basion to the tip of the dens (normal range 2–12 mm).	Unstable injury from disruption of ligaments between the occiput, C1, and upper dens from high kinetic energy injuries (usually motor vehicle collisions). Often associated with traumatic injuries to brainstem and cranial nerves. More common in children than adults.
Jefferson C1 fracture ▷ *Fig. 10.69*	Rough edge fractures of the arch of C1, often multiple fracture sites.	Compression burst fracture of the arch of C1, often stable, can be unstable when there is disruption of transverse or posterior ligament or comminution of anterior arch, often associated with fractures at other cervical vertebrae.
C2 dens fracture ▷ *Fig. 10.70a, b* ▷ *Fig. 10.71*	**Type I:** Fracture at the upper portion of dens above transverse ligament (unstable) from avulsion at the alar ligament. **Type II:** Transverse fracture through the lower portion of the dens (may be unstable). **Type III:** Oblique fracture involving the dens and body of C2 (usually stable).	Traumatic fracture involving the upper, middle to lower portions of the dens.

(continues on page 452)

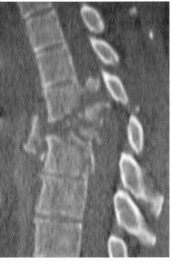

Fig. 10.66   Traumatic fracture. Sagittal image shows comminuted fractures of adjacent thoracic vertebrae involving all three columns (unstable).

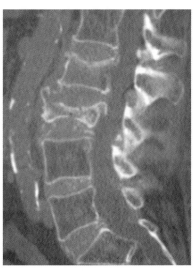

Fig. 10.67   Osteopenic fracture. Sagittal image shows compression fracture deformities at the L2 and L3 vertebral bodies in the setting of osteopenia.

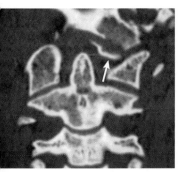

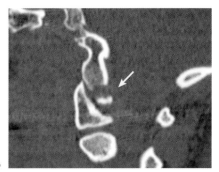

b

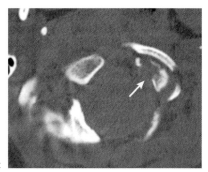

c

Fig. 10.68a–c   Occipital condyle fracture. Coronal (**a**), sagittal (**b**), and axial (**c**) images show fracture of the left occipital condyle (arrows).

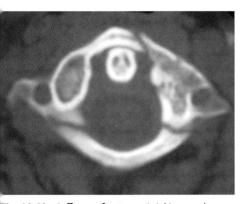

Fig. 10.69   Jefferson fracture. Axial image shows fractures at the anterior and posterior arches of C1.

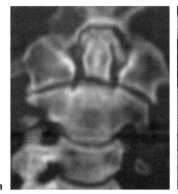

a

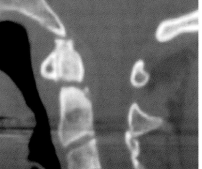

b

Fig. 10.70a, b   C2 dens fracture, type II. Coronal (**a**) and sagittal (**b**) images show a fracture through the base of the dens.

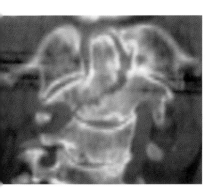

Fig. 10.71   C2 dens fracture, type III. Coronal image shows an oblique fracture involving the dens and body of C2.

Table 10.5   (Cont.) Spine: Traumatic lesions

Lesions	CT Findings	Comments
C2 body fracture type I ▷ *Fig. 10.72*	Fracture of the inferior end plate of C2 with teardrop fragment.	Extension injury with teardrop fracture of anteroinferior vertebral end plate of the C2 vertebra.
C2 body fracture type II	Horizontal fracture plane through the lower body of C2.	Horizontal shear fracture through the lower portion of the C2 body (lower than C2 dens type III fracture).
C2 body fracture type III (burst fracture)	Comminuted fracture of C2 body with or without separation of body from posterior arch (hangman's fracture). Fracture fragments of C2 body are often displaced peripherally, with or without extension of fragments into spinal canal compression.	Traumatic comminuted fracture of the C2 body from axial compression force. Often unstable, especially with associated hangman's fracture; with or without spinal cord contusion.
C2 body fracture type IV	Sagittal plane fracture through C2.	Severe unstable fracture in the sagittal plane through C2.
C2 hangman's fracture ▷ *Fig. 10.73a–d*	Disrupted ring of C2 from bilateral pedicle fractures separating the C2 body from the posterior arch of C2. Skull, C1, and C2 bodies are displaced anteriorly with respect to C3.	Unstable injury from traumatic bilateral pedicle fractures from hyperextension and distraction mechanisms with separation of the C2 body from the posterior arch of C2. Fractures can extend into C2 body and/or through foramen transversarium with injury/occlusion of vertebral artery. Often associated with spinal cord injury.
Hyperflexion cervical spine injury ▷ *Fig. 10.74a, b* ▷ *Fig. 10.75*	Sagittal plane fracture associated with compression of the anterior portion of the vertebral body, with teardrop fracture at the anteroinferior portion of the vertebral body or quadrangular fracture extending from the inferior end plate to the anterosuperior cortical margin. A portion of the fractured vertebral body is usually subluxed anteriorly with respect to the vertebral body below with resultant kyphosis. Facet joints are widened due to disruption. Narrowing of the disk height seen below the vertebral body fracture from disk injury. Typically, prevertebral soft tissue swelling is seen, with widened interspinous distance.	Flexion compression injuries that account for up to 15% of cervical vertebral fractures and often occur from motor vehicle collisions, falls, and diving into shallow water. Fractures involve the anterior portion of the vertebral body with fractures also involving the posterior elements in 50%, with or without tearing of posterior ligaments. Teardrop hyperflexion injuries result in disruption of all ligaments, facet joints, and disks. Quadrangular fractures extend from the inferior to superior cortical margins with disruption of the anterior and posterior longitudinal ligaments and disks.
Hyperextension injury cervical fracture	Fractures of vertebral bony arch (laminae, facets, and spinous process) on axial CT images. Sagittal CT images show malalignment of facets and/or spondylolisthesis.	Extension injury from posterior displacement of the head and upper cervical spine resulting in fractures of the arch (laminae) and/or posterior elements, with or without disruption of anterior longitudinal ligament. Disruption of posterior column results in instability. Can be associated with spinal cord contusion, vertebral artery injury (dissection/occlusion), and other vertebral fractures.

(continues on page 454)

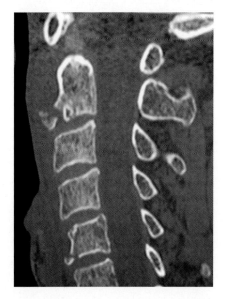

Fig. 10.72   C2 body fracture, type I. Sagittal image shows a fracture of the inferior end plate of C2 with teardrop fragment.

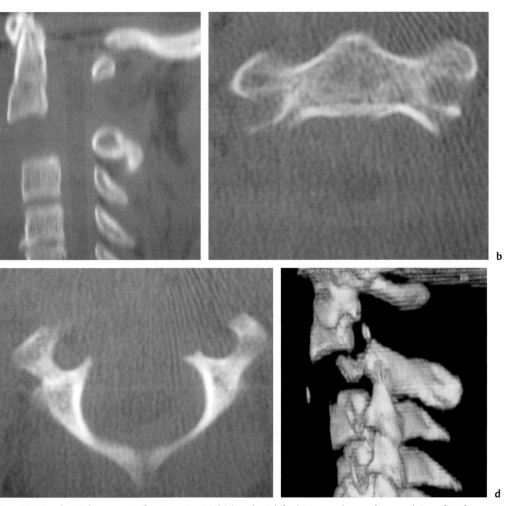

Fig. 10.73a–d   C2 hangman's fracture. Sagittal (**a**) and axial (**b,c**) images show a disrupted ring of C2 from bilateral pedicle fractures separating the C2 body from the posterior arch of C2. C1 and C2 bodies and skull are displaced anteriorly with respect to C3, as seen on a sagittal volume-rendered image (**d**).

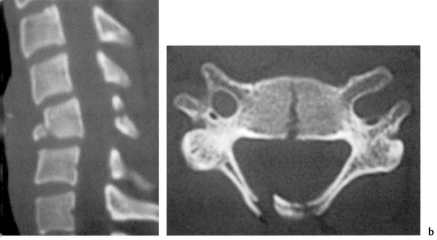

Fig. 10.74a, b   Hyperflexion cervical spine fracture, teardrop type. Sagittal (**a**) and axial (**b**) images show a sagittal plane fracture with compression of the anterior portion of the vertebral body, with a teardrop fracture at the anteroinferior portion of the vertebral body. Posterior fractures involving the laminae are also seen. Facet joints are widened due to disruption. Prevertebral soft tissue swelling is seen, as well as a widened interspinous distance.

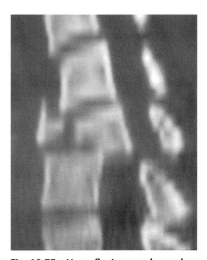

Fig. 10.75   Hyperflexion quadrangular fracture. Sagittal plane fracture associated with compression of the anterior portion of the vertebral body is visible with quadrangular fracture extending from the inferior end plate to the antero-superior cortical margin. The fractured vertebral body is subluxed with respect to the vertebral body below with resultant kyphosis. Facet joints are widened due to disruption. Narrowing of the disk height below the vertebral body fracture from disk injury is seen.

III Spine

Table 10.5 (Cont.) Spine: Traumatic lesions

Lesions	CT Findings	Comments
Hyperflexion-rotation cervical injuries ▷ *Fig. 10.76a, b*	Rotatory subluxation of vertebral body and posterior elements, with or without jumped or perched facets, with or without fractures at facets, with or without fracture of the vertebral body. For unilateral locked facet, axial CT image shows rotatory subluxation with absence of normal facet articulation (naked facet sign). Sagittal CT images show perched or jumped facets.	Hyperflexion-rotation force resulting in traumatic disruption of spinal ligaments (facet-capsular, annular, and/or longitudinal ligaments) with subluxation involving the facet joints with or without fracture. Can occur as unilateral or bilateral locked facets.
Hyperextension-rotation cervical injuries	Unilateral fracture of articular pillar, pedicle, and/or lamina, with or without injury/occlusion of vertebral artery.	Unilateral laminar or facet fracture with ligament disruption (anterior annular and capsular ligaments) from combined hyperextension and rotation mechanism of injury.
Cervical vertebral burst fracture ▷ *Fig. 10.77a, b*	Comminuted fracture extending through both end plates of vertebral body; associated fractures at the posterior elements.	Comminuted fractures involving the superior and inferior end plates of a cervical vertebral body secondary to axial compression mechanism without fractures involving the posterior elements. Can be unstable if both anterior and middle columns involved.
Cervical vertebral fracture/ dislocation ▷ *Fig. 10.78a, b*	Comminuted fractures of posterior elements (laminae, facets, and spinous processes) associated with anterior, lateral, and/or posterior subluxations; with or without fractures involving vertebral bodies, disks, and transverse processes.	Highly unstable fractures involving all three columns from shear, rotation, and distraction mechanisms. Subluxed fracture components involving the vertebral body usually also involve tearing of the disk. Lateral flexion mechanism of injury resulting in unilateral fracture of articular pillar, with or without fractures of vertebral body, transverse process.
Cervical lateral flexion injury	Sagittal plane fracture or articular pillar with malalignment, with or without fracture of vertebral body, transverse process.	
Clay shoveler's fracture	Avulsion fracture from the spinous processes of C6 and C7. Occasionally occurs at other levels.	Stable fracture from avulsion of bone from the C6 or C7 spinous processes by the posterior supraspinous ligaments as a result of strong shear forces secondary to lifting heavy weights with arms extended.
Thoracic/lumbar anterior compression fracture ▷ *Fig. 10.79a, b*	Anterior wedge-shaped vertebral body from fractures involving the superior end plate and anterior cortical margin. Multiple fracture lines often seen within the vertebral body. Decrease in height of vertebral body with normal bone density up to 50%. Usually no subluxation because of lack of significant injury to posterior column.	Flexion-induced fracture of anterior portion of vertebral body from axial load injury involving only the anterior column and sparing the middle and posterior columns. Can occur from trauma in normal or osteoporotic bone. Fractures in the setting of osteoporosis can have delayed or inadequate healing, resulting in progressive height loss. Typically stable because of lack of involvement of the middle and posterior columns. Can involve more than one level.

(continues on page 456)

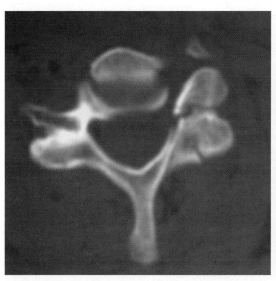
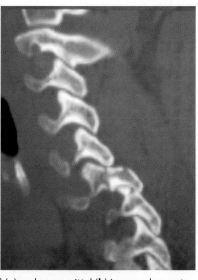

a   b

Fig. 10.76a, b   Rotatory injury, C-spine facet fracture. Axial (**a**) and parasagittal (**b**) images show rotatory subluxation of the vertebral body and left posterior elements, jumped left facet, with fractures.

III Spine

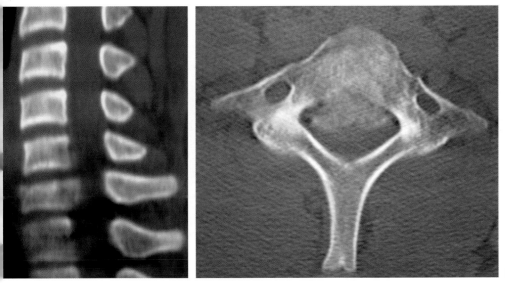

Fig. 10.77a, b Cervical vertebral burst fracture. Sagittal (**a**) and axial (**b**) images show a burst fracture with retropulsed fragment into the spinal canal.

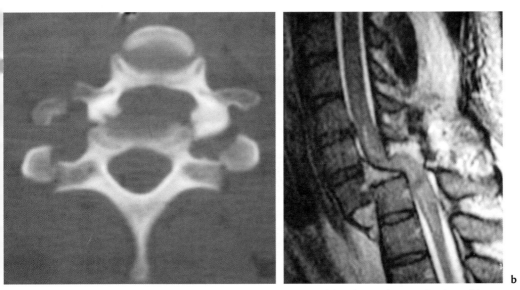

Fig. 10.78a, b Cervical vertebral fracture/dislocation. Axial CT image (**a**) and sagittal T2-weighted MRI (**b**) show fracture dislocation at C7–T1 with disruption of all three columns and ligaments with spinal cord transection.

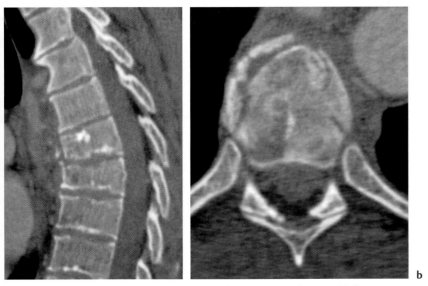

Fig. 10.79a, b Thoracic anterior compression fracture. Sagittal image (**a**) shows anterior wedge deformities of two adjacent thoracic vertebral bodies. Axial image (**b**) shows a fracture of the anterior portion of one of the vertebral bodies.

Table 10.5 (Cont.) Spine: Traumatic lesions

Lesions	CT Findings	Comments
Thoracic/lumbar lateral compression fracture	Lateral wedge-shaped vertebral body from fractures involving the superior end plate and lateral cortical margin. Typically spares the posterior cortical margin of the vertebral body without retropulsed fragments. Commonly occur at T12 to L2 and at T6 and T7; multiple vertebrae involved in 20%.	Asymmetric fracture involving superior and anterior end plates of vertebral body from asymmetric axial load with or without flexion. Can occur from trauma in normal or osteoporotic bone. Fractures in the setting of osteoporosis can have delayed or inadequate healing resulting in progressive height loss. Typically stable because of lack of involvement of the middle and posterior columns. Can involve more than one level.
Thoracic/lumbar burst fracture ▷ *Fig. 10.80a, b*	Comminuted fracture of vertebral body involving both superior and inferior end plates, decrease in vertebral body height at anterior and posterior cortical margins, often with bone fragments displaced into the spinal canal, widened pedicles; with or without malalignment of fractured vertebral body and/or facets.	Unstable comminuted compression fractures involving the vertebral body from axial compression mechanism without fractures involving the posterior elements. Can be unstable if both anterior and middle columns involved.
Thoracic/lumbar facet–lamina fracture	Fractures involving laminae and facet joints with widened neural arch/pedicles, with or without vertebral body and/or facet subluxation/dislocation, with or without comminution of vertebral body.	Fractures involving the posterior column from extension, flexion-distraction, or flexion-rotation mechanisms. Often occur between T11 and L4. Unstable fractures occur when all three columns are involved. Can be stable when one or two columns are involved.
Thoracic/lumbar chance fracture ▷ *Fig. 10.81a, b*	Fractures involving the anterior, middle, and posterior columns; anterior wedging of vertebral body with decrease in height of vertebral body often > 50% even with normal bone density. Horizontally oriented fracture planes through vertebral body and posterior elements, disruption/separation of facet joints and interspinous ligaments with widening of the interspinous distance; with or without comminuted fractures of vertebral body, with or without retropulsed fracture fragments from vertebral body into spinal canal; widened interspinous distance; with or without anterior displacement of vertebrae above fracture (distraction fracture).	Unstable flexion-distraction injury from high-velocity collision or fall causing compression of the anterior column and distraction of middle and posterior columns. Often occurs between T11 and L3.
Thoracic/lumbar fracture-dislocation	Comminuted fractures of posterior elements (laminae, facets, and spinous processes) associated with anterior, lateral, and/or posterior subluxations; with or without fractures involving vertebral bodies, disks, transverse processes, and/or ribs.	Highly unstable fractures involving all three columns from shear, rotation, and distraction mechanisms. Subluxed fracture components involving the vertebral body usually also involve tearing of the disk.
Fracture/ankylosing spondylitis ▷ *Fig. 10.82a, b*	Rigidity of the spine caused by ossification of the anterior and posterior longitudinal ligaments, syndesmophytes, and osteoporosis; increases the predisposition to spinal fractures with minor trauma. Fractures can occur through the vertebral body and/or disk. Also associated with atlantodens instability.	Autoimmune inflammatory disorder associated with HLA-B27. Inflammation involves the sacroiliac joints, diskovertebral junctions, spinal ligaments, apophyseal joints, costovertebral joints, and atlantoaxial joints. Findings include osteitis, sydesmophytosis, diskovertebral erosions, calcifications along the anterior and posterior longitudinal ligaments, osseous fusion across joints, and osteoporosis.

(continues on page 458)

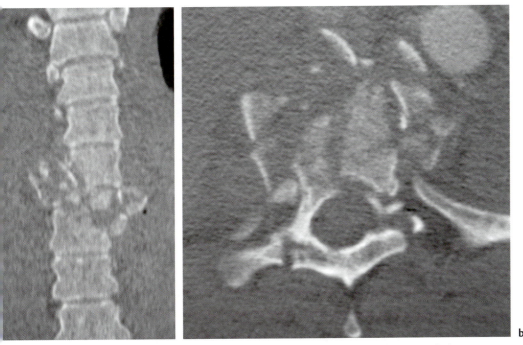

b

Fig. 10.80a, b   Thoracic burst fracture. Coronal (**a**) and axial (**b**) images show burst fractures of adjacent thoracic vertebrae.

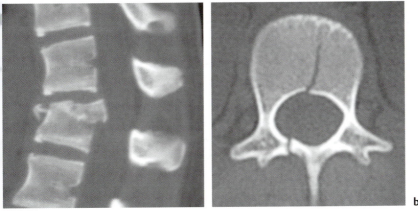

b

Fig. 10.81a, b   Chance fracture. Sagittal (**a**) and axial (**b**) images shows horizontally oriented fracture planes through the vertebral body and posterior elements.

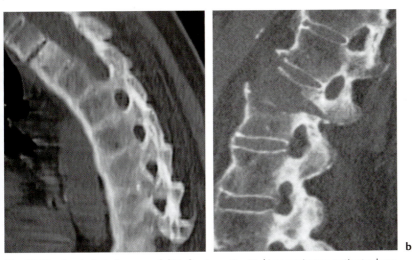

b

Fig. 10.82a, b   Ankylosing spondylitis fracture. Sagittal images in two patients show horizontally oriented fracture planes through the vertebral body and posterior elements in patients with ankylosing spondylitis ("bamboo spines").

III Spine

Table 10.5 (Cont.) Spine: Traumatic lesions

Lesions	CT Findings	Comments
Fracture (malignancy-related) ▷ *Fig. 10.83*	Fractures often associated with destructive changes at cortical margins of vertebrae, with or without convex outward-bowed configuration of compressed vertebral bodies, with or without paravertebral mass lesions, with or without destructive lesions in other vertebrae.	Neoplasms in bone are associated with bone destruction and decreased capability for maintaining integrity with axial loading, as well as lowering the threshold for fracture with minor trauma.
Epidural hematoma	Epidural collection with low to intermediate and/or slightly high attenuation, with or without spinal cord compression, with or without minimal peripheral pattern of enhancement at hematoma.	The CT appearance of epidural hematoma depends on the age, hematocrit, and degree of clot formation and retraction. Can be spontaneous or result from trauma or complication (coagulopathy, lumbar puncture, myelography, and surgery).
Disk herniation ▷ *Fig. 10.84*	**Disk herniation/protrusion:** Disk herniation in which the head of the protruding disk is equal in size to the neck on sagittal reconstructed images. **Disk herniation/extrusion:** Disk herniation in which the head of the disk herniation is larger than the neck on sagittal reconstructed images. **Disk herniation/extruded disk fragment:** Disk herniation that is not in contiguity with disk of origin.	Represents a disk herniation (focal > broad-based) that results from inner annular disruption or subtotal annular disruption with extension of nucleus pulposus toward annular injury with expansive deformation. Represents a disk herniation (focal > broad-based) with extension of nucleus pulposus through zone of annular disruption with expansive deformation. **Disk herniation/extruded disk fragment–herniation/extrusion:** Herniated fragment of nucleus pulposus without connection to disk of origin. Disk herniations can be midline, off-midline in lateral recess, posterolateral within intervertebral foramen, lateral, or anterior. Can extend superiorly, inferiorly, or both directions; with or without associated epidural hematoma, with or without compression or displacement of thecal sac and/or nerve roots in lateral recess and/or foramen. Disk herniations can occur into the end plates of vertebral bodies, Schmorl nodes.

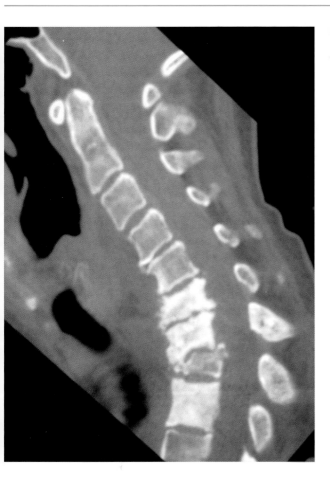

Fig. 10.83 Pathologic fracture from neoplastic disease. Sagittal image shows an osteosclerotic and osteolytic metastatic lesion, as well as a pathologic fracture involving the T1 vertebral body.

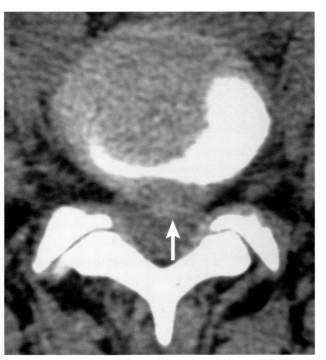

Fig. 10.84 Disk herniation. Axial image shows a posterior disk herniation centrally and on the left (arrow).

Table 10.6 Intradural extramedullary lesions

Lesions	CT Findings	Comments
Dural ectasia	Scalloping of the dorsal aspects of vertebral bodies, dilation of optic nerve sheaths, dilation of intervertebral and sacral foraminal nerve sheaths, lateral meningoceles.	Dural dysplasia associated with NF1. Can also be seen with connective tissue disease, such as Marfan syndrome.
Tarlov cysts (perineural cysts)	Well-circumscribed cysts with attenuation comparable to cerebrospinal fluid (CSF) involving nerve root sleeves associated with chronic erosive changes involving adjacent bony structures. Sacral (with or without widening of sacral foramina) > lumbar nerve root sleeves. Usually range from 15 to 20 mm in diameter but can be larger.	Typically represent incidental asymptomatic anatomical variants.
Dorsal dermal sinus	Epithelial-lined tube extending internally from the dorsal skin of lower back, with or without extension into spinal canal through the median raphe or spina bifida, with or without associated dermoid or epidermoid in spinal canal (~50%).	Abnormality resulting from lack of normal developmental separation of superficial and neural ectoderm. Lumbar region > occipital region. Potential source of infection involving spine and spinal canal.
Dermoid ▷ *Fig. 10.85a, b*	Well-circumscribed, spheroid or multilobulated, intradural extramedullary or intramedullary lesions, usually with low to intermediate attenuation. No contrast enhancement. Lumbar region most common location in spine. Can cause chemical meningitis if dermoid cyst ruptures into the subarachnoid space. Commonly located at or near midline.	Nonneoplastic congenital or acquired ectodermal inclusion cystic lesions filled with lipid material, cholesterol, desquamated cells, and keratinaceous debris; usually mild mass effect on adjacent spinal cord or nerve roots; adults: M > F; with or without related clinical symptoms.
Epidermoid	Well-circumscribed, spheroid or multilobulated, intradural or extramedullary lesion with low to intermediate attenuation No contrast enhancement.	Nonneoplastic extramedullary epithelial-inclusion lesions filled with desquamated cells and keratinaceous debris; usually mild mass effect on adjacent spinal cord and/or nerve roots. May be congenital (with or without associated with dorsal dermal sinus, spina bifida, and hemivertebrae) or acquired (late complication of lumbar puncture).
Neurenteric cyst ▷ *Fig. 10.86a–c*	Circumscribed intradural extramedullary structures with low to intermediate attenuation. Usually no contrast enhancement. Location: thoracic > cervical > posterior cranial fossa > craniovertebral junction > lumbar; usually midline in position and often ventral to the spinal cord. Typically associated with anomalies of the adjacent vertebrae.	Results from developmental failure of separation the notochord and foregut; observed in patients older than 40 y.
Neoplasm and other masses		
Ependymoma	Intradural, circumscribed, lobulated lesions at conus medullaris and/or cauda equina/filum terminale, rarely in sacrococcygeal soft tissues; lesions usually have intermediate attenuation, with or without hemorrhage.	Ependymomas at conus medullaris or cauda equina/filum terminale usually are myxopapillary type, thought to arise from ependymal glia of filum terminale. Slight male predominance. Usually are slow-growing neoplasms associated with long duration of back pain, sensory deficits, motor weakness, and bladder and bowel dysfunction; with or without chronic erosion of bone with scalloping of vertebral bodies and enlargement of intervertebral foramina.
Schwannoma (neurinoma)	Circumscribed or lobulated extramedullary lesions, intermediate attenuation, with contrast enhancement. Large lesions can have cystic degeneration and/or hemorrhage.	Encapsulated neoplasms arising asymmetrically from nerve sheath; most common type of intradural extramedullary neoplasms; usual presentation in adults with pain and radiculopathy, paresthesias, and lower extremity weakness. Multiple schwannomas seen with NF2.
Meningioma	Extra- or intradural extramedullary lesions, intermediate attenuation, with contrast enhancement, with or without calcifications.	Usually benign neoplasms, typically occurs in adults (> 40 y), F > M; multiple meningiomas seen with NF2; can result in compression of adjacent spinal cord and nerve roots, rarely invasive/malignant types.

(continues on page 462)

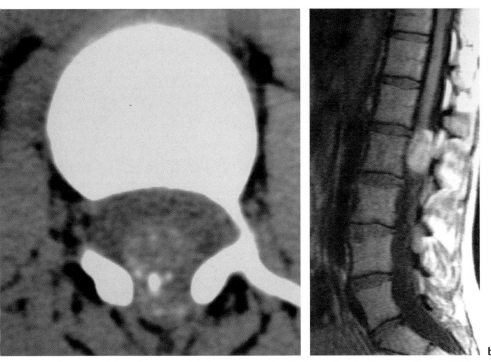

Fig. 10.85a, b   Dermoid. Axial CT image (**a**) shows an intradural lesion with mixed intermediate and high attenuation, which has high signal on sagittal T1-weighted MRI (**b**).

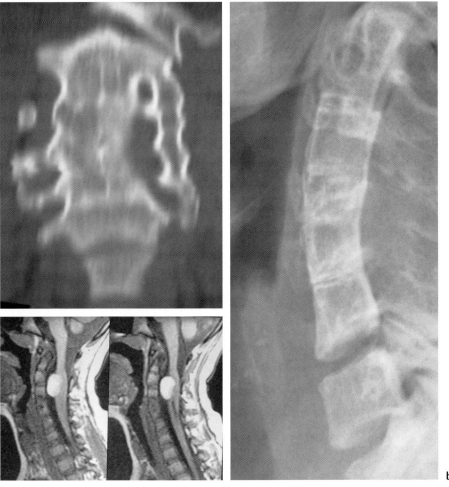

Fig. 10.86a–c   Neurenteric cyst. Coronal CT image (**a**) and lateral radiograph (**b**) show segmentation anomalies involving multiple cervical vertebrae. An intradural extramedullary lesion with high signal is seen on sagittal T1-weighted MRI (**c**).

III Spine

Table 10.6   (Cont.) Intradural extramedullary lesions

Lesions	CT Findings	Comments
Neurofibroma ▷ *Fig. 10.87*	Lobulated extramedullary lesions with or without irregular margins, with or without extradural extension of lesion with dumbbell shape, with contrast enhancement; with or without erosion of foramina, with or without scalloping of dorsal margin of vertebral body (chronic erosion or dural ectasia/NF1).	Unencapsulated neoplasms involving nerve and nerve sheath; common type of intradural extramedullary neoplasms often with extradural extension; usual presentation in adults with pain and radiculopathy, paresthesias, and lower extremity weakness. Multiple neurofibromas seen with NF1.
Paraganglioma	Spheroid or lobulated intradural-extramedullary lesion with intermediate attenuation, with or without tubular vessels, with contrast enhancement, with or without foci of hemorrhage; usually located in region of cauda equina and filum terminale.	Paragangliomas are neoplasms that arise from paraganglion cells of neural crest origin and usually occur at carotid body, jugular foramen, middle ear, and along vagus nerve. Rarely occur in spine.
Leptomeningeal metastases ▷ *Fig. 10.88a, b*	Single or multiple nodular lesions and/or focal or diffuse abnormal subarachnoid disease along pial surface of spinal cord. Leptomeningeal tumor is best seen on postmyelographic CT images.	Disseminated tumor in the subarachnoid space (leptomeninges) usually is associated with significant pathology (neoplasm vs inflammation and/or infection). Primary neoplasms commonly associated with disseminated subarachnoid tumor include primitive neuroectodermal tumors (e.g., medulloblastoma), glioblastoma, ependymoma, and choroid plexus papilloma/carcinoma. Metastases within CSF can result from direct extension through the dura or by hematogenous dissemination or via the choroid plexus. The most frequent primary neoplasms outside CNS within subarachnoid metastases are lung carcinoma, breast carcinoma, melanoma, lymphoma, and leukemia.
Arachnoid cyst	Well-circumscribed intradural extramedullary lesions with attenuation similar to CSF, no contrast enhancement.	Nonneoplastic congenital, developmental, or acquired extra-axial lesions filled with CSF; usually mild mass effect on adjacent spinal cord or nerve roots.
Teratoma	Circumscribed lesions with variable low, intermediate, and/or high attenuation; with or without contrast enhancement. May contain calcifications and cysts, as well as fatty components that can cause chemical meningitis if ruptured.	Composed of derivatives of ectoderm, mesoderm, and/or endoderm.
Leptomeningeal infection/inflammation	Single or multiple nodular subarachnoid lesions or thickened nerve roots on postmyelographic CT images. Leptomeningeal inflammation often best seen on postcontrast MRI.	Contrast enhancement in the subarachnoid space (leptomeninges) on MRI is usually associated with significant pathology (inflammation and/or infection vs neoplasm). Inflammation and/or infection of the leptomeninges can result from pyogenic, fungal, or parasitic diseases, as well as tuberculosis. Neurosarcoid results in granulomatous disease in the leptomeninges, producing similar patterns of subarachnoid enhancement.
Adhesive arachnoiditis	Clumping of nerve roots within the thecal sac and/or peripheral positioning of nerve roots within the thecal sac, "empty sac" sign on postmyelographic CT images.	Adhesive arachnoiditis is a chronic disorder that results in aggregation of nerve roots within the thecal sac or adhesion of nerve roots to the inner margin of the thecal sac. Can result from prior surgery, hemorrhage, radiation treatment, meningitis, or myelography (pantopaque).
Arachnoiditis ossificans ▷ *Fig. 10.89a, b*	Irregular zones with high attenuation in the subarachnoid space.	Chronic inflammatory disorder that results in metaplastic ossification changes in the subarachnoid space; usually occurs in the thoracic and lumbar regions. Can be associated with prior infection, prior myelography, and surgery.
Pyogenic arachnoiditis	Nerve root enlargement with or without clumping of nerve roots within the thecal sac on postmyelographic CT. Contrast enhancement on MRI involving one or more nerve roots within the thecal sac.	Pyogenic arachnoiditis can result from surgical complication, extension of intracranial meningitis, epidural abscess, vertebral osteomyelitis, or immunocompromised status.

(continues on page 464)

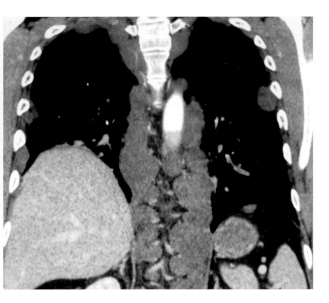

Fig. 10.87   Neurofibroma. Coronal image shows multiple paraspinal neurofibromas in a patient with neurofibromatosis type 1.

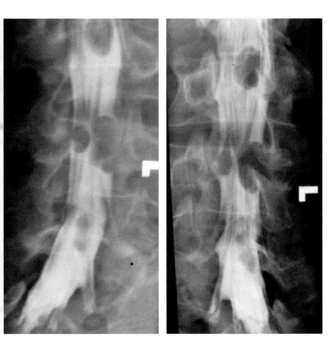

b

Fig. 10.88a, b   Leptomeningeal metastases. Myelographic images show multiple intradural nodular lesions from drop metastases.

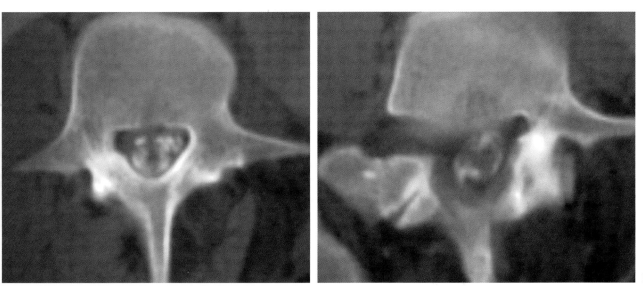

b

Fig. 10.89a, b   Arachnoiditis ossificans. Axial CTs (not postmyelography) show amorphous intrathecal calcifications/ossifications.

III Spine

Table 10.6   (Cont.) Intradural extramedullary lesions

Lesions	CT Findings	Comments
Vascular		
Arteriovenous malformation (AVM)	Lesions with irregular margins that can be located in the spinal cord (white and/or gray matter), dura, or both locations. AVMs contain multiple tortuous vessels, as well as areas of hemorrhage in various phases, calcifications, gliosis, and myelomalacia. The venous portions often show contrast enhancement.	Intracranial AVMs much more common than spinal AVMs. Annual risk of hemorrhage. AVMs can be sporadic, congenital, or associated with a history of trauma.
Other		
Hemorrhage within CSF	Hemorrhage into CSF can result in transient amorphous increased attenuation.	Hemorrhage into CSF from cranial or spinal surgery, trauma, vascular malformation, or neoplasm can result in leptomeningeal enhancement.
Intradural herniated disk	Amorphous structure with intermediate attenuation.	Disk herniations rarely extend through dura into the thecal sac.

Table 10.7   Spine: Intradural intramedullary lesions

Lesions	CT Findings	Comments
Inflammatory		
Demyelinating disease		
Multiple sclerosis	Intramedullary lesion or multiple lesions in spinal cord. MRI is the optimal test to evaluate for lesions in the spinal cord. CT myelography may show focal zones of atrophy in the spinal cord at old plaques.	Multiple sclerosis is the most common acquired demyelinating disease usually affecting women (peak ages 20–40 y). Plaques in spinal cord associated with atrophy often associated with relapsing/remitting type of multiple sclerosis (MS). Devic disease is a variant of MS that consists of optic neuritis and progressive demyelination of spinal cord without evidence of demyelination in the brain.
Acute disseminated encephalomyelitis (ADEM)	Intramedullary lesion or multiple lesions in spinal cord. MRI is the optimal test to evaluate for lesions in the spinal cord. CT myelography may show focal zones of atrophy in the spinal cord at remote sites of demyelination.	ADEM is a noninfectious monophasic inflammatory/demyelination process involving the spinal cord and/or brain that occurs several weeks after viral infection or vaccination. Children > adults. Associated with various bilateral motor and sensory deficits.
Transverse myelitis	Intramedullary lesion or multiple lesions in spinal cord. MRI is the optimal test to evaluate for lesions in the spinal cord. CT myelography may show focal zones of atrophy in the spinal cord at remote sites of demyelination.	Transverse myelitis is a noninfectious inflammatory process involving both halves of the spinal cord, as well as gray and white matter; multiple causes: demyelination after viral infection or vaccination (possibly a variant of ADEM), autoimmune diseases/collagen vascular diseases (systemic lupus erythematosus), paraneoplastic syndromes, atypical multiple sclerosis, idiopathic; can be diagnosis of exclusion; M > F, mean age 45 y. Associated with various bilateral motor and sensory deficits. Pathologic changes considered to be a combination of demyelination and arterial or venous ischemia.
Other noninfectious inflammatory diseases involving the spinal cord		
Sarcoid	Intramedullary lesion or multiple lesions in spinal cord. MRI is the optimal test to evaluate for lesions in the spinal cord. CT myelography may show focal zones of enlargement of the spinal cord.	Sarcoidosis is a multisystem, noncaseating, granulomatous disease of uncertain etiology that involves the CNS in ~5% to 15%. Rarely involves the spinal cord. Association with severe neurologic deficits if untreated. May mimic intramedullary neoplasm.

(continues on page 465)

Table 10.7 (Cont.) Spine: Intradural intramedullary lesions

Lesions	CT Findings	Comments
Infectious diseases of the spinal cord		
Abscess	Intramedullary lesion in spinal cord best seen with MRI. CT myelography may show focal zone of enlargement of the spinal cord at the site of abscess.	Infection can result from hematogenous dissemination or spread within CSF. Organisms reported to result in spinal cord abscess or nonviral myelitis include *Streptococcus milleri, Streptococcus pyogenes, Mycobacterium tuberculosis,* atypical mycobacteria, syphilis, *Schistosoma mansoni,* and fungi (*Cryptococcus, Candida,* and *Aspergillus*); seen in immunocompromised patients.
Parasitic	Intramedullary lesion in spinal cord best seen with MRI. CT myelography may show focal zones of enlargement of the spinal cord at the site of abscess; with or without leptomeningeal lesions. Concurrent lesions in brain are usually present.	Parasitic infection of the spinal cord is rare. The most common type of parasite to involve the spinal cord is *Toxoplasma gondii* in immunocompromised patients. Toxoplasmosis rarely involves the spinal cord unlike cerebral infection. *S. mansoni* can involve the spinal cord in immunocompetent patients in Asia/Africa. Associated with rapid decline in neurologic function related to site of lesion in spinal cord.
Vascular		
Intramedullary hemorrhage	Intramedullary lesion in spinal cord best seen with MRI. CT myelography may show focal zone of enlargement of the spinal cord at the site of hematoma.	Can result from trauma, vascular malformations, coagulopathy, amyloid angiopathy, infarction, metastases, abscesses, viral infections (herpes simplex, cytomegalovirus [CMV]).
Arteriovenous malformation	Lesions with irregular margins that can be located in the spinal cord (white and/or gray matter), dura, or both locations. AVMs contain multiple tortuous tubular vessels as calcifications, as seen on CT and CT myelography. Not usually associated with mass effect unless there is recent hemorrhage or venous occlusion.	Intracranial AVMs much more common than spinal AVMs. Annual risk of hemorrhage. AVMs can be sporadic, congenital, or associated with a history of trauma. Multiple AVMs can be seen in syndromes: Rendu–Osler–Weber: AVMs in brain and lungs and mucosal capillary telangiectasias; Wyburn–Mason: AVMs in brain and retina, with cutaneous nevi.
Syringohydromyelia ▷ *Fig. 10.90a–c*	Enlarged spinal cord with intramedullary fluid-filled zone that is central or slightly eccentric.	Hydromyelia refers to distention of the central canal of the spinal cord (lined by ependymal cells). Syringomyelia refers to dissection of CSF into the spinal cord (not lined by ependymal cells). Syringohydromyelia refers to combination of both. May be secondary to congenital/developmental anomalies (Chiari I, Chiari II malformations, and basilar invagination) and also secondary to neoplasms of the spinal cord (astrocytoma, ependymoma, and hemangioblastoma).

(continues on page 466)

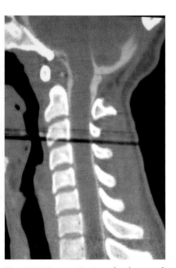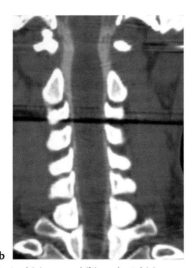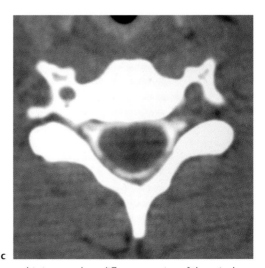

Fig. 10.90a–c   Syringohydromyelia. Sagittal (**a**), coronal (**b**), and axial (**c**) postmyelographic images show diffuse expansion of the spinal cord secondary to a syrinx.

III Spine

Table 10.7 (Cont.) Spine: Intradural intramedullary lesions

Lesions	CT Findings	Comments
Neoplastic		
Astrocytoma ▷ *Fig. 10.91a, b*	Intramedullary expansile lesions as seen on CT myelography. Lesions often extend multiple vertebral segments. Locations: cervical spinal cord > upper thoracic spinal cord > conus medullaris.	Most common intramedullary tumor in children, second most common in adults. Occurs more frequently in children than adults. Most are low-grade tumors (90% children, 75% adults). Anaplastic astrocytomas account for most of the rest, glioblastomas account for only 1%.
Ependymoma	Intramedullary circumscribed expansile lesion, often midline/central location in spinal cord. Intramedullary locations: cervical spinal cord (44%), both cervical and upper thoracic spinal cord (23%), thoracic spinal cord (26%). Lesions often extend three or four vertebral segments. With or without scoliosis, chronic bone erosion.	Most common intramedullary tumor in adults (60% of glial neoplasms). Adults > children. Intramedullary ependymomas involving the upper spinal cord often are cellular or mixed histologic types, whereas ependymomas at the conus medullaris or cauda equina usually are myxopapillary. Slight male predominance. Usually are slow-growing neoplasms associated with long duration of neck or back pain, sensory deficits, motor weakness, bladder and bowel dysfunction.
Ganglioglioma	Circumscribed intramedullary tumors. Association with scoliosis (44%) and bone erosion (93%).	Rare tumors involving the spinal cord (1% of spinal neoplasms). May extend inferiorly from lesion in cerebellum, ganglioglioma (contains glial and neuronal elements), ganglioneuroma (contains only ganglion cells), gangliocytoma (contains only neuronal elements). Uncommon tumors, patients younger than 30 y, slow-growing neoplasms.
Hemangioblastoma ▷ *Fig. 10.92a, b*	Circumscribed tumors usually located in the superficial portion of the spinal cord; small contrast-enhancing nodule, with or without cyst, or larger lesion with prominent heterogeneous enhancement with or without vessels within lesion or at the periphery. Usually associated with syrinx. Locations: thoracic spinal cord (50%–60%), cervical spinal cord (40%–50%).	Represent ~5% of spinal cord neoplasms. Usually intramedullary lesion but occasionally extends into the intradural space or extradural location. Sporadic lesions usually occur in patients younger than 40 y. Multiple lesions occur in adolescents with von Hippel–Lindau disease.
Metastasis	Intramedullary lesion or superficial lesions on the spinal cord, with or without leptomeningeal tumor nodules. Often extend two or three vertebral segments.	Rare intramedullary lesions that can present with pain, bladder or bowel dysfunction, and paresthesias. Location: cervical spinal cord (45%), thoracic spinal cord (35%), lumbar region (8%). Usually solitary lesions, occasionally multiple; spread hematogenously via arteries or direct extension into leptomeninges with invasion of pial surface or central canal of the spinal cord. Primary CNS tumors include primitive neuroectodermal tumor/medulloblastoma, glioblastoma. Primary tumors outside CNS: lung carcinoma (70%), breast carcinoma (11%), melanoma (5%), renal cell carcinoma (4%), colorectal carcinoma (3%), lymphoma (3%), others (4%).

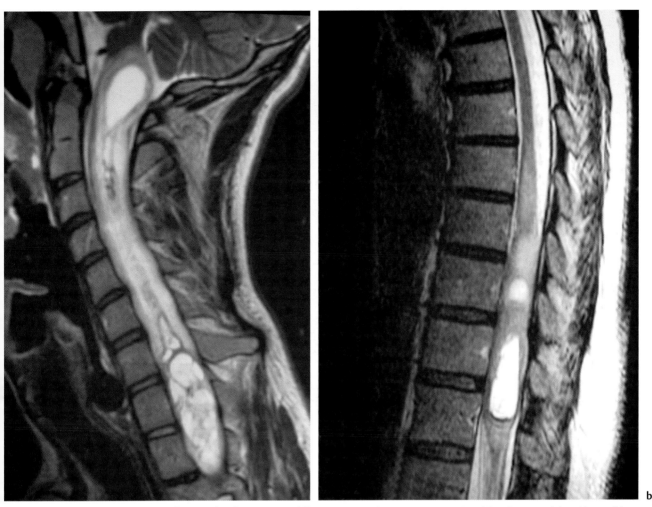

b

Fig. 10.91a, b Astrocytoma. Sagittal T2-weighted MRIs in two different patients show astrocytomas involving the upper (**a**) and lower (**b**) spinal cord.

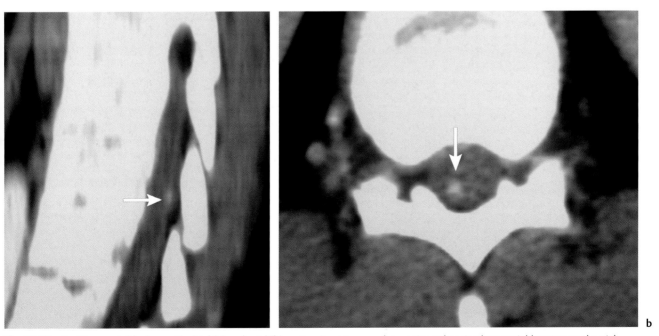

b

Fig. 10.92a, b Hemangioblastoma. Sagittal (**a**) and axial (**b**) postcontrast images show a tiny enhancing hemangioblastoma on the pial surface of the spinal cord in this patient with von Hippel–Lindau disease (arrows).

IV Musculoskeletal System

11 Soft Tissue Disease

Francis A. Burgener

Magnetic resonance imaging (MRI) is far superior to computed tomography (CT) for the visualization of soft tissue pathology because of greater soft tissue contrast and an overall improved tissue characterization based on signal behavior on different pulse sequences and relaxation parameters. Compared with MRI, CT is more sensitive for the diagnosis of both tiny soft tissue calcifications and air collections and facilitates differentiation between the two.

For CT, the contrast characteristics of soft tissue disease depend on the relative proportions of fat, water, and mineral. Normal muscles are of soft tissue density and are separated from each other by fatty septa. In many muscle diseases, the muscle fibers become necrotic and degenerate or are replaced by fat and connective tissue. Fatty replacement of muscle may be complete and homogeneous or incomplete and inhomogeneous, but it is not characteristic for a specific disease. It is observed with muscular dystrophies, neuropathies, ischemias, and metabolic and systemic myopathies, as well as idiopathically (**Fig. 11.1**). CT is of little use in the differentiation of these conditions, but it may play an important role in the localization, distribution, and assessment of the extent of muscular involvement.

CT is useful in the evaluation of soft tissue masses. It allows definition of the exact dimensions of a lesion and its relationship to nearby neurovascular structures and bone. Certain limitations of CT in the evaluation of soft tissue masses, however, must be recognized. With the exception of a few lesions, such as lipomas (**Fig. 11.2**) and cysts (**Fig. 11.3**), CT rarely allows a specific histologic diagnosis based on attenuation values and appearance. Besides lipomas and cysts, other lesions may contain adipose tissue or fluid, respectively. The density of fat ranges from −50 to −100 HU. A fluid-containing lesion appears

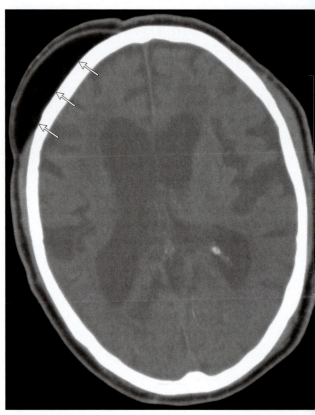

Fig. 11.2 Lipoma. A fatty lesion (arrows) between the scalp and skull is seen.

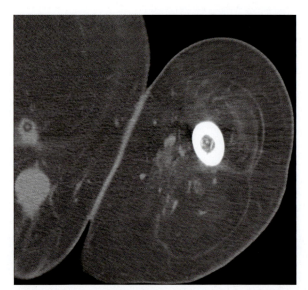

Fig. 11.1 Muscular dystrophy. Complete fatty replacement of all muscles in the thigh is seen.

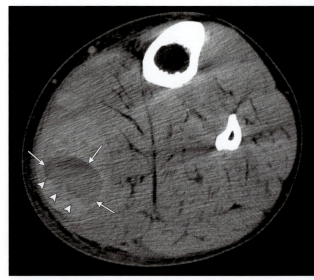

Fig. 11.3 Baker (popliteal) cyst. A fluid-containing lesion (arrows) hypodense to the surrounding muscles is seen. The poorly defined border on the posteroinferior border (arrowheads) indicates that the cyst is ruptured.

Table 11.1   Fat-containing soft tissue lesions

Lipoma (subcutaneous, intermuscular, intramuscular, and synovial)
Lipoma arborescens (diffuse synovial lipoma in the knee)
Neural fibrolipoma (fibrolipomatous hamartoma usually of the median nerve in the wrist)
Macrodystrophia lipomatosa (neural fibrolipoma with macrodactyly)
Lipoblastoma (lipoma in infancy and early childhood)
Hibernoma (brown fat tumor, typically involving the shoulder region, chest wall, or thigh)
Hemangioma
Elastofibroma (between the inferior margin of the scapula and chest wall)
Liposarcoma

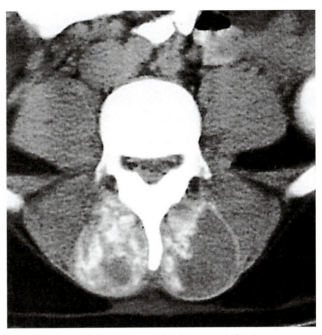

Fig. 11.4   Renal failure. Paraspinal soft tissue calcifications are seen.

hypodense to muscle and has a density similar to water or slightly above it (range 0–20 HU). Fat-containing lesions are summarized in **Table 11.1** and cystic lesions in **Table 11.2**.

Overestimation of a soft tissue mass with CT is possible because of adjacent soft tissue edema. Differentiation of actual invasion of neighboring structures such as the neurovascular bundle and bone from simple distortion and pressure defects by the adjacent mass is not always feasible.

Soft tissue calcifications can easily be appreciated by CT. They can be classified as metabolic (metastatic), dystrophic, or idiopathic.

Metabolic (metastatic) calcifications are associated with a disturbance in calcium/phosphorous metabolism, resulting in the deposition of calcium in normal tissues (**Fig. 11.4**). Such conditions include renal osteodystrophy (less commonly, primary hyperparathyroidism), hypoparathyroidism, hypervitaminosis D, milk–alkali syndrome (prolonged excessive intake of milk and alkali for heartburn in peptic ulcer disease, often associated with renal insufficiency), sarcoidosis, and processes associated with massive bone destruction (e.g., metastases, multiple myeloma, and leukemia).

Dystrophic calcifications represent calcium deposits in damaged tissue without metabolic derangement. They are associated with traumatic, ischemic, neuropathic, infectious, and neoplastic conditions. Besides calcification of a hematoma, other traumatic causes include sequelae of previous surgery, irradiation, and thermal injuries. Foreign body and injection

granulomas also frequently calcify. Subcutaneous fat necrosis resulting in calcification of the subcutaneous adipose tissue is found with pancreatic disorders, Weber–Christian disease (nonsuppurative nodular panniculitis with subsequent necrosis and fibrosis in the subcutaneous fat and all visceral adipose tissues), and vascular insufficiency, in which calcified varicose veins or arteriosclerotic arteries are frequently also present. In the infectious group, calcified abscesses and granulomas are encountered. Soft tissue calcifications are also found in a variety of parasitic infestations, such as cysticercosis and echinococcosis. Tumor calcifications occur in both benign and malignant neoplasms. In benign tumors, the calcifications may be central (e.g., in lipomas [**Fig. 11.5**] and hemangiomas) or peripheral (e.g., in myxomas and xanthomas). In malignant neoplasms, such as synovial sarcoma, and less commonly in other soft tissue sarcomas, such as malignant fibrous histiocytoma, leiomyosarcoma, and rhabdomyosarcoma, both necrosis and hemorrhage may lead to secondary calcifications. Extraskeletal chondrosarcomas and osteosarcomas may demonstrate irregular, poorly marginated calcific deposits, whereas calcifications in their benign counterparts (chondromas and osteomas) tend to be well defined.

Table 11.2   Cystic soft tissue lesions

Synovial cyst (cystic lesion lined by synovial membrane that may or may not communicate with the neighboring joint)
Ganglion or ganglionic cyst (arising from tendon sheaths, tendon, and muscles)
Meniscal (parameniscal) cyst (associated with chronic meniscal tears)
Labral (paralabral) cyst (associated with glenoid and acetabular labral tears)
Distended bursa (commonly associated with chronic mechanical irritation, trauma, rheumatoid arthritis, and gout)
Cystic lymphangioma or hygroma (may be associated with Turner or Noonan syndrome and several trisomies)
Branchial cleft cyst (limited to the head and neck area)
Myxoma (benign subcutaneous or intramuscular cystic neoplasm, either thin-walled or thick-walled, sometimes with septation)
Chronic (liquefied) hematoma (pseudocapsule and "hematocrit effect" caused by settling of cellular elements at the bottom of the cystic lesion may occasionally be observed)
Abscess (irregular, thick-walled or, less commonly, thin-walled cystic lesion with considerable wall enhancement and surrounding edema)
Necrotic tumor (irregular, thick-walled, usually malignant)
Aneurysm and pseudoaneurysm (most common in popliteal artery)

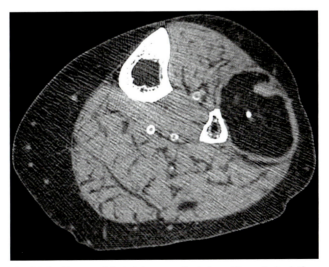

Fig. 11.5   Lipoma. A fatty intramuscular lesion with central calcification is seen.

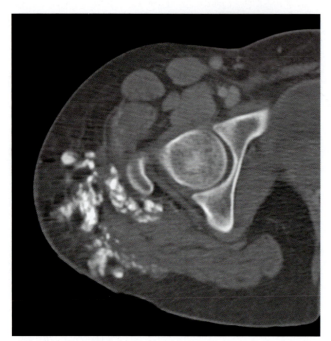

Fig. 11.6   Scleroderma. Irregular calcifications about the trochanter are seen.

Phleboliths are dystrophic calcifications in organizing thrombi. They present as circular or elliptical calcifications with radiolucent centers measuring <1 cm in their longest diameter. They are commonly found in hemangiomas and varicosities. They are quite characteristic but may occasionally be simulated by extra-articular (tenosynovial) chondromatosis, cysticercosis, and the calcified fatty deposits in Ehlers–Danlos syndrome (connective tissue disease with joint hyperextensibility and multiple musculoskeletal and other anomalies).

Idiopathic soft tissue calcifications are limited to the connective tissue disorders (e.g., scleroderma [**Fig. 11.6**], dermatomyositis, and occasionally systemic lupus erythematosus) and idiopathic calcinosis (**Fig. 11.7**). In the latter conditions, the calcifications

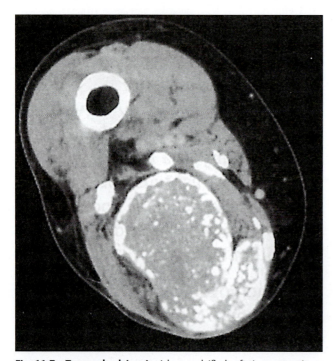

Fig. 11.7   Tumoral calcinosis. A large calcified soft tissue mass is seen in the right thigh.

Table 11.3   Soft tissue calcifications

Metabolic (metastatic) calcifications
    Hyperparathyroidism (primary; more commonly secondary, due to chronic renal disease; and, rarely, ectopic, caused by lung or kidney tumors)
    Hypoparathyroidism
    Hypervitaminosis D
    Williams syndrome (idiopathic hypercalcemia of infancy)
    Milk–alkali syndrome
    Sarcoidosis
    Conditions associated with massive bone destruction (e.g., metastases, multiple myeloma, and leukemia)
Dystrophic calcifications
    Trauma* (hematoma, surgery, irradiation, thermal injuries, foreign bodies, and injection granulomas)
    Ischemia/necrosis*
    Vascular disorders* (atherosclerosis, Mönckeberg sclerosis, and diabetes mellitus)
    Phleboliths
    Neurologic disorders*
    Tumors* (synovial sarcoma, lipoma, hemangioma, cartilaginous and osteoblastic tumors, and necrotic tumors)
    Infection and infestation* (abscess, granuloma, tuberculosis, leprosy, cysticercosis, echinococcosis, dracunculiasis, and loiasis)
    Articular/para-articular disorders (calcific tendinosis and bursitis, gout) (see also **Table 11.4**)
Idiopathic calcifications
    Connective tissue disorders (scleroderma, dermatomyositis, and systemic lupus erythematosus)
    Calcinosis (universalis, tumoralis, and circumscripta)

* Indicates that condition may progress to ossification.

may be widespread and arranged in longitudinal bands (calcinosis universalis) or in multiple, well-demarcated masses of calcium often about articulations (tumoral calcinosis), or they may be localized (circumscript calcinosis, or calcinosis circumscripta). In tumoral and circumscript calcinosis, calcium–fluid levels are sometimes observed. Soft tissue calcifications are summarized in **Table 11.3**; **Table 11.4** lists soft tissue calcifications commonly found in para-articular distribution.

Soft tissue ossification is diagnosed when cancellous bone is surrounded by cortical bone. Because only a limited number of diseases presenting initially with soft tissue calcification may eventually progress to soft tissue ossification, the differential diagnosis of the latter is accordingly smaller. A common cause of soft tissue ossification is traumatic myositis ossificans. It is characterized by a peripheral ring of ossification ("eggshell" calcification) surrounding a more lucent center (**Fig. 11.8**). Furthermore, the lesion is typically separated in its entire

Table 11.4   Para-articular soft tissue calcifications

Calcific tendinosis and bursitis
Connective tissue disease (especially scleroderma)
Idiopathic calcinosis (tumoral and circumscripta)
Hyperparathyroidism (primary and particularly secondary)
Hypoparathyroidism
Hypervitaminosis D
Milk–alkali syndrome
Articular disorders (calcium pyrophosphate deposition disease [CPPD], hydroxyapatite crystal deposition disease [HADD], gout, trauma,* neurologic disorders,* infections,* synovial chondromatosis*)
Sarcoidosis
Tumors (especially synovial sarcoma and soft tissue chondrosarcoma)

* May be ossified.

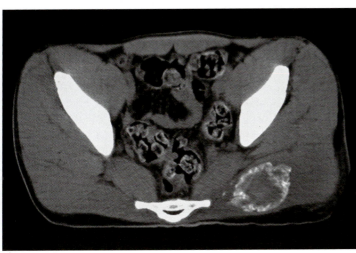 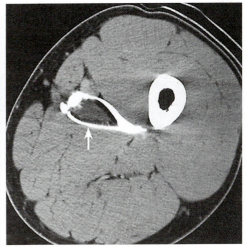

b

Fig. 11.8a, b Traumatic myositis ossificans (two cases). (a) Early stage: A ring of calcification/ossification is seen in the periphery of a hematoma in the left gluteus maximus muscle. (**b**) Late stage: An ossified hematoma is seen in the left thigh (arrow).

length from the adjacent cortex when located near a bone. In the absence of a history of trauma, the same lesion is often referred to as a pseudomalignant osseous tumor of soft tissue. A parosteal osteosarcoma presents as a radiodense lesion attached in a sessile fashion to the external cortex (**Fig. 11.9a**). In contrast to myositis ossificans, ossification of the tumor proceeds from the base of the lesion to its periphery. An osteochondroma is composed of a medullary cavity that is contiguous with the bone from which it arose and is surrounded by sharply defined cortical bone and a thin cartilaginous cap with varying degrees of calcifications (**Fig. 11.9b**). Soft tissue ossifications with a predilection for the para-articular regions are found in melorheostosis, a condition in which the bony alterations are diagnostic. Heterotopic bone formation occurs commonly after surgery, especially after insertion of hip

prostheses and in a variety of neurologic disorders, especially paraplegia. Venous insufficiency and thermal injuries may lead to soft tissue ossification in the extremities. Myositis ossificans progressiva (fibrodysplasia ossificans progressiva) is a rare cause of soft tissue ossification associated with anomalies and hypoplasias of the great toes and thumbs, exostoses, and progressive fusion of primarily the axial skeleton. Soft tissue ossifications are summarized in **Table 11.5**.

The hallmark of *necrotizing fasciitis* (**Fig. 11.10**) is the presence of soft tissue gas, but this finding is not universally present. Gas in this life-threatening condition is commonly produced by a mixture of both aerobic and anaerobic bacteria. CT features include, besides soft tissue gas, marked edematous thickening of both the superficial and deep fasciae often associated with fluid collections, whereas the edematous

IV Musculoskeletal System

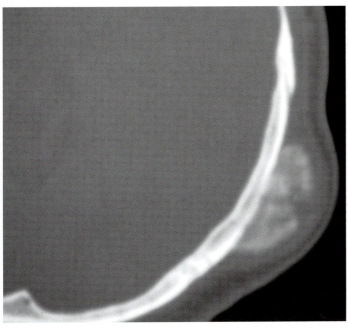 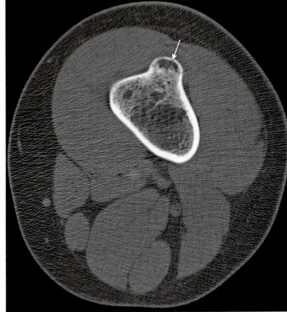

b

Fig. 11.9a, b Parosteal sarcoma and osteochondroma. An ossified parosteal sarcoma (**a**) is attached in sessile fashion to the outer table of the skull. The medullary cavity of an osteochondroma (**b**, arrow) is contiguous with the femur from which it arose and surrounded by sharply defined cortical bone. The cartilaginous cap without calcifications is not appreciated.

Table 11.5 Soft tissue ossification (heterotopic bone formation)

Hematoma (e.g., following total hip prosthesis)
Myositis ossificans traumatica
Myositis (fibrodysplasia) ossificans progressiva
Thermal injuries
Surgical scars
Venous insufficiency
Infection
Tumors (synovial osteochondromatosis, pseudomalignant osseous soft tissue tumor, and parosteal and extraskeletal osteosarcoma)
Melorheostosis
Neurologic disorders (paraplegia, cerebrovascular accident, poliomyelitis, and multiple sclerosis)

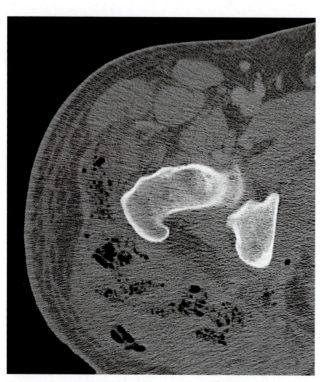

Fig. 11.10 Necrotizing fasciitis. Extensive soft tissue gas is seen in the gluteal and obturator internus muscles. The edematous changes in the adjacent subcutaneous fat are only relatively mild.

changes in the muscle and adipose tissue are often less severe. *Cellulitis,* a streptococcal or, less commonly, a staphylococcal infection, can be differentiated from necrotizing fasciitis by the predominant involvement of the subcutaneous fat and superficial fascial tissues and the absence of soft tissue gas. *Pyomyositis* typically affects otherwise healthy children and young adults, especially in tropical regions, but it is also recognized with increasing frequency in malnourished and immunodeficient patients. Gas bubbles are occasionally seen in this intramuscular abscess caused by a *Staphylococcus aureus* infection in about 90% and by a streptococcal infection in the remaining cases.

Soft tissue contamination with *gas gangrene* occurs in devitalized tissues in which the arterial blood supply has been compromised. Predisposing factors for this clostridial infection include contaminated wounds, burns, decubitus ulcers, and diabetes mellitus. Gas in the subcutaneous tissue presents in this condition typically as linear or netlike lucent areas, whereas in the muscles, it characteristically produces circular collections of varying sizes. Conditions associated with soft tissue gas are summarized in **Table 11.6.**

Differentiation between a benign and malignant soft tissue lesion is not always possible either. Features for a benign process are small size; smooth, well-defined borders; and the absence of invasion of the adjacent muscles and bones. Criteria for a malignant process include a large size, poor definition, inhomogeneous density, blurring of the adjacent fat, and invasion of the adjacent muscles and bone.

The differential diagnosis of soft tissue lesions is discussed in **Table 11.7.**

Table 11.6 Soft tissue gas

Skin defects (e.g., decubitus ulcer and surgical defects)
Sinus tracts and fistulas
Iatrogenic interventions
Penetrating trauma (e.g., gunshot wound)
Perforation of gas-containing structures (e.g., rib fracture with lung injury, fractured trachea)
Pyomyositis and abscess formation
Gangrene (gas phlegmon)
Necrotizing fasciitis

Table 11.7   Soft tissue lesions

Disease	CT Findings	Comments
Cyst ▷ *Fig. 11.11* ▷ *Fig. 11.12*	Sharply marginated, homogeneous, unilocular or multilocular mass of water density. Higher attenuation values after intracystic hemorrhage. No enhancement after intravenous (IV) contrast administration. Occasionally, minimal enhancement of the thin cystic wall occurs. Differential diagnosis: para-articular meniscal and labral cysts are associated with chronic tears and degeneration of the corresponding joint structures.	Cystic lesions in the vicinity of a joint usually represent a **synovial cyst** (herniation of the synovial membrane through the joint capsule) or a **distended bursa** (with or without communication with the adjacent articulation). These conditions are of traumatic, degenerative, or inflammatory origin. Rheumatoid arthritis is the most common cause of a large synovial cyst. A **ganglion (ganglion cyst)** is a cystic, tumorlike lesion that is commonly attached to a tendon sheath. A **myxoma** is a cystic connective soft tissue lesion, often with intratumoral septa in intramuscular, subcutaneous, or aponeurotic location.

(continues on page 476)

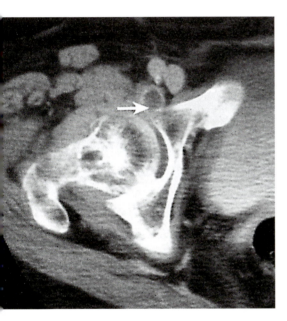

Fig. 11.11   Synovial cyst in rheumatoid arthritis. Small cyst (arrow) connecting with the right hip joint projects anterior to the acetabulum.

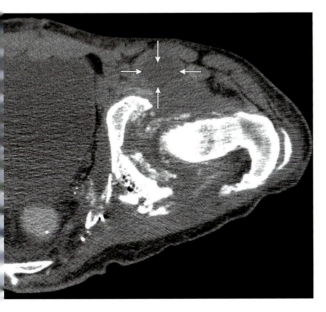

Fig. 11.12   Iliopsoas bursitis. An enlarged iliopsoas bursa containing serous fluid is seen (arrows). An infected hemorrhagic and destroyed hip with numerous loose fracture fragments secondary to gunshot injury is also present.

IV   Musculoskeletal System

Table 11.7   (Cont.) Soft tissue lesions

Disease	CT Findings	Comments
Lipoma ▷ *Fig. 11.13a, b* ▷ *Fig. 11.14* ▷ *Fig. 11.15*	Well-defined, homogeneous, fatty soft tissue mass (−50 to −100 HU) without significant contrast enhancement is virtually diagnostic. Thin septations or vessels and calcifications or ossifications within the tumor are occasionally observed. Lipomas located close to bone (**parosteal lipomas**) may incite a localized hyperostosis. Invasion into the surrounding soft tissue or areas of soft tissue within the lesion suggest the possibility of a liposarcoma, although these findings might also be found with rare infiltrating varieties of lipomas and angiolipomas or with necrosis and hemorrhage occurring within a lipoma.	Most common benign soft tissue tumor. Predilection for the subcutaneous fat (superficial lipomas) in patients between 30 and 50 y of age, with female predominance. Multiple in 5% of all patients. Deep lipomas arise in the subfascial tissue or within muscle and may reach considerable size. Variants of fatty tumors include **(neural) fibrolipoma, mesenchymoma** (lipoma with significant chondroid and osseous metaplasia), **lipomatosis** (diffuse infiltrative overgrowth of mature adipose tissue), **hibernoma** (hypervascular tumor of brown fat usually in the shoulder region, chest wall, or thigh) (▷ *Fig. 11.16*), **lipoblastoma** (superficial infiltrating lipomatous lesion in the extremities occurring usually in infancy and early childhood), **lipoma arborescens** (fatty infiltration beneath synovial joint lining, usually in the knee), and **macrodystrophia lipomatosa** resulting in grotesque enlargement of one or more digits in the same extremity.
Hemangioma ▷ *Fig. 11.17* ▷ *Fig. 11.18*	Inhomogeneous, usually relatively well-defined mass that may contain phleboliths. Hemangiomas have a density of 30 to 40 HU and enhance markedly following IV contrast medium administration. Occasionally, phleboliths are found within the lesion. When adjacent to bone, erosions and solid periosteal reactions are occasionally observed. Capillary, cavernous, venous, and arteriovenous hemangiomas are differentiated. Cavernous hemangiomas may contain a large amount of fat.	Most common vascular tumor with a predilection for the skin. Deep soft tissue hemangiomas are usually asymptomatic. Conditions associated with multiple hemangiomas include consumption coagulopathy (Kasabach–Merritt syndrome), cardiac decompensation, gangrene, massive osteolysis of Gorham, Klippel–Trenaunay syndrome (varicose veins, soft tissue and bone hypertrophy), Parkes–Weber syndrome (Klippel–Trenaunay with arteriovenous fistulas), Sturge-Weber syndrome (meningofacial angiomatosis), or Maffucci syndrome (enchondromatosis) with hemangioma.
Lymphangioma ▷ *Fig. 11.19*	Similar to hemangioma but without phleboliths and less contrast enhancement. **Branchial cleft cysts** in the head and neck area must be differentiated from a cystic lymphangioma.	Rare. Cystic lymphangioma (hygroma) may be associated with Turner and Noonan syndromes and several trisomies.

(continues on page 478)

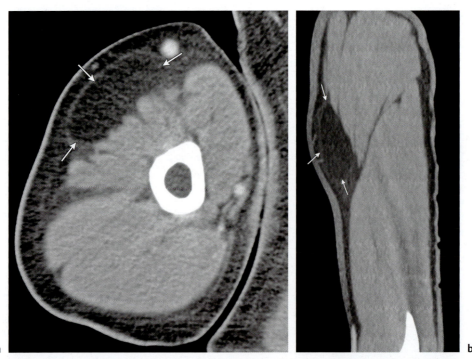

Fig. 11.13a, b   Subcutaneous lipoma. A fatty lesion (arrows) is seen in the upper arm that is difficult to demarcate from the normal surrounding adipose tissue (**a**, axial; **b**, sagittal).

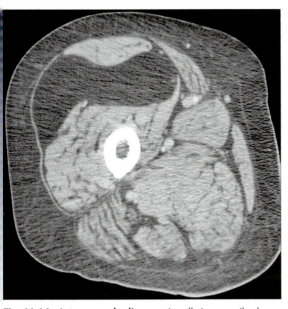

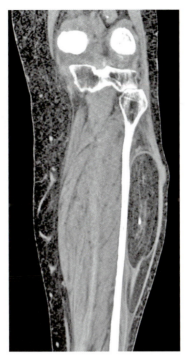

Fig. 11.15   Lipoma. A fatty lesion with central calcification is seen in the lower leg.

Fig. 11.14   Intramuscular lipoma. A well-circumscribed fatty lesion is seen in the quadriceps femoris muscle of the thigh.

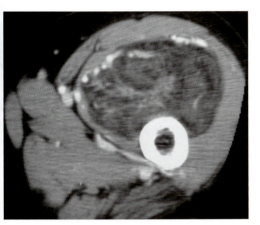

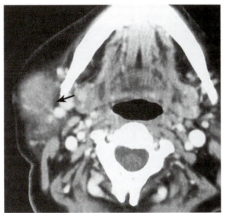

Fig. 11.16   Hibernoma. A fatty lesion containing soft tissue components is seen in the thigh. The lesion cannot be differentiated radiographically from a liposarcoma.

Fig. 11.17   Hemangioma (capillary). An enhancing mass is seen in the right lateral face (arrow).

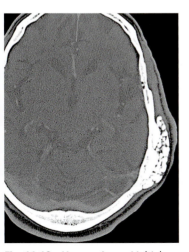

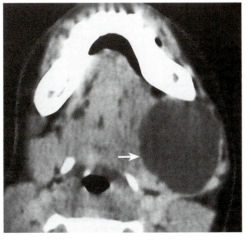

Fig. 11.18   Hemangioma. Multiple calcifications (phleboliths) are seen in a scalp lesion with induction of new bone formation in the adjacent outer table of the skull.

Fig. 11.19   Lymphangioma. A large cystic mass projects behind the left mandibular angle.

IV   Musculoskeletal System

Table 11.7 (Cont.) Soft tissue lesions

Disease	CT Findings	Comments
Neurofibroma and neurilemoma (schwannoma) ▷ *Fig. 11.20*	Well-defined, homogeneous lesions with marked enhancement after IV contrast administration. **Plexiform (cirsoid) neurofibromas**, found only in neurofibromatosis, present as poorly circumscribed inhomogeneous lesion with potential for malignant transformation.	Solitary neurofibromas and neurilemoma (benign schwannoma, neurinoma) are slow-growing lesions found most commonly in the third to fifth decades of life. The CT appearance of neurofibrosarcomas (▷ *Fig. 11.21*) and malignant schwannomas (▷ *Fig. 11.22*) is similar to their benign counterparts. They occur in approximately 50% of patients with neurofibromatosis.
Morton neuroma	Well-defined, often dumbbell-shaped lesion between metatarsal heads, frequently associated with intermetatarsal bursitis.	Fibrous response to mechanical impingement of an interdigital plantar nerve most often between the heads of the third and fourth metatarsals. Female predominance (high-heel shoes).
Elastofibroma ▷ *Fig. 11.23*	Unilateral or bilateral (25%), subscapular lesion of lenticular shape typically located between the inferior scapula and chest wall.	Benign, usually asymptomatic, tumorlike, fibrous lesion secondary to mechanical friction. Found in middle-aged and elderly persons with female predominance. May contain adipose tissue.
Chondroma	Well-demarcated soft tissue mass containing curvilinear, ringlike or nodular calcifications. Intracapsular chondromas arise most often in the knee.	Occurs predominantly in the third and fourth decades of life, especially in hands and feet.
Other benign soft tissue tumors ▷ *Fig. 11.24*	Well-defined, homogeneous soft tissue masses with usually moderate, uniform enhancement after IV contrast administration.	Fibroma, benign fibrous histiocytoma, giant cell tumor of the tendon sheath (hands and feet), rhabdomyoma, and mesenchymoma.
Fibromatosis ▷ *Fig. 11.25a, b*	Variety of benign fibrous proliferation presenting as well or more commonly poorly defined homogeneous soft tissue lesions. May simulate a malignant lesion by infiltrating into the adjacent tissues and even bone. Recurrences are frequent.	**Desmoid** (▷ *Fig. 11.26a, b*) arises in abdominal and extraabdominal musculature (especially the shoulder area). **Nodular and proliferative fasciitis** occurs in the extremities of adults. **Recurring digital fibromas** occur in the fingers and toes of infants. **Palmar and plantar fibromatosis** are fibrous proliferations of the palmar and plantar fascia. **Juvenile aponeurotic fibroma** arises in the aponeurotic tissues of the hands and feet of young children. May calcify. **Congenital generalized fibromatosis** occurs in infants and may affect not only soft tissues but also viscera and bone.

(continues on page 480)

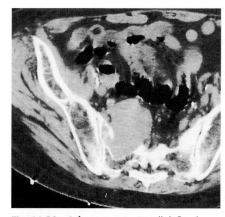

Fig. 11.20 Schwannoma. A well-defined homogeneous mass is eroding the adjacent sacral foramen.

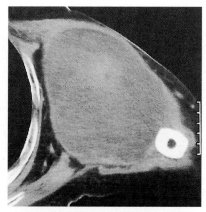

Fig. 11.21 Neurofibrosarcoma. A well-defined, huge, hypodense soft tissue mass arising from the left armpit is seen in this patient with neurofibromatosis.

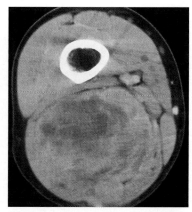

Fig. 11.22 Malignant schwannoma. A relatively poorly defined mass with inhomogeneous, hypodense central areas is evident in the thigh.

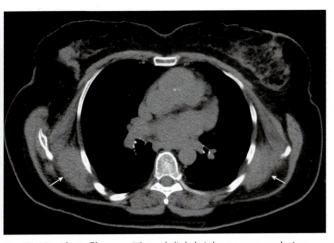

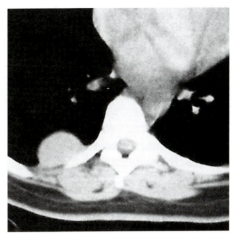

Fig. 11.23 Elastofibroma. Bilateral slightly inhomogeneous lesions (arrows) adjacent to the posterolateral chest wall just beneath the inferior scapular angles are seen.

Fig. 11.24 Pleural fibroma (benign mesothelioma). A well-defined homogeneous mass arises from the posterior pleura.

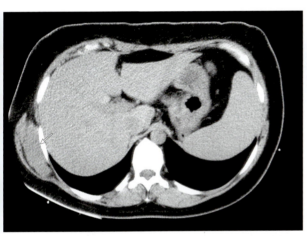

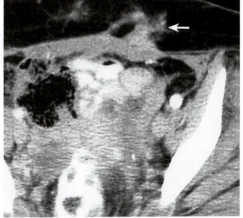

b

Fig. 11.25a, b Fibromatosis (two cases). A well-defined oblong soft tissue mass (**a**) is seen in the right posterolateral abdominal wall (arrow). A more aggressive lesion (**b**) is evident as a poorly defined soft tissue density in the left anterior abdominal wall (arrow).

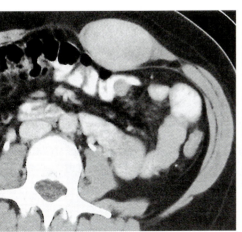

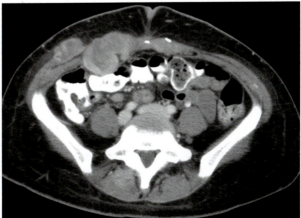

b

Fig. 11.26a, b Desmoid (two patients). An oval-shaped, homogeneous mass (**a**) is seen in the left anterior abdominal wall. Well-circumscribed, somewhat irregular outlined lesions (**b**) with hypodense centers are seen in the right anterior abdominal wall.

IV Musculoskeletal System

Table 11.7   (Cont.) Soft tissue lesions

Disease	CT Findings	Comments
Liposarcoma ▷ *Fig. 11.27a–c*	Well- or poorly defined, heterogeneous mass with a variable amount of fatty tissue. Because of their fibrous, myxomatous, and vascular elements, liposarcomas have a higher attenuation than lipomas and enhance with IV contrast. Calcification or ossification may be seen in well-differentiated sarcomas.	Common soft tissue malignancy of the middle-aged and elderly. Frequent involvement of the lower extremity. Histologically, five different types (well-differentiated, embryonal, myxoid, pleomorphic, and round cell) are recognized. With the exception of the well-differentiated liposarcoma, these neoplasms are highly malignant.
Malignant fibrous histiocytoma ▷ *Fig. 11.28*	Well- or poorly defined, inhomogeneous soft tissue mass, often with necrotic (hypodense) areas and considerable contrast enhancement. Erosion/destruction of an adjacent bone occurs. A periosteal reaction is, however, rare unless a pathologic fracture has occurred. Intratumoral calcifications are unusual.	Most common primary malignant soft tissue tumor. Occurs at all ages, most often around age 50 y. Slight male predominance. Lower extremity is the most frequent location. **Fibrosarcomas** have similar radiologic and histologic features but appear overall slightly less malignant. **Dermatofibrosarcoma protuberans** (▷ *Fig. 11.29*) presents as single or multiple nodules in the skin or subcutaneous tissue of the trunk and, less commonly, the extremities and the head and neck.
Rhabdomyosarcoma ▷ *Fig. 11.30*	Fairly well to poorly defined soft tissue mass. Erosion or invasion of the adjacent bone common. Inhomogeneous appearance after necrosis, hemorrhage, and cystic degeneration. **Leiomyosarcomas** (▷ *Fig. 11.31*) present in similar fashion, but large areas of tumor necrosis, which may eventually calcify, are common. These neoplasms are most often found in the retroperitoneum or thigh or may be associated with major blood vessels (e.g., saphenous vein).	Occurs usually under the age of 50 y. In adults, the tumor is usually located in the deeper tissues of the extremities and torso. In children, the tumor predominates in the head, neck, and urogenital tract. The benign **rhabdomyoma** is an extremely rare tumor of benign striated muscle cells.
Synovial sarcoma ▷ *Fig. 11.32a, b*	Relatively poorly defined, usually inhomogeneous mass with calcifications in 30% and erosion/destruction of adjacent bone without reactive sclerosis in 20% of cases.	Most frequently seen in the thigh and lower extremity, usually in young adults, but all ages can be affected. Calcified metastases are not uncommon, especially in the lungs, but they may be late (several years after initial diagnosis).

(continues on page 482)

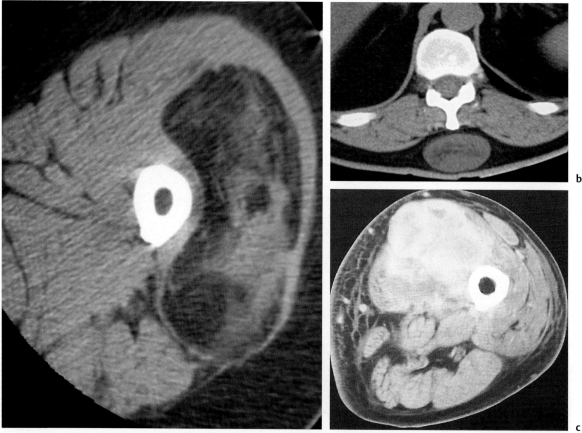

Fig. 11.27a–c   Liposarcoma (three different patients). A fatty mass (**a**) containing irregular soft tissue components is seen in the thigh. A well-circumscribed ovoid mass (**b**) containing only small amounts of fatty tissue in its center is seen posterior of the spine. A relatively well-defined heterogeneous mass (**c**) containing only a small amount of fatty tissue is seen in the anterior thigh.

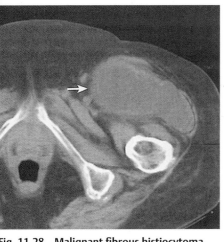

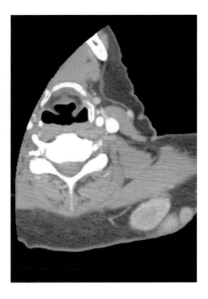

Fig. 11.29 Dermatofibrosarcoma protuberans. A subcutaneous lesion with a hypodense center and adjacent nodular thickening of the skin is seen.

Fig. 11.28 Malignant fibrous histiocytoma. A relatively poorly defined homogeneous soft tissue mass is evident (arrow).

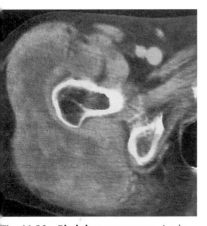

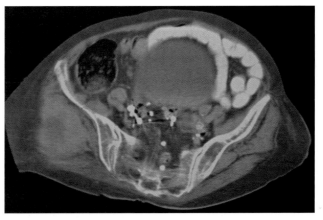

Fig. 11.30 Rhabdomyosarcoma. A relatively well-defined inhomogeneous mass surrounds the right proximal femur.

Fig. 11.31 Leiomyosarcoma. A large pear-shaped mass with a hypodense (necrotic) center is seen lateral to the right pelvis.

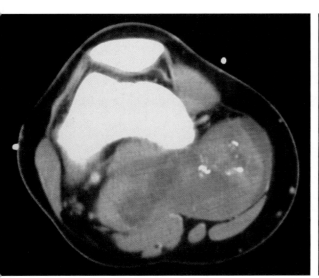

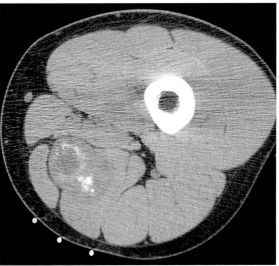

b

Fig. 11.32a, b Synovial sarcoma (two cases). A poorly defined mass with multiple irregular calcifications and slightly lower attenuation than the adjacent muscles is seen posterior to the knee (**a**) and in the semimembranosus muscle of the thigh (**b**).

IV Musculoskeletal System

Table 11.7 (Cont.) Soft tissue lesions

Disease	CT Findings	Comments
Other malignant soft tissue sarcomas ▷ *Fig. 11.33* ▷ *Fig. 11.34* ▷ *Fig. 11.35* ▷ *Fig. 11.36*	Well- or poorly defined mass lesions that may erode or invade the adjacent bone.	**Metastases, melanomas, lymphomas, extraosseous plasmacytomas, angiosarcomas, clear cell sarcomas** (also known as **malignant melanomas of soft parts**; arise in vicinity of tendons and aponeuroses, most commonly in the foot and ankle), **alveolar soft tissue sarcomas** (**malignant granular cell myoblastoma**) originating in muscles, **epithelioid sarcomas** (arising primarily in fingers, hands, and forearms of young adults), **Askin tumors** (neuroectodermal small cell tumors arising from intercostal nerves), and **primary soft tissue osteosarcomas, Ewing sarcomas, primitive neuroectodermal tumor (PNET),** and **chondrosarcomas.**
Abscess/pyomyositis ▷ *Fig. 11.37* ▷ *Fig. 11.38* ▷ *Fig. 11.39*	Poorly defined, isodense or slightly hypodense mass (early stage) or, more commonly, well-defined cystic lesion with a relatively thick wall and occasionally septation. The attenuation value of the liquefied content frequently exceeds 25 HU. Enhancement of the nonliquefied components after contrast administration. Presence of soft tissue gas in the absence of surgical or percutaneous intervention is rare but virtually diagnostic.	Common causes of soft tissue abscesses include penetrating traumas, iatrogenic interventions, IV drug abuse, spread from a contiguous infection, and septic embolism. In **tuberculous spondylitis,** a fusiform psoas abscess with amorphous or teardrop-shaped calcifications is often associated (▷ *Fig. 11.40*).
Hematoma/ hemorrhage ▷ *Fig. 11.41* ▷ *Fig. 11.42*	Homogeneous enlargement of the involved muscle, which might be hyperdense in the acute stage. In the subacute stage, the hematoma may be poorly defined and is either isodense or slightly hypodense. With liquefaction, it progresses to a patchy or inhomogeneous appearance. When completely liquefied, the hematoma again has a homogeneous density that is lower than muscle and may be surrounded by a pseudocapsule that enhances after contrast administration. A "hematocrit effect" caused by settling of the cellular elements within the liquefied hematoma is occasionally observed. Calcification and ossification (myositis ossificans) can occur in a later stage.	Soft tissue hemorrhage occurs spontaneously, following trauma or surgery, with a variety of bleeding disorders, and during anticoagulation therapy. Bleeding into a tumor or abscess is quite common.
Aneurysm/ pseudoaneurysm	Round soft tissue density with occasionally curvilinear calcification in the vicinity of a major artery. Inhomogeneous appearance when partially thrombosed. IV contrast administration is diagnostic.	Popliteal artery aneurysm is the most common aneurysmatic lesion found in the extremities and presents as a pulsatile mass.

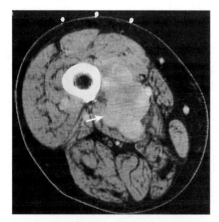

Fig. 11.33 Alveolar soft tissue sarcoma. A lobulated, relatively well-defined soft tissue mass is seen in the thigh (arrow).

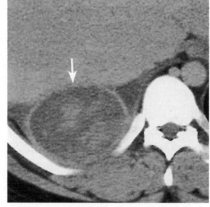

Fig. 11.34 Askin tumor. A well-defined, slightly inhomogeneous mass arising from the intercostal nerve projects between the posterior chest wall and liver (arrow).

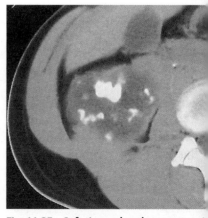

Fig. 11.35 Soft tissue chondrosarcoma. A relatively well-defined soft tissue mass with scattered calcifications is seen.

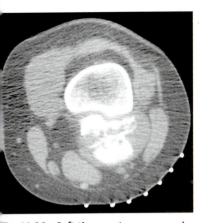

Fig. 11.36   Soft tissue osteosarcoma. An irregular ossified mass not attached to the distal femur is seen.

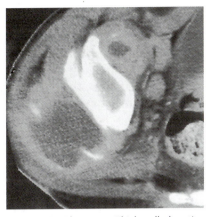

Fig. 11.37   Abscesses. Thick-walled cystic lesions are seen projecting medially and laterally to the ischium in this paraplegic patient with decubitus ulcers. Note also the thick periosteal reaction along the lateral aspect of the ischium.

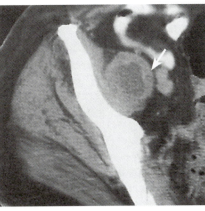

Fig. 11.38   Abscess. The iliopsoas abscess presents a cystic lesion with an irregular thick wall (arrow).

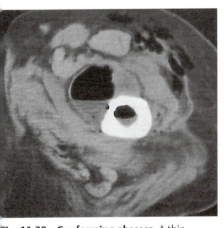

Fig. 11.39   Gas-forming abscess. A thin-walled cystic lesion with air–fluid level projects anteromedial to the left femur. A second fluid level is seen in the femur. Note also the irregular gas collections in the anterolateral soft tissues of the thigh.

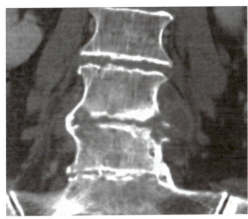

Fig. 11.40   Psoas abscess in tuberculous spondylitis. Disk space narrowing with erosion of the adjacent end plates most apparent at the adjacent corners of the L4–L5 vertebral bodies is seen. On the right side, the tuberculous infection is sealed off by a bridging periosteal reaction; on the left side, a tuberculous psoas abscess presenting as an oblong soft tissue mass containing loculated hypodense foci and two small calcifications is seen.

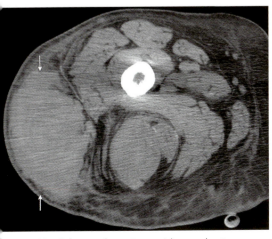

Fig. 11.41   Subacute hematoma. A large subcutaneous mass (arrows) isodense to muscle is seen.

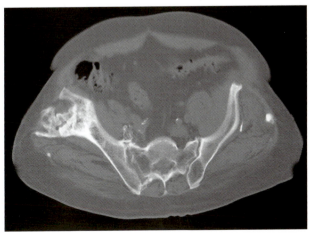

Fig. 11.42   Traumatic myositis ossificans. A healing right iliac crest fracture with extensive surrounding heterotopic bone formation is seen.

IV   Musculoskeletal System

12 Joint Disease

Francis A. Burgener

The diagnosis of articular disorders is primarily made by conventional radiography. Computed tomography (CT) is useful to assess the extent of both bone and soft tissue involvement. Para-articular soft tissue masses such as synovial cysts and abscesses are readily depicted by CT (**Fig. 12.1**). In skeletal trauma with joint involvement, CT can be very valuable to accurately define fractures and dislocations and to delineate intra-articular osteochondral fragments that may escape detection by plain film radiography. This is particularly true for the evaluation of joints that either have a complex anatomy or are difficult, if not impossible, to visualize in two perpendicular planes by conventional radiography. An example of the latter is the diagnosis of a *sternoclavicular joint dislocation* that is difficult to ascertain by conventional imaging technique but is easily documented by CT, as the dislocated clavicle is usually located anteriorly or occasionally posteriorly to the adjacent sternum (**Fig. 12.2**).

Each *sacroiliac joint* consists of two articulations: the posterosuperior two thirds of the joint are syndesmotic, and the anteroinferior one third is synovial. Sacroiliac joints are difficult to analyze on plain films, and their interpretation is greatly facilitated by CT. The normal synovial sacroiliac joint measures 2 to 4 mm in width; the ligamentous portion of the joint is more variable and wider. Normal sacroiliac joints are symmetric and without erosions, sclerosis, and fusions. Widening of the sacroiliac joints is commonly found in *traumatic diastasis* (**Fig. 12.3**), where it can be unilateral or bilateral, and in *primary or secondary hyperparathyroidism* (**Fig. 12.4**). Unilateral widening of a sacroiliac joint associated with erosions, destruction, and sclerosis suggests an infectious process (**Fig. 12.5**). Occasionally, widening of the sacroiliac joints is also observed in the early (erosive) stage in a variety of inflammatory diseases, such as ankylosing spondylitis, enteropathic spondyloarthropathy, Reiter syndrome, psoriasis, and rheumatoid arthritis. These conditions, however, tend to progress to a more characteristic joint space narrowing and eventual fusion. Associated erosions and

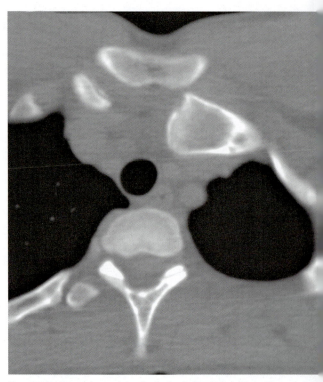

Fig. 12.2 Posterior sternoclavicular joint dislocation. The medial end of the left clavicle is posteromedially displaced with regard to the sternal manubrium.

particularly sclerosis are always more pronounced on the iliac side of the joint.

Sacroiliitis can be differentiated by both distribution and morphology of the articular changes. A bilateral and symmetrical involvement of the sacroiliac joints with poorly defined erosions and adjacent sclerosis, joint space narrowing, intra-articular

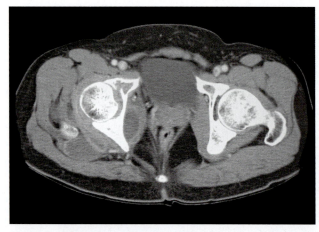

Fig. 12.1 Tuberculous arthritis. A destructive lesion in the anterior wall of the right acetabulum and several hypodense soft tissue abscesses surrounding the right hip are seen.

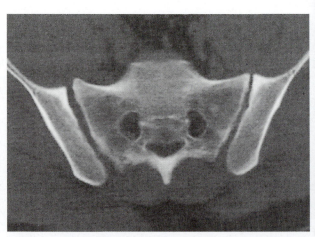

Fig. 12.3 Traumatic diastasis of the right sacroiliac joint. Compared with the normal left side, the right sacroiliac joint is widened.

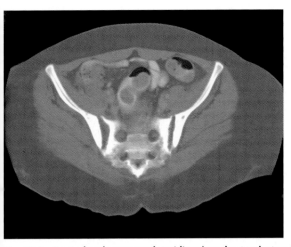

Fig. 12.4   Secondary hyperparathyroidism (renal osteodystrophy). Symmetric widening of both sacroiliac joints with adjacent sclerosis is caused by extensive subchondrial bony resorption.

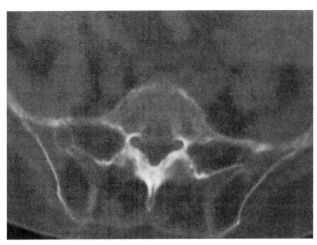

Fig. 12.6   Ankylosing spondylitis. Complete symmetric osseous fusion of both sacroiliac joints is seen.

osseous fusion, and ligamentous ossification is characteristic for *ankylosing spondylitis* (**Fig. 12.6**) and *enteropathic spondyloarthropathy*. In *psoriasis* and *Reiter syndrome,* the sacroiliac joint involvement is usually bilateral but characteristically asymmetric and associated with extensive sclerosis, particularly on the ilium, and occasional fusion. Both conditions must be differentiated from *osteitis condensans ilii* (**Fig. 12.7**), where a symmetric triangular sclerosis of the inferior aspect of the ilium is not associated with any sacroiliac joint abnormality. In *rheumatoid arthritis,* sacroiliac joint manifestations occur only late in the disease and include bilateral superficial erosions with minimal sclerosis but usually without bony ankylosis. In *primary* and *secondary hyperparathyroidism (renal osteodystrophy),* subchondral bone resorption results in symmetric widening of the sacroiliac joints with adjacent sclerosis (**Fig. 12.8**). Unilateral sacroiliac joint involvement suggests infectious or posttraumatic joint disease. *Pyogenic sacroiliitis* occurs commonly in intravenous drug abusers, and CT may demonstrate an associated soft tissue abscess besides erosive and sclerotic changes in the involved sacroiliac joint (**Fig. 12.9**). *Degenerative sacroiliac joint disease* is relatively frequently seen in patients older than 40 y.

Narrowing of the joint space, sclerosis with usually smooth subchondral bone margins, and anterior osteophytes progressing occasionally to complete bony bridging of the sacroiliac joint can be encountered. Rarely, small subchondral cysts that may simulate erosions are also present. Occasionally, these cysts contain air (pneumatocysts) (**Fig. 12.10**). Many other arthritic processes such as gout and calcium pyrophosphate deposition disease (CPDD) may rarely affect the sacroiliac joints also, but they have no characteristic features. *Sacroiliitis circumscripta* (**Fig. 12.11**) is a nonspecific localized inflammatory process of unknown etiology presenting initially with superficial erosions with subsequent sclerosis and eventually a bridging osteophyte anteriorly.

Pelvic trauma may involve the sacroiliac joint and can be difficult to detect with conventional radiographs. Diastasis of one or both sacroiliac joints (**Fig. 12.12**) may be associated with separation of the pubic symphysis ("pelvic dislocation"). Unilateral sacroiliac joint dislocation associated with a fracture of the ipsilateral superior and inferior pubic rami is termed a *Malgaigne-type pelvic fracture/dislocation,* whereas the sacroiliac joint dissociation with fracture of the contralateral pubic rami

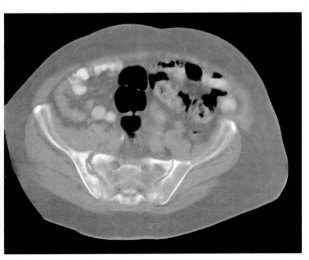

Fig. 12.5   Pyogenic sacroiliitis. Irregular erosion is seen in the right sacroiliac joint. A small bony fragment projects within the joint. Note also the soft tissue swelling anterior to the right sacroiliac joint.

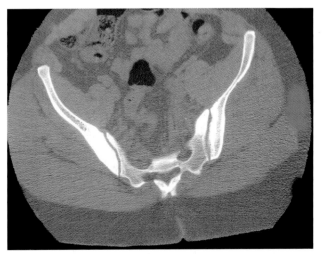

Fig. 12.7   Osteitis condensans ilii. The bilateral sclerosis of the ilium adjacent to the sacroiliac joints is not associated with any arthritic changes. On the left side, beginning sclerosis of the sacrum is also evident, which is not unusual in this condition.

IV Musculoskeletal System

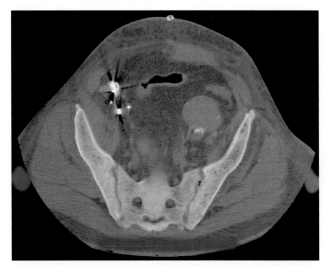

Fig. 12.8 Secondary hyperparathyroidism (renal osteodystrophy). Widening of both sacroiliac joints is caused by bony resorption. Diffuse bone sclerosis is also evident.

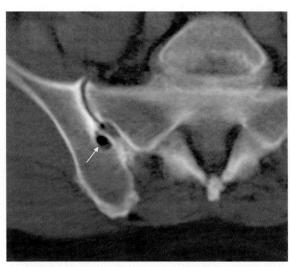

Fig. 12.10 Degenerative sacroiliac joint disease. Sclerosis of the subchondral bone, especially on the anterior iliac side, tiny osteophyte formations, and a pneumatocyst (arrow) are seen.

is a bucket handle–type injury. The pelvic ring is formed by the pelvis and sacrum. All conditions with at least two complete interruptions of the pelvic ring such as fractures or dislocations are unstable and require open or closed stabilization to prevent complete pelvic collapse.

The hip is a ball-and-socket joint consisting of the femoral head and the acetabulum. The latter is composed of the acetabular roof, the anterior and posterior wall, the quadrilateral lamina, and the anterior and posterior labrum. In contrast to conventional radiography, these parts can readily be discerned by CT with the exception of the fibrocartilaginous labrum and therefore assessed individually for disease involvement (**Fig. 12.13**).

Fractures involving various components of the acetabulum and femoral head can be diagnosed with high accuracy with proper anteroposterior, lateral, and oblique (Judet) views of the hip. However, in a multitrauma patient, adequate conventional radiographs cannot always be obtained. In these conditions, CT is useful in the detection of acetabular and femoral head fractures.

Compared to conventional radiography, the greatest contribution of CT consists of the accurate depiction of the fracture-dislocation pattern in the hip that dictates whether a particular injury will subject to open or closed reduction and treatment. This decision is largely dependent on the number and size of intra-articular bone fragments, fracture fragment displacement, and congruity between femoral head and acetabulum (**Fig. 12.14**). Usually these questions cannot be satisfactorily answered by conventional radiography.

Osteochondral fractures of the femoral head (capital fractures) are frequently associated with posterior hip dislocations caused by a pull of the ligamentum capitis femoris connecting the fovea of the femoral head with the transverse ligament at the bottom of the acetabulum (**Fig. 12.15**). These avulsion fractures are often difficult to diagnose by conventional technique and may eventually result in a clinical and radiographic picture that is impossible to differentiate from avascular necrosis of the femoral head.

Avascular necrosis (AVN) of the femoral head is caused by obstruction or disruption of its blood supply. The most common

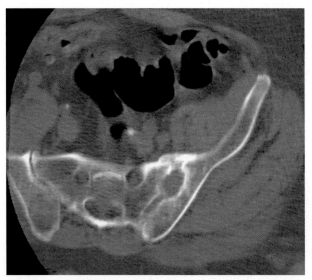

Fig. 12.9 Pyogenic sacroiliitis. A destructive lesion with surrounding sclerosis is seen in the anterior aspect of the left sacroiliac joint. Small hypodense foci in the adjacent enlarged iliopsoas muscle represent small abscesses.

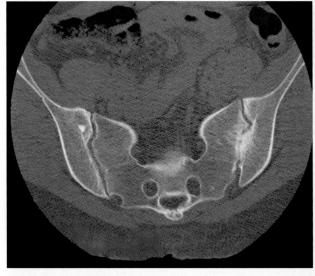

Fig. 12.11 Sacroiliitis circumscripta. Focal joint space narrowing with small erosions and adjacent sclerosis are seen in the midportion of the left sacroiliac joint.

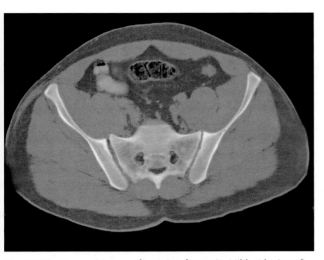

Fig. 12.12   Traumatic sacroiliac joint diastasis. Mild widening of the right sacroiliac joint with intact subchondral bone is seen.

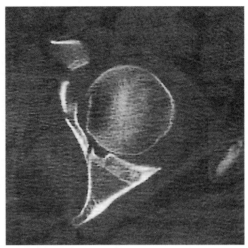

Fig. 12.14   Acetabular fracture. Fractures of the anterior osseous labrum, anterior wall, and quadrilateral lamina are seen, whereas both the posterior wall and osseous labrum are intact.

causes include sequelae of a femoral neck fracture, steroid therapy, sickle cell disease, and collagen vascular diseases (especially lupus erythematosus and rheumatoid arthritis). Less common causes of AVN include human immunodeficiency virus (HIV) infection, alcoholism, pancreatitis, a variety of vascular diseases, including arteriosclerosis, caisson disease (dysbaric osteonecrosis), Gaucher disease, amyloidosis, radiation therapy, and pregnancy. An idiopathic form of AVN of the hip can occur at any age, but it is most common in children between 4 and 7 y of age, where it is termed *Legg–Calvé–Perthes disease* (**Fig. 12.16**).

CT is less sensitive in diagnosing AVN of the hip than either nuclear medicine or magnetic resonance imaging (MRI). Compared with conventional radiography, CT upgrades the stage of AVN in approximately one third of cases, which may have consequences for the selection of the optimum therapy. In the normal hip, an asterisk-like condensation of bone in the center of the femoral head is seen on transaxial CT images at the level of the fovea caused by the crossing of compressive and tensile trabeculae (asterisk or star sign, **Fig. 12.17**). In early AVN, the well-defined and centrally located asterisk appears smudged by focal sclerosis and bone resorption, or, in slightly more advanced cases, the radiodense zone reaches the articular surface of the femoral head (**Fig. 12.18**). The following stages of AVN of the hip can be recognized: (1) minimal focal sclerosis and osteopenia; (2) distinct sclerosis and focal lucencies or cyst formation; (3) subchondral lucency (crescent sign) but without flattening (collapse) of the femoral head; (4) subchondral fracture and/or flattening of the femoral head; and (5) marked collapse of the femoral head with secondary arthritic changes, including joint space narrowing and acetabular involvement.

Femoroacetabular impingement (FAI) is caused by abnormal abutment between the proximal femur and adjacent acetabular rim in flexion and internal rotation, resulting in damaging of the acetabular labrum and cartilage with subsequent osteoarthritis.

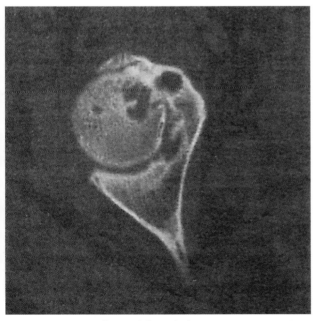

Fig. 12.13   Osteoarthritis of the right hip. Joint space narrowing, sclerosis, and geode formations are affecting almost exclusively the anterior part of the joint.

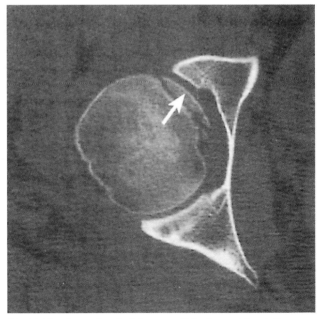

Fig. 12.15   Osteochondral fracture of the femoral head. Fracture was caused by a posterior hip dislocation, which is now reduced (arrow).

IV Musculoskeletal System

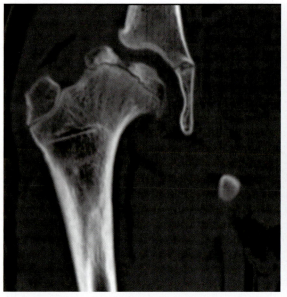
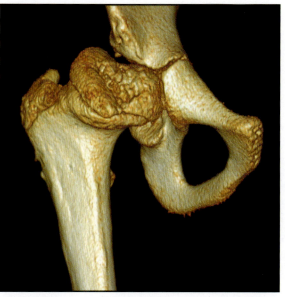

a   b

Fig. 12.16a, b Legg–Calvé–Perthes disease. An irregular flattened and fragmented femoral head epiphysis is associated with a wide femoral neck and a slightly dysplastic acetabulum (**a**, coronal; **b**, three-dimensional reconstruction).

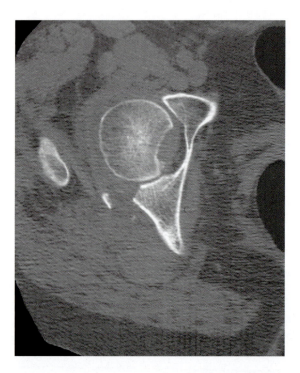

Fig. 12.17 Normal asterisk or star sign. An asterisk-like condensation of bone is seen in the center of the femoral head that is caused by the crossing of compressive and tensile trabeculae. Sequelae of complete reduction of a posterior hip dislocation are also evident and include an avulsion fracture of the posterior osseous acetabular rim and a fracture of the femoral head evident as a crescent-shaped defect in its medial aspect.

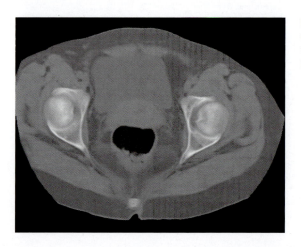

Fig. 12.18 Avascular necrosis of both femoral heads. The normal asterisk (see Fig. 12.17) is smudged by focal sclerosis that reaches the articular surface of the femoral head. Beginning fragmentation of the left femoral head in its medial portion is also suspected.

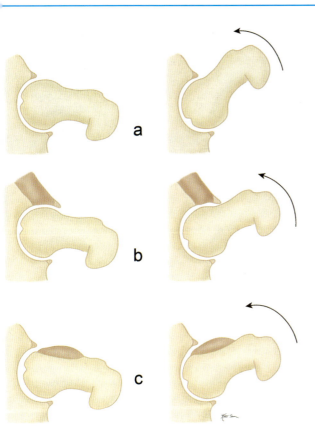

Fig. 12.19a–c   Femoral acetabular impingement (FAI). (a) Normal (axial). Sufficient joint clearance allows unrestricted range of motion. **(b)** Pincer impingement. Excessive acetabular overcoverage (shaded area) results in contact at the femoral head–neck junction and acetabular rim. **(c)** Cam impingement. Aspherical portion of the femoral head–neck junction (shaded area) is jammed into the acetabulum. (Modified from Tannast M, Siebenrock KA, Anderson SE. Femoroacetabular impingement: radiographic diagnosis—what the radiologist should know. AJR Am J Roentgenol 2007;188:1540–1552.)

A cam-type impingement caused by a bony prominence or bump of the anterolateral femur head–neck junction is differentiated from a pincer-type impingement caused by overcoverage of the femoral head by the acetabulum. Acetabular overcoverage results from acetabular retroversion (posteriorly rotated acetabulum), coxa profunda (deep acetabular socket extending on conventional radiographs medial to the ilioischial line), or protrusio acetabuli (acetabular protrusion into the pelvis). FAI is most commonly caused by a combination of both types (mixed cam–pincer type) (**Figs. 12.19, 12.20**).

CT findings of the cam-type FAI may also include, besides the bony bump at the anterolateral femur head–neck junction (sometimes referred to as a "pistol grip" deformity), a femoral osteophyte posterolateral to the osseous bump (bump–osteophyte complex), herniation pit (synovial or fibrocartilaginous defect with thin sclerotic border anterolateral in the proximal femur neck), and thickened iliofemoral ligament. Acetabular findings in the pincer-type impingement may include, besides retroversion, coxa profunda, or protrusio acetabuli, acetabular rim osteophytes, an os acetabuli, subchondral sclerosis, and labral (paralabral) cysts. FAI typically presents in young, physically active patients and if untreated may progress to premature full-blown osteoarthritis with its characteristic imaging findings.

Plain-film radiography and MRI are the main imaging methods for evaluation of the knee. MRI is far superior to CT in the assessment of ligamentous, meniscal, and articular cartilage pathology.

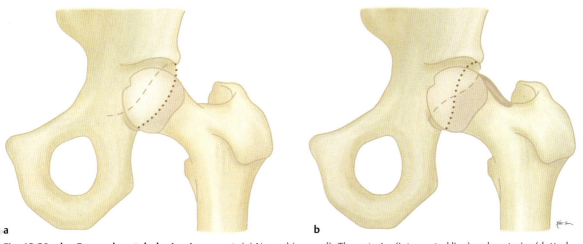

Fig. 12.20a, b   Femoral acetabular impingement. (a) Normal (coronal). The anterior (interrupted line) and posterior (dotted line) osseous rim of the acetabulum do not cross over. The contour of the femoral head–neck junction is normal. **(b)** Mixed pincer and cam impingement (combined type). Because of acetabular retroversion, the anterior (interrupted line) and posterior (dotted line) osseous acetabular rim do cross over, producing the cross-over sign or the "figure 8" configuration. In addition, a "pistol grip" deformity is evident in the proximal femur, produced by bone apposition of the superolateral aspect of the femoral head–neck junction (shaded area).

IV Musculoskeletal System

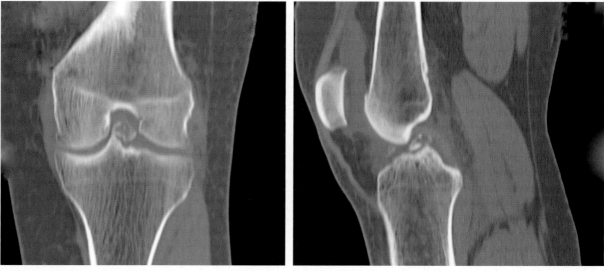

a   b

Fig. 12.21a, b   Loose intra-articular bodies. Coronal (**a**) and sagittal (**b**) views show several small loose bodies in the intercondylic notch of the distal femur.

CT might be useful in identifying intra-articular loose bodies in such conditions as osteochondritis dissecans, osteochondromatosis, and a variety of arthritic joint diseases (e.g., degenerative, neuropathic, posttraumatic, infectious, CPDD, hydroxyapatite crystal deposition disease [HADD], and ochronosis) (**Fig. 12.21**).

Spontaneous osteonecrosis of the knee (SONK, Ahlbäck disease) (**Fig. 12.22**) typically affects elderly, predominantly female patients with acute medial joint pain. It characteristically involves the weight-bearing surface of the medial femoral condyle, although the lateral femoral condyle and the tibia plateau may occasionally be affected. More recently, an insufficiency fracture in an osteoporotic patient has also been implicated as

etiology besides the vascular pathogenesis. Mild flattening of the weight-bearing aspect of the femoral condyle associated with an area of radiolucency with sclerosis proximal to it precedes the full-blown picture of a radiolucent focus surrounded by a sclerotic halo associated with a collapsed subchondral bone. In contrast, *osteochondritis dissecans* (**Fig. 12.23**) most commonly affects the non–weight-bearing portion of the medial femoral condyle in the intercondylic notch area and occurs primarily in young male patients.

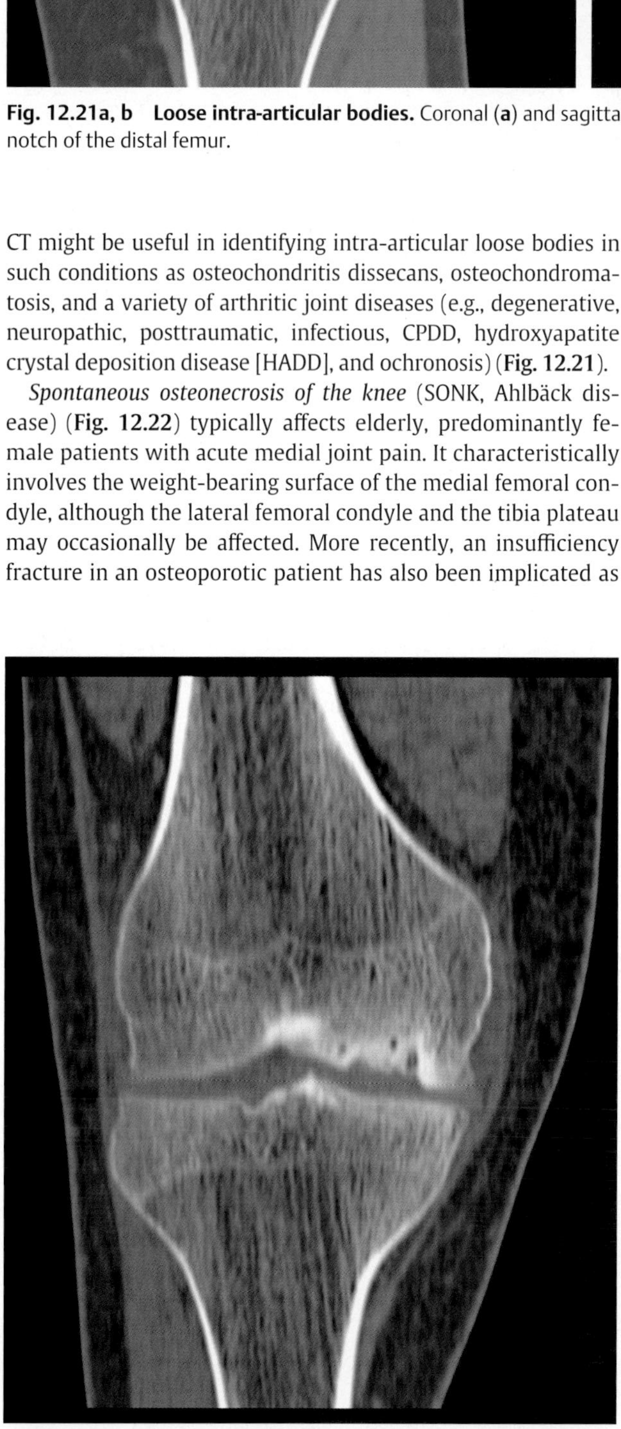

CT, including reformatted coronal and sagittal scans, can be useful in the accurate delineation of fractures of both the femur condyles and tibial plateau (**Fig. 12.24**). The degree of subchondral depression and fracture fragment displacement are crucial factors in the selection of the treatment modality (e.g., conservative vs surgical intervention).

Fractures of the ankle and foot are reliably diagnosed with conventional radiography. CT may be useful in these cases to assess fragment displacement and joint involvement and to identify the number and position of loose bodies (**Fig. 12.25**). CT may also depict subtle fractures and subluxations, especially in the tarsal bones, that may escape detection with conventional technique. For both therapeutic and prognostic reasons, an accurate fracture assessment is particularly important in the tibial plafond, the dome of the talus, the subtalar joints, and the tarsometatarsal joints (Lisfranc joint). Accompanying soft tissue injuries, including trapped soft tissue structures and lacerated ligaments and tendons, may also be diagnosed, but their CT evaluation is inferior to MRI. Nevertheless, the bony structures in the ankle and foot are well suited for CT evaluation, as images in different planes can be obtained by reformation of the axial images.

CT is effective in diagnosing *tarsal coalitions* that may be complete or incomplete and composed of fibrous (40%), cartilaginous (10%), or osseous (50%) tissue. Coalitions commonly occur between the calcaneus and navicular and between the talus and calcaneus, less frequently between the talus and navicular, and rarely between the calcaneus and cuboid (**Figs. 12.26, 12.27**). Occasionally, more than two tarsal bones are affected. Fusion between the talus and calcaneus most frequently occurs at the level of the sustentaculum tali (**Fig. 12.28**) and may be difficult to demonstrate by plain film radiography. Coalition of the posterior subtalar facet joint is not uncommon either. Reformatted coronal images are most useful for the unequivocal

Fig. 12.22   Spontaneous osteonecrosis of the knee (SONK, Ahlbäck disease). An irregular osteochondral defect with secondary sclerosis is seen in the weight-bearing portion of the medial femoral condyle.

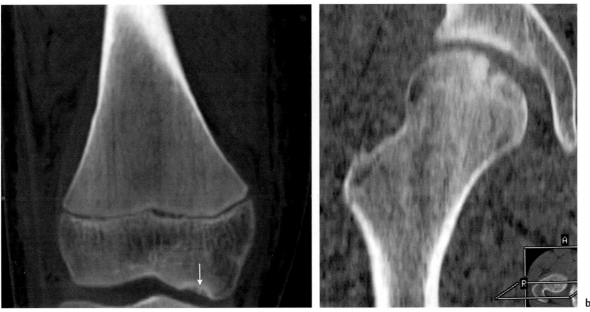

Fig. 12.23a, b   Osteochondritis dissecans. An osteochondral lesion is seen in the medial femur condyle (**a**) and the femoral head (**b**).

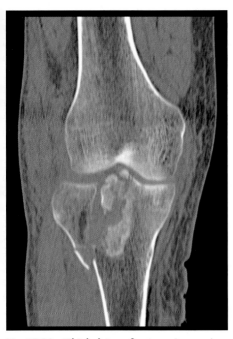

Fig. 12.24   Tibial plateau fracture. A comminuted intra-articular fracture with several loose fracture fragments is seen involving both the medial and lateral tibial plateau and the intercondylic area.

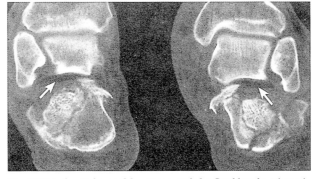

Fig. 12.25a, b   Calcaneal fractures with fat-fluid levels. Bilateral comminuted calcaneal fractures with fat–fluid levels (arrows) in both subtalar joints are seen.

IV Musculoskeletal System

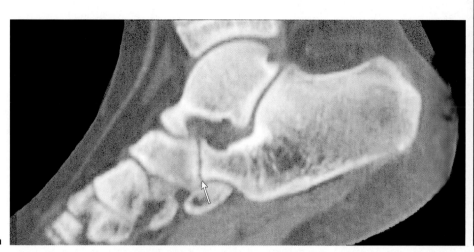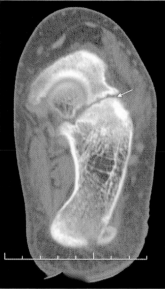

a

Fig. 12.26a, b   Fibrous calcaneonavicular coalition. Sagittal (**a**) and coronal (**b**) views demonstrate what appears to be a joint between the calcaneus and navicular (arrow) with severe degenerative changes.

demonstration of this coalition. In case of a fibrous or cartilaginous union, secondary changes such as close apposition of the involved joints, sclerosis of the articular margins, and cortical irregularities may be evident. Hypoplasia of the talar head and/ or a talar beak arising characteristically at the talonavicular joint may also be associated with tarsal coalitions. This talar beak has to be differentiated from the more common degenerative talar spur that originates at the insertion of the talonavicular joint capsule and is therefore not directly contiguous with the distal articular surface of the talus.

CT is useful for displaying various shoulder fractures, including Hill–Sachs compression fractures, involving the posterolateral humeral head, and osseous Bankart lesions, involving the anteroinferior glenoid rim, both of which are commonly associated with anterior glenohumeral dislocations (**Fig. 12.29**). The glenoid labrum is best evaluated with CT double-contrast arthrography. The normal glenoid labrum is a fibrocartilaginous structure with smooth margins. It is triangular-shaped anteriorly and more rounded and thicker posteriorly. With shoulder instability pattern and recurrent dislocations, the labrum may be blunted, frayed, embedded with iodinated contrast material, and partially or completely torn. CT arthrotomography demonstrates associated capsular and rotator cuff tears, loose bodies, joint cartilage abnormalities, synovial hypertrophy, and anomalies of the intra-articular portion of the long biceps tendon, which may be either displaced from its normal location in the bicipital groove or completely absent, indicating a complete tear.

In the complex articulations of the elbow and wrist, CT may be useful for the identification of subtle fractures and subluxations that are not recognized by conventional methods (**Fig. 12.30**). Fracture complications such as nonunion and avascular necrosis (e.g., in the scaphoid) are also effectively evaluated by CT (**Figs. 12.31, 12.32**).

The *temporomandibular joint* is divided by a disk that may dislocate, usually in an anterior direction. CT is comparable to arthrography in diagnosing this condition, as the disk can be accurately localized because of its relatively high CT density in excess of 60 HU. However, MRI is the imaging procedure of choice in this condition, as it demonstrates disk displacement as well as other joint pathology far better than CT.

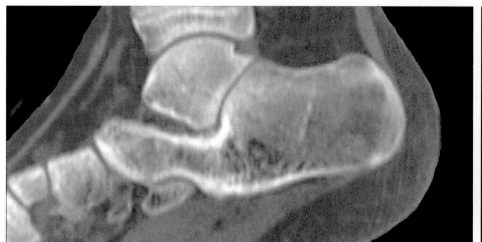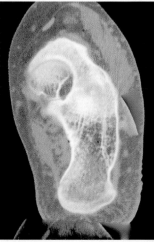

a

Fig. 12.27a, b   Osseous calcaneonavicular coalition. Sagittal (**a**) and coronal (**b**) views demonstrate an osseous connection between the calcaneus and navicular.

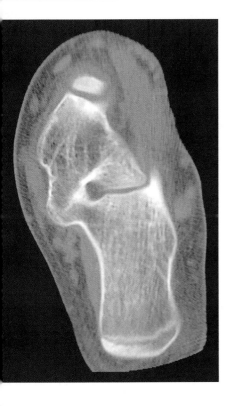

Fig. 12.28 Osseous talocalcaneal coalition. An osseous connection at the level of the sustentaculum tali is seen. The posterior subtalar facet joint projecting laterally of the sustentaculum tali remains open.

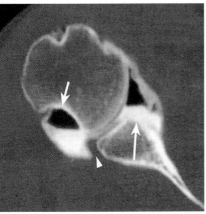

Fig. 12.29 Shoulder arthrotomography. A Hill–Sachs defect (short arrow) and a Bankart lesion (torn anterior glenoid labrum, long arrow) are seen in this patient with a history of anterior shoulder dislocations. Note the normal posterior glenoid labrum (arrowhead).

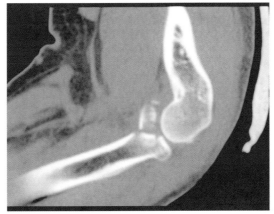

Fig. 12.30 Radial head fracture. A comminuted fracture with several loose intra-articular fragments is seen.

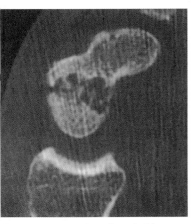

Fig. 12.31 Nonunion of scaphoid fracture. An irregular widened fracture line without evidence of bony bridging is seen.

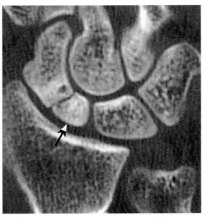

Fig. 12.32 Avascular necrosis of the scaphoid. Both sclerosis and collapse of the proximal scaphoid fracture fragment are diagnostic (arrow).

IV Musculoskeletal System

13 Generalized Bone Disease

Francis A. Burgener

Bone consists of three major components: the mineralized structure, the red marrow, and the yellow marrow. In the mineral component, cancellous or trabecular bone is surrounded by compact or cortical bone. Computed tomography (CT) is an excellent method to analyze the mineralized component, whereas magnetic resonance imaging (MRI) is the method of choice for the evaluation of red and yellow marrow.

Diseases affecting either the mineralized structure or the bone marrow may increase or decrease the bony mass. *Osteosclerosis* is caused by an increased activity of osteoblasts or by osteogenic or chondrogenic tumor cells forming bonelike tissue. Diffuse osteosclerosis is most commonly associated with sickle cell disease (**Fig. 13.1**) and renal osteodystrophy (secondary hyperparathyroidism) (**Fig. 13.2**). Other causes are myelofibrosis (**Fig. 13.3**), fluorosis (with preferential axial skeletal involvement and ligamentous calcifications), mastocytosis, osteopetrosis, and pyknodysostosis. Diffuse osteosclerosis is common in extensive metastatic disease, especially from breast and prostatic carcinomas (**Fig. 13.4**), lymphoma (especially Hodgkin disease) (**Fig. 13.5**), and Paget disease (**Fig. 13.6**), but in these conditions, it is usually not uniform even with extensive involvement. Major causes of widespread or diffuse osteosclerosis in the adult are summarized in **Table 13.1**.

Osteopenia is defined as a decrease in bone density regardless of its etiology. The bone density correlates with both osteoid matrix mass and its calcification. Causes of generalized osteopenia include osteoporosis, osteomalacia, hyperparathyroidism, and bone marrow hyperplasia. In osteoporosis, the osteoid matrix is reduced but normally calcified. In osteomalacia, the osteoid matrix is inadequately mineralized. In hyperparathyroidism, bone resorption is accelerated by an increased osteoclast to osteoblast ratio that is often associated with insufficient matrix calcification. In myeloproliferative disorders (e.g., thalassemia, leukemia, and multiple myeloma), the bone mass is partially replaced by the hypercellular bone marrow

(**Table 13.2**). CT can also be used to accurately measure bone mineral content. A description of this technique is beyond the scope of this chapter, especially because this method has largely been replaced by dual energy x-ray absorptiometry (DEXA-scan).

Generalized osteoporosis is characterized by cortical thinning and reduction in both the number and thickness of, preferentially, the non–weight-bearing trabeculae (**Fig. 13.7**). The disease is most prominent in the axial skeleton, particularly the vertebral column. The involved vertebral bodies may be wedge-shaped, biconcave ("fish vertebrae"), or compressed. Protrusion of portions of the intervertebral disk through the end plates into the vertebral body (Schmorl nodes) may also be present.

A spotty osteoporosis is occasionally found in the appendicular skeleton near a joint and indicates a more acute process. It is usually associated with disuse and immobilization or found with reflex sympathetic dystrophy (RSD, also known as complex regional pain syndrome), transient regional osteoporosis, and rheumatoid or septic arthritis. In these conditions, the osteoporosis may also present either as homogeneous juxta-articular loss of bone density or as bandlike lucent areas in the subchondral and metaphyseal bone. Spotty and bandlike osteoporosis may at times be difficult to differentiate from malignancy, although the latter condition tends to primarily involve the cancellous bone and spare the cortical bone, with the exception of endosteal scalloping. **Table 13.3** summarizes disorders with regional or localized osteoporosis.

Osteoporosis is often complicated by fractures commonly involving the lower thoracic and lumbar spine, hips, distal radius, and ribs. *Insufficiency fractures* may present as poorly defined irregular sclerotic bands or radiolucent lines, preferably in the pubic rami and symphysis, the supra-acetabular area, sacrum, femoral neck, and proximal and distal tibia. A cortical break is not always appreciated in these conditions. Insufficiency fractures presenting in the diametaphyses of long tubular bones as poorly defined sclerotic bands have to be differentiated from

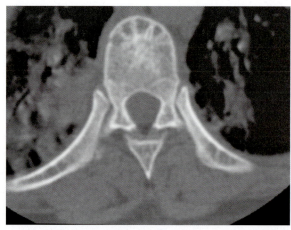
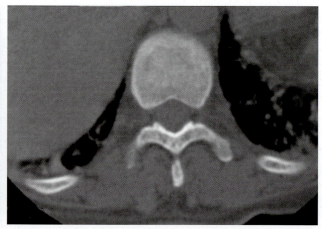

Fig. 13.1a, b Sickle cell disease. A diffuse increase in bone density is seen in T10 (**a**) and L1 (**b**) vertebrae. The cystic changes in the anterior aspect of T10 and the adjacent poorly defined localized sclerosis are likely the sequelae of osteonecrosis.

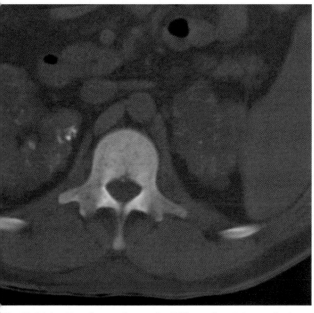

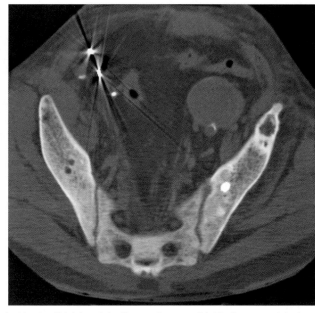

b

Fig. 13.2a, b   Renal osteodystrophy. Diffuse sclerosis is seen in the vertebral body of L1 (**a**) and the ilium and sacrum (**b**). The larger cystic lesion with sclerotic border in the left iliac crest represents a brown tumor. Note also the bone resorption in the sacroiliac joints, especially on the left side.

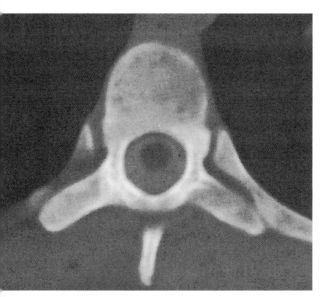

Fig. 13.3   Myelofibrosis. Diffuse sclerosis of the entire vertebral body and adjacent ribs is seen.

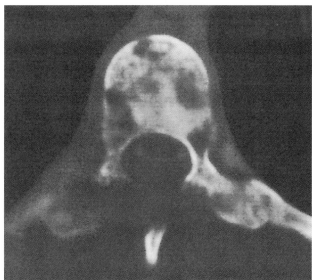

Fig. 13.4   Osteoblastic metastasis from breast carcinoma. Nonhomogeneous sclerosis with destructive lesions in the posterior elements and adjacent ribs is seen.

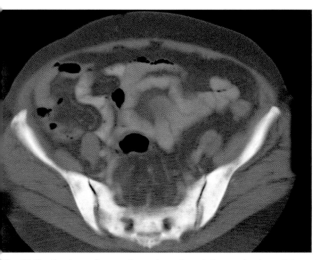

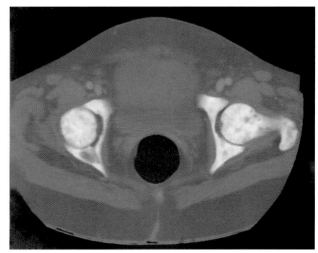

b

Fig. 13.5a, b   Lymphoma. Extensive sclerosis is seen in the pelvis and sacrum (**a**) and both hips (**b**).

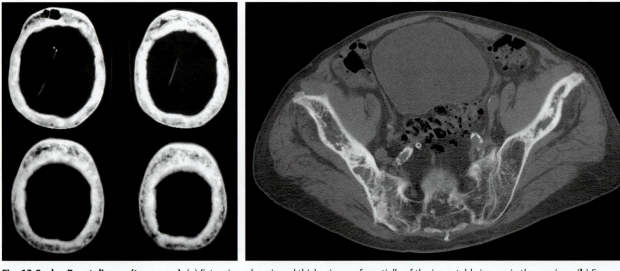

a

Fig. 13.6a, b   Paget disease (two cases). (a) Extensive sclerosis and thickening preferentially of the inner table is seen in the cranium. **(b)** Expansion of the ilium bilaterally associated with cortical thickening, coarse trabeculation, and scattered sclerotic foci is evident. Similar but less conspicuous findings are seen in the sacrum.

Table 13.1   Widespread or diffuse osteosclerosis

Sickle cell disease

Renal osteodystrophy

Metastases (especially from breast and prostatic carcinomas)

Lymphoma (especially histiocytic [large B-cell] and Hodgkin lymphoma)

Myelofibrosis and myeloid metaplasia

Fluorosis

Paget disease

Fibrous dysplasia (polyostotic form)

Mastocytosis

Tuberous sclerosis

Sarcoidosis

Oxalosis

Heavy metal poisoning (chronic)

Engelmann–Camurati disease (predominantly diaphyses of long bones, which may be spindle-shaped)

Van Buchem disease (diffuse sclerosis and cortical thickening of predominantly the tubular bones)

Erdheim–Chester disease (patchy or diffuse osteosclerosis and cortical thickening of major long bones with relative sparing of the epiphyses)

Vitamin D–resistant rickets (sclerosis of mainly the axial skeleton in the adult)

Hypoparathyroidism and pseudohypoparathyroidism

Hereditary hyperphosphatasia (juvenile Paget disease)

Osteopetrosis

Pyknodysostosis

Osteopoikilosis

Melorheostosis

Healing osteolytic process (e.g., metastases, multiple myeloma, leukemia, osteomalacia, rickets, and hyperparathyroidism)

Table 13.2   Generalized osteopenia

Osteoporosis

Postmenopausal, senile

Immobilization, disuse

Medication (chronic steroids and heparin)

Osteogenesis imperfecta

Nutritional deficiency (scurvy, malnutrition, nephrosis, chronic liver disease, and alcoholism)

Endocrinopathy (Cushing disease, hypogonadism, hyperthyroidism, Addison disease, acromegaly, diabetes mellitus, and pregnancy)

Connective tissue disease (e.g., rheumatoid arthritis)

Homocystinuria

Idiopathic (e.g., juvenile osteoporosis)

Osteomalacia

Vitamin D deficiency (rickets and osteomalacia)

Malabsorption (diseases of gastrointestinal tract, hepatobiliary system, and pancreas)

Dietary calcium deficiency

Vitamin D–resistant rickets (x-linked hypophosphatemia)

Renal tubular acidosis

Fanconi syndrome

Chronic anticonvulsant drug therapy (e.g., phenytoin [Dilantin])

Hypophosphatasia

Hyperparathyroidism

Primary, secondary, and tertiary

Bone marrow hyperplasia

Hemolytic anemias (e.g., thalassemia major)

Leukemia

Multiple myeloma

Extensive osteolytic metastases

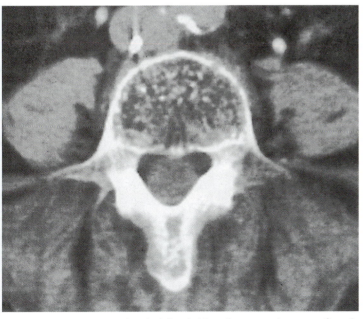

Fig. 13.7   Osteoporosis. Sharply defined, thinned cortex and accentuation of vertical trabeculae are characteristic.

Table 13.3   Regional or localized osteoporosis

Immobilization, disuse

Reflex sympathetic dystrophy (RSD, complex regional pain syndrome [CRPS])

Transient regional osteoporosis (transient bone marrow edema, including transient osteoporosis of the hip and regional migratory osteoporosis of lower extremities)

Radiation therapy (early stage)

Burns and frostbites

Infection and inflammation (e.g., early acute osteomyelitis, tuberculosis, septic arthritis, and rheumatoid arthritis)

Paget diesase (lytic phase)

Fibrous dysplasia (purely lytic or "ground glass" appearance)

Neoplasm (e.g., osteolytic metastases, multiple myeloma, lymphoma, rarely other benign or malignant bone tumors)

reinforcement lines (bone bars) presenting as well-defined, thin sclerotic lines with a horizontal or oblique course.

In *osteomalacia,* the loss of bone mass is associated with indistinct trabeculae and a fuzzy interface between cortical and medullary bone. Osseous deformities (e.g., acetabular protrusions) and pseudofractures (Looser zones) in the pubic rami, medial aspect of the femoral neck, axillary margin of the scapula, and ribs may be observed. *Rickets* (osteomalacia in infants and children) is diagnosed by the characteristic changes in the tubular bones that include both poorly defined and poorly calcified epiphyses, widening of the physis, and widened, cupped, and frayed metaphyses.

In *hyperparathyroidism,* the loss of bone density is radiographically similar to osteomalacia. Subperiosteal bone resorption (especially the radial aspect of the proximal and middle phalanges of the second and third fingers and the medial margins of the proximal tibia) is, however, virtually diagnostic. Other associated features include cortical striations ("tunneling of the cortex"), subchondral bone resorption (e.g., widening of the sacroiliac, sternoclavicular, and acromioclavicular joints and pubic symphysis), subligamentous bone resorption (trochanters, ischial and humeral tuberosities, calcanei, and distal clavicles), chondrocalcinosis, brown tumors, soft tissue calcifications (especially arterial and para-articular), nephrocalcinosis, and nephroureterolithiasis. In *secondary hyperparathyroidism (renal osteodystrophy),* diffuse osteosclerosis, rather than osteopenia, is usually present.

Both bone marrow hyperplasia and neoplasia may induce generalized osteopenia and/or sclerosis. In *thalassemia major,* a reticulated or cystic trabecular pattern with widened medullary spaces and thinned cortices is characteristic (**Fig. 13.8**). Other typically associated features are Erlenmeyer flask deformities (flaring of the metaphyses and epiphyses of the long bones, especially distal femora), expanded posterior aspects of the ribs, widening of the diploic space of the skull with thinning of the outer table and dense radial striations traversing the thickened calvarium ("hair on end" appearance) with sparing of the base of the occiput, and poor pneumatization of the paranasal sinuses and mastoids.

In *sickle cell disease,* generalized osteosclerosis may be the dominant feature, mainly involving the axial skeleton. Signs of bone infarction in the long tubular bones are commonly associated with this condition. In other anemias (e.g., iron-deficiency anemia and hereditary spherocytosis), the skeletal abnormalities caused by marrow hyperplasia are generally less severe and usually inconspicuous.

The radiologic manifestations of many *lipid storage diseases* (e.g., Gaucher and Niemann–Pick diseases) are similar to bone marrow hyperplasia in anemias and include a generalized osteopenia, often with coarse trabecular pattern, cortical thinning and scalloping, and Erlenmeyer flask deformities. However, in *Gaucher disease,* avascular necrosis of the femoral heads, calcified bone infarcts, and discrete lytic lesions with or without sclerotic margins are characteristically associated.

Leukemias are divided into acute and chronic forms. Acute forms occur in both children (peak age 2–5 y) and adults, whereas chronic forms are prevalent in patients between 35 and 60 y of age. Skeletal manifestations are most common in acute childhood leukemia and least common in chronic forms. Diffuse osteopenia may be associated with radiolucent metaphyseal bands, irregular lytic foci with or without periosteal reaction, and occasionally increased thickness of

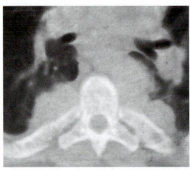 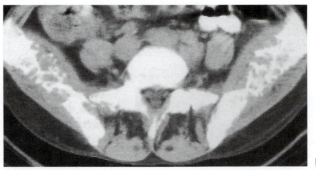

a   b

Fig. 13.8a, b   Thalassemia major. (a) A cystic trabecular pattern in the vertebra and adjacent widened ribs is associated with extramedullary hematopoiesis evident as bilateral paravertebral soft tissue masses. **(b)** A symmetric reticular pattern associated with soft tissue masses (extramedullary hematopoiesis) is found in both iliac wings.

bone trabeculae and areas of osteosclerosis. Because leukemia arises from the red bone marrow, bony manifestations in adults are largely limited to the axial skeleton, whereas in children, involvement occurs frequently in both the axial and appendicular bones.

Multiple myeloma (**Fig. 13.9**) characteristically presents as widespread osteolytic lesions with discrete margins of rather uniform size, more frequently involving the axial skeleton. Endosteal scalloping of the cortical bone is frequently observed with involvement of the appendicular skeleton. In the spine, preferential involvement of the vertebral bodies with paraspinal extension and sparing of the posterior elements is characteristic. Diffuse skeletal osteopenia without well-defined lytic foci, however, is the most common manifestation of the disease that simulates the appearance of osteoporosis. Primary focal or diffuse sclerotic lesions are rare in multiple myeloma. They are more often the consequence of irradiation, chemotherapy, or pathologic fracture of initially lytic multiple myeloma lesions.

Diffuse osteolytic skeletal metastases (**Fig. 13.10**) may at times be difficult to differentiate from multiple myeloma. Lytic bony metastases tend to be more variable in size and less well defined. In the spine, both vertebral bodies and posterior elements are involved with equal frequency, whereas in the long tubular bones, endosteal scalloping is not as commonly observed as in multiple myeloma.

Diffuse osteolytic, mixed, or sclerotic lesions similar to metastatic involvement may also be encountered in both Hodgkin disease and non–Hodgkin lymphoma (**Fig. 13.11**). It is normally a manifestation of generalized disease, although primary bony lesions occasionally occur with non–Hodgkin lymphoma. Approximately 20% of patients with widespread lymphoma

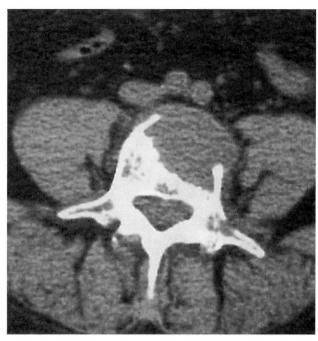

Fig. 13.10 Osteolytic metastasis from thyroid carcinoma. A lytic lesion is seen in the left anterior aspect of the vertebral body.

have skeletal involvement. In Hodgkin disease, the spine, pelvis (including the hips), ribs, and sternum are most commonly affected and tend to be sclerotic, whereas in non–Hodgkin lymphoma, the lesions predominate in the appendicular skeleton and are more often osteolytic.

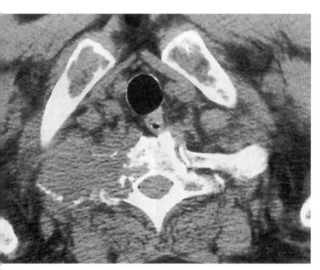

Fig. 13.9 Multiple myeloma. Lytic destructive lesions are evident in the vertebral body and transverse processes. An expansile lytic mass with virtually complete destruction of the bone is evident in the right posterior rib. Erosive and lytic lesions are also present in the left posterior rib and the sternal ends of both clavicles.

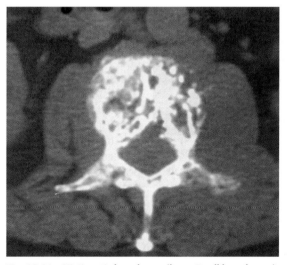

Fig. 13.11 Histiocytic lymphoma (large B-cell lymphoma). A coarse hemangioma-like pattern with extension into the posterior elements is characteristic. Paraspinal soft tissue involvement is also evident.

14 Localized Bone Disease

Francis A. Burgener

Most skeletal lesions are initially evaluated by conventional radiography, which has an intermediate sensitivity but a high specificity. Computed tomography (CT) has a higher sensitivity than conventional radiography in the diagnosis of a localized bone lesion and is also superior to the latter in the assessment of the osseous and soft tissue extent of the process.

In specific instances, however, CT has definite diagnostic value. Because of its superior contrast resolution, CT allows differentiation between cystic and solid lesions and the demonstration of fat within a lesion (e.g., intraosseous lipoma, **Fig. 14.1**).

Demonstration of a radiolucent nidus within surrounding bone sclerosis strongly suggests the diagnosis of an osteoid osteoma (**Fig. 14.2**), but it may also be encountered with a cortical abscess. A linear radiolucency running perpendicular to a cortex that is locally thickened is characteristic of a stress fracture. Intraosseous gas is found in osteonecrosis, gas-forming infections (**Fig. 14.3**), and occasionally pneumatocysts (**Fig. 14.4**).

Fluid levels in osseous lesions are most frequently associated with aneurysmal bone cysts, but they are also not uncommon in simple (unicameral) bone cysts and may occasionally be found in giant cell tumors, chondroblastomas, telangiectatic osteosarcomas, and a variety of other bone lesions (**Table 14.1**).

Fat–fluid levels within a bony lesion are indicative of acute osteomyelitis.

Sequestra (**Fig. 14.5**) can be readily identified by CT as radiodense foci and are highly suggestive of chronic osteomyelitis, but occasionally they are also found in tumors, such as fibrosarcomas and metastases, as well as in eosinophilic granulomas. They have to be differentiated from a centrally displaced cortical fracture fragment in a complex chronic fracture or a pathologic fracture (e.g., "fallen fragment" sign in a simple [unicameral] bone cyst, **Fig. 14.6**). A partially calcified nidus of an osteoid osteoma can also mimic osteomyelitis with a sequestrum. In healing fractures, osteonecrotic loose bone fragments may at times be impossible to differentiate from a sequestrum of an osteomyelitis complicating the fracture.

A radiodense focus within a lytic cranial lesion is termed *button sequestrum* (**Fig. 14.7**). Button sequestra are found with eosinophilic granulomas, metastases (especially from breast carcinoma), epidermoids, osteomyelitis (including tuberculosis and syphilis), radiation necrosis, bone flaps undergoing avascular necrosis, and bur holes.

The differential diagnosis of localized bone lesions is outlined in **Table 14.2**.

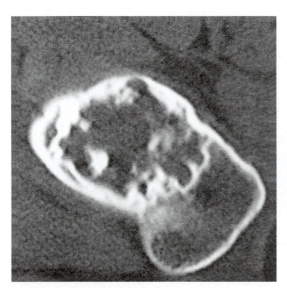

Fig. 14.1 Intraosseous lipoma. Sclerotic, fat-containing lesion just proximal to the intertrochanteric line in the left femoral neck is diagnostic. A similar lesion, but without fat, is characteristic for fibrous dysplasia.

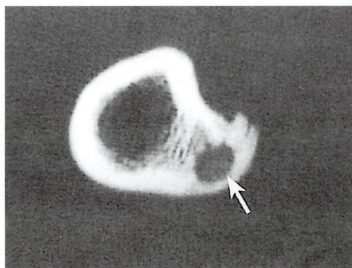

Fig. 14.2 Osteoid osteoma. A radiolucent nidus surrounded by sclerosis (arrow) is characteristic for an osteoid osteoma.

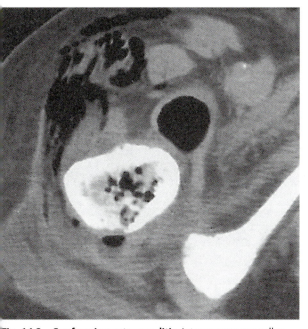

Fig. 14.3 Gas-forming osteomyelitis. Intraosseous gas collections are seen in the proximal femur. Note also the gas collections in the surrounding soft tissue.

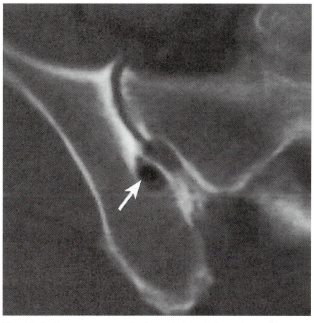

Fig. 14.4 Pneumatocyst. Gas in a subchondral cyst (arrow) is usually found in degenerative sacroiliac joint disease with vacuum phenomenon, both of which were also present in this case.

Table 14.1 Bone lesions with fluid levels

Aneurysmal bone cyst

Simple (unicameral) bone cyst

Giant cell tumor

Chondroblastoma

Intraosseous ganglion

Posttraumatic cyst

Fibrous dysplasia

Osteomyelitis (abscess)

Osteoblastoma

Brown tumor

Telangiectatic osteosarcoma

Fibrosarcoma

Plasmacytoma

Metastases

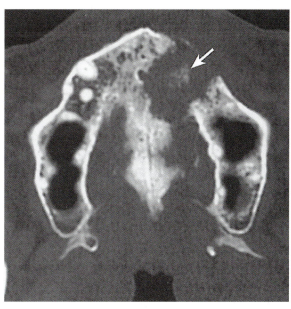

Fig. 14.5 Osteomyelitis with bone sequestrum. A destructive lesion with sequestrum (arrow) is seen in the hard palate.

IV Musculoskeletal System

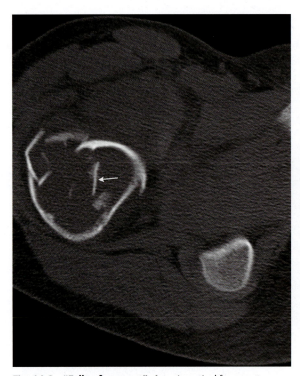

Fig. 14.6 **"Fallen fragment" sign.** A cortical fragment (arrow) is seen in an expansile lytic lesion (simple bone cyst) with pathologic fracture.

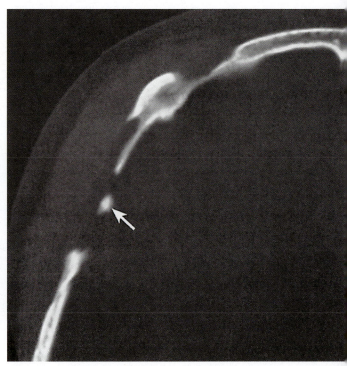

Fig. 14.7 **Eosinophilic granuloma with button sequestrum.** A button sequestrum (arrow) is seen in a large lytic skull lesion. The asymmetric destruction of the outer and inner tables at the anteromedial border of this lesion results in the "beveled-edge" appearance on conventional radiography. A second osteolytic lesion is visible more medially.

Table 14.2 Localized bone lesions

Disease	CT Findings	Comments
Subchondral cyst (geode) ▷ *Fig. 14.8*	Solitary or multiple lytic defects measuring up to 3 cm in diameter with typically a thin sclerotic border. Communication with the adjacent arthritic joint is often identifiable. Gas is occasionally found in these lesions (pneumatocysts), especially about the sacroiliac joints.	Associated with osteoarthritis (primary and posttraumatic), rheumatoid arthritis, avascular necrosis, and calcium pyrophosphate deposition disease (CPDD). Differential diagnosis: An intraosseous tophus in chronic gouty arthritis that may or may not be calcified must be differentiated.
Intraosseous ganglion ▷ *Fig. 14.9a, b* ▷ *Fig. 14.10*	Unilocular or, less commonly, multilocular, well-defined lytic epiphyseal lesion, often with a sclerotic margin. It may be associated with an extraosseous component of near-water to soft tissue density (soft tissue ganglion). Preferred locations are the medial malleolus of the tibia, femoral head, acetabulum, and carpal bones. Characteristically, the lesion does not communicate with the adjacent joint and is not associated with an arthritic process.	A *herniation pit* (▷ **Fig. 14.11**) is a well-circumscribed radiolucent defect usually measuring < 1 cm in diameter with a thin sclerotic border in the anterolateral aspect of the proximal femoral neck, which may represent an incidental finding or is associated with femoroacetabular impingement (FAI).
Echinococcosis	Complex, expansile, trabeculated, osteolytic lesion(s). Cortical violation and adjacent soft tissue mass formation, often with calcification, may be associated. Vertebral column, pelvis, long bones, adjacent ribs, and skull are most frequently involved.	Caused by *Echinococcus granulosus* (hydatid disease) or, less commonly, *Echinococcus multilocularis*. Cysts may develop in various viscera, particularly the liver and the lungs. Calcification of the cyst wall is common except in the lung.

(continues on page 504)

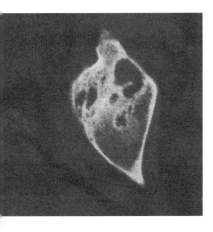

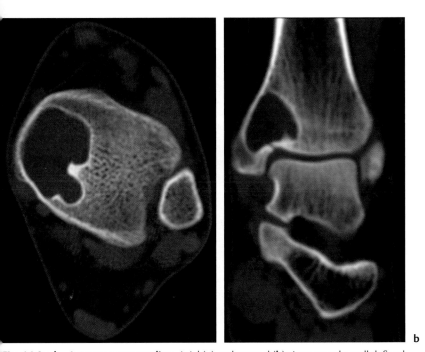

Fig. 14.8   Subchondral cysts (geodes). Subchondral cysts surrounded by sclerosis are seen in the acetabular dome of the right hip with advanced osteoarthritis.

b

Fig. 14.9a, b   Intraosseous ganglion. Axial (**a**) and coronal (**b**) views reveal a well-defined lytic lesion with sclerotic margin in the medial malleolus.

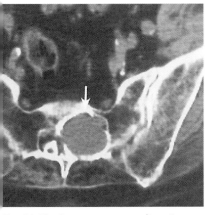

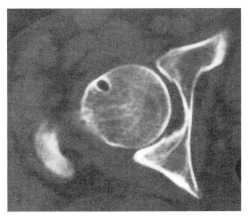

Fig. 14.10   Intraosseous ganglion. A round lesion with a thin sclerotic margin is seen in the sacrum (arrow). The diagnosis was confirmed by percutaneous CT–guided biopsy.

Fig. 14.11   Herniation pit. A small defect in the anterolateral femoral head-neck junction is characteristic.

Table 14.2   (Cont.) Localized bone lesions

Disease	CT Findings	Comments
Simple (unicameral) bone cysts ▷ *Fig. 14.12* ▷ *Fig. 14.13*	Centrally located, slightly expansile osteolytic lesion with cortical thinning. A central component of near-water density is characteristic but not always appreciated. Preferred locations in children are the metaphyses of long tubular bones (especially humerus and femur) and in adults the calcaneus and the ilium of the pelvis. Diaphyseal cysts in long bones are frequently large, expansile, and multiloculated. Fluid levels may be present.	In long tubular bones of children, the metaphyseal cyst is juxtaposed to the physis and frequently has an elongated shape paralleling the bone axis. A pathologic fracture is common. The fracture fragment within the cyst drops to the dependent portion of the lesion ("fallen fragment" sign). A pneumatocyst is diagnosed in the presence of either intralesional gas or a gas–fluid level.
Aneurysmal bone cyst ▷ *Fig. 14.14* ▷ *Fig. 14.15*	Presents most commonly either as an eccentric, expansile, osteolytic lesion with thin cortical shell or with extraosseous soft tissue component located in the metaphysis of a long tubular bone. Sclerosis at the site where the periost is lifted by the lesion ("buttressing") is common. Fine trabeculation and fluid levels within the lesion are characteristic. Other common locations are the posterior elements of the spine and the innominate bone, where a large soft tissue component may simulate a malignancy.	Primary lesions are found in 80% of patients younger than age 20 y. Secondary aneurysmal bone cysts arise in preexisting bone lesions, such as giant cell tumors, osteoblastomas, chondroblastomas, telangiectatic osteosarcomas, malignant fibrous histiocytomas, fibrous dysplasia, and Paget disease.
Epidermoid (inclusion cyst) ▷ *Fig. 14.16* ▷ *Fig. 14.17*	Intraosseous lesions present as well-defined osteolytic defects often with thin sclerotic margin occurring in the terminal phalanges of the hand and in the skull. Lesions may be expansile with thinning or destruction of the cortex. The cyst content consists of thick, waxy material rich in cholesterol varying from −5 to 20 HU. A button sequestrum is frequently seen in calvarial lesions.	Usually observed in the second to fourth decades of life. A history of trauma is frequently present, suggesting intraosseous implantation of ectodermal tissue with subsequent development of an epidermoid. The cysts are lined with a stratified squamous epithelium shedding keratin debris that breaks down and forms cholesterol.
Glomus tumor ▷ *Fig. 14.18*	Osteolytic lesions with marked contrast enhancement occurring in the terminal phalanges of the hand and temporal bone.	In the fingertips, the lesion is indistinguishable on plain radiographs from an epidermoid (inclusion cyst).
Lipoma ▷ *Fig. 14.19* ▷ *Fig. 14.20*	Well-circumscribed osteolytic lesion, often surrounded by a sclerotic border. May contain a central calcified nidus (especially in the calcaneus). Low attenuation of the fatty tissue is virtually diagnostic.	Rarely, fatty degeneration secondary to infarction and lesion containing histiocytes with fat vacuoles may also demonstrate negative CT values. **Liposclerosing myxofibroma** is a rare benign, well-defined lytic lesion typically surrounded by a sclerotic border in the pretrochanteric or intertrochanteric region of the proximal femur. However, fat is not invariably demonstrated by CT. Liposarcomas rarely arise in bone.

(continues on page 506)

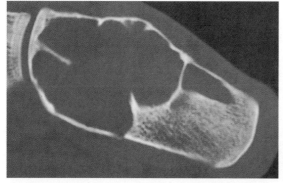

Fig. 14.12   Simple (unicameral) bone cyst. A slightly expansile osteolytic lesion of water density is seen in the calcaneus.

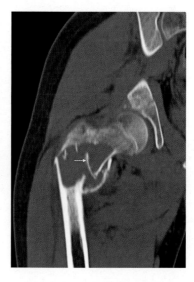

Fig. 14.13   Simple (unicameral) bone cyst. A well-defined osteolytic lesion with pathologic fracture depicting a "fallen fragment" (arrow) is seen in the intratrochanteric/subtrochanteric area.

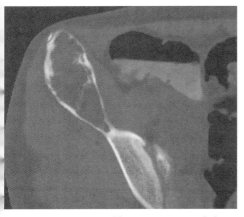

Fig. 14.14   Aneurysmal bone cyst. Expansile lytic lesion with fine trabeculation and a thin cortical shell is seen in the iliac bone.

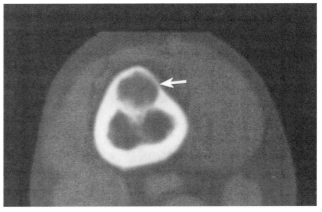

Fig. 14.15   Aneurysmal bone cyst in Paget disease. A cystic lesion (arrow) originates from the femur shaft that demonstrates cortical thickening due to Paget disease.

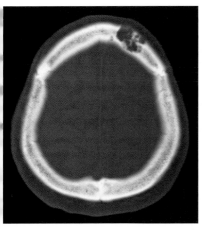

Fig. 14.16   Epidermoid. A lytic lesion with destruction of the outer table containing a small bony fragment (button sequestrum) is seen in the left frontal bone.

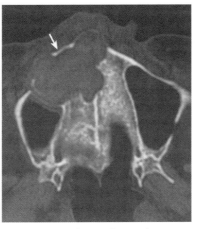

Fig. 14.17   Epidermoid. Irregular expansile lytic lesion involving the hard palate and anterior base of the right maxillary antrum (arrow) is seen.

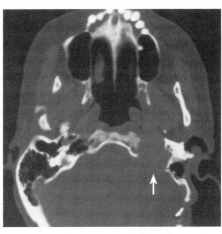

Fig. 14.18   Glomus tumor. A large destructive lesion is seen in the petrous bone (arrow).

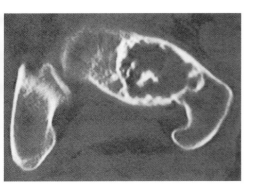

Fig. 14.19   Lipoma. Sclerotic lesion just proximal to the intertrochanteric line containing fat and small central calcifications is characteristic.

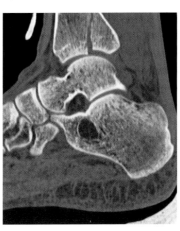

Fig. 14.20   Lipoma. A fatty lesion with barely perceptible sclerotic margin is seen in the anterior calcaneus. A pilon fracture is also evident in the tibial plafond.

Table 14.2 (Cont.) Localized bone lesions

Disease	CT Findings	Comments
Hemangioma ▷ *Fig. 14.21* ▷ *Fig. 14.22* ▷ *Fig. 14.23*	**Spine:** Small focal osteolytic lesion with trabeculae often arranged in a honeycomb or "cartwheel" configuration to coarse, vertical trabecular pattern ("corduroy" appearance) involving the vertebral body. The diameter of thickened vertical trabeculae is rather uniform. (Differential diagnosis: Multiple myeloma, metastases, and Paget disease, which may present with irregular, coarse trabecular thickening.) Extension into the posterior elements, paraspinal soft tissues, and spinal canal occurs but is not common. **Skull:** Slightly expansile osteolytic lesion with lattice-like ("cartwheel") or radiating ("sunburst") pattern. **Pelvis and tubular bones:** Poorly defined osteolytic lesion with lattice-like trabecular pattern. Involvement is uncommon.	Usually found in patients older than 40 y, with female predominance. Occasionally non–Hodgkin lymphoma (especially the histiocytic type) and metastases (e.g., breast carcinoma) may simulate a hemangioma in the spine. Cystic angiomatosis (▷ *Fig. 14.24*) is characterized by widespread cystic bone lesions that are frequently combined with visceral involvement.
Osteochondroma ▷ *Fig. 14.25* ▷ *Fig. 14.26* ▷ *Fig. 14.27*	Bony protuberance demonstrating cortical and medullary contiguity with parent bone is diagnostic in tubular bones. The lesion may be pedunculated (with narrow stalk and bulbous tip) or sessile (with broad, flat base). Osteochondromas characteristically originate from the metaphyses and point away from the nearby articulation. The tip of the osteochondroma is covered by a hyaline cartilage cap that may contain regular stippled calcifications. A large cartilaginous cap thicker than 2 cm often with irregular calcifications is suspicious for malignant transformation. The thickness of the cartilage cap is best assessed with MRI. In the pelvis, osteochondromas are frequently large and difficult to differentiate from lesions that have undergone malignant transformation. In the ribs, osteochondromas frequently occur at the costochondral junction.	Osteochondromas occur in children and adolescents as a slow-growing, painless mass. They are intimately related to the physis and cease to enlarge with fusion of the adjacent growth plates. Rarely osteochondromas may develop in adults after trauma. Differential diagnosis: 1. **Supracondylar process of the humerus:** Spur originating from the anteromedial aspect of the distal humerus pointing toward the elbow (phylogenetic vestige). 2. **Pes anserinus spur** in the medial aspect of the proximal tibia (enthesophyte, occasionally associated with anserinus bursitis). 3. **Posttraumatic spurs** secondary to healed avulsion fractures. 4. **"Tug" lesions** at tendinous attachment sites in the lower extremity. 5. See also periosteal (juxtacortical) chondroma and bizarre parosteal osteochondromatous proliferation (BPOP) in this table. Hereditary multiple exostoses (▷ *Fig. 14.28*) present with multiple, usually bilateral, and symmetric osteochondromas in the axial and appendicular skeleton associated with bone modeling deformities.

(continues on page 508)

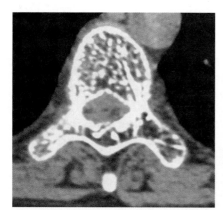

Fig. 14.21 Hemangioma. Uniform thickening of the vertical trabeculae of the entire vertebra resulting in a "polka dot" appearance is seen.

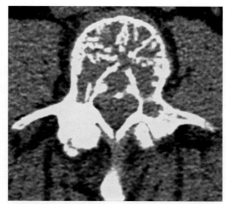

Fig. 14.22 Hemangioma. Thickened trabeculae in the vertebral body are evident, resulting in a "cartwheel" appearance. This finding is more commonly associated with a hemangioma of the skull.

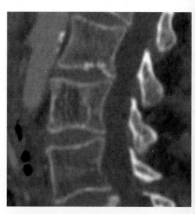

Fig. 14.23 Hemangioma. A lytic lesion with sclerotic margin is seen in the anterior two thirds of a vertebral body containing prominent vertical trabeculae ("corduroy" appearance).

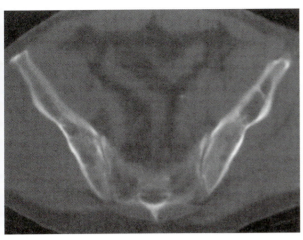

Fig. 14.24   Cystic angiomatosis. Multiple well-defined osteolytic lesions of variable size with or without sclerotic margins are seen in the pelvis and sacrum.

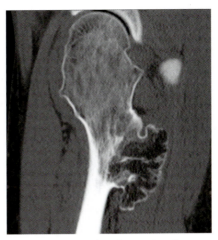

Fig. 14.25   Osteochondroma. A pedunculated lesion with irregular outline is seen in the subtrochanteric area.

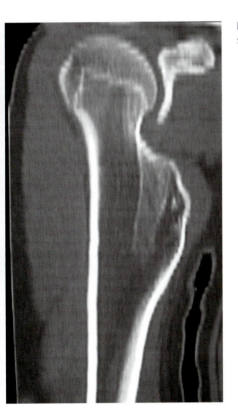

Fig. 14.26   Osteochondroma. A sessile lesion with a broad, flat base is seen in the subtrochanteric area.

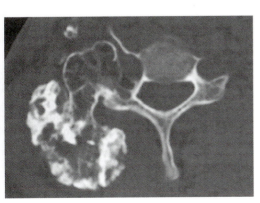

Fig. 14.27   Osteochondroma. A large pedunculated osteochondroma with extensive cap calcification arises from a cervical vertebral body. This lesion cannot be differentiated from a peripheral chondrosarcoma.

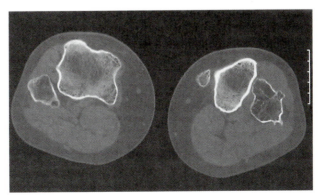

Fig. 14.28   Hereditary multiple exostoses. Deformed proximal tibia and fibula bilaterally with multiple osteochondromas are characteristic.

Table 14.2   (Cont.) Localized bone lesions

Disease	CT Findings	Comments
Dysplasia epiphysealis hemimelica (Trevor disease)	Lobulated osseous mass (articular chondroma) originating in an epiphysis, carpal, or tarsal bone. Presents initially in infants with irregular calcifications/ossifications on one side of an enlarged epiphysis or a carpal/tarsal bone. Preferential involvement is the medial side of a lower extremity epiphysis (e.g., distal femur, proximal and distal tibia) or the medial side of a tarsal bone (e.g., talus). Multiple bones in a single extremity are affected in two thirds of cases.	Presents in children and young adults with swelling, pain, and deformity localized to one side of the body. Histologically, the pedunculated mass with cartilaginous cap is indistinguishable from an osteochondroma.
Enchondroma ▷ *Fig. 14.29* ▷ *Fig. 14.30*	Well-circumscribed lesion, often with endosteal scalloping composed of hyaline-type cartilage with varying degrees of calcifications. Preferred locations are the metaphyses of the long tubular bones and the diaphyses in the short tubular bones of the hands and feet. In the long tubular bones, larger lesions with sizable areas of uncalcified matrix should suggest the possibility of malignant transformation or a low-grade chondrosarcoma. Other imaging features in long tubular bones suggesting low-grade malignancy include extensive endosteal scalloping (more than two thirds of the cortical thickness or more than two thirds of the length of the lesion) and solid periosteal reaction/localized cortical thickening about the lesion. Frank cortical destruction and associated soft tissue mass are virtually diagnostic for a chondrosarcoma.	Enchondromas are usually discovered in the third or fourth decade of life as incidental findings or painless swelling. The presence of pain should arouse suspicion of malignant transformation. **Enchondromatosis (Ollier disease)** is characterized by multiple, asymmetrically distributed enchondromas often in deformed tubular bones and the pelvis. In **Maffucci syndrome**, multiple soft tissue cavernous hemangiomas with phleboliths are associated with enchondromatosis with predilection for tubular bones of the hands and feet.
Periosteal (juxtacortical) chondroma ▷ *Fig. 14.31*	Soft tissue mass with erosion of the adjacent cortex and varying degrees of periosteal new bone formation, including buttressing (thickening of the cortex at the distal and proximal margins of the lesion) is typical. Matrix calcification is evident in the majority of cases and may be extensive. Metaphyses of the long tubular bones and hands are most commonly affected.	All ages are affected, but usually diagnosed under the age of 30 y. Slight male predominance.
Bizarre parosteal osteochondromatous proliferation (BPOP)	Well-marginated sessile or pedunculated mass of heterotopic ossification arising from the cortical surface without medullary contiguity between lesion and adjacent bone is characteristic.	Occurs usually in the hands and feet (occasionally in long tubular bones) without age and gender predilection. A history of trauma is evident in some patients. **Florid reactive periostitis** involving most commonly the proximal or middle phalanges of the hands is best considered a variant of traumatic myositis ossificans.
Chondroblastoma ▷ *Fig. 14.32*	Well-defined lytic epiphyseal or apophyseal lesion with or without a sclerotic border and matrix calcifications. A solid periosteal reaction in the adjacent metaphyseal shaft may be induced by bone marrow edema. Approximately 10% of chondroblastomas occur in the hands and feet with predilection for the talus and calcaneus.	Uncommon benign cartilaginous lesion occurring between the ages of 5 and 25 y with slight male predominance.
Chondromyxoid fibroma	Eccentric metaphyseal osteolytic lesion with cortical expansion, coarse trabeculation, endosteal scalloping, and scalloped sclerotic medullary border is a typical presentation. Destruction of the cortex resulting in a hemispherical osseous defect or "bite" without periosteal reaction is a characteristic finding in larger lesions. Predilection for the long tubular bones, especially of the lower extremity, but occasionally also found in the pelvis, foot, and hand.	Uncommon benign cartilaginous lesion occurring between the ages of 5 and 25 y with slight male predominance. Slowly progressive pain, tenderness, swelling, and restriction of motion are typical. **Fibrocartilaginous mesenchymoma** is a very rare benign solitary expansile osteolytic lesion with spotty or ringlike calcifications, cortical destruction, and soft tissue invasion originating most often in the metaphysis of a long tubular bone. Age distribution is similar to chondromyxoid fibroma.
Periosteal (juxtacortical) desmoid	Saucer-like defect in the posteromedial cortex of the distal femur, often associated with adjacent sclerosis, periostitis, and soft tissue swelling.	Occurs between the ages of 15 and 20 y. Considered to be a sequela of trauma at the insertion of the adductor magnus muscle.

(continues on page 510)

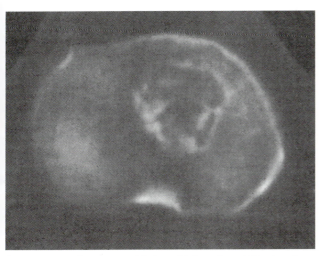

Fig. 14.29   Enchondroma. A lesion with irregular calcifications is seen in the distal femur.

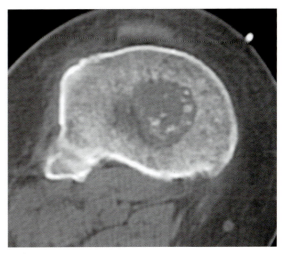

Fig. 14.30   Enchondroma. An osteolytic lesion with punctate calcification is seen in the proximal tibia.

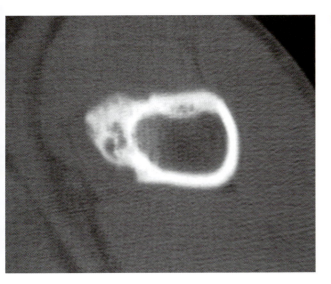

Fig. 14.31   Periosteal (juxtacortical) chondroma. An irregular ossified mass containing osteolytic foci originates from the femoral shaft cortex.

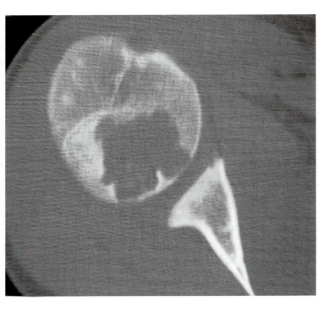

Fig. 14.32   Chondroblastoma. An irregular osteolytic lesion in the humeral head is seen. A few faint punctate calcifications within the lesion are present but difficult to appreciate with this window setting.

Table 14.2   (Cont.) Localized bone lesions

Disease	CT Findings	Comments
Nonossifying fibroma ▷ *Fig. 14.33a, b*	Small lesions present as round or oblong, well-delineated, radiolucent areas in the cortex with normal or sclerotic adjacent bone. They typically arise in the metaphysis at a short distance from the physis. Larger lesions present as a well-delineated, eccentric, oblong osteolytic area in the diametaphysis. They frequently have a multiloculated appearance, and both cortical expansion and thinning may be evident. The long tubular bones, especially the tibia and femur, are most frequently affected. With time the lesions may spontaneously disappear or become sclerotic.	Usually diagnosed in patients younger than 20 y. Smaller lesions are referred to as *benign fibrous cortical defects*. They are asymptomatic and diagnosed as an incidental finding on routine radiography and occasionally are multifocal. They usually regress spontaneously or less commonly enlarge and migrate with growth into the diaphyses, eventually being referred to as nonossifying fibromas. Pathologic fractures in larger lesions are not uncommon. **Jaffe–Campanacci syndrome** consists of multiple nonossifying fibromas associated with café-au-lait spots, mental retardation, and hypogonadism. **Benign fibrous histiocytomas** (fibroxanthoma) are histologically identical to nonossifying fibromas but present as slightly more aggressive lesions in patients older than 20 y without site predilection.
Desmoplastic fibroma ▷ *Fig. 14.34*	Central, often trabeculated (soap bubble or honeycomb pattern) osteolytic lesion in the metaphyses of long tubular bones, mandible, and pelvis. Slight bony expansion with endosteal erosion and limited periosteal bone formation may be associated.	Rare benign neoplasm occurring in the second and third decades of life. Pain and swelling are the leading clinical symptoms, or a pathologic fracture may be the presenting feature.
Bone island (enostosis) ▷ *Fig. 14.35*	Single or multiple intraosseous foci of homogeneously dense bone most often found in the pelvis, proximal femurs, and spine. They may be round, ovoid, or oblong and are aligned with the long axis of the trabecular architecture. Tiny bone spicules radiating from the periphery of the lesion are characteristic. A somewhat radiolucent center may occasionally be encountered. Range in size from a few millimeters to a few centimeters.	Incidental finding in all age groups. Lesions may slowly increase or decrease in size over years. Bone scintigraphy is usually negative. Differential diagnosis: osteoblastic metastases. A curettaged and *methylmethacrylate cemented bone lesion* may resemble a large enostosis. **Osteopoikilosis** (▷ *Fig. 14.36*): Numerous small sclerotic foci with symmetric distribution in periarticular locations.
Osteoma ▷ *Fig. 14.37a, b* ▷ *Fig. 14.38*	Mass of either uniformly dense compact bone or less dense cancellous bone protruding from the skull and facial bones (especially the paranasal sinuses). Rarely, osteomas arise from the cortical surface of the clavicle, pelvis, and tubular bones.	**Gardner syndrome:** Autosomal dominant disease consisting of multiple osteomas, colonic polyposis, and soft tissue tumors (especially desmoids). **Tuberous sclerosis:** Multiple osteoma-like lesions may be associated, especially in the metacarpals and metatarsals. **Melorheostosis:** Partial or circumferential cortical thickening of a tubular bone ("wax flowing down the side of a candle"). Osteoma-like protrusions and soft tissue ossifications may be associated (▷ *Fig. 14.39*).

(continues on page 512)

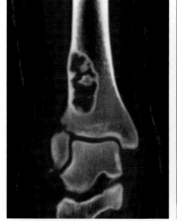
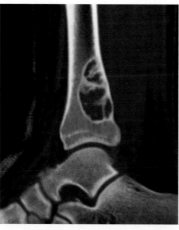

Fig. 14.33a, b   Nonossifying fibroma. Coronal (**a**) and sagittal (**b**) views show an eccentric lesion with sclerotic margins and irregular trabeculation.

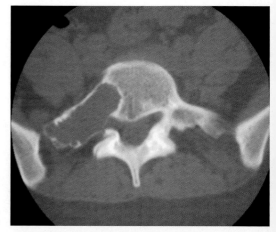

Fig. 14.34   Desmoplastic fibroma. An expansile osteolytic lesion with beginning cortical destruction is seen in the right transverse process.

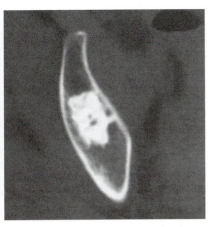

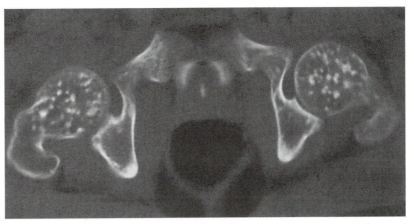

Fig. 14.35   Bone island (enostosis). A large sclerotic focus is seen within the right ilium.

Fig. 14.36   Osteopoikilosis. Numerous small sclerotic foci with symmetric distribution in both femoral heads are seen.

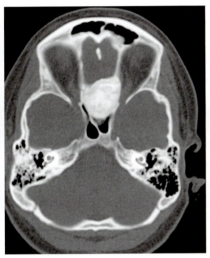

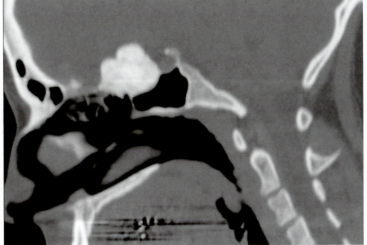

b

Fig. 14.37a, b   Osteoma. Axial (**a**) and sagittal (**b**) views reveal a well-circumscribed sclerotic mass in the sphenoid sinus.

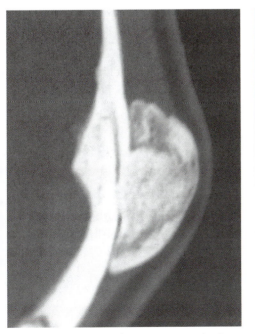

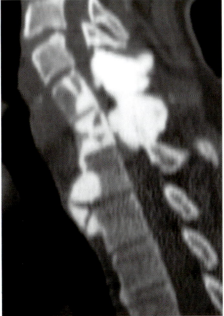

Fig. 14.38   Osteoma. A bony mass protrudes from the vault of the skull.

Fig. 14.39   Melorheostosis. An irregular sclerotic lesion expands over four vertebral bodies of the lower cervical spine and extends into the prevertebral soft tissue space at the C6–C7 level.

Table 14.2 (Cont.) Localized bone lesions

Disease	CT Findings	Comments
Osteoid osteoma ▷ *Fig. 14.40* ▷ *Fig. 14.41*	**Diaphysis of long tubular bones:** Cortical radiolucent lesion (nidus) measuring < 1 cm in diameter surrounded by a zone of uniform bone sclerosis (elliptical thickening of the cortex) is virtually diagnostic. The nidus enhances after intravenous (IV) contrast administration and occasionally has a calcified center. **Intra-articular location:** A nonconspicuous small radiolucent focus often without significant reactive sclerosis may be present. A synovial inflammatory response including a joint effusion is commonly associated and may mimic an infectious arthritic process. **Carpal and tarsal bones:** A partially or completely calcified lesion with or without only mild reactive sclerosis is characteristic. **Spine:** A small osteolytic focus surrounded by extensive sclerosis in the posterior elements is the most common presentation. A scoliotic deformity is usually associated with the lesion that is located near its apex on the concave side of the curvature.	Occurs in patients between 7 and 25 y of age, with a male predominance (3:1). Pain is the hallmark of the disease, usually more dramatic at night and ameliorated by aspirin. Bone scintigraphy shows an unusual intense uptake in the center of the lesion (nidus) surrounded by the less intense uptake of the adjacent sclerotic bone (double density sign), differentiating it from chronic cortical osteomyelitis with small abscess formation. Localized cortical thickening caused by a stress fracture typically is associated with a transverse linear radiolucency. In the lumbar spine, a unilateral osteosclerotic focus about a pedicle is frequently caused by a hypertrophied interarticular pars caused by unilateral spondylolysis of the contralateral side.
Osteoblastoma ▷ *Fig. 14.42a, b* ▷ *Fig. 14.43*	**Long tubular bones:** Osteoblastomas typically originate in either the medullary or cortical bone of the diaphysis and present as expansile osteolytic lesions, often with areas of calcification or ossification, surrounding bone sclerosis and frequently exuberant solid periosteal reaction. **Spine:** Well-defined expansile osteolytic lesion that may be partially or extensively calcified and surrounded by mild sclerosis at best is commonly found in the posterior elements. **Hands, feet, and pelvis:** Slightly expansile lytic lesion with varying degrees of matrix calcification/ossification and surrounding reactive sclerosis is the most common presentation.	Usually diagnosed in the second and third decades of life, with a male predominance (2:1) and similar clinical presentation as in osteoid osteomas. The size of the nidus (actual size of the osteolytic lesion, which, however, at times may be partially to completely calcified/ossified), is used to differentiate between osteoblastomas (> 2 cm) and osteoid osteomas (< 2 cm). *Aggressive (malignant) osteoblastomas* are differentiated from the typical (conventional) osteoblastomas by a more aggressive pattern of tumor behavior, including a much greater likelihood to recur. The radiologic features of both types are similar, but cortical violation with tumor extension into the neighboring soft tissues is suggestive of an aggressive osteoblastoma.

(continues on page 514)

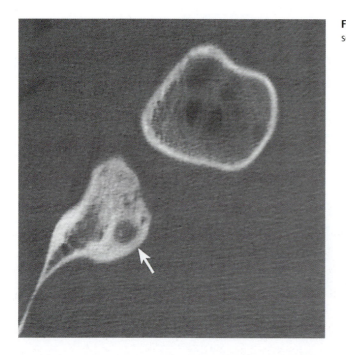

Fig. 14.40 Osteoid osteoma. A radiolucent nidus surrounded by sclerotic bone seen in the glenoid (arrow) is characteristic.

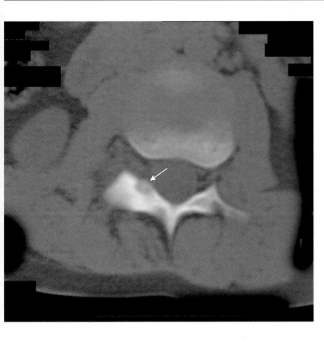

Fig. 14.41   Osteoid osteoma. A small osteolytic nidus with tiny central calcification (arrow) and extensive surrounding sclerosis is seen in the lamina.

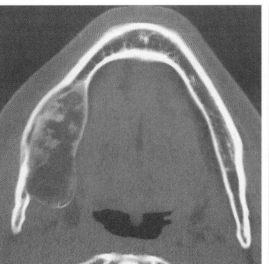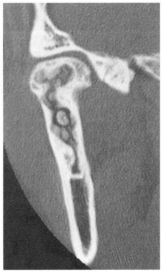

b

Fig. 14.42a, b   Osteoblastoma (two cases). (a) An expansile osteolytic lesion with areas of calcification/ossification is seen in the body of the mandible. **(b)** A lesion with irregular, thick sclerotic margins containing several round ossifications is seen in the condylar process of the mandible.

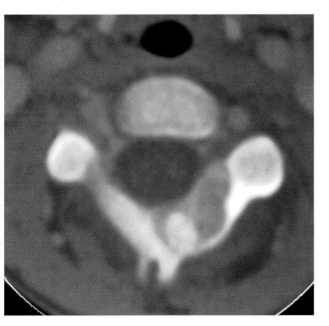

Fig. 14.43   Osteoblastoma. A large, slightly expansile, lytic lesion > 2 cm in length and containing an ovoid ossification in its medial aspect is seen in the left lamina.

Table 14.2   (Cont.) Localized bone lesions

Disease	CT Findings	Comments
Giant cell tumor ▷ *Fig. 14.44* ▷ *Fig. 14.45* ▷ *Fig. 14.46a–c*	In the long tubular bone (85%), a giant cell tumor presents as an eccentric expansile osteolytic lesion, often with a delicate trabecular pattern ("soap bubble" appearance), extending from the metaphysis to the subchondral bone. The margins of the lesion may be well or poorly defined, but sclerosis and periosteal reactions are typically absent. Cortical breakthrough with spread into the adjacent soft tissues occurs. Fluid levels within the lesion may be evident. Occasionally, the tumor is found in the pelvis, sacrum, ribs, vertebral bodies, hands, and feet.	Occurs usually in the third and fourth decades of life, with equal gender distribution. Tumor recurrence is about 50% in excised and grafted lesions but markedly reduced when cemented with methylmethacrylate instead of bone grafts. Malignant giant cell tumors (including malignant transformation of a benign giant cell tumor) account for approximately 5%. **Giant cell (reparative) granuloma** has a more benign course and similar histologic and radiologic features as a giant cell tumor, although cortical violation with spread into neighboring soft tissues does not occur, and a predilection for facial bones and short tubular bones of the hands and feet exists.
Chordoma ▷ *Fig. 14.47a, b*	Destructive expansile osteolytic lesion with large soft tissue mass and intratumoral calcifications in up to 90% of cases is characteristic. Calcifications found in the tumor periphery can also represent sequestered bone fragments. Originates from the sacrum and coccyx (60%), clivus (30%), and spine, especially C2 (10%). Sacral lesions typically grow anteriorly and may contain cystic areas. In the spine vertebral collapse, sclerosis ("ivory" vertebrae) and erosion of the posterior aspect of the vertebral body and neural foramina are additional manifestations. Involvement of two contiguous vertebrae is not uncommon.	Sacrococcygeal chordomas occur in 40- to 60-y-old patients, with male predominance. Spheno-occipital chordomas are usually diagnosed in 20- to 40-y-old patients without gender predilection. The **chondroid chordoma** is a variant comprising one third of all clivus chordomas with better prognosis and particularly prominent calcifications. Hematogenous metastases may eventually develop in about one third of all chordomas.
Adamantinoma (angioblastoma)	Single or multiple, central or eccentric, multilocular, slightly expansile, sharply or poorly delineated osteolytic lesions with or without reactive sclerosis in the diaphysis of the tibia (85%) with preferential involvement of its anterior cortex or, rarely, in other long tubular bones. Cortical destruction, exuberant periostitis, and a soft tissue mass may be associated.	Usually diagnosed in the third and fourth decades of life with slight male predominance. History of trauma is frequent. Local swelling is the major clinical finding. Differential diagnosis: Osteofibrous dysplasia. See under fibrous dysplasia at the end of this table.
Ameloblastoma ▷ *Fig. 14.48a, b*	Presentation ranges from unilocular cyst to multilocular, often trabeculated lesion with cortical expansion or destruction and occasionally a large soft tissue mass in the mandible or, much less commonly, the maxilla.	Usually diagnosed in the fourth and fifth decades of life without gender predilection.

(continues on page 516)

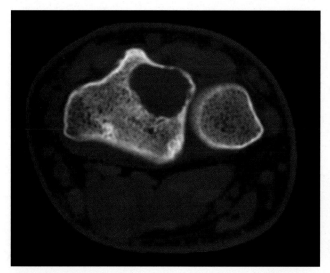

Fig. 14.44   Giant cell tumor. An eccentric, slightly expansile osteolytic lesion without a sclerotic border is seen in the distal radius.

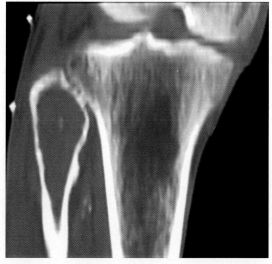

Fig. 14.45   Giant cell tumor. An expansile osteolytic lesion is seen in the proximal fibula.

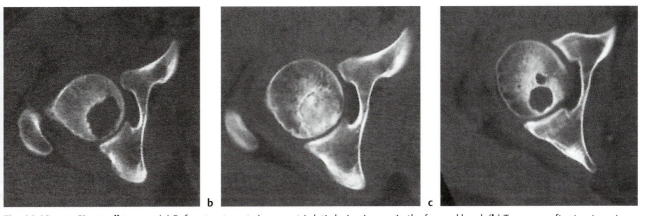

Fig. 14.46a–c   Giant-cell tumor. (**a**) Before treatment. An eccentric lytic lesion is seen in the femoral head. (**b**) Two years after treatment with curettage and bone chips impaction. The treated lesion presents as sclerotic focus without lucencies. (**c**) Two years later, tumor recurrence is evident by the appearance of new lytic areas within the treated lesion.

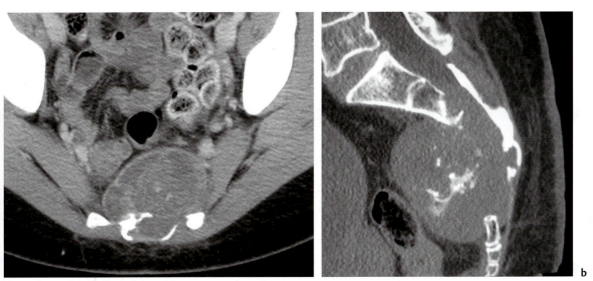

Fig. 14.47a, b   Chordoma (two cases). Axial (**a**) and sagittal (**b**) views show a large destructive lesion originating in the sacrum and growing anteriorly into the presacral space. The lesion contains calcifications or ossifications, the latter representing displaced bony fragments.

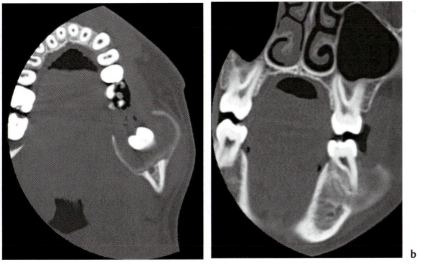

Fig. 14.48a, b   Ameloblastoma. Axial (**a**) and coronal (**b**) views reveal a large expansile cystic lesion in the mandible with disrupted margins containing a molar with a partially resorbed root.

IV Musculoskeletal System

Table 14.2 (Cont.) Localized bone lesions

Disease	CT Findings	Comments
Fibrosarcoma ▷ *Fig. 14.49*	Well or poorly marginated osteolytic lesion with general lack of both periosteal reaction and osteosclerosis is typical. Irregular thin or thick intratumoral septation, cortical violation, and soft tissue mass are frequently associated. Dystrophic calcifications and sequestered bone fragments are occasionally seen within the tumor. Preferential involvement of the metaphyses of the long tubular bones (70%) with frequent extension into the diaphyses and epiphyses.	Rare malignant bone tumor occurring in the third to sixth decades of life without gender predilection. The histologic spectrum of fibrosarcomas ranging from well differentiated to poorly differentiated lesions is reflected in the greatly variable radiologic presentation. May complicate Paget disease, bone infarcts, radiation necrosis, and chronic osteomyelitis.
Malignant fibrous histiocytoma ▷ *Fig. 14.50*	A poorly defined osteolytic lesion with cortical destruction, large soft tissue mass, and absence of both periosteal reaction and new bone formation is the most common presentation. The ends of long tubular bones from diaphysis to epiphysis are affected in 75% of cases with strong predilection for the lower extremity. Osseous expansion is unusual but may be observed in flat bones, such as pelvis, ribs, scapula, and sternum.	Occurs at any age, but the majority of cases are diagnosed in the fifth, sixth, and seventh decades of life, with slight male predominance. The lesion cannot be radiographically differentiated from a highly malignant fibrosarcoma. May develop in abnormal bone such as Paget disease and bone infarcts or secondary to radiation therapy.
Chondrosarcoma, central ▷ *Fig. 14.51* ▷ *Fig. 14.52* ▷ *Fig. 14.53*	A slightly expansile, often multilobulated osteolytic lesion with cortical thickening, endosteal erosion, and scattered stippled or irregular calcifications is characteristic. Matrix calcification representing the most specific finding is only present in about two thirds of the cases. Lesions without matrix calcifications are virtually impossible to differentiate from fibrosarcomas. Demonstration of a poorly defined osteolysis, cortical violation, and large soft tissue mass indicate a highly aggressive lesion, but an interrupted periosteal reaction typically is absent. However, more often a geographic destruction pattern is present, suggesting a less malignant process. The tumor has a predilection for the metaphyses of the long tubular bones (especially femur and humerus) and flat bones (especially pelvis) and the vertebrae.	Occurs usually between 30 and 60 y of age, with male predominance. The tumor arises de novo in the medullary cavity or is caused by malignant transformation of an enchondroma. Low-grade chondrosarcomas are extremely difficult to differentiate from enchondromas. Irregular matrix calcifications (as opposed to punctate, ring, and arclike calcifications), large areas of noncalcified tumor matrix, poorly defined osteolysis, extensive endosteal scalloping, and cortical thickening (even solid) suggest malignancy.
Chondrosarcoma, peripheral ▷ *Fig. 14.54a, b* ▷ *Fig. 14.55*	Malignant transformation of a benign osteochondroma is suggested by demonstration of a bulky cartilaginous cap measuring > 2 cm in width, scattered and irregular calcifications within the cartilaginous cap, associated soft tissue mass, focal soft tissue areas within the bony component of the lesion, and destruction or pressure erosion of the adjacent bone. Differentiation of an osteochondroma from a peripheral chondrosarcoma is not always possible with CT, and supplementation with other imaging techniques, such as bone scintigraphy and MRI, is often required.	Local pain and growth of an osteochondroma in adulthood suggest clinically malignant transformation. The risk of malignant transformation in patients with hereditary multiple exostoses is estimated to be up to 25%, whereas in a solitary osteochondroma, it is < 1%. Rarely, a peripheral chondrosarcoma develops de novo from the periost (periosteal or juxtacortical chondrosarcoma).

(continues on page 518)

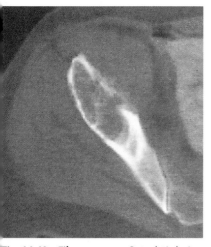

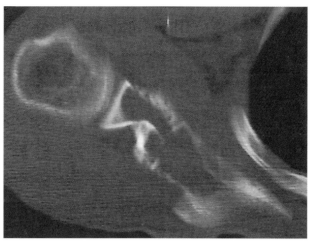

Fig. 14.49 Fibrosarcoma. Osteolytic lesion with cortical violation and a soft tissue mass is seen in the right iliac wing.

Fig. 14.50 Malignant fibrous histiocytoma. Osteolytic lesion with cortical destruction is seen in the scapula.

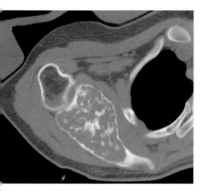

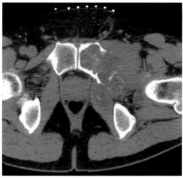

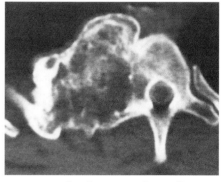

Fig. 14.51 Chondrosarcoma (central). An expansile osteolytic lesion with a thinned but intact cortex containing multiple irregular calcifications is seen in the scapula. Findings are consistent with a low-grade malignancy.

Fig. 14.52 Chondrosarcoma (central). A destructive osteolytic lesion with a large associated soft tissue mass containing numerous tiny calcifications is seen in the left pubic bone.

Fig. 14.53 Chondrosarcoma (central). An expansile mass with irregular calcifications, thick sclerosis on its lateral margin, and cortical violations on its anterior and posterior margins is seen in a thoracic vertebra.

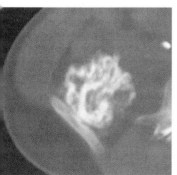

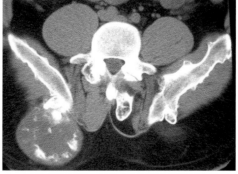

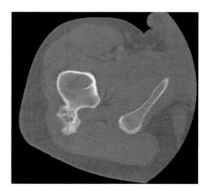

b

Fig. 14.54a, b Chondrosarcoma (peripheral) (two cases). A large, irregular, extensively calcified mass (**a**) originates from the right iliac wing. A large soft tissue mass (**b**) containing multiple irregular calcifications originates from the posterior aspect of the right iliac wing. Enthesopathy ("whiskering") of the anterior iliac wing is incidentally seen caused by diffuse idiopathic skeletal hyperostosis (DISH).

Fig. 14.55 Chondrosarcoma (peripheral). An irregular calcified cap is seen in a pedunculated exostosis consistent with malignant transformation of an osteochondroma.

IV Musculoskeletal System

Table 14.2 (Cont.) Localized bone lesions

Disease	CT Findings	Comments
Clear cell chondrosarcoma ▷ *Fig. 14.56*	Poorly or well-defined (sclerotic borders), slightly expansile epiphyseal lesion with central calcifications in about one third of the cases is characteristic. Most frequent locations are the proximal ends of the femur, humerus, and tibia.	Rare cartilaginous bone tumor occurring between ages 25 and 50 y, with slight male predominance. Imaging features are virtually identical to a chondroblastoma.
Dedifferentiated chondrosarcoma	Features of both a low-grade chondrosarcoma (nonexpansile osteolytic lesion with intact cortex and matrix calcifications) and a highly anaplastic sarcoma (expansile, poorly defined osteolytic lesion with cortical destruction and large soft tissue mass, but usually without calcification) are characteristic. The transition between these two tumor components is usually abrupt. Distribution of the tumor is similar to conventional chondrosarcoma, with femur, humerus, and pelvis being the most frequent sites of involvement.	Occurs in patients older than 50 y without gender predilection. Presents with pain, soft tissue swelling, or pathologic fracture (one third of patients). The prognosis is very poor.
Mesenchymal chondrosarcoma ▷ *Fig. 14.57*	Features are indistinguishable from a high-grade conventional chondrosarcoma and include poorly defined osteolysis, matrix calcifications, cortical expansion and violation, and soft tissue mass. Most frequent sites of involvement are femur, ribs, and spine.	Occurs usually between age 20 and 40 y and has a poor prognosis. Metastases to lymph nodes and other bones are not unusual. Approximately 50% of mesenchymal chondrosarcomas arise in the soft tissues. **Myxoid chondrosarcoma** is the most common extraskeletal chondrosarcoma type and has a relatively low-grade malignancy.
Osteosarcoma ▷ *Fig. 14.58a, b* ▷ *Fig. 14.59* ▷ *Fig. 14.60* ▷ *Fig. 14.61*	Conventional osteosarcoma presenting as a poorly defined intramedullary lesion most often originating in the metaphyses of long tubular bones with varying degrees of osteolysis and osteosclerosis is most characteristic. The tumor may be purely osteolytic or osteoblastic. Cortical destruction associated with an interrupted periosteal reaction in the form of a Codman triangle (laminated triangular elevation of the periost at the tumor periphery) or with perpendicular ("hair on end" or "sunburst"), laminated ("onion skin"), or amorphous appearance is most characteristic. Large soft tissue masses are commonly found in tumors with cortical violation. Surrounding tumor edema and hemorrhage may result in overestimation of the actual tumor size. "Skip" metastases (areas of tumor separated from the main neoplasm) can be identified in the medullary canal by their higher attenuation values than the normal bone marrow. Most common sites of involvement are the long tubular bones (80%), especially the femur, tibia, and humerus. Osteosarcomas are relatively infrequent in the pelvis, spine, and facial bones and rare in the remaining skeleton. **Telangiectatic osteosarcomas** commonly present as large, multilocular, expansile, and predominantly lytic lesions, often with cortical violation and tumor extension into the soft tissues, but without significant periosteal reaction and sclerosis. Fluid levels are often also evident. **Small cell osteosarcomas** commonly present as large predominantly osteolytic lesions, extending from the metaphysis to the diaphysis of a long tubular bone associated with interrupted periosteal reaction and large soft tissue masses. They resemble Ewing sarcomas. **Intraosseous low-grade osteosarcomas** present as purely sclerotic and mixed osteolytic/osteoblastic lesions often limited to the medullary portion of the diametaphyses of long tubular bones, especially of the tibia and femur. Irregular cortical thickening may be associated. The tumor is frequently mistaken for a benign osteosclerotic process.	Osteosarcomas most commonly present in the second and third decades of life with pain, swelling, restriction of motion, and pyrexia. Men are more frequently affected than women. In the elderly, they may be a complication of Paget disease or radiation therapy. **Gnathic osteosarcomas** present as purely osteoblastic, osteolytic, or mixed lesions in the mandible or less frequently maxilla, occur in the middle-aged and elderly, and have a relatively benign course. **Intracortical osteosarcomas** are rare and originate in the cortices of the tibia and femur, presenting as slightly expansile osteolytic lesions with surrounding sclerosis. **Osteosarcomatosis** refers to simultaneous involvement of more than one skeletal site. It has to be differentiated from a unicentric lesion with distal skeletal metastases.

(continues on page 520)

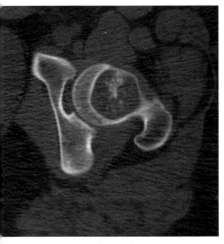

Fig. 14.56   Clear cell chondrosarcoma. An osteolytic lesion with sclerotic margins containing punctate calcifications is seen in the left femoral head. The lesion cannot be differentiated radiographically from a chondroblastoma.

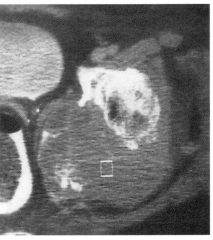

Fig. 14.57   Mesenchymal chondrosarcoma. A large soft tissue mass with scattered calcifications and destruction of the left hip is seen.

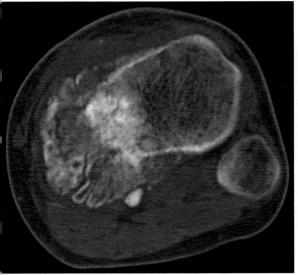

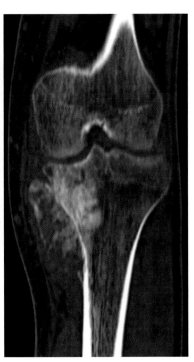

b

Fig. 14.58a, b   Osteosarcoma. Axial (**a**) and coronal (**b**) views show a mixed osteolytic and osteoblastic lesion originating in the medial metaphysis of the proximal tibia with a large soft tissue component depicting amorphous periosteal new bone formation.

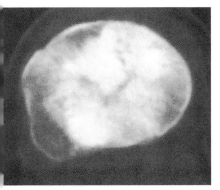

Fig. 14.59   Osteosarcoma. Poorly defined osteosclerotic foci are seen in the distal femur without cortical violation and soft tissue mass.

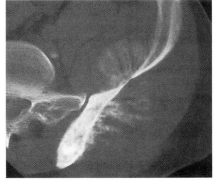

Fig. 14.60   Osteosarcoma. Poorly defined osteosclerotic lesion in the left ilium adjacent to the sacroiliac joint is associated with perpendicular periosteal reaction and a large soft tissue mass.

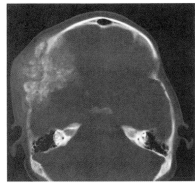

Fig. 14.61   Osteosarcoma. Large osteosclerotic mass with destruction of the skull is seen in the right frontoparietal region of the skull.

IV Musculoskeletal System

Table 14.2   (Cont.) Localized bone lesions

Disease	CT Findings	Comments
Periosteal osteosarcoma	Oblong, dense lesion arising from the diaphyseal surface of a long tubular bone with irregular thickening and occasionally saucerization of the adjacent cortex is typical. A Codman triangle and radiating or cloud-like osseous proliferation are frequently associated. Femur, tibia, and humerus are the most common sites of involvement. The medullary cavity is typically not involved.	Usually diagnosed in the second and third decades of life with better prognosis than conventional osteosarcomas, but worse than parosteal osteosarcomas. Radiologic and histologic features of periosteal osteosarcomas and periosteal (juxtacortical) chondrosarcomas are similar if not identical. A **high-grade surface osteosarcoma** (▷ *Fig. 14.62*) arises from the external surface of the cortex with clinical, histologic, and radiologic features comparable to a conventional osteosarcoma.
Parosteal osteosarcoma ▷ *Fig. 14.63a, b*	A large radiodense oval or round mass with smooth, lobulated, or irregular margins attached in sessile fashion to the external metaphyseal cortex of a long tubular bone is characteristic. A thin radiolucent line may separate the lesion outside its attachment (pedicle) from the cortex, which itself may be thickened. With progressive enlargement, the tumor tends to wrap around the bone. Ossification within the tumor proceeds from its base to the periphery and may be homogeneous or contain radiolucent areas. Tumor extension into the medullary bone is unusual. The most characteristic location is the posterior surface of the distal femur.	Most common type of osteosarcoma arising on the surface of a bone. Affected patients are adults most often in the third and fourth decades of life. Symptoms are typically insidious and include pain, swelling, and a palpable mass. The prognosis is better than in both conventional and periosteal osteosarcomas. Differential diagnosis: Posttraumatic myositis ossificans can be differentiated from a parosteal osteosarcoma by the demonstration of a fine radiolucent line separating the lesion in its entire length from the adjacent bone. Furthermore, the ossification in myositis ossificans is evenly radiodense throughout the lesion, and its periphery is sharply delineated, representing cancellous bone surrounded by a cortex.
Ewing sarcoma ▷ *Fig. 14.64* ▷ *Fig. 14.65*	A poorly defined osteolytic lesion with cortical violation and large soft tissue mass is characteristic. In tubular bones, an interrupted periosteal reaction of the laminated ("onion skin") or, less commonly, perpendicular ("sunburst" or "hair on end") pattern is typically associated. Saucerization of the cortex is a rare but relatively characteristic manifestation of the disease. In flat and irregular bones, osteosclerosis can be the dominant radiographic feature. The tumor can affect any bone but has a predilection for the diametaphysis of long tubular bones and overall the lower half of the skeleton. The most common locations include femur, tibia, humerus, pelvis, and sacrum.	Usually diagnosed between the ages of 5 and 30 y (peak 10–15 y), with slight male predominance. Involvement of the tubular bones occurs more often in children, whereas involvement of the flat bones is more commonly found in young adults. Patients present with localized pain and swelling, occasionally combined with fever and leukocytosis. The tumor is rare in blacks. **Primitive neuroectodermal tumors (PNETs)** (▷ *Fig. 14.66a*) have similar histologic and imaging features, but epiphyseal involvement, pathologic fractures, and distant metastases occur more frequently when compared with Ewing sarcoma. **Askin tumor** is a PNET variant arising from the intercostal nerves or ribs, usually in young Caucasian female patients (▷ *Fig. 14.66b*).

(continues on page 522)

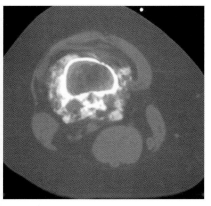

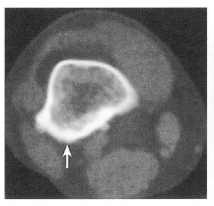

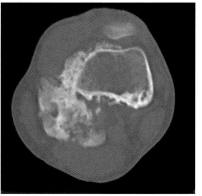

a

b

Fig. 14.62   High-grade surface osteosar-coma. A mass with highly irregular new bone formation surrounds the distal femur.

Fig. 14.63a, b   Parosteal osteosarcoma (two cases). (a) Irregular cortical thickening is seen in the posterior aspect of the distal femur in this low-grade malignancy. **(b)** A large ossified soft tissue mass is attached to the posteromedial aspect of the distal femur.

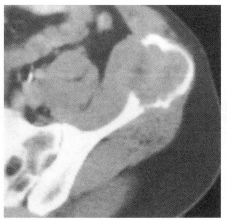

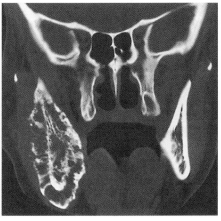

Fig. 14.64   Ewing sarcoma. Expansile destructive lesion with a large soft tissue mass is seen in the left iliac wing.

Fig. 14.65   Ewing sarcoma. Expansile osteolytic lesion with interrupted periosteal reaction is seen in the right ramus of the mandible.

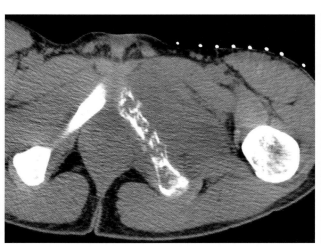

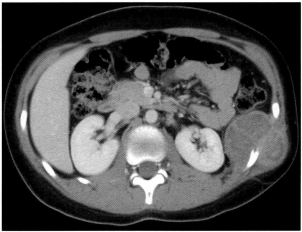

b

Fig. 14.66a, b   (a) Primitive neuroectodermal tumor (PNET). A permeative destructive lesion associated with a large soft tissue mass is evident in the left ischiopubic ramus. **(b) Askin tumor.** A large soft tissue mass is seen in the posterolateral aspect of the left abdominal wall originating from the adjacent rib.

Table 14.2   (Cont.) Localized bone lesions

Disease	CT Findings	Comments
Angiosarcoma ▷ *Fig. 14.67*	Solitary or multiple, poorly or well-demarcated lesions most commonly located in the medulla or cortex of long tubular bones, pelvis, spine, and skull. Cortical thinning or violation and/or mild expansion without periostitis is occasionally associated.	Occurs in the fourth and fifth decades, with male predominance. If multicentric, it may simulate multiple myeloma, metastases, cystic angiomatosis, and cystic osteomyelitis (e.g., tuberculous or fungal). **Hemangioendothelioma** (▷ *Fig. 14.68*) refers to a low-grade malignant angiosarcoma. **Hemangiopericytoma** is a borderline malignant tumor with similar imaging features.
Plasmacytoma ▷ *Fig. 14.69*	Presents either as an expansile (blow-out) trabeculated osteolytic lesion with cortical thinning and violation measuring up to several centimeters in diameter or as a well marginated, purely osteolytic focus with endosteal scalloping. Rarely, it may present as a sclerotic lesion (e.g., "ivory" vertebra). Most common locations are spine and pelvis. Complications in the spine include transdiscal tumor spread and pathologic fractures resulting sometimes in complete dissolution of a vertebral body.	Plasmacytoma may be considered a solitary manifestation of multiple myeloma with conversion to the latter occurring as late as 20 y after initial diagnosis. Plasmacytoma affects younger patients than multiple myeloma, with about half the patients being 50 or younger at the time of diagnosis. It frequently presents with neurologic symptoms and radiographically may be mistaken for a giant cell tumor.
Multiple myeloma ▷ *Fig. 14.70a, b*	Multiple well-marginated ("punched out") or poorly delineated osteolytic lesions of relatively uniform size are characteristic. Endosteal scalloping is typically present with larger lesions in the long tubular bones. Diffuse osteopenia without well-defined areas of osteolysis is, however, the most common presentation. Periosteal new bone formation is exceedingly rare. Focal or multiple sclerotic lesions are an unusual initial presentation but may develop after chemotherapy, irradiation, or pathologic fracture. Preferred locations in order of decreasing frequency are spine, ribs, skull, pelvis, long tubular bones, and clavicles (distal end). Spine: Generalized osteopenia with or without osteolytic foci is characteristic. Associated findings may include irregular thickening of the vertical trabeculae, relative sparing of the posterior elements, scalloping of the anterior margins of the vertebral bodies (pressure erosions from adjacent soft tissue lesions), and paraspinal or extradural tumor extension. Pathologic compression fractures are a frequent complication.	Occurs in patients older than 40 y with male predominance, presenting with bone pain, anemia, hypercalcemia, proteinuria (including Bence–Jones proteins), and monoclonal gammopathy (high erythrocyte sedimentation rate [ESR], abnormal electrophoresis). **Waldenström macroglobulinemia** presents with similar clinical and radiographic findings, but the radiographic features are usually less conspicuous. **Plasma cell granuloma:** Solitary or scattered, slow-growing osteoblastic foci consisting histologically of a dense infiltrate of normal plasma cells. Considered to be a variant of **chronic recurrent multifocal osteomyelitis (CRMO)** or **SAPHO** (synovitis, acne, pustulosis, hyperostosis, and osteitis). **POEMS syndrome** (polyneuropathy, organomegaly, endocrinopathy, M-protein, skin changes): Solitary or multiple osteosclerotic lesions and fluffy spiculated hyperostotic areas preferentially at sites of ligamentous attachments in axial and para-axial locations.

(continues on page 524)

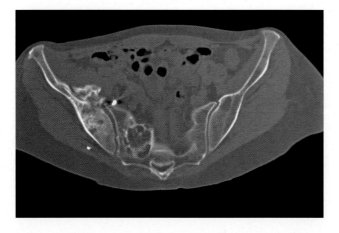

Fig. 14.67   Angiosarcoma. Multiple irregular osteolytic lesions, some with cortical violations, are seen in the right ilium and right sacral wing.

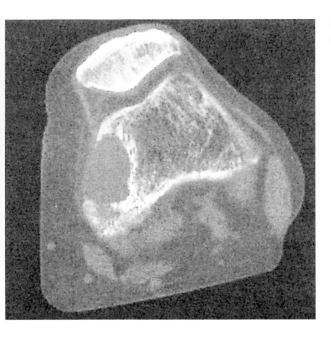

Fig. 14.68   Malignant hemangioendothelioma. A lytic lesion is seen in the medial aspect of the left distal femur.

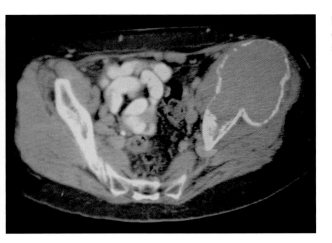

Fig. 14.69   Plasmacytoma. A large expansile ("blow-out") osteolytic lesion with a markedly thinned, partially intact cortical rim is seen in the left ilium.

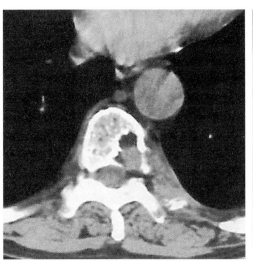

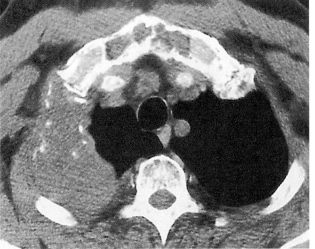

b

Fig. 14.70a, b   Multiple myeloma (two cases). (a) A sharply demarcated osteolytic lesion is seen in the left posterolateral aspect of the thoracic vertebral body with extension into the adjacent lateral paraspinal soft tissue. (**b**) A large soft tissue mass is seen in the right lateral chest wall originating from an almost completely destroyed rib. Expansile lytic lesions are also present in the sternum and adjacent ribs.

Table 14.2 (Cont.) Localized bone lesions

Disease	CT Findings	Comments
Metastases ▷ *Fig. 14.71a, b* ▷ *Fig. 14.72* ▷ *Fig. 14.73* ▷ *Fig. 14.74*	Solitary or, more commonly, multiple osteolytic, osteoblastic, or mixed osteolytic-osteoblastic lesions with preferential involvement of the red marrow containing skeleton (spine, pelvis, ribs, skull, proximal femora, and humeri) is characteristic. Osteolytic metastases may be well or poorly marginated. Osteoblastic metastases may be focal or diffuse. In the spine, besides the vertebral bodies, the posterior elements, including the pedicles, are frequently also involved (differential diagnosis: multiple myeloma). Purely osteolytic metastases commonly arise from carcinomas of lung, kidney, thyroid, and lymphoma. Purely osteoblastic metastases are most often associated with prostatic and breast carcinomas, but also with Hodgkin lymphoma, carcinoids, and medulloblastomas. Periosteal reactions are highly unusual in metastatic disease except in prostatic and breast carcinomas, gastrointestinal (GI) malignancies, and neuroblastomas. Neither osseous expansion nor soft tissue masses are typically associated with bone metastases except in rib lesions, osteolytic metastases from carcinomas originating in the kidney, thyroid, lung, and liver, and osteoblastic metastases from prostatic and breast carcinomas. One or more sclerotic vertebral body ("ivory" vertebra) is most often caused by prostatic or breast carcinoma metastases, but also found with Hodgkin lymphoma and Paget disease. Pathologic fractures are a frequent complication, especially in the spine. Response of an osteolytic metastasis to treatment (e.g., chemotherapy or radiation therapy) is evident by progressive sclerosis proceeding from the periphery toward the center of the lesion with eventual reduction in size or disappearance of the osteolytic focus. The appearance of osteosclerotic foci during therapy is usually caused by progression of the disease, but it may also indicate a healing response of preexisting osteolytic metastases that could initially not be identified on imaging examinations. A positive treatment response of osteoblastic lesions is evident by decrease and eventual disappearance of the sclerotic focus.	Bone metastases are by far the most common skeletal malignancy occurring either by hematogenous spread or direct tumor extension. They most frequently originate from carcinomas of breast, prostate, lung, kidney, thyroid, and GI tract. Breast carcinoma metastases tend to be mixed or, less commonly, purely osteolytic or osteoblastic, often extensive and frequently associated with pathologic fractures. Prostate carcinoma metastases are characteristically osteoblastic, may be expansile (simulating Paget disease), or associated with periostitis. Bronchogenic carcinoma metastases are typically osteolytic or mixed and occasionally expansile. An eccentric erosion of the external cortex of a long tubular bone ("cookie bite" sign) and an intracortical osteolytic lesion are rare in metastatic disease but when present strongly suggest a bronchogenic or GI primary tumor. Kidney and thyroid carcinoma metastases are often solitary, purely osteolytic lesions and may be expansile and depict a septated (bubbly) appearance. GI tract metastases cover the whole spectrum from purely osteolytic to purely osteoblastic. Metastases from colon or rectum carcinoma may occasionally resemble an osteosarcoma and depict a sunburst periosteal reaction. Metastatic bone disease with unknown primary most often originates from prostate, lymphoma, breast, lung, kidney, thyroid, or colon.

(continues on page 526)

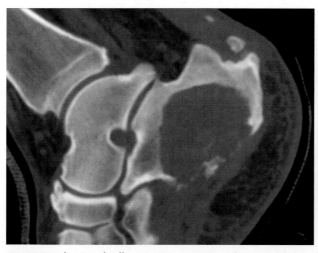
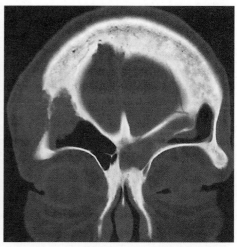

a   b

Fig. 14.71a, b Renal cell carcinoma metastases (two cases). (a) A large expansile, purely osteolytic metastasis with cortical disruption is seen in the calcaneus. **(b)** A large osteolytic lesion is seen in the right frontal bone.

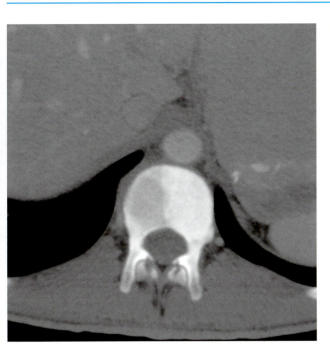

Fig. 14.72 Squamous cell carcinoma metastasis. A poorly defined osteolytic lesion is seen in the right half of the vertebral body.

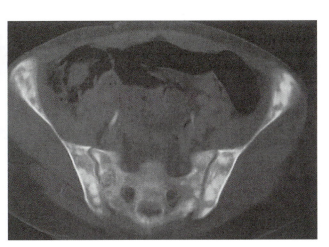

Fig. 14.73 Prostatic carcinoma metastases. Generalized osteoblastic metastases with a patchy sclerotic appearance in the ilium and a more diffuse sclerotic pattern in the sacrum are seen.

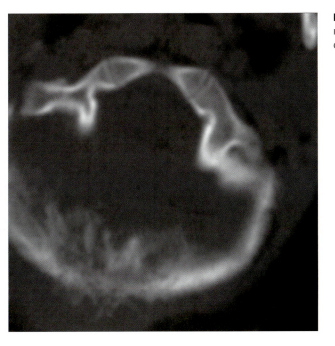

Fig. 14.74 Neuroblastoma metastasis. A predominantly osteolytic metastasis with extensive fluffy new bone formation is seen in the occiput.

Table 14.2   (Cont.) Localized bone lesions

Disease	CT Findings	Comments
Lymphoma ▷ *Fig. 14.75a–d* ▷ *Fig. 14.76*	Preferential sites of involvement include spine, pelvis, scapula, and ribs. In long tubular bones, involvement of the diametaphysis of the femur and tibia about the knee is most common. **Non–Hodgkin lymphoma** typically presents as solitary or, more often, multiple poorly defined osteolytic lesions. **Histiocytic lymphoma** (large B-cell lymphoma) frequently has a mixed osteolytic-osteoblastic appearance and may resemble Paget disease without bony expansion. Purely osteoblastic lesions are uncommon in non–Hodgkin lymphoma. **Hodgkin disease** of the bone is caused by secondary involvement. Its presentation ranges from purely osteolytic to purely osteoblastic lesions. Diffuse sclerosis of a vertebral body ("ivory" vertebra) is not an unusual manifestation. Osteolytic lesions tend to be poorly defined and are associated with periostitis in one third of the cases.	Secondary involvement of bone caused by hematogenous spread or, less frequently, by direct invasion occurs in one third of patients with non–Hodgkin lymphoma and in 10% with Hodgkin disease. Primary bone lymphoma is much less common, accounting for about 5% of all primary malignant bone tumors, is almost exclusively limited to non–Hodgkin lymphoma (especially the histiocytic [large B-cell] type), and typically occurs in older patients, with a 2:1 male predominance. **Burkitt lymphoma** presents as expansile osteolytic lesions associated with a soft tissue mass. Involvement of the facial bones (especially the maxilla) is most characteristic in children in tropical Africa. Nonendemic Burkitt lymphoma may be associated with immunodeficiency (e.g., organ transplantation and acquired immunodeficiency syndrome [AIDS]). **Mycosis fungoides** is a T-cell lymphoma with primary involvement of the skin. Discrete or poorly defined osteolytic lesions may be associated in the appendicular skeleton.
Leukemia	Diffuse osteopenia with medullary widening and cortical thinning in tubular bones and vertebral compressions are the most common presentation. Moth-eaten or permeative osteolysis may be found in both tubular and flat bones. Radiolucent and/or radiodense metaphyseal bands, as well as periosteal new bone formation, are particularly common in children. Complications may include intra-articular and subperiosteal hemorrhages, septic arthritis, osteomyelitis, osteonecrosis, and secondary gout. **Granulocytic sarcomas** (chloromas) present as single or multiple, often expansile lytic lesions in the skull, spine, ribs, sternum, and long tubular bones, usually in acute myelogenic leukemia.	Leukemias are classified based on cell maturity (acute with immature or blastic cells versus chronic with mature cells), cell morphology (myeloid versus lymphoid) or cell origin (thymus derived T cells versus blood marrow derived B cells). Skeletal abnormalities are similar for all forms of leukemias, but are most common in acute childhood leukemias, where they occur in over 50% of cases, and least common in chronic leukemias.

(continues on page 528)

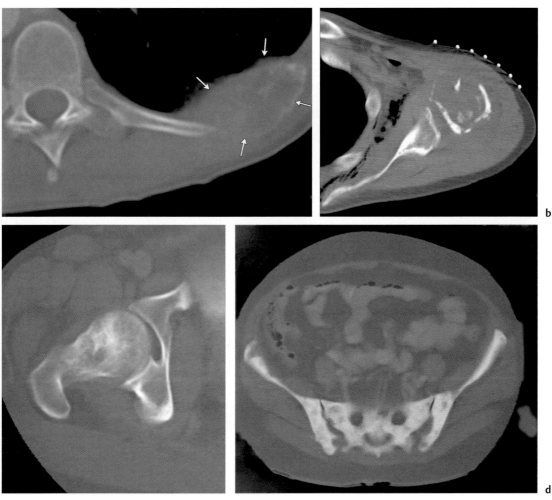

Fig. 14.75a–d   Lymphoma. Osseous manifestations vary from a chest wall soft tissue mass (arrows) secondary to a completely destroyed rib (**a**), to a solitary osteolytic humeral head lesion (**b**), to a mixed osteolytic and osteoblastic lesion in the femoral neck (**c**), and diffuse osteoblastic manifestations (**d**).

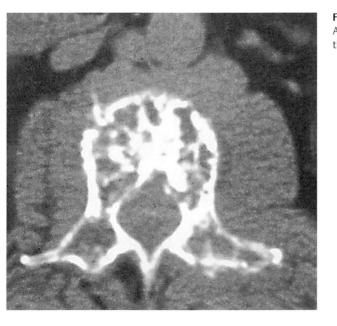

Fig. 14.76   Histiocytic lymphoma (large B-cell lymphoma). A coarse trabecular pattern that can mimic a hemangioma is seen in this vertebral body. A paraspinal soft tissue mass is also evident.

Table 14.2   (Cont.) Localized bone lesions

Disease	CT Findings	Comments
Langerhans cell histiocytosis (histiocytosis X) ▷ *Fig. 14.77* ▷ *Fig. 14.78* ▷ *Fig. 14.79a–c*	**Eosinophilic granuloma** presents as solitary or, less commonly, multiple lesions with preferential involvement of skull, mandible, spine, ribs, and the diametaphyses (rarely epiphyses) of long tubular bones. Relatively well-defined radiolucent areas with endosteal scalloping with or without slight bone expansion and varying degrees of periosteal new bone formation and sclerosis are typical in the long bones. More aggressive lesions with cortical violation and interrupted laminated periosteal reaction may mimic acute osteomyelitis or Ewing sarcoma. Well-defined lytic lesions with or without sclerotic borders may be found in the skull and pelvis. A radiodense focus (button sequestrum) is frequently observed in skull lesions. Larger osteolytic areas in the skull typically depict beveled edges caused by the uneven destruction of the inner and outer tables. In the mandible, radiolucent lesions about the teeth may lead to the "floating teeth" appearance. In the spine, a collapsed vertebral body (vertebra plana) with intact intervertebral spaces or, less frequently, a lytic and occasionally slightly expansile lesion involving the vertebral body and/or the posterior elements may be found.	Langerhans cell histiocytosis comprises three major conditions. 1. **Eosinophilic granuloma** is both the most common and most benign variant, representing about 70% of cases. It is usually diagnosed between age 5 and 20 y. Spontaneous healing of a solitary lesion occurs, typically progressing from the periphery toward its center, and eventually resulting in its disappearance or transformation into a sclerotic focus. 2. **Hand–Schüller–Christian disease** is characterized by the triad of exophthalmos, diabetes insipidus, and large lytic skull lesions ("geographic skull"). 3. **Letterer–Siwe disease** is the acute disseminated variant in children younger than 2. Bone lesions are less common but may include multiple widespread lytic lesions in the skull ("raindrop" pattern). Hepatosplenomegaly, lymphadenopathy, and nonitching eczematous skin lesions are commonly associated.
Amyloidosis	Osteolytic lesions of variable size with endosteal scalloping simulating multiple myeloma preferentially located in the proximal humerus or proximal femur is the most common presentation. Subchondral amyloid deposition may result in avascular necrosis caused by perivascular amyloid deposition with subsequent vascular occlusion. Pathologic fractures are a relatively common complication. Subchondral cyst formation and erosions in the hand and wrist (especially carpal bones) associated with periarticular or diffuse osteoporosis may simulate rheumatoid arthritis, although extensive nodular soft tissue masses, well-defined cystic lesions with or without surrounding sclerosis and preservation of the joint space are more characteristic for amyloidosis.	Musculoskeletal abnormalities are the result of amyloid deposition in bone, synovium, and soft tissue. Primary amyloidosis occurs in patients older than 40, with male predominance. It may be associated with multiple myeloma. Secondary amyloidosis is associated with chronic renal disease, rheumatoid arthritis, lupus erythematosus, ulcerative colitis, chronic suppurative disease, and lymphoproliferative disorders.
Brown tumor in hyperparathyroidism ▷ *Fig. 14.80*	Single or multiple, occasionally expansile, well- to poorly defined osteolytic lesions of the axial and appendicular skeleton. Eccentric or cortical location is not unusual. Common sites of involvement are facial bones, pelvis, ribs, and femora. Brown tumors may undergo necrosis and liquefaction, producing cysts, or with proper treatment (removal of the parathyroid adenoma) become increasingly sclerotic.	Brown tumors are more commonly associated with primary than secondary hyperparathyroidism. Other manifestations of hyperparathyroidism are usually also apparent and include osteopenia, subperiosteal, endosteal, and subchondral bone resorption, intracortical tunneling, chondrocalcinosis, and paraarticular calcifications and vascular calcifications. Bone sclerosis is common in secondary hyperparathyroidism.
Hemophilic pseudotumor ▷ *Fig. 14.81*	Central (intraosseous) or eccentric (subperiosteal), well-demarcated osteolytic lesion, often associated with cortical violation, a solid or interrupted periosteal reaction, and a large soft tissue mass is a common presentation. Minimal to massive calcification within the lesion is occasionally also encountered. Rarely, more than one bone contains a pseudotumor. Preferred locations are pelvis, femur, tibia, and hand.	Lesions are late sequelae of intramedullary or periosteal hemorrhage/hematoma occurring in < 2% of hemophiliacs. Hemophilic arthropathy, including dense joint effusions and joint contractures, avascular necrosis, especially of the femoral head and talus, spontaneous fractures, and soft tissue hematomas, may also be evident. Knee, ankle, and elbow are most frequently affected.
Intraosseous tophus in gout	One or more cystic lesions often with partial calcification may be found in the subchondral and deeper osseous areas simulating enchondromas. Larger intraosseous calcifications may mimic bone infarcts. These findings are most frequently seen in the hands and feet. Association with characteristic findings of gouty arthropathy is diagnostic.	Occurs in about 5% of patients with chronic gouty arthritis. Intraosseous urate deposition with subsequent calcifications usually originates from the adjacent joint, penetrates the cartilaginous surface, and extends into the spongiosa.

(continues on page 530)

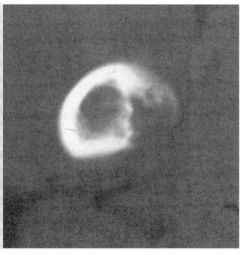

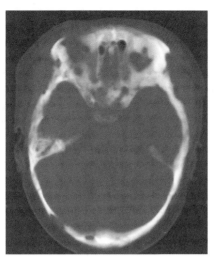

Fig. 14.77   Langerhans cell histiocytosis. An eccentric lesion is seen in the midshaft of the femur with cortical destruction, soft tissue extension, and periosteal reaction.

Fig. 14.78   Langerhans cell histiocytosis. Diffuse lytic and sclerotic involvement of the vault and base of the skull is seen.

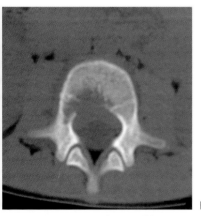

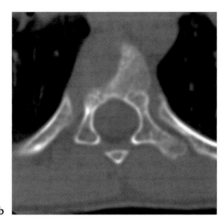

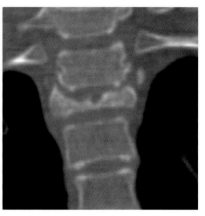

Fig. 14.79a–c   Langerhans cell histiocytosis. Vertebral manifestations include a poorly defined osteolytic lesion (**a**), a well-demarcated osteolytic lesion with a sclerotic border (**b**), and a vertebra plana (**c**).

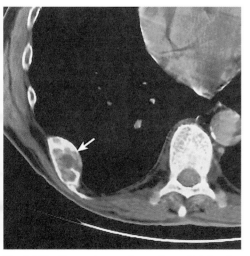

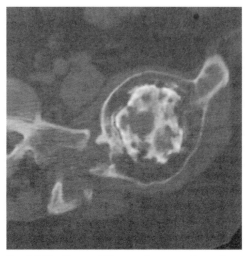

Fig. 14.80   Brown tumor. Expansile, well-defined osteolytic lesion is seen in a rib (arrow).

Fig. 14.81   Hemophilic pseudotumor. Expansile lesion with central calcification is seen in the left ilium of a patient with von Willebrand disease.

Table 14.2   (Cont.) Localized bone lesions

Disease	CT Findings	Comments
Osteonecrosis (bone infarct and avascular necrosis) ▷ *Fig. 14.82*	Early signs are nonspecific and include mottled osteopenia, poorly defined osteolytic lesion(s), or patchy osteopenic and sclerotic areas. Findings are more characteristic in a more advanced later stage. In the diametaphyses, they include serpiginous peripheral rim of calcification or sclerosis surrounding an oblong area of bone rarefaction. Periostitis and matrix calcifications are frequently associated. Intramedullary calcifications are often the only finding and are typically shell-like and peripheral, whereas the calcifications in chondroid matrix tumors tend to be punctate, ringlike or irregular and central and are surrounded by a rim of noncalcified, radiolucent tumor matrix. Solid periosteal reactions and cortical thickening may be associated with both conditions, but in the case of chondroid matrix tumor suggest a low-grade chondrosarcoma rather than enchondroma. Typical findings of osteonecrosis in the epiphyses (avascular necrosis) include curvilinear subchondral sclerosis, subchondral cyst(s) with sclerotic rim, arclike subchondral radiolucency (crescent sign), subchondral fragmentation, and eventually collapse of the articular surface, with considerable sclerosis and secondary degenerative changes in the affected joint.	Osteonecrosis can be divided into bone infarction, occurring more frequently in the metadiaphyseal regions of long bones (e.g., femur, humerus, and tibia) than in the axial skeleton, and avascular necrosis involving the subarticular bone. Solitary bone infarcts are frequently diagnosed as an incidental finding. Scintigraphy and MRI are far more sensitive than CT in the diagnosis of early avascular necrosis. Osteonecrosis may be idiopathic (25%) or associated with hematological and reticuloendothelial diseases (e.g., sickle cell and Gaucher disease), connective tissue diseases (e.g., lupus erythematosus), trauma (e.g., subcapital hip fracture), human immunodeficiency virus [HIV] infection, renal transplantation, alcoholism, steroid use, pancreatitis, gout, amyloidosis, hemophilia, irradiation, and caisson disease. **Radiation osteitis (osteonecrosis)** (▷ *Fig. 14.83*) presents with a mixture of osteopenia, osteosclerosis, and coarse trabeculation (pagetoid bone). Round to ovoid radiolucent lesions within the cortex of long tubular bones are characteristic as opposed to endosteal scalloping caused by tumor recurrence. Bony changes are dose-dependent, with a minimal dose of 3000 cGy required, and occur at the earliest 1 y after irradiation, at a time, when a nuclear medicine scan no longer depicts an increased uptake. **Calcified intraosseous hematomas** may present on CT similar to a calcified bone infarct.
Healing fracture/stress fracture ▷ *Fig. 14.84*	Osteosclerosis and localized callus formation in the cortex of long tubular bones may simulate chronic cortical osteomyelitis and osteoid osteoma, respectively. Demonstration of a fracture line in an area of localized elliptical cortical thickening of a long tubular bone (as opposed to a round or ovoid intracortical abscess or a nidus) is diagnostic.	CT is useful in the assessment of fracture healing and the diagnosis of complications, such as delayed union, nonunion, osteomyelitis, osteonecrosis, and posttraumatic myositis ossificans.
Pigmented villonodular synovitis (PVNS) ▷ *Fig. 14.85*	Intra-articular/periarticular soft tissue mass and joint effusion with often slightly increased attenuation values due to varying degrees of hemosiderin deposition are characteristic. Subchondral pressure erosions with or without sclerotic margins may be found in "tight" joints, such as hip, ankle, and wrist. Calcifications, osteoporosis, and joint space narrowing are typically absent. Pressure erosions in the knee (most commonly involved joint) are uncommon.	Monoarticular proliferative synovial disorder presenting with insidious onset of swelling, pain of long duration, and decreased range of motion occurring typically in young adults. A hemorrhagic (chocolate brown) joint effusion in the absence of trauma is characteristic. Differential diagnosis: synovial (osteo)chondromatosis in which calcified/ossified loose bodies are characteristic.

(continues on page 532)

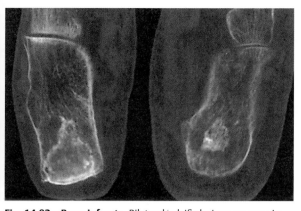

Fig. 14.82 Bone infarcts. Bilateral calcific lesions are seen in both calcanei.

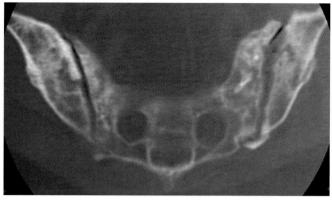

Fig. 14.83 Radiation osteitis. Mixed lytic and sclerotic lesions are seen in both ilia and adjacent sacrum.

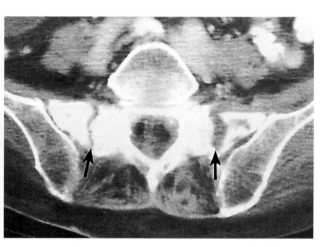

Fig. 14.84 Insufficiency fractures. Symmetric bilateral fracture lines (arrows) with considerable adjacent sclerosis are seen in the sacrum.

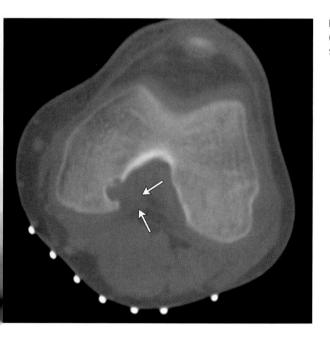

Fig. 14.85 Pigmented villonodular synovitis. A soft tissue mass (arrows) is seen in the intercondylic area causing an erosion with sclerotic margin in the medial femoral condyle.

Table 14.2   (Cont.) Localized bone lesions

Disease	CT Findings	Comments
Osteomyelitis (acute) ▷ *Fig. 14.86* ▷ *Fig. 14.87* ▷ *Fig. 14.88* ▷ *Fig. 14.89*	**Hematogenous osteomyelitis** presents initially in the medullary space with focal osteoporosis, endosteal scalloping, and osteolysis due to hyperemia, edema, abscess formation, and trabecular destruction. Progression of the disease to the Haversian and Volkmann canals results in cortical fissuring with subsequent destruction and subperiosteal abscess formation. A periosteal reaction (laminated or, less commonly, spiculated) is a characteristic finding at this stage. After 1 month, a sequestrum (detached necrotic cortical bone) presenting as a radiodense bony spicule surrounded by granulation tissue and newly formed cortical bone (involucrum) may be evident. An opening in the involucrum is termed a cloaca. Sinus tracts leading to the skin surface are often evident. Occasionally, intraosseous gas or fat–fluid (pus) levels may be seen. In both infants and adults, extension of the disease process into the adjacent joint is common, whereas in childhood (1–16 y), the open growth plate represents an effective barrier to the spread of the infection from the metaphysis to the epiphysis and joint, respectively. **Osteomyelitis from a contiguous soft tissue infection** typically presents as focal osteoporosis due to edema with subsequent cortical erosion. Periostitis is another less frequent initial finding. Cortical destruction and bone marrow infection with abscess formation may ensue.	Affects all ages, but is commonly found in children, diabetics, and IV drug abusers. Occurs by hematogenous route, spread from contiguous infection, or direct implantation (punctures, penetrating injury, and postoperative infection). Pyogenic osteomyelitis in children is most often caused by *Staphylococcus aureus, Streptococci, Escherichia coli,* and *Haemophilus influenzae.* Gram-negative organisms are not uncommon in adults and IV drug abusers. **Tuberculous osteomyelitis** occurs mainly by the hematogenous route. Spinal involvement accounts for about 50% of skeletal tuberculosis. Paraspinal abscess formation (e.g., in psoas muscle) is common and frequently contains calcifications. Compared with pyogenic osteomyelitis, osteoporosis is more pronounced, whereas new bone formation is less extensive. **Tuberculous dactylitis** (spina ventosa) refers to cystic expansion of the short tubular bones of the hands and feet of young children with varying degrees of periostitis. **Cystic tuberculosis** presents as one or multiple well-defined osteolytic foci without sclerosis, preferentially in the peripheral skeleton. **Fungal osteomyelitis** resembles a tuberculous infection. Solitary or multiple osteolytic lesions with discrete margins, mild surrounding sclerosis, and little or no periosteal reaction are a common presentation.
Brodie abscess ▷ *Fig. 14.90*	Usually solitary, lytic, and often elongated lesion with sclerotic border typically in the metaphyses of long bones. Epiphyses, diaphyses, and flat and irregular bones (e.g., carpus and tarsus) are less common locations. In the epiphysis, a circular well-defined osteolytic lesion is typical. In the diaphysis, the abscesses may be found in central, subcortical, or cortical locations. In the cortex, the abscess is surrounded by periosteal new bone formation, simulating an osteoid osteoma or a stress fracture.	Subacute pyogenic osteomyelitis (smoldering indolent infection), usually of *staphylococcal origin,* is common in children, in whom the lesion is typically located in the proximal or distal tibia metaphysis and sometimes connected to the growth plate by a tortuous channel. Histologically, a central purulent or mucoid fluid collection is surrounded by inflammatory granulation tissue and spongy bone eburnation. The lesion may occasionally contain a central sequestrum.
Osteomyelitis, chronic ▷ *Fig. 14.91*	Thick, irregular sclerotic bone with radiolucencies and extensive periosteal new bone formation is characteristic. Signs of remaining activity or reactivation include a change from the previous exam, poorly defined areas of osteolysis, laminated periosteal reaction, poorly defined bony excrescences, and demonstration of a sequestrum, sinus tract, or soft tissue abscess. **Sclerosing osteomyelitis of Garré** is a low-grade infection without purulent exudate presenting as focal or circumferential cortical thickening and sclerosis in the mandible (most commonly) or diaphyses of long tubular bones. In the latter location, osteoid osteoma, stress fracture, and **Ribbing disease** (hereditary multiple diaphyseal sclerosis with typically asymmetric distribution) must be considered in the differential diagnosis.	Late acquired **syphilis** resembles chronic osteomyelitis. Thickened sclerotic long bones caused by endosteal and periosteal new bone formation and ill-defined lytic lesions (gumma formation) are characteristic. **CRMO (chronic recurrent multifocal osteomyelitis, chronic plasma cell osteomyelitis)** presents most commonly in children with a protracted clinical course and often symmetric involvement of the medial ends of the clavicles or the metaphyses of long bones with a combination of osteolysis and osteosclerosis and extensive periosteal reaction and new bone formation. **SAPHO syndrome** may be a related condition. **Epidermoid carcinoma** occurs in 1% of osteomyelitis at the site of a chronically draining sinus and is evident as an enlarging soft tissue mass eroding the osteomyelitic bone.

(continues on page 534)

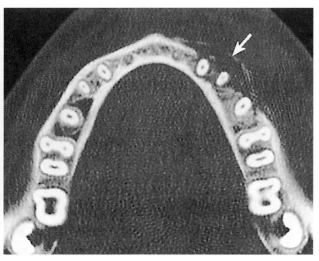

Fig. 14.86 Osteomyelitis. Destructive lesion is seen in the mandible with a thin, laminated periosteal reaction (arrow).

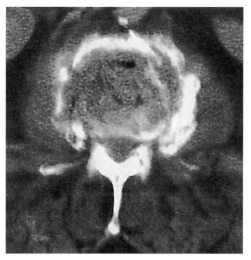

Fig. 14.87 Gas-forming osteomyelitis. Destructive lesion with scattered areas of gas collection is seen in the lumbar vertebral body.

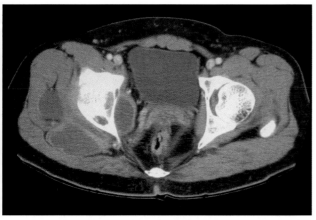

Fig. 14.88 Tuberculous osteomyelitis. Osteolytic lesions in the right acetabular roof are associated with three large abscesses in the surrounding soft tissues.

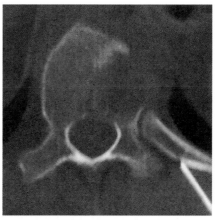

Fig. 14.89 Fungal osteomyelitis. Focal destructive lesion is seen in the thoracic vertebral body. CT-guided biopsy revealed blastomycosis.

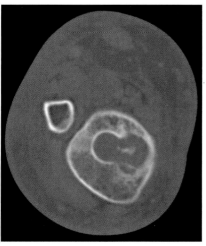

Fig. 14.90 Brodie abscess. A figure 8–shaped osteolytic lesion with a central bone sequestrum and thin sclerotic margins is seen in the tibia.

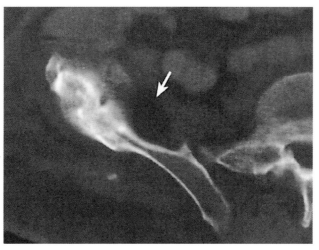

Fig. 14.91 Chronic osteomyelitis. Osteolytic defects surrounded by sclerosis are evident in the right iliac wing. An iliopsoas abscess (arrow) is also evident as a low-density soft tissue lesion.

Table 14.2 (Cont.) Localized bone lesions

Disease	CT Findings	Comments
Gorham disease (vanishing bone disease) ▷ *Fig. 14.92*	Progressive, often massive osteolysis without attempt of repair (no periosteal or osteosclerotic reaction) spreading across joints or intervertebral spaces is characteristic. Preferential locations are the hip and shoulder regions, although any bone can be affected. Tapering or "pointing" of the long bones at the sites of osteolysis is typical. In the pelvis, a rapidly destructive arthropathy of the hip presenting with destruction of primarily the femoral head and to a lesser degree the acetabulum must be differentiated. This condition may represent an unusual aggressive form of osteoarthritis (rapidly progressive destructive osteoarthritis), osteonecrosis, CPPD, or hydroxyapatite crystal deposition disease (HADD), or may occur after intra-articular corticosteroid injections. **Proximal femoral focal deficiency (PFFD)** characterized by partial absence of the proximal femur is diagnosed in infancy.	Occurs sporadically at any age, without gender predilection, but is usually diagnosed before the age of 40 y. Histologically, a nonmalignant proliferation of angiomatous and fibrous tissue is evident. Other osteolysis syndromes diagnosed in infancy or childhood include acro-osteolysis of Hajdu and Cheney, Joseph, or Shinz, carpal-tarsal osteolysis (hereditary or associated with nephropathy), Farber disease (elbows, wrists, knees, and ankles), and Winchester syndrome (carpal and tarsal areas and elbows).
Fibromatosis	Solitary or multiple soft tissue masses with erosions of the adjacent bone or osteolytic lesions. Cortical hyperostosis may be associated with bone involvement.	Variety of benign, but often aggressive fibrous proliferations presenting in both children and adults as tumorlike soft tissue lesions. Involvement of the adjacent bone is not uncommon in infantile forms of the disease.
Membranous lipodystrophy (polycystic lipomembranous osteodysplasia)	Symmetric and slowly progressive lytic lesions are found in the carpal and tarsal bones and the ends of long and short tubular bones. Bone deformities may eventually occur from pathologic fractures.	Rare hereditary disorder of adipose tissue affecting primarily the bones and brain. Presents commonly in the second or third decade of life with painful bones and joints and subsequently with presenile dementia.
Paget disease (osteitis deformans) ▷ *Fig. 14.93* ▷ *Fig. 14.94* ▷ *Fig. 14.95* ▷ *Fig. 14.96*	Monostotic or more commonly polyostotic asymmetric lesions with preferential involvement of the pelvis, femur, tibia, spine, skull, scapula, and humerus. The pattern of involvement ranges from purely osteolytic (e.g., osteoporosis circumscripta in the calvarium, and V- or flame-shaped defect in the diaphyses of long bones) to purely osteosclerotic (e.g., "ivory" vertebra). The mixed pattern (e.g., "picture frame" vertebra and "cotton wool" appearance of the skull) that is usually associated with bony enlargement, cortical thickening, and coarse trabeculation represents the most common manifestation. In long bones, the disease characteristically progresses from an epiphysis to the diaphysis. Bone softening may result in bowing deformities of the long bones, acetabular protrusion, biconcave compression of vertebral end plates, and basilar invagination. Complications include cortical stress fractures, single or multiple horizontal radiolucent lines in the convex aspect of the deformed bone (lateral aspect of the femoral neck and shaft, anterior aspect of tibia), transverse pathologic fractures, and sarcomatous degeneration.	Common disorder of middle-aged and elderly patients that is often diagnosed as an incidental finding on radiographs obtained for unrelated purposes. The disease is present in 10% of patients over the age of 80 y and rare in patients under 40. Laboratory findings include elevated alkaline phosphatase and hydroxyproline levels in the serum and abnormally high hydroxyproline urine levels. Serum acid phosphatase values are normal. Neoplastic involvement in Paget disease includes sarcomatous degeneration, giant cell tumor, aneurysmal bone cyst, and superimposition of metastases, multiple myeloma, and lymphoma. Sarcomatous degeneration occurs in about 1% of patients usually older than 55 y. Predominantly osteolytic osteosarcomas (60%), malignant fibrous histiocytoma/fibrosarcomas (25%), and chondrosarcomas (10%) are the most frequent tumors found in sarcomatous degeneration. **Calvarial hyperostosis interna** (frontalis or generalisata) must be differentiated from Paget disease. Both conditions affect primarily the inner table, but in calvarial hyperostosis, it is irregularly thickened or nodular in outline and predominates in elderly women (▷ *Fig. 14.97*).

(continues on page 536)

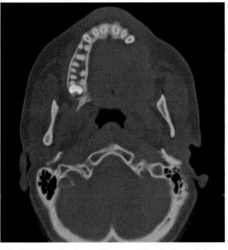

Fig. 14.92   Gorham disease. Dissolution of the mandible without any bony response such as periosteal reaction is seen.

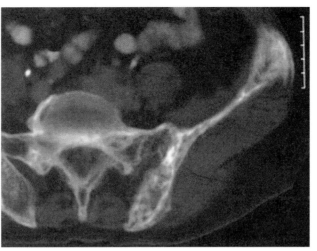

Fig. 14.93   Paget disease. Coarse trabeculation, sclerotic foci, and cortical thickening are seen in the left hemipelvis.

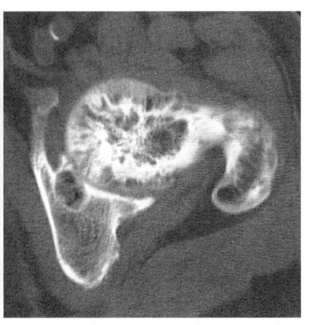

Fig. 14.94   Paget disease. Coarse trabeculation with sclerotic and lytic changes is seen in the proximal femur. Note also the synovial cyst in the posterior wall of the acetabulum.

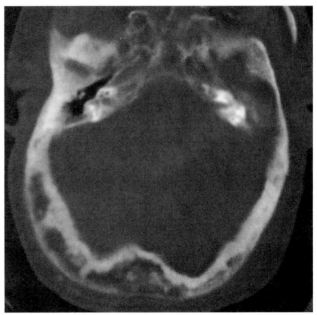

Fig. 14.95   Paget disease. Irregular thickening with both sclerotic and lytic changes involves preferentially the inner table and the diploic space.

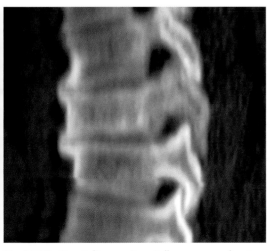

Fig. 14.96   Paget disease. A partially compressed vertebral body with "picture frame" appearance is seen in the thoracic spine.

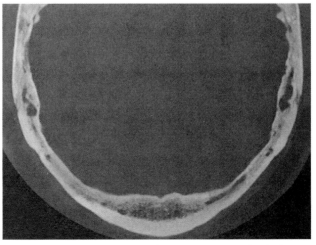

Fig. 14.97   Hyperostosis generalisata interna. Irregular thickening of the cranial vault is largely confined to the inner table.

IV Musculoskeletal System

Table 14.2 (Cont.) Localized bone lesions

Disease	CT Findings	Comments
Fibrous dysplasia ▷ *Fig. 14.98* ▷ *Fig. 14.99a, b* ▷ *Fig. 14.100* ▷ *Fig. 14.101* ▷ *Fig. 14.102*	Solitary or multiple, often slightly expansile radiolucent lesions that may have a hazy quality ("ground glass" appearance). The matrix may also be uniformly dense, partially calcified or ossified, or thick, dense bands may be present. A curvilinear sclerotic rim may outline lytic lesions. Purely sclerotic lesions occur in the skull and facial bones. The monostotic form (75%) commonly involves a rib, femur, tibia, humerus, and mandible, whereas the polyostotic form (25%) frequently involves the skull and facial bones, pelvis, spine, and shoulder girdle besides the long tubular bones. Polyostotic fibrous dysplasia may be unilateral or bilateral and may affect several bones of a single limb, both limbs, or all four extremities besides the axial skeleton. Solitary lesions in the long bones are located in the diaphyses or, less commonly, metaphyses. Bowing deformities are frequent in the polyostotic form.	Usually diagnosed before the age of 30. In **McCune-Albright syndrome**, precocious female sexual development and café-au-lait spots are associated with the polyostotic form. Differential diagnosis: Neurofibromatosis, where more irregularly contoured and darker café-au-lait spots are frequently associated with similar bone lesions. **Ossifying fibromas** are closely related to fibrous dysplasia and occur in the facial bones (especially mandible) and tubular bones (especially anterior aspect of the tibia). In the latter location, they are also referred to as **osteofibrous dysplasia** (▷ *Figs. 14.103, 14.104 [p. 538]*). Skeletal abnormalities in **neurofibromatosis 1 (von Recklinghausen disease)** may simulate polyostotic fibrous dysplasia. A unilateral enlarged orbit with absent lesser and greater sphenoid wings is **diagnostic** (▷ *Fig. 14.105, p. 538*). Severe kyphoscoliosis, associated with vertebral body wedging and scalloping, and foraminal enlargement are typical findings in the spine. Congenital pseudoarthrosis in the distal tibia and fibula is another manifestation.
Sarcoidosis	Solitary or multiple osteolytic lesions with a coarsened or lacework trabecular pattern that may be associated with endosteal scalloping or cortical violation without periosteal reaction is the most common presentation. Purely osteolytic ("punched out") cystic lesions or purely osteosclerotic foci are less common presentations. The hand is the predominant site of involvement where acrosclerosis or acro-osteolysis may also be present.	Osseous sarcoidosis is usually associated with either skin lesions or pulmonary disease.
Particle disease (foreign body granuloma) ▷ *Fig. 14.106, p. 538*	Presents typically as scalloped osteolytic lesions with or without sclerotic margins about a prosthetic component. Larger expansile lesions may become trabeculated and eventually break through cortex without inciting a periosteal reaction.	Foreign body reaction to prosthetic components such as polymethylmethacrylate cement, polyethylene, and silicone. Rarely, an intraosseous foreign body granuloma is found that is not associated with joint replacement surgery or any other known cause of accidental foreign body implantation. If the foreign body is located in the cortex, the lesion may mimic a chronic cortical abscess or osteoid osteoma/osteoblastoma, respectively.

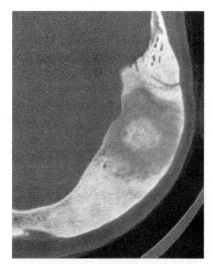

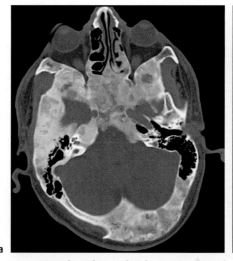

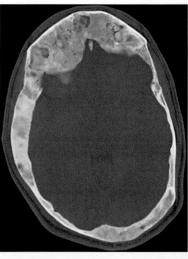

Fig. 14.98 Fibrous dysplasia. Localized thickening of the calvarium with a radiolucent lesion containing a sclerotic center is evident.

Fig. 14.99a, b Fibrous dysplasia. Irregular enlargement of the bone with "ground glass" appearance interrupted by scattered osteolytic lesions is seen in the base (**a**) and vault (**b**) of the skull.

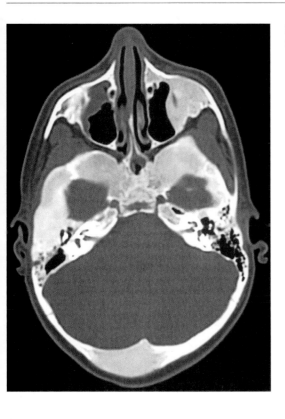

Fig. 14.100   Fibrous dysplasia. "Ground glass" appearance is evident in all enlarged bony structures of the skull.

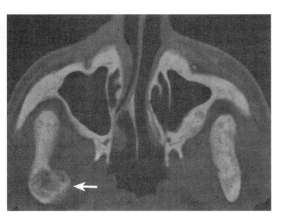

Fig. 14.101   Fibrous dysplasia. Variable sclerotic thickening of all facial bones is seen with scattered radiolucent lesions, the largest being located in the posterior aspect of the right mandible (arrow).

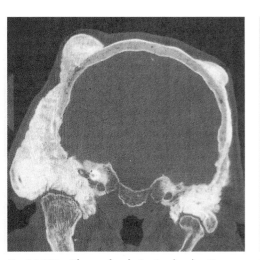

Fig. 14.102   Fibrous dysplasia. Purely sclerotic changes with irregular bone thickening are limited to the skull base and outer tables of the cranial vault. Abnormal condylar processes of the mandible are also evident.

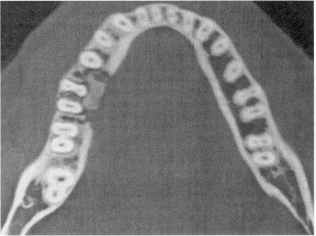

Fig. 14.103   Ossifying fibroma. Sclerotic and lytic changes are seen in the right mandible.

IV Musculoskeletal System

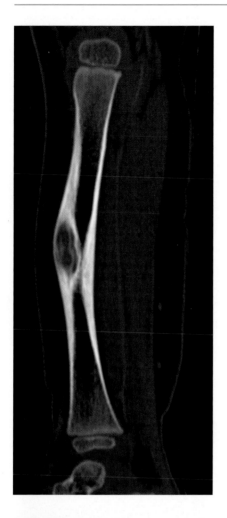

Fig. 14.104 Ossifying fibroma (osteofibrous dysplasia). An expansile, elliptical osteolytic lesion with intact margins is seen in the anterior cortex of the tibial shaft.

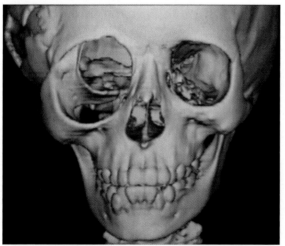

Fig. 14.105 Neurofibromatosis. An enlarged and deformed right orbit with absent sphenoid wings is diagnostic.

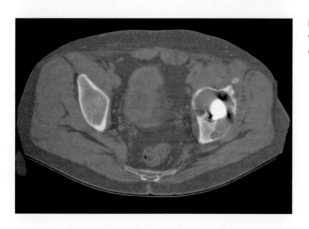

Fig. 14.106 Particle disease. A slightly expansile osteolytic lesion with thinning and scalloping of the cortex is seen about the acetabular component of the left total hip prosthesis.

15 Trauma and Fractures

Francis A. Burgener

Conventional radiography remains the primary diagnostic imaging modality for assessing fractures and dislocations. However, the role of computed tomography (CT) in fracture evaluation increased greatly with the introduction of helical multislice scanners, allowing shortening of examination time and display of images in multiple planes with superb resolution or three-dimensional reconstruction, respectively. Compared with conventional radiography, CT is overall superior to visualize skeletal pathology, but drawbacks of the latter imaging modality include greater expense, increased radiation dose, and both motion and metal artifacts.

The radiologic diagnosis of an acute fracture is usually not associated with any problems. A sharply demarcated fracture line is the hallmark of an acute fracture. Occasionally, however, a frank fracture line cannot be demonstrated in nondisplaced fractures even when conventional images in several projections are taken. In this condition, high-resolution CT usually allows arrival at the correct diagnosis by demonstration of a cortical break or disruption of the normal spongiosa pattern that could not be appreciated with the conventional radiographic examination. Because of its high sensitivity, magnetic resonance imaging (MRI) however, is the image modality of choice for identifying occult fractures for which correct early diagnosis is essential (e.g., femoral neck and scaphoid fractures).

CT is useful in the evaluation of all complex fractures, but the most common indications include fractures of the spine, scapula, and pelvis, fractures of long tubular bones extending into an articular surface, and fractures/dislocations involving carpal and tarsal bones. In all these locations, fractures are missed or underestimated in up to 50% of cases when conventional radiography is compared with CT, resulting not infrequently in a change of the patient's management based on the additional information provided by CT. CT is often inevitable in the evaluation of the reduction of complex fractures and dislocations and is of considerable value in the assessment of complications in fracture healing.

Fracture healing begins with an inflammatory response resulting in the organization of the fracture hematoma by invasion of fibrovascular tissue. Bone resorption along the fracture margins becomes evident and in undisplaced fractures may allow at this stage (several days after the injury incidence) an unequivocal radiographic diagnosis. Periosteal and endosteal callus formation usually becomes visible 2 to 3 weeks after injury and is first evident as a thin periosteal reaction and irregular mottled calcifications about the fracture, increasing with time in density and finally developing bone texture. The healing process of a noncomplicated fracture from injury to consolidation takes one to several months. Fracture healing progresses more rapidly in oblique or spiral fractures, in a single fracture, and in younger patients. The healing process is slower in larger bones, in transverse fractures, in the presence of multiple fractures, in osteopenia, and with increasing age of the patient. *Malunion* refers to a fracture that is healed with significant fracture fragment displacement and/or angulation.

A *delayed union* is found with poor reduction, incomplete immobilization, in the presence of infection, in vitamin C and/or D deficiencies, and in areas of preexisting bone disease (pathologic fractures). Infections are particularly common in *compound* (open) *fractures*, where extensive soft tissue damage is caused by either a fracture fragment piercing through the skin or by an object (e.g., a projectile) penetrating from the outside.

Assessing partially united and nonunited fractures is especially improved by CT when compared with conventional radiography. *Nonunion* (**Figs. 15.1, 15.2**) is characterized by failure of fracture healing 6 to 9 months after injury. The fracture margins are well delineated and often sclerotic, and a frank area of intervening translucency is present. Nonunion may result from the same complications associated with delayed union or by interposition of soft tissue between the fracture fragments. Hypertrophic nonunion is commonly caused by continued motion at the fracture site. In these cases, the fracture line persists or excessive and prolonged bone resorption at the fracture margins occurs. Eventually the bone ends become sclerotic, and there is a varying degree of non-bridging external callus formation. Atrophic nonunion is thought to result from extensive bone death. The radiographic appearance is that of a persistent fracture line without demonstrable callus formation (**Fig. 15.3**). Nonunion may eventually progress to pseudoarthrosis formation.

Fracture healing in osteogenesis imperfecta is complicated by *pseudoarthrosis* formations with a higher incidence than in normal bone. Pseudarthrosis is also a common feature in neurofibromatosis, where it is most often found in the lower two thirds of the tibia. Pseudoarthrosis occurs also in fibrous dysplasia, which often demonstrates bone changes radiographically similar to neurofibromatosis. The two disorders can, however, often be differentiated by their skin manifestations. The café-au-lait spots in fibrous dysplasia are irregularly outlined, whereas they are smoothly outlined in neurofibromatosis. Furthermore, the presence of cutaneous fibromas is characteristic for the latter condition. "Congenital pseudoarthrosis" involving the distal tibia and/or fibula shaft is a rare condition that may or may not be related to neurofibromatosis or fibrous dysplasia (forme fruste?).

A fracture may be complete or incomplete. The former implies complete disruption in the continuity of a bone. In an incomplete fracture, only some of the bony trabeculae are completely severed, whereas others are bent or remain intact. Incomplete fractures occur predominantly in elastic bones of children and young adults.

A *dislocation* is a complete disruption of a joint with the articular surfaces no longer in contact with each other. A *subluxation* is a less severe disruption of a joint in which some articular contact remains. Traumatic, habitual, pathologic (secondary to joint disease), paralytic, and congenital dislocations are differentiated.

Depending on their radiographic appearances, fractures are classified into different types (**Fig. 15.4**). Fracture alignment refers to the relationship of one fragment to another. Unless stated differently, the fracture displacement always refers to the distal fragment with regard to the proximal one. A fracture may be displaced in the transverse (horizontal) or longitudinal (vertical) plane, angulated, and/or rotated. Displacement in the transverse plane may be medial or lateral and anterior

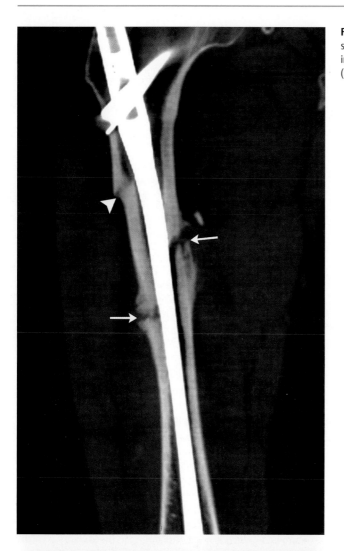

Fig. 15.1   Nonunion. A segmental fracture of the femur shaft is seen 1 y after the accident. The proximal fracture (arrowhead) is healing, whereas no signs of healing are evident in the distal fractures (arrows).

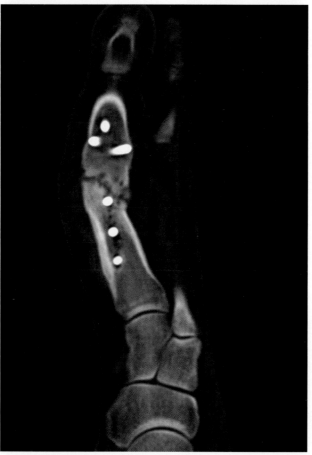

Fig. 15.2   Nonunion. An oblique fracture with irregular sclerotic margins is seen in the great toe.

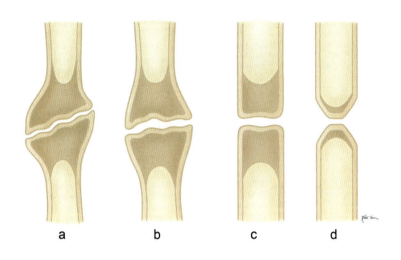

Fig. 15.3a–d Nonunion. (**a**) Hypertrophic (elephant foot). (**b**) Hypertrophic (horse foot). (**c**) Oligotrophic. (**d**) Atrophic.

a   b   c   d

or posterior. Displacement in the longitudinal plane results in either fracture distraction or impaction. When the fracture fragments are completely separated, overriding of the fracture fragments with corresponding foreshortening of the bone (bayonet deformity) may occur. Fracture angulation may be medial (the distal fragment is angulated toward the midline, and the apex of the fracture is lateral, corresponding to varus deformity) or lateral (the distal fragment is angulated away from the midline, and the apex of the fracture is medial, corresponding to valgus deformity) and anterior (the apex of the fracture is posterior) or posterior (the apex of the fracture is anterior). Fracture rotation may be internal (distal fracture fragment rotates medially) or external (distal fracture fragment rotates laterally).

Fractures in children may present with special features. Greenstick fractures are incomplete fractures of the relatively soft growing bone perforating only one cortex and ramifying within the medullary cavity. Bowing fractures present as bending of the radius, ulna, or fibula without evidence of a bony break. Comparison radiographs of the opposite side are often required for correct diagnosis. Torus (buckling) fractures produce a buckling of the metaphyseal cortex in children and osteopenic adults (**Fig. 15.5**).

Trauma to the bone in children and adolescents often involves the cartilage (growth) plate, as long as the epiphyses are not closed. These injuries can be classified into different types using the Salter–Harris method (**Fig. 15.6**). A Salter–Harris type III fracture in

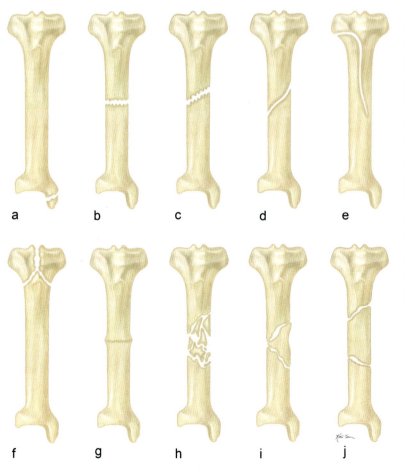

Fig. 15.4a–j Classification of fractures according to their radiographic appearance. (**a**) Avulsion fracture (secondary to forcible tearing of a ligament or tendon attachment, e.g., medial malleolar fracture). A chip fracture has the same radiographic appearance but is caused by direct impact. (**b**) Transverse fracture (secondary to shearing force to opposite sides of a bone or to impact force along the transverse axis). (**c**) Oblique fracture (secondary to impact along an oblique axis). (**d**) Spiral fracture (secondary to a rotary-type injury). (**e**) Longitudinal fracture (secondary to impact force along the longitudinal axis). (**f**) T-, V-, or Y-shaped fracture in proximity of joints (secondary to impact force along the longitudinal axis). (**g**) Impacted fracture or compression fracture (secondary to impact force along the longitudinal axis). A depressed fracture refers to an articular surface (transchondral fracture). (**h**) Comminuted fracture (secondary to severe external trauma or shattering effect of a projectile). (**i**) Fracture with butterfly fragment (wedge fracture). (**j**) Segmental fracture.

a   b   c   d   e

f   g   h   i   j

IV Musculoskeletal System

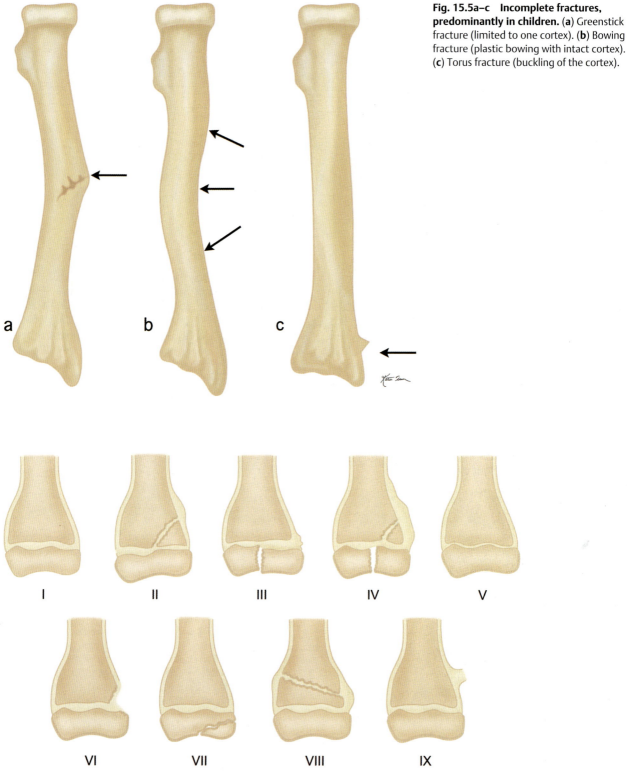

Fig. 15.5a–c Incomplete fractures, predominantly in children. (a) Greenstick fracture (limited to one cortex). **(b)** Bowing fracture (plastic bowing with intact cortex). **(c)** Torus fracture (buckling of the cortex).

a

b

c

I

II

III

IV

V

VI

VII

VIII

IX

Fig. 15.6 Salter–Harris classification of growth plate injuries (types I–V) with Rang and Ogden's additions (types VI–IX). Type I: Injury limited to the cartilage plate, which shows complete transverse laceration. The fracture may not be appreciated without epiphyseal displacement. The bone itself is intact. Prognosis is good. **Type II:** Incomplete transverse laceration of the cartilage plate associated with oblique fracture of the metaphysis. Triangular fracture fragment remains attached to the epiphysis. Prognosis is good. **Type III:** Incomplete transverse laceration of the cartilage plate associated with longitudinal fracture through the epiphysis. Prognosis is bad if the fracture is not reduced with smooth joint surface. **Type IV:** Oblique longitudinal fracture through the epiphysis, cartilage plate, and metaphysis. Prognosis is bad if the fracture is not perfectly reduced. **Type V:** Crushing of the cartilage plate with intact bone. Premature closure of the plate and stoppage of growth are relatively common. **Type VI:** Trauma to the perichondrium with tethering of the growth plate. **Type VII:** Fracture of the epiphysis. **Type VIII:** Fracture of the metaphysis. **Type IX:** Avulsion injury of the periosteum.

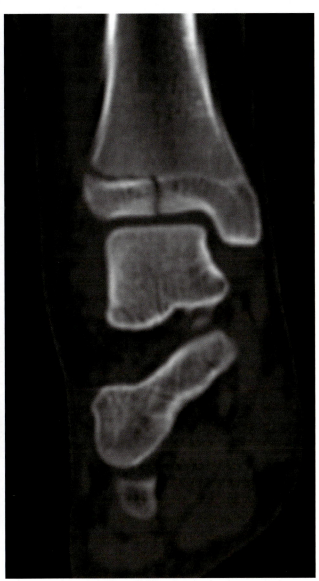

Fig. 15.7 Juvenile Tillaux fracture. A fracture of the anterolateral aspect of the distal tibial epiphysis is seen.

the lateral distal tibia epiphysis is referred to as a juvenile Tillaux fracture (**Figs. 15.7, 15.8**). A triplane (triplanar) fracture of the distal tibia in adolescents represents a variation of a Salter–Harris type IV injury (**Figs. 15.9, 15.10**). Two, three, or four fragments (parts) may result, with two fragments being most common.

A tibial tubercle avulsion fracture in the immature skeleton is divided by the Ogden classification system into three types: avulsion through the secondary ossification center, extension of the fracture into the proximal tibial epiphysis, and extension through the tibial epiphysis into the knee joint (**Fig. 15.11**).

A traumatic epiphysiolysis of the femur head is particularly common in boys between 10 and 15 y of age, although a history of acute trauma is often not available. In these cases of slipped capital femoral epiphyses (SCFE), repeated low-grade trauma is believed to be the triggering mechanism (**Fig. 15.12**). Regardless of its etiology, SCFE represents a Salter–Harris type I fracture. The displacement of the femoral head in relation to the metaphysis is almost always in a posterior, inferior, and medial direction, and the physis appears blurred and widened. Sequelae of SCFE include remodeling and reactive bone formation in the femoral neck that may create a protuberance on its superolateral aspect known as Herndon hump. It is indistinguishable from the "pistol grip" deformity in femoroacetabular impingement (FAI).

In the pelvis, avulsion fractures at tendinous attachment sites such as the anterosuperior and anteroinferior iliac spines and ischial tuberosity are common before these secondary ossification centers are fused.

Multiple fractures and dislocations in an infant should raise the suspicion of an abused (battered) child syndrome (shaken baby syndrome). More subtle findings in this condition include injuries to the cartilage plate, metaphyseal fragmentation and avulsions (metaphyseal corner fractures), the latter producing a characteristic "bucket handle" deformity, posttraumatic metaphyseal cupping, and cortical thickening.

Selection of the appropriate fracture management requires accurate fracture classification that in complex cases is best accomplished with multiplanar CT. In most instances, the fracture staging system currently used in CT was originally devised for conventional radiography. A generic or universal classification system that can be applied to any bone within

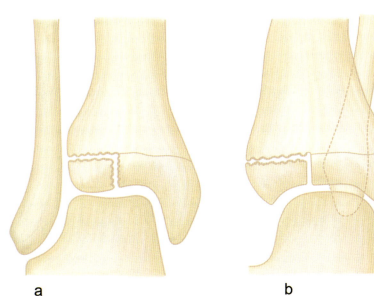

a   b

Fig. 15.8a, b Juvenile Tillaux fracture. Anteroposterior (**a**) and lateral (**b**) views reveal a Harris–Salter type III fracture involving the anterolateral aspect of the distal tibial epiphysis.

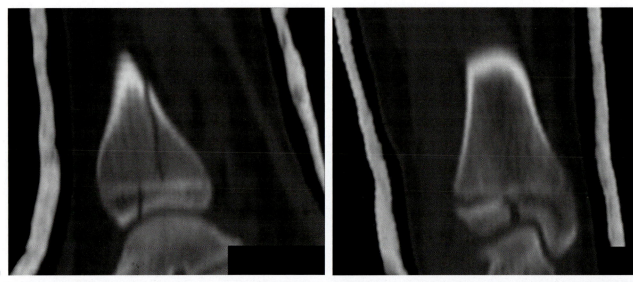

Fig. 15.9a, b Triplane (triplanar) fracture. (a) Sagittal view shows a fracture originating in the posterior distal metaphysis that extends into the closed physis medially and progresses from there through the epiphysis into the ankle. **(b)** Coronal view shows a detached anterolateral epiphyseal fragment.

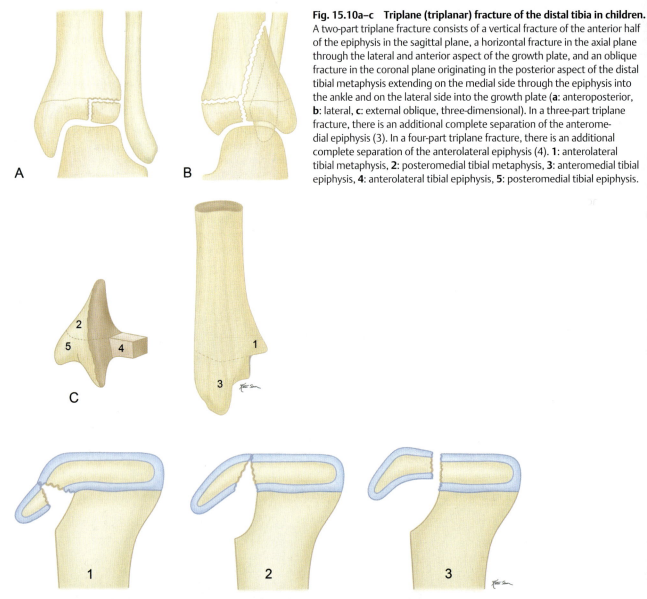

Fig. 15.10a–c Triplane (triplanar) fracture of the distal tibia in children. A two-part triplane fracture consists of a vertical fracture of the anterior half of the epiphysis in the sagittal plane, a horizontal fracture in the axial plane through the lateral and anterior aspect of the growth plate, and an oblique fracture in the coronal plane originating in the posterior aspect of the distal tibial metaphysis extending on the medial side through the epiphysis into the ankle and on the lateral side into the growth plate (**a**: anteroposterior, **b**: lateral, **c**: external oblique, three-dimensional). In a three-part triplane fracture, there is an additional complete separation of the anteromedial epiphysis (3). In a four-part triplane fracture, there is an additional complete separation of the anterolateral epiphysis (4). **1**: anterolateral tibial metaphysis, **2**: posteromedial tibial metaphysis, **3**: anteromedial tibial epiphysis, **4**: anterolateral tibial epiphysis, **5**: posteromedial tibial epiphysis.

Fig. 15.11 Ogden classification of tibial tubercle avulsion fractures in the immature skeleton. 1: Fracture of the avulsed tibial tubercle does not extend into the epiphysis. **2**: Fracture extends/involves the proximal tibial epiphysis, but the articular surface is intact. **3**: Fracture extends through the articular surface of the proximal tibial epiphysis.

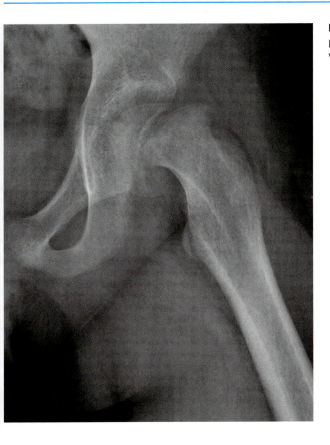

Fig. 15.12 Slipped capital femoral epiphysis (SCFE). A widened physis and posteroinferior displacement of the femoral head are visible (conventional radiograph).

the body was designed by the Arbeitsgemeinschaft für Osteo-synthesefragen/Orthopaedic Trauma Association (AO/OTA). Each fracture is identified by four numbers and one letter. The first number identifies the bone (e.g., 1: humerus, 2: forearm, 3: femur, 4: tibia, etc.). The second number identifies the location within the bone (1: proximal end, 2: shaft (diaphysis), 3: distal end). The fracture type is identified by a letter (A: two fragments only, B: comminuted, C: highly comminuted or segmental). The third number defines the group the fracture belongs to (fracture groups are different for each fracture type, with a scale ranging from 1 to 3). The fourth number defines the subgroup (most detailed fracture determination differing from bone to bone, with a scale ranging from 1 to 3). A complete description of this classification system is beyond the scope of this text. A simplified AO/OTA classification system may be applied for all shaft (diaphyseal) fractures where three types (1: noncomminuted, 2: comminuted but with contact between the main proximal and distal fragments [e.g. wedge fracture with butterfly fragment], and 3: comminuted but without contact between the main fragments [e.g., segmental fracture]) are differentiated. The fracture pattern (e.g., transverse, oblique, or spiral) should also be indicated. Furthermore, in the forearm and lower leg, the presence of subluxation/dislocation at the end of a fractured bone (e.g., proximal and distal radioulnar and tibiofibular joints, respectively) must also be assessed.

A fracture classification system adapted for specific sites appears more useful in clinical practice. Unfortunately, several different classification systems exist for virtually every fracture location, and there is no consent among orthopedic surgeons on the one to be most relevant for the patient's management. In the following section, we have limited our discussion to the fracture classification systems that are preferred by the orthopedic surgeons at our institution.

Shoulder Girdle and Upper Extremity

Scapula fractures are classified according to their anatomical location. Fractures of the body and spine, acromion, coracoid, extra-articular glenoid, and intra-articular glenoid are differentiated. Acromial fractures are classified as minimally displaced (type 1), displaced but without encroachment of the subacromial space (type 2), and displaced with encroachment of the subacromial space (type 3). An os acromiale (**Fig. 15.13**) should not be confused with a distal nondisplaced acromion fracture. Coracoid fractures proximal (type 1) and distal (type 2) to the coracoclavicular ligament are differentiated. Extra-articular glenoid neck fractures may involve either the anatomical neck (distal glenoid) or the surgical neck (proximal glenoid) and are divided in fractures without (type 1) or with (type 2) associated clavicle fracture or acromioclavicular (AC) separation. Accurate classification of the intra-articular glenoid fractures is most important for the selection of the appropriate treatment modality (**Fig. 15.14**).

Clavicle fractures are classified into three types according to the anatomical segment involved. Fractures of the proximal (medial) third (5%), middle third (80%), and distal (lateral) third (15%) are distinguished. The proximal fracture fragment is commonly elevated, whereas the distal fragment may be medially and caudally displaced. Fractures of the distal clavicle have been classified by Neer into three types. Type 1 consists of a nonarticular fracture without significant displacement, indicating intact coracoclavicular ligaments. Type 2 is a displaced nonarticular fracture with detached conoid component of the coracoclavicular ligament from the medial segment and intact

trapezoid component of this ligament attached to the distal (lateral) segment. Type 3 fracture extends into the AC joint.

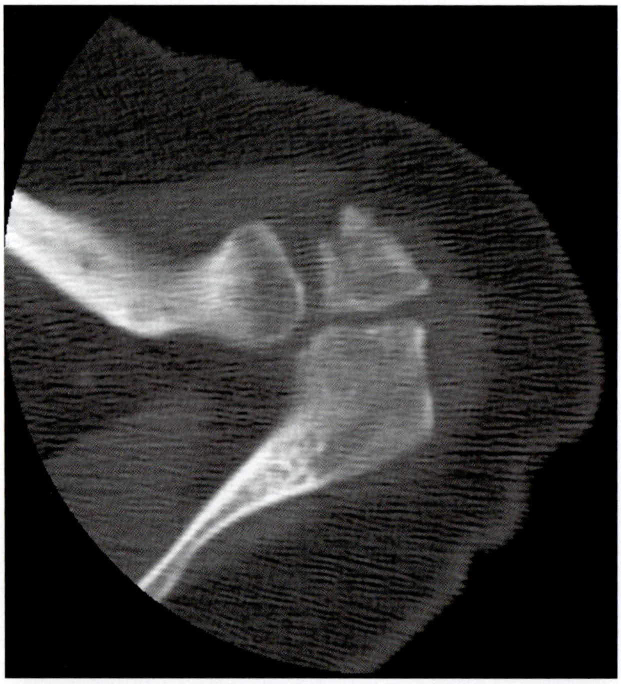

Sternoclavicular joint dislocations (**Fig. 15.15**) essentially occur in an anteroposterior direction and thus are virtually impossible to assess with conventional radiography unless some subluxation in the craniocaudal plane is associated, resulting in asymmetry of the medial clavicle ends on chest radiographs. CT is the imaging modality of choice in the evaluation of the sternoclavicular joint. Anterior (presternal) subluxation and dislocation are most common, with the medial end of the clavicle displaced anteriorly or anterosuperiorly. Except for a "cosmetic bump," they are not associated with serious complications. Posterior (retrosternal) dislocations and subluxations are uncommon. The medial end of the clavicle is displaced posteriorly or posteromedially, and injuries to the adjacent neurovascular structures and airways are frequently associated. Sternoclavicular trauma may be accompanied with fractures of the clavicle and dislocations of the AC joint.

AC joint injuries are assessed radiographically by the width and displacement in this joint and the coracoclavicular distance. The width of a normal AC joint ranges from 0.3 to 0.8 cm, and the normal coracoclavicular distance measures 1.0 to 1.2 cm. These measurements, however, are not completely reliable because of an enormous variation in the normal population. Therefore, in borderline cases, comparison with the normal contralateral side should be obtained. Six types of AC joint injuries can be differentiated. In type 1 injury, the AC joint is normal or minimally widened. Para-articular soft tissue swelling may be the only abnormality. In type 2 separation, the distal end of the clavicle is slightly elevated (subluxed), the width of the AC joint widened between 1 and 1.5 cm, and the coracoclavicular distance typically varying between 1.3 and 1.5 cm. Type 3 injury represents a complete dislocation (separation) of the AC joint, with the lateral end of the clavicle projecting completely above the superior border of the acromion. The coracoclavicular distance measures 1.6 cm or more; otherwise, a fracture of the coracoid process is also suspected. Type 4 injury appears similar to a type 3 separation, but posterior displacement of the distal clavicle is also present. Type 5 injury appears like a severe type 3 separation, but instead of the clavicle being displaced superiorly, the finding is caused by marked inferior displacement of the scapula. Type 6 injuries represent an inferior dislocation of the distal clavicle with either a decreased coracoclavicular distance (subacromial type) or a reversed coracoclavicular distance (subcoracoid type).

In *glenohumeral joint dislocations,* anterior, posterior, superior, and inferior dislocations are differentiated. Anterior dislocations may be associated with a compression fracture on the posterolateral aspect of the humeral head (Hill–Sachs lesion) and less frequently with a fracture of the anteroinferior rim of the glenoid (Bankart lesion), which may be limited to the cartilaginous labrum and not involve the osseous structures (**Fig. 15.16**). Posterior dislocations (**Fig. 15.17**) are much less common and often not recognized on conventional radiographs. A compression fracture on the humeral head ("reverse Hill–Sachs lesion") may be evident. Both anterosuperior (subcoracoid) and inferior

Fig. 15.13 Os acromiale. The detached distal end of the acromion is a normal variant.

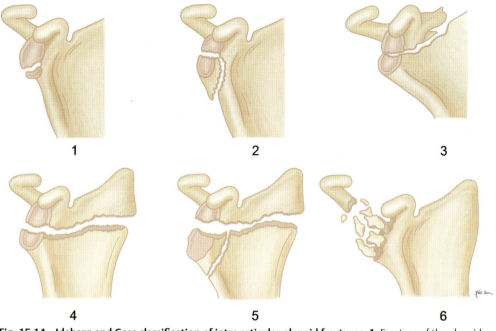

Fig. 15.14 Ideberg and Goss classification of intra-articular glenoid fractures. 1: Fracture of the glenoid rim. **2**: Transverse or oblique fracture through the glenoid fossa with inferior fragment displaced with the subluxed humeral head. **3**: Oblique fracture through the glenoid exiting at the midsuperior border of the scapula. **4**: Horizontal fracture of the glenoid exiting through the medial border of the scapula. **5**: Similar to 4, but with complete separation of the inferior glenoid. **6**: Severe comminution of the articular surface of the glenoid.

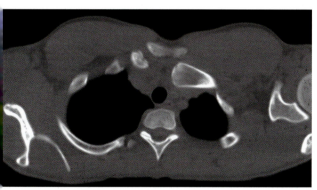

Fig. 15.15 Posterior sternoclavicular joint dislocation. The medial end of the left clavicle is displaced posteromedially under the manubrium of the sternum.

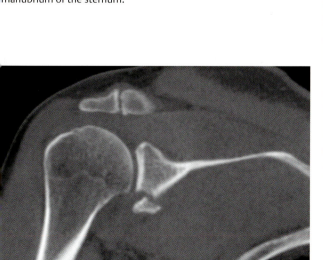

Fig. 15.16 Osseous Bankart lesion. A fracture of the inferior glenoid is seen.

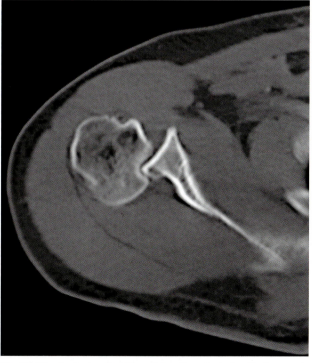

Fig. 15.17 Posterior shoulder dislocation. Posterior displacement of the humeral head depicting a compression fracture (reverse Hill–Sachs lesion) caused by compression of the posterior glenoid is seen.

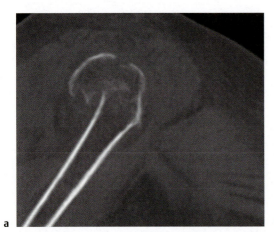 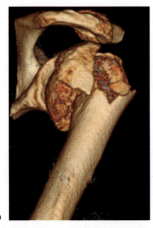 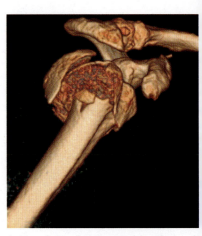

a   b   c

Fig. 15.18a–c Proximal humerus fracture. Coronal (**a**) and three-dimensional reconstruction (**b,c**) views show a fracture involving the surgical neck and the greater and lesser tuberosities. The fractures of the surgical neck and greater tuberosity are considerably displaced, whereas the lesser tuberosity fracture is not significantly displaced.

(luxatio erecta) dislocations are very rare. An inferior subluxation (drooping shoulder) is associated with hemarthrosis in proximal intra-articular humerus fractures, but it is also seen with neuromuscular disease involving the rotator cuff and hemiparesis.

Fractures of the proximal humerus (**Fig. 15.18**) occur between one or all four major segments, which include the articular segment (anatomical neck fracture), the proximal humerus shaft (surgical neck fracture), the greater tuberosity, and the lesser tuberosity. The modified Neer four-segment classification (**Fig. 15.19**) is based on the number of displaced segments. Any fracture that is not displaced or only minimally displaced (< 1 cm) and is not angulated or only minimally angulated (< 45°) is disregarded. A one-part fracture may involve any or all four anatomical segments, but there is no displacement or angulation between fracture fragments. A two-part fracture indicates that only one segment is displaced in relation to the three that remain undisplaced or are intact. A two-part surgical neck fracture is also diagnosed in the absence of any angulation or horizontal displacement when the fracture is either impacted or comminuted. A three-part fracture commonly consists of a displaced greater or lesser tuberosity fracture combined with a surgical neck fracture. A four-part fracture typically involves both greater and lesser tuberosities in addition to the surgical neck with displacement of all four segments. Two-, three-, and four-part fractures may be associated with either anterior or posterior glenohumeral joint dislocation.

If a single tuberosity fracture is present in an anterior shoulder dislocation, it invariably involves the greater tuberosity, whereas in a posterior dislocation, it involves the lesser tuberosity. Fractures of the surgical neck and the second tuberosity, however, may also be associated in these conditions. Furthermore, the fracture may involve the articular surface, resulting in "head-splitting" and "impression" fractures caused by severe impaction of the humeral head into the glenoid. Head-splitting fractures caused by central impact are not always associated with dislocations. In impression fractures, the defect in the humeral head is anterior and represents a severe reverse Hill–Sachs lesion extending into the articular surface of the humeral head, resulting from a traumatic posterior dislocation. In both conditions, loose intra-articular fracture fragments are a frequent finding.

Humerus shaft fractures are best classified into three types: noncomminuted; comminuted, but with contact between the main proximal and distal fragments; and comminuted, but without contact between the main fragments. In addition, the fracture pattern (e.g., transverse, oblique, or spiral) should be indicated.

Fractures of the elbow (**Fig. 15.20**) may involve the distal humerus, proximal radius, and proximal ulna. Extra-articular fractures of the distal humerus may involve the epicondyles or supracondylar area. Intra-articular fractures of the distal humerus may involve either the trochlea or the capitellum alone (transcondylar or unicondylar fractures) or both (bicondylar or intercondylar fractures with or without supracondylar comminution) (**Fig. 15.21**). Supracondylar fractures are the most common elbow fracture in children younger than 10.

Fractures of the radial head are common in adults, but when nondisplaced or minimally displaced, they may be difficult to demonstrate with conventional radiography. Radial head fractures with extension into the articular surface must be differentiated from extra-articular radial neck fractures. Radial head fractures are classified in four types: nondisplaced or minimally displaced fractures; marginal fractures with partial displacement of the radial head, including impaction, depression, or angulation; comminuted fractures involving the entire head; and fracture and dislocation of the radial head (**Fig. 15.22**). An Essex–Lopresti fracture consists of a comminuted displaced fracture of the radial head associated with posterior subluxation of the distal ulna secondary to a tear of the entire interosseous membrane of the forearm. Fractures of the proximal ulna may involve the coronoid process or the olecranon, but the former rarely occurs as an isolated injury and is often associated with a posterior elbow dislocation.

Olecranon fractures may be classified according to their location in the proximal, middle, or distal third of the olecranon. The proximal olecranon fracture may be extra-articular (avulsion fracture) or intra-articular, whereas the remaining fractures are all intra-articular. Transverse or oblique fractures in the middle third of the olecranon are most common. A more useful classification for the patient's management is based on displacement, comminution, and ulnohumeral instability (**Fig. 15.23**).

Simple elbow dislocations without associated fractures may involve the ulna alone, the radius alone, or both the ulna and radius. Posterior and posterolateral dislocations of both ulna and radius account for 80% to 90% of all elbow dislocations. Anterior dislocations without associated fractures are exceedingly rare. Medial and lateral dislocations are likely to represent incompletely reduced posterior dislocations.

A *Monteggia fracture* (**Fig. 15.24a**) is the association of a proximal ulnar shaft fracture with dislocation of the radial head. Both the apex of angulation of the ulnar fracture and the dislocation of the radial head are anterior in type 1 (60%), posterior in type 2 (15%), lateral in type 3 (20%), and similar to type 1 but associated with a radius shaft fracture at the level of the ulnar fracture in type 4 (5%). A *Galeazzi fracture* (**Fig. 15.24b**) consists of

Anatomical segment	One-part	Two-part	Three-part	Four-part
Nondisplaced segments (1 to 4)	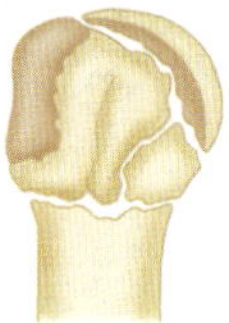			
Anatomical neck		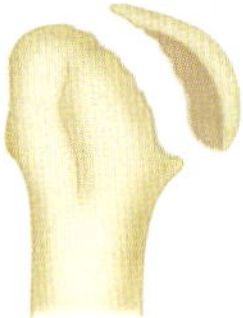		
Surgical neck		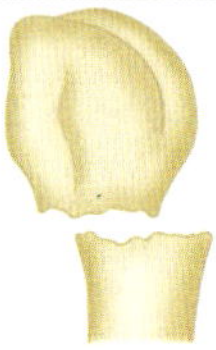		
Greater tuberosity		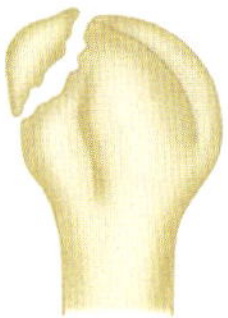	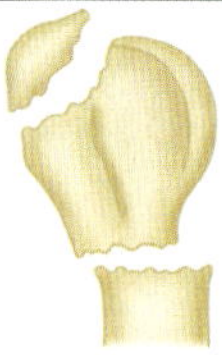	
Lesser tuberosity		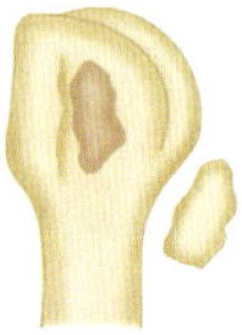	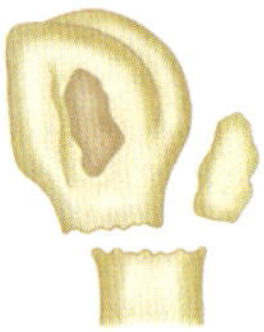	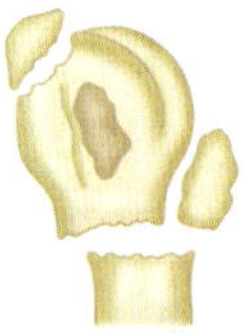
Anterior fracture-dislocation		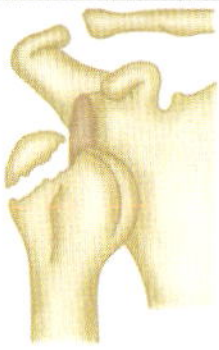	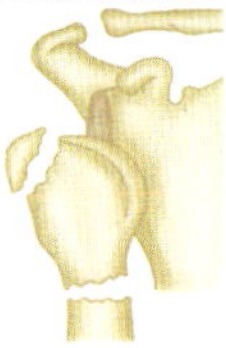	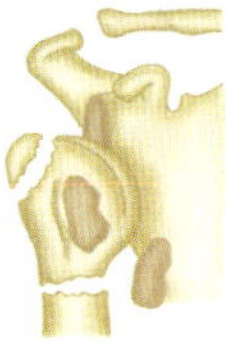
Posterior fracture dislocation		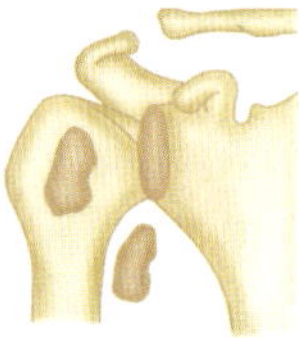	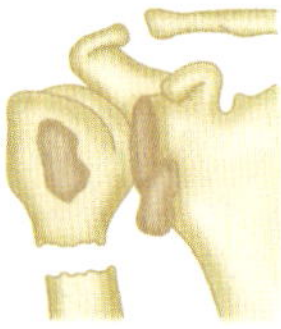	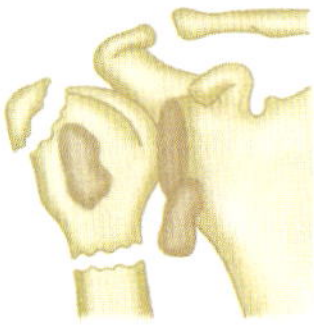
Dislocation with articular surface involvement		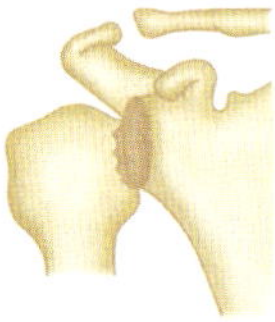 impression	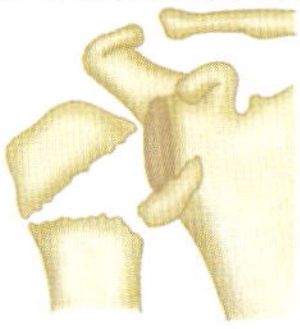 head-splitting	

Fig. 15.19 Modified Neer four-segment classification of proximal humerus fractures. Two-part surgical neck fractures may also be comminuted or impacted. "Head-splitting" fractures are not always associated with a shoulder dislocation. "Impression" fractures correspond to a severe reverse Hill–Sachs defect extending into the articular surface associated with traumatic posterior dislocation.

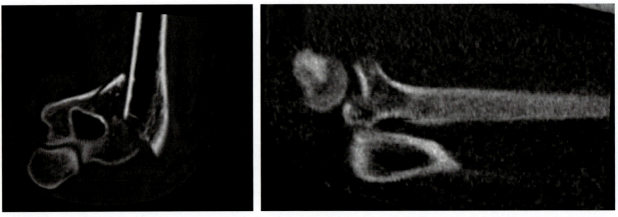

a   b

Fig. 15.20a, b   Elbow fractures (two cases). (a) A comminuted supracondylar fracture is seen. **(b)** A comminuted radial head fracture is evident.

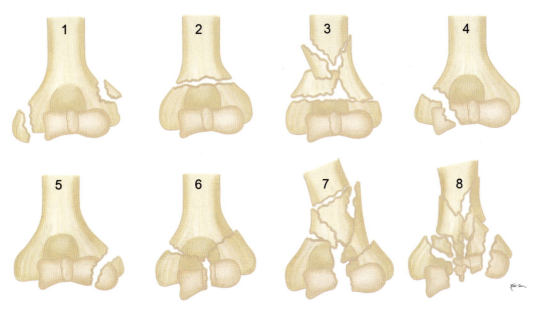

Fig. 15.21   Müller classification of distal humerus fractures. 1–3: Extra-articular (epicondylar or supracondylar). **4–9** Intra-articular (transcondylar, bicondylar, or intercondylar). **1**: Avulsion of medial or lateral epicondyle. **2**: Simple supracondylar fracture. **3**: Comminuted supracondylar fracture. **4**: Fracture of trochlea. **5**: Fracture of capitellum. **6**: Y-shaped bicondylar fracture. **7**: Y-shaped intercondylar fracture with supracondylar comminution. **8**: Comminuted intercondylar and supracondylar fracture (complex comminuted fracture).

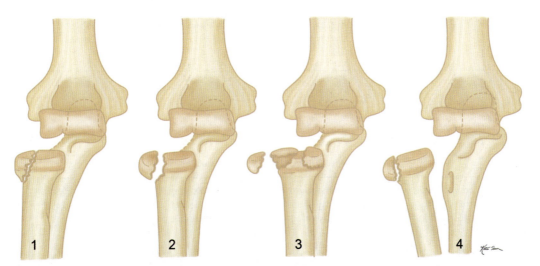

Fig. 15.22   Modified Mason classification of radial head fractures. 1: Nondisplaced. **2**: Displaced (including impaction, depression, and angulation). **3**: Comminuted with involvement of the entire head. **4**: Fracture and dislocation of the radial head.

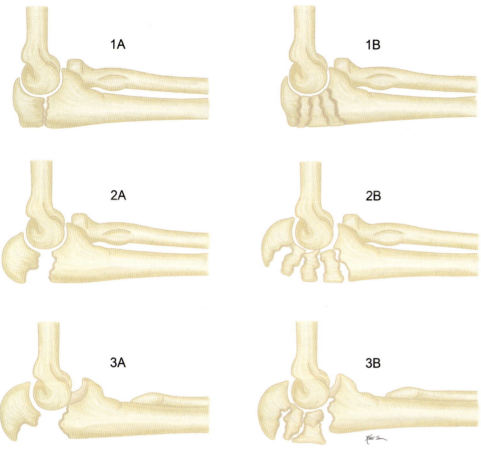

Fig. 15.23 Mayo classification of olecranon fractures. Classification assesses displacement, comminution, and subluxation/dislocation. **1A**: Undisplaced, noncomminuted. **1B**: Undisplaced, comminuted. **2A**: Displaced, noncomminuted. **2B**: Displaced, comminuted. **3A**: Noncomminuted, unstable (subluxed) ulnohumeral joint. **3B**: Comminuted, unstable (subluxed) ulnohumeral joint.

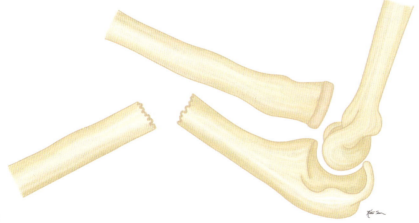

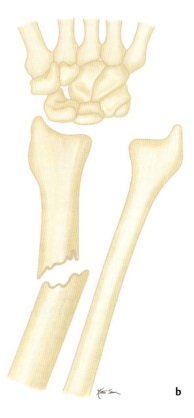

a

Fig. 15.24a, b   (a) **Monteggia fracture (type 1).** Fracture of proximal ulnar shaft with angulation apex anterior and anterior dislocation of the radial head. For types 2 to 4, see text. (b) **Galeazzi fracture.** Fracture of distal radius with angulation apex posterior and medial and posteromedial dislocation of the ulna in the distal radioulnar joint. The radius fracture fragments may also overlap.

b

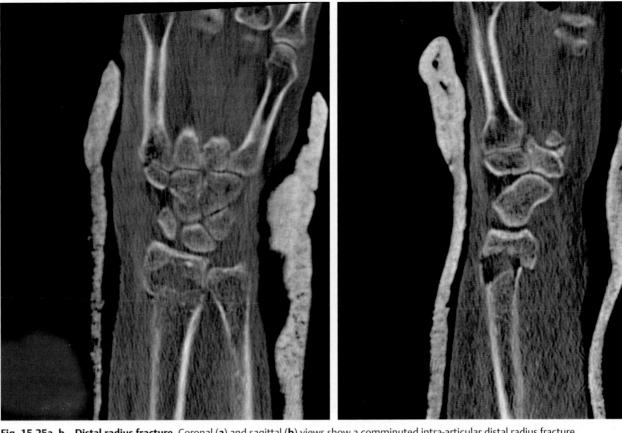

a

Fig. 15.25a, b Distal radius fracture. Coronal (**a**) and sagittal (**b**) views show a comminuted intra-articular distal radius fracture.

a fracture of the distal third of the radius with angulation apex dorsal and medial (ulnar) associated with dorsal and medial dislocation of the ulna in the distal radioulnar joint. A *Piedmont fracture* is an isolated fracture of the distal radius shaft without involvement of the distal radioulnar joint. A *nightstick fracture* is an isolated ulnar shaft fracture caused by a direct blow to the forearm.

Distal radius fractures (**Fig. 15.25**) include (1) *Colles fracture* (extra-articular, usually occurring about 2–3 cm from the articular surface with typically radial and dorsal displacement and angulation apex volar associated frequently with an ulnar styloid fracture; in another definition of a Colles fracture, an intra-articular extension is also acceptable), (2) *Smith fracture* (extra- or intra-articular fracture with volar displacement of the distal fragment), (3) *Barton fracture* (intra-articular oblique fracture of the dorsal distal radius), (4) reverse (volar) Barton fracture (intra-articular oblique fracture of the volar distal radius), and (5) *Hutchinson* or *chauffeur's fracture* (fracture of the radial styloid process).

A more useful classification system of distal radius fractures was devised by Frykman that takes into consideration the involvement of both the radiocarpal and distal radioulnar joints, besides the ulnar styloid (**Fig. 15.26**).

Isolated intra-articular fractures of the distal ulna, including the ulnar styloid, are uncommon. Posttraumatic symptoms in the distal ulna are frequently caused by an injury to the triangular fibrocartilage complex (TFCC) that is best evaluated by MRI. The TFCC is the main stabilizing structure of the distal radioulnar joint. Subluxations and dislocations in this joint are therefore invariably associated with a disruption in the TFCC that besides being traumatic may also be inflammatory or degenerative in nature. An isolated injury to the TFCC or ulnar styloid fracture may be associated with a distal radioulnar joint subluxation or dislocation. The latter occurs frequently in combination with a

radius fracture, for example, the radius shaft (Galeazzi fracture) or the radial head (Essex–Lopresti fracture).

To diagnose a *distal radioulnar joint instability,* the wrist has to be imaged in pronation, neutral position, and supination of the forearm. In the normal wrist, the articulating surfaces of the distal radius and ulna are congruent in pronation and neutral position, but not in supination due to the normal configuration of the distal ulna (**Fig. 15.27**). Furthermore, minimal dorsal (posterior) subluxation of the ulna in pronation and minimal volar (anterior) subluxation of the ulna in supination may occur in the normal wrist. Comparison views of the opposite side are therefore helpful for diagnosing minor degrees of instability.

Severe wrist injuries may result in a positive or negative ulnar variance, which, however, is more commonly a normal variant. A positive ulnar variance (long ulna) may be associated with ulnar impaction (abutment) syndrome, in which the chronic impaction of the ulnar head against the TFCC and the ulnar-sided carpal bones results in progressive degeneration of these structures. This condition has to be distinguished from the ulnar impingement syndrome, which is associated with a negative ulnar variance. It is caused by a short distal ulna that impinges on the distal radius proximal to the sigmoid notch, resulting in scalloping of the distal radius or pseudoarthrosis formation at that site. A negative ulnar variance may also be associated with Kienböck disease.

The scaphoid is the most commonly fractured carpal bone, accounting for approximately two thirds of all carpal fractures (**Fig. 15.28**). *Scaphoid fractures* can be classified according to the direction of the fracture line (e.g., horizontal, oblique, or vertical) or by anatomical location (**Fig. 15.29**). Waist fractures account for 80% of scaphoid fractures, proximal pole fractures for 15%, tuberosity fractures for 4%, and distal articular pole fractures for 1%. The vascular blood supply of the scaphoid occurs by volar and dorsal branches of the radial artery entering the

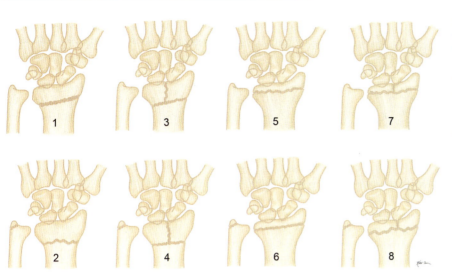

Fig. 15.26 Frykman classification of distal radius fractures. Classification is based on the involvement of ulnar styloid, radiocarpal joint (RCJ), and distal radioulnar joint (DRUJ). Ulnar styloid is fractured in 2, 4, 6, and 8. Fracture extension into the RCJ is present in 3, 4, 7, and 8. Fracture extension into the DRUJ is present in 5, 6, 7, and 8.

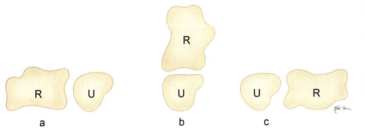

Fig. 15.27a–c Normal alignment in the right distal radioulnar joint. Pronation (**a**) and neutral (thumb up) (**b**) position. In these positions, the joint is congruent. Supination (**c**). The joint is not congruent, but the ulna is centered within the sigmoid notch of the radius.
R radius
U ulna

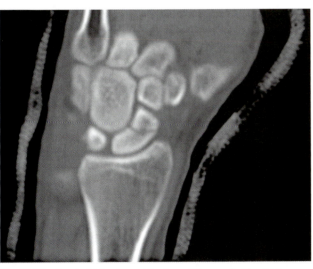

Fig. 15.28 Scaphoid fracture. A fracture of the scaphoid waist is seen.

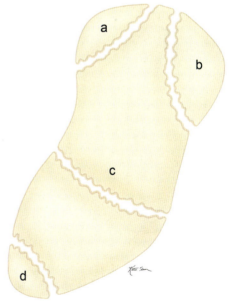

Fig. 15.29 Scaphoid fractures may involve the distal pole (**a**, 1%), tubercle (**b**, 4%), waist (**c**, 80%), or proximal pole (**d**, 15%).

bone in its distal half. Because of the retrograde vascular supply, the risk of complications markedly increases with fractures involving the proximal half of the scaphoid. Common complications of the scaphoid waist and even more so of proximal pole fractures include nonunion and avascular necrosis of the proximal fracture fragment.

The *triquetrum* is the second most fractured carpal bone, accounting for almost 20%. Most fractures of this bone are avulsion fractures associated with ligamentous damage. Transverse fractures may be associated with perilunate dislocation. Fractures in the remaining carpal bones are rare. In the lunate osteochondral and transverse body fractures as well as avulsions of the dorsal and palmar horns occur. Lunate fragmentation associated with Kienböck disease should not be confused with an acute fracture. The majority of trapezium fractures are either avulsions or vertical fractures of the body. Capitate fractures may be isolated or combined with other carpal fractures or fracture-dislocations. Complications in these fractures are rare, and they may heal even without immobilization. Hamate fractures are frequently associated with fractures of the fifth or less frequently fourth metacarpals. Fracture of the hook of the hamate is the most common hamate fracture. Fractures of the pisiform and trapezoid are the rarest carpal bone fractures.

Carpal instability can be classified into static or dissociative and dynamic or nondissociative types. Imaging of the latter may be difficult and usually requires a functional study, such as fluoroscopy or cineradiography. Triquetrohamate instability presents with painful clicking caused by abnormal motion between the triquetrum and hamate. Static instability patterns include volar, dorsal, or ulnar translocation (subluxation) of the carpus with regard to the distal radius. Instabilities within the proximal carpal row include scapholunate and lunotriquetral dissociations and scapholunate advanced collapse (SLAC). Two other major carpal instability patterns are dorsal (DISI) and volar (VISI) intercalated segmental instability (**Fig. 15.30**). In sagittal projection with the wrist in neutral flexion-extension, the angle between the axes of the scaphoid and lunate ranges from 30° to 60°. In DISI, the lunate is tilted dorsally 15° or more, and the scapholunate angle measures > 60°. In VISI, the lunate is tilted volarly 15° or more, and the scapholunate angle measures < 30°. DISI is associated with rotary subluxation of the scaphoid (distal pole of the scaphoid is tilted toward the palm) and scapholunate dissociation (scapholunate distance at the site of ligamentous insertion measures > 4 mm in coronal plane). In VISI, the capitate is often tilted dorsally, resulting in a capitolunate angle > 30° (normal 0–30°), and lunotriquetral dissociation may be associated. Scapholunate dissociation and rotary subluxation of the scaphoid represent stage 1 of four sequential stages of dislocations involving the lunate. Stage 2 (perilunate dislocation) represents a dorsal dislocation of the capitate (**Fig. 15.31**).

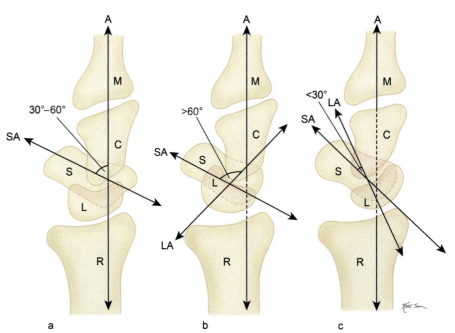

a   b   c

Fig. 15.30a–c   Dorsal intercalated segmental instability (DISI) and volar intercalated segmental instability (VISI), sagittal projection with the wrist in the neutral position. (**a**) Normal. A continuous line can be drawn through the longitudinal axis of the third metacarpal, capitate, lunate, and radius. This line intersects a second line through the longitudinal axis of the scaphoid at an angle of 30° to 60°. (**b**) DISI. The lunate is tilted dorsally at an angle of 15° or more, and the scaphoid is tilted volarly, resulting in a scaphoid-lunate angle > 60°. The longitudinal axis connecting the third metacarpal with the radius is interrupted at the lunate (*dashed line*). (**c**) VISI. The lunate is tilted volarly at an angle of 15° or more, resulting in a scaphoid-lunate angle < 30°. The longitudinal axis connecting the third metatarsal with the radius is interrupted (*dashed line*) at the lunate and the dorsally tilted capitate (not shown in drawing).

A longitudinal axis connecting third metacarpal with radius
C capitate
L lunate
LA longitudinal axis through lunate
M third metacarpal
R radius
S scaphoid
SA longitudinal axis through scaphoid

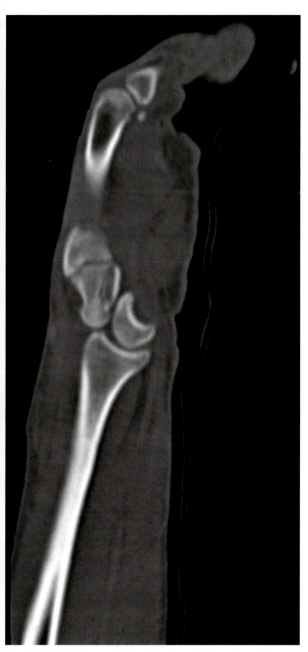

Fig. 15.31   Perilunate dislocation. Dorsal dislocation of the capitate is seen.

Stage 3 (midcarpal dislocation) consists of an anterior subluxation of the lunate associated with a dorsal dislocation of the capitate. Stage 4 (lunate dislocation) represents a complete anterior lunate dislocation associated with a dorsal dislocation of the capitate (**Fig. 15.32**). These four sequential stages of lunate injuries are also referred to as the lesser arc pattern, whereas a greater arc injury involves fracture of any carpal bones adjacent to a dislocated lunate (usually a perilunate dislocation). In these cases, the prefix *trans* indicates which bone is fractured. The most common carpal fracture-dislocation is the transscaphoid perilunate dislocation. A pure albeit rare greater arc injury consists of a transscaphoid, transcapitate, transhamate or transtriquetral perilunate dislocation.

Scaphoid dislocation is rare. An isolated radiovolar dislocation of the scaphoid with intact distal carpal row has to be differentiated from the same scaphoid dislocation associated with disruption of the distal carpal row evident by proximal migration of the radial half of the carpus including radial dislocation in the capitolunate joint.

The majority of *first carpometacarpal injuries* are fracture dislocations rather than pure dislocations, which are almost always dorsoradial. *Bennett* and *Rolando fractures* are intraarticular fractures of the base of the first metacarpal frequently associated with dorsoradial subluxation/dislocation of the shaft. In the noncomminuted Bennett fracture, a small fragment on the volar and ulnar aspect of the base of the first metacarpal remains in articulation with the trapezium, whereas the remaining first metacarpal is dorsally and radially displaced. The Rolando fracture (**Fig. 15.33**) is a comminuted Bennett fracture, often with a Y, V, or T configuration that is not infrequently associated with small, loose intra-articular bony fragments that are readily appreciated by CT and almost impossible to diagnose with conventional radiography. Dislocation in the second through fifth carpometacarpal joints are rare high-energy injuries, almost always dorsal, and usually associated with fractures of the adjacent carpal and metacarpal bones.

Metacarpal fractures can be differentiated according to their anatomical location in head, neck, shaft, and base fractures. A boxer fracture is a metacarpal neck fracture with apex dorsal angulation. It may occur in any metacarpal with the exception of the thumb but is most common in the fifth. Residual angular deformity with apex dorsal is of less serious consequence in the metacarpals of the fourth and fifth finger, in which there is some mobility at the carpometacarpal joints, than in the second

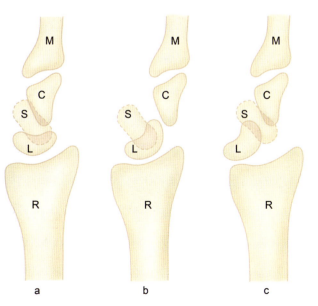

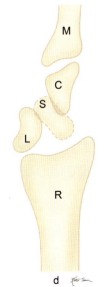

Fig. 15.32a–d   Perilunate, midcarpal, and lunate dislocation. Normal (**a**), perilunate (**b**), midcarpal (**c**), and lunate (**d**) dislocations.
C capitate
L lunate
M third metacarpal
R radius
S scaphoid

IV Musculoskeletal System

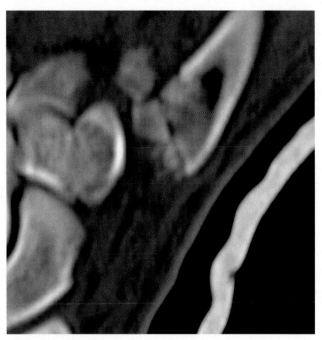

Fig. 15.33   Rolando fracture. A comminuted intra-articular fracture of the base of the thumb with several small loose fracture fragments is seen.

and third fingers, where there is no mobility in the corresponding joints, resulting in protrusion of the metacarpal heads in the palm that may be associated with a painful grip.

Gamekeeper's (skier's) thumb is an injury to the ulnar collateral ligament of the first metacarpophalangeal joint with or without a bony avulsion from the base of the proximal phalanx resulting from a violent abduction of the thumb, most often a skiing accident. A sesamoid fracture must be differentiated in the presence of volar tenderness. Dorsal dislocations are the most common in metacarpophalangeal joints 2 to 5. They are really subluxations, as some contact remains in these joints. The volar plate stays volar or distal to the metacarpal head.

Phalangeal fractures are classified based on their anatomical location within the bone (head, neck, shaft, and base) and further modified by the direction of the fracture plane (transverse, oblique, spiral, or comminuted) and the measurable degree of displacement and angulation. Dorsal base fractures include a mallet fracture, in which an avulsion injury at the base of the dorsal aspect of the distal phalanx is associated with damage to the extensor mechanism, producing a flexion (mallet) deformity in the distal interphalangeal joint. The most common volar plate fracture represents an intra-articular avulsion fracture in the base of the middle phalanx at the volar plate attachment site, usually secondary to dorsal dislocation of the proximal interphalangeal joint.

Pelvis and Lower Extremity

Pelvic fractures must be assessed for both stability and acetabular involvement. Stable pelvic fractures (**Fig. 15.34**) do not disrupt the osseous ring formed by the pelvis and sacrum (type 1 injuries) or disrupt it in only one place (type 2 injuries), whereas unstable fractures (**Fig. 15.35**) completely disrupt the ring in two or more places (type 3 injuries). Type 1 injuries include avulsion fractures that occur at tendinous attachment sites, such as the anterosuperior and anteroinferior iliac spines, ischial tuberosity, and iliac crest. These fractures occur commonly in children before closure of the corresponding physis (cartilage plate) and athletes secondary to forcible muscular contraction. Avulsions from the symphysis pubis at the origin of the adductor longus and brevis and the gracilis ("sports hernia") may be associated with subtle osseous fragments. Another common type 1 injury represents a unilateral pubic ramus fracture (usually in the superior ramus) occurring in elderly patients after a fall or prosthetic hip replacement surgery and in athletes as stress fracture. Isolated transverse or vertical sacral fractures (**Fig. 15.36**) are rare and have to be differentiated from insufficiency fractures in osteopenia that have usually both a vertical and horizontal course. Type 2 injuries (single break in the pelvic ring) include ipsilateral fractures of the superior and inferior pubic (ischiopubic) rami, fracture of the pubic body adjacent to the symphysis, subluxation of one sacroiliac joint (**Fig. 15.37**) or the pubic symphysis, and a fracture paralleling the sacroiliac joint (**Fig. 15.38**). The likelihood of a second break in the pelvic ring (type 3 injury) increases with a greater degree of joint diastasis or fracture displacement at the primary injury site. It should be kept in mind that spontaneous recoil of a separated sacroiliac joint may occur that may result in underestimation of the pelvic injury. Type 3 injuries (double breaks in the pelvic ring) include straddle fractures (vertical fractures of both superior pubic and ischiopubic rami or unilateral vertical rami fractures associated with symphyseal diastasis) (**Fig. 15.39**) and injuries with complete disruption of both the anterior and posterior pelvic ring (e.g., Malgaigne fracture, bucket handle fracture, and pelvic "dislocation") (**Fig. 15.40**). More extensive disruptions of the pelvis result from massive crush injuries in which the osseous ring is completely shattered. In the unstable jumper's fracture (**Fig. 15.41**), dissociation of the central portions of the sacrum from its lateral portions occurs by bilateral vertical sacral fractures, most commonly through the neural foramina representing the weakest points in the sacrum. Pelvic fractures are frequently associated with severe soft tissue injuries, including vascular lacerations, compression or disruption of peripheral nerves, and perforation of the urinary bladder, urethra, rectosigmoid, and anus.

Classification systems of pelvic fractures combining the direction of the force that created the injury with the fracture pattern seen radiographically allow a highly specific injury description and are preferred by orthopedic surgeons (**Table 15.1**). Four underlying mechanisms of injury that produce a distinctive radiographic pattern are discerned by the Young–Burgess classification:

1. *Lateral compression (LC):* A lateral force vector characteristically causes transverse fractures of the pubic rami, vertical compression fractures of the sacrum, and fractures of the iliac wings, as well as pelvic instability caused by rotation of one or both hemipelvises (rotational instability). In a "windswept" pelvis, anterior rotation of the hemipelvis at the side of the impact is associated with posterior rotation of the contralateral hemipelvis.

2. *Anteroposterior compression (AC):* An anteroposterior or posteroanterior force vector produces vertically oriented pubic rami fractures and disruption of the pubic symphysis and the sacroiliac joints, resulting in pelvic "dislocation" ("sprung" pelvis or "open book" injury).

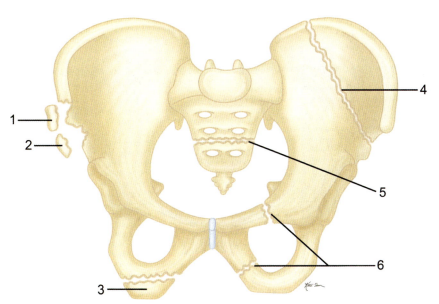

Fig. 15.34 Stable pelvic fractures. 1: Avulsion of anterosuperior iliac spine. **2:** Avulsion of anteroinferior iliac spine. **3:** Avulsion of ischial tuberosity. **4:** Iliac wing fracture. **5:** Sacral fracture. **6:** Unilateral superior and ischiopubic rami fractures (in addition, a fracture of the contralateral superior or ischiopubic ramus may be associated). Differential diagnosis: straddle fracture (see **Fig. 15.35**).

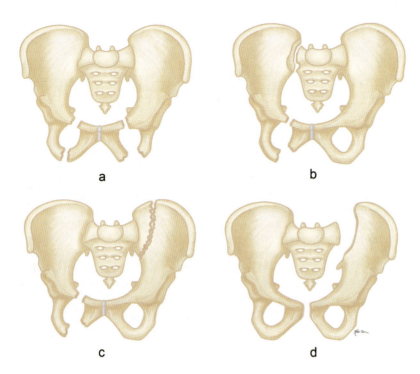

Fig. 15.35a–d Unstable pelvic fractures.
(**a**) Straddle fracture. Both the superior and ischiopubic rami are fractured bilaterally.
(**b**) Malgaigne fracture. Instead of the ipsilateral sacral wing fracture, the ipsilateral sacroiliac joint may be disrupted, or the ilium along the ipsilateral sacroiliac joint may be fractured. (**c**) Bucket handle fracture. (**d**) Pelvic "dislocation" (pubic diastasis associated with unilateral or bilateral sacroiliac joint disruption).

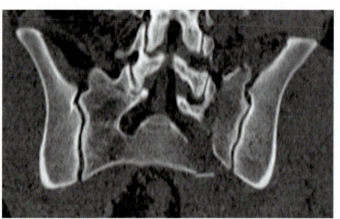

Fig. 15.36 Unilateral sacral fracture. A fracture through the left sacral wing is seen.

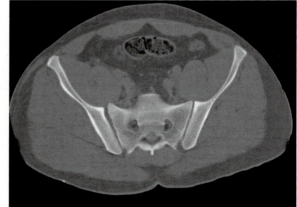

Fig. 15.37 Subluxation of the sacroiliac joint. Mild widening of the right sacroiliac joint is seen.

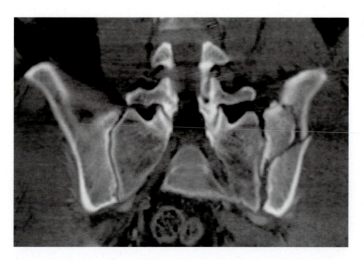

Fig. 15.38 Ilial fracture. A fracture of the left ilium with extension into the sacroiliac joint that is slightly widened is evident.

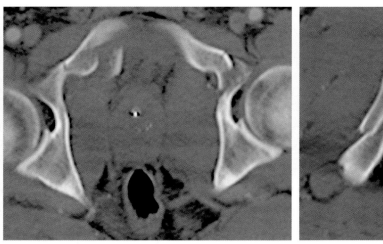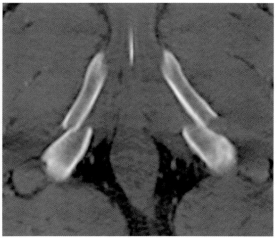

Fig. 15.39a, b   Straddle fracture. Fractures of bilateral superior pubic rami (**a**) and bilateral ischiopubic rami (**b**) are visible.

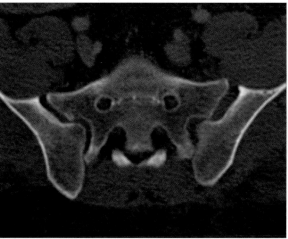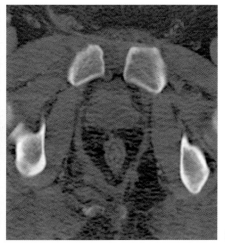

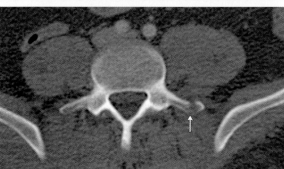

Fig. 15.40a–c   Unstable pelvic fractures.
The pelvis ring is completely disrupted anteriorly and posteriorly. (**a**) Markedly widened
left and slightly widened right sacroiliac joint.
(**b**) Widened pubic symphysis. (**c**) Fracture of
the left transverse process of L5 (*arrow*). This
finding is frequently associated with unstable
pelvic fractures.

Fig. 15.41   Jumper's fracture. Bilateral vertical sacral fractures (arrows)
separate the central portion of the sacrum from its wings.

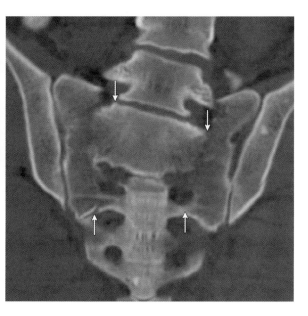

Table 15.1 Dynamic classification of pelvic injuries (modified from Tile)

Type A	Stable Fractures of the pelvis without ring disruption Fractures of the pelvis with single ring disruption and minimal displacement
Type B	Rotationally unstable Lateral compression (LC) with transverse fractures of the superior pubic and ischiopubic rami (anterior ring) and either ipsilateral or contralateral posterior ring injury Anteroposterior compression (APC) with symphyseal diastasis or vertical rami fractures with unilateral or bilateral anterior widening of the sacroiliac joints
Type C	Rotationally and vertically unstable LC with bilateral posterior ring disruption APC with complete disruption (dislocation) of one sacroiliac joint and lateral displacement of the hemipelvis Vertical shear fractures (VS) with complete disruption of both the anterior ring (unilateral or bilateral superior pubic and ischiopubic rami fractures or symphyseal diastasis) and posterior ring (sacral fracture or sacroiliac joint dislocation) associated with superior displacement of the hemipelvis Combination (complex) mechanism fractures, such as combination of LC and VS and crush injuries

3. *Vertical shear (VC):* An inferosuperior force vector produces vertically oriented fractures of the pubic rami and disruption of the sacroiliac joints and sacral or ilial fractures, paralleling this joint. The involved hemipelvis typically is displaced superiorly. Because all ligaments stabilizing the osseous pelvic ring (e.g., iliolumbar, anterior and posterior sacroiliac, and sacrospinous and sacrotuberous ligaments) are affected in this type of injury, the pelvic instability is most severe and both rotationally and vertically unstable. Fracture of the transverse process of L5 where the iliolumbar ligament attaches is a harbinger of an unstable pelvic injury.

4. *Combined (complex) mechanism:* Two or more different force vectors have been delivered to the pelvis. Lateral compression and vertical shear are the most common combination.

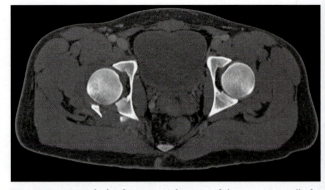

Fig. 15.43 Acetabular fracture. A fracture of the posterior wall of the right acetabulum is seen.

Pelvic fractures may extend into the acetabulum, where the dome (acetabular roof), the anterior (iliopubic) wall and column, the quadrilateral lamina (surface), or the posterior (ilioischial) wall and column may be involved (**Fig. 15.42**). Anterior and posterior wall fractures (**Figs. 15.43, 15.44**) are limited to the acetabulum and affect only a portion of the corresponding column, including its articular surface, whereas anterior and posterior column fractures separate the entire column from the innominate bone and are almost always associated with an ischiopubic ramus fracture. Rarely an anterior column fracture extends only into the superior pubic ramus and spares the ischiopubic ramus. In this case, the fracture has to originate in the ilium above the anteroinferior iliac spine of the pelvis; otherwise, it is by definition an anterior wall fracture. The most widely used acetabular fracture classification was devised by Letournel and Judet in which five simple (elementary) and five complex (associated) patterns are distinguished (**Table 15.2, Fig. 15.45**).

Hip dislocations can be classified as anterior, central (medial), and posterior. In anterior dislocation, the femoral head lies medial and inferior to the acetabulum, projecting into the suprapubic or obturator region, and the femur is abducted, externally rotated, and sometimes flexed. Central dislocation (traumatic protrusio acetabuli) is always associated with an

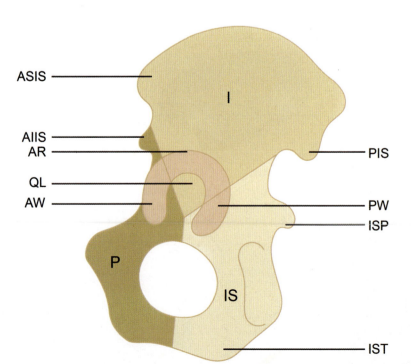

Fig. 15.42 Lateral pelvis.

AIIS	anteroinferior iliac spine
AR	acetabular roof
ASIS	anterosuperior iliac spine
AW	anterior acetabular wall
I	ilium
IS	ischium
ISP	ischial spine
IST	ischial tuberosity
PIS	posteroinferior iliac spine
PW	posterior acetabular wall
QL	quadrilateral lamina
Dark shaded area	anterior column
Light shaded area	posterior column

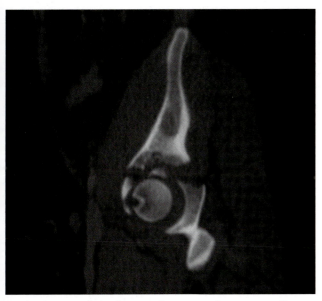

Fig. 15.44 Acetabular fracture. A transverse fracture extending from the anterior to posterior acetabular wall with loose intra-articular fragments is evident.

Table 15.2 Acetabular fracture classification of Letournel and Judet	
Elementary fractures	
Posterior wall	30%
Posterior column	4%
Anterior wall	1%
Anterior column	4%
Transverse	10%
Associated fractures	
Posterior column and wall	4%
Anterior column or wall and posterior hemitransverse	7%
Transverse and posterior wall	20%
T-shaped	7%
Both columns	13%

acetabular fracture, with the femoral head protruding into the pelvic cavity (**Fig. 15.46**). Posterior dislocation (**Fig. 15.47**) is by far the most common type, accounting for almost 90% of all hip dislocations. In posterior dislocation, the femoral head lies lateral and superior to the acetabulum, and the femur usually is internally rotated and adducted. Dislocations are commonly associated with fractures of the pelvis, especially the acetabulum, and fractures of the femoral head and, less commonly, neck. The Thompson and Epstein classification of posterior hip dislocations incorporates associated fractures (**Table 15.3**). Femoral head fractures (**Fig. 15.48**) associated

with posterior hip dislocations may be subdivided into four types (**Table 15.4**). In posterior hip dislocations with the femoral head being displaced superolaterally, the ligamentum teres (ligamentum capitis femoris) originating in the fovea of the femoral head and inserting into the transverse acetabular ligament at the floor of the acetabulum invariably ruptures or causes an avulsion fracture at the fovea. This avulsion fracture may extend cephalad in the weight-bearing articular surface of the femoral head (Pipkin type 2 fracture) that eventually may result in a deformed femoral head radiographically indistinguishable from sequelae of avascular necrosis.

Fractures of the proximal femur (commonly referred to as hip fractures) may be classified as capital, subcapital, midcervical (transcervical), basicervical, intertrochanteric, and subtrochanteric (**Fig. 15.49**). *Capital fractures* are uncommon and usually associated with posterior hip dislocations. *Femoral neck* fractures (**Fig. 15.50**) commonly occur in osteoporotic patients (e.g., elderly white women) after minor trauma. Common complications include nonunion, especially in the presence of severe

IV Musculoskeletal System

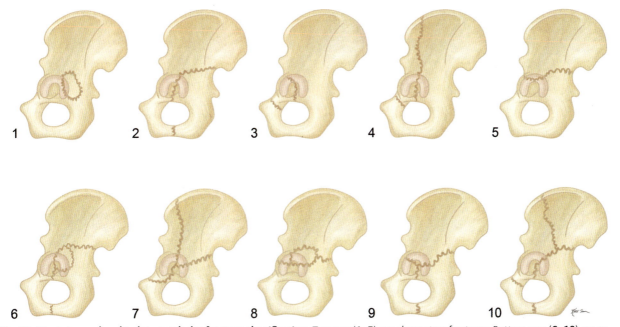

Fig. 15.45 Letournel and Judet acetabular fracture classification. Top row (**1–5**) are elementary fractures. Bottom row (**6–10**) are associated fractures. **1:** Posterior wall fracture. **2:** Posterior column fracture. **3:** Anterior wall fracture. **4:** Anterior column fracture. **5:** Transverse fracture. **6:** Posterior column and wall fracture. **7:** Anterior column or wall fracture and posterior hemitransverse fracture. **8:** Transverse and posterior wall fracture. **9:** T-shaped fracture. **10:** Both anterior and posterior column fracture. Note that both the anterior wall (**3**) and anterior column (**4**) fractures are associated with a superior pubic ramus fracture, but the difference is that the former originates below and the latter above the anteroinferior iliac spine. More often the anterior column fracture is associated with an ischiopubic fracture. In that case, the anterior column fracture may also originate below the anteroinferior iliac spine.

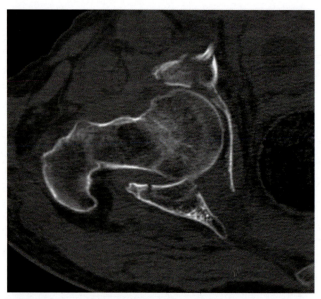

Fig. 15.46 Central (medial) hip dislocation (traumatic protrusio acetabuli). Medial displacement of the femoral head is associated with fractures of the anterior and posterior acetabular wall and the quadrilateral lamina.

osteoporosis, and avascular necrosis of the femoral head, because its main blood supply derives from branches of the circumflex femoral arteries entering the bone distal to the fracture line at the base of the femoral neck. Fractures of the femoral neck can be classified according to their anatomical location (see **Fig. 15.49**), the angle the fracture line in the neck forms

Table 15.3 Classification of posterior hip dislocations (Thompson and Epstein)	
Type 1	Dislocation with or without minor acetabular fracture
Type 2	Dislocation with single large fracture of the posterior acetabular wall
Type 3	Dislocation with comminuted fracture of the acetabulum
Type 4	Dislocation with comminuted acetabular fracture extending to the acetabular floor
Type 5	Dislocation with fracture of the head or neck of the femur

with the horizontal plane (Pauwels classification, **Fig. 15.51**), and the displacement of the fracture fragments (Garden classification, **Fig. 15.52**). Garden 1 is an impacted ("incomplete") fracture with valgus deformity, Garden 2 a nondisplaced fracture with varus deformity, Garden 3 a displaced fracture with varus deformity, and Garden 4 a fracture with cephalad displacement (foreshortening) of the femur shaft. Garden 1 and 2 fractures are commonly treated with internal fixation using multiple cancellous lag screws, Garden 3 and 4 with hemiarthroplasty.

In *intertrochanteric fractures,* differentiation between a stable and unstable fracture pattern is largely based on the integrity of the posteromedial cortex (**Fig. 15.53**), where the calcar is located. In stable fractures, the posteromedial cortex remains intact or has minimal comminution with cortical opposition of the fracture fragments. Intertrochanteric fractures can be classified based on the number of fracture fragments (**Fig. 15.54**). Two- and three-part fractures in this system tend to be stable, whereas four- and multipart fractures are unstable. Both a two-part intertrochanteric fracture with varus deformity and a two-part fracture of the proximal femur shaft extending into the lesser trochanter (reverse obliquity pattern) are always unstable, the latter because of the tendency for medial displacement of the femoral shaft. Sliding (dynamic) hip screw devices such as gamma nails are used for the operative treatment of intertrochanteric and extracapsular basicervical neck fractures.

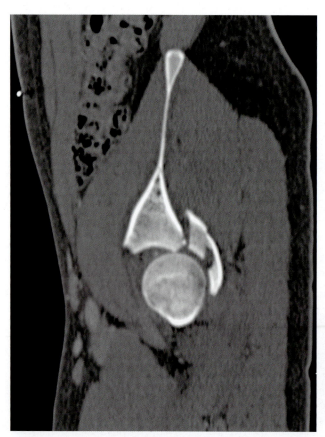

Fig. 15.47 Posterior hip subluxation. Posterior displacement of the femoral head with fracture of the posterior acetabular wall is seen.

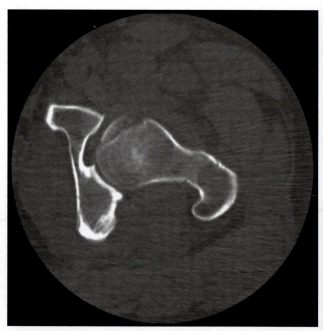

Fig. 15.48 Femoral head fracture. A crescent-shaped avulsion fracture of the femoral head resulted from a posterior hip dislocation that had been reduced.

Table 15.4 Classification of femoral head fractures associated with posterior hip dislocations (modified from Pipkin)

Type 1	Femoral head fracture caudad to the fovea
Type 2	Femoral head fracture cephalad to the fovea
Type 3	Femoral head and neck fracture
Type 4	Femoral head fracture associated with acetabular fracture
Subtypes:	4.1: Femoral head fracture caudad to fovea 4.2: Femoral head fracture cephalad to fovea 4.3: Femoral head and neck fracture

Subtrochanteric fractures are classified according to the level of the fracture line (**Fig. 15.55**) or both location and degree of comminution affecting the stability of the fractures (**Fig. 15.56**). It is generally accepted that both a more distally located fracture and a greater comminution result in a higher incidence of complications, which include malunion, nonunion, hardware failure, and infection.

Femur shaft fractures are best classified by location (proximal, middle, and distal third or junction between these regions) and fracture morphology, including degree and type of comminution. A simplified AO/OTA classification differentiates between two-part fractures (type A), wedge fractures with butterfly fragments of varying size and possible comminution (type B), and complex fracture, including segmental and multipart comminuted fractures without contact between the proximal and distal diaphyseal segments (type C).

Fractures of the distal femur (**Fig. 15.57**) are classified as extra-articular supracondylar and intra-articular unicondylar and bicondylar fractures (**Fig. 15.58**). The severity of the fracture, which is inversely related to the prognosis, progressively increases in this classification system from one type or subgroup

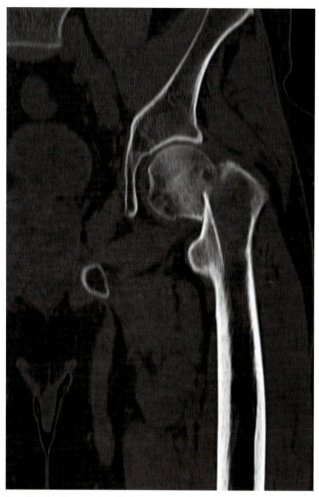

Fig. 15.50 Femoral neck fracture. A subcapital fracture with superior displacement (foreshortening) of the femoral shaft is evident.

to the next. Complications include vascular injuries, infection, painful internal fixation devices (e.g., screws protruding outside the cortex), hardware failure, nonunion, malunion, and post-traumatic osteoarthritis. Loose intra-articular bodies may be the sequelae of osteochondral and meniscal fractures.

Patellar fractures are classified for a treatment-directed approach as either nondisplaced or displaced (**Fig. 15.59**). A displaced fracture is defined by fracture fragment separation of 4 mm or more or an articular incongruity of 2 mm or more. Descriptive terms such as transverse, vertical, stellate (comminuted), marginal (medial or lateral side), proximal or

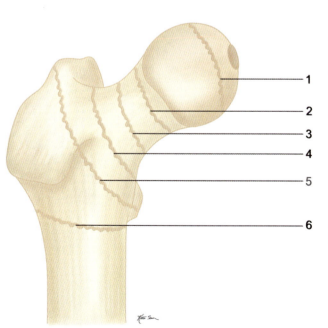

Fig. 15.49 Proximal femur fractures. 1: Capital. **2**: Subcapital. **3**: Midcervical. **4**: Basicervical. **5**: Intertrochanteric. **6**: Subtrochanteric. Fractures **1** to **3** are intracapsular and **4** to **6** extracapsular. Fractures **2, 3,** and **4** are femur neck fractures.

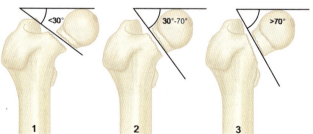

Fig. 15.51 Pauwels classification of femoral neck fractures. The classification is based on the angle the fracture forms with the horizontal plane. As the fracture progresses from type 1 to type 3, the obliquity of the fracture line increases, resulting in increased shearing forces at the fracture site with corresponding increased risk of nonunion.

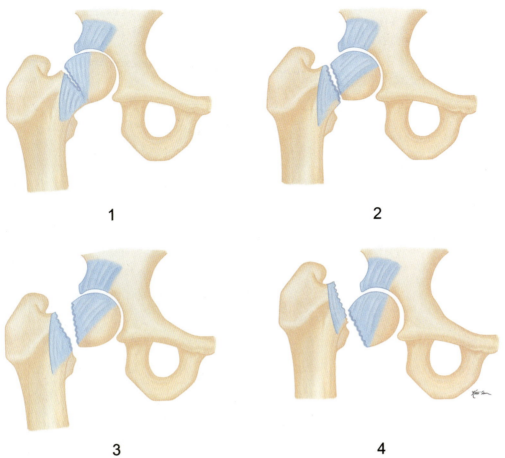

Fig. 15.52 Garden classification of femoral neck fractures. Displacement is graded according to the alignment and angulation of the compressive trabeculae in the femoral neck fracture. Garden 1 is an impacted ("incomplete") fracture with valgus deformity. Garden 2 is a nondisplaced fracture with varus deformity. Garden 3 is a displaced fracture with varus deformity. Garden 4 is a fracture with cephalad displacement (foreshortening) of the femur shaft. External rotation is present in 1, 3, and 4. The compressive trabeculae (blue) between femoral head and neck at the fracture site form a valgus angle in Garden 1 and a varus angle in Garden 2 and 3.

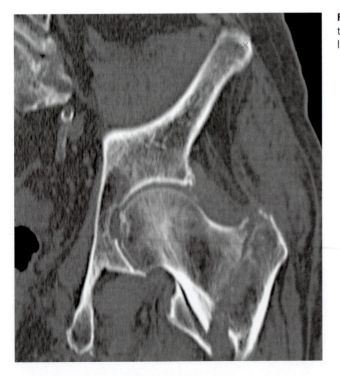

Fig. 15.53 Intertrochanteric fracture. A fracture extending from the greater to the lesser trochanter with complete separation of the latter is seen.

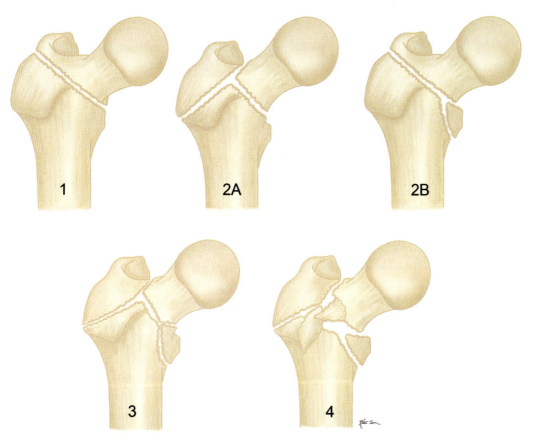

Fig. 15.54 Classification of intertrochanteric fractures. Nondisplaced two- and three-part fractures (top row) are stable. Four- and multipart fractures (bottom row) are unstable. **1**: Two-part fracture (linear intertrochanteric, greater or lesser trochanter). **2**: Three-part fracture: intertrochanteric with comminution of greater trochanter (**2A**) or lesser trochanter (**2B**). **3**: Four-part fracture: intertrochanteric with comminution to both trochanters. **4**: Multipart: comminuted intertrochanteric fracture with separation of both trochanters. Two-part fractures involving either the greater or lesser trochanter are always stable. Intertrochanteric fractures with varus deformity are always unstable.

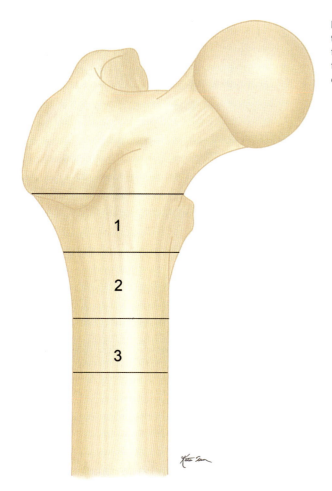

Fig. 15.55 Fielding classification of subtrochanteric fractures. The classification is based on the fracture level. Type 1 fractures (most common) occur at the level of the lesser trochanter; type 2, up to 2.5 cm below the lesser trochanter; type 3 (least common), between 2.5 and 5 cm below the lesser trochanter.

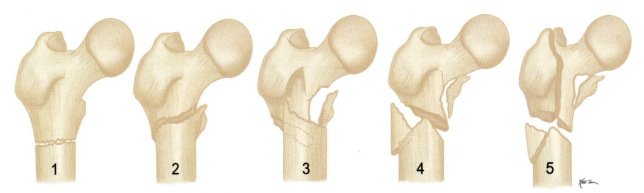

Fig. 15.56 Modified Seinsheimer classification of subtrochanteric fractures. Type 1: Nondisplaced. Type 2: Two-part: transverse, oblique, or spiral fracture with or without extension into the lesser trochanter. Type 3: Three-part: oblique or spiral fracture with either detached lesser trochanter or butterfly fragment posterior. Type 4: Oblique or spiral fracture with detached lesser trochanter and butterfly fragment posterior. Type 5: Subtrochanteric and intertrochanteric fractures.

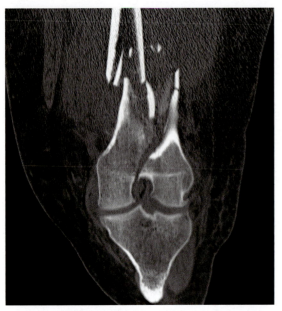

Fig. 15.57 Distal femur fracture. A comminuted distal femoral metaphysis fracture with extension into the knee is seen.

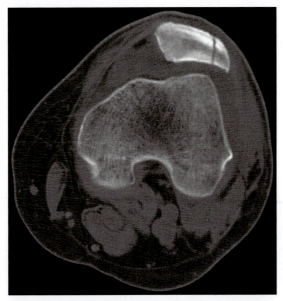

Fig. 15.59 Patellar fracture. A nondisplaced vertical fracture of the lateral aspect of the patella is seen. Also evident is lateral subluxation of the patella.

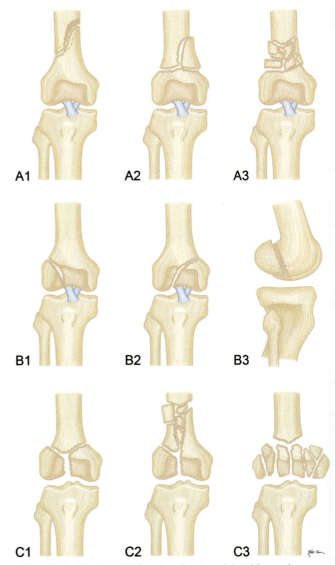

Fig. 15.58 Modified Müller classification of distal femur fractures.
A: Supracondylar (extra-articular). **B**: Unicondylar. **C**: Bicondylar.
A1: Simple (two-part). **A2**: Metaphyseal wedge (butterfly fragment, three-part). **A3**: Metaphyseal complex (comminuted, multipart).
B1: Lateral condyle (sagittal plane). **B2**: Medial condyle (sagittal plane). **B3**: Lateral or medial condyle (coronal plane). **C1**: Simple bicondylar and simple metaphyseal T- or Y-fracture. **C2**: Simple bicondylar and comminuted (multifragmentary) metaphyseal fractures. **C3**: Comminuted (multifragmentary) bicondylar.

distal pole, and osteochondral can be used to further describe patellar fractures. Bipartite and, rarely, multipartite patella with the fragments representing accessory ossification center(s) with a smoothly rounded margin are characteristically located in the superolateral aspect of the patella and must be differentiated.

Tibial plateau fractures (**Fig. 15.60**) are the most common proximal tibia fractures involving either the medial or lateral plateau or both. Schatzker's classification of tibial plateau fractures is most widely used and differentiates between medial and lateral involvement (**Fig. 15.61**). Type 1 (split fracture) is a pure cleavage fracture of the lateral tibial plateau. Type 2 (split-depression) is a cleavage fracture of the lateral tibial plateau in which the remaining articular surface is depressed into the metaphysis. Type 3 (depression) is a central depression fracture of the lateral tibial plateau. Type 4 involves the medial tibial plateau either as a split (4A), depression (4B), or split-depression (4C) fracture. Tibial spine fractures are frequently associated. Type 5 is a bicondylar fracture in which the fracture line often forms an inverted Y with intact junction between metaphysis and diaphysis. Type 6 is a tibial plateau fracture in which there is complete dissociation between the metaphysis and the diaphysis. These fractures may have varying degrees of comminution of one or both tibial condyles and the articular surface. Late complications include painful hardware (up to 50%), malunion, and posttraumatic osteoarthritis.

A *Segond fracture* is an avulsion from the lateral aspect of the proximal tibia just distal to the joint line at the insertion of the reinforced capsule. This fracture is frequently associated with tears of the anterior cruciate ligament and lateral meniscus secondary to varus stress with internal rotation of the flexed knee. The Segond fracture has to be differentiated from an avulsion of the *Gerdy tubercle* (insertion of the iliotibial tract) that is located anterior and slightly more distal to the former. A *reverse Segond-type fracture* consists of an avulsion fracture of the medial aspect of the proximal tibia at the insertion of the medial collateral ligament associated with tears of the posterior cruciate ligament and medial meniscus secondary to valgus stress and external rotation of the flexed knee.

Knee dislocation is a relatively rare injury that, besides extensive ligamentous damage and avulsions, is also frequently associated with a neurovascular insult (popliteal artery, peroneal nerve). In order of decreasing frequency anterior, posterior, medial, and lateral dislocations are differentiated. Spontaneous reduction is not uncommon, resulting in underdiagnosis of this injury. Disruption of all four major ligaments of the knee (both cruciate and collateral ligaments) is highly suggestive that a dislocation has occurred. MRI is the imaging modality of choice for the evaluation of knee dislocations.

Patellar dislocation is usually lateral, but it may be transient (spontaneous reduction of a traumatic dislocation). In this case,

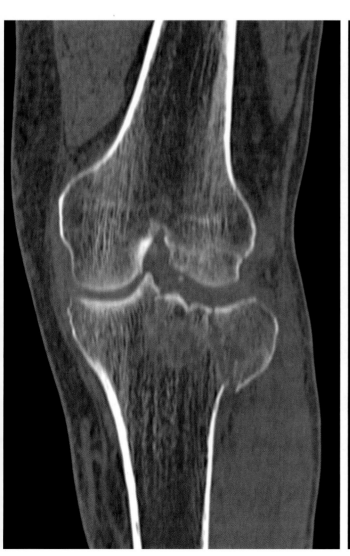
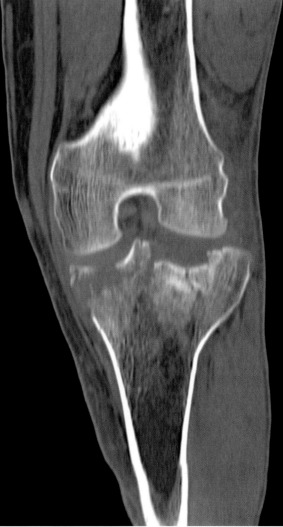

b

Fig. 15.60a, b   Tibial plateau fractures (two cases). (a) Lateral tibial plateau fracture without significant depression. **(b)** Bilateral tibial plateau fractures with considerable depression on the lateral side.

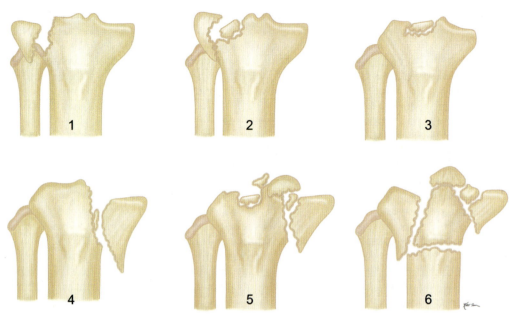

Fig. 15.61   Schatzker classification of tibial plateau fractures. Type 1: Split fracture (cleavage fracture) of lateral plateau. Type 2: Split-depression fracture (combined cleavage and compression fracture) of lateral plateau. Type 3: Central depression fracture of lateral plateau. Type 4: Medial plateau fracture with split and/or depression. Type 5: Bicondylar fracture with intact metaphyseal and diaphyseal junction. Type 6: Plateau fracture with complete dissociation between metaphysis and diaphysis. Proximal fibular fractures may be associated with all types.

an osteochondral fracture of the medial patellar facet and lateral femoral condyle may be the clue for the correct diagnosis. Predisposing factors include a patella alta, deficient height of the lateral femoral condyle, shallowness of the patellofemoral groove, and genu valgum or recurvatum.

Proximal tibiofibular joint dislocation occurs anteriorly or, less frequently, posteriorly. Peroneal nerve injury may be associated with the posterior dislocation.

Tibia and fibula shaft fractures occur isolated or together. An isolated fibular shaft fracture is uncommon and results from a direct blow. More typically, an apparently isolated fibular fracture is actually a component of an ankle injury (e.g., Maisonneuve fracture). Because of the subcutaneous location of the anteromedial surface of the tibia, an open (compound) fracture is not uncommon, resulting in a relatively high incidence of infection with nonunion. The AO/OTA classification of diaphyseal tibial fractures differentiates between two-part fractures (type A), wedge fracture with butterfly fragment (type B), and complex fractures (segmental or multipart fractures, type C). In type A fractures, spiral (A1), oblique (A2), and transverse (A3) fractures are differentiated. In type B fractures, an intact spiral wedge or butterfly fragment (B1), an intact nonspiral wedge in which the butterfly fragment is separated from the tibial shaft by oblique (not spiral) fracture lines (B2), and a fractured wedge (B3) are discerned. Furthermore, for both type A and B fractures, it must be assessed if the fibula is intact or if the tibia and fibula fractures are at the same or a different level. Type C fractures are further subdivided by the number of fracture fragments. *Compartment syndrome* occurs in about 4% of all tibial shaft fractures, but it is most common in male patients under 35 y of age. The syndrome may affect all four compartments of the lower leg, but it is always present in the anterior compartment. The diagnosis is made by monitoring the compartment pressure and can be supported by MRI.

In the *ankle,* axial-loading injuries resulting in tibial plafond (pilon) fractures and rotational ankle injuries resulting in malleolar fractures are differentiated. It has to be kept in mind, however, that axial load and rotational forces may coexist in an ankle injury, resulting in a more complex fracture pattern.

Tibial plafond (pilon) fractures (**Fig. 15.62**) typically result from motor vehicle accidents or falls from heights. Classifying these fractures by description, the displacement of the talus and articular fragments should be noted. The talus is frequently proximally displaced, but it may translate in any direction. The degree of comminution of both the articular surface and the metaphyseal area of the distal tibia must be assessed. The presence or absence of an associated fibula fracture and, if present, its location and degree of comminution also need to be evaluated. All these factors are essential in treatment planning and outcome prediction. Distal tibia fractures are divided by the AO/OTA classification system into the following categories: type A, nonarticular fractures; type B, partial articular fractures (these fractures are similar to rotational ankle fractures with extension into the tibial plafond and will be discussed later in this chapter); and type C, total articular fracture. Intra-articular tibial plafond (pilon) fractures are classified into three types. Type 1 is a nondisplaced cleavage fracture, type 2 a minimally comminuted and displaced fracture with articular incongruity but without depression of any articular fracture fragment, and type 3 a highly comminuted and displaced fracture (**Fig. 15.63**).

Rotational ankle fractures can be classified by location as unimalleolar, bimalleolar, trimalleolar, or complex (comminuted intra-articular fracture of the distal tibia associated with a distal fibular fracture, indistinguishable from a pilon fracture). Rotational injuries of the ankle are commonly caused by supination (inversion, adduction) or pronation (eversion, abduction) of the foot and may be associated with external (lateral) rotation of the foot. These injuries may be ligamentous, osseous, or a combination of both. Rotational ankle fractures can be classified by either anatomical location or injury mechanism. The Weber classification is based on the level of the fibular fracture: type A fracture is at or below the level of the ankle joint line, type B fracture originates at the level of the joint line or slightly above it and progresses superiorly, and type C fracture is located 2 cm or higher above the ankle joint line (**Fig. 15.64**). Type C fractures correspond to the pronation-external rotation (PER) fracture of the Lauge–Hansen classification (**Fig. 15.65**), which is based on

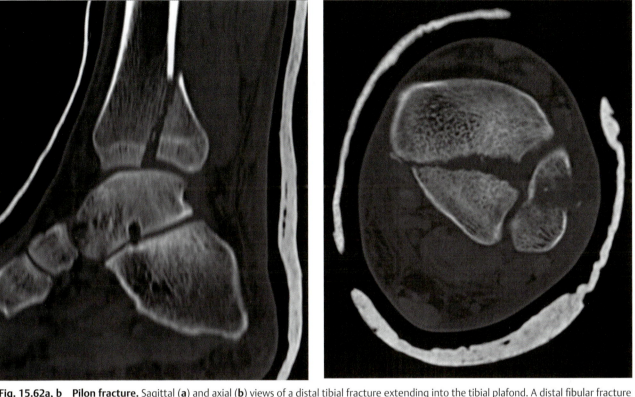

b

Fig. 15.62a, b   Pilon fracture. Sagittal (**a**) and axial (**b**) views of a distal tibial fracture extending into the tibial plafond. A distal fibular fracture is also evident in **b.**

IV   Musculoskeletal System

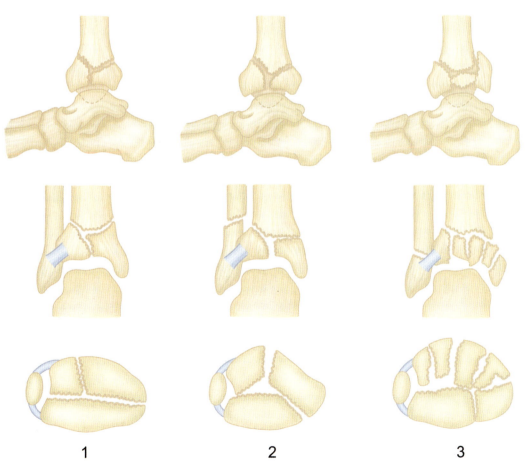

| | **1** | | **2** | | **3** |

Fig. 15.63   Modified Müller classification of pilon fractures. Sagittal, coronal, and axial illustrations through the tibial plafond. Type 1: Nondisplaced fracture of the articular surface of the tibial plafond. Type 2: Minimally displaced and comminuted fracture with articular incongruity. Type 3: Highly comminuted and displaced fracture commonly with impacted articular fracture fragments.

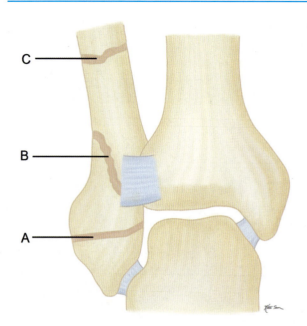

Fig. 15.64 Weber classification of ankle fractures. The classification is based on the anatomical location of the fracture line in the fibula. Type A: Fracture originates at or below the ankle joint line and corresponds to supination or pronation injuries of the ankle without external rotation. Type B: Fracture originates at the joint line and progresses superiorly and posteriorly. It corresponds to a supination–external rotation (SER) injury. Type C: Fracture originates 2 cm or higher above the joint line and corresponds to a pronation–external rotation (PER) injury. See **Fig. 15.65** for correlation between anatomical fracture location and injury mechanism.

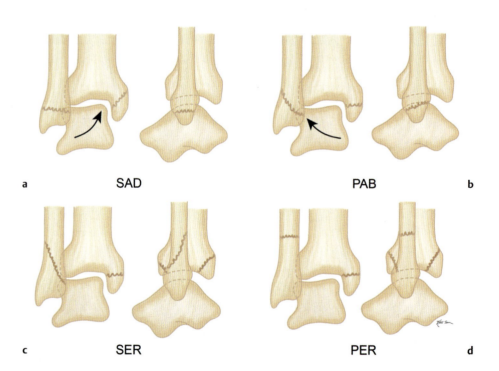

Fig. 15.65a–d Lauge-Hansen classification of ankle fractures. (a) Supination–adduction (SAD) injury (20%). Transverse (avulsion fracture of the lateral malleolus and oblique (talar impaction) fracture of the medial malleolus, both originating at or below the joint line. **(b)** Pronation–abduction (PAB) injury (10%). Transverse (avulsion) fracture of the medial malleolus and oblique (talar impaction) fracture of the lateral malleolus, both originating at or below the joint line. **(c)** SER injury (60%). Spiral fracture of the distal fibula originating at or up to 1.5 cm above the joint line and extending in a dorsal and proximal direction. Fractures of the medial and posterior malleolus and the anterior tibial (Chaput) tubercle may be associated. **(d)** PER injury (10%). Fracture of the medial malleolus associated with a transverse supramalleolar (2 cm or higher above the joint line) fibula fracture. Fractures of the posterior malleolus and anterior tibial (Chaput) tubercle may be associated. Note that instead of a malleolar fracture, the corresponding medial (deltoid) or lateral collateral ligament may be torn. Widening of the mortise (injury to the tibiofibular syndesmosis consisting of the anterior and posterior tibiofibular ligaments, inferior transverse ligament [immediately distal to the latter], and interosseous membrane) can be diagnosed when the distal tibiofibular joint measures ≥ 4 mm in width or when there is a joint incongruity. With conventional radiography, there is no longer an overlap between the distal tibia and fibula on the mortise view in this condition. Avulsion fractures of the anterior tibial (Chaput) tubercle and posterior malleolus indicate an injury to the anterior and posterior tibiofibular ligaments, respectively, and are found only with injuries associated with an external rotational component, such as SER and PER.

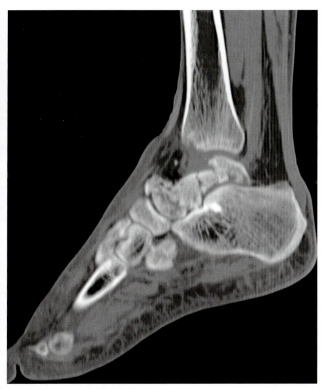

Fig. 15.66   Talar fracture. Comminuted fracture of the talus involving the head, neck, and body is seen.

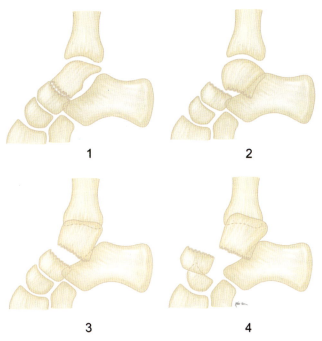

Fig. 15.67   Modified Hawkins classification of talar neck fractures. Type 1: Undisplaced fracture without associated joint subluxation or dislocation. Type 2: Talar neck fracture with dislocation of the talocalcaneal joint. Type 3: Talar neck fracture with dislocation of the ankle and the talocalcaneal joint. Type 4: Talar neck fracture with dislocation of the ankle, talocalcaneal, and talonavicular joint.

the injury mechanism. These fibular shaft fractures associated with ankle injuries are often better known by their eponym. A *Maisonneuve fracture* is a pronation external rotation type injury consisting of a proximal fibula fracture, disruption of the tibiofibular syndesmosis distal to this fracture, and a medial malleolar fracture or a torn medial collateral (deltoid) ligament. A *Dupuytren fracture* consists of a distal fibula fracture 2 to 7 cm above the ankle joint line associated with disruption of the distal tibiofibular syndesmosis and the medial collateral (deltoid) ligament. The same injury with intact tibiofibular syndesmosis is termed a *Pott fracture*.

Avulsion fractures predominate in the *talus* and occur in the superior aspect of the head and neck and in the lateral, medial, and posterior aspects of the body. These fractures are frequently associated with ankle injuries. Major talar fractures may involve the head, neck, body, and the lateral or posterior process (**Fig. 15.66**). Of these, talar neck fractures are the most common and typically depict a vertical fracture course. The modified Hawkins classification differentiates four types of talar neck fractures. Type 1 is an undisplaced fracture without dislocation. Type 2 refers to a talar neck fracture with associated dislocation of the subtalar joint. This is the most common type. Type 3 is a talar neck fracture with dislocation of both the ankle and subtalar joint. Type 4 is also associated with subluxation or dislocation in the talonavicular joint (**Fig. 15.67**). Osteonecrosis of the proximal fracture fragment is a common complication of talar neck fracture. It is relatively rare in Hawkins type 1 fractures but may reach close to 100% in type 4 fractures. The appearance of a linear subchondral lucent area (Hawkins sign) in the talar dome after 1 to 3 months relates to hyperemia and continuity of blood supply and should not be misinterpreted as a crescent sign of osteonecrosis. At this stage, osteonecrosis manifests itself as relatively increased density in the proximal talar fragment when compared with the distal one.

Besides rare talar body fractures (**Fig. 15.68**) presenting in a variety of fracture patterns, osteochondral fractures of the talar

dome and fractures involving either the lateral or posterior process of the talar body are more common and must be recognized as separate entities. The lateral talar process is a large, broad-based, wedge-shaped prominence of the talar body and includes two articular surfaces. Dorsolaterally, it articulates

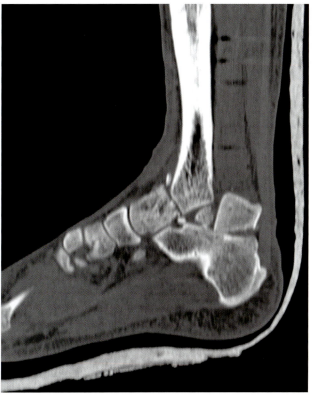

Fig. 15.68   Talar body fracture. A comminuted fracture of the talus with numerous loose fragments and displacement of the rotated talar body posteriorly is seen.

IV Musculoskeletal System

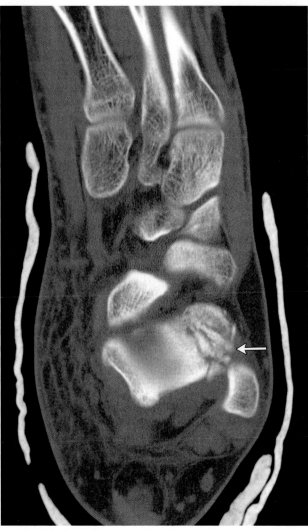

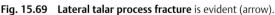

Fig. 15.69 **Lateral talar process fracture** is evident (arrow).

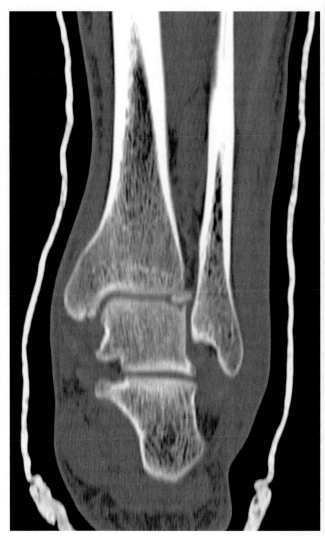

Fig. 15.70 **Osteochondral fracture** of the lateral talar dome is seen.

with the fibula and inferomedially with the anterior portion of the posterior facet of the calcaneus. CT is frequently required for the diagnosis of a lateral process fracture (**Fig. 15.69**). Differentiation of an os trigonum from a posterior process fracture may be difficult at times, particularly when the former is diseased. Osteochondral fractures (**Fig. 15.70**) of the medial or lateral talar dome result from shearing or rotatory forces applied to the articular surface in conjunction with an ankle injury. Differentiation of an osteochondral fracture from osteochondritis dissecans is not always possible based on imaging examinations alone. A chondral fracture limited to the joint cartilage without involvement of the subchondral bone is not appreciated by CT and requires CT arthrography or MRI for diagnosis.

Dislocation of the talus can occur with or without major talar fractures. A subtalar (peritalar) dislocation has to be differentiated from a total talar dislocation. *A subtalar dislocation* involves simultaneous dislocations of the talocalcaneal and talonavicular joint. Subtalar dislocations occur in any direction. Up to 85% of dislocations are medial, in which the calcaneus and the rest of the foot are displaced medially. The navicular is located medial and sometimes dorsal to the head and neck of the talus. Lateral subtalar dislocations are second in frequency, followed by anterior and posterior subtalar dislocations. In the total talar dislocation, the ankle is, besides the talocalcaneal and talonavicular joint, also completely dislocated (not only subluxed), resulting in a "floating talus." Talar osteonecrosis is a frequent complication in this condition.

Calcaneal fractures (**Fig. 15.71**) are the most common tarsal fractures. They can be intra-articular (75%) or extra-articular (25%). Extra-articular calcaneal fractures are typically caused by either twisting forces, resulting in fractures of the tuberosity, sustentaculum tali, or anterior process, or a pull by the Achilles tendon, resulting in a beaklike avulsion fracture of the posterosuperior aspect of the calcaneus. Intra-articular fractures occur in vertical falls in which the talus is driven into the calcaneus. This injury mechanism is bilateral in 10%. Calcaneal fractures can be classified based on both anatomical location and injury mechanism (**Fig. 15.72**). A specific calcaneal fracture classification system for CT was devised by Sanders (**Fig. 15.73**). Based on the oblique coronal plane perpendicular to the posterior facet, this structure is divided into three equal segments, defined as lateral (A), central (B), and medial (C). All nondisplaced articular fractures (< 2 mm), regardless of the number of fracture lines, are designated as type 1 fractures. Type 2 are two-part fractures of the posterior facet. Three types are differentiated, depending on the location of the fracture line in the lateral segment (2A), central segment (2B), or medial segment (2C). Type 3 are three-part fractures that usually feature a centrally depressed fragment. Based on the location of the two fracture lines in the posterior facet, the following fracture can be identified: 3AB, 3AC, and 3BC. Type 4 are four-part or multipart highly comminuted fractures of the posterior facet.

In the *navicular bone,* dorsal avulsion fractures related to the talonavicular or naviculocuneiform ligament insertion are

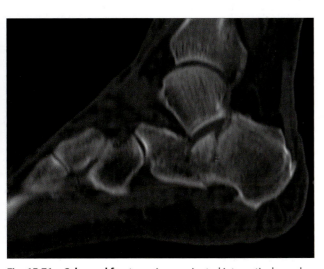

Fig. 15.71 Calcaneal fracture. A comminuted intra-articular and depressed calcaneal fracture is seen.

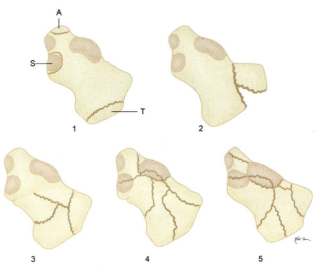

Fig. 15.72 Rowe classification of calcaneal fractures. Type 1: Fractures of the tuberosity (T), sustentaculum tali (S) containing the middle subtalar facet, or anterior process (A). Type 2: Beak fracture or avulsion fracture at the insertion of the Achilles tendon. Type 3: Comminuted fracture not involving the subtalar joint. Type 4: Comminuted fracture involving the subtalar joint. Type 5: Comminuted depressed subtalar joint fracture.

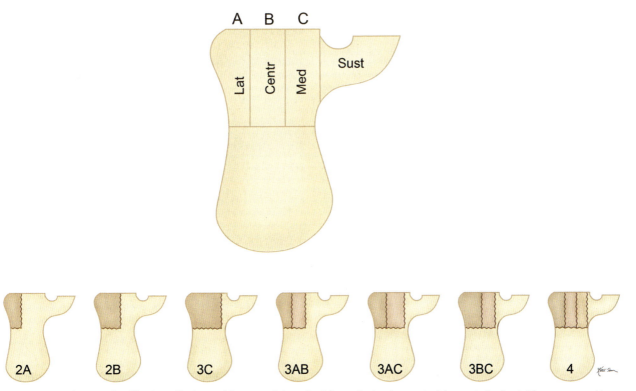

Fig. 15.73 Sanders CT classification of calcaneal fractures is based solely on the involvement of the posterior facet. The assessment is made on the oblique coronal image in the plane of the posterior facet. For this purpose, the posterior facet is divided into three equal parts, defined as lateral (A), central (B), and medial (C) segments. Type 1 fractures include all nondisplaced (< 2 mm) fractures of the posterior facet. Type 2 fractures are two-part or split fractures, typically with lateral displacement of the lateral fracture fragment. Depending on the location of the primary fracture line, three types—2A, 2B, and 2C—are differentiated. Type 3 fractures are three-part fractures that usually have a depressed central fracture fragment. Depending on the location of the two fracture lines, three types—3AB, 3AC, and 3BC—are differentiated. Type 4 fractures are highly comminuted four- or multipart fractures involving all three segments (A, B, and C) of the posterior facet. Shaded areas indicate fracture fragments. Sust: sustentaculum tali.

IV Musculoskeletal System

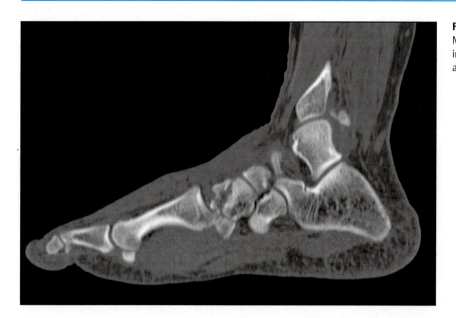

Fig. 15.74 Lisfranc fracture–dislocation. Multiple fractures involving the medial and intermediate cuneiforms and dorsal subluxation of the first metatarsal are visible.

most common. An os supranaviculare or os infranaviculare, respectively, must be differentiated from these avulsion fractures. Fracture of the navicular tuberosity at the insertion of the tibialis posterior is another traction type injury that should not be confused with an os tibiale externum (os naviculare secundarium). Body fractures of the navicular are horizontal (splitting the navicular into dorsal and plantar segments), vertical (resulting in medial and lateral segments), or comminuted. An isolated dislocation or subluxation of the navicular is usually associated with a neuropathic foot.

Cuboidal fractures and dislocations rarely occur as an isolated entity, but they are not uncommon in association with other tarsal bone injuries and complex Lisfranc joint disruptions. Avulsion fractures and, less frequently, two-part or comminuted body fractures are recognized. A fracture of the os peroneum, a sesamoid within the peroneus longus tendon, can clinically simulate an isolated cuboid injury. A bipartite os peroneum has to be differentiated from a fracture of this sesamoid.

Fractures of the cuneiforms are usually associated with tarsometatarsal joint injuries. The spectrum of these injuries ranges from simple sprains to complex tarsometatarsal dislocations, also referred to as Lisfranc fracture-dislocations (**Fig. 15.74**). Severe injuries with instability occur from high-energy trauma, such as a fall from a height or motor vehicle collision. Three types of Lisfranc joint instability can be differentiated in severe injuries: (1) first ray separation, evident as medial subluxation of the first metatarsal as an isolated finding or associated with widening of the space between the medial and intermediate cuneiforms; (2) homolateral dislocation of the first to fifth metatarsal; and (3) divergent dislocation, with lateral displacement of the second through the fifth metatarsal and medial or absent displacement of the first metatarsal (**Fig. 15.75**). Dorsal (rarely plantar) subluxation/dislocation in the tarsometatarsal joints is frequently associated. Fractures may be present in all tarsometatarsal joints, but they are most common in the base of the second metatarsal, followed by the third metatarsal and the medial and intermediate cuneiforms. Metatarsal fractures involving the shaft or neck may be transverse, oblique, spiral, or comminuted. Fractures of the metatarsal head are uncommon and, when present, usually associated with more typical fractures of adjacent metatarsals. In the fifth metatarsal, an intra-articular avulsion of the tuberosity at the peroneus brevis insertion has to be differentiated from a Jones fracture, which refers to an extra-articular transverse fracture of the proximal shaft. Jones fractures have a high incidence of nonunion.

Metatarsophalangeal injuries most commonly occur in the first metatarsophalangeal joint. Dislocations can occur in any direction, but in the first metatarsophalangeal joint they

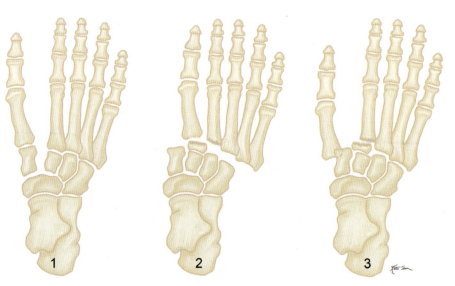

Fig. 15.75 Lisfranc fracture–dislocation. Type 1: First ray separation: medial subluxation of the first metatarsal with or without widening of the space between medial and intermediate cuneiforms. Type 2: Homolateral form: metatarsals 1 through 5 are all subluxed or dislocated laterally. Type 3: Divergent form: the first metatarsal stays in place or is medially subluxed or dislocated. Metatarsals 2 to 5 are laterally subluxed or dislocated. In types 2 and 3, a fracture of the base of the second metatarsal is virtually always associated. Other metatarsal fractures (especially the base of the third) and cuneiforms (especially medial and intermediate) may also be present.

typically occur in dorsal or plantar direction. Hyperdorsiflexion injuries of the first metatarsophalangeal joint include both a turf toe and a sesamoid fracture (**Fig. 15.76**). These conditions are best assessed with MRI. A sesamoid fracture may be difficult to differentiate from a partite sesamoid. On CT, a fractured sesamoid has rough, irregular borders, and there is only minimal separation of the fragments unless the plantar plate is torn. The partite sesamoid has smooth sclerotic edges, and the sum of the partite sesamoids makes a sesamoid larger than a normal one (**Fig. 15.77**).

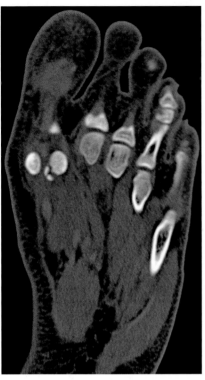

Fig. 15.76 Sesamoid fracture. Fracture of the lateral sesamoid of the great toe is seen with two small fracture fragments projecting proximal and medial to the lateral sesamoid.

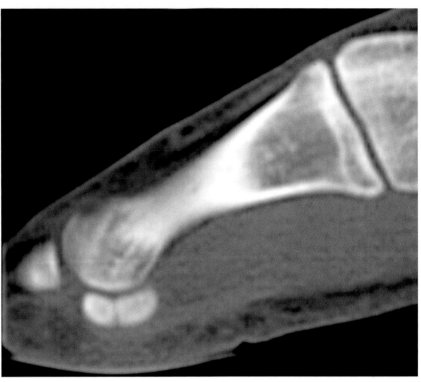

Fig. 15.77 Bipartite sesamoid. In contrast to a sesamoid fracture, the bipartite sesamoid has smooth and sclerotic margins.

IV Musculoskeletal System

Spine

Cervical (C) spine injuries are caused by hyperflexion (e.g., anterior wedge or compression fracture, teardrop fracture, anterior subluxation, and bilateral jumped facets with anterior subluxation of the superior vertebra), hyperextension (e.g., avulsion anteroinferior corner of a vertebral body, typically at C2, or C3, and hangman's fracture), hyperrotation (e.g., rotary atlantoaxial subluxation), hyperflexion and rotation (e.g., unilateral jumped facet), lateral hyperflexion (e.g., unilateral pillar fracture), and vertical compression (e.g., Jefferson fracture and burst fractures C3–C7). Differentiation between stable and unstable cervical spine injuries is of utmost importance (**Table 15.5**).

Occipital condyle fractures were classified into three types by Anderson and Montesano. Type 1 is an impacted comminuted condylar fracture with minimal displacement secondary to axial loading. It is usually stable. Type 2 injuries are potentially unstable injuries caused by a shear mechanism that results in an oblique fracture extending from the condyle into the skull base. Type 3 fractures are unstable avulsion injuries secondary to rotation and lateral bending, presenting with a transverse fracture line through the occipital condyle (**Fig. 15.78**). Any occipital condylar fracture associated with craniocervical dissociation is unstable.

Craniocervical dissociation is considered unstable with translation or distraction > 2 mm in any plane. *Occipitocervical dislocations* can be classified according to the direction of displacement of the occiput with regard to C1 in anterior (type 1), vertical (distraction, type 2), and posterior (type 3) plane. The degree of instability may be underestimated with CT, as spontaneous reduction occurs, and the vast majority of lesions are ligamentous involving the three main craniocervical stabilizers, that is, the alar ligaments (occipital condyles to dens), the tectorial membrane (clivus to C2 portion of the posterior longitudinal ligament), and the transverse ligament crossing behind the dens between the lateral masses of the atlas. MRI is the imaging modality of choice for these injuries.

Fractures of the atlas (C1) may be classified into (1) stable posterior arch fractures caused by hyperextension; (2) isolated anterior arch fractures ranging from minimally displaced to comminuted, which may be unstable; (3) unilateral comminuted

Table 15.5 Stability assessment of cervical spine injuries
Stable injuries:
Fracture of posterior arch of C1
Rotary subluxation C1–C2
Odontoid fracture (type 1)
Extension teardrop fracture
Compression fracture (anterior two thirds of vertebral body)
Laminar fracture
Transverse process fracture
Spinous process fracture (including clay shoveler's fracture)
Unilateral perched or locked facet
Subluxation (≤ 2 mm)
Stable or unstable injuries:
Occipital condyle fracture
C1 anterior arch or lateral mass fractures
Atlantoaxial subluxation
Odontoid fracture (type 3)
Facet and pillar fractures
Subluxation (3 and 4 mm)
Unstable injuries:
Jefferson fracture
Odontoid fracture (type 2)
Hangman's fracture
Flexion teardrop fracture
Hyperextension fracture-dislocation
Burst fracture (C3–C7)
Occipitocervical subluxation (> 2 mm)
Bilateral jumped (perched or locked) facets
Subluxation (≥ 5 mm)
Dislocation

or lateral mass fractures caused by rotation or lateral flexion forces, which are frequently unstable; and (4) burst (Jefferson) fractures, which are unstable. In the Jefferson fracture (**Fig. 15.79**), the axial load resulting from a blow to the vertex of the head drives the lateral masses outward, resulting in bilateral symmetrical fractures of the anterior and posterior arches of C1, which are invariably associated with disruption of the transverse ligament.

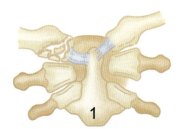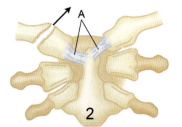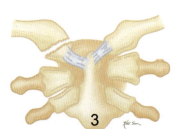

Fig. 15.78 Anderson and Montesano classification of occipital condyle fractures. Type 1: Comminuted impaction fractures, usually stable. Type 2: Shear fractures (occasionally impaction fractures) extending into the base of the skull (arrow), usually unstable. Type 3: Alar ligament avulsion fracture secondary to distraction, usually unstable.
A alar ligaments

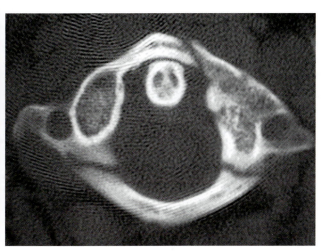

Fig. 15.79 Jefferson fracture (burst fracture of C1). Left anterior and bilateral posterior arch fractures are seen.

Atlantoaxial subluxations may be rotational or transitional and are frequently nontraumatic (e.g., rheumatoid arthritis and Down syndrome [trisomy 21]). Rotational injuries range from mild subluxation to complete dislocation of the atlantoaxial lateral masses. Anterior C1–C2 subluxation is diagnosed when the distance between the anterior arch of C1 and the dens measures 3 mm or more in adults and 5 mm or more in children. Distraction atlantoaxial injuries are considered to be a variant of craniocervical dissociation. A distraction injury in either the occiput–C1 or C1–C2 joint is present when the vertical separation is > 2 mm. At times cranial traction is required for the proper diagnosis.

Injuries to the axis (C2) include fractures of the odontoid process (dens) and traumatic spondylolisthesis of C2 (hangman's fracture). *Dens fractures* are classified based on the anatomical location of the fracture line (**Fig. 15.80**). Type 1 is an oblique fracture near the tip of the dens representing an avulsion at the insertion of the alar ligament. This fracture must be differentiated from an unfused ossification center at the tip of the dens (ossiculum terminale of Bergman), typically separated from the dens by a transverse lucent line. Type 2 injuries are unstable transverse fractures through the base of the dens and carry a high risk of nonunion. An unfused dens (os odontoideum) characteristically has a rounded inferior border with a smooth, thin

cortical margin. Nonunion of a dens fracture may present in a similar fashion. Type 3 fractures extend from the base of the dens into the vertebral body and have a wider fracture surface (**Fig. 15.80**). These fractures tend to be stable but are not invariably so. Hangman's fractures (**Fig. 15.81**) occur most commonly in motor vehicle accidents, when the face strikes the windshield, forcing the neck into hyperextension. Type 1 injury is a nondisplaced fracture through the pedicles (interarticular pars) of C2 extending between the superior and inferior facets. Type 2 fracture is a displaced interarticular pars fracture without (2A) or with (2B) disruption of the discoligamentous complex at C2–C3. Type 3 injury is a type 2 fracture with dislocation of the C2–C3 facet joints (**Fig. 15.82**).

Subaxial (middle and lower cervical spine) injuries are classified based on injury mechanism, anatomical location, or a combination thereof. There are four basic types of injury mechanism in the subaxial spine: hyperflexion, compression, hyperextension, and lateral hyperflexion. Depending on the severity of the trauma, stable and unstable injuries occur with each of the four aforementioned injury mechanisms. Combination injury patterns, such as compression (axial loading) with either hyperflexion or hyperextension, however, are common. Hyperflexion injuries are typically associated with some degree of compression in the anterior column (anterior aspect of the vertebrae) and some degree of distraction in the posterior column, whereas the opposite applies for hyperextension injuries. Anterior or posterior translation may further complicate these injury patterns.

In the subaxial cervical spine, stable hyperflexion injuries include compression (anterior wedge) fractures and clay shoveler's fractures, predominantly unstable injuries, such as subluxations and dislocations of the facet joints, and highly unstable injuries, such as teardrop fractures (**Fig. 15.83**). In a compression (anterior wedge) fracture, there is anterior compression of the vertebral body, and although the posterior ligament complex is stretched, it remains intact (**Fig. 15.84a**). The highly unstable flexion teardrop fracture in the middle and lower C spine most commonly involves C5. The vertebral body is split into a smaller anteroinferior teardrop fragment and a larger posterior fragment that is displaced posteriorly into the spinal canal. The anterior and posterior longitudinal ligaments, ligamentum flavum, and interspinous ligaments are all disrupted, resulting in widening of the facet joints ("facet gapping"), and fractures of the posterior elements, most frequently of the spinous process, are associated (**Fig. 15.84b**).

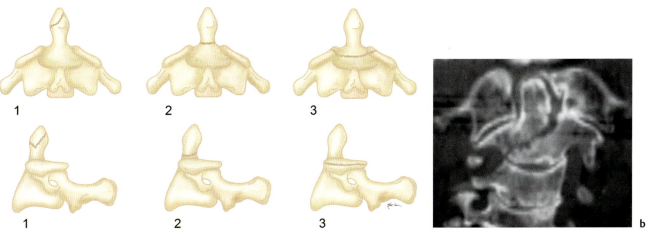

Fig. 15.80a, b Classification of dens fractures (Anderson and D'Alonzo). Type 1: Usually oblique fracture of the upper part of the dens (alar ligament avulsion fracture), stable. Type 2: Transverse fracture through the base of the dens above body and lateral masses of C2, unstable. Type 3: Fracture extending below the base of the dens into the body and lateral masses of C2, usually stable. (**b**) A fracture extending from the base of the dens into the vertebral body is seen.

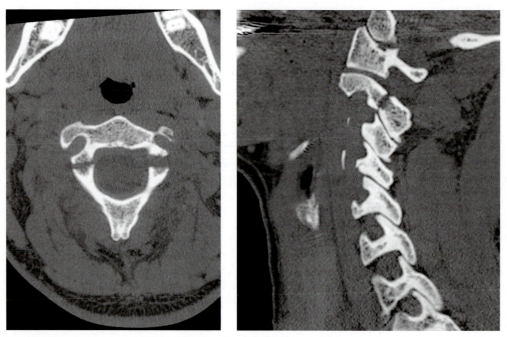

Fig. 15.81a, b   Hangman's fracture. Axial (**a**) and sagittal (**b**) views of a bilateral interarticular pars fracture of C2.

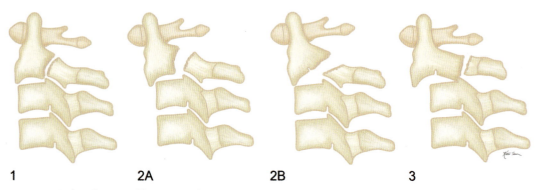

1   **2A**   **2B**   **3**

Fig. 15.82   Classification of hangman's fractures (C2–arch fractures or traumatic spondylolisthesis of C2). Type 1: Nondisplaced fractures through the pedicles of C2 extending between the superior and inferior facets. Type 2: Displaced fractures through the pedicles of C2 extending between the superior and inferior facets. 2A: Without disruption of the discoligamentous complex at C2–C3. 2B: With disruption of the discoligamentous complex at C2–C3 evident by a widened C2–C3 disk space posteriorly and anterior angulation of C2 against C3. Anterior subluxation of C2 is usually minimal. Type 3: Bilateral arch fractures of C2 with dislocation of the C2–C3 facet joints (jumped facets).

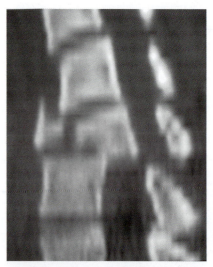

Fig. 15.83   Flexion teardrop fracture. The vertebral body of C5 is split into a smaller anteroinferior teardrop fragment and a larger posterior fragment that is displaced posteriorly into the spinal canal.

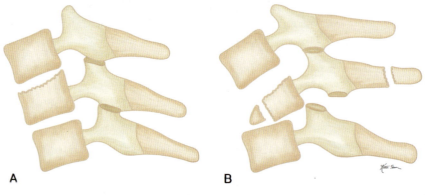

A   **B**

Fig. 15.84a, b   Hyperflexion injuries. (**a**) Compression (anterior wedge) fracture: anterior wedging with compression of the superior end plate. Stable. (**b**) Teardrop fracture: smaller anteroinferior teardrop fragment and larger posterior fragment that is displaced posteriorly into the spinal canal. The anterior and posterior longitudinal ligaments, ligamentum flavum, and interspinous ligaments are all torn, resulting in widening of the facet joints ("facet gapping") and widened interspinous distance. Fractures of the posterior elements, most frequently of the spinous process, are commonly associated. Highly unstable.

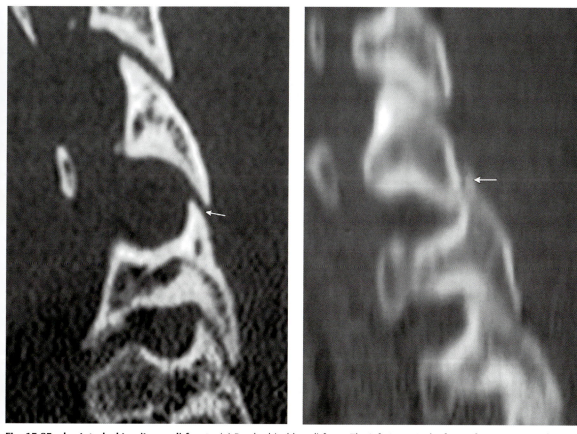

b

Fig. 15.85a, b   Interlocking (jumped) facets. (a) Perched (subluxed) facet. The inferior articular facet of C4 is positioned on top of the superior facet of C5 (arrow). **(b)** Locked facet. The inferior articular facet of C5 is positioned anterior of the superior facet of C6 (arrow).

Subluxed (perched) and dislocated (locked) facet joints are unilateral or bilateral hyperflexion (distraction) injuries with tearing of the corresponding joint capsules and ligamentous complex (**Fig. 15.85**). An isolated hyperflexion sprain evident by widening of both the interspinous distance and the posterior aspect of the facet joints can be considered the mildest form of a posterior column distraction injury. In bilateral interlocking (jumped) facets, the inferior articular facets of the upper vertebra are positioned either on top (perched facets) or in front (locked facets) of the superior facets of the lower vertebra

(**Fig. 15.86**). This condition is associated with anterior subluxation of the involved upper vertebra and extensive injuries of all spinous ligaments at that level. In a unilateral locked facet, a rotational force component is also present besides the hyperflexion. In the absence of disk space widening or anterior subluxation, this injury is considered mechanically stable. A clay shoveler's fracture is an oblique or vertical avulsion fracture of the spinous process of C6 or C7 (less commonly, T1 to T3) caused by a sudden load on the flexed spine. Occasionally, more than one spinous process is involved.

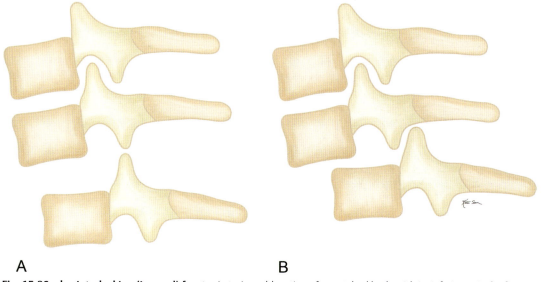

A   B

Fig. 15.86a, b   Interlocking (jumped) facets. Anterior subluxation of a vertebral body with its inferior articular facets either on top (**a**, perched facets) or in front (**b**, locked facets) of the superior facets of the lower vertebra.

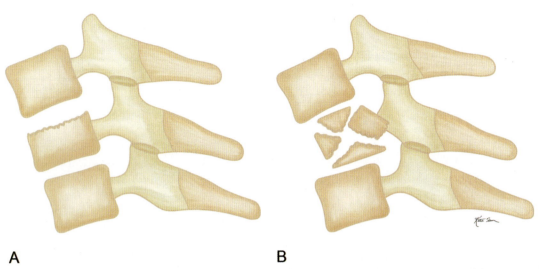

A   **B**

Fig. 15.87a, b   Axial loading (vertical compression) injuries. (a) Compression fracture: compression of the superior plate with mild anterior wedging. Stable. **(b)** Burst fracture: comminuted fracture of the vertebral body with height loss and retropulsion, preferentially the posterosuperior aspect of the fractured vertebral body. Unstable.

Compression (axial loading) injuries in the subaxial cervical spine vary from stable compression fracture to unstable burst fractures (**Fig. 15.87**). Compression fractures resulting from axial loading are similar in appearance to compression (anterior wedge) fractures secondary to hyperflexion, although the latter may demonstrate more anterior wedging. Burst fractures characteristically demonstrate extensive vertebral body comminution, varying degrees of height loss, and, most importantly, posterior vertebral involvement with retropulsion, preferentially of the posterosuperior aspect of the fractured vertebral body.

Hyperextension injuries in the middle and lower C spine result in distraction injuries in the anterior column and compression fractures of the posterior elements (**Fig. 15.88**). They occur most commonly during motor vehicle accidents involving rear-end collisions (whiplash injuries). An extension teardrop fracture (**Fig. 15.89**) is a stable avulsion fracture arising from the anteroinferior corner of a vertebral body and is typically located in the upper C spine (e.g., C2 and C3). The vertical height of this teardrop fracture fragment usually exceeds its horizontal dimension. No other fracture or subluxation is associated with this injury. Hyperextension fracture-dislocation injuries may be highly unstable injuries despite the fact that they may produce only very subtle bony abnormalities. These injuries with torn anterior longitudinal ligaments may present with an anteriorly widened disk space and small avulsion fractures at the insertion site of the anulus fibrosus. Retrolisthesis of the vertebra above the discal injury is

frequently also present, but it may be only minimal. Other manifestations include unilateral or bilateral arch fractures (pedicle, facet, and lamina), which may be associated with varying degrees of anterolisthesis. Involvement may be at multiple levels.

Lateral hyperflexion injuries occur by compression of one side of the spine. With further energy, the contralateral side may fail under tension. The most common fracture produced is unilateral wedging of the vertebral body and its associated lateral mass. Fractures of the arch similar to those occurring in hyperextension injuries are also present in the majority of cases that may result in lateral translation of the fracture fragments (floating lateral mass).

Fractures in the thoracolumbar spine can be classified based on the injury mechanism in compression fractures, burst fractures, Chance fractures (distraction fractures or seat-belt injuries), and fracture-dislocations. To assess fracture stability, Denis introduced the concept of the three columns in the thoracolumbar spine (**Fig. 15.90**). The anterior column comprises the anterior two-thirds of both the vertebral body and the disk and the anterior longitudinal ligament. The middle column consists of the posterior third of both the vertebral body and the disk, the posterior longitudinal and the pedicles. The posterior column includes the posterior portion of the neural arch (lamina) with all its appendices (transverse process, superior and inferior articular process, and spinous process) and the ligamentum flavum, the supraspinous and interspinous ligaments, and the capsule of the facet joints. It is the opinion of the author of this chapter, how-

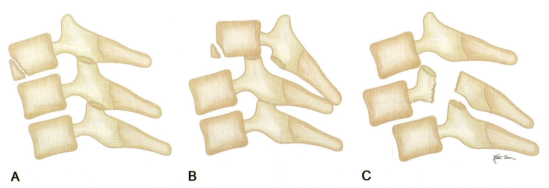

A   **B**   **C**

Fig. 15.88a–c   Hyperextension injuries. (a) Extension teardrop fracture: Stable avulsion fracture arising from the anteroinferior corner of a vertebral body, commonly C2 or C3. **(b)** Unstable extension distraction injury: Anteriorly widened disk space with small avulsion fracture at the anteroinferior corner (insertion of anulus fibrosus) and posterior subluxation of the vertebra above the discal injury. **(c)** Unstable extension compression injury: neural arch fractures (facet, pedicle, or lamina) with anterolisthesis, involvement frequently at multiple levels.

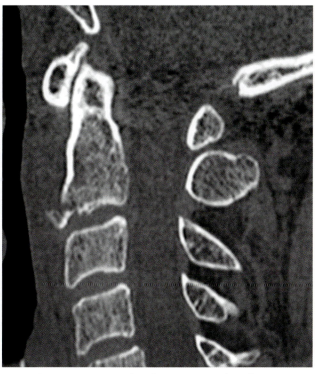

Fig. 15.89 Extension teardrop fracture. An avulsion fracture arising from the anteroinferior corner of C2 is seen.

Table 15.6 Column involvement of thoracolumbar spine fractures			
Type of Fracture	**Column Involvement**		
	Anterior	**Middle**	**Posterior**
Compression	Compression	None or compression (in severe cases)	None or distraction (in severe cases)
Burst	Compression	Compression	None or compression
Chance	None or compression	Distraction	Distraction
Fracture-dislocation	Shear, compression, rotation	Shear, distraction, rotation	Shear, distraction, rotation

ever, that reducing the middle column from the posterior third of the vertebral body to its posterior cortex is more appropriate for the differentiation between stable and unstable injuries. Any fracture involving the middle column defined in this way must be considered unstable, as an isolated fracture involvement of the middle column is not possible. In the original three-column classification system, one-column fractures are considered stable and three-column fractures unstable, whereas two-column fractures may be stable or unstable (**Table 15.6**).

Compression fractures (**Fig. 15.91**) occur from anterior or, less commonly, lateral flexion with axial loading. Typically, the compression fracture is a stable injury with involvement limited to the anterior column. Buckling of the cortex near the upper end plate (rarely the lower end plate or both end plates) or an arc of

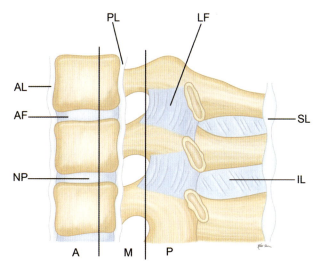

Fig. 15.90 Three-column concept of Denis. Method is used to assess the stability of thoracolumbar spinal injuries. **A:** Anterior column consisting of the anterior two thirds of the vertebral body and disk and the anterior longitudinal ligament. **M:** Middle column consisting of the posterior third of the vertebral body and disk, as well as the posterior longitudinal ligament and pedicles. **P:** Posterior column, consisting of the posterior portion of the neural arch (lamina) with all its appendices (transverse process, superior and inferior articular process, and spinous process) and the posterior ligament complex, including the ligamentum flavum, the supraspinous and interspinous ligaments, and the capsule of the facet joints. One-column fractures are stable, two-column fractures stable or unstable, and three-column fractures unstable.

A	anterior column	**M**	middle column
AF	anulus fibrosus	**NP**	nucleus pulposus
AL	anterior longitudinal ligament	**P**	posterior column
IL	interspinous ligament	**PL**	posterior longitudinal ligament
LF	ligamentum flavum	**SL**	supraspinous ligament

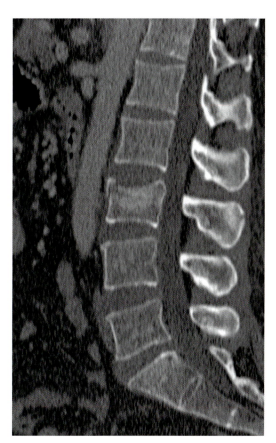

Fig. 15.91 Compression fracture. An L3 fracture is visible with compression of its superior end plate and detachment of the anterosuperior corner of the vertebra.

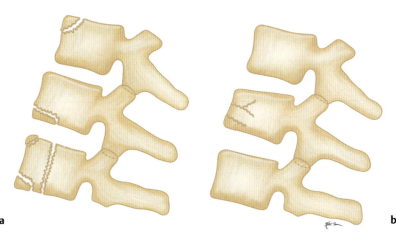

a

b

Fig. 15.92a, b   Compression fractures resulting from anterior flexion (anterior wedge fractures). (**a**) Buckling of the cortex near the superior end plate (**top**), inferior end plate (**center**), or both end plates (**bottom**). A vertical fracture of the vertebral body may be associated. (**b**) Compression (anterior wedge) fracture of the anterior aspect of the vertebral body. All four fractures are considered stable, as they are confined to the anterior column. In severe cases, the fractures may extend to the middle column, and partial failure of the posterior column due to distraction may be associated.

irregular bony fragments displaced circumferentially around the vertebral body may be the only finding. However, a loss of height of the anterior vertebral body ranging from minimal to < 50% is the typical presentation. Preferential involvement is the superior aspect of the vertebral body (**Fig. 15.92**). Severe compression fractures may extend into the middle column, and distraction injuries in the posterior ligamentous complex may be associated, resulting in unstable compression fractures. The most common site of involvement is the lower thoracic and upper lumbar spine, in order of frequency affecting L1, L2, T12, T7, and L3.

All *burst fractures* (**Fig. 15.93**) should be considered unstable, although this assessment is not unanimously shared in the orthopedic literature. They result from axial loading that may be associated with flexion. The thoracolumbar junction with T12, L1, and L2 is the most common site of involvement. The burst

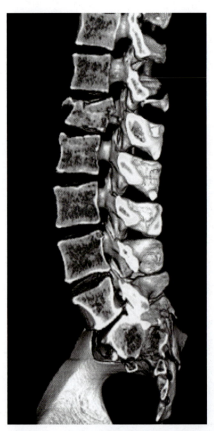

Fig. 15.93   Burst fracture. Compression of the superior end plate with retropulsion of the posterosuperior fracture fragment into the spinal canal is evident at L1. Minimal retrolisthesis of L1 is also present. Mild compression of the superior end plate of L2 and a fracture of the spinous process of T12 are also seen.

fracture is a comminuted fracture with centrifugal fragment displacement, resulting in an increased vertebral body diameter (especially in the sagittal plane), increased interpedicular distance, and splaying of the facet joints. The anterior vertebral wedging is similar to a compression fracture, but the burst fracture differs from the latter by the characteristic retropulsion of the posterosuperior corner of the fractured vertebral body into the spinal canal. Posterior column fractures may be associated with burst fractures and include vertical fractures of one or both laminae and the spinous process (**Fig. 15.94**).

Chance fractures (distraction fractures, seat-belt injuries) are hyperflexion injuries subjecting the posterior and middle vertebral columns, or all three columns, to distraction forces (**Fig. 15.95**). Such injuries occur most frequently at the thoracolumbar junction, particularly at L1 or L2. They rarely occur through bone alone and are most commonly the result of osseous and ligamentous failure beginning posteriorly and propagating anteriorly. The imaging findings depend on whether the injury is predominantly osseous or ligamentous. Horizontal fractures originating in the spinous process or lamina with or without involvement of the transverse processes, extending through the pedicles into the vertebral body without significant damage to ligamentous structures, is a typical presentation of a primarily osseous manifestation. Its constant feature is transverse fracture without dislocation or subluxation. Occasionally, there is also mild compression of the anterior aspect of the vertebral body. A primarily soft tissue injury presents with disruption of the posterior ligamentous complex, resulting in interspinous widening and increased height of the intervertebral foramina; widening, superior subluxation, perching, or locking of the facet joints may be evident. With disruption of the posterior fibers of the anulus fibrosus, widening of the posterior portion of the disk space may be apparent. In a two-level injury, distraction of the posterior ligamentous complex occurs at one level, while the disk involvement affects the next level farther down (**Fig. 15.96**).

Fracture-dislocations of the thoracolumbar spine are highly unstable injuries involving all three columns (**Fig. 15.97**). Transitional deformity, which can occur in the sagittal and/or coronal planes, is the hallmark of this injury. This intervertebral subluxation or dislocation is typically not associated with loss of height of a vertebral body. The spinal distribution of the injury is bimodal, with one peak at the T6–T7 level and the second peak at the thoracolumbar junction. Fracture-dislocations result from various forces, including shear, rotation, and distraction (**Fig. 15.98**). In shear injuries, anterior, posterior, and/or lateral subluxation/dislocation of the spine is associated with severely comminuted fractures in the posterior column, including the facet joints, transverse and spinous processes, and laminae, which may be free-floating. Rotational injuries

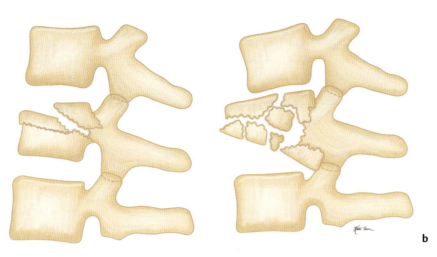

Fig. 15.94a, b   Burst fractures. (a) Compression of the superior end plate with retropulsion of a fracture fragment posterosuperiorly into the spinal canal is characteristic. A coronal image will show widening of the interpedicular distance and splaying of the facet joints. A similar fracture involving the inferior end plate is much less common. **(b)** Highly comminuted burst fracture with involvement of both end plates and retropulsion of more than one fracture fragment. These fractures are considered unstable. Posterior column fractures (e.g., lamina and spinous process) are frequently associated.

b

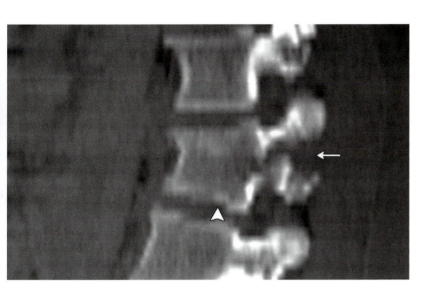

Fig. 15.95   Chance fracture. A horizontal fracture with splitting of the posterior elements of L2 (arrow) extends through the pedicle into the vertebral body and exits in the inferior end plate (arrowhead). Mild compression of the anterosuperior end plate of L2 is also evident.

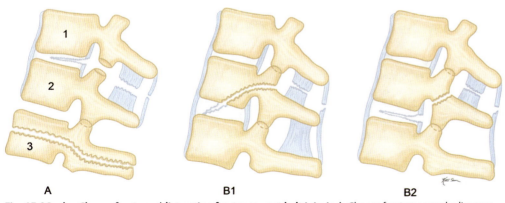

A   B1   B2

Fig. 15.96a, b   Chance fractures (distraction fractures, seat-belt injuries). Chance fractures may be ligamentous, osseous, or a combination of both, and one- or two-level injuries are discerned. **(A)** One-level injury. **1** and **2:** Rupture of all ligaments of the posterior column and the posterior longitudinal ligament of the middle column with extension into the disk. **3:** Horizontal splitting of a vertebral body without ligament disruption (true Chance fracture). **(B)** Two-level injury. **B1:** Rupture of all ligaments of the posterior column with a transverse fracture of the vertebral arch and body with extension into the disk one level below the ligamentous involvement in the posterior column. **B2:** Rupture of all ligaments of the posterior column, fracture of the vertebral arch, and rupture of the posterior longitudinal ligament and disk on the next lower level. All seat-belt injuries are unstable. They are not associated with anterior or posterior translation. Differential diagnosis: Fracture-dislocations (see **Fig. 15.51**).

are associated with a slice fracture of the vertebral body, multiple rib and/or transverse process fractures, dislocations of the costotransverse joints, usually unilateral displaced fractures of the articular facets, and rotary malalignment of two vertebrae located above and below the injury. The rotational slice fracture is a horizontal fracture involving the superior end plate. This fragment is displaced as a unit together with the adjacent intervertebral disk and upper vertebra pivoting relative to the caudal vertebra below the slice fracture. A fracture-dislocation of the distraction type differs from a Chance fracture (seatbelt injury) by the fact that the entire disk is torn, allowing the vertebra above to translate on the vertebra below. A traumatic spondylolisthesis can be considered a manifestation of a fracture-dislocation injury, but it is rare when compared with other nontraumatic conditions, such as degenerative changes in the disk and facet joints and chronic defects of the pars interarticularis (spondylolysis). These conditions are dealt with in greater detail in the spine section.

Isolated transverse process fractures in the lumbar spine result from lateral hyperflexion injuries or, less commonly, from a direct blow. They may be multiple, most commonly involve the levels of L3 and L4, and are stable. L5 transverse process fractures are frequently associated with unstable pelvic fractures.

Traumatic fractures of the spine have to be differentiated from subacute or chronic compression fractures associated with osteopenia (insufficiency fractures). These fractures are frequently located in the midthoracic spine, whereas traumatic fractures are preferentially located in the thoracolumbar region. A narrow zone of increased density below the fractured end plate, produced by impacted trabeculae and/or attempted fracture healing, is commonly present in compression fractures associated with osteoporosis (**Fig. 15.99**).

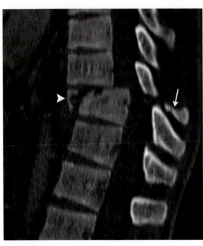

Fig. 15.97 Fracture-dislocation. Anterolisthesis of the intact vertebral body of T12 with fractured posterior elements (arrow) against the anteriorly compressed L1 is seen. Note that the anterosuperior fracture fragment of L1 (arrowhead) is perfectly aligned with the anterior end plate of T12 indicating that the disk between T12 and L1 is intact anteriorly.

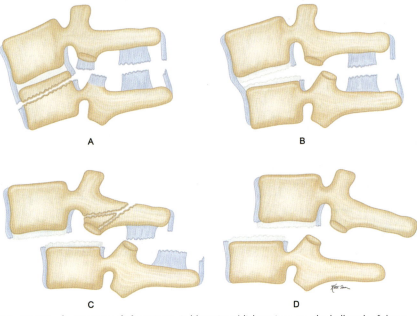

A

B

C

D

Fig. 15.98a–d Fracture-dislocations. Subluxations/dislocations are the hallmark of these injuries which may be purely ligamentous. (**A**) Flexion-rotation injury. The rotational slice fracture involving the superior end plate is characteristic. This fragment is displaced as a unit together with the adjacent disk and upper vertebra pivoting relative to the caudal vertebra below the slice fracture. Fracture of the superior articular process of the same vertebra and rupture of the ligaments of the posterior column, as well as both the anterior and posterior longitudinal ligament, are also present. (**B**) Flexion-distraction injury. Disruption of all spinal ligaments except the anterior longitudinal ligament and complete rupture of the disk with anterolisthesis and dislocations of the facet joints are evident. Differential diagnosis: Ligamentous one-level seat-belt injury, where there is an incomplete disk rupture without anterolisthesis. (**C,D**) Shear injuries. Traumatic anterolisthesis (**C**) and posterolisthesis (**D**) with disruption of all spinous ligaments and dislocations of the facet joints. Multiple fractures in the posterior column including lamina, articular facets, and spinous process are commonly associated with traumatic anterolisthesis. All fracture-dislocation injuries are highly unstable.

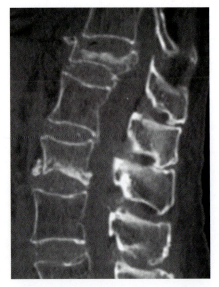

Fig. 15.99 Insufficiency compression fractures. A zone of increased density below the fractured superior end plate of T12 and above the fractured inferior end plate of L2 is suggestive of nontraumatic compression fractures associated with osteoporosis.

Nonacute Trauma

Osteochondritis dissecans appears to be caused in a great majority, if not all cases, by stress, usually of a chronic nature. The knee is the most common site of involvement, with preferential involvement of the medial femoral condyle, followed by the lateral femoral condyle and patella. The disease has also been observed in the distal tibia (tibia plafond), the talar dome, the capitulum of the humerus, and the heads of the femur, humerus, and metatarsals, especially the first (**Fig. 15.100**). The bony fragment may still be located in the corresponding defect of the articular surface or may have become completely separated from the latter and form a loose intra-articular body. The differential diagnosis of loose intra-articular bodies is shown in **Table 15.7**.

Stress fractures can be subdivided into fatigue fractures and insufficiency fractures. *Fatigue fractures* occur in normal bones with the application of an abnormal stress or torque caused by

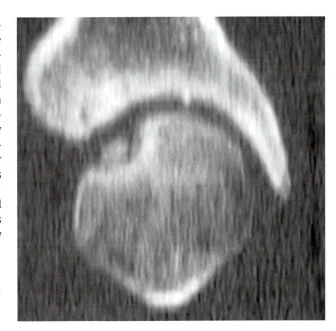

Fig. 15.100 Osteochondritis dissecans. The bony fragment is seen in the corresponding defect with sclerotic margin of the articular surface of the femoral head.

IV Musculoskeletal System

Table 15.7 Differential diagnosis of loose intra-articular bodies

Disease	Preferred Location	Number of Loose Bodies	Other Imaging Findings	Comments
Osteochondritis dissecans	Knee, ankle, capitulum humeri	One	Defect (pit) in articular surface at the site of origin	Preponderant in young men
Synovial chondromatosis/osteochondromatosis (juvenile or idiopathic)	Large joints, bursae	Multiple (often > 10), relatively uniform in size, one third not calcified	Joint effusion common	Preponderant in young to middle-aged men. Hypertrophic cartilaginous synovial growths that may become detached, calcified, and eventually ossified
Trauma (chondral and osteochondral fractures)	None	One or more, not always calcified	Evidence of trauma	Secondary to bone and/or cartilage fractures (articular surface, meniscus)
Septic or tuberculous arthritis	None	One or more	Evidence of joint destruction and deformity	Rare. Characteristic clinical history
Degenerative joint disease	Weight-bearing joints	One or more detached spurs	Osteophytosis, sclerosis, subchondral cysts, and joint space narrowing	Usually in elderly patients; synovial (osteo)chondrometaplasia may ensue that is indistinguishable from juvenile (osteo)chondromatosis
CPDD arthropathy	Large joints of upper and lower extremities	One or more	Similar to degenerative joint disease, but more destructive and progressive. Chondrocalcinosis and subchondral cyst formation are common and often prominent	Middle-aged and elderly patients
Avascular necrosis	Hip, knee, shoulder	One or more	Advanced stage with flattened or collapsed articular surface	Bone infarcts may also be present. May simulate osteochondritis dissecans in the knee, but is often bicondylar or bilateral
Neuropathic arthropathy (hypertrophic form)	Weight-bearing joints	Multiple, varying size	Marked sclerosis, disintegration of articular surfaces and subluxation	Loss of pain sensation (diabetes, syphilis [Charcot joint], and other neurologic disorders)

Table 15.8   Stress fractures (see Fig. 15.101)

Location	Activity
1. Lower cervical or upper thoracic spinous process	Shoveling
2. Clavicle	Postoperative (radical neck dissection)
3. Coracoid process of scapula	Trap shooting
4. Ribs	Carrying heavy pack (first rib), golf, coughing
5. Humerus: distal shaft	Throwing a ball
6. Ulna: coronoid process, shaft	Pitching a ball, throwing a javelin, pitchfork work, propelling wheelchair
7. Hook of hamate	Holding golf club, tennis racket, baseball bat
8. Lumbar vertebra: pars interarticularis (spondylolysis)	Ballet, lifting heavy objects, scrubbing floors
9. Femur: neck or shaft	Ballet, marching, running, gymnastics
10. Pelvis: obturator ring	Stooping, bowling, gymnastics
11. Patella	Hurdling
12. Tibia	Running (proximal shaft in children, mid- and distal shaft in adults)
13. Fibula: proximal or distal shaft	Jumping, parachuting, running
14. Calcaneus	Jumping, parachuting, prolonged standing, recent immobilization
15. Navicular	Stamping on ground, marching, running
16. Metatarsals	Marching, stamping on ground, prolonged standing, ballet, postoperative (bunionectomy)
17. Sesamoids of great toe	Prolonged standing, ballet, turf toe

a new strenuous or repeated activity. *Insufficiency fractures* occur when normal stress is placed on an abnormal (osteopenic) bone. Stress fractures are usually symptomatic. They begin as small cortical cracks and may progress to subcortical infraction and eventually a fracture running transversely across the bone. If the fracture line cannot be demonstrated by CT, MRI or a radionuclide examination is always positive and may provide an early diagnosis. MRI has comparable sensitivity and superior specificity to bone scintigraphy in the assessment of stress fractures. Osteomyelitis and bone tumors such as osteoid osteomas can be differentiated from a stress fracture on the basis of both characteristic location and the typical history of stress fractures (**Table 15.8, Fig. 15.101**). At a later stage, periosteal reactions with subsequent localized callus formation and cortical thickening obscuring the fracture line are found in the diaphyses of tubular bones. A healing stress fracture limited to the cortex may present as localized cortical thickening that may at times be difficult to differentiate from an osteoid osteoma or healing cortical abscess. However, in the latter two conditions, a central radiolucency may be evident representing the nidus or the abscess, respectively, whereas in the stress fracture, a transverse fracture line may be visible. In an epiphyseal and metaphyseal location (e.g., tibia plateau) and cancellous bone (e.g., calcaneus), a bandlike focal sclerosis usually without appreciable periosteal reaction is more characteristic.

Osteoporosis and rheumatoid arthritis are the two most common conditions in which *insufficiency fractures* are encountered. Reinforcement lines (bone bars) presenting as well-defined, usually thin sclerotic lines extending partially or completely across the marrow cavity in patients with osteopenia have to be differentiated from poorly defined, bandlike insufficiency fractures. Reinforcement lines can be considered as unmasking of growth arrest lines occurring in childhood, although their pathogenesis is unclear. They are incidental findings without clinical relevance.

Pathologic fractures occur at sites of preexisting abnormalities and are often caused by a minor trauma that would not fracture healthy bone (**Fig. 15.102**). The differential diagnosis between pathologic and nonpathologic fracture can at times be difficult, particularly when the injury occurred several days to weeks

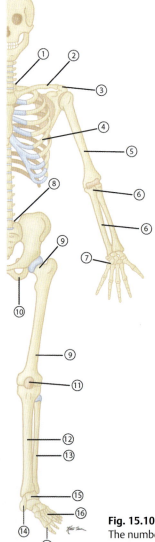

Fig. 15.101   Locations of stress fractures. The numbers in the figure correspond to the numbers in **Table 15.8**.

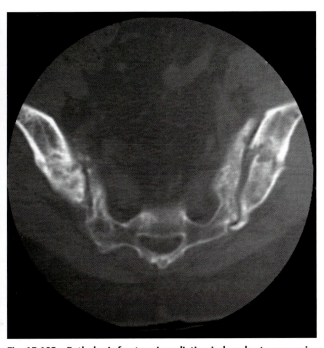

Fig. 15.102 Pathologic fracture in radiation-induced osteonecrosis. Mixed lytic and sclerotic changes are seen in both ilia and adjacent sacral wings several years past irradiation. A frank pathologic fracture is seen in the left iliac wing, with an imminent pathologic fracture evident in the corresponding location of the right iliac wing.

prior to the first imaging examination. In these cases, bone resorption occurring at the site of a nonpathologic fracture may simulate an underlying pathologic lesion and the posttraumatic hematoma a soft tissue extension of the bone lesion. Furthermore, a smaller underlying lytic or sclerotic bone lesion can also be missed by CT, particularly in the presence of displacement at the fracture site. In these cases, the demonstration of other lytic or sclerotic lesions, as well as the absence of a history of trauma or the lack of fracture pain, should suggest the possibility of a pathologic fracture. Pathologic fractures can also occur as early as 5 months after radiation therapy, that is, at a time when the bone does not reveal any radiation-induced changes.

Avulsion fractures at the site of ligament and tendon attachments can be differentiated from accessory ossicles by the lack of a clearly defined cortical margin around the entire bone typical of the latter condition. Furthermore accessory bones have characteristic anatomical locations (**Figs. 15.103, 15.104**). The diagnosis of an avulsion fracture can be further supported by the demonstration of a cortical defect or irregularity in the adjacent bone. Avulsion injuries are caused by either a single violent traumatic event or repetitive injuries. They are particularly common in children, as the physeal cartilage of an apophysis is considerably weaker than tendinous or ligamentous tissue. Several avulsion injuries about the pelvis and hips occur in young athletes, including the anterosuperior or anteroinferior iliac spine, iliac crest, ischial tuberosity, pubic symphysis (adductor muscle insertion sites), and greater or lesser trochanter.

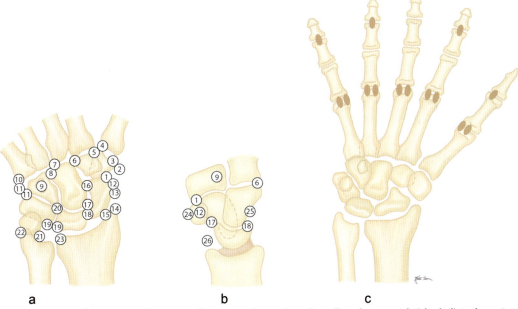

a   b   c

Fig. 15.103a–c Characteristic locations of accessory bones (numbered) and sesamoids (shaded) in the wrist and hand. Anteroposterior (**a,c**) and lateral (**b**) projections of the hand.

1. Epitrapezium
2. Calcification (bursa, flexor carpi radialis)
3. Paratrapezium
4. Trapezium secundarium
5. Trapezoides secundarium
6. Os styloideum (ninth carpal bone or carpe bossu)
7. Ossiculum Gruberi
8. Capitatum secundarium
9. Os hamuli proprium
10. Os vesalianum
11. Os ulnare externum (calcifications in bursa or tendon)
12. Os radiale externum
13. Avulsion of the scaphoid, not an accessory bone
14. Persisting center of ossification of the radial styloid process
15. Accessory bone between scaphoid and radius (paranaviculare)
16. Os centrale carpi
17. Hypolunatum
18. Epilunatum
19. Accessory bone between lunatum and triquetrum
20. Epipyramis
21. Avulsion of the styloid process of the ulna (os triangulare)
22. Persistent nucleus of the styloid process of the ulna
23. Small osseous element in the radioulnar joint
24. Calcification of the pisiform
25. Avulsion of the triquetrum, not an accessory bone
26. Tendon or bursal calcification

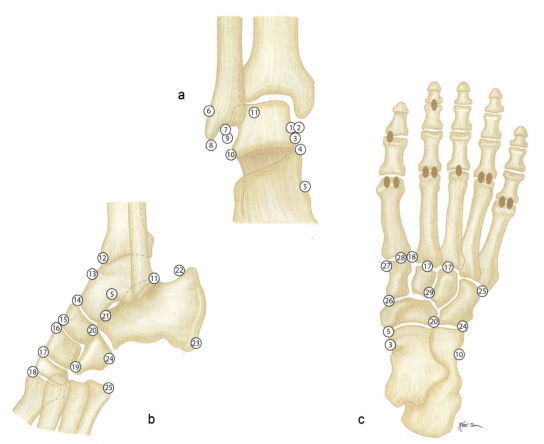

Fig. 15.104a–c   Characteristic locations of accessory bones (numbered) and sesamoids (shaded) in the ankle and foot. (a) Anteroposterior projection of the ankle. **(b)** Lateral projection of the ankle. **(c)** Anteroposterior projection of the foot.

1. Accessory bone (or sesamoid) between the medial malleolus and the talus
2. Os subtibiale
3. Talus accessorius
4. Os sustentaculi
5. Os tibiale externum (os naviculare secondarium)
6. Os retinaculi
7. Accessory ossicle (or sesamoid) between the lateral malleolus and the talus
8. Os subfibulare
9. Talus secundarius
10. Os trochleare calcanei
11. Os trigonum
12. Os talotibiale
13. Os supratalare
14. Os supranaviculare
15. Os infranaviculare
16. Os intercuneiforme
17. Os cuneometatarsale
18. Os intermetatarsale
19. Os unci
20. Secondary cuboid
21. Calcaneus secundarius
22. Os accessorium supracalcaneum
23. Os subcalcis
24. Os peroneum (a sesamoid bone)
25. Os vesalianum
26. Os cuneonaviculare mediale
27. Sesamum tibiale anterius
28. Os cuneometatarsale/plantare
29. Os intercuneiforme

Calcifications and *ossifications* developing in a ligament after acute or repeated low-grade trauma can be impossible to differentiate from an ossicle, as both may be well corticated. A characteristic location (e.g., Pellegrini–Stieda ossification in an old medial collateral ligament injury of the knee) or the patient's history (e.g., "rider's bone" in the adductor muscles of the thigh) may suggest the correct diagnosis.

Heterotopic bone formation in soft tissues following trauma is often termed *posttraumatic myositis ossificans* (**Fig. 15.105**), because it occurs most commonly in muscle but is also found in tendons, ligaments, periosteum, and other connective tissues. It frequently develops after insertion of a joint prosthesis, particularly in the hip, and in paraplegic patients. Occasionally, myositis ossificans can mimic a parosteal sarcoma. It can be distinguished from the latter by the fact that its entire periphery is smoothly marginated by a thin cortex ("eggshell" calcification) and by the demonstration of a fine radiolucent line separating

the lesion in its entire length from the adjacent bone. A central amorphous calcification associated with a soft tissue mass is not consistent with myositis ossificans and suggests a synovial sarcoma or extraosseous osteogenic sarcoma, where it is present in 30% and 50% of cases, respectively.

Excessive callus formation following a fracture may occasionally have a tumorlike appearance. It is found in fractures that have not been properly immobilized. These fractures may not have been diagnosed because of a decreased sensitivity to pain secondary to a neurologic disorder. Because fractures are not immobilized in abused (battered) child syndrome, excessive callus formation is common in that condition too. Excessive callus formation is also associated in both traumatic and insufficiency fractures of patients with elevated steroid blood concentrations (e.g., Cushing syndrome and steroid therapy). Finally, fractures occurring in osteogenesis imperfecta may heal with excessive callus formation.

Fractures extending to the articular surface result in a joint effusion (hemarthrosis). A hematocrit effect may be evident in a hemarthrosis characterized by a fluid level caused by the separation of the serum on top of the cellular components of the blood. The demonstration of a fat–fluid level (lipohemarthrosis) in any joint is presumptive evidence of an intra-articular fracture (**Fig. 15.106**). Pseudofractures (Looser zones, Milkman syndrome) are assumed to be incomplete stress (insufficiency) fractures, presenting radiographically as narrow (2–3 mm) radiolucent bands lying perpendicular to the cortex. At a later stage, sclerosis develops around these lesions, making them more readily detectable. Pseudofractures are present in vitamin D deficiency (osteomalacia and rickets), vitamin D–resistant rickets, hypophosphatasia, renal osteodystrophy, Paget disease, fibrous dysplasia, and hereditary hyperphosphatasia (juvenile

Paget disease) or are rarely idiopathic. They are located in the femur (neck and shaft), pubic and ischial rami, scapula, clavicle, ribs, ulna (proximal shaft), radius (distal shaft), metacarpals, metatarsals, and phalanges.

Nutrient arteries pierce the diaphyses of tubular bones obliquely. Their site of entry and angulation are fairly constant, and, characteristically, the vessels point away from the dominant growing end of the bone (the end with the epiphyseal center in short tubular bones or the end with the later fusing epiphysis in long bones). In the long tubular bones of the upper extremity, they run toward the elbow, whereas in the lower extremity, they run away from the knee ("to the elbow they go, from the knee they flee"). Nutrient arteries may be evident as oblique radiolucent cortical channels that should not be confused with fracture lines.

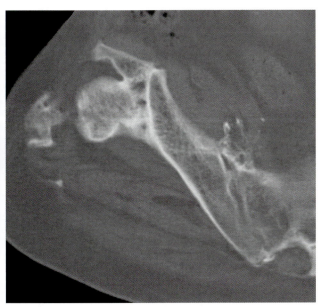

Fig. 15.105 Posttraumatic myositis ossificans. Irregular heterotopic bone formation is seen about an anterior iliac crest fracture.

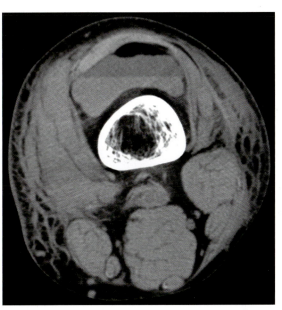

Fig. 15.106 Lipohemarthrosis. A joint effusion in the suprapatellar recess consisting of three layers is visible. The density of the layers from top to bottom increase, representing fat (yellow bone marrow), serum, and cellular components of the blood.

V Thorax

16 Lungs

Christopher Herzog and Francis A. Burgener

Conventional radiographs are the imaging modality of choice for the initial assessment of diseases of the lung or chest. Unfortunately, projection effects and a limited density resolution often restrict their informational value. Computed tomography (CT), particularly high-resolution CT, due to its high-contrast resolution and ability to depict even anatomical structures of submillimeter thickness, is regarded as a highly valuable complementary imaging method in the workup of pathologic processes of the thorax.

With the introduction of multislice CT and an isotropic voxel size of up to 0.4 m³, the image quality of multiplanar reconstructions has finally equaled that of transverse scans; thus, multiplanar assessment has become a standard approach in CT chest imaging. However, most diagnoses can still be made on simple 5-mm transverse slices reconstructed at 5-mm increments and acquired during inspiratory breath hold. A high-resolution CT scan, if needed, typically is done in addition to the 5/5-mm spiral scan, usually as a 1-mm slice thickness/10-mm increment sequence. Though this approach still represents the gold standard, on multislice CT scanners allowing for detector collimations < 1 mm, high-resolution images may alternatively be reconstructed directly from the spiral scan. Thus, the patient is exposed to a lower radiation dose without the two additional scans. However, a second CT scan may still be useful to identify air trapping, for example (i.e., when an additional expiratory scan is needed). In such circumstances, the additional scan may be acquired as a 1-mm slice thickness/10-mm increment sequence. High-resolution CT typically is required in the presence of diffuse lung disease to detect and quantify subtle parenchymal changes and for morphological characterization, respectively.

On CT scans, attenuation values of normal lung parenchyma range from −700 to −900 HU. In the dependent portions of the lung, attenuation values usually are lower (less negative) due to orthostatic effects (i.e., increased blood flow). Because the most dependent portion of the lung on transverse CT images is the dorsal aspect of the lower lobe, this region physiologically often shows an ill-defined, up to 4-cm-thick band of higher attenuation. Likewise, attenuation values decrease (become more negative) when the amount of intrapulmonary air increases. This is observed during labored inspiration but also in several diseases with air trapping (e.g., emphysema).

Bilateral hyperlucency is most often caused by chronic obstructive pulmonary disease (COPD) (**Fig. 16.1**). Other diseases typically associated with emphysema are alpha-1-antitrypsin deficiency, Marfan syndrome, Ehlers–Danlos syndrome, intravenous (IV) drug use, and human immunodeficiency virus (HIV) infection. Attenuation of emphysematous lung parenchyma amounts to values < −950 HU. Primary bullous lung disease (vanishing lung) is an accelerated form of paraseptal emphysema found in young men who usually become symptomatic only if a spontaneous pneumothorax occurs. Pulmonary interstitial emphysema, a complication of enforced respiratory therapy, similarly presents with bilateral hyperlucent lungs, which is often associated with a pneumomediastinum. Revers-

ible conditions of air trapping resulting in bilateral hyperlucency include asthmatic attacks and acute bronchiolitis, especially in children younger than 3 y. Other causes of a bilateral hyperlucent lung are decreased pulmonary blood flow due to thromboembolism (Westermark sign), pulmonary arterial hypertension, and a right-to-left shunt.

A *unilateral or lobular hyperlucency* is most often caused by air trapping due to extrinsic or intrinsic obstruction of a major bronchus. A unilateral hyperlucent lung with decreased lung volume despite air trapping, a small ipsilateral pulmonary hilus, and tubular or varicose bronchiectasis is diagnostic of the Swyer–James or Macleod syndrome. Compensatory emphysema is evident in the remaining lung after lobectomy or due to lobular atelectasis. Other causes of unilateral hyperlucency are one-sided emphysema/thromboembolic disease and rare congenital conditions, such as a hypogenetic lung, absent pulmonary artery (usually right), anomalous origin of the left pulmonary artery, and congenital lobular emphysema (usually upper or middle lobe), as well as scimitar syndrome. The latter is a combination of a hypoplastic hyperlucent right lung, small ipsilateral hilus, right shift of the heart and mediastinum, and a partial anomalous pulmonary venous return resembling a scimitar.

Normal major and minor fissures are usually not visible on CT scans, but their location can be assumed from a 2- to 3-cm-thick band of hyperlucent lung tissue, corresponding to relatively avascular parenchyma on each side of the fissure. Occasionally, a poorly defined ribbonlike zone of increased density is evident in the avascular area adjacent to the fissure, caused by volume averaging of the latter. In high-resolution CT, the fissures are usually visible as pencil-thin white lines.

The pulmonary acinus (**Fig. 16.2**) is defined as the portion of lung distal to a terminal bronchiole and consists of respiratory bronchioles, alveolar ducts, alveolar sacs, and alveoli. The *primary pulmonary lobule* comprises all alveolar ducts, alveolar sacs, and alveoli together with their accompanying blood vessels, nerves, and connective tissues distal to the last respiratory bronchiole. The secondary pulmonary lobule is defined as the smallest discrete portion of lung that is surrounded by a connective tissue septum. It is composed of 3 to 5 terminal bronchioles or 30 to 50 primary lobules. It has an irregular polyhedral shape and ranges from 1 to 2.5 cm in diameter. On high-resolution CT scans, the secondary pulmonary lobule can be identified in both normal and pathologic states. It is surrounded by interlobular septa containing the peripheral tributaries of pulmonary veins and lymphatics. Because of the hydrostatic dilation of the intraseptal veins, the septa are most prominent in the dependent portions of the lung. Subtle changes of the secondary pulmonary lobule are first seen in the subpleural space of dependent lung portions.

Even on high-resolution CT scans terminal bronchioles and accompanying pulmonary arterioles are only rarely evident in healthy individuals. If visible, they appear as small dots or tiny branching structures in the centers of secondary lobules and are often referred to as centrilobular arteries and bronchioles.

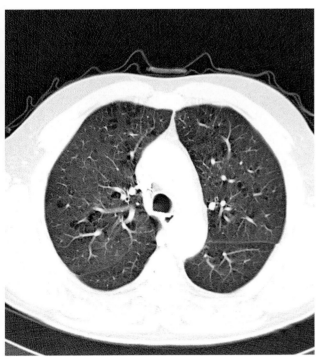

Fig. 16.1 Panlobular emphysema. Bilateral hyperlucent lungs are evident with rarefaction of the peripheral pulmonary structures and relative prominence of central pulmonary vasculature.

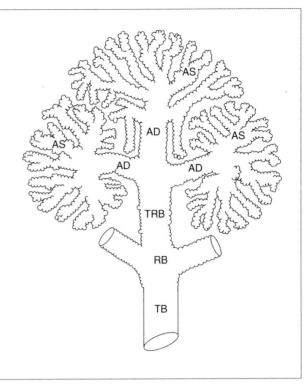

Fig. 16.2 Pulmonary acinus topography. The pulmonary acinus begins at the termination of the terminal bronchiole (TB) and measures ~8 mm at its widest diameter. Alveoli are tiny outpouchings found in the walls of an acinus.
AD alveolar duct
AS alveolar sac
RB respiratory bronchiole
TRB terminal respiratory bronchiole

An increase in lung density occurs when air is replaced by liquid or solid material. A partially hyperdense lung lobule is found in early atelectasis and a completely collapsed lobule in atelectasis. The hallmarks of atelectasis are a loss in lung volume and a displacement of fissures (**Fig. 16.3**). The upper lobes collapse upward, medially, and anteriorly. A totally collapsed right upper lobe may eventually simulate an anterior paramediastinal mass. A right middle lobe collapse appears as a wedge-shaped density, with one side of the wedge abutting the mediastinum. The lower lobes collapse medially and inferiorly, maintaining contact with the posterior mediastinum.

Atelectasis may be divided into obstructive and nonobstructive forms. Obstructive (resorption) atelectasis occurs when the communication between the trachea and the lung periphery is obstructed by either an endobronchial lesion or extrinsic compression. The cause of obstruction is often identified on CT scans. The collapsed airless lung parenchyma distal to the obstruction is of soft tissue density, obliterating normal vascular structures. Bronchi are typically fluid-filled and thus air bronchograms are usually absent.

Nonobstructive atelectasis forms include relaxation, compression, round, adhesive, and cicatrization.

Relaxation (passive) atelectasis is observed in the presence of a pneumothorax or pleural effusion causing retraction of the lung from the chest wall toward the hilum. Compression atelectasis refers to the loss of lung volume adjacent to a large pulmonary or pleural space-occupying lesion.

Round (helical) atelectasis (labeled *R* in **Fig. 16.3**) is caused by contracting pleural fibrosis, resulting in compression and often folding of contiguous lung parenchyma. It is associated primarily with asbestos-related pleural disease and is most commonly located in the posterior portion of a lower lobe. The characteristic CT appearance consists of a rounded subpleural opacity that is densest at its periphery. The bronchovascular bundle entering the lesion appears curvilinear ("comet tail" sign) and often contains

an air bronchogram. Linear bands radiating from the mass into the lung parenchyma are also characteristic ("crow's feet").

In adhesive atelectasis, alveolar collapse occurs in the presence of patent airways and is likely caused by a lack of surfactant. It is found in respiratory distress syndrome of the newborn, acute radiation pneumonitis, and viral pneumonia.

Cicatrization (scar) atelectasis is associated with pulmonary fibrosis that may be localized or generalized. Localized disease is the sequela of chronic infection (e.g., tuberculosis) or inflammation (e.g., radiation). In these conditions, parenchymal fibrosis results not only in atelectasis, but also by traction on airway walls in bronchiectasis. The combination of severe loss of volume associated with extensive air bronchograms in normal or dilated bronchioles is characteristic.

Bronchiectasis (**Fig. 16.4**) is an irreversible bronchial dilation and, depending on the severity of the disease, can be classified into cylindrical, varicose, and cystic forms. Cylindrical (tubular) bronchiectasis is characterized by uniform mild dilation of the bronchi; in varicose bronchiectasis, the bronchial dilation is further increased and alternates with areas of localized constriction; in cystic (saccular) bronchiectasis, the bronchial dilation increases progressively toward the periphery, resulting in cystic spaces measuring up to a few centimeters in diameter.

High-resolution CT is more accurate than CT in the diagnosis of bronchiectasis and has completely replaced bronchography. Cylindrical bronchiectases are recognized on CT as dilated thick-walled bronchi extending toward the lung periphery, whereas normal intraparenchymal bronchi are usually not visualized in the lung periphery. If cut perpendicular to their longitudinal

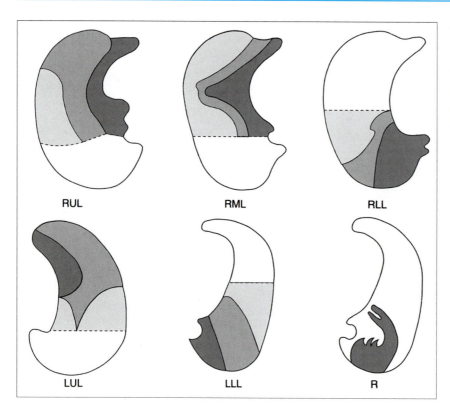

Fig. 16.3 Atelectasis. Patterns of progressive atelectasis pattern are shown for the right upper lobe (RUL), right middle lobe (RML), right lower lobe (RLL), left upper lobe (LUL), and left lower lobe (LLL). The dashed line presents the pertinent interlobular fissure in a normal position. Characteristic features of a round atelectasis (R) include a "comet tail" and "crow's feet."

axis, bronchi appear as ring-shaped bronchiectases accompanied by a much smaller pulmonary artery branch, producing a characteristic "signet ring" sign (**Fig. 16.5**). Bronchiectases may be filled completely with secretions or mucus, evident as large homogeneous tubular structures within the lung periphery. More advanced varicose bronchiectasis assumes a beaded configuration. Cystic bronchiectasis presents as thick-walled cystic spaces measuring up to 2 cm and often grouped together in a cluster. Fluid levels of varying sizes within these cysts are often evident and characteristic.

Acquired bronchiectasis is the late sequela of bronchial wall damage. Diseases that predispose to bronchial wall infection and subsequent bronchiectasis formation include immunologic deficiency states such as agammaglobulinemia, chronic granulomatous disease, and allergic pulmonary aspergillosis.

In children, typical underlying diseases are measles, pertussis, and bronchiolitis obliterans, the latter often resulting in the Swyer–James syndrome. Bronchiectases are also a constant feature in cystic fibrosis and Kartagener syndrome (i.e., dyskinetic endobronchial cilia).

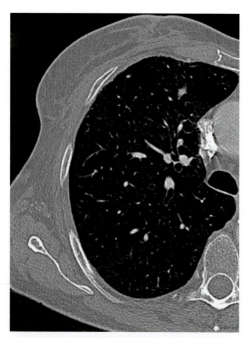

Fig. 16.4 Bronchiectasis. View of cylindriform bronchiectasis (parahilar) in the middle lobe of the right lung.

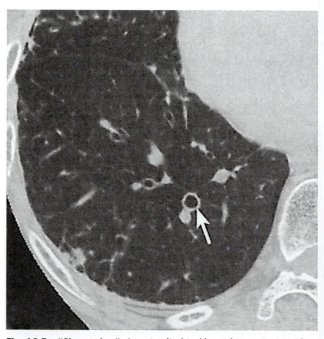

Fig. 16.5 "Signet ring" sign. A cylindrical bronchiectasis viewed end on with the accompanying considerably smaller pulmonary artery branch produces the characteristic "signet ring" sign (arrow).

In adults, bronchiectases are typically associated with chronic aspiration, inhalation of toxic fumes, extrinsic and intrinsic bronchial obstruction (e.g., neoplasms or aspiration of foreign bodies), and emphysema.

Cicatricial (traction) bronchiectases develop as a result of retractile forces of the fibrotic lung on the bronchial wall and are observed in chronic tuberculosis, radiation pneumonitis, and some interstitial diseases such as sarcoidosis. Congenital abnormalities of the bronchial wall such as bronchomalacia are other, though rare, causes of traction bronchiectasis.

Chronic bronchitis is a clinical diagnosis based on excessive mucus production. On high-resolution CT, concentric bronchial wall thickening ("tram lines") without bronchial dilation or the signet ring sign (as characteristic of bronchiectasis) is evident. These findings correspond to prominent lung markings or the "dirty chest" appearance of a lung seen on plain film radiography.

Emphysema (**Fig. 16.6**) is defined as an absolute permanent enlargement of any or all parts of the acinus associated with destruction of alveolar parenchyma but without fibrosis. It is a typical end-stage of COPD, a state of irreversibly obstructed airways without known mechanism, but it is also observed in patients with asthma, bronchiolitis, and alpha-1-antitrypsin deficiency. COPD has a male predominance ($\sim$10:1), and cigarette smoking is a major factor.

Four different types of emphysema are recognized: centrilobular, panlobular or panacinar, paraseptal, and irregular (**Fig. 16.7**).

In centrilobular emphysema, the respiratory bronchioles (the central or proximal portions of the acinus) are destroyed. It is observed primarily in the upper lung lobes and is commonly associated with smoking. CT findings range from scattered punctate dark holes via a moth-eaten pattern to larger areas of destroyed lung. Pulmonary vascular pruning and distortion are evident in more advanced stages.

In panlobular (panacinar) emphysema, the acinus and secondary lobules are uniformly destroyed, leading to a homogeneously distributed diminishment of the interstitium without zonal preference. On CT, widespread areas of low attenuation are characteristic. However, despite some differences in the distribution patterns, it is often impossible to differentiate a panlobular from an advanced centrilobular emphysema. In addition, differentiation between normal and diseased lung often is difficult. Panlobular emphysema is characteristic for alpha-1-antitrypsin deficiency, but it can also be found in smokers.

Paraseptal emphysema selectively involves the alveolar ducts and sacs in the periphery of the acinus or lobules. It is characteristically seen adjacent to the pleura and interlobular

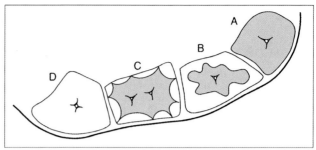

Fig. 16.7 Emphysema pattern. Schematic display of four secondary pulmonary lobules with barely visible centrilobular arteries and bronchioles. Normal secondary pulmonary lobule (A). Centrilobular emphysema (B). The respiratory bronchi (central or proximal portions of the acinus) are destroyed. Paraseptal emphysema; only alveolar ducts and sacs (peripheral portion of the acinus) are destroyed (C). Panlobular (panacinar) emphysema; note that the acinus and secondary lobule are destroyed in full (D).

septa. It may represent an early form of bullous lung disease that may progress to bullous emphysema. Typical findings on CT scans are subpleural emphysematous spaces < 5 mm and larger subpleural bullae, both usually in the vicinity of the mediastinal pleura. Paraseptal emphysema is limited in extent and usually not associated with clinical disease, with the exception of a spontaneous pneumothorax.

Irregular (paracicatricial or scar) emphysema is always associated with localized (e.g., tuberculosis) or generalized pulmonary fibrosis (e.g., sarcoidosis and pneumoconiosis). Clinical abnormalities in this form of emphysema are mainly related to the underlying lung disease.

Bullae are frequently associated with emphysema but may also be found as a localized process in otherwise normal lungs (primary bullous disease). A bulla is defined as an air-filled thin-walled ("hairline") intrapulmonary cavity > 1 cm in diameter.

The pulmonary interstitium is the supporting structure of the lung and can be divided into two compartments: (1) the central or axial interstitial space, consisting of the connective tissue surrounding major airways and pulmonary vessels, and (2) the peripheral interstitial space, including the connective tissue of interlobular septa, as well as around the centrilobular arterioles and bronchioles. From an anatomical point of view, any distinction between the central and peripheral interstitium is arbitrary. However, in high-resolution CT, several interstitial diseases are first seen in the peripheral (subpleural) but not in the central interstitial spaces (**Fig. 16.8**).

A key finding of interstitial lung disease is thickening of interlobular septa (reticular thickening), primarily visible in the peripheral (i.e., subpleural and basal) space. Normal interlobular septa are usually below the spatial resolution of high-resolution CT. Depending on the underlying disease, other typical findings include nodular and nonnodular thickening of interlobular septa, centrilobular nodules, and honeycombing.

Nodular thickening of interlobular septa and peribronchial noduli are commonly associated with interstitial diseases affecting the lymphatics, such as metastatic spread (i.e., lymphangiosis carcinomatosa), sarcoidosis, and silicosis. Nonnodular thickening is more typical of infectious diseases or fibrosis.

Centrilobular noduli may show a bronchocentric or a lymphatic pattern.

A bronchocentric pattern affects the acinus, including all structures distal to the end-terminal bronchiole. It is initiated through inhalation of particles and subsequent mural infection/inflammation. High-resolution CT shows multiple < 5-mm nodules, often Y or V shaped ("tree-in-bud" sign). The peripheral

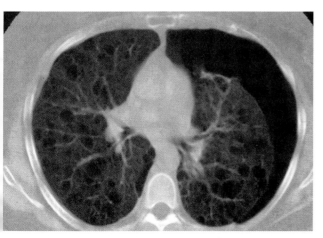

Fig. 16.6 Emphysema. Hyperlucent lungs with numerous black holes (small bullae). Also seen is a concomitant left pneumothorax.

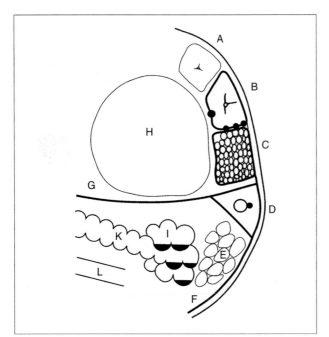

Fig. 16.8 Peripheral interstitial disease pattern. Normal secondary pulmonary lobule (A). Thickening of the interlobular septa, which may be nodular (B); note also the thickening of the centrilobular artery and bronchiole. Honeycombing (C). "Signet ring" sign (D). Also evident are tubular bronchiectasis and the adjacent pulmonary arterial branch cut perpendicular. Thin-walled cystic spaces (E), which may become confluent. Thickened subpleural line (F). Parenchymal bands or scars terminating in interlobular septa at the pleural surface (G). Bulla (H). Cystic bronchiectases (I), commonly with fluid levels. Varicose bronchiectasis (K). Tubular bronchiectasis (L).

subpleural space typically is spared (differential diagnosis to lymphatic pattern). Expiratory scans show mosaic perfusion (thickening of paper-thin bronchioles leading to regional air trapping). Differential diagnoses include respiratory bronchiolitis, viral bronchiolitis, hypersensitivity pneumonitis, coal workers' pneumoconiosis, COPD, and centrilobular emphysema.

The lymphatics form two pulmonary networks: a central network along arteries and airways down to the respiratory bronchioles and a peripheral network along pulmonary veins, interlobular septa, and pleura. In the lymphatic pattern, centrilobular nodules < 5 mm are found in a peribronchiolar, periseptal, and subpleural distribution. However, it may still be initiated through inhalation of particles; thus, differentiation between a bronchocentric and lymphatic pattern often is difficult. Involvement of the subpleural space is highly indicative of the latter. A lymphatic pattern is observed in diseases with a predominantly lymphatic spread, including sarcoidosis, lymphangiosis carcinomatosa, metastatic spread, pneumoconiosis, lymphocytic interstitial pneumonia (LIP), and cardiogenic pulmonary edema.

Honeycombing is an advanced stage of pulmonary interstitial fibrosis. Uniform cystic spaces ranging in diameter from 5 to 10 mm with thick walls are characteristic.

Honeycombing is caused by a limited number of diseases, including idiopathic pulmonary fibrosis, scleroderma, rheumatoid lung disease, eosinophilic granuloma, lymphangioleiomyomatosis, pneumoconiosis (e.g., silicosis, coal workers' pneumoconiosis, and asbestosis), and sarcoidosis. It is particularly evident in both lower lobes except for eosinophilic granuloma, sarcoidosis, and silicosis, which show upper zone predominance of honeycombing. In idiopathic pulmonary fibrosis and scleroderma, the lung volume is characteristically decreased, whereas in pneumoconiosis and sarcoidosis, it is increased. This is due to

a coexistence of pulmonary fibrosis and obstructive airway disease with cystic spaces varying from 1 to 10 cm in diameter.

Extensive fibrosis results in architectural distortion. Occasionally, traction bronchiectasis and conglomerate masses (progressive massive fibrosis [PMF]) preferentially located in the upper lobes may occur, especially in pneumoconiosis and sarcoidosis.

Typically observed in patients with asbestosis, but also those with pulmonary fibrosis and lymphangitic carcinomatosis, are thin subpleural lines, 2 to 10 cm long, paralleling the chest wall (curvilinear subpleural lines), as well as nontapering bands of fibrous tissue radiating from the lung periphery.

Central peribronchial interstitial edema, infiltrates, and fibrosis manifest on CT as apparent bronchial wall thickening. Irregular and serrated thickening of bronchi and vessels suggests fibrosis, whereas a smooth thickening of these structures favors edema and infiltrates. Besides these edematous and infectious processes, central interstitial thickening is associated with lymphangitic carcinomatosis, lymphoma, and sarcoidosis.

In *air-space (alveolar) disease,* the air in peripheral airways is replaced by fluid, cells, or solid substances, resulting in an increased regional lung density.

The following conditions may be underlying causes: (1) low osmotic blood pressure (e.g., hypoproteinemia), (2) high capillary blood pressure (e.g., congestive heart failure), (3) defective alveolocapillary barrier (e.g., shock, lung contusion, and inhalation of noxious gases), (4) aspiration, (5) secretion of abnormal substances (e.g., cystic fibrosis), (6) deposition of abnormal substances (e.g., alveolar proteinosis), (7) invasion of cells (e.g., infectious and inflammatory conditions), and (8) intra-alveolar cell growth (e.g., neoplasm).

As indicated above, air-space disease (**Fig. 16.9**) presents in its early stages as poorly defined bronchocentric nodularities, measuring about 0.5 to 1 cm in diameter. With progression of the disease, these nodules coalesce and form larger areas of consolidation, obscuring pulmonary vessels and causing characteristic air bronchograms (**Fig. 16.10**). However, air bronchograms are also encountered in atelectasis and, rarely, in extensive interstitial disease, such as sarcoidosis.

Diffuse air-space disease tends to involve central portions of the lungs, whereas diffuse interstitial processes are predominantly observed in the lung periphery. CT attenuation values do not permit differentiation between different air-space consolidations. Relatively high attenuation values are found in acute pulmonary hemorrhage and chronic renal failure, possibly due to dystrophic microcalcifications.

Diffuse interstitial and/or micronodular densities with increased attenuation are associated with mitral stenosis or other conditions with chronically elevated left atrial pressure, as well as with healed disseminated infections, such as tuberculosis, histoplasmosis and varicella pneumonitis, silicosis, radiopaque dust inhalation, amyloidosis, and alveolar microlithiasis. Occasionally,

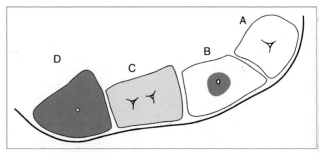

Fig. 16.9 Air-space disease pattern. Normal secondary pulmonary lobule (A). Centrilobular consolidation (B). Ground-glass opacity (C). Air-space consolidation (D).

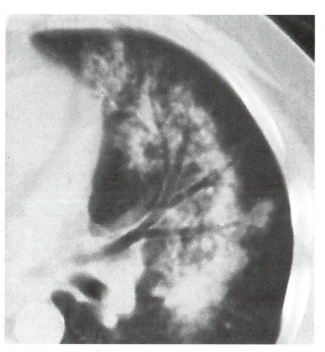

Fig. 16.10 Air bronchograms. Bronchi are contrasted by the surrounding air-space disease (uremic pneumonia).

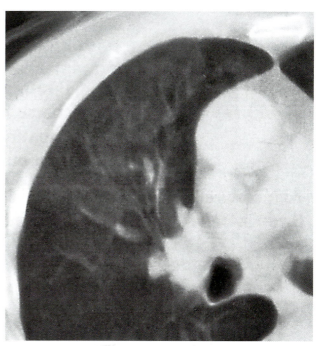

Fig. 16.11 Ground-glass infiltrate. A hazy pulmonary density is caused by pneumocystic pneumonia.

they are also found in pulmonary fibrosis (idiopathic or long-term busulfan therapy), deposition of iodine-containing drugs (e.g., amiodarone therapy or postlymphography), idiopathic pulmonary hemosiderosis, and Goodpasture syndrome.

These densities are observed in conditions in which either air in the acini is only partially replaced by soft tissue-equivalent material or the walls of the acini are diffusely thickened. This appearance is nonspecific and can be found with any early manifestation of a diffuse acinar or interstitial process. Interstitial pneumonias (e.g., viral and pneumocystic [*Pneumocystis carinii*, PCP]), desquamative interstitial pneumonitis, and alveolar proteinosis frequently present in this fashion.

Ground-glass opacity (**Fig. 16.11**) refers to a subtle, hazy increase in lung density on high-resolution CT. It is a nonspecific finding and differs from true air-space disease in that it does not obscure pulmonary vessels. It may likewise result from either alveolar or parenchymal abnormalities. Thus, ground-glass opacities can be caused by intra-alveolar fluid/inflammation, and simply represent an alveolitis, or be affected by mild thickening of the septal or alveolar interstitium (e.g., due to an edema, inflammation, infection or neoplasmatic infiltration). Ground-glass opacities are also often associated with a mosaic pattern, air trapping, "crazy paving," and fibrosis (e.g., honeycombing). A mosaic pattern simply describes regional differences in parenchymal density due to either air trapping or zones of increased consolidation. Air trapping is highly indicative of an airway disease and appears as normal parenchyma on inspiratory scans and low attenuating regions on expiratory scans. By contrast, zones of increased consolidation remain unaltered during expiratory scans. Crazy paving describes a pattern in which thickened, polygonal interlobular septa are superimposed on ground-glass opacities. This pattern is observed in pulmonary alveolar proteinosis, PCP, acute respiratory distress syndrome (ARDS), hemorrhage, and acute exogenous lipoid pneumonia.

Compared with conventional radiography, pulmonary nodules are detected much earlier and more easily on CT scans. Differentiation between benign and malignant lesions remains a major problem, however. Small peripheral metastases cannot be differentiated from granulomas or intrapulmonary lymph nodes, which are also found in a subpleural location. In case

of sepsis or metastatic spread, usually numerous similar-sized pulmonary lesions are found. A vessel entering a small nodule is suggestive of a hematogenous metastasis, but it may also be associated with septic emboli.

A solitary pulmonary nodule can be assumed benign if it remains stable in volume over a 2-y period. Also, a mean density > 200 HU on noncontrast CT scans is an indicator of a benign lesion. The high attenuation value reflects subtle calcifications within the lesion that are not discernible on the images. In general, visible calcifications are highly suggestive of a benign lesion. Benign calcifications (including histoplasmoma) tend to be either centrally located or diffusely distributed throughout the lesion, whereas eccentric calcifications can also be found in malignant lesions (e.g., scar carcinoma originating from a granuloma or metastases from osteoblastoma). Lack of contrast uptake (< 20 HU increase after bolus injection) is another indicator of a benign lesion. The demonstration of fat within the lesion usually suggests a benign hamartoma or, less commonly, a lipomatous lesion, fat embolus, or lipoid pneumonia. Thus, any solitary nodule with smooth borders measuring < 2 cm in diameter in an a-symptomatic patient younger than 40 y is likely to be benign and should be monitored. Usually a follow-up CT examination within 6 to 9 months and a thorough clinical review and patient history allow further validation.

Malignant lesions frequently exceed 2 cm in diameter, have a spiculated margin, and a mean attenuation value < 150 HU on precontrast CT scans, as well as eccentric cavitations and, if present, intratumoral calcifications. A bronchovascular bundle converging toward the lesion may be visible, and usually enhancement of the mass is > 20 HU after contrast injection. Additional findings include a notch in the mass, heterogeneity of the lesion, and a surrounding halo of lower density (hemorrhage/lymphangiosis). In a subpleural location, retraction of the pleura toward the mass may produce a pleural tag that is caused by a desmoplastic reaction. All these signs, however, are not specific for a malignancy and may also be found in a variety of benign conditions.

The differential diagnosis of diffuse lung disease is discussed in **Table 16.1** and solitary and multiple focal pulmonary lesions in **Table 16.2**.

Table 16.1 Diffuse lung disease

Disease	CT Findings	Comments
Vascular		
Disseminated intravascular coagulation (DIC)	Minimal scattered parenchymal densities to massive pulmonary edema. **Diagnostic pearls:** Massive pulmonary edema and the course of the disease often are indistinguishable from those of adult respiratory distress syndrome (ARDS).	Always occurs in the wake of other disorders, such as shock, sepsis, cancer, obstetric complications, burn injuries, and hepatic disease.
Diffuse alveolar hemorrhage ▷ *Fig. 16.12*	Poorly defined consolidations to widespread bilateral air-space opacities often with air bronchograms. **Diagnostic pearls:** A coarse reticular pattern may become evident during resolution, which may last between a few days to a week.	Spontaneous pulmonary hemorrhage is associated with several bleeding disorders and vasculitides, such as systemic lupus erythematosus (SLE), polyarteritis nodosa, Henoch–Schönlein purpura, and Wegener granulomatosis.
Pulmonary fat embolism ▷ *Fig. 16.13*	Minimal to widespread air-space consolidations with predilection for the peripheral zones of the lower lung fields. On high-resolution CT, bilateral ground-glass opacities and thickening of interlobular septa are seen. **Diagnostic pearls:** Micronodular (< 5 mm) centrilobular and subpleural opacities representing alveolar edema or hemorrhage; fat-attenuating pulmonary artery filling defects on contrast-enhanced CT.	Typical complication of (surgery of) long bone fractures. Onset 1 to 2 days after trauma/surgery. Resolution may take 1 to 4 weeks. Clinical presentation is classified into major and minor symptoms according to Gurd. Major criteria comprise subconjunctival/axillary petechia, mental changes, hypoxemia, and pulmonary edema. Minor symptoms include fat globuli in sputum or urine, tachycardia, emboli in retina, increasing sedimentation rate, drop in hematocrit or platelet values, and temperatures > 38.5°C (101.3°F). Diagnosis requires at least one major and four minor symptoms.
Cardiogenic pulmonary edema ▷ *Fig. 16.14*	From smooth thickening of interlobular septa (interstitial edema) via ground-glass opacities in the dependent lung portions (alveolar edema) to (partial) atelectasis of the lung (often with air bronchograms). Pleural effusions are common. **Diagnostic pearls:** Changes tend to be more peripheral.	Transudation of fluid into the central and peripheral interstitial space constitutes interstitial edema as the first stage of pulmonary edema. This is followed by transudation of fluid into the air-space (alveolar edema). With progression, completely opacified acini coalesce, producing a "patchwork quilt" appearance of atelectatic lung portions.
Noncardiogenic pulmonary edema ▷ *Fig. 16.14*	Similar appearance as in cardiogenic edema, but findings tend to be more centrally located. **Diagnostic pearls:** "Butterfly wing" congestion of central lung portion.	Noncardiogenic pulmonary edema with elevated microvascular pressure is associated with renal failure (see **Fig. 16.10**), hypervolemia, hyperinfusion, hypoproteinemia, and neurologic disorders (e.g., head trauma and increased intracranial pressure).
Goodpasture syndrome ▷ *Fig. 16.15*	Bilateral patchy to diffuse ground-glass opacities with or without consolidations with air bronchograms; usually more prominent in the perihilar area, as well as middle and lower lung zones (acute phase). Within a few days, ground-glass opacities are replaced by a reticular pattern with smooth septal thickening. Asymmetric pulmonary fibrosis with coarse reticular pattern and eventually honeycombing is typical for the chronic phase. **Diagnostic pearls:** Sparing of costrophrenic angles and subpleural space. Pleural effusions are unusual.	Rare disease; M > F. Hemoptysis typically precedes the clinical manifestations of renal disease (glomerulonephritis) by several months. Hemorrhagic episodes cause bilateral ground-glass opacities, which are soon replaced by interstitial thickening. Ten to 12 days after onset, interstitial changes typically resolve. Recurrent bleeding episodes cause progressive interstitial fibrosis. Hilar lymph node enlargement may be observed during acute stage.
Idiopathic pulmonary hemosiderosis (IPH) ▷ *Fig. 16.15*	Similar pattern as in Goodpasture syndrome. **Diagnostic pearls:** Lack of renal involvement and thus absence of antineutrophil cytoplasmic antibody (ANCA) and antibasal membrane antibodies.	Chronic IPH usually presents with malaise, iron deficiency anemia, finger clubbing, hepatosplenomegaly, and bilirubinemia. Acute IPH is relatively rare and presents with pulmonary hemorrhage and fever.

(continues on page 600)

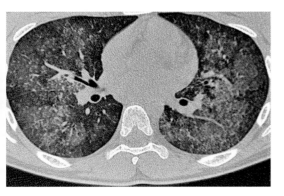

Fig. 16.12 Diffuse alveolar hemorrhage. Widespread bilateral air-space opacities.

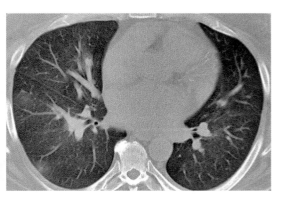

Fig. 16.13 Pulmonary fat embolism. Discrete form with bilateral ground-glass opacities in a subpleural location.

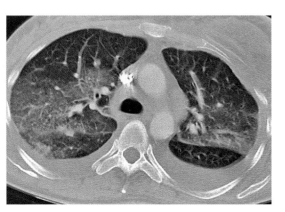

Fig. 16.14 Cardiogenic pulmonary edema. Smooth thickening of interlobular septa, along with ground-glass opacities, in the dependent lung portions and air bronchograms. Bilateral pleural effusion.

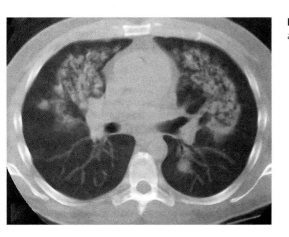

Fig. 16.15 Goodpasture syndrome. Bilateral dense air-space consolidations are visible, sparing the lung periphery (butterfly distribution).

Table 16.1 (Cont.) Diffuse lung disease

Disease	CT Findings	Comments
Inflammation		
Lymphocytic interstitial pneumonia (LIP) ▷ *Fig. 16.16*	Diffuse septal thickening through lymphocytic infiltrates and formation of thin-walled cysts with a preference of basal parts of the lung. **Diagnostic pearls:** *Diffuse disease:* Classic example for lymphatic distribution pattern of micronoduli (i.e., centrilobular and subpleural micronoduli < 5 mm) within the secondary lobule. "Tree-in-bud" sign not due to bronchiolitis but secondary to thickening of bronchovascular bundles. Thin-walled (1–25 mm) cysts involving < 10% of the lung parenchyma are the most characteristic finding. Associated with diffuse ground-glass opacities/consolidations, septal thickening. *Focal disease:* Air-space consolidations with air bronchograms (pseudolymphoma). Partly enlarged hilar lymph nodes may initially appear as a focal central mass or simulating central pneumonia. Usually there are no pleural effusions.	Diffuse disease commonly referred to as LIP, focal disease referred to as pseudolymphoma. Primarily affects middle-aged women. Histologically, a diffuse hyperplasia of bronchus-associated lymphoid tissue (BALT), which is a subset of mucosa-associated lymphoid tissue (MALT). LIP is triggered through recurrent antigen exposure, such as viral infections (Epstein–Barr virus, human immunodeficiency virus [HIV], etc.), autoimmune diseases (Sjögren syndrome, rheumatoid arthritis, myasthenia gravis, Hashimoto thyroiditis, etc.), immunodeficiency (graft-vs-host reaction [GvHR]), and drugs. Treatment depends on stimulating antigen/agent. Lymphatic distribution pattern of micronoduli is also observed in patients with pneumoconiosis, sarcoidosis, lymphangitis carcinomatosa (usually pleural effusions), and amyloidosis.
Acute interstitial pneumonia (AIP, Hamman–Rich syndrome) ▷ *Fig. 16.17*	Rapid progressive diffuse alveolar damage of unknown etiology. **Diagnostic pearls:** Diffuse bilateral, almost symmetrical ground-glass densities in the lower lung. May develop into architectural distortion and honeycombing with dense air space opacifications with or without bronchiectasis. Crazy paving is observed.	Rare idiopathic lung fibrosis. Histological diffuse alveolar damage rapidly progresses through three stages (exudative, proliferative, and fibrotic). Acute onset of clinical symptoms, which are similar to ARDS or a viral pneumonia. Poor prognosis (mortality > 50% within 8 weeks).
Idiopathic pulmonary fibrosis (IPF)/usual interstitial pneumonia (UIP) ▷ *Fig. 16.18a, b*	Interstitial fibrosis with a subpleural and basal preponderance. **Diagnostic pearls:** Initially distinct reticular inter-lobular thickening is seen with presence of ground-glass opacifications (thickened interstitium of the secondary pulmonary lobule). With progression of the disease, a coarse reticulonod-ular pattern, honeycombing, irregular subpleural thickening, fibrous bands (frequently originating from the pleural surface), traction bronchiectases, and eventually severe architectural distortion. Often accompanied by centrilobular/paraseptal emphysema.	Histologically, an interstitial inflammation with presence of fibroblasts, lymphocytes, and histiocytes. Typical onset between 40 and 70 y of age, with slight male predominance. Symptoms include progressive dyspnea, nonproductive cough, weight loss, and fatigue. Clinical symptoms include digital clubbing, breathlessness, and noncoughing. Digital clubbing is common and may precede clinical symptoms. Moderate progression with overall poor prognosis. Drug reaction may have similar lung patterns and clinical symptoms, which stop immediately after drug abstinence.
Nonspecific interstitial pneumonia (NSIP) ▷ *Fig. 16.19a, b*	May not be an entity of its own, but rather a pattern that is observed in a variety of pulmonary and systemic diseases. **Diagnostic pearls:** Ill-defined bilateral patchy ground-glass opacifications. May additionally show overlying diffuse interstitial disease ("crazy paving") that presents initially as a fine reticular pattern and later progresses to a coarser reticulation and, rarely, honeycombing. Fibrotic changes may lead to architectural distortion.	Observed particularly in combination with or as a pulmonary pattern in collagen vascular disease, systemic sclerosis, rheumatoid arthritis, drug-induced pulmonary disease, and hypersensitivity pneumonia, as well as after radiation therapy.
Desquamative interstitial pneumonia (DIP)	Chronic idiopathic interstitial pneumonia often observed in smokers. **Diagnostic pearls:** Irregular linear opacities and diffuse ground-glass opacities with a slight preference of the periphery of lower lung zones; some presence of thin-walled small cysts (< 3 cm in diameter). Honeycombing is unusual.	Histologically, macrophage filling of alveolar spaces. May be the end stage of a chronic respiratory bronchiolitis after having progressed to a respiratory bronchiolitis-associated interstitial lung disease (RB-ILD). DIP and UIP may reflect different stages of the same disease process. The clinical course thus can be benign and may completely stop after cessation of smoking with or without steroid treatment. Without treatment, DIP may progress to UIP.

(continues on page 602)

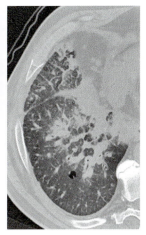 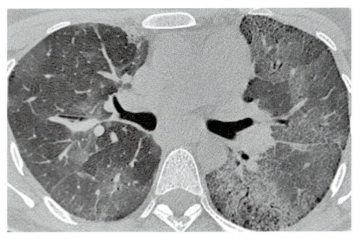

Fig. 16.16 Lymphocytic interstitial pneumonia. Focal disease (pseudolymphoma) of the right lung, simulating pneumonia. Also visible are diffuse ground-glass opacities, loose subpleural centrilobular micronoduli, septal thickening, and formation of a thin-walled cyst. Note the absence of pleural effusions. Sjögren syndrome would present with bilateral rather than focal disease.

Fig. 16.17 Acute interstitial pneumonia. Diffuse bilateral ground-glass opacities. Note the marked "crazy paving" and signs of architectural distortion, including honeycombing and dense air-space opacifications, particularly affecting the left lung.

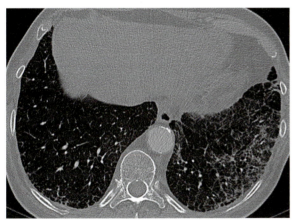 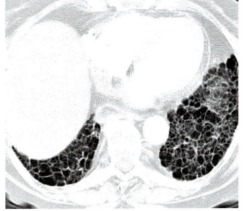

b

Fig. 16.18a, b Idiopathic pulmonary fibrosis. Initially distinct reticular interlobular thickening with the presence of ground-glass opacifications (**a**). End-stage disease with a coarse reticulonodular pattern, honeycombing, irregular subpleural thickening, fibrous bands (frequently originating from the pleural surface), traction bronchiectases, and accompanying centrilobular emphysema (**b**).

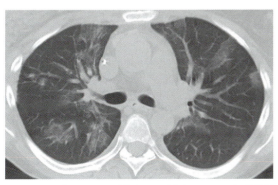 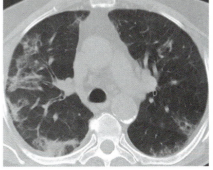

b

Fig. 16.19a, b Nonspecific interstitial pneumonia (NSIP). Initially ill-defined bilateral patchy ground-glass opacifications (**a**), progressing in later stages to a coarser reticulation (**b**). This pattern is also observed in collagen vascular diseases, rheumatoid arthritis, drug-induced pulmonary disease, and hypersensitivity pneumonia, as well as after radiation therapy.

V Thorax

Table 16.1 (Cont.) Diffuse lung disease

Disease	CT Findings	Comments
Bronchiolitis ▷ *Fig. 16.20*	Multiple small centrilobular nodules and ground-glass opacities with relative sparing of the subpleural space (bronchocentric pattern). **Diagnostic pearls:** V- or Y-shaped tubular opacities ("tree-in-bud" sign) and sharply marginated regions of increased lung attenuation ("air trapping") on expiratory high-resolution CT.	Ground-glass opacities represent centrilobular nodules within secondary lobule. Spread of disease is bronchogenic. Involvement of subpleural space is indicative of lymphatic or hematogenous spread (lymphatic pattern). Bronchiolitis typically associated with toxic smoke/gas inhalation (i.e., respiratory bronchiolitis); viral or mycoplasmatic infections, particularly in children younger than 3 y (infectious bronchiolitis); connective tissue disease (e.g., rheumatoid disease); cryptogenic organizing pneumonia (COP); hypersensitivity pneumonitis; aspiration; pneumoconiosis; and as a late complication after organ transplantation (months to years).
Cystic fibrosis (mucoviscidosis) ▷ *Fig. 16.21a, b*	Diffuse bronchiectasis, peribronchial cuffing, and mucous plugging, primarily affecting upper lobes. **Diagnostic pearls:** Subsegmental, segmental, or lobular atelectasis with right upper lobe predilection and recurrent focal pneumonitis (air-trapping, tree-in-bud sign, mosaic perfusion). Prominent hili may be caused by a combination of peribronchial cuffing, mild adenopathy, and enlarged pulmonary arteries (secondary pulmonary hypertension).	Autosomal recessive disease with 1:2000 incidence, almost exclusively observed in Caucasians. Positive sweat test (abnormally high chloride concentrations) is diagnostic. Peribronchial thickening and prolonged mucous plugging result in hyperinflation with subsequent development of bullae and both tubular and cystic bronchiectases.
Silicosis/coal workers' pneumoconiosis ▷ *Fig. 16.22*	Micronodular (1–10 mm) thickening of the interstitium predominantly affecting the middle and upper portions of the lung. **Diagnostic pearls:** Typical features are thickened interlobular septa, subpleural lines and nodular pleural irregularities, radiating fibrous bands, honeycombing, and traction bronchiectases. In 10% of cases, nodules may calcify centrally (especially in silicosis). Hilar adenopathy is frequently present and may in 5% of cases show calcifications in a characteristic "eggshell" pattern (especially in silicosis). Nodules may aggregate into progressive massive fibrosis (PMF), presenting as bilateral dense opacities most often observed in the dorsal aspect of the upper lobes. PMF may cavitate.	Silica is more fibrogenic than coal. Silica/coal particles are inhaled into respiratory bronchioles and subsequently digested by macrophages and lymphocytes. These macrophages transport the particles to hilar and mediastinal lymph nodes, forming granulomas. It usually takes 10 to 20 y of exposure before radiologic abnormalities become evident. However, acute silicosis of sandblasters may present in < 1 y as diffuse air-space disease. Caplan syndrome: rheumatoid arthritis associated with pneumoconiosis, especially coal workers' pneumoconiosis.
Asbestosis ▷ *Fig. 16.23* ▷ *Fig. 16.24*	Peripheral interstitial fibrosis usually located in lower parts of the lung and presenting with thickened interlobular septa, centrilobular nodules, curvilinear subpleural lines, fibrous bands, and honeycombing. **Diagnostic pearls:** Nodular pulmonary pattern and hilar adenopathy are unusual and not characteristic. May be associated with asbestos-related pleural disease, round atelectasis, pulmonary or interlobular fissural fibrous masses, bronchogenic carcinoma, and mesothelioma. A round atelectasis is a round or lentiform subpleural density with a "comet tail" produced by the curvilinear bronchovascular bundle entering the lesion.	Asbestos fibers are very thin, heat resistant, and durable. After inhalation, they travel into lower lung zones and are deposited into respiratory bronchioles. They are too large to be removed by lymphocytes or macrophages and thus lead to a distinct local fibrosis. Pleural disease usually is induced after penetration of these fibers through the lung into the pleural space. Asbestos-related pleural disease consists of focal pleural plaques (70%), diffuse pleural thickening (20%), pleural calcifications (20%), and pleural effusions (20%). **Talcosis** resembles asbestosis and asbestos-related pleural disease. **Aluminium (bauxite) pneumoconiosis:** Coarse reticulonodular pattern often associated with pleural thickening.
Berylliosis	Sarcoidosis-like lung pattern in patients with exposure to beryllium (nuclear power plants, electronic/aerospace industries). **Diagnostic pearls:** Nodular to reticulonodular pattern sparing apices and bases, sometimes associated with hilar and mediastinal adenopathy. Pulmonary nodules may calcify (differential diagnosis: sarcoidosis).	Probably a type IV hypersensitivity reaction to beryllium dust. Acute berylliosis is rare and presents as pulmonary edema following an overwhelming exposure.

(continues on page 604)

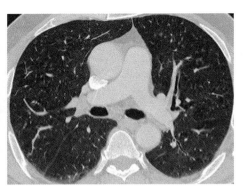

Fig. 16.20   Bronchiolitis. Multiple small V- and Y-shaped centrilobular opacities ("tree-in-bud" sign) and ground-glass opacities with relative sparing of the subpleural space (bronchocentric pattern), as well as implied regions of air trapping.

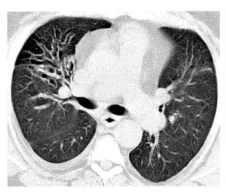 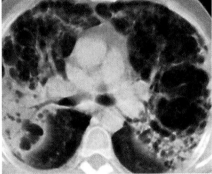

b

Fig. 16.21a, b   Cystic fibrosis. Varicose bronchiectasis with peribronchial cuffing and mucous plugging, particularly affecting the middle lobe of the right lung (**a**). Advanced disease with architectural distortion and extensive chronic pulmonary infiltrates (**b**).

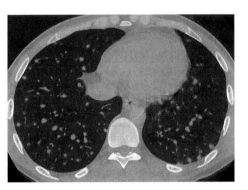

Fig. 16.22   Silicosis. Multiple well-defined nodules with middle and upper lung zone predominance.

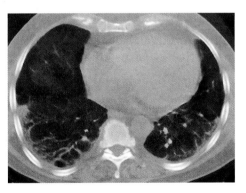

Fig. 16.23   Pulmonary asbestosis. Peripheral coarse interstitial thickening mostly involving the lower lung zones.

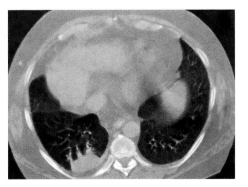

Fig. 16.24   Round atelectasis in pulmonary asbestosis. A subpleural mass with three irregular bands radiating from the mass into the lung parenchyma (crow's feet) is visible in the right posterior chest. Note the bilateral peripheral interstitial thickening as an early sign of pulmonary asbestosis.

V Thorax

Table 16.1 (Cont.) Diffuse lung disease

Disease	CT Findings	Comments
Radiopaque dust inhalation (iron, tin, barium, antimony, and rare-earth compounds)	Dense granular stippling uniformly distributed over both lung fields. **Diagnostic pearls:** Density of the tiny nodules correlates with the atomic number of the inhaled element.	Usually lack of clinical symptoms, as these substances are not fibrogenic. In mixed dust disease (e.g., in association with silica) pulmonary granulomas and fibrosis may occur (e.g., siderosilicosis).
Silo filler's disease (NO$_2$ inhalation)	Acute bronchiolitis with bilateral reticulonodular or patchy infiltrates in the middle and lower lung fields that may progress rapidly to massive air-space disease within 24 hours. **Diagnostic pearls:** Complete resolution typically occurs within a few days if not fatal. After 2 to 5 weeks, bronchiolitis obliterans develops with multiple discrete nodular opacities of varying size scattered throughout both lung fields.	NO$_2$ inhalation injuries may also be associated with industrial exposure to fuming nitric acid or the use of explosives in mining operations. Exposure to other toxic gases such as SO$_2$, H$_2$S, ammonia, chlorine, and phosgene causes similar pulmonary abnormalities.
Pulmonary alveolar proteinosis ▷ *Fig. 16.25*	Bilateral peripheral air-space disease, occasionally with ground-glass appearance and mildly thickened interlobular septa. **Diagnostic pearls:** Thickened interstitium affects polygonal opacities with central ground-glass appearance (crazy paving). Also seen: geographic distribution of ground-glass opacities on high-resolution CT. A coarse reticular pattern simulating honeycombing is less common. Pleural effusions are absent.	Age peak: 20 to 50 y. Often observed in immunocompromised patients. M > F (3:1). Fungal infections such as from *Nocardia*, *Aspergillus*, and *Cryptococcus* are typical and often associated.
Alveolar microlithiasis	Bilateral atypical dense appearance of lung. **Diagnostic pearls:** Superimposition and summation of discrete and extremely sharply defined microliths measuring < 1 mm in diameter. On high-resolution CT, characteristically micronodular calcifications are superimposed on ground-glass opacities.	Rare disorders of obscure etiology with familial occurrence in over 50% of cases. Typically without clinical symptoms. Usually found in patients between 30 and 50 y of age but may also be observed in infants. May eventually result in cardiac/lung failure.
Smoke and fume inhalation	Bilateral patchy parenchymal densities (transient pulmonary edema) developing within hours after exposure. **Diagnostic pearls:** Patchy lung densities may resolve within a few days or progress to severe pulmonary air-space disease with atelectasis, hemorrhage, necrosis, and pneumonia. May eventually result in ARDS.	Characteristic pulmonary parenchymal disease in patients with burn injuries. May be caused by three mechanisms: toxic combustion products, direct trauma from heat, and shock and sepsis.
Extrinsic allergic alveolitis (hypersensitivity pneumonitis) ▷ *Fig. 16.26a–c*	Allergic lung disease caused by a variety of organic and chemical antigens. **Diagnostic pearls:** Always compare inspiratory with expiratory high-resolution CT. *Acute stage:* Bilateral air-space consolidations and ill-defined centrilobular micronodules, predominantly affecting the middle and lower portions of the lung. *Subacute stage:* Patchy ground-glass opacities, ill-defined centrilobular micronodules, mosaic perfusion (air trapping), and cyst formation (middle and lower portions of the lung). *Chronic stage:* Diffuse interstitial fibrosis characterized by a coarse reticular pattern, honeycombing architectural distortion, and formation of traction bronchiectases. Often associated with loss of volume, especially in the upper lobes, and compensatory inflation of the least-affected lung zones. Typically sparing of costophrenic angles.	Acute or insidious onset of progressive dyspnea. Radiographic findings usually parallel clinical symptoms but are also observed in symptom-free patients. Both type III (immune complex) and type IV (cell-mediated) reactions are regarded as inducing mechanisms. Sources of exposure include moldy hay (farmer's lung), pigeons, canaries, parakeets, chickens (bird fancier's lung), moldy sugar cane residuals (bagassosis), moldy cheese (cheese washer's lung), air conditioning, humidifiers, damp walls or floors, and hot tubs (humidifier lung). Treatment of choice is avoidance of antigen exposure and steroids (during the acute stage).

(continues on page 606)

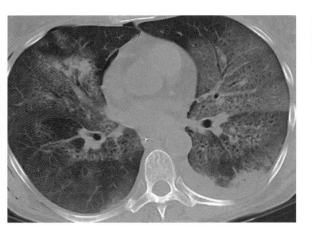

Fig. 16.25 Pulmonary alveolar proteinosis. Bilateral peripheral air-space disease with ground-glass appearance and mildly thickened interlobular septa ("crazy paving"). The pleural effusion on the left is uncommon.

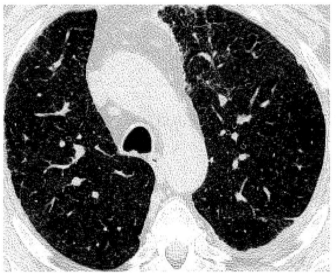

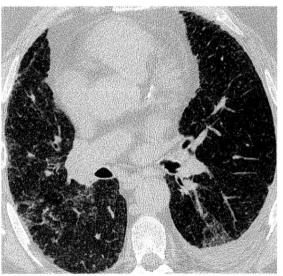

b

Fig. 16.26a–c Extrinsic allergic alveolitis. Acute stage with bilateral air-space consolidations and ill-defined centrilobular micronodules (**a**). Subacute stage with patchy ground-glass opacities, ill-defined centrilobular micronodules, and air-trapping (**b**). Chronic stage with a coarse reticular pattern, honeycombing, architectural distortion, and formation of traction bronchiectases (**c**).

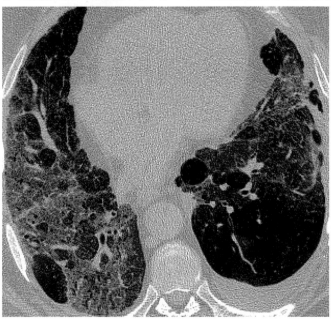

Table 16.1 (Cont.) Diffuse lung disease

Disease	CT Findings	Comments
Drug-induced pulmonary disease ▷ **Fig. 16.27a, b**	A heterogeneous pattern of air-space and interstitial changes in patients with long-lasting exposure to a variety of drugs. **Diagnostic pearls:** Lung manifestations range from pulmonary edema (e.g., heroin, intravenous [IV] contrast agents, salicylates) and patchy air-space disease (e.g., amiodarone, chlorpromazine) to an interstitial disease of a reticular or reticulonodular nature (e.g., chemotherapeutic agents, nitrofurantoin) that may progress to honeycombing (see also **Fig. 16.19**).	The time span for development and resolution of pulmonary changes depends on the mechanism involved and thus is extremely variable, ranging from a few hours to several months. Pulmonary disease is caused by drug hypersensitivity or toxicity. Typical concomitant clinical manifestations are spasmodic asthma, noncardiogenic edema, Löffler syndrome, interstitial and alveolar pneumonitis, SLE-like syndromes, and pulmonary vasculitis.
Rheumatoid lung ▷ **Fig. 16.28**	Diffuse interstitial pneumonitis and fibrosis presenting as reticulonodular to coarse reticular pattern and honeycombing with more frequent involvement of the lower lung fields. **Diagnostic pearls:** COP-like pattern, mosaic perfusion with air trapping on expiratory high-resolution CT, and bronchocentric pattern of nodules (granulomas) (see also **Figs. 16.18, 16.19**). Nodules range from 5 mm to 5 cm in diameter and may cavitate. Large nodules often are found in a subpleural location, may be lobulated, and resemble neoplasms. Concomitant pleuritis and fibrobullous changes in the upper lobes are other rare manifestations.	More common in middle-aged women with rheumatoid arthritis. Complications such as superimposed infections, amyloidosis, and respiratory failure may lead to death. Unilateral or bilateral pleural effusion is the most frequent manifestation of rheumatoid disease in the thorax. In the majority of cases, it is the sole thoracic abnormality and precedes other lung abnormalities. These pleural abnormalities may help to differ rheumatoid arthritis–related lung disease from usual interstitial pneumonia (UIP). Treatment of choice is classic rheumatoid arthritis medication.
Pulmonary scleroderma	Generalized connective tissue disease affecting several organ systems, including the gastrointestinal (GI) tract, lung, skin, heart, and kidneys. **Diagnostic pearls:** Nonspecific interstitial pneumonitis (NSIP) with ground-glass opacifications and diffuse interstitial disease, presenting initially as a fine reticular pattern, progressing to coarser reticulation and rarely, honeycombing. Changes particularly affect lower lung zones. Progressive loss of lung volume with worsening of the disease. Absent pleural reactions characteristic (see **Figs. 16.18, 16.19**).	Histologically, an overproduction and tissue deposition of collagen. Particularly affects middle-aged (30–50 y) women. Pulmonary findings may resemble idiopathic pulmonary fibrosis. An air-filled dilated esophagus due to aperistalsis and/or soft tissue calcinosis (e.g., around the shoulders) may be associated and is pathognomonic. Poor prognosis, with ~70% 5-y survival rate. Typical cause of death is aspiration pneumonia.
Systemic lupus erythematosus (SLE) ▷ **Fig. 16.29**	Discrete bilateral pleural effusions/pleural thickening in young female patients with a history of SLE. **Diagnostic pearls:** Pleural and pericardial effusions; bilateral subpleural reticular opacities with or without honeycombing; bronchocentric micronodular pattern (tree-in-bud); bronchiectasis/bronchial wall cuffing; lupus pneumonitis with coarse linear bands and patchy ground-glass opacities in the periphery of the lung. Seldom edema or hemorrhage (see also **Fig. 16.19**).	Radiographic manifestations of drug-induced and idiopathic SLE are identical. Differential diagnosis: Goodpasture syndrome, NSIP, UIP, rheumatoid arthritis lung, pneumonia.
Pulmonary dermatomyositis (polymyositis) ▷ **Fig. 16.30a, b**	Interstitial lung manifestations similar to scleroderma, but less frequent and less severe. Pathologic changes typically resemble NSIP, COP, or UIP, or a combination of the three. **Diagnostic pearls:** Patchy symmetric bilateral subpleural consolidations in combination with reduced lung volumes; bilateral symmetric basal ground-glass opacities; reticular opacities with coarse parenchymal bands and irregular thickening of the bronchovascular bundle. May finally result in honeycombing and architectural distortion (see also **Figs. 16.18, 16.19**).	Rare autoimmune disease affecting particularly middle-aged women (twice as often as men). Paralysis of pharyngeal and respiratory muscles may result in aspiration and diaphragmatic elevation, respectively. Bilateral symmetric basal ground-glass opacities are a sign of an ongoing, active inflammation process. Steroids are treatment of choice. Bilateral basal linear densities may be residual findings after steroid treatment.
Sjögren syndrome	Interstitial disease of reticulonodular nature and patchy infiltrates, sometimes associated with small effusions. **Diagnostic pearls:** Similar findings as observed in diffuse LIP: centrilobular and subpleural micronoduli (lymphatic pattern), thin-walled (1–25 mm) cysts, bronchiolitis (tree-in-bud sign), and diffuse ground-glass opacities or consolidations (see **Fig 16.16**).	Particularly affects middle-aged women. Occurs in 90% of patients presenting with sicca syndrome (i.e., keratoconjunctivitis sicca, xerostomia, and recurrent parotid gland swelling). Secondary Sjögren syndrome is associated with rheumatoid arthritis and other connective tissue diseases, transplant recipients, and acquired immunodeficiency syndrome (AIDS).

(continues on page 608)

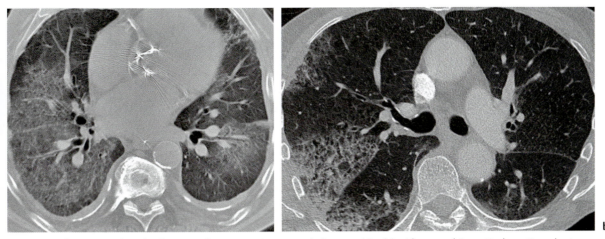

Fig. 16.27a, b   Drug-induced pulmonary disease. Distinct ground-glass opacities (**a**) with an overlying reticular pattern due to amiodarone. Reticulonodular pattern with patchy subpleural air-space opacifications (**b**) that partly progress to honeycombing due to methotrexate.

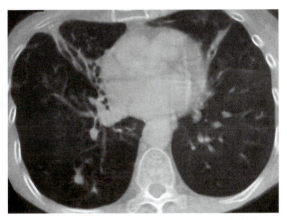

Fig. 16.28   Rheumatoid lung. Nonspecific septal thickening and honeycombing in the middle lobe of the right lung. A singular, slightly lobulated nodule apical is seen in the right lower lobe.

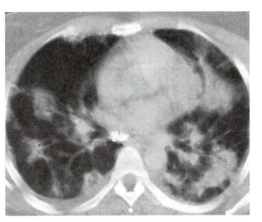

Fig. 16.29   Systemic lupus erythematosus. Pleural effusions and dominant pneumonitis with poorly defined patchy air-space opacities involving predominantly the periphery of both lower lobes.

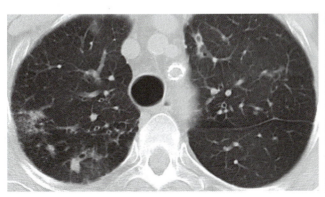

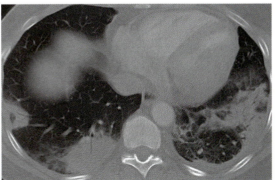

Fig. 16.30a, b   Cryptogenic organizing pneumonia (COP). Randomly distributed ground-glass opacities and nodules (**a**) that soon progress to irregular consolidations in a predominantly subpleural location that apparently ignores the lobular structure of the lung (**b**).

Table 16.1   (Cont.) Diffuse lung disease

Disease	CT Findings	Comments
Cryptogenic organizing pneumonia ▷ *Fig. 16.30a, b, p. 607*	Formerly termed bronchiolitis obliterans organizing pneumonia (BOOP). **Diagnostic pearls:** Irregular consolidations in predominantly subpleural location, randomly distributed ground-glass opacities, and nodules. Consolidations appear to ignore lobular structure of the lung. Typically affects middle and lower portions of the lung.	Idiopathic alveolar disease extends into small airways. Contrary to macroscopic appearance, lung architecture is preserved (no fibrosis). Histologically, chronic inflammatory and fibroblastic tissue. Clinical symptoms are chronic cough, dyspnea, and fever over a 3- to 6-month period prior to diagnosis. Important differential diagnosis to pneumonia, lymphoma, and sarcoidosis. Treatment of choice: oral steroids.
Histiocytosis X (eosinophilic granuloma ▷ *Fig. 16.31a, b*	Diffuse bilateral reticular pattern with upper and mid-zone predominance and consisting of multiple small irregular nodules and small cysts embedded within normal lung parenchyma. **Diagnostic pearls:** Centrilobular, peribronchial nodules (1–5 mm in diameter). Larger nodules may occasionally exceed 10 mm and cavitate. Thin-walled cysts (< 10 mm), equally distributed through the central and peripheral lung zones. Pulmonary fibrosis with interlobular septal thickening, honeycombing, and enlarging cystic spaces (up to several centimeters in diameter) may become evident with progression of the disease. Hilar adenopathy and pleural effusions are unusual in adults.	Occurs usually in middle-aged Caucasian patients, typically with a history of nicotine abuse. Histologically, a diffuse destruction of distal airways induced by granulomas containing large mononuclear cells with characteristic cytoplasmic inclusions (Langerhans cells). At the time of diagnosis, ~25% of patients are asymptomatic. Nonproductive cough is the most common presentation in the remaining patients. Spontaneous pneumothorax is a frequent complication in advanced stages. Disease may regress, resolve completely, stabilize, or progress to advanced fibrosis. Treatment includes smoking cessation and steroids. Severe forms may require lung transplantation.
Pulmonary sarcoidosis ▷ *Fig. 16.32a–c*	Symmetric mediastinal and hilar lymphadenopathy with or without micronodular lung opacities, involving preferentially the middle and upper portions of the lung. **Diagnostic pearls:** *Interstitial pattern (common):* In early stages, multiple micronoduli (< 5 mm) with perivascular, centrilobular, perilymphatic (i.e., along bronchovascular bundles) distribution. In advanced stages, a coarse reticulonodular pattern with thickened interlobular septa. Nodules > 1 cm in diameter are rare, and cavitation is unusual. Progression of the disease results in fibrosis with honeycombing, long linear bands extending to the pleural surface, cicatricial bronchiectases, progressive massive fibrosis, and large bullae (up to 10 cm). *"Alveolar" pattern (uncommon):* Indistinctly defined peripheral densities, sometimes with ground-glass appearance, resembling an active alveolitis. Coalescence of these densities produces large opacities, often with air bronchograms, located either centrally or peripherally in the lung.	Highest incidence in black women between 20 and 40 y of age. Approximately half of patients are asymptomatic at time of diagnosis. Histologically, well-defined granulomas with a rim consisting of fibroblasts and lymphocytes. Hilar and mediastinal (azygos and aortopulmonic window) adenopathy is by far the most common intrathoracic manifestation (80%). Pleural effusions are uncommon. **Staging:** 0: No demonstrable abnormality 1: Hilar and mediastinal adenopathy 2: Adenopathy associated with pulmonary disease 3: Pulmonary disease without adenopathy 4: Pulmonary fibrosis
Lymphangioleiomyomatosis ▷ *Fig. 16.33*	Progressive cystic destruction of the lung induced by proliferating atypical muscle cells. **Diagnostic pearls:** Well-defined, uniformly thin-walled cysts distributed diffusely throughout both lungs, slightly prominent at the lung bases, as well as scattered ground-glass opacities. Cysts enlarge and coalesce (up to several centimeters in diameter) with progression of the disease.	Rare disease, exclusively found in women of child-bearing age. May be a forme fruste of tuberous sclerosis that can present with identical pulmonary CT findings. Mediastinal lymphadenopathy, chylous pleural with or without pericardial effusions, and recurrent pneumothorax are common associated findings.
Radiation-induced lung disease ▷ *Fig. 16.34*	Radiation pneumonitis is observed during acute stage, radiation fibrosis during chronic stage. **Diagnostic pearls:** Pulmonary findings are strictly confined to the radiated area of the lung. *Radiation pneumonitis:* Ground-glass opacities, patchy consolidations often with air bronchograms, and occasionally loss of volume (due to loss of surfactant or bronchiolar plugging). *Radiation fibrosis:* Severe shrinkage of the radiated lung, fibrous bands, traction bronchiectasis, solid consolidations (fibrosis) with spiculated borders, and localized pleural thickening.	Radiation damage to the lung increases with the dose and is lessened by fractionation. Pulmonary changes are not observed for a fractionated dose of < 3000 rads. Pulmonary manifestations may occur at any time within the first 6 months after cessation of the radiotherapy. Though delayed changes are common, any pulmonary changes occurring > 1 y after radiotherapy are highly unlikely to be caused by the radiotheraphy.

(continues on page 610)

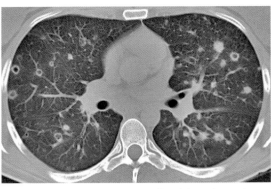
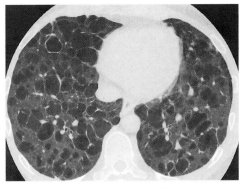

Fig. 16.31a, b   Histiocytosis X. Diffuse bilateral irregular nodules (**a**) that cavitate and become thick-walled cysts. In the end, patients present with numerous thin-walled cysts (> 10 mm), which are equally distributed throughout the lung (**b**).

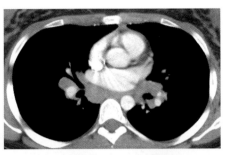
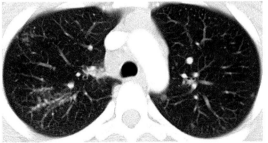
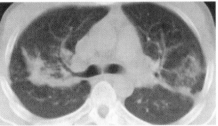

Fig. 16.32a–c   Pulmonary sarcoidosis. Symmetric mediastinal lymphadenopathy (**a**) with perilymphatic (i.e., along bronchovascular bundles) micronodular lung opacities involving the upper portion of the right lung (**b**). Progression of the disease results in progressive massive fibrosis (**c**).

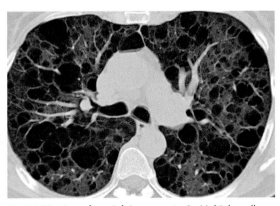
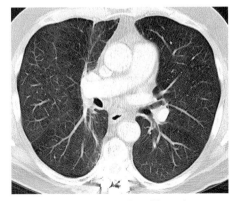

Fig. 16.33   Lymphangioleiomyomatosis. Multiple well-defined, uniformly thin-walled cysts distributed diffusely throughout both lungs.

Fig. 16.34   Radiation-induced lung disease. Paramediastinal fibrosis restricted to those parts of the lung that had been irradiated (due to a mediastinal lymphoma).

V Thorax

Table 16.1   (Cont.) Diffuse lung disease

Disease	CT Findings	Comments
Thromboembolic disease ▷ *Fig. 16.35a, b*	Parenchymal changes due to a thromboembolic disease of the pulmonary arteries. **Diagnostic pearls:** CT density of the lung distal to occluded arteries may be either decreased (oligemia or Westermark sign) or increased (atelectasis, edema, or hemorrhage). Peripheral wedge-shaped areas of consolidation with neither air bronchograms nor cavitation represent either atelectasis or infarcts, the latter corresponding to a Hampton hump on conventional radiographs. Small pleural effusions are common.	Dyspnea, pleuritic chest, and deep vein thrombosis are a common clinical presentation. Laboratory findings include electrocardiogram (ECG) changes and abnormal blood gas levels. Septic emboli present as multiple, ill-defined, round or wedge-shaped opacities with frequent cavitation in the lung periphery. Predisposing factors are IV drug abuse, immune deficiency, IV catheters, alcoholism, and congenital heart disease.
Trauma		
Pulmonary contusion ▷ *Fig. 16.36*	Predominantly trauma-induced contusion of lung parenchyma. **Diagnostic pearls:** Irregular patchy air-space opacities to diffuse consolidations and discrete pleural effusions. Rib fractures may be absent.	Parenchymal contusion zones appear within 6 hours after injury (usually blunt chest trauma) and resolve within 3 days. They consist of edema and blood in the absence of substantial tissue disruption. Differential diagnosis: pulmonary fat embolism.
Aspiration pneumonia ▷ *Fig. 16.37*	Aspiration of solid or fluid material into large airways. **Diagnostic pearls:** Patchy infiltrates to homogeneous consolidations; usually symmetric bilateral gravitational distribution, which may also be asymmetric (depending on position of patient at time of aspiration) and segmental to lobular atelectasis. Superinfection may lead to necrotizing pneumonia with abscess formation and central cavitation.	Chronic aspiration pneumonia is associated with Zenker diverticulum, esophageal stenosis, achalasia, tracheoesophageal fistula, and neuromuscular disorders involving the pharynx. May eventually lead to residual scarring of lung parenchyma. Lung changes in nonchronic aspiration usually resolve within 7 to 10 days after proper treatment (steroids and antibiotics).
Aspiration of amniotic fluid	Diffuse ubiquitous pulmonary consolidations, often rapidly increasing in size and density with lethal outcome.	Affects exclusively neonates at birth. Predisposing factors include difficult labor, intra-uterine fetal death, advanced maternal age, and multiparity.
Aspiration due to near drowning	Symmetrical widespread pulmonary edema that may occasionally be delayed up to 2 days.	Edema usually resolves completely within 3 to 5 days, but may also last up to 10 days.
Infectious		
Pneumonia, bacterial ▷ *Fig. 16.38*	Focal parenchymal consolidation in patients with fever. **Diagnostic pearls:** Focal patchy air-space consolidations, often associated with areas of consolidations and air bronchograms. Discrete pleural effusions, atelectasis, and cavitation are common. On contrast-enhanced CT, differential diagnosis to simple compression atelectasis is possible due to a lack of contrast media uptake in pneumonic parenchyma.	Bronchogenic; usually spread by inhalation (e.g., *Staphylococcus*), aspiration (anaerobics), or direct invasion (i.e., abscesses, cavities; e.g., in tuberculosis [TB]). Hematogenous spread usually through anaerobics (e.g., *Pseudomonas*). Old compression atelectasis may not show contrast media uptake due to the Euler–Liljestrand mechanism.
Pneumonia, mycobacterial ▷ *Fig. 16.39*	Most commonly, pneumonia due to an infection with mycobacteria TB. **Diagnostic pearls:** In *primary TB* localized micronodular airspace opacities usually confined to one lobe in the upper part of the lung. May in advanced stages spread bronchogenically to other lobes and thus lead to numerous bronchocentric air-space consolidations (tree-in-bud sign). Often concomitant hilar and/or mediastinal adenopathy. In secondary or miliary TB, hematogenous spread and thus lymphatic distribution pattern of uniform micronodules (involving the subpleural space). Pleural effusions are common.	Usually secondary to mycobacteria TB. In rare cases, pneumonia may be due to *Mycobacterium avium* infection (MAI). A pathognomonic pattern in these patients is the presence of widespread centrilobular micronodules in combination with ventral bronchiectasis in the middle lobe with or without lingula. Lymphatic pattern in miliary TB is due to hematogenic seeding.
Pneumonia, viral and mycoplasma	Diffuse interstitial thickening in patients with fever. **Diagnostic pearls:** Variable appearance depending on virus type. Typical is interstitial thickening with or without presence of centrilobular nodules. Ground-glass opacities usually only superimposed in advanced stages.	Most common in children and young adults. Signs of myoplasma pneumonia are usually not discernible from those of viral pneumonia.

(continues on page 612)

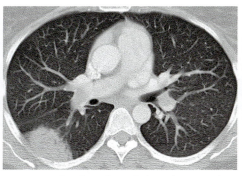
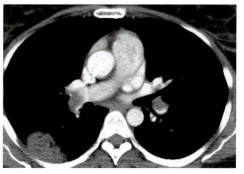

b

Fig. 16.35a, b   Thromboembolic pulmonary disease. Large thrombus within the right pulmonary artery with a peripheral wedge-shaped area of consolidation representing infarcted lung.

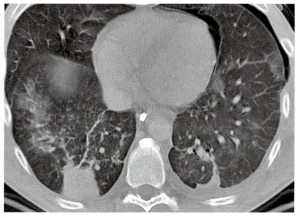

Fig. 16.36   Pulmonary contusion. Trauma-induced dorsal contusion of both lungs with irregular patchy air-space opacities, discrete pleural effusions, and ventral pneumothorax on the left side.

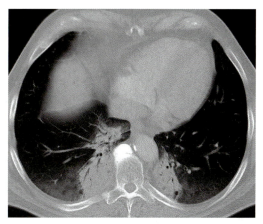

Fig. 16.37   Aspiration pneumonia. Symmetric bilateral segmental atelectasis with air bronchograms and discrete ground-glass opacities.

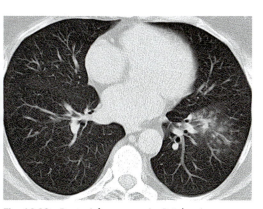

Fig. 16.38   Bacterial pneumonia. Patchy air-space consolidations in the apical left lower lobe.

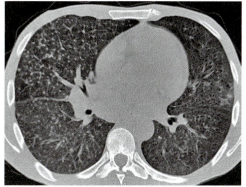

Fig. 16.39   Mycobacterial pneumonia. Miliary tuberculosis (TB) with a lymphatic distribution pattern (involvement of the subpleural space) of multiple equally sized micronoduli.

Table 16.1 (Cont.) Diffuse lung disease

Disease	CT Findings	Comments
Cytomegalovirus (CMV) ▷ *Fig. 16.40*	Diffuse interstitial thickening in immunocompromised patients with fever. **Diagnostic pearls:** Thickened interlobular septa and centrilobular micronodules, usually involving lung periphery, and diffuse ground-glass opacities (less prominent than in pneumocystic pneumonia). Small pleural effusions are frequently associated.	Particularly affects neonates and immunocompromised patients (especially organ transplant recipients). Diffuse ground-glass opacities predominant findings in Hantavirus and severe acute respiratory syndrome (SARS). Lobular ground-glass opacities also observed in herpes simplex and influenza. Segmental consolidations observed in adenovirus.
Pneumonia, fungal	Discrete air-space consolidations in immunocompromised patients with fever. **Diagnostic pearls:** Patchy, homogeneous, poorly defined peribronchial ground-glass opacities with or without centrilobular nodular pattern.	Disseminated disease is an early appearance of acute fungal sepsis and is found particularly in immunocompromised patients. Patients may still be symptom-free. Focal consolidations and cavitations are much more typical for fungal infections but are typically observed only in subsequent stages. The most common fungi are *Candida* and *Aspergillus*.
Pneumocystis pneumonia ▷ *Fig. 16.41a, b*	Opportunistic fungal infection affecting particularly immunocompromised patients. **Diagnostic pearls:** Bilateral ground-glass opacities with sparing of the subpleural space are the dominant finding. Also characteristic are superimposed intra- and interlobular septal thickening leading to crazy paving, lack of tree-in-bud sign, often mosaic pattern caused by alternating involvement and sparing of subsegmental areas. Thin-walled cysts are frequently associated, especially in the upper lobes, and may lead to spontaneous pneumothorax. Pleural effusions and hilar adenopathy are not characteristic. May evolve into asymmetric consolidations and reticular opacities if not treated.	In immunocompromised patients, particularly those with AIDS, pneumocystic pneumonia is the most frequent pulmonary complication. Presents with an abrupt onset of dyspnea, hypoxemia, and nonproductive cough. Diagnosis is made with bronchoalveolar lavage in > 90% of cases. Symptoms in AIDS patients usually subacute, developing within weeks. Symptoms in non-HIV patients usually rapid, evolving over 5 to 10 days. Cysts are observed only in HIV-associated pneumocystic pneumonia. Medical treatment is therapy of choice.

Metabolic

Disease	CT Findings	Comments
Adult respiratory distress syndrome (ARDS) ▷ *Fig. 16.14, p. 599*	Bilateral diffuse air-space opacities. **Diagnostic pearls:** Ground-glass opacities (interstitial and alveolar edema and hemorrhagic fluid) and dense parenchymal consolidations (atelectasis) in the dependent lung in combination with normally aerated lung. Can be differentiated from cardiogenic pulmonary edema by a normal heart size, more diffuse lung involvement, extensive and conspicuous air bronchograms, a cystic or "bubbly" appearance of the parenchymal involvement after 7 days, and the absence of significant pleural effusion.	ARDS is defined as noncardiogenic pulmonary edema with normal microvascular pressure and increased capillary permeability. It may be due to direct injury to the lung (i.e., primary or pulmonary ARDS) or capillary leakage (i.e., indirect or extrapulmonary ARDS). ARDS may occur secondary to trauma, shock, sepsis, aspiration, and a variety of other direct or indirect pulmonary insults. In premature infants, a "spongy" lung pattern is associated with bronchopulmonary dysplasia due to prolonged high oxygen therapy.
Centrilobular emphysema ▷ *Fig. 16.42a, b*	Clearly demarcated cavities in the centrilobular portion of the secondary pulmonary lobule. **Diagnostic pearls:** Primarily affects upper portions of lung zones (apex, apica segment of lower lobules). Margins of the secondary pulmonary lobule are preserved. Emphysematous cavities lack a wall and are surrounded by normal lung parenchyma.	Histologically, an enlargement and destruction of alveolar walls. Strongly associated with nicotine abuse; also observed after inhalation of industrial dust. Slight male predominance; peak age between 40 and 75 y. Smoking abstinence may stabilize or slow down the disease. More severe cases require medical therapy (bronchodilators) or surgery (lung volume reduction/lung transplantation).
Panlobular emphysema ▷ *Fig. 16.43a, b*	Ill-defined diminishing of lung parenchyma without fibrosis. **Diagnostic pearls:** Homogeneously distributed diminishment of the interstitium due to acinar enlargement without zonal preference. Differentiation of normal and diseased lung often difficult. Lung with a threshold HU density < −960 is emphysematous.	Histologically, destruction of alveolar tissue with abnormal enlargement of all parts of the acinus. Commonly associated with alpha-1-antitrypsin deficiency. Slight male predominance. Only symptomatic in patients with advanced disease. No therapy may be necessary, but severe cases may require surgical lung volume reduction or even lung transplantation.

(continues on page 614)

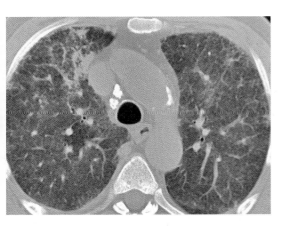

Fig. 16.40   Cytomegalovirus. Thickened interlobular septa and centrilobular micronodules, particularly involving the lung periphery. Also note the concomitant diffuse ground-glass opacities.

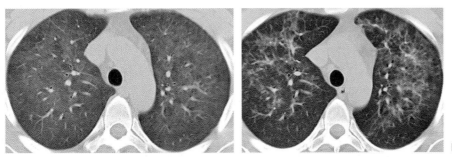

b

Fig. 16.41a, b   Pneumocystis pneumonia. Acute stage showing bilateral ground-glass opacities with sparing of the subpleural space (**a**). A 4-month follow-up examination in the same patient without treatment shows progression into asymmetric reticular consolidations (**b**).

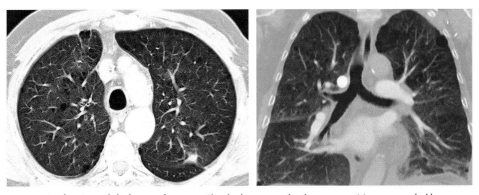

b

Fig. 16.42a, b   Centrilobular emphysema. Clearly demarcated pulmonary cavities surrounded by normal lung parenchyma (**a**), which primarily affects the upper portions of lung zones (**b**).

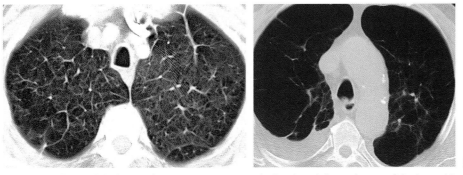

b

Fig. 16.43a, b   Panlobular emphysema. Homogeneously distributed diminishment of the interstitium (**a**), resulting in bullous emphysema (**b**).

V Thorax

Table 16.1 (Cont.) Diffuse lung disease

Disease	CT Findings	Comments
Neoplasms		
Pulmonary Kaposi sarcoma ▷ *Fig. 16.44a, b*	AIDS-associated bilateral pulmonary neoplasm with concomitant involvement of skin, lymph nodes, and GI tract. **Diagnostic pearls:** Bilateral ill-defined noduli and coarse reticulonodular opacities with basilar preference, as well as thickening of the bronchovascular bundle with ill-defined perihilar consolidations.	Abnormal endothelial vascular channels embedded within spindle-shaped stromal cells. Herpes virus associated disease; > 90% occur in male AIDS patients with low CD4 count and concomitant skin and/or mouth lesions. Hilar adenopathy and pleural effusions are associated in ~25% of cases.
Alveolar cell (bronchoalveolar) carcinoma ▷ *Fig. 16.45a, b*	Pneumonia-like progressive regional/lobular consolidation of the lung. **Diagnostic pearls:** Uni- to bilateral focal or multifocal air-space opacities; increased volume of affected lobe (no atelectasis); ill-defined lobulated and/or spiculated peripheral nodules; ground-glass-opacities with or without reticulonodular pattern (crazy paving). After contrast administration, vessels typically opacify within consolidations (CT angiogram sign). Pleural effusions and local lymph node involvement are uncommon.	Histologically, cancer arising from bronchiolar epithelium and type II pneumocytes. Cancer cells typically spread bronchogenically via the tracheobronchial tree (cancer pneumonia). Any antibiotic-resistant pneumonia-like consolidation is highly suspicious. Local form presenting as a well-circumscribed peripheral mass is more common. Diffuse form presenting as bilateral chronic consolidations with air bronchograms is rare. Overall poor prognosis.
Pulmonary lymphoma ▷ *Fig. 16.46*	Concomitant pulmonary involvement of lymphoma. **Diagnostic pearls:** Typically ill-defined consolidations with air bronchograms (nodules ranging from diffuse miliary pattern to only a few large lesions); coarse perihilar reticulonodular pattern (caused by direct extension from hilar lymph nodes); and peripheral interstitial disease with irregular thickened subpleural lines, interlobular septa, and lymphatic nodular distribution pattern (centrilobular nodules involving the subpleural space) (see also **Fig. 16.19, p. 601**).	Lung infection in patients with lymphoma is more often due to drug reactions, concomitant pneumonia, or hemorrhage rather than the underlying disease itself. Pulmonary manifestation of lymphoma is usually associated with or subsequent to hilar and mediastinal lymph node involvement. Similar pulmonary manifestations may be observed in patients with leukemia.
Pulmonary metastases ▷ *Fig. 16.47*	Pulmonary involvement due to lymphatic or hemorrhagic spread of neoplasm. **Diagnostic pearls:** Classic lymphatic nodular distribution pattern (i.e., clusters of similar-sized centrilobular nodules, which are diffusely distributed throughout the entire lung and involving also the subpleural space). Arterial feeders entering single lesions are common but not specific (differential diagnosis: septic emboli and other hematogenous infections).	Nodular pulmonary metastases are commonly associated with neoplasms of the lung, kidney, colon, gonads, uterus, bone, head, and neck (including thyroid), melanomas, and soft tissue sarcomas. An important differential diagnosis is pulmonary septicemia, which may not be discernible from hematogenous spread of metastases on imaging findings alone.
Lymphangitic carcinomatosis ▷ *Fig. 16.48a, b*	Lymphatic spread of neoplastic cells. **Diagnostic pearls:** Usually asymmetric nodular septal thickening confined to one lung/lobe (may also involve both lungs; may resemble edema: Kerley B lines on radiographs); centrilobular micronodules involving the subpleural space (lymphatic distribution pattern); nonspecific patchy ground-glass opacities with or without septal thickening (crazy paving). Pleural effusions and associated hilar/mediastinal lymph nodes are common.	Typical clinical syndrome is shortness of breath. Commonly observed in breast, prostate, stomach, pancreas, and lung cancer. Poor prognosis.

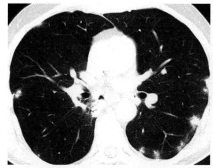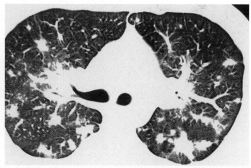

a   b

Fig. 16.44a, b Pulmonary Kaposi sarcoma. Bilateral ill-defined noduli and coarse reticulonodular opacities with basilar preference (**a**). Another patient with thickening of the bronchovascular bundle and ill-defined perihilar consolidations (**b**).

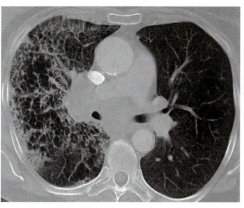
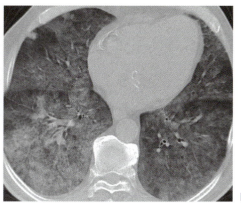

Fig. 16.45a, b   Alveolar cell (bronchoalveolar) carcinoma. Examples of unilateral growth with a predominantly reticulonodular pattern (**a**) and multifocal growth with ground-glass opacities (**b**).

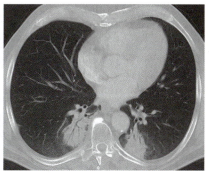

Fig. 16.46   Pulmonary lymphoma. Ill-defined large consolidations with air bronchograms.

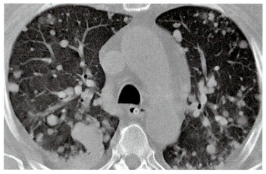

Fig. 16.47   Pulmonary metastases (renal cell carcinoma). Multiple pulmonary nodules with a lymphatic distribution pattern (i.e., distal to vessel endings due to a hematogenous spread).

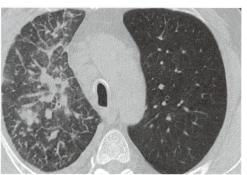
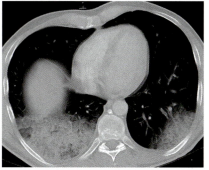

Fig. 16.48a, b   Appearance pattern of lymphangitic carcinomatosis. Unilateral asymmetric nodular septal thickening (**a**), with centrilobular micronodules involving the subpleural space, patchy ground-glass opacities, and discrete pleural effusion on the right. Bilateral edema-like appearance with "crazy paving" (**b**).

Table 16.2   Focal lung lesions

Disease	CT Findings	Comments
Vascular		
Arteriovenous malformation (AVM) ▷ *Fig. 16.49*	Pulmonary arteriovenous fistula. **Diagnostic pearls:** Solitary (two thirds) or multiple (one third) round to oval nodules 1 to 5 mm in size. Nodules are well-defined, homogeneous, and typically slightly lobulated. Nodules are surrounded by normal lung tissue. Often feeding arteries and draining veins are visible; thus, sequential contrast enhancement on dynamic CT is diagnostic. Predilection for the medial third of the lung and for lower lobes.	Symptomatic only in the presence of multiple AVMs. Diagnosed usually in early adulthood either as an isolated anomaly or associated with Rendu–Osler–Weber syndrome (hereditary hemorrhagic telangiectasia). The latter presents with telangiectatic changes in the skin and mucous membranes, epistaxis, and GI bleeding.
Pulmonary infarction ▷ *Fig. 16.50a, b*	Vascular occlusion due to a thromboembolic disease often associated with an underlying cardiopulmonary disease. **Diagnostic pearls:** Wedge-shaped, initially ill-defined, pleura-based consolidation with apex pointing toward the hilum (Hampton hump). "Melting ice block" sign: over time, consolidation becomes well defined and shrinks. May occasionally cavitate. After IV contrast administration often peripheral rim-like contrast enhancement of normal lung tissue.	Other findings supporting the diagnosis of pulmonary embolism include loss of lung volume with elevated ipsilateral diaphragm, ipsilateral oligemia (Westermark sign), ipsilateral pleural effusions, and enlarged central pulmonary arteries with evidence of intravascular clots on postcontrast scans.
Varices of pulmonary veins ▷ *Fig. 16.51*	Varicose enlargement of a pulmonary vein. **Diagnostic pearls:** Well-defined, round or lobulated mass in close proximity to the left atrium, as well as contrast enhancement simultaneous with the left atrium.	Histologically, a tortuous dilation of a pulmonary vein just before entering the left atrium. May be acquired due to pulmonary venous hypertension or be congenital.
Inflammation		
Amyloidosis	A variety of conditions in which amyloid proteins are abnormally deposited in the lung. **Diagnostic pearls:** *Tracheobronchial type:* Endobronchial nodules with obstructive airway disease. *Nodular type:* Solitary or multiple nodules, partly with cavitation and/or calcification. *Diffuse parenchymal type:* Diffuse interstitial disease of miliary or reticulonodular nature.	Histologically, deposition of fibrils of light-chain immunoglobulins in perivascular distribution. Primary amyloidosis (amyloid L) associated either with no disease or with multiple myeloma. Secondary amyloidosis (amyloid A) associated with rheumatoid arthritis, TB, bronchiectasis, and Hodgkin disease. Senile amyloidosis affects several organs, including lungs in elderly patients. Familial amyloidosis is rare.
Progressive massive fibrosis (PMF) ▷ *Fig. 16.52*	Conglomerate masses ranging in the middle and upper lung zones and associated with a variety of pneumoconiosis. **Diagnostic pearls:** Often bilateral but usually asymmetric. Size ranges from 1 to 10 cm. Lateral margin often sharply defined, medial margin usually ill-defined. Mass appears spindle-shaped, with a shorter anteroposterior and a longer mediolateral diameter. Cavitation occurs due to either ischemic necrosis or superimposed TB. Shrinkage of PMF affects compensatory surrounding emphysema with multiple centripetal pseudopodia originating from the mass.	Aggregation of smaller nodules indicates PMF. It is found exclusively with pneumoconiosis, especially coal workers' pneumoconiosis and silicosis, and less commonly with asbestosis. However, in sarcoidosis, massive fibrosis may also present as a central homogeneous mass or large nodular lesions with irregular margins.

(continues on page 618)

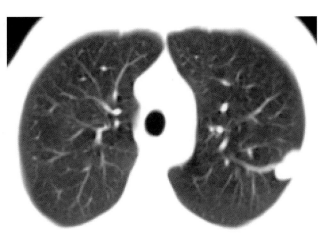

Fig. 16.49 Arteriovenous malformation. A slightly lobulated subpleural mass is seen on the left side with a feeding vessel.

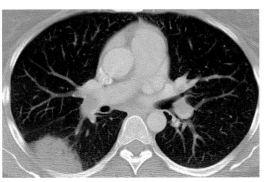
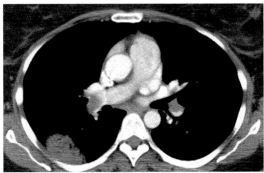

b

Fig. 16.50a, b Pulmonary infarction. Wedge-shaped pleura-based consolidation dorsally in the right lower lobe (**a**) with corresponding pulmonary artery embolus (**b**).

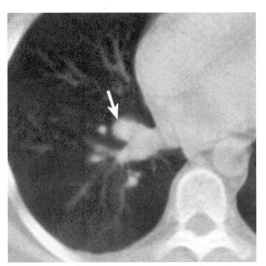
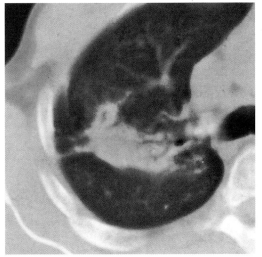

Fig. 16.51 Pulmonary varix. Note the enlarged pulmonary vein (arrow).

Fig. 16.52 Progressive massive fibrosis (PMF) in sarcoidosis. A poorly marginated dense conglomerate mass is evident in the right midlung.

Table 16.2 (Cont.) Focal lung lesions

Disease	CT Findings	Comments
Wegener granulomatosis ▷ *Fig. 16.53*	A form of necrotizing vasculitis affecting the lungs, kidneys, and other organs. **Diagnostic pearls:** Multiple, usually sharply defined, bilateral nodules ranging from < 1 to 10 cm and commonly found in the lower lung zones; presence of "feeding" vessels entering the nodules; often thick-walled and nonregular cavitation that may progress into thin-walled cavities. Pleural effusions occur, but lymphadenopathy is rare. Endobronchial lesions cause segmental, lobular, and total lung atelectasis. Diffuse pulmonary hemorrhage may occur.	The limited form affects only the lungs. The full mold also affects the kidneys and upper airways (nose and sinuses). The lymphomatoid variant of Wegener granulomatosis typically spares the paranasal sinuses. Allergic granulomatosis (Churg–Strauss syndrome) presents as either multinodular disease or nonsegmental air-space consolidation in peripheral distribution, similar to eosinophilic pneumonia. Differential diagnosis: polyarteritis nodosa and necrotizing sarcoid granulomatosis, which may also present as multinodular disease.
Rheumatoid necrobiotic nodules ▷ *Fig. 16.54*	A rare manifestation of rheumatoid lung disease. **Diagnostic pearls:** Solitary or multiple, well-circumscribed, peripheral nodules measuring from 5 mm to 5 cm in diameter. Cavitation is common and may be thick or thin walled with a smooth inner lining.	Subcutaneous and pulmonary nodules may wax and wane simultaneously. Caplan syndrome: Necrobiotic nodules and rheumatoid arthritis in patients with coal workers' pneumoconiosis. These nodules may calcify.
Pneumatoceles ▷ *Fig. 16.55*	Solitary or multiple cystic lesions due to obstructive overinflation associated with acute pneumonia. **Diagnostic pearls:** May occur and even enlarge during healing phase. Usually resolve within weeks or months.	In children, most commonly observed in the wake of staphylococcal pneumonia. In adults, typically associated with pneumocystic pneumonia in AIDS and other types of atypical pneumonia. Traumatic pneumatoceles (pneumatocysts) may occur after toxic gas inhalation or blunt chest trauma.
Lipoid pneumonia ▷ *Fig. 16.56*	Distal chronic bronchial obstruction. **Diagnostic pearls:** Irregular mass or areas of consolidation containing regions of fat; often referred to as inflammatory pseudotumor. May persist over months and mimic bronchogenic carcinomas.	May be exogenous (i.e., chronic aspiration of oil) or endogenous (cholesterol pneumonia). Similar inflammatory mass lesions but without fat entrapment are found with solid or liquid aspirations other than oil and in postobstructive pneumonitis.
Congenital		
Bronchopulmonary sequestration (intralobular/ extralobular) ▷ *Fig. 16.57* ▷ *Fig. 16.58*	Lung tissue separated from normal lung with blood supply from symmetric arteries and without participation in ventilation. **Diagnostic pearls:** Well-defined heterogeneous mass in a posterior basal lower lobe segment, typically contiguous with the diaphragm; abnormal feeding vessels arise from the aorta, its side branches, or intercostal arteries. Often single multicystic with or without air–fluid levels due to infection resulting from communication with the bronchial tree. Sequestered segments may show air trapping (left: 66%; right: 33%).	Intralobular sequestration usually presents in adulthood and is associated with other congenital anomalies (10%). Extralobular sequestration (20% of all sequestrations) characteristically presents as a homogeneous noncavitating mass in neonates often associated with other congenital anomalies. Venous drainage via systemic veins to the right heart. Differential diagnosis: venous drainage of intralobular sequestration via pulmonary veins.
Cystic adenomatoid malformation (CAM) ▷ *Fig. 16.59*	A rare developmental anomaly of the lower respiratory tract. **Diagnostic pearls:** Solitary or multiple, thin- or less commonly, thick-walled cystic mass; occasional presence of air–fluid levels; in the majority of cases, unilateral lung involvement with contralateral shift of the mediastinum. Absence of abnormal feeding and draining vessels may differentiate this condition from sequestration.	Intralobular mass of disorganized pulmonary tissue (mesenchymal and epithelial) with or without gross cyst formation. The pathogenesis of these tumors remains unknown. Type I (50%): Single or multiple large cysts of variable size, often > 20 mm. Type II (40%): Multiple small cysts of uniform size measuring < 12 mm. Type III (10%): Solid mass without gross cyst formation (only microscopic cysts). Diagnosed in neonates and children. Associated in 25% with renal and GI abnormalities (especially types II and III). Multilobular involvement in 20%; middle lobe, however, is rarely affected.

(continues on page 620)

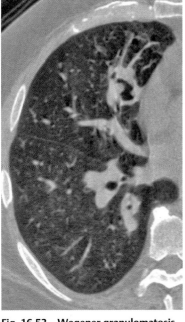

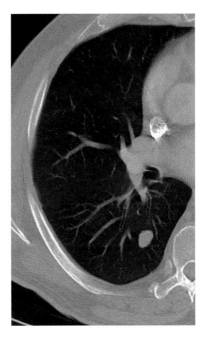

Fig. 16.54 Rheumatoid necrobiotic nodule. A well-circumscribed, solitary peripheral nodule, which was removed and histologically proven. Cavitation is absent.

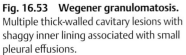

Fig. 16.53 Wegener granulomatosis. Multiple thick-walled cavitary lesions with shaggy inner lining associated with small pleural effusions.

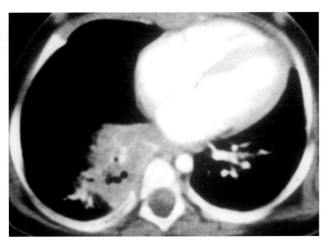

Fig. 16.55 Pneumatocele. Solitary cystic lesion in the basal right lung due to obstructive overinflation associated with an acute pneumonia.

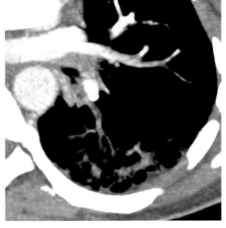

Fig. 16.56 Lipoid pneumonia. Chronic bronchial obstruction of the left lower lobe with a pneumonia-like consolidation containing regions of fat (dark spots within consolidation).

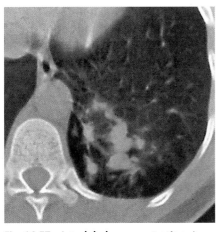

Fig. 16.57 Intralobular sequestration. A cluster of abnormal vessels in the posterobasal segment of the left lower lobe.

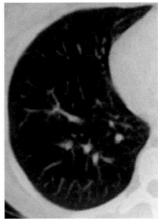

Fig. 16.58 Intralobular seques-tration. Irregular multiloculated cystic mass in the posterobasal segment of the left lower lobe.

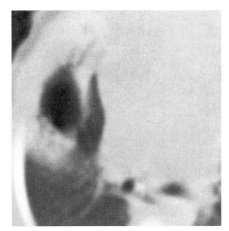

Fig. 16.59 Cystic adenomatoid malforma-tion (type I). A large cystic mass in the anter-obasal right upper lobe.

V Thorax

Table 16.2   (Cont.) Focal lung lesions

Disease	CT Findings	Comments
Congenital bronchial atresia ▷ *Fig. 16.60a, b*	Congenital atresia of a segmental bronchus with otherwise normal distal architecture. **Diagnostic pearls**: Classic triad: Mucus-filled bronchocele with hyperdistended and hypoperfused distal lung segment. Mucus-filled bronchocele appears as a round/ovoid or lobulated well-defined perihilar mass. Bronchocele nonenhancing on postcontrast scans.	Usually asymptomatic and discovered in screening chest radiographs in children and young adults. CT clearly demonstrates the anomaly and may be used to confirm the diagnosis. Characteristically affects apicoposterior segment of left upper lobe (< 50%), but also right upper lobe (20%), lower lobes (each 15%), and rarely right middle lobe (5%). Differential diagnosis: Intralobular pulmonary sequestration.
Trauma		
Pulmonary hematoma/ traumatic lung cyst ▷ *Fig. 16.61*	Typically resulting from blunt chest trauma. **Diagnostic pearls:** Single or multiple oval to spherical lesions ranging from 2 to 14 cm in diameter and presenting either as blood-isointense cystic lesions or thin-walled cavities with or without air–fluid level.	Typically observed in children and young adults after severe blunt chest trauma, but also after partial lung resection. Lesions usually develop immediately in the area of maximum impact, but may also occur hours to days after the trauma. Findings may persist for months.
Infection		
Tuberculosis (TB) ▷ *Fig. 16.62*	Focal lesion particularly in the apical/posterior segment of the upper lobes and associated with a TB infection. **Diagnostic pearls:** *Tuberculoma:* Smooth, well-defined, partly lobulated, round or oval nodule ranging in size from 1 to 4 cm. Small satellite lesions in the immediate vicinity of the lesion are common. Calcification occurs frequently. *Cavitary tuberculosis:* Thin- to moderately thick-walled cavity with smooth inner lining. Fluid levels are rare. Surrounded by either air-space consolidation (i.e., local, exudative TB) or fibrotic changes with loss of volume and bronchiectasis (local fibroproductive TB). Pleural thickening (apical cap) is commonly associated.	Complication of cavitary TB includes bronchogenic spread of infectious material resulting in an exudative bronchopneumonia. Miliary TB due to hematogenous dissemination. In 30% of adults with primary TB, cavitation is evident as air-space consolidation without site predilection, ipsilateral hilar adenopathy, and pleural effusion. In atypical mycobacterial infections (e.g., MAI), cavities are more common and usually multiple.
Histoplasmosis	A fungal disease of the lung. **Diagnostic pearls:** Histoplasmomas are one or several well-circumscribed nodules up to 3 cm in diameter with lower lobe predilection. Central calcification ("target lesion") is characteristic.	Airborne spores of the fungus *Histoplasma capsulatum* are inhaled in the lungs, affecting local granulomatous reaction. In case of cavitation, granulomas resemble tuberculomas and thus may be indistinguishable. TB has an upper lobe predilection.
Echinococcosis (hydatid disease)	Solitary round to oval cystic mass measuring up to 10 cm in diameter. **Diagnostic pearls:** Wall calcifications are not observed in lung lesions. "Crescent" sign due to air dissecting between cyst wall and surrounding lung tissue. "Water lily" sign: Cyst membrane may float on top of an air–fluid level or lie at the bottom after rupture of a cyst into a bronchus.	Infection with the larval form of *Echinococcus multilocularis* causing alveolar echinococcosis.
Amebiasis ▷ *Fig. 16.63*	A complication of a GI infection with *Entamoeba histolytica*. **Diagnostic pearls:** Right lower lobe consolidation often progressing into an abscess with a thick-walled cavity and irregular inner surface, as well as right pleural effusion.	An infectious disease caused by *Entamoeba histolytica* (a parasitic one-celled microorganism). Pulmonary manifestation is a direct extension from a liver abscess through the diaphragm.

(continues on page 622)

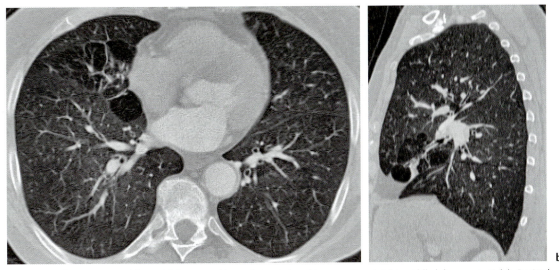

b

Fig. 16.60a, b   Congenital bronchial atresia. Hyperdistended and hypoperfused right middle lobe segment (**a**). Sagittal multiplanar reconstruction shows a mucus-filled bronchocele (**b**).

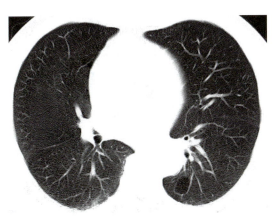

Fig. 16.61   Lung cyst. Single thin-walled oval cavity without air–fluid level in the apical left lower lobe.

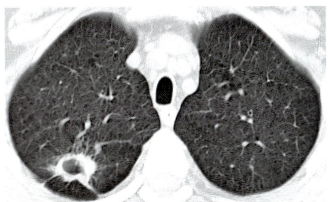

Fig. 16.62   Cavitary tuberculosis. An ill-defined, thick-walled cavitary lesion in the posterior segment of the right upper lobe. The lesion is indistinguishable from a cavitating (squamous cell) bronchogenic carcinoma.

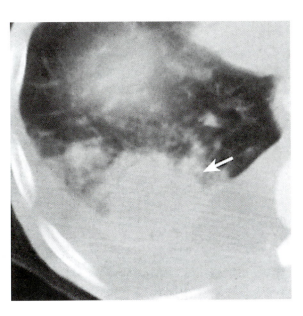

Fig. 16.63   Amebiasis. A poorly marginated right lower lobe consolidation (arrow) surrounded by patchy parenchymal infiltrations and associated with a pleural effusion.

Table 16.2 (Cont.) Focal lung lesions

Disease	CT Findings	Comments
Aspergillosis ▷ *Fig. 16.64* ▷ *Fig. 16.65* ▷ *Fig. 16.66*	Aspergillosis covers a large spectrum of diseases, including pulmonary aspergilloma, allergic bronchopulmonary aspergillosis, and invasive aspergillosis. **Diagnostic pearls:** *Aspergilloma:* Round, solid, or spongelike mass within a preexisting cavity. Frequently found in the upper lobes. Scattered or fine rimlike calcifications occur. *Allergic bronchopulmonary aspergillosis (ABPA):* Mucous plugs within dilated (sub-)segmental bronchi producing a "cluster of grapes" or an inverted Y or V appearance. Often postobstructive airway disease. *Invasive aspergillosis:* One, more often several ill-defined pulmonary nodules sitting at the distal end of a bronchus. Surrounding halo of low attenuation due to hemorrhage (invasion of vessels). Cavitation may affect an air crescent sign (air surrounding a sequestrum of necrotic lung) or a large empty cavity.	Aspergillomas are associated with chronic cavitary lung disease, particularly TB. May cause hemoptysis. ABPA is common in patients with asthma and cystic fibrosis. May result in widespread bronchiectasis and fibrosis. Invasive aspergillosis develops particularly in immunocompromised patients. Bronchocentric granulomatosis may be considered a variant of ABPA and appears both clinically and radiologically in a similar fashion.
Coccidioidomycosis ▷ *Fig. 16.67*	Fungal infection caused by *Coccidioides immitis*. **Diagnostic pearls:** Solitary or multiple nodules between 0.5 and 5 cm in size (coccidioidomas). Predilection for middle and upper lung zones. May evolve into thin-walled cavities, typically located in the anterior segment of the upper lobes.	Primary coccidioidomycosis presents as consolidation preferentially in lower lobes with ipsilateral hilar adenopathy and small pleural effusion in 20% each. Disseminated coccidioidomycosis presents with a miliary pattern.
Actinomycosis, nocardiosis, blastomycosis, cryptococcosis, mucormycosis ▷ *Fig. 16.68*	Rare granulomatous pulmonary infections. **Diagnostic pearls:** Large consolidation or mass measuring up to 10 cm in diameter with primarily lower lobe involvement. Development of large thick-walled cavities is a common feature.	Usually in debilitated or immunocompromised patients. A common complication of actinomycosis and nocardiosis is empyema with subsequent rib and chest wall involvement.
Septic emboli ▷ *Fig. 16.69a, b*	Multiple well- or ill-defined, round or wedge-shaped subpleural lesions, more often with lower lobe predilection. **Diagnostic pearls:** Involvement of the subpleural space and/or vessels entering the lesion is indicative of hematogenous spread. Thin-walled cavitation is frequent. Target sign: Air–fluid level and central hypoattenuation representing necrotic tissue highly suspicious of superinfection.	Most commonly caused by *Staphylococcus* or *Streptococcus*. Often affects patients younger than 40. Predisposing factors include IV drug abuse, indwelling catheters, hemodialysis shunts, septic thrombophlebitis, endocarditis, osteomyelitis, and pharyngeal and pelvic infections.
Round pneumonia	Rare appearance of pneumonia. **Diagnostic pearls:** Spherical air-space consolidation with air bronchograms and fluffy borders. Always in a posterior location, typically affecting the lower lobe.	Caused by *Haemophilus*, *Streptococcus*, or *Pneumococcus*. Predominantly observed in children.

(continues on page 624)

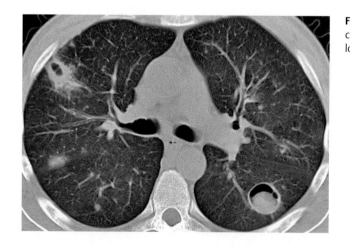

Fig. 16.64 Aspergilloma. Round, solid mass within a preexisting cyst in the apical left lower lobe. Also visible is an invasive aspergillosis with central cavitation in the middle lobe.

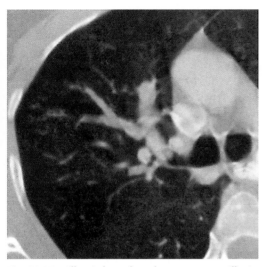

Fig. 16.65 Allergic bronchopulmonary aspergillosis (ABPA). Mucus plugs within dilated middle lobe bronchi producing an inverted Y or V appearance.

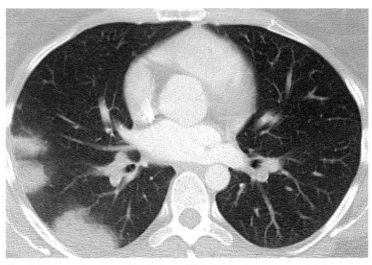

Fig. 16.66 Invasive aspergillosis. Several ill-defined pulmonary consolidations at the distal end of right upper lobe bronchi. Note the surrounding halo of low attenuation due to hemorrhage (see also **Fig. 16.63**).

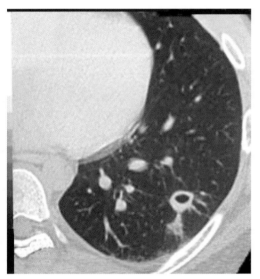

Fig. 16.67 Coccidioidomycosis. Thick-walled solitary cavity located in the upper segment of the left lower lobe.

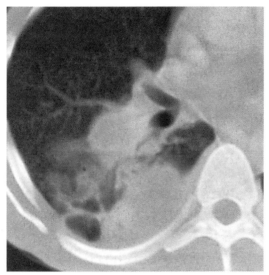

Fig. 16.68 Nocardiosis. Large consolidation consisting of different-sized nodular lesions in the dorsal right lower lobe partly evolving into thick-walled cavities.

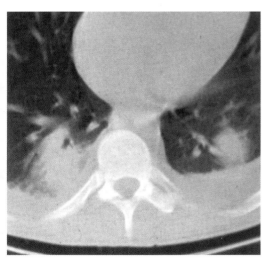
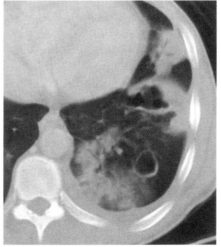

b

Fig. 16.69a, b Septic emboli. Bilateral presence of ill-defined round to wedge-shaped subpleural lesions in the lower lobes (**a**). Ill-defined peripheral lesions and a small thin-walled cavitary lesion in the left lower lobe (**b**). Pleural effusions are present in both patients.

Table 16.2 (Cont.) Focal lung lesions

Disease	CT Findings	Comments
Lung abscess ▷ *Fig. 16.70*	Necrosis of pulmonary tissue and formation of cavities (> 2 cm) containing necrotic debris or fluid caused by microbial infection. **Diagnostic pearls:** Locally decreased CT density surrounded by a consolidation is characteristic prior to cavitation. Also characteristic are a hyperattenuating wall and a hypoattenuating (necrotic) center on postcontrast scans; and thick-walled cavitation with a shaggy inner lining in the acute stage, becoming smoother over time. Intracavitary air–fluid levels are common. Occasionally strands of residual lung tissue traversing the cavity may be present.	Often due to aspiration, which may occur during altered consciousness. Alcoholism is the most common condition predisposing to lung abscesses. Other causes include necrotizing pneumonias, bronchial obstruction with infection, and infected pulmonary infarcts. Lung abscess is considered primary (60%) when it results from an existing lung parenchymal process and is termed secondary when it complicates another process (e.g., vascular) or follows rupture of an extrapulmonary abscess into the lung.

Benign neoplasms

Disease	CT Findings	Comments
Hamartoma ▷ *Fig. 16.71*	Benign neoplasm composed of cartilage, connective tissue, muscle, fat, and bone. **Diagnostic pearls:** Solitary, well-defined, often lobulated lesion in the lung periphery, measuring up to 10 cm in diameter. Endobronchial location in 10%. In 30%, stippled or conglomerate ("popcorn") calcifications. Focal intratumoral fat collections in 50%.	The most common benign neoplasm of the lung and the most common cause of solitary pulmonary nodule (5%–8%). More common in men (preponderance 2:1 to 3:1). Peak incidence 60 to 70 y. Usually asymptomatic and discovered incidentally. May rarely be associated with hemoptysis and cough. Multiple pulmonary fibroleiomyomata hamartomas is a related but extremely rare condition.
Papilloma (papillomatosis)	A benign lesion of the larynx and trachea. **Diagnostic pearls:** Multiple or, less commonly, solitary endotracheal and endobronchial lesions with frequent cavitation. Obstructive pneumonitis and atelectasis are often associated with endobronchial location.	Usually arise in the larynx and spread distally In children and young adults, presenting with hoarseness and occasionally hemoptysis. Associated with human papilloma virus (HPV). Recurrent respiratory papillomatosis is a rare, but acknowledged, risk factor for pulmonary squamous cell carcinoma.
Bronchiectasis ▷ *Fig. 16.72* ▷ *Fig. 16.73*	A disease state defined by localized, irreversible dilation of part of the bronchial tree. **Diagnostic pearls:** *Cystic/saccular:* Thick-walled cystic spaces measuring up to 3 cm in diameter, usually with variable fluid levels. Cysts are either grouped together in a cluster or strung together in a linear fashion. *Tubular/cylindrical:* Thick-walled, dilated, nontapering crowded tubular structures ("tram lines"). "Gloved finger" appearance when filled with mucus. "Signet ring" appearance when viewed in cross section with a dilated, thick-walled bronchus producing the ring and the accompanying pulmonary artery branch the signet. *Varicose:* Thick-walled, dilated bronchi with beaded contour.	Bronchiectasis is classified as an obstructive lung disease, along with emphysema, bronchitis, and cystic fibrosis. **Congenital:** Kartagener or immotile cilia syndrome (situs inversus, sinusitis, and bronchiectasis), cystic fibrosis, chronic granulomatosis disease of childhood, alpha-1-antitrypsin deficiency. **Postinfectious:** Chronic granulomatous disease (e.g., TB), measles, pertussis, Swyer–James syndrome (unilateral hyperlucent lung with decreased volume, air trapping, small ipsilateral hilum, and varicose bronchiectasis). **Postobstructive:** Aspiration and fumes inhalation. **Cicatricial bronchiectasis** is associated with advanced pulmonary fibrosis. **Reversible bronchiectasis** refers to temporary dilation during pneumonia.
Bullae ▷ *Fig. 16.74*	Bullae are cystic spaces > 1 cm in diameter confined by a hairline-thin wall that is visible in its entire circumference. **Diagnostic pearls:** May be isolated or a component of advanced fibrotic lung disease or emphysema. Single large bulla occasionally isolated in the upper lobe. May also be secondary to an evacuated pulmonary hematoma, old abscess, or bronchial cyst.	Pneumothorax is a frequent complication. Differential diagnosis: focal emphysema *Blebs* are cystic spaces, within the visceral pleura, usually above the apices, and not associated with lung destruction. They are rare and often the cause of a spontaneous pneumothorax.
Bronchogenic cyst ▷ *Fig. 16.75*	Developmental foregut anomalies usually located within the mediastinum. **Diagnostic pearls:** Solitary, well-defined, round or oval, homogeneous mass of water density (50%) or higher. Measuring up to several centimeters in diameter. Most commonly located in the central (perihilar) portions of a lower lobe. Communication with the bronchial system occurs in 30% of cases, resulting in a thin-walled cystic lesion with or without an air–fluid level.	Although typically asymptomatic, infection or compression of adjacent structures may become prominent. Communication with the adjacent airways typically results in an infection, in which case the cyst fluid is replaced by pus and air. Infected congenital and acquired cysts (e.g., following lung abscess) cannot be differentiated except for a more widespread distribution of the latter.

(continues on page 626)

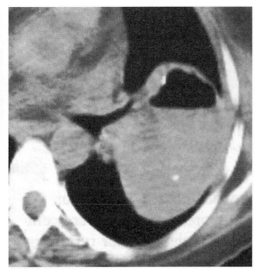

Fig. 16.70   Lung abscess. A thin-walled, smooth cavity with an air–fluid level in the left lower lobe.

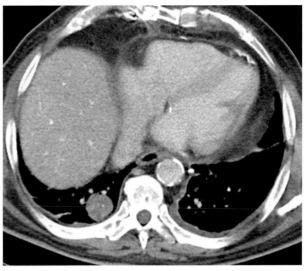

Fig. 16.71   Hamartoma. A peripheral pulmonary nodule with a discrete calcification and focal intratumoral fat collections.

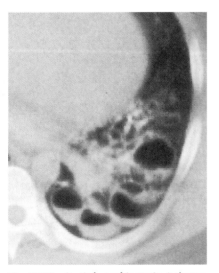

Fig. 16.72   Cystic bronchiectasis. A cluster of thick-walled cysts in the left lower lobe with variable fluid levels.

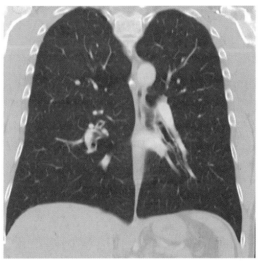

Fig. 16.73   Tubular bronchiectasis. The bronchiectasis appears as a thick-walled, dilated, nontapering tubular structure in the lingula resembling "tram lines."

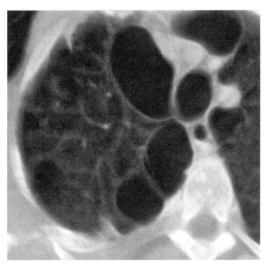

Fig. 16.74   Bullae. Large cystic spaces are evident along the mediastinal pleura. They are confined by a hairline-thin wall, which is visible in its entire circumference.

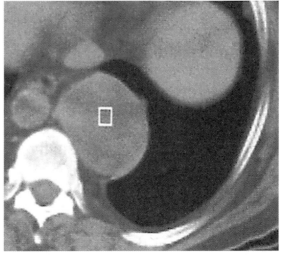

Fig. 16.75   Bronchogenic cyst. A solitary, well-defined, homogeneous round mass of water density is seen adjacent to the mediastinal pleura.

V Thorax

Table 16.2   (Cont.) Focal lung lesions

Disease	CT Findings	Comments
Mesenchymal tumors	A group of endobronchial or small peripheral neoplasms with similar CT features but different histologic origin. **Diagnostic pearls:** Well-defined small endobronchial or small peripheral nodules. Except for endobronchial lipomas (fat), findings are nonspecific.	Endobronchial lesions include granular cell myoblastomas, lipomas, leiomyomas, and lack of extrabronchial extension. Small peripheral nodules comprise fibromas, neurogenic tumors, and leiomyomas. Malignant variants of these tumors may very rarely also originate in the lung but usually represent hematogenous spread metastases from another region of the body.

Malignant neoplasms		
Bronchial adenoma ▷ *Fig. 16.76* ▷ *Fig. 16.77*	A group of bronchial neoplasms that resemble each other grossly but are microscopically different. **Diagnostic pearls:** Eighty percent arise within lobular, or (sub-) segmental bronchi, presenting as an endobronchial mass with frequent extension beyond the bronchial wall. Postobstructive atelectasis and pneumonitis are the most common presentations. Postobstructive hyperinflation is less common. Peripheral adenomas (20%) are well-defined round lesions measuring 2 to 5 cm in diameter. Contrast enhancement may be considerable.	Diagnosed usually in patients between 30 and 50 y of age, often presenting with hemoptysis. Comprise a variety of histologic subtypes, including carcinoids (90%), cylindromas (adenoid cystic carcinomas), mucoepidermoid carcinomas, and pleomorphic adenomas. These locally invasive, low-grade malignant tumors metastasize to regional lymph nodes and even distant sites. Kulchitsky cells are found in several of theses neoplasms, including carcinoids, atypical carcinoids, and small cell carcinomas in order of increasing malignancy.
Bronchogenic carcinoma ▷ *Fig. 16.78* ▷ *Fig. 16.79* ▷ *Fig. 16.80* ▷ *Fig. 16.81* ▷ *Fig. 16.82*	A group of primary lung neoplasms with similar staging system but different histologic architecture. **Diagnostic pearls:** Characterized by solitary peripheral or central mass, usually with irregular or spiculated border. Thick-walled cavitation with an irregular inner lining most commonly occurs with squamous cell carcinoma (15%). Eccentric calcifications are found in 5% and are caused by engulfment of a calcified granuloma or tumor necrosis. Diffusely calcified mucinous adenocarcinomas are extremely rare. Distal airway obstruction presenting as segmental, lobular, or lung atelectasis, and obstructive pneumonitis is found in 30% of the cases. Air bronchograms are absent. Endobronchial lesions or circumferential bronchial narrowing/occlusion are commonly demonstrated in central tumors. Pulmonary vessels may be occluded or contain tumor thrombi. Unilateral hilar adenopathy with or without mediastinal involvement is common and may be the only manifestation in 5% of cases, especially in small cell carcinomas. Pleural effusions are present in 10% of cases at presentation. Localized or diffuse pleural thickening is occasionally found with peripheral tumors. Direct tumor extension into the chest wall, ribs, and vertebrae may also be evident in more advanced cases.	**Classification:** 1. Squamous cell (epidermoid) carcinoma (35%): Endobronchial lesion with airway obstruction (two thirds) or peripheral nodule (one third). 2. Adenocarcinoma (35%): Peripheral mass. 3. Small cell carcinoma (20%): Often small lung lesion with large hilar and mediastinal adenopathy. 4. Large cell carcinoma (15%): Large bulky peripheral mass. **TNM staging:** **T0:** No evidence of tumor **T1:** Tumor < 3 cm **T2:** Tumor > 3 cm or tumor with visceral pleural invasion or associated with obstructive pneumonia/atelectasis **T3:** Tumor < 2 cm from carina, or invasion of parietal pleural, chest wall, diaphragm, mediastinal pleura, or pericardium **T4:** Invasion of carina, heart, great vessels, trachea, esophagus, vertebral body, or malignant effusion **N0:** No lymph node metastases **N1:** Peribronchial and/or ipsilateral hilar node involvement **N2:** Ipsilateral mediastinal node involvement **N3:** Contralateral hilar and/or mediastinal node involvement **M0:** No distant metastases **M1:** Distant metastases (bone, adrenals, liver, kidneys, brain, lungs, etc.) **Staging (1–3A) resectable, 3B-4 nonresectable):** **1:** T12, N0, M0 **2:** T1–2, N1, M0 **3A:** T3, or T1–3, N2, M0 **3B:** T1–3, N3, T4, N0–2, M0 **4:** T4, N3, M0, or M1 **Pancoast tumor** (superior pulmonary sulcus tumor (▷ *Fig. 16.82*) (4%): Presents classically with pain, rib destruction, Horner syndrome, and atrophy of hand muscles.

(continues on page 628)

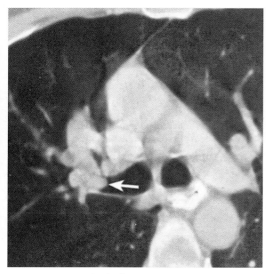

Fig. 16.76   Bronchial adenoma, endobronchial type (carcinoid). The adenoma causes enlargement of the right upper lobe bronchus (arrow) and may be indistinguishable from other endobronchial lesions, such as papilloma and metastasis (see also **Fig. 16.86**).

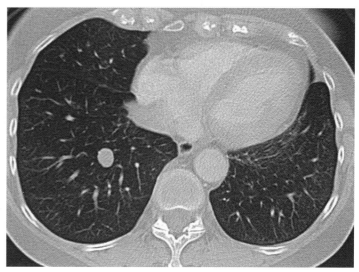

Fig. 16.77   Bronchial adenoma, peripheral type (carcinoid). The adenoma appears as a well-defined, peripheral round lesion.

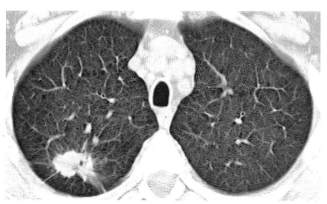

Fig. 16.78   Peripheral bronchogenic carcinoma (squamous cell carcinoma). Tumor < 3 cm in diameter. Also noted are beginning central cavitation, the presence of a pleural tail, and peritumoral carcinomatosis, all typical signs of malignancy (T1N0M0).

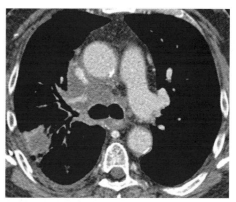

Fig. 16.79   Peripheral bronchogenic carcinoma (adenocarcinoma). Tumor infiltration of the visceral pleural and extensive ipsilateral mediastinal lymphadenopathy. Pleura effusion separates visceral from parietal pleura (T2N2M0).

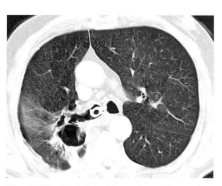

Fig. 16.80   Peripheral bronchogenic carcinoma (squamous cell carcinoma). A large irregular cavitating mass in the apical right lower lobe, < 2 cm from the carina, with distinct peritumoral carcinomatosis and invasion of the parietal pleural (T3N0M0).

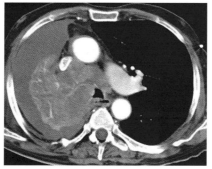

Fig. 16.81   Central bronchogenic carcinoma (small cell carcinoma). Large endobronchial mass is evident within the right main bronchus, already bulging into the trachea. Associated with this are complete atelectasis of the right lung, infiltration and occlusion of the pulmonary artery, extensive mediastinal lymphadenopathy, and concomitant pleural effusion (T4N3M0).

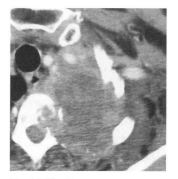

Fig. 16.82   Pancoast tumor. A large inhomogeneous mass in the apex of the left lung with destruction of the adjacent vertebral body and posterior rib.

V Thorax

Table 16.2 (Cont.) Focal lung lesions

Disease	CT Findings	Comments
Alveolar cell (bronchoalveolar) carcinoma ▷ *Fig. 16.83*	The least common of primary pulmonary carcinomas, and controversial as to its cell of origin. **Diagnostic pearls:** The local form (75%) presents as a peripheral well-defined nodule when small (1–4 cm). Linear strands (pleural tags) may extend from a subpleural nodule to the pleura, representing a desmoplastic reaction with pleural indrawing. Larger lesions (> 4 cm) appear heterogeneous with air bronchograms and irregular margins (sunburst appearance). Often opacified vessels visible within the lesion on postcontrast scans. May be multifocal.	Ultrastructurally, all tumors are similarly composed of large cells with abundant cytoplasm and small nuclei in close contact with each other. Pleural effusions and metastases to local lymph nodes and distant sites occur but are uncommon. Diffuse form (25%) presents as air-space consolidation often involving both lung fields.
Metastases ▷ *Fig. 16.84* ▷ *Fig. 16.85* ▷ *Fig. 16.86* ▷ *Fig. 16.87* ▷ *Fig. 16.88*	Focal nodules primarily found in the presence of a hematogenous spread. **Diagnostic pearls:** Pulmonary nodules range in size from miliary lesions to large well-defined masses ("cannonball" metastases). Vessels entering the lesions are observed in ~30% of the cases. Hilar or mediastinal lymphadenopathy is usually absent. Cavitation is rare, but it is characteristic of squamous cell carcinoma originating from the head, neck, or cervix. Calcifications are also rare and occur typically in mucinous adenocarcinomas, osteosarcomas, synovial sarcomas, thyroid carcinomas (papillary and medullary), and malignant germ cell tumors.	A miliary pattern is usually associated with highly vascular metastases originating from carcinoma of the breast, thyroid, kidney, prostate, soft tissue, and chorion or bone sarcomas. "Cannonball" metastases are typically associated with renal and colonic carcinomas, melanomas, and sarcomas. Ill-defined metastases due to hemorrhage are common in Kaposi sarcoma and choriocarcinoma. Endobronchial metastases presenting with airway obstruction occur with bronchogenic, renal, breast, and colon carcinomas and melanomas. Solitary metastases are uncommon and typically originate from carcinomas of the colon (especially rectosigmoid area), kidney, testicles, and breast, sarcomas (especially bone), and melanoma.
Lymphoma ▷ *Fig. 16.89*	Primary pulmonary disease is a rare disease, more often secondary pulmonary lymphoma. **Diagnostic pearls:** The most common pulmonary manifestation is a coarse bilateral reticulonodular pattern resembling lymphangitis carcinomatosis (see also **Fig. 16.46, p. 615**). Alternatively, multiple rather than solitary, poorly defined nodules or air-space consolidation with air bronchograms are found. Pulmonary findings are usually associated with or subsequent to hilar and mediastinal lymph node involvement. Endobronchial lesions that may be associated with obstructive airway disease are rare. Pleural effusion occurs in 30% of cases and may be associated with circumscribed subpleural thickening. **Primary pulmonary lymphoma:** Nodules with irregular margins or focal areas of consolidation, with air bronchograms. **Secondary pulmonary lymphoma:** Thickening of interlobular septa, discrete pulmonary nodules, and areas of consolidation. **Hodgkin disease:** Thin- or thick-walled cavities.	Primary pulmonary lymphoma is usually non-Hodgkin type; secondary pulmonary lymphoma is more common in patients with recurrent disease. Recurrent or secondary pulmonary involvement may result from direct mediastinal nodal extension, from lymphatic or hematogenous dissemination from distant sites, or from foci of parenchymal lymphoid tissue. **Pseudolymphoma** presents as localized interstitial or air-space disease with air bronchograms but without lymphadenopathy. It is a benign lymphomatous infiltration and can be considered as a localized form of LIP. **Plasmacytoma** (primary of the lung) and secondary multiple myeloma manifestations are rare (1%) and similar to lymphoma.

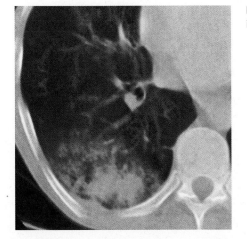

Fig. 16.83 Local alveolar cell carcinoma. An ill-defined, patchy peripheral consolidation is seen in the right lower lobe.

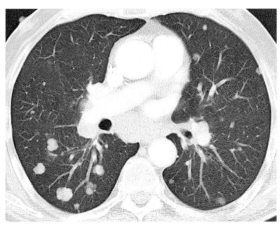

Fig. 16.84 Multiple lobulated metastases. Multiple lobulated metastases seen in a patient with breast carcinoma.

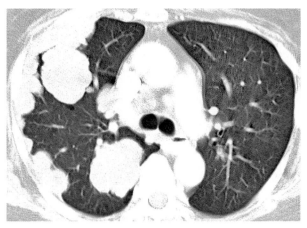

Fig. 16.85 Cannonball metastases. Cannonball metastases seen in a patient with soft tissue sarcoma.

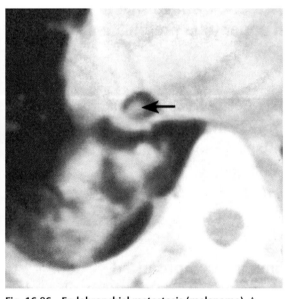

Fig. 16.86 Endobronchial metastasis (melanoma). A nodular lesion in the right lower lobe bronchus (arrow). Densities in the right lower lobe are caused by obstructive pneumonia (melanoma).

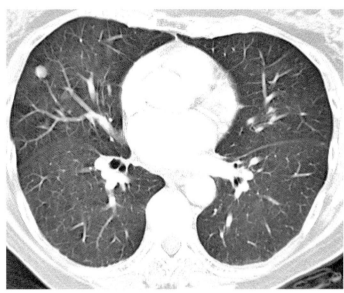

Fig. 16.87 Solitary metastasis (colon carcinoma). Well-defined round lesion in the right middle lobe.

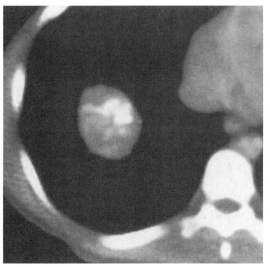

Fig. 16.88 Calcified pulmonary metastasis. A nodule with irregular calcifications is seen in the right lower lobe (chondrosarcoma).

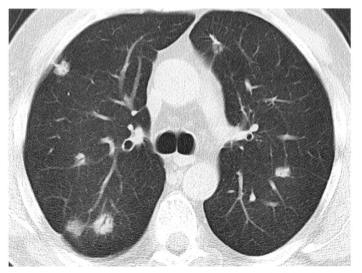

Fig. 16.89 Primary pulmonary lymphoma. Several poorly defined nodular densities with air bronchograms.

17 Pleura, Chest Wall, and Diaphragm

Christopher Herzog and Francis A. Burgener

On computed tomography (CT) scans, the pleura appears as a 1- to 2-mm-thick line between lung parenchyma and visualized ribs. Starting from the inside, this line represents the visceral and parietal pleura, extrapleural fat, endothoracic fascia, and innermost intercostal muscle. The latter is absent in the paravertebral region, resulting in a distinctly thinner lining. On axial scans, the most posterior ribs are always the lowest in the thoracic cage, with each more anterior rib arising from the level of a vertebral body above. The pleural line may be distinctly thicker in obese patients due to excessive extrapleural fat. This condition can usually be differentiated from pleural disease by its perfect symmetry.

A *pneumothorax* (**Fig. 17.1**) is easily diagnosed on CT scans even in the presence of extensive soft tissue emphysema. Other air collections, such as subpleural blebs, pneumopericardium, and mediastinal emphysema, can also readily be differentiated from an adjacent loculated pneumothorax with CT.

Pleural effusions (transudative, exudative, and chylous) have a homogeneous, near-water density and cannot be differentiated by CT (**Fig. 17.2**). An acute hemothorax, by contrast, commonly appears rather inhomogeneous, with a CT density greater than water, especially in its most dependent locations (hemoglobin). Pleural fluid initially collects in the most dependent portion of the pleural space, which is posteromedial and caudal to the lung base in the supine position. Small amounts of fluid usually appear crescent- or lenticularlike, but it may also be impossible to differentiate a discrete pleural effusion from pleural thickening. In these cases, freely mobile fluid can be diagnosed by obtaining an additional set of images in a prone or lateral decubitus position. Furthermore, after intravenous contrast medium administration, a thickened, inflamed, or neoplastic pleura enhances, whereas purely fibrotic pleural thickening and pleural fluid do not. Larger pleural effusions extend toward the lateral chest wall and may enter the major fissure, where the fluid tapers medially, producing a characteristic "beak" sign. Large pleural effusions may also compress the lower lobe and displace it

anteriorly. The collapsed lower lobe thus seems to float on the pleural fluid. In this situation, the noninflated posterior edge of the lower lobe may easily be mistaken for the diaphragm with pleural fluid posteriorly and peritoneal fluid anteriorly. Similarly, inversion of a hemidiaphragm by massive pleural effusion may also simulate intra-abdominal fluid. However, a correct diagnosis usually is possible by analyzing the relationship of both fluid collection and the lower lobe on subsequent transverse images and multiplanar reformations.

Both pleural and peritoneal fluid presents as an arcuate or semilunar density displacing liver and spleen inward from the adjacent chest wall (**Figs. 17.2, 17.3**). The entity of the fluid collections can be assessed based on a variety of different criteria. Fluid outside (i.e., peripheral to) the diaphragm is always pleural, whereas fluid inside the diaphragm is peritoneal. Pleural fluid may surround the lung, whereas peritoneal fluid may be surrounded by the lung bases. In the posterior costophrenic angle, pleural fluid is posterior to the diaphragm, causing anterolateral displacement of the crus, whereas peritoneal fluid is anterior to the diaphragm. When scrolling through transverse images in a craniocaudal direction, pleural fluid gradually diminishes, whereas peritoneal fluid increases in size, progressively extending lateral to the liver and spleen. Fluid seen posterior to the liver is within the pleural space, as the peritoneal space does not extend into this region (the bare area of the liver is not covered by peritoneum). The interface of pleural fluid with the liver or spleen is hazy, whereas with peritoneal fluid, it is sharp.

Unilateral or bilateral pleural effusions not associated with any other signs of intrathoracic disease are often tuberculous in younger patients and predominantly neoplastic in the elderly. Neoplastic effusions are found with metastases, lymphoma, and leukemia and in the Meigs–Salmon syndrome. The latter describes a nonmalignant pleural effusion and ascites in the presence of benign or malignant ovarian tumors, or occasionally a uterine leiomyoma. Pleural effusions may also be the sole finding of viral or

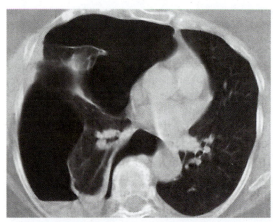

Fig. 17.1 Pneumothorax. A large right tension pneumothorax with shifting of heart and mediastinum to the left. The collapsed right lung still adheres locally to the lateral and posterior chest wall. There is a discrete fluid level in the posterior right pleural cavity.

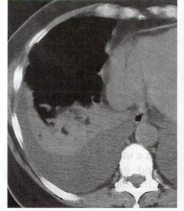 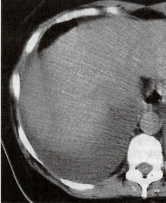

Fig. 17.2a, b Pleural effusion. Right pleural effusion presents as a low-density, crescent-shaped lesion posterior to the lung base that has a higher density because of compression atelectasis and edema (**a**). More caudally, the pleural effusion encircles the posteromedial aspect of the liver, creating a hazy interface (**b**).

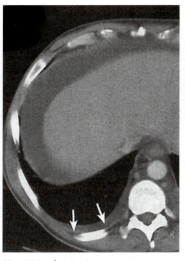 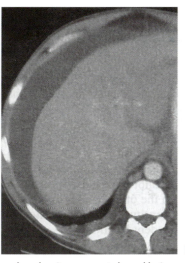

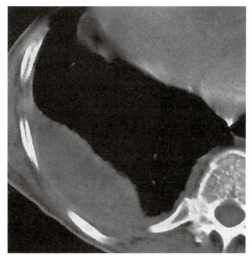

b

Fig. 17.3a, b   Ascites. Ascites presents as a low-density, crescent-shaped lesion anteromedial to the liver with sharp interface (**a**). Note also a small right pleural effusion (arrows). More caudally, the ascites extends to the right side of the liver but spares its posteromedial margin (**b**).

Fig. 17.4   Loculated empyema. A low-density, lenticular-shaped lesion between high-attenuating thickened layers of parietal and visceral pleura ("split pleura" sign).

mycoplasmatic infections. Regarding collagen vascular diseases, both rheumatoid disease and systemic lupus erythematosus (primary and drug-induced) often present with pleural effusion as the only intrathoracic manifestation. Congestive heart failure is the most common cause of pleural effusion, but it usually is associated with an enlarged cardiac silhouette and other signs of cardiac decompensation. In Dressler syndrome, pericardiac and pleural effusions typically develop 2 to 3 weeks after myocardial infarction or pericardial surgery. However, occasionally they may occur months or even years after the causative episode.

Traumatic and postsurgical pleural effusions are common, but both history and associated findings are usually diagnostic. Patients with asbestos exposure occasionally present with pleural effusion alone. A variety of abdominal diseases, such as pancreatitis, subphrenic abscess, ascites of any etiology, renal failure, and cirrhosis, are frequently associated with pleural effusion, but in these conditions, the primary cause is usually clearly evident on CT. Myxedema, familial Mediterranean fever (familial paroxysmal polyserositis), and primary lymphedema are rare inherited conditions presenting with pleural effusion as the only intrathoracic abnormality.

Empyema is a purulent pleural infection usually secondary to a bacterial pneumonia. Other less frequent extrapulmonary sources include bacteremia, subphrenic abscess, spondylitis, thoracotomy, and penetrating chest trauma. An empyema has to be differentiated from a parapneumonic effusion, which is an uninfected (sympathetic) serous exudate in pneumonia that resolves spontaneously. It results from increased permeability of the inflamed visceral pleura. Pulmonary infections that frequently extend beyond the pleural space into the chest wall include actinomycosis and nocardiosis, and occasionally tuberculosis (TB), blastomycosis, and coccidioidomycosis. Large empyemas may compress the neighboring lung, resulting in gradual displacement and bowing of the adjacent pulmonary vessels and bronchi. The visceral and parietal pleural layer appears relatively thin, smooth, and of uniform thickness but strongly enhances on postcontrast scans. Nonenhancing pus thus becomes clearly visible between both pleural layers ("split pleura" sign). The shape of the empyema, as well as a possible air–fluid level, changes when moving the patient from a supine to a prone or decubitus position.

A *loculated empyema* (**Fig. 17.4**) is trapped between the visceral and parietal pleura and thus is lenticular, elliptical, or round on cross-sectional images. It is sharply demarcated from lung parenchyma and forms an obtuse angle with the chest wall.

In an organizing empyema, the walls may become thickened and eventually even calcified. Demonstration of fluid collections within the thickened pleural peel is highly suspicious of a still ongoing and active infection.

An empyema has to be differentiated from a peripheral lung abscess abutting the pleural surface (**Fig. 17.5**). Lung abscesses tend to be spherical without change in shape and with equidimensional air–fluid level when the patient is scanned in different positions. The margins of a lung abscess are irregularly

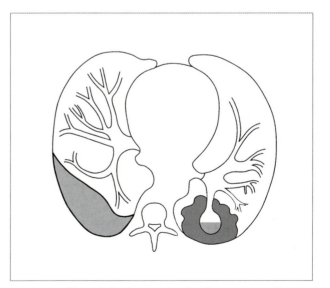

Fig. 17.5   Differentiation between loculated empyema and lung abscess. An empyema (right lung base) is lenticular-shaped and well-defined by smooth, uniform margins (split pleura sign). It thus creates obtuse angles with the chest wall and displaces lung parenchyma. A lung abscess (left lung base) has a more spherical shape, typically presents with one or more cavities, and usually shows an air–fluid level. It creates acute angles with the chest wall, and the outer margin appears ill-defined and irregular. Often vessels can be observed entering the lesion.

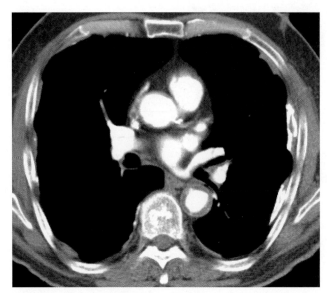

Fig. 17.6   Asbestos-related pleural disease. Calcified plaques are attached to the left pleura and noncalcified plaques to the right pleura. On soft tissue CT scans, calcified plaques may easily be mistaken for ribs.

shaped, poorly defined, and may contain areas of cavitation. The lesion characteristically forms an acute angle with the chest wall. Pulmonary vessels and bronchi seem to enter the abscess rather than being displaced by it. On postcontrast scans, the walls of a lung abscess usually strongly contrast with the necrotic low-density material in the center.

Pleural thickening is primarily caused by fibrosis and neoplasia. Pleural fibrosis is a common sequela of hemothorax, empyema, TB, and exposure to asbestos or talc. In all these conditions, focal to extensive pleural calcifications are frequent, and, with the exception of asbestos and talc inhalation, the pleural fibrosis predominantly affects the visceral pleura. Other causes of nonneoplastic pleural thickening are fungal infections, chronic polyarthritis, radiation therapy, organizing pleural effusions, sarcoidosis, and, rarely, splenosis (posttraumatic implantation of splenic tissue on the left pleura). Neoplastic pleural thickening is associated with mesotheliomas (benign and malignant), metastasis, lymphoma, local invasion

from bronchogenic carcinomas (especially Pancoast tumors), and malignant thymomas.

Extensive pleural thickening caused by fibrosis may result in encasement of the lung, resulting in restriction and loss of volume. A thickened layer of extrapleural fat often becomes visible at this stage, separating the parietal pleura, which may be calcified, from the rib cage.

Asbestos-related pleural disease (**Figs. 17.6, 17.7**) is almost invariably bilateral. Pleural plaques (smooth focal thickening of the parietal pleura) are characteristically visible adjacent to the posterior and lateral inner surface of the sixth to tenth ribs. The pleura between adjacent ribs is often spared ("skip lesions"). Diffuse, more or less uniform pleural thickening in the lower hemithorax is another less frequent manifestation. Focal visceral pleural fibrosis may occur and cause interlobular fissural thickening, occasionally simulating pulmonary nodules or arousing a round atelectasis. Pleural plaques with or without calcifications frequently are evident in the diaphragmatic pleura but typically spare the costophrenic angles. Calcifications range from punctate, nodular, or linear densities to complete encirclement of the lower portions of the lung. Diaphragmatic plaques may occasionally be missed on transverse CT slices if they lie in the scanning plane. Mediastinal and paravertebral pleural plaques and thickening also are common CT findings.

Benign (fibrous) mesotheliomas (**Fig. 17.8**) usually arise from the visceral pleura. They present as a localized, sharply defined soft tissue mass, sometimes with slightly lobulated margins, ranging from 2 to 14 cm in diameter. Smaller lesions are homogeneous on CT, whereas larger lesions may have an inhomogeneous appearance, particularly on postcontrast scans, due to necrosis, hemorrhage, cyst formation, and calcification. Occasionally, a small pleural effusion is associated.

Malignant mesothelioma (**Figs. 17.9, 17.10**) is a highly malignant neoplasm and carries an extremely poor prognosis. The majority of cases are found in patients with known asbestos exposure. It presents as diffuse nodular or plaquelike pleural thickening that eventually encases the entire lung. Hemorrhagic pleural effusions are commonly associated and may mask irregular, nodular pleural thickening caused by the malignancy. CT images obtained from different scan positions (e.g., prone and supine or lateral decubitus) usually allow pleural fluid collection to be differentiated from mesothelioma. In the presence of malignant

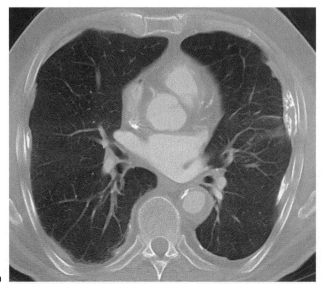

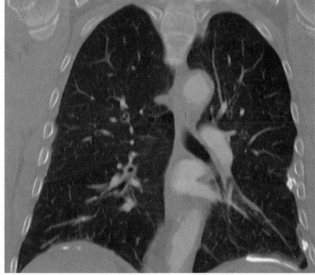

a

Fig. 17.7a, b   Asbestos-related pleural disease. Same patient as in **Fig. 17.6.** Calcified pleural plaques become more evident when applying a lung window (**a**). Coronal multiplanar reconstruction shows involvement not only of the left lateral chest wall but also the left diaphragmatic pleura (**b**).

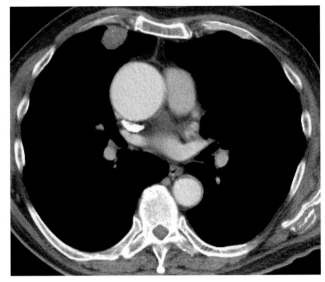

Fig. 17.8 Benign mesothelioma. A localized, well-defined soft tissue mass adheres to the visceral pleural.

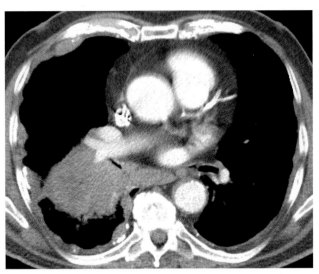

Fig. 17.10 Malignant mesothelioma. A bandlike soft tissue mass spreads along the dorsal and lateral circumference of the pleura. High-attenuation of some of the plaques indicates malignant transformation. Concomitant near-atelectasis of the right lower lobe is due to mediastinal tumor infiltration.

mesothelioma, even large effusions frequently do not cause significant mediastinal shifting to the contralateral side, most likely due to tumor encasement of the affected hemithorax. Significant contrast enhancement of mesotheliomas is often helpful to differentiate tumor from both asbestos-related pleural thickening and loculated pleural effusions. The tumor typically spreads by local invasion into fissures and adjacent structures, such as the ipsilateral lung, mediastinum, pericardium, diaphragm, lateral chest wall, and contralateral hemithorax. Hematogenous metastases are uncommon.

Pleural metastases (**Figs. 17.11, 17.12**) presenting with nodular pleural thickening and effusions are often indistinguishable from malignant mesothelioma. Bilateral involvement, as well as the absence of both asbestos-related pleural disease and pulmonary asbestosis, favors metastatic disease. Besides bronchogenic carcinoma (especially Pancoast tumor) and malignant

thymoma, which both invade the pleura by contiguous spread, hematogenous pleural metastases most frequently originate from carcinoma of the breast, kidney, ovary, and gastrointestinal tract. Pleural lymphoma may present as a localized, broad-based pleural mass, usually associated with pleural effusion, but is rarely an initial manifestation of the disease.

An *apical cap* is a crescent-shaped soft tissue equivalent mass at the lung apex with or without a superior sulcus lesion that may be caused by a variety of conditions. Pleural fluid tends to accumulate over the pulmonary apex, especially in the supine position. Apical pleural thickening not associated with a soft tissue mass may result from chronic TB (usually bilateral but often asymmetric), healed empyema, hemothorax, or radiation therapy. Any irregular soft tissue mass with involvement of the brachiocephalic plexus and vessels and/or invasion of the adjacent ribs and vertebral bodies is suspicious of a malignant neoplasm.

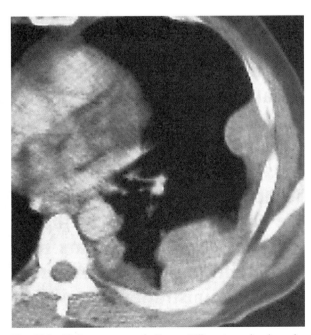

Fig. 17.9 Malignant mesothelioma. Diffuse, irregular-shaped nodular soft tissue masses sit along the left laterodorsal chest wall.

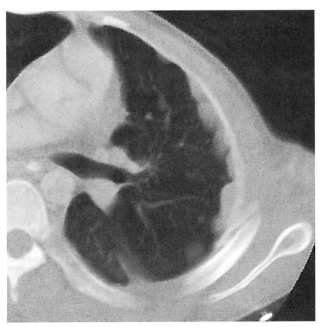

Fig. 17.11 Pleural metastases (renal carcinoma). Multiple nodular densities spread along the left lateral chest wall.

V Thorax

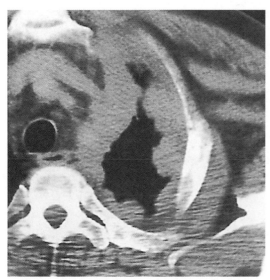

Fig. 17.12   Pleural metastases (gastric carcinoma). Similar appearance as in **Fig. 17.11** with encasement of the left lung by an irregular, bandlike soft tissue pleural mass.

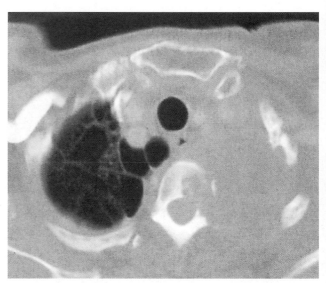

Fig. 17.14   Breast carcinoma metastasis. A large mass lesion is seen in the apex of the left hemithorax with destruction of the adjacent vertebral body and ribs. Bullous changes are incidentally noted in the right upper lobe.

The most common superior sulcus malignancy is a Pancoast tumor (**Fig. 17.13**), but metastases (e.g., from breast carcinoma; **Fig. 17.14**) and, rarely, lymphoma can present in a similar fashion. Benign tumors are rare and may be of either neural (e.g., neurofibroma and schwannoma) or mesenchymal (e.g., fibroma, desmoid, and lipoma) origin. Hematomas and hemorrhages in the superior sulcus are either associated with rib, clavicle, and spine fractures, secondary to aortic or great vessel rupture, or iatrogenic (e.g., catheter perforation). Atelectasis of the upper lobe and normal variants, such as excessive periapical fat or vascular anomalies (e.g., elongation or dilation of the subclavian artery), may also produce apical densities, but they are easily differentiated on CT scans due to their characteristic features.

Extrapleural chest wall lesions commonly originate from the ribs or intercostal soft tissues, including vessels and nerves. Displacing the overlying parietal and visceral pleura centrally, these lesions typically form an obtuse angle with the chest wall (**Fig. 17.15**). Associated chest wall abnormalities (e.g., rib destruction) support their extrapleural origin. Rib lesions are most commonly caused by traumatic, neoplastic, and infectious processes and do not differ from their presentation in other skeletal locations. Common rib lesions include healed fractures, metastases (**Fig. 17.16**), multiple myeloma (**Fig. 17.17**), osteomyelitis (bacterial, tuberculous, or fungal), and benign conditions, such as fibrous dysplasia, bone cyst, enchondroma, osteochondroma, eosinophilic granuloma, brown tumors, and extramedullary hematopoiesis (**Fig. 17.18**).

The axillary space is confined by the pectoralis major and minor muscles anteriorly; the latissimus dorsi, teres major, and subscapularis muscles posteriorly; the chest wall and serratus anterior muscle medially; and the coracobrachialis and biceps muscles laterally. When scanning is performed in a supine position, both arms are lifted above the head, and the axilla is thus bare to the side.

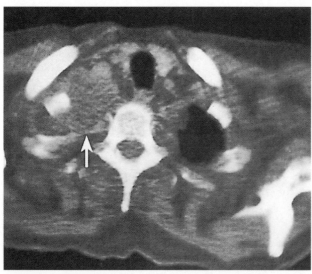

Fig. 17.13   Pancoast tumor. A mass lesion (arrow) is visible in the right superior sulcus.

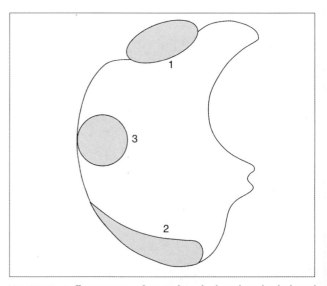

Fig. 17.15   Differentiation of extrapleural, pleural, and subpleural lesions. Extrapleural lesions (**1**) usually form obtuse angles with the chest wall by displacing the overlying pleura centrally. Pleural lesions (**2**) may form obtuse angles with the chest wall when the lesion remains confined between both pleural layers or acute angles when the lesion protrudes into the lung parenchyma. Subpleural (peripheral lung) lesions (**3**) typically form acute angles with the chest wall.

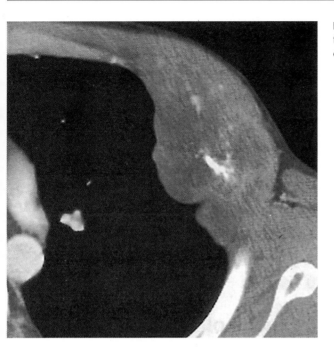

Fig. 17.16   Chest wall metastasis (renal carcinoma). A large soft tissue mass in the left anterior chest wall with an almost completely destroyed rib.

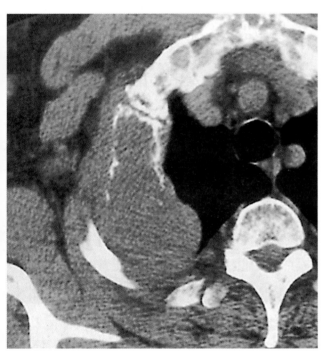

Fig. 17.17   Multiple myeloma. A large soft tissue mass originating from a swollen lytic rib lesion.

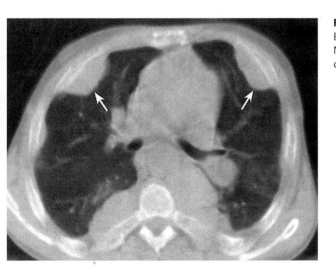

Fig. 17.18   Extramedullary hematopoiesis in thalassemia. Bilateral soft tissue densities (arrows) originating from anterior ribs. Note bilateral paraspinal soft tissue masses and cystic reticular bony changes, both due to extramedullary hematopoiesis.

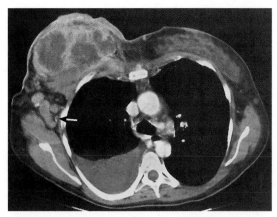

Fig. 17.19   Breast carcinoma with axillary lymph node metastases. Large exulcerating necrotic tumor of the right breast with a cluster of enlarged right axillary lymph nodes (arrow) and right pleural effusion.

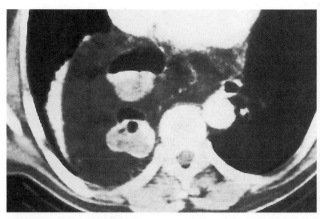

Fig. 17.20   Bochdalek hernia. A large posterior diaphragmatic hernia containing fat and bowel loops is seen on the right side. Usually these hernias occur on the left side.

The axilla contains the axillary artery and vein, branches of the brachial plexus, and a large number of lymph nodes all embedded within the fatty tissue. The axillary vein lies physiologically anterior and caudal to the axillary artery, whereas the brachial plexus is located cephalad and posterior to the artery. Normal axillary lymph nodes are oval shaped, measure < 10 mm in size, and contain a central fatty hilus. Ovoid lymph nodes measuring between 1.5 and 2 cm in diameter suggest inflammation (reactive hyperplasia). Lymph nodes exceeding 2 cm in diameter are indicative of metastatic or lymphomatous disease. A common origin of axillary and parasternal (internal mammary) lymph node metastases is breast carcinoma (**Fig. 17.19**). However, lymph nodes may appear rather small but still bear micrometastases. As a general rule, the ratio between smallest and largest lymph node diameter should be ≤ 0.5. Any ratio approaching 1—and thus corresponding to a rounding of the node—is highly suspicious of inflammatory, infectious, or metastatic affection. Lack of central fat is likewise pathognomonic, but it may be observed in asymptomatic persons.

The diaphragm is a large, dome-shaped muscle that incompletely divides the thorax from the abdomen. The diaphragmatic crura are tendinous structures arising from the anterolateral surface of the upper lumbar spine. The right crus is larger and longer than the left crus and originates from the first three lumbar vertebral bodies, whereas the left crus arises from the first two lumbar vertebrae. The nodular appearance of the diaphragmatic crura should not be mistaken for enlarged retrocrural lymph nodes, which normally are small (< 6 mm in diameter).

Diaphragmatic hernias may be either congenital or acquired. Hiatal hernia (herniation of the stomach through the esophageal hiatus) is by far the most common type and does not require CT for diagnosis. Bochdalek hernias (**Fig. 17.20**) are commonly left-sided and occur anywhere along the posterior costodiaphragmatic margin. They tend to be rather large and may contain omental or retroperitoneal fat, bowel, spleen, liver, kidney, stomach, and pancreas. Morgagni hernias are rare and usually right-sided; tend to be small; occur through an anteromedial

parasternal defect; may contain liver, omentum, or bowel; and are often associated with a pericardial defect.

Traumatic diaphragmatic hernias (**Fig. 17.21**) are found with both blunt and penetrating trauma, but they can be asymptomatic for months and even years. Over 90% of these hernias are located on the left side, usually in the central or posterior portion of the diaphragm. Omentum, stomach, bowel, spleen, and kidney may herniate through the ruptured diaphragm; thus, strangulation is a common complication.

A diaphragmatic eventration is caused by a congenitally weak diaphragm with cephalad displacement of the corresponding abdominal content. The eventration occurs more frequently on the right side, where it involves the anteromedial portion of the diaphragm. In this situation, the liver is displaced superiorly and should not be confused with a peripheral pulmonary or pleural mass. On the left side, the eventration usually involves the entire hemidiaphragm and mimics diaphragmatic paralysis.

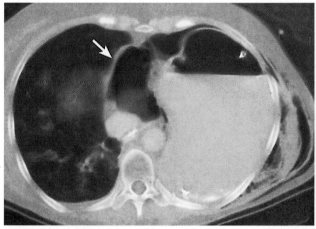

Fig. 17.21   Traumatic diaphragmatic hernia. A large hernia containing distended stomach is seen in the left hemithorax. Concomitant pneumopericardium (arrow), pneumothorax, and soft tissue emphysema are seen in the left lateral chest wall.

18 Heart and Mediastinum

Christopher Herzog

Mediastinum describes a space that extends between the thoracic inlet and the diaphragm and may be divided into an anterior, middle, and posterior compartment. *Anterior* refers to the space between the sternum and ventral pericardium, posterior to the space between the dorsal pericardium and posterior thoracic wall and middle to the remaining space in between, excluding the pericardium and pleural space. Although this subdivision is consistent in the lower mediastinum, it becomes arbitrary in the upper mediastinum (i.e., above the level of the heart), where many pathologic processes involve two or all mediastinal compartments. **Tables 18.1** and **18.2** list all pathologic mediastinal processes. Any preferential or typical location is referred to in the comment section.

A typical, though most often nonvisible, mediastinal structure is the thymus, which lies ventrally to the anterior aortic arch. Being isodense to musculature in young children and adolescents, its density becomes fat equivalent after the age of 20 y. Thus, in older patients, the thymus is masked by mediastinal fat. On transverse scans, its maximum size should not exceed 1.8 cm in patients younger than 20 y and 1.3 cm in older patients. Thymic enlargement in adults commonly is observed along with hyperthyroidism, but it may also occur as a rebound phenomenon following steroid treatment and chemotherapy. The right and left lobes may be separate structures or be fused together; thus, the shape of the thymus is highly variable.

The pulmonary hilum is anatomically ill-defined and represents a depression on the mediastinal pulmonary surface where bronchus, blood vessels, and nerves enter the lung. The left and right pulmonary hila are asymmetrical and thus, because of vessel opacification, it is necessary to systematically analyze both to differentiate between vasculature, lymph nodes, and hilar masses.

Differentiation may be difficult, as masses and hilar or mediastinal lymph nodes often coexist. Nonpathologic mediastinal lymph nodes show a large central fat hilum and thus are barely visible on computed tomography (CT) scans. If visible, they appear as small oval structures, with a smallest to longest diameter ratio of < 1. Any cross-sectional diameter > 1 cm, nodal rounding, or diminishing of central fat is suspicious.

If correctly planed and performed, CT usually allows proper assessment of mediastinal and hilar structures. Any multidetector-row CT with ≥ 4 detector rows, ≤ 500 ms rotation time, and ≤ 2.5 mm collimator width is suitable. Sixty to 80 mL of ≥ 350 mg U/mL contrast media, injected at a rate of ≥ 3.5 mL/s and initiation of image acquisition 30 seconds after starting of contrast material injection, usually leads to sufficient vessel opacification. Although this approach usually allows for screening of pulmonary artery embolism, bolus triggering on the pulmonary artery is preferable in these patients.

With these technical requirements, adequate differentiation between nonvascular (**Fig. 18.1**) and vascular (**Table 18.2**) mediastinal diseases usually is easily achieved.

Many cardiac diseases may also be visible on conventional CT scans; thus, familiarity with normal cardiac anatomy is necessary for comprehensive assessment of the mediastinum.

Small amounts (> 25 mL) of pericardial fluid are typically observed in the retroaortic pericardial recess as a sickle-shaped, discretely hypodense finding dorsal to the root of the aorta (**Fig. 18.1**). Pericardial fluid may occasionally also be seen around the right cardiac auricles and in the vicinity of the apex of the heart.

Fluid collections > 50 mL constitute a pericardial effusion. Serous transudates are observed in congestive heart failure, hypoalbuminemia, or after irradiation: Lymph fluid may be secondary to neoplasm, cardiothoracic surgery, or obstruction of the hilum or superior vena cava. Fibrinous exudates occur in the presence of infections, uremia, collagen diseases, and hypersensitivity conditions. Hemorrhagic fluid collections may be iatrogenic following surgery or catheterization, traumatic, secondary to myocardial infarction (MI), metabolic (coagulopathy), or neoplastic (metastatic/primary cardiac neoplasms). CT attenuation values of hemorrhagic fluid approaches blood density (20–40 HU) and may show fluid–fluid levels (i.e., sedimentation of hemoglobin). The latter is indicative of a subacute/chronic state. Differentiation between serous and fibrinous effusions is usually not possible.

The contours of the heart are smoothed by a variable amount of subepicardial fat (**Figs. 18.2, 18.3**), which must be differentiated from mediastinal lipomatosis (**Fig. 18.23**).

Conventional axial CT scans can be used to assess (1) overall size and shape of the heart and its chambers, (2) thickness of the myocardium, (3) presence of cardiac valve and coronary vessel calcifications, (4) topographic relationship between cardiac chambers and large vessels, (5) larger intracavitary masses, and (6) global patency of aortocoronary venous bypasses (ACVBs). **Table 18.3** discusses cardiac abnormalities relevant to CT examinations of the chest.

Any further cardiac assessment requires dedicated CT scan protocols, which are beyond the scope of this book and may be found elsewhere in more detail. The most important technical requirement is coregistration of an electrocardiogram (ECG) signal during image acquisition, which can be done either retrospectively (ECG gating) or prospectively (ECG triggering). ECG gating provides continuous spiral CT datasets in combination with continuous ECG traces, and thus allows retrospective image reconstruction from any phase of the cardiac cycle. This strategy not only is robust in relation to cardiac motion artifacts, but also gives way for assessment of myocardial function. ECG triggering—or the step-and-shoot technique—provides prospective single-image acquisition from a predefined heart phase and thus a much lower radiation dose (up to < 1 mSv for a complete CT dataset of the heart) as compared with ECG gating (3–5 mSv). However, in arrhythmic or noncompliant patients, additional scanning may be required.

Coronary artery calcifications may be assessed and quantified with any multidetector-row CT scanner offering ≥ 4 detector rows, ≤ 500 ms rotation time, and ECG-gating or -triggering capability. Semimanual evaluation programs allow the calcium load to be quantified either according to the method described by Agatston or by simply determining total calcium volume. It is important to always consider the normal distribution of calcified plaques in patients of similar age and gender.

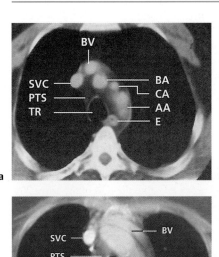

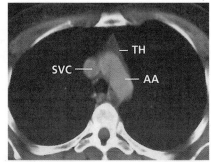

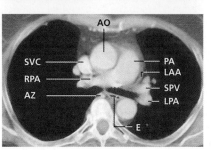

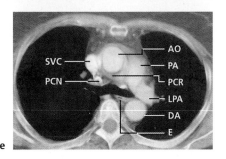

Fig. 18.1a–e   Normal topography of the upper mediastinum as visualized after intravenous (IV) contrast administration. Structures just above the aortic arch (**a**). Thymus (**b**). Structures at the level of the aortic arch (**c**). Structures at the level of the tracheal bifurcation (**d**). Structures at the level of the left pulmonary artery, below the tracheal bifurcation (**e**).

AA	aortic arch
AO	aorta
AZ	azygos vein
BA	brachiocephalic artery
BV	brachiocephalic vein
CA	carotid artery
DA	descending aorta
E	esophagus
LAA	left atrial appendage
LPA	left pulmonary artery
PA	pulmonary artery
PCN	precarinal calcified nodes
PCR	pericardial recess
PTS	pretracheal space (with nodes)
RPA	right pulmonary artery
SPV	superior pulmonary vein
SVC	superior vena cava
TH	thymus
TR	trachea

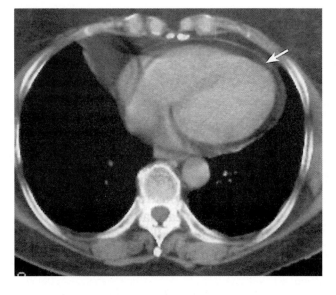

Fig. 18.2   Normal pericardiac fat. The amount of fat (arrow) between the myocardium and pericardium varies.

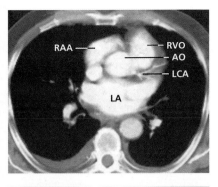

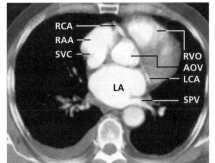

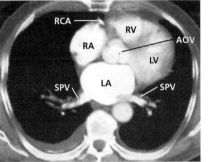

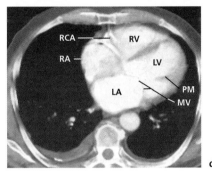

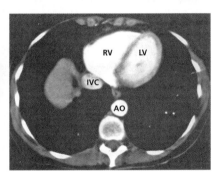

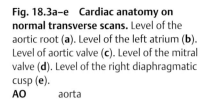

Fig. 18.3a–e Cardiac anatomy on normal transverse scans. Level of the aortic root (**a**). Level of the left atrium (**b**). Level of aortic valve (**c**). Level of the mitral valve (**d**). Level of the right diaphragmatic cusp (**e**).

AO	aorta
AOV	aortic valve
IVC	inferior vena cava
LA	left atrium
LCA	left coronary artery
LV	left ventricle
MV	mitral valve
PM	papillary muscle
RA	right atrium
RAA	right atrial appendage
RCA	right coronary artery
RV	right ventricle
RVO	right ventricle outflow tract
SPV	superior pulmonary vein
SVC	superior vena cava

Table 18.1   Mediastinal and hilar lesions

Disease	CT Findings	Comments
Vascular		
See **Table 18.2 Mediastinal vascular disease**		
Inflammatory		
Pancreatic pseudocyst ▷ *Fig. 18.4*	Fibrous encapsulated fluid collection of inflammatory pancreatic exudate. **Diagnostic pearls:** On precontrast scans, well-defined hypodense mediastinal cystic lesion is seen. Cyst walls may calcify. Low-density intracystic gas bubbles are seen in cases of secondary infection.	Evidence of pancreatitis may be present on abdominal CT in a patient with signs of chronic pancreatitis or following pancreas surgery/interventions. Usually extends through the esophageal hiatus from the abdomen.
Nonspecific lymph node hyperplasia ▷ *Fig. 18.5*	Lymph node hyperplasia in association with a variety of pulmonary or generalized infections. **Diagnostic pearls:** Slightly enlarged, sharply marginated lymph nodes with homogeneous contrast attenuation.	CT appearance of hilar and mediastinal lymph nodes lacks specific morphologic appearance to serve diagnostic purposes.
Sarcoidosis ▷ *Fig. 18.6*	Symmetric mediastinal and hilar lympadenopathy in patients with suspected sarcoidosis. **Diagnostic pearls:** Enlargement of the paratracheal and preaortic lymph nodes in the upper mediastinum and symmetrical hilar lymphadenopathy are characteristic. Large conglomerates may occur. Calcifications are rare and occur late. Lympadenopathy may occur with or without micronodular lung opacities, involving preferentially the middle and upper portions of the lung.	Histologically, well-defined granulomas with a rim consisting of fibroblasts and lymphocytes. In the absence of characteristic pulmonary parenchymal changes, malignant lymphoma is an important differential diagnosis.
Pneumoconiosis	Inflammatory lung disease caused by a variety of organic and chemical antigens. **Diagnostic pearls:** Lung manifestations often with associated minor enlargement of hilar and mediastinal lymph nodes. In patients with chronic exposition setting, lymph nodes show centripetal ringlike calcifications.	Lymph node changes are nonspecific, but pulmonary parenchymal findings are usually diagnostic.
Chronic granulomatous or sclerosing mediastinitis	Separate ends of a spectrum of chronic granulomatous inflammation of the mediastinum. **Diagnostic pearls:** Lobulated, elongated soft tissue mass may be detected in any part of the mediastinum. Commonly contains calcification and is predominantly right-sided.	Caused by a long-standing inflammation of the mediastinum leading to growth of acellular collagen and fibrous tissue within the chest and around the central vessels and airways. Major airway or superior vena cava compression may be present. May be associated with tuberculosis (TB), sarcoidosis, or a manifestation of idiopathic fibrosclerosis. Has a different cause, treatment, and prognosis than acute infectious mediastinitis.
Megaesophagus ▷ *Fig. 18.7* ▷ *Fig. 18.8*	Characterized by > 10 cm luminal widening of the esophagus. **Diagnostic pearls:** Often contains fluid or air–fluid level. Wall thickness > 3 mm when distended.	Underlying cause of megaesophagus is chronic or recurrent inflammation, such as achalasia, Chagas disease, scleroderma, and candidiasis in immunocompromised patients.
Tracheomalacia ▷ *Fig. 18.9* ▷ *Fig. 18.10*	Flaccidity of the tracheal support cartilage leading to focal tracheal collapse and concomitant cranial widening, especially when increased airflow is demanded. **Diagnostic pearls:** Focal narrowing of the medial and distal trachea with dilation cranially to it; sometimes thickened walls within dilated tracheal segment.	Tracheomalacia has a variety of etiologies, including polychondritis, complication of tracheal intubation, tumors, foreign bodies, and congenital tracheal stenosis. Physiologically, the trachea slightly dilates during inspiration and narrows during expiration. These processes are exaggerated in tracheomalacia, leading to airway collapse on expiration. The usual symptom of tracheomalacia is expiratory stridor or laryngeal crow.

(continues on page 642)

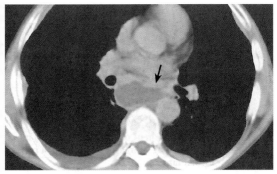

Fig. 18.4   Pancreatic pseudocyst in the posterior mediastinum. Cyst mimics megaesophagus but is nonattenuating after oral contrast medium. The esophagus appears as a small, compressed slit ventrally to the pseudocyst (arrow).

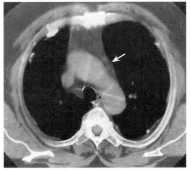

Fig. 18.5   Nonspecific enlargement of preaortic lymph nodes in a patient with pleural changes due to asbestos exposure.

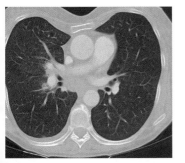

Fig. 18.6   Sarcoidosis. Enlarged hilar lymph nodes on the right side with concomitant perilymphatic noduli in the lung parenchyma.

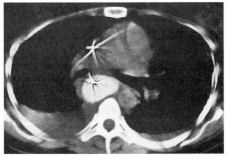

Fig. 18.7   Megaesophagus. Dilated esophageal diameter with thickening of the esophageal wall.

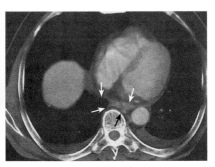

Fig. 18.8   Periesophageal fibrosis. Periesophageal fibrosis due to chronic ulcerating esophagitis appears as a subtle fibrosis in the region of the distal esophagus (arrows). Like varices, it enhances less strongly.

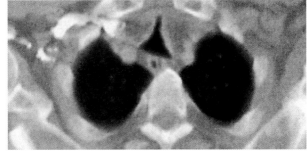

Fig. 18.9   Tracheomalacia. Narrowing of the tracheal lumen and thickened tracheal wall.

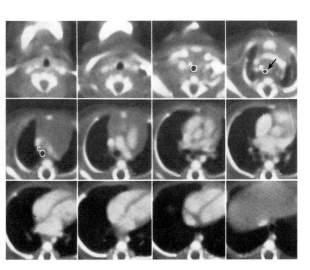

Fig. 18.10   Congenital tracheal stenosis simulating vascular ring-induced airway compression. The series of CT images shows no vascular ring but a fixed stenosis of 14 mm^2 (arrow).

V Thorax

Table 18.1   (Cont.) Mediastinal and hilar lesions

Disease	CT Findings	Comments
Congenital		
Bronchogenic cyst ▷ *Fig. 18.11*	A usually spherical cyst arising as an embryonic outpouching of the foregut or trachea. **Diagnostic pearls:** Round or oval, well-defined, very thin-walled, nonenhancing near-water-density mass. Characteristic location is just below the carina, protruding toward the right. Contour may be affected by contact with more solid structures. Rarely calcifies.	Also referred to as bronchial cyst and usually asymptomatic unless it becomes infected. Seen in different age groups from infants through adults. Can potentially be life-threatening, as cysts can lead to compression, hemorrhage, rupture, or infection. Most common in the middle mediastinum; may occur in the posterior and occasionally in the anterior mediastinum. May contain viscous material and have a density up to 60 HU but usually does not enhance.
Pericardial cyst ▷ *Fig. 18.12*	Usually asymptomatic, rare benign congenital anomaly in the middle mediastinum. **Diagnostic pearls:** Round, smooth, thin-walled, nonenhancing mass of near-water density, most commonly located in the right cardiophrenic angle (middle or anterior mediastinum). May change shape when the patient is turned from supine to prone position. Near-water attenuation differentiates pericardial cysts from lipomas and fat pads.	Incidence rate: 1/100,000. Occurs most frequently in the third or fourth decade of life and equally among men and women. Pericardial cysts represent 6% of mediastinal masses, 33% of mediastinal cysts. Other cysts in the mediastinum are bronchogenic (34%), enteric (12%), thymic and others (21%). In the middle mediastinum, 61% of presenting masses are cysts. Pericardial and bronchogenic cysts share the second most common etiology after lymphomas.
Neurenteric cyst, gastroenteric cyst ▷ *Fig. 18.13*	A combination of an endodermal cyst with a vertebral dysplasia. **Diagnostic pearls:** Smooth, thin-walled, nonenhancing mass of near-water density in the posterior mediastinum. May contain viscous material and have a density near soft tissue but does not enhance.	Neurenteric cysts, along with Rathke cleft and colloid cysts, are endodermally derived lesions of the central nervous system (CNS). Spine anomalies may be associated.
Thoracic meningocele ▷ *Fig. 18.14*	A closing disorder of the neural tube with herniation of the meninges through a vertebral column defect. **Diagnostic pearls:** Well-defined, solitary or multiple, water-density paravertebral posterior mediastinal lesion. May appear bilateral. No enhancement after intravenous (IV) contrast administration. Enhances only after intrathecal contrast administration.	Most meningoceles occur in the lower lumbar region and manifest after birth. Occult meningoceles manifest later. Widening of the spinal canal and vertebral erosion is often associated.
Lymphangioma	Congenital malformation of lymphatic channels. **Diagnostic pearls:** Anterosuperior mediastinal mass usually adjunctive with a larger component in the neck; multiloculated, homogeneous, smooth mass near-water density; often appears cystic. May compress nearby structures. Usually no attenuation on postcontrast scans.	Histologically, lymphatic sacs lined with endothelial cells, cavernous or cystic. Three to 10% of all cervical lymphangiomas extend into the mediastinum. Classified into three subtypes: simple, cavernous, or cystic. May be asymptomatic in middle-aged persons. More common in male children/infants. Cystic hygroma occurs in children and may be clinically apparent at birth or within 2 y.
Bochdalek herniation	Herniation through the lumbocostal triangle. **Diagnostic pearls:** A low left-sided, rarely bilateral, posterior mediastinal mass is seen at a paravertebral location; enters into the chest between the chest wall and the spleen (see also **Fig. 17.20**). May contain fat only, or rarely also bowel loops.	The most common congenital defect of the diaphragm. Bochdalek foramen is a lumbocostal triangle located posterolaterally. A hernia occurs in the presence of an incomplete closure of the pericardioperitoneal canals by the pleuroperitoneal membrane. A large Bochdalek hernia may be a rare cause of acute respiratory distress in neonates.
Traumatic		
Pneumomediastinum ▷ *Fig. 18.15a, b*	Extraluminal/pulmonary air within the mediastinum. **Diagnostic pearls:** Mediastinal streaks or bubbles of air, often extending from/to the neck. May be associated with subcutaneous or pulmonary interstitial emphysema and/or pneumothorax.	More often spontaneous than traumatic.
Fracture of vertebra with hematoma	Paravertebral soft tissue mass associated with vertebral fracture(s). **Diagnostic pearls:** Similar findings as in mediastinal hemorrhage or hematoma but usually confined to the posterior mediastinum.	Typically high-speed car accidents or falls.

(continues on page 644)

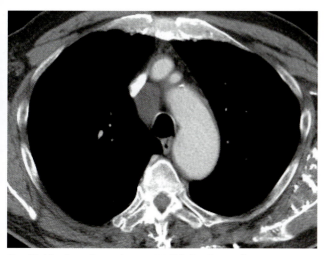

Fig. 18.11 Bronchogenic cyst. Well-defined, round, very thin-walled, nonenhancing mass of near-water density outpouching ventrally of the trachea.

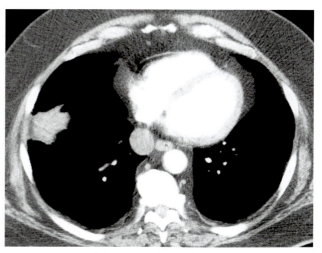

Fig. 18.12 Pericardial cyst. Round, smooth, thin-walled, nonenhancing mass of near-water density located in the right cardiophrenic angle. Note the large subpleural bronchogenic carcinoma in the right lung.

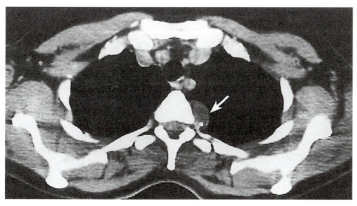

Fig. 18.13 Neurenteric cyst. Water-density, thin-walled, nonattenuating mass in the upper posterior mediastinum near the neural foramen (arrow).

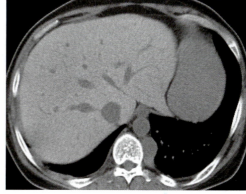

Fig. 18.14 Thoracic meningocele. Well-defined, solitary, water-density paravertebral lesion on the left. Note a discrete tail extending into the neuroforamen.

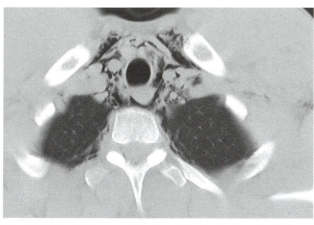

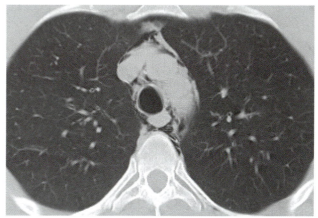

Fig. 18.15a, b Pneumomediastinum. Mediastinal streaks of air, extending from/to the neck (**a**) throughout the complete mediastinum (**b**).

Table 18.1   (Cont.) Mediastinal and hilar lesions

Disease	CT Findings	Comments
Infectious		
Tuberculosis (TB)	Lymph node enlargement due to an infection with mycobacteria tuberculosis. **Diagnostic pearls:** Asymmetrically enlarged paratracheal and tracheobronchial lymph nodes in the acute phase. On postcontrast scans, lymph nodes often show peripheral enhancement and central areas of necrosis-related hypodensity. In subacute/chronic TB, lymph nodes may conglomerate and show speckled calcifications.	Characteristic pulmonary parenchymal changes are typically present (see also **Fig. 16.39**).
Acute mediastinitis, mediastinal abscess ▷ **Fig. 18.16**	Acute mediastinitis is usually caused by bacterial overgrowth following a rupture of either the trachea or esophagus. It may progress rapidly into a mediastinal abscess. **Diagnostic pearls:** Hypoattenuating diffuse, mediastinal widening associated with small gas bubbles. Discrete cavity with a shaggy, slightly enhancing wall represents an abscess.	Esophageal rupture is the most common cause and is associated with larger amounts of mediastinal gas. Any infection in the neck may also spread into the mediastinum. After sternotomy, gas bubbles and fluid in the anterior mediastinum are indicative of an infection.
Acute anthrax	Acute infection caused by *Bacillus anthracis*. **Diagnostic pearls:** Symmetric widening of the anterior and middle mediastinum resulting from hemorrhagic, diffuse edema of lymph nodes. Patchy pulmonary opacities and pleural effusion are also seen.	*B. anthracis* is a rod-shaped, gram-positive aerobic bacterium that is about 1×9 μm in length. There are 89 known strains of the bacteria. They produce two powerful exotoxins and a lethal toxin. Most common among sorters and combers in the wool industry. Pulmonary changes are more prominent than mediastinal ones.
Spondylitis	Either an inflammation or infection of the vertebrae depending on the underlying cause. **Diagnostic pearls:** Fusiform, ill-defined, low-density paravertebral mass. Erosion or destruction of vertebral bodies at the level of the mass; usually in the inferior thoracic spine. Distinct attenuation on postcontrast scans.	Pyogenic spondylitis usually affects one disk space only. Involvement of multiple disk spaces and large calcified paraspinal masses suggest spinal tuberculosis (Pott disease), marked by stiffness of the vertebral column, pain on motion, tenderness on pressure, prominence of certain vertebral spines, and occasionally abdominal pain, abscess formation, and paralysis. Ankylosing spondylitis is a human leukocyte antigen (HLA) B27–associated autoimmune inflammation involving the spine and sacroiliac joints.
Neoplastic/thymic tumors		
Thymic hyperplasia, thymic rebound hyperplasia ▷ **Fig. 18.17**	Diffuse symmetric enlargement of the thymic gland. **Diagnostic pearls:** Particularly the anteroposterior thickness of the gland is increased with preservation of the normal shape. Attenuation remains unchanged. Differentiation from thymic carcinoma usually not possible.	In adults, normal thymus measures < 1.3 cm. Thymic hyperplasia (i.e., thymoma) may be associated with hyperthyroidism as in Graves disease, acromegaly, Addison disease, and myasthenia gravis. Rebound hyperplasia occurs in children and young adults recovering from severe illness, after treatment for Cushing disease, or chemotherapy. Rebound may simulate recurrence of neoplasm on CT but is actually a transient overgrowth that resolves with time or after steroid treatment.
Lipoma, thymolipoma ▷ **Fig. 18.18a, b**	Rare benign mediastinal masses. **Diagnostic pearls:** Large, smooth, or lobulated fat-density mass within the anterior mediastinum. Usually indistinguishable from lipomas, but may contain components of soft tissue density.	Asymptomatic benign mass predominantly composed of fat (50%–80%). Lipoma may also occur in other parts of the mediastinum. Thymolipoma is found only in the anterior mediastinum. Liposarcoma of the mediastinum is extremely rare, generally has a higher postcontrast attenuation than fat, and is more commonly found in the posterior mediastinum.
Thymic cyst ▷ **Fig. 18.19**	Solitary or multiloculated, water-density, thin-walled anterior mediastinal lesion. **Diagnostic pearls:** Near-water density attenuation of the cyst. Size ranges from some mm to > 12 cm. Usually no mural enhancement. Thin intracystic septations, hemorrhage and (subsequent), calcifications are observed.	Constitutes 1% of all mediastinal masses. Usually congenital, but may also be inflammatory or neoplastic. Often found in patients with Hodgkin disease either concomitantly or following radiation therapy. It may persist after therapy and thus usually does not reflect a residue or recurrent lymphoma.

(continues on page 646)

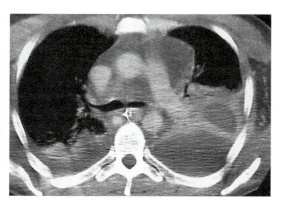

Fig. 18.16   Acute mediastinitis in a 38-year-old man, as a complication of a peritonsillary abscess. The mediastinum is widened and contains low-density pus. Note bilateral concomitant pleural empyema.

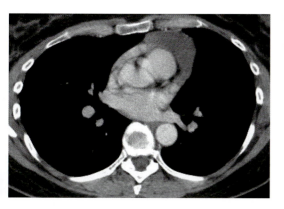

Fig. 18.17   Thymic rebound hyperplasia after chemotherapy. Diffuse symmetric enlargement of the thymic gland. Differentiation from thymic carcinoma is not possible.

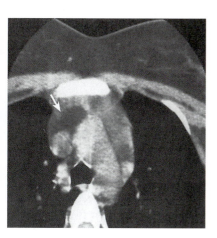
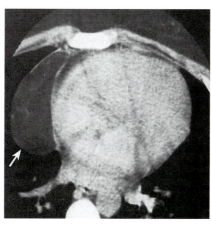

b

Fig. 18.18a, b   Mediastinal lipoma. Fatty tumor (arrow) extending from the upper anterior mediastinum (**a**) along the right side of the pericardium (**b**). Subtle soft tissue density stranding is seen within the neoplasm.

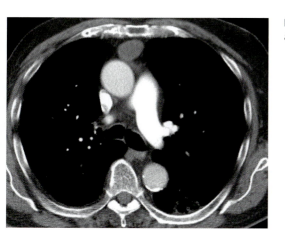

Fig. 18.19   Thymic cyst. Near-water-density lesion in the anterior mediastinum at the level of the pulmonary artery. No attenuation is evident after IV contrast.

Table 18.1   (Cont.) Mediastinal and hilar lesions

Disease	CT Findings	Comments
Thymoma ▷ *Fig. 18.20*	Epithelial thymic neoplasm in the anterior mediastinum. **Diagnostic pearls:** Round, oval, or lobulated well-defined mass of thymic density without a visible capsule; 25% show focal calcifications. Contrast uptake may be homogeneous in small lesions and heterogeneous in larger lesions. Convex shape and lobulation favor thymoma over thymic rebound or persistent thymic tissue. Invasive thymoma (35%) has a muscle-equivalent density and shows a mild enhancement, but can also be heterogeneous and have eggshell calcifications. Pleural or pericardial deposits are indicative of malignancy.	Shows a variable amount of lymphocytes. The most common primary mediastinal tumor (20%) usually seen in adults. Predominantly in patients 50 to 70 y of age; no gender preponderance. Fifty percent of patients are asymptomatic, 30% present with myasthenia gravis, 20% with symptoms due to mediastinal infiltration or compression. Ten to 15% of patients with myasthenia gravis and hypogammaglobulinemia also have a thymoma. Thymic carcinoid is not distinguishable from thymoma. Thymic carcinoma is a poorly defined large anterior mediastinal mass that commonly invades adjacent structures. Thymic Hodgkin lymphoma may be difficult to distinguish from thymoma even histologically. Chest wall invasion and lymphadenopathy suggest lymphoma (nodular sclerosis).
Neoplastic/germ cell tumors (GCTs)		
Teratoma ▷ *Fig. 18.21*	The vast majority (70%) of benign to low-malignant mediastinal GCTs. **Diagnostic pearls:** Mature and immature teratomas are well-defined, multiloculated, cystic, middle mediastinal masses with irregular capsular walls and septa, which may enhance. Mature tumors often are completely solid. Ossification, calcification, and fat deposits, often visible as a fat–fluid level, are observed in 50%. Teratoma with additional malignant components (TAMC) typically is an ill-defined, large, thick-capsulated mediastinal mass. Heterogeneous attenuation is indicative of hemorrhage and necrosis. Infiltration of mediastinal fat, vessels, and airways is often observed.	Teratoma is a GCT of young adults (20—30 y). It represents > 70% of all GCTs and occurs as three subtypes. Mature teratoma is a well-differentiated benign tumor and is the most common type. Immature teratoma consists of < 10% mesenchymal and neuroectodermal tissue. TAMC is a very aggressive subtype. Its primary denomination as "malignant teratoma" or "teratocarcinoma" is no longer used. Mature teratomas are usually asymptomatic and have an excellent prognosis. Immature teratoma is equally asymptomatic but may be a little more aggressive. TAMC is a very aggressive neoplasm with poor prognosis due to an insufficient response to chemotherapy. All types are occasionally also found in the anterior and posterior mediastinum.
Seminoma (germinoma)	GCT, histologically consisting of uniform sheets of lymphocytes and round cells. **Diagnostic pearls:** Large, well-defined lobulated mass in the middle or anterior mediastinum. May be homogeneous or contain low-attenuation areas. Tends to extend to the left of midline. Calcification, necrosis, or invasion is uncommon. Discrete attenuation on postcontrast scans.	Represents 15% to 20% of all GCTs; has a peak in the third decade of life and is almost exclusively restricted to men. It is the most common malignant mediastinal GCT. Chest pain or respiratory symptoms are typical clinical complaints. Metastases to bone and lungs are common. Highly radiosensitive.
Nonseminomatous germ cell tumor (NSGCT) (embryonal cell carcinoma, choriocarcinoma, mixed cell tumors, etc.)	NSCGT is a nomenclature for all GCTs that are not teratomas or seminomas. **Diagnostic pearls:** Large, ill-defined, lobulated anterior mediastinal mass with heterogeneous attenuation depending on predominant soft tissue component. Central hypodensities and calcification may occur with heterogeneous contrast enhancement. May displace or infiltrate mediastinal structures. Often concomitant pleural or pericardial effusion.	GCTs are a mixed group of neoplasms. They have a common histologic origin from the three primitive germ cell layers. Histologic features depend on tumor subtype. About 15% of patients with NSGCTs present clinically with Klinefelter syndrome. Patients often have an elevated serum alpha fetoprotein level. Clinical symptoms include chest pain and dyspnea. Overall prognosis is poor, particularly in the presence of mediastinal invasion or pleural/pericardial effusion.
Neoplastic/thyroid and parathyroid tumors		
Goiter ▷ *Fig. 18.22a, b*	Also denominated mediastinal or substernal goiter. **Diagnostic pearls:** Well-defined heterogeneous mass. May deviate the trachea and displace mediastinal vessels. Focal calcification is common. Precontrast attenuation is over 100 HU; enhances intensely.	Primary goiter due to migration anomaly and thus separate from thyroid gland. Secondary due to diffuse enlargement of thyroid gland and thus contiguous with the organ. Represents 10% of all mediastinal masses; 75% to 80% in the anterior mediastinum, 20% to 25% in the posterior mediastinum.
Intrathoracic thyroid carcinoma	Substernal/mediastinal expansion of a primary thyroid malignancy. **Diagnostic pearls:** Well- to ill-defined anterior mediastinal mass, slightly hyperdense on precontrast scans with a heterogeneous or peripheral postcontrast attenuation. May contain calcifications and hemorrhage (like benign lesions). Necrosis is present in > 50% and lymphadenopathy in 75% of cases.	Papillary thyroid carcinoma is the most common malignancy. It spreads locally via lymphatics. Follicular thyroid carcinoma occurs in adults and metastasizes hematogenously. Anaplastic thyroid carcinoma represents 4% to 15% of thyroid malignancies in the seventh decade of life. It is a rapidly enlarging mass causing tracheal obstruction and symptoms at an early stage.

(continues on page 648)

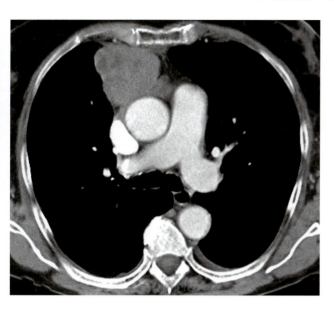

Fig. 18.20 Thymoma. Lobulated well-defined mass of thymic density without a visible capsule and with heterogeneous attenuation after IV contrast.

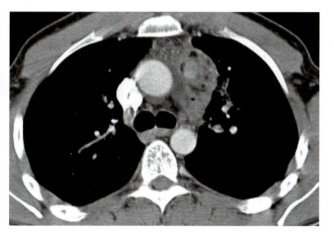

Fig. 18.21 Teratoma. Well-defined, multiloculated cystic anterior mediastinal mass with irregular heterogeneous attenuation and fat deposits.

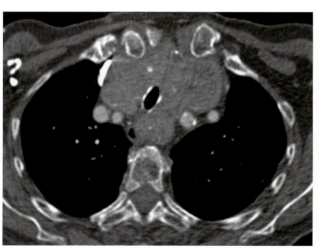
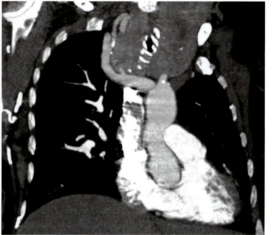

Fig. 18.22a, b Retrosternal goiter. Posterior mediastinal mass with intense but inhomogeneous enhancement and the presence of subtle intralesional calcifications (**a**). Distinct anterior displacement of supra-aortal vessels is seen on coronal multiplanar reconstruction (MPR) (**b**).

Table 18.1 (Cont.) Mediastinal and hilar lesions

Disease	CT Findings	Comments
Medullary carcinoma of the thyroid	Medullary carcinoma of the thyroid is a distinct thyroid carcinoma originating in the parafollicular C cells of the thyroid gland. **Diagnostic pearls:** On postcontrast scans, a low-density mediastinal nodule is seen; visible within strongly enhancing thyroid tissue if the gland extends as far caudally.	C cells produce calcitonin. Often occurs in conjunction with multiple endocrine neoplasia syndrome II (MEN II). Tumor measures between 2 and 26 mm and may occur anywhere from the neck to the mediastinum.
Ectopic parathyroid gland	Ectopic location of the parathyroid gland. **Diagnostic pearls:** Well-defined round and on precontrast scans hypodense mass of 1 to 2 cm resembling a lymph node. On postcontrast scans, homogeneous attenuation between 60 and 70 HU as compared with lymph nodes with either > 90 and attenuation or a clearly visible central fat pad.	Of patients undergoing surgery for hyperparathyroidism, 22% present with an ectopic parathyroid gland. Eighty-one percent of those are localized in the anterior mediastinum. The tumor size usually correlates with the level of hypercalcemia. Technetium 99m-labeled sestamibi and tetrofosmin tomography are the imaging modalities of choice, but CT may be useful for surgical planning.

Neoplastic/other primary tumors and tumorlike lesions

Disease	CT Findings	Comments
Lipomatosis ▷ *Fig. 18.23*	Excessive fat deposition within the mediastinum. **Diagnostic pearls:** Diffusely enlarged mediastinum due to smooth, symmetric, sometimes lobulated accumulation of fat in the mediastinum. Pleuropericardial fat pads are commonly enlarged.	Usually associated with Cushing syndrome or long-term corticosteroid therapy, occasionally with simple obesity.
Lymphoma ▷ *Fig. 18.24* ▷ *Fig. 18.25*	Mediastinal lymphadenopathy due to Hodgkin (HL) or non–Hodgkin (NHL) lymphoma. **Diagnostic pearls:** HL presents as a slightly inhomogeneous bulky mass in the anterior mediastinum. Attenuation on postcontrast scans is discrete. Involvement of multiple nodal groups is characteristic. NHL presents as a bulky mediastinal bilateral hilar mass with predilection of the superior mediastinum. Lymph node enlargement is more prominent in paratracheal, retrocrural, and paravertebral locations. Postcontrast attenuation of enlarged lymph nodes may be normal or decreased.	Mediastinal involvement is more common in HL (> 50%) than in NHL (20%). Cervical and upper anterior lymph nodes are involved more often in HL. Involvement of paracardiac or lower posterior mediastinal nodes in HL is rare.
Leukemia	Comcomitant lymph node enlargement in leukemic patients. Usually symmetric, modest enlargement of mediastinal and bronchopulmonary lymph nodes. **Diagnostic pearls:** Round, homogeneous lymph nodes with slightly increased attenuation on postcontrast scans.	More often observed in lymphocytic than in myelocytic leukemia. Often associated with pleural effusion and pulmonary parenchymal involvement.
Lymph node metastases ▷ *Fig. 18.26* ▷ *Fig. 18.27*	Lymph node enlargement due to lymphatic spread of malignant neoplasties. **Diagnostic pearls:** Size of lymph nodes not indicative of presence or absence of metastases. Calcifications are observed in metastases from cartilaginous or osseous tumors, mucinous adenocarcinoma, or bronchoalveolar carcinoma. On postcontrast scans, pronounced enhancement is observed in metastatic lymph nodes of renal, thyroid, and choriocarcinoma.	Bronchogenic carcinoma typically shows early spread to mediastinal lymph nodes. Even lymph nodes < 10 mm may contain micrometastases. Skip metastases (e.g., sparing of hilar lymph nodes)/contralateral lymph node metastases are observed. Any (near) round lymph node with a ratio of shortest/longest diameter near 1 and without central fat pad is highly suspicious, particularly if measuring > 10 mm in size. Other common primaries are head and neck tumors, breast cancer, renal carcinoma, and malignant melanoma.
Giant cell lymph node hyperplasia (Castleman disease) ▷ *Fig. 18.28*	Rare benign lymphoproliferative hyperplasia of lymph nodes. **Diagnostic pearls:** *Localized type:* Well-defined or lobulated enlarged lymph nodes with strong homogeneous attenuation on postcontrast scans. Inhomogeneous or ring enhancement is indicative of necrosis. No pulmonary involvement. *Multicentric type:* Several large, sharply demarcated mediastinal and hilar lymph nodes, with concomitant abdominal and/or cervical lymphadenopathy, with moderate postcontrast enhancement. Lymphogenic pulmonary pattern (i.e., ill-defined centrilobular nodules, nodular septal thickening, ground-glass opacities).	Histologically, hyaline vascular (90%), plasma cell (9%), or mixed types. Observed in middle-aged adults without any gender preponderance. Clinically, differentiation into a localized and multicentric type. Hyaline vascular types are usually localized and asymptomatic; plasma cell types, multicentric and symptomatic. In > 70% of cases, involvement of only the thorax; in 15%, also in the neck and/or abdomen. Localized forms may be treated by surgical resection; multicentric forms may need chemotherapy.

(continues on page 650)

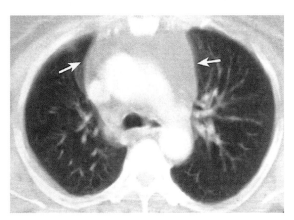

Fig. 18.23 Mediastinal lipomatosis. Smooth, symmetric accumulation of fat within the anterior mediastinum (arrows).

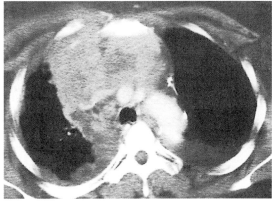

Fig. 18.24 Mediastinal lymphoma. Large cell lymphoma involving the anterior, middle, and posterior mediastinum, as well as the chest wall. Note the inhomogeneous enhancement and massive displacement of blood vessels.

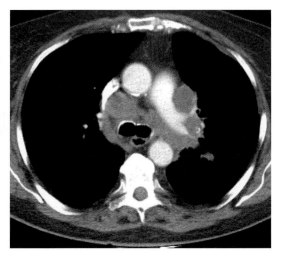

Fig. 18.25 Mediastinal non–Hodgkin lymphoma. A bulky mediastinal bilateral hilar mass with prominent enlargement of paratracheal lymph nodes.

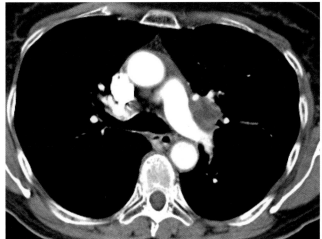

Fig. 18.26 Hilar lymph node metastasis (melanoma). Metastatic left hilar lymph node is well contrasted against the pulmonary artery.

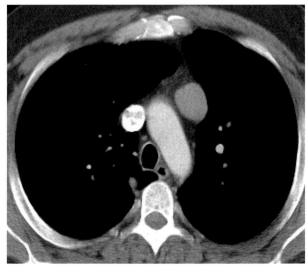

Fig. 18.27 Para-aortal lymph node metastasis (breast cancer).

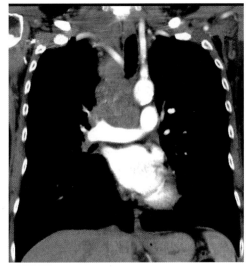

Fig. 18.28 Castleman disease. Multicentric-type tumor with multiple large but sharply demarcated mediastinal and cervical lymph nodes. Diagnosis was made based on histologic results. CT appearance is indistinguishable from lymphoma or metastatic disease.

V Thorax

Table 18.1   (Cont.) Mediastinal and hilar lesions

Disease	CT Findings	Comments
Neurogenic tumors ▷ *Fig. 18.29*	Well-defined, round to oval posterior mediastinal mass. **Diagnostic pearls:** *Nerve sheath tumors:* Low-attenuation, well-defined, paravertebral soft tissue mass. Calcifications and dumbbell appearance with a dilated neural foramen (extension into spinal canal) are observed in 10% to 15% of cases. Neoplasms usually show distinct, homogeneous enhancement, but may also have hypodense areas due to local necrosis. *Sympathetic ganglion tumors:* Ill-defined, typically longitudinally elongated paravertebral mass. Heterogeneous attenuation due to calcifications (ganglioneuromas/neuroblastomas), necrosis, hemorrhage, and cystic degeneration. Paragangliomas show strong homogeneous enhancement on postcontrast scans.	Histologic differentiation between nerve sheath tumors (neurinoma, neurofibroma, schwannoma, peripheral nerve sheath tumor, etc.) and sympathetic ganglion tumors (paraganglioma, ganglioneuroma, neuroblastoma). Neurofibromas and neurinomas occur in young adults, sympathicoblastomas during early childhood. Except for the rare paragangliomas (localized along the sympathetic chain, vagus nerve, intracardial, etc.), all other neoplasms are found exclusively in the posterior mediastinum. Paragangliomas are a form of extraadrenal pheochromocytoma and thus may present with a hypertonic crisis. Bone destruction, invasion of mediastinal structures, and pleural effusion suggest malignancy; otherwise, CT features lack histologic specificity.
Esophageal neoplasm ▷ *Fig. 18.30* ▷ *Fig. 18.31a, b*	Localized bulging of the esophagus. **Diagnostic pearls:** Short- to long-segment wall thickening and passage obstruction often associated with prestenotic dilation. Any eccentric wall thickening > 3 to 5 mm in a distended esophagus is highly suspicious of a neoplasm. Ill-defined periesophageal fat planes suggest spread into surrounding structures. Contrast enhancement often is discrete but may improve the tumor delineation.	Most commonly squamous cell carcinoma. Leiomyoma is located in the submucosa and thus typically appears as a smoothly marginated, homogeneously enhancing focal wall thickening. Inflammatory wall thickening of the esophagus may mimic a neoplasm but is usually more generalized. An esophageal diverticulum can be differentiated from a duplication cyst or necrotic neoplasm by oral contrast administration: a diverticulum is filled, but not a duplication cyst/neoplasm. Exact assessment of localization and longitudinal extension of the tumor, involvement of regional lymph nodes, local invasion (i.e., periesophageal fat stranding), and distant metastases is highly important for planning further therapeutic procedures.
Miscellaneous		
Diaphragmatic hernias ▷ *Fig. 18.32 a–c*	Hernia through either the foramen of Morgagni or Bochdalek hernia. Morgagni hernia is characterized by a fat-density mass in the right cardiophrenic angle. Contains fine linear densities, which represent omental vessels. Bochdalek hernia typically is left posterolateral (> 80%), large, and associated with organs (kidney, spleen, bowel, stomach, liver, etc.).	Uncommon diaphragmatic hernias through the foramen of Morgagni, which is a small triangular sternocostal zone lying between the costal and sternal attachments of the thoracic diaphragm. Demonstration of omental vessels helps in distinguishing Morgagni hernia from a pericardial fat pad. Bochdalek hernia accounts for > 80% of all nonhiatal hernias and is caused by a failure of closure of the pleuroperitoneal cavity.
Esophageal hiatal hernia	Protrusion of (part) of the stomach through the esophageal hiatus of the diaphragm. **Diagnostic pearls:** Axial hernias often resemble esophageal masses. A second contrast-filled lumen lateral to the distal esophagus is always indicative of paraesophageal hernia. Best visualized on coronal reformations. Rule out other cystic mediastinal masses (see also **Fig. 24.9, p. 745**).	Common in elderly and overweight patients. Perigastric fat may herniate through the esophageal hiatus without the stomach proper. Axial (sliding) hernias must be differentiated from paraesophageal hernias. In axial hernias, the gastroesophageal (GE) junction and the cardia are displaced intrathoracically. In paraesophageal hernias, the fundus with or without the GE junction is displaced intrathoracically.
Extramedullary hematopoiesis ▷ *Fig. 18.33*	Hematopoiesis occurring outside the medulla of the bone. **Diagnostic pearls:** Paravertebral soft tissue masses in the lower half of the thorax. May appear as fat-density masses.	More frequently associated with pathologic processes, such as myelofibrosis. Extramedullary hematopoiesis occurs typically with a characteristic purpura ("blueberry muffin" baby) in congenital hemolytic anemias (hereditary spherocytosis, thalassemia, sickle cell anemia, or TORCH [toxoplasmosis, other agents, rubella, cytomegalovirus, herpes simplex] infections).

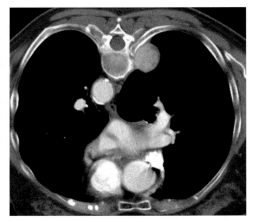

Fig. 18.29   Neurinoma. Well-defined, low-attenuation, paravertebral soft tissue mass on the right with distinct homogeneous enhancement.

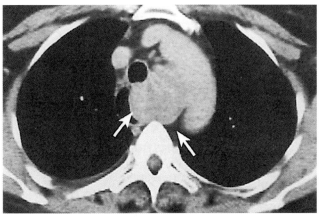

Fig. 18.30   Esophageal neurilemoma. Radiographically, the tumor is indistinguishable from a leiomyoma.

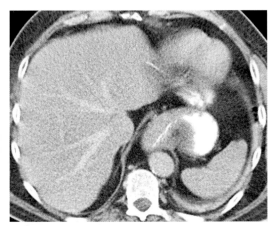
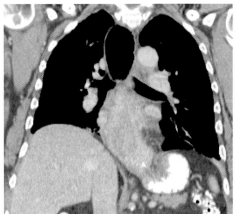

Fig. 18.31a, b   Distal esophagus carcinoma. Marked circular thickening of the distal esophagus and the cardia of the stomach (**a**). Multiplanar reconstruction (MPR) shows various paraesophageal and right hilar lymph nodes (**b**).

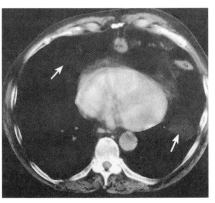
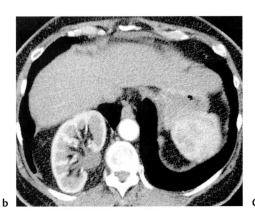
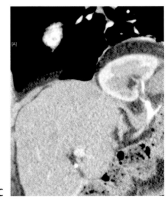

Fig. 18.32a–c   Diaphragmatic hernias. Large fat-density mass ventral to the heart (arrows). Linear densities represent omental vessels (**a**). Herniated right kidney through large Bochdalek hernia in the left posterolateral angle (**b**). Sagittal MRI shows defect in the posterior diaphragm (**c**).

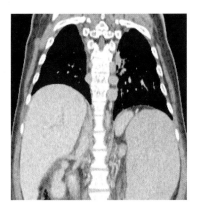

Fig. 18.33   Extramedullary hematopoiesis. Multiple well-defined paravertebral soft tissue masses in a patient with thalassemia major. Note hemachromatosis of the liver and concomitant splenomegaly. Same patient as in **Fig. 18.34.**

V Thorax

Table 18.2 Mediastinal vessels

Disease	CT Findings	Comments
Vascular		
Dilation of the pulmonary artery ▷ *Fig. 18.34*	Dilated pulmonary artery. **Diagnostic pearls:** On precontrast scans, may mimic large hilar masses.	Common causes include congenital pulmonary valvular stenosis and cor pulmonale; > 28 mm pulmonary trunk diameter is indicative of pulmonary hypertension.
Kinking/aneurysm of the innominate artery (right) or the subclavian artery (left)	Unusually wide lumen of the involved vessel.	May be associated with atherosclerosis or coarctation of the aorta.
Superior vena cava (SVC) dilation	Widened SVC in the right middle mediastinum.	Secondary to elevated central venous pressure (heart failure) or compression/obstruction due to a mediastinal mass.
Azygos or hemiazygos dilation	**Diagnostic pearls:** Unusually large enhancing vessel at the normal posterior mediastinal location of the corresponding vessel.	Usually of no significance, but may be associated with elevated central venous pressure or with azygos continuation of the inferior vena cava (IVC).
Mediastinal varices	Increased dilation, number, and/or tortuosity of mediastinal veins. **Diagnostic pearls:** *Paraesophageal varices:* Collateral mediastinal vessels adjacent to the esophagus. *Esophageal varices:* Collateral mediastinal vessels within the esophagus.	Varices classified as uphill or downhill, depending on underlying pathology. Uphill varices occur due to portal hypertension. Downhill varices mainly occur due to SVC obstruction.
Aortic surgery ▷ *Fig. 26.3, p. 779*	History of previous interventional stent or surgical graft placement. **Diagnostic pearls:** Initially high attenuation, later (> 2 wk) low-attenuation, homogeneous perigraft mass indicative of hematoma. Fluid–fluid levels show sedation of hemoglobin in time. Irregular, septated periaortic fluid or gas collection indicates an infected graft. Irregular periaortic fat stranding on nonenhanced CT and moderate attenuation of aortic wall and periaortic fat on postcontrast scans are typical of stent/graft infection. Septated periaortic fluid or gas collection highly suspicious of abscess formation. Lack of luminal contrast enhancement observed in thrombosis. A blood-equivalent mass lesion with rim enhancement with or without septations may be a pseudoaneurysm.	Aortic graft may be end-to-side, end-to-end, or intra-aneurysmal. Ascending aorta grafts may include aortic valve replacement. Ventral collections of perigraft gas and fluid shortly after surgery may be a normal postoperative finding. Differential diagnosis: Seroma, lymphocele. A common complication of endovascular aneurysm repair (EVAR) is endoleaks, which may continue to perfuse and pressurize the aneurysm sac, thereby conferring an ongoing risk of aneurysm enlargement and/or rupture. Endoleaks are classified by the source of blood flow and organized into five categories. **I:** Attachment site leaks **II:** Collateral vessel leaks **III:** Graft failure (i.e., midgraft hole, junctional leak, or disconnection) **IV:** Graft wall porosity **V:** Endotension (with or without endoleak)
Inflammatory		
Aortic atherosclerosis ▷ *Fig. 18.35a, b*	Degenerative arterial disease. **Diagnostic pearls:** Semicircular, smooth to irregular aortic wall thickening and hypoattenuation of plaques, which are usually wall adherent and may or may not be partly calcified or not. Calcifications occur as curvilinear hyperdensities on the outer side of the plaque (i.e., within the aortic wall).	Atherosclerotic risk factors (see Framingham risk factors) initiate vascular stress with subsequent local vascular inflammation, progressive intimal thickening, and finally stenosis; may also lead to formation of an intravasal thrombus or an aneurysm. Plaques may be calcified (stable) or noncalcified (more prone to rupture, e.g., atheromas). Eccentric array of calcifications is an important differentiator from aortic dissection (centrally displaced intima).

(continues on page 654)

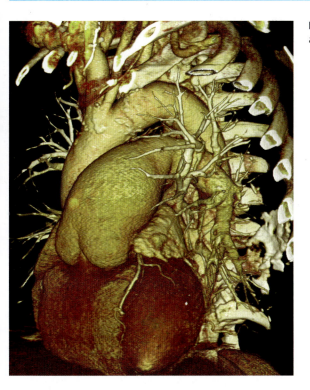

Fig. 18.34   Pulmonary hypertension. Marked dilation of the pulmonary artery. Same patient as in **Fig. 18.33**.

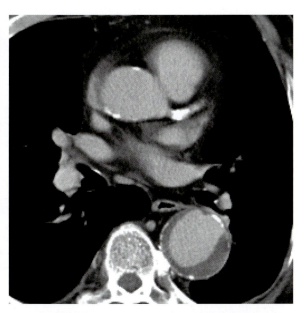

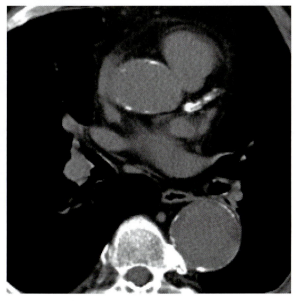

Fig. 18.35a, b   Aortic atherosclerosis. Semicircular, smooth aortic wall thickening on contrast-enhanced CT angiography (**a**). Nonenhanced CT shows that calcifications are located on the outer side of the plaque (i.e., within the aortic wall) (**b**).

Table 18.2   (Cont.) Mediastinal vessels

Disease	CT Findings	Comments
Aortic aneurysm ▷ *Fig. 18.36a, b* ▷ *Fig. 18.37a, b* ▷ *Fig. 18.38a, b* ▷ *Fig. 18.39*	Segmental to total saccular or fusiform aortic dilation. **Diagnostic pearls:** Fusiform or saccular dilation of the aorta and pear shape of sinus of Valsalva in case of anuloaortic ectasia. Curvilinear calcification of the dilated aortic wall is common. Any thrombus, if present, lies centrally to these calcifications. An intimal flap indicates dissecting aneurysm, which may be present without significant dilation of the aorta. Aneurysm may extend into abdomen and may involve ascending aorta, aortic arch, and/or descending aorta (see Crawford classification). Normal ascending aorta measures < 4 cm in diameter; normal descending aorta measures < 3 cm in diameter. Signs of an imminent aortic aneurysm rupture are soft tissue stranding of perianeurysmal fat and local lung atelectasis.	Common conditions associated with aortic aneurysm are atherosclerosis, cystic medial necrosis (including Marfan disease), trauma, and mycotic infection. An aneurysm just distal to the origin of the left subclavian artery is likely due to closed trauma. **Crawford classification for staging:** **Type 1:** Aneurysm from left subclavian artery to renal arteries **Type 2:** Aneurysm from left subclavian artery to aortic bifurcation **Type 3:** Aneurysm from descending aorta to aortic bifurcation **Type 4:** Aneurysm from upper abdominal aorta and all or none of the infrarenal aorta Surgical/interventional repair required for 1 cm/y diameter growth rate or diameters > 5.5 cm (ascending aorta) and > 6.5 cm (descending aorta). Any sign of an imminent aortic aneurysm rupture is an emergency situation.
Aortic dissection ▷ *Fig. 18.40a–c* ▷ *Fig. 18.41a, b*	Spontaneous intimal tear with continuous mucosal wall separation. **Diagnostic pearls:** Nonenhanced CT: Calcified intima displaced centrally Contrast-enhanced CT (arterial phase): Contrast-filled double (true and false lumen) channel with an intervening intimal flap spirals down the aorta Indicators of false lumen: Usually the larger lumen has delayed contrast. "Beak" sign: Acute angle between dissected flap and outer wall Presence of cobwebs: Thin mucosal strands crossing false lumen Intraluminal thrombus with centrally displaced intima (calcifications) In general, eccentric array of calcifications is an important differentiator to aortic dissection (centrally displaced intima).	Histologically, a cystic media necrosis from either atherosclerosis or congenital disorders. May be due to collagen disorders (Ehlers–Danlos syndrome, Marfan syndrome, Turner syndrome, osteogenesis imperfecta, etc.), trauma, hypertension, or pregnancy (> 50% of dissections in women). **Stanford classification of dissections:** **Type A:** Entry of dissection in ascending aorta (70%) **Type B:** Entry of distal to left subclavian artery (30%) Intimo-intimo intussusception is observed in case of complete circumferential dissection. Typical complications include occlusion of aortic side branches and continuation into iliac arteries. Multiplanar reconstruction (MPR) is useful for assessment of exact dimension of dissection. Look out for distal reentry. Typical pitfalls are streaks (i.e., motion artifacts in the ascending aorta). When in doubt, perform electrocardiogram- (ECG-)triggered CT.

(continues on page 656)

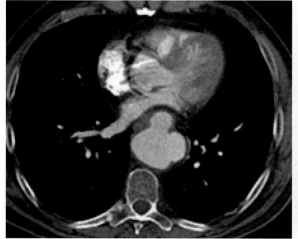
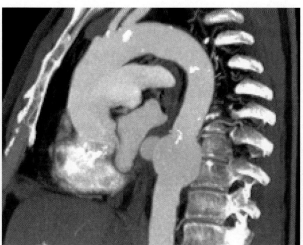

Fig. 18.36a, b   Saccular aortic aneurysm. Crawford type 3 saccular aortic aneurysm of the descending aorta on transverse CT scan (**a**) and maximum intensity projection (MIP) (**b**).

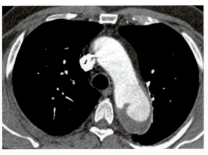
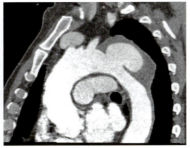

Fig. 18.37a, b   Saccular aortic aneurysm of the descending aorta (Crawford type 1). On transverse scan, an intimal flap is seen (**a**), but sagittal MPR shows true saccular aneurysm with no dissection (**b**).

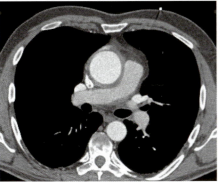
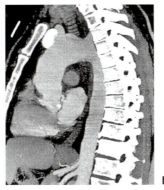

Fig. 18.38a, b   Fusiform aneurysm. Fusiform aneurysm of the ascending aorta (**a**) without involvement of the aortic arch or supra-aortic vessels (**b**).

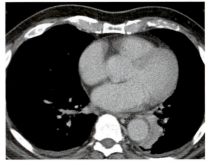

Fig. 18.39   Imminent rupture of aortic aneurysm. Soft tissue stranding of perianeurysmal fat and local lung atelectasis are highly suspicious of an imminent aortic rupture. This is an emergency situation.

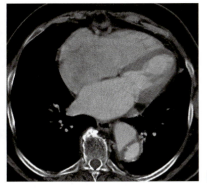
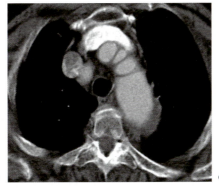
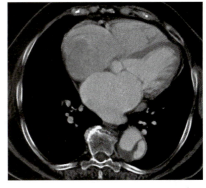

Fig. 18.40a–c   Aortic dissection. Calcified intima displaced centrally (**a**). A contrast-filled double channel spirals down the entire aorta and also involves supra-aortic vessels (Stanford type A) (**b**). The false lumen is the smaller lumen, recognizable by the beaklike angulation with the aortic wall and presence of intraluminal cobwebs (**c**).

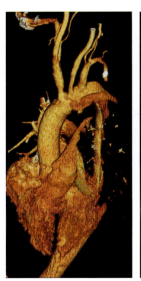
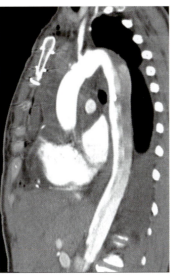

Fig. 18.41a, b   Aortic dissection. Stanford type B aortic dissection (**a**) with a partly thrombosed larger false lumen (**b**).

V Thorax

Table 18.2   (Cont.) Mediastinal vessels

Disease	CT Findings	Comments
Intramural hemorrhage (IMH) ▷ *Fig. 18.42a–c*	Localized hemorrhage within the aortic media. **Diagnostic pearls:** IMH usually presents as focal crescenteric, high-attenuation thickening of the aortic wall with internal displacement of intimal calcifications. Hyperattenuation is usually far better appreciated on unenhanced images. Protocols for aortic imaging should always begin with noncontrast helical images of the chest. On postcontrast scan, hypoattenuating as compared with hyperattenuating aortic lumen ("flip-flop" pattern) is common. Unlike atherosclerotic plaque, IMH generally creates a smooth margin with the contrast-enhanced aortic lumen.	The natural history of IMH is not completely evident. Several causes for the formation of IMH include: 1. Rupture of the vasa vasorum resulting in weakening of the aortic wall 2. Spontaneous thrombosis of the false lumen of an aortic dissection 3. Penetrating atherosclerotic ulcer induced by rupture of an intimal atherosclerotic plaque, allowing blood to gain access to the aortic media (**Fig. 18.42c**). It is unclear which mechanism predominates, but most likely all of the above mechanisms play some role in the development of IMH. Pathologically, IMH results in weakening of the aortic wall, which may predispose to dissection or rupture of the aorta.
Takayasu arteritis ▷ *Fig. 18.43*	Widespread smooth wall thickening and narrowing of the aorta and adjacent major vessels. **Diagnostic pearls:** Concentric smooth wall thickening and local aortic and arterial stenosis. Dystrophic wall calcifications may occur, also homogeneous involvement of large supra-aortic arteries. Plaques may enhance on postcontrast scans.	Disease of unknown etiology, which is typically observed in Asian countries/populations. Histologically, the inflammation starts with a mononuclear infiltration of the adventitia, followed by granulomatous changes in the media and subsequent fibrosis and thickening of the intima and media. Type I affects predominantly young adults ($< 20–30$ y) without any gender preponderance. Complications occur mainly due to stroke and hypertension. Steroids are the treatment method of choice. Angioplasty may be applied in the presence of stenosis.
Occlusion of superior vena cava (SVC) ▷ *Fig. 18.44*	Total or near total occlusion of the SVC. **Diagnostic pearls:** Diagnosed by visualization of underlying cause and the exact level of the occlusion, as well as display of collateral pathways.	May result from thrombus formation, external compression, IV growth, or a combination of all three. Collateral pathways include the posterior system (azygos-hemiazygos vein/paravertebral veins), the anterolateral system (internal mammary veins/anterior thoracic veins), and the superior system (anterior jugular venous system/external jugular vein/transverse arch).
Congenital		
Aortic coarctation ▷ *Fig. 18.45*	Localized stenosis of the distal aortic arch or descending aorta. **Diagnostic pearls:** Narrowing of the distal aortic arch and/or descending aorta. Tortuous intercostal arteries serve as collaterals and thus lead to marked inferior rib notching.	Occurs in $< 1\%$ of neonates. CT may allow diagnosis before clinical symptoms and bone erosions. Occasionally, an incidental finding on CT. MPRs in parasagittal/para-aortic orientation are useful for diagnosis.
Double aortic arch	Two aortic arches form a complete vascular ring that can compress the trachea and/or esophagus. **Diagnostic pearls:** The arches may compress both sides of the trachea, usually more on the right side. Most commonly, there is a larger (dominant) right arch behind and a hypoplastic left aortic arch in front of the trachea/esophagus. The two arches join posteriorly to form the descending aorta which is usually on the left side (but may also be right-sided or in the midline). The right subclavian and common carotid arteries arise from the right arch and the left from the left arch.	A rare congenital abnormality but one of the two most common forms of vascular ring, a class of congenital anomalies of the aortic arch system in which the trachea and esophagus are completely encircled by connected segments of the aortic arch and its branches. Although the double aortic arch has various forms, the common defining feature is that both the left and right aortic arches are present. Usually asymptomatic, but may cause stridor, dyspnea, or recurrent pneumonia. Seventy-five percent occur in the left descending aorta, and the smaller arch is usually (80%) anterior.
Left aortic arch/aberrant right subclavian artery	The right subclavian artery arises as the last branch of the aortic arch and crosses the mediastinum from left to right behind the trachea and the esophagus. **Diagnostic pearls:** Tubular opacity behind the esophagus in contiguity with the aberrant right subclavian artery, which is seen on the right posterior aspect of the trachea.	The most common anomaly of the aortic arch, with an incidence of 0.4% to 2%. Also known as arteria lusoria. Mirror image of right aortic arch (RAA) in **Fig. 18.44.** May cause dysphagia.

(continues on page 658)

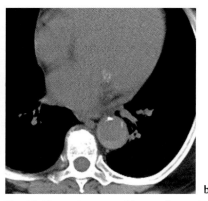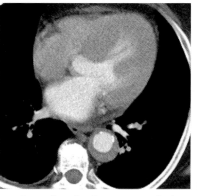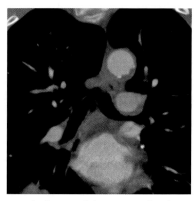

Fig. 18.42a–c   Intramural hemorrhage. On nonenhanced CT, focal crescenteric, high-attenuation thickening of the aortic wall with internal displacement of intimal calcifications (**a**). After IV contrast, typical flip-flop pattern (**b**). Penetrating atherosclerotic ulcer of the aorta: hypodense atheroma with central ulceration at the flow of the aortic arch (**c**).

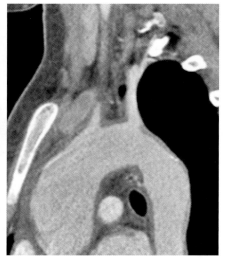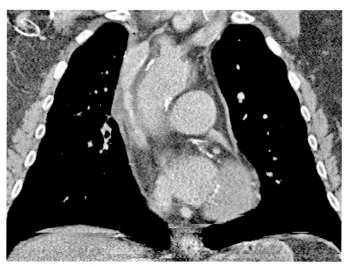

Fig. 18.43   Takayasu arteritis in a 20-year-old female patient. Widespread smooth wall thickening of the aorta, dystrophic wall calcifications in the aortic arch, local stenosis of the distal aorta, and homogeneous involvement of large supra-aortic arteries.

Fig. 18.44   Bronchogenic carcinoma. Near occlusion of the superior vena cava due to infiltration of central bronchogenic carcinoma with collateral flow through an enlarged azygos vein (visible on the left side, just above the left atrial appendage).

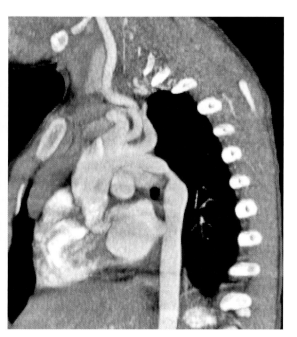

Fig. 18.45   Aortic coarctation. Localized stenosis of the distal aortic arch clearly visible on sagittal MPR.

V Thorax

Table 18.2 (Cont.) Mediastinal vessels

Disease	CT Findings	Comments
Right aortic arch (RAA) ▷ *Fig. 18.46*	Two types: RAA with either aberrant left subclavian artery or mirror imaging branching. **Diagnostic pearls:** In both types, the aortic arch passes and descends to the right of the trachea. In case of an RAA with aberrant left subclavian artery, there are four supra-aortic vessels (left and right carotid and subclavian artery). The left common carotid artery is the first branch, whereas the left subclavian artery is the last, taking a retropharyngeal course. In case of RAA with mirror imaging branching, there are only three supra-aortic branches (left innominate, right carotid, and subclavian artery). The left innominate artery originates as the first branch of the aorta, and there is no visible retroesophageal vessel.	RAA is due to a partial regression of the left fourth aortic arch. In case of an RAA with aberrant left subclavian artery, the left arch is interrupted between the left carotid and subclavian artery. It may form a vascular ring with the left ductus arteriosus. In 5% to 12% of cases, there is an association with congenital heart disease (i.e., tetralogy of Fallot, truncus arteriosus, transposition of great vessels). In some cases, the left subclavian artery may arise from the aortic diverticulum. In case of an RAA with mirror imaging branching, it is interrupted dorsally to the left subclavian artery. Tetralogy of Fallot is present in 98% of cases.
Circumflex right aortic arch/ left descending aorta	A rare anomaly of the aortic arch. **Diagnostic pearls:** Transversely oriented right aortic arch causes impression of the posterior trachea and descends on the left side.	May mimic double aortic arch.
Persistent left superior vena cava (SVC) ▷ *Fig. 18.47*	Persistent left anterior and common cardinal vein that drains via the coronary sinus into the right atrium. **Diagnostic pearls:** In 80% of cases, the right SVC is also present.	The most common anomaly of the systemic venous return to the heart, with an incidence of 0.3% in normal patients and 4.4% in patients with congenital heart disease. Increased incidence in asplenia syndrome.
Left superior vena cava (SVC) ▷ *Fig. 18.48*	Persistence of left common cardinal vein. **Diagnostic pearls:** Large mediastinal vein that descends left of the aortic arch and drains into the coronary sinus; absence of SVC on the right side. Often associated with absent left brachiocephalic vein.	No known genetic predisposition. Higher prevalence in patients with congenital heart disease.
Azygos continuation of the inferior vena cava (IVC)	Congenital anomaly with multiple variants. **Diagnostic pearls:** Dilated azygos and hemiazygos veins in their paravertebral course associated with nonvisualization of the intrathoracic IVC.	Systemic venous return to the heart is via azygos and hemiazygos veins. Hepatic veins drain independently by a venous confluence into the right atrium. Often associated with heart anomaly, abnormal situs, and asplenia or polysplenia.
Traumatic		
Mediastinal hemorrhage or hematoma	Diffuse mediastinal widening, commonly in upper mediastinum. **Diagnostic pearls:** Ill-defined mediastinal mass with direct relationship to larger vessels. In an acute setting hyperdense, on nonenhanced CT. Hyperdense contrast streaks/pools on postcontrast scans are indicative of an Hb-relevant bleeding. Subacute hematomas become iso- to hypodense (0–20 HU) within weeks and show no attenuation on postcontrast scans. Sometimes sedimentation levels are visible.	Associated with trauma, surgery, or dissecting aneurysm of the aorta. May require urgent surgical/ interventional repair.
Neoplasms		
Hemangioma	Congenital malformation of vascular channels. **Diagnostic pearls:** Anterior mediastinal mass sometimes with presence of phleboliths; well-defined mass with heterogeneous attenuation; small ringlike or round calcifications (phleboliths) in one third of cases; on postcontrast scans, heterogeneous (often delayed) attenuation.	Histologically, hemangiomas are endothelial-lined vascular channels with admixed fibrosis and sclerosis. Classified into three subtypes: capillary, cavernous, and venous. If not asymptomatic, patients usually present with chest pain. More common in children. May increase in size over time. Surgery recommended only if lesions become symptomatic.

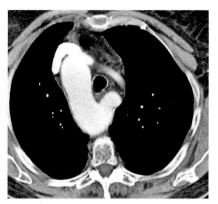

Fig. 18.46 Right aortic arch. The aortic arch passes and descends to the right of the trachea, aberrant left subclavian, taking a retropharyngeal course.

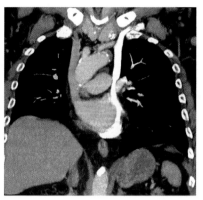

Fig. 18.47 Persistent left superior vena cava. Persistent left anterior and common cardinal vein that drains via the coronary sinus into the right atrium.

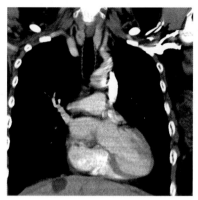

Fig. 18.48 Left superior vena cava (SVC). Large left mediastinal vessel that drains into the coronary sinus. Note the absence of the SVC on the right side.

CT coronary angiography is prone to motion artifacts; thus, spatial and temporal resolutions are key. It is advisable to use (ECG-gated/-triggered) CT scanners that provide at least ≥ 40 detector rows, ≤ 0.5 mm collimation width, and ≤ 180 ms rotation time. In addition, proper patient preparation and use of bolus triggering or test bolus calculation at the level of the aortic root are critical for sufficient image quality.

However, even with current state-of the-art CT scanners that fulfill these technical requirements, the best image quality is still achieved at heart rates < 60 bpm and in the presence of maximal distended coronary arteries. Intravenous (IV) beta blockage and sublingual nitro application prior to scanning thus are highly recommended. Motion or reconstruction artifacts and/or vessel calcifications are typical reasons to overcall the degree of coronary artery stenosis. Assessment of CT coronary arteriograms therefore requires not only a thorough understanding of coronary anatomy but also sufficient experience in the interpretation of coronary atherosclerosis. Readers are advised to use center-line multiplanar reconstruction (MPR) stenosis assessment and should be aware that the degree of stenosis on CT scans is usually calculated as area of stenosis, whereas on angiograms, it is determined by diameter of stenosis. Calcified lesions tend to be overcalled by up to 30%. Thus, it is useful to apply near-bone window/level settings for better appreciation of these lesions. According to the American Heart Association (AHA), there are eight different plaque types based on five phases of atherosclerosis, but CT can only reliably differ between calcified and noncalcified plaques. **Figure 18.51** is a schematic drawing of coronary artery segments according to the AHA.

Assessment of functional parameters remains a domain of echocardiography or magnetic resonance imaging (MRI) due to their much higher temporal resolution. However, it may be roughly estimated from retrospectively gated CT data sets.

New scanner generations, such as dual-source CT, which combines two-scan detectors and x-ray tubes in one gantry, allow for rotation times of < 160 ms (i.e., image acquisition times of < 80 ms) and thus may challenge these established non-CT image modalities. In addition, radiation dose, scan times, and systolic motion artifacts are significantly reduced as compared with single-source CT scanners. Functional assessment is usually done by using short- or long-axis reformations, which are cut perpendicular to each other, the level of atrial valves, and the myocardial septum. Short-axis views also allow segmental allocation of myocardial vascular supply. **Figure 18.53** is a schematic drawing of left ventricle (LV) myocardial segments according to the AHA.

Table 18.3 outlines differential diagnoses of cardiac abnormalities that may be visible on conventional CT scans. However, due to didactic reasons, several cases not only derive from ECG-gated/-triggered data sets, but also are shown as volume rendering threshold (VRT) reformations, short-/long-axis views, or center-line MPRs.

Intrathoracic nonvascular calcifications are usually harmless sequelae of bygone processes. They occur in the lung parenchyma, mediastinum, hilar and mediastinal lymph nodes, pleura, and chest wall, or in any combination of these structures. The cause of calcifications may be determined by means of the location and pattern of calcifications, as well as knowledge of associated clinical features. Apart from vascular lesions, the most common cause of thoracic calcifications is a previous infection. Less often they may be due to neoplasms, metabolic disorders, occupational exposure, or previous medical therapy. Small calcifications may be visible on CT or high-resolution CT but not on conventional chest radiographs. Thoracic calcifications are discussed in **Table 18.4.**

Table 18.3 Heart

Disease	CT Findings	Comments
Vascular		
Coronary artery atherosclerosis ▷ *Fig. 18.49a–c* ▷ *Fig. 18.50*	Degenerative arterial disease with intramural accumulation of fatty substance, cholesterol, calcium, and cellular waste products. **Diagnostic pearls:** Luminal narrowing of coronary arteries. Usually the plaque is nicely visualized as a hypodense area within hyperdense vessel. An overall hazy appearance of the lumen indicates total occlusion. Exact stenosis localization may be described in the report according to the AHA classification (**Fig. 18.51**).	Atherosclerotic risk factors (see Framingham risk factors) initiate vascular stress with subsequent local vascular inflammation, progressive intimal thickening, and finally stenosis. Presence of contrast material distal to a total occlusion may be due to collateral flow and not indicative of a remaining lumen.
Coronary artery aneurysm ▷ *Fig. 18.52a, b*	More than 1.5 times dilated coronary artery diameters as compared with adjacent vascular segment. **Diagnostic pearls:** May be fusiform or saccular, thrombosed or dissected. Calcifications occur in the presence of atherosclerosis.	May be congenital, procedural (percutaneous transluminal coronary angioplasty [PTCA], etc.), or due to atherosclerosis, Kawasaki disease, or connective tissue disease (Marfan syndrome, systemic lupus erythematosus [SLE], etc.).

(continues on page 662)

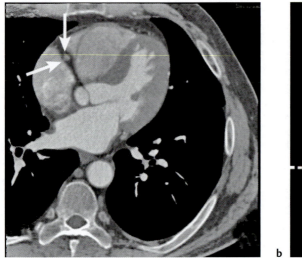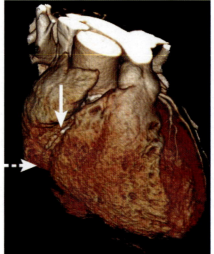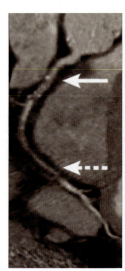

Fig. 18.49a–c   Coronary artery atherosclerosis. On a transverse CT scan, a distinct hypodense area (**a**) within an otherwise hyperdense proximal right coronary artery (RCA) represents > 50% stenosis (arrow). Three-dimensional overview shows > 50% proximal stenosis (white arrow) and medial total occlusion (break-off; dashed arrow) of the RCA (**b**). Corresponding CPR shows partly calcified proximal > 50% stenosis (white arrow) and an overall hazy mid-RCA lumen (**c**), which is pathognomonic for a total occlusion (dashed arrow).

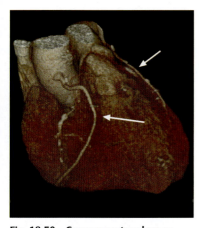

Fig. 18.50 Coronary artery bypass grafting (CABG). Venous graft to the RCA (bottom arrow). Left internal mammary artery (LIMA) graft to the left coronary artery (LCA) (top arrow). Note metal clips on the LIMA graft.

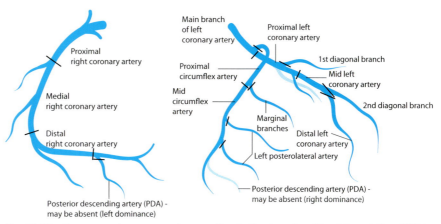

Fig. 18.51 Coronary artery segments according to the American Heart Association (AHA). (With kind permission from Springer Science+Business Media: Diagnostische und Interventionelle Radiologie, Kap. 21, Herz und Gefaesse, 2010, Vogl TJ, Reith W, Rummeny EJ. Figure 21.17.)

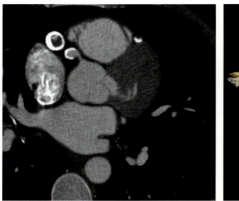
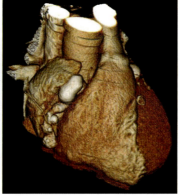

Fig. 18.52a, b Coronary artery aneurysm of the right coronary artery (RCA). Saccular, partly thrombosed, and calcified aneurysms in the complete RCA (**a**). Three-dimensional reconstruction shows additional aneurysms of the left coronary artery (**b**).

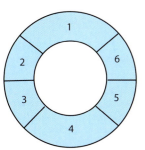
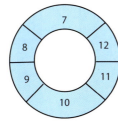
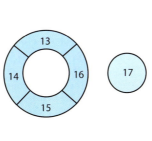
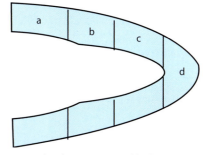

Fig. 18.53 Schematic drawing of left ventricle (LV) myocardial segments according to the AHA. On the short-axis views (**a**), the anterior wall is at 12 o'clock; the lateral wall is at 3 o'clock; the inferior wall is at 6 o'clock; and the septal wall is at 9 o'clock. Short-axis views are cut perpendicular to the long axis (**b**): segments 1 to 6 on short-axis views are located near the base of the heart (zone a on long axis drawing); segment 18 represents the apex (zone d). Segments 7 to 12 (zone B9) and 13–16 (zone c) lie within both. (With kind permission from Springer Science+Business Media: Diagnostische und Interventionelle Radiologie, Kap. 21, Herz und Gefaesse, 2010, Vogl TJ, Reith W, Rummeny EJ. Figure 21.24.)

V Thorax

Table 18.3   (Cont.) Heart

Disease	CT Findings	Comments
Myocardial ischemia ▷ *Fig. 18.54*	Myocardial hypoperfusion due to obstructive coronary artery disease. **Diagnostic pearls:** Ill-defined hypodensity within subendocardial myocardium. Restricted to myocardial segments that are supplied by the near-occluded vessel.	May be visible on non-ECG-gated CT of the chest. Indicative of a > 70% diameter (i.e., > 90% area) stenosis and thus a first sign of imminent MI.
Acute myocardial infarction (MI) ▷ *Fig. 18.55*	Acute coronary artery occlusion leading to ischemic myocyte damage. **Diagnostic pearls:** Vascular filling defect on CT angiograms, ill-defined transmural hypodensity. Restricted to myocardial segments (see **Fig. 18.53, p. 661**) that are supplied by the occluded vessel.	Usually due to atherosclerotic plaque rupture followed by thrombosis. May present with typical clinical symptoms such as acute chest pain, elevated cardiac enzymes (troponin, creatine kinase myocardial band fraction [CK-MB]), and ST elevation, but also without any of these findings (non–ST elevation MI).
Chronic myocardial infarction (MI) ▷ *Fig. 18.56* ▷ *Fig. 18.57*	Myocardial damage and scar formation due to prolonged ischemia or previous MI. **Diagnostic pearls:** Thinning of myocardium with diminished transmural perfusion, often presence of fatty deposits in subendocardial myocardium. Myocardial aneurysm or calcifications may occur. Restricted to myocardial segments that were supplied by the occluded vessel.	Secondary findings include enlarged left atrium and ventricle with or without findings of pulmonary hypertension. Fast-rotating CT scanners (dual-source CT) may also show myocardial hypokinesis/akinesis/dyskinesis. On late-enhancement scans, typically intramural/transmural contrast accumulation (contrast material pools within extracellular matrix, which is enlarged due to scar formation).
Myocardial aneurysm ▷ *Fig. 18.58*	Segmental outward bulging of thinned, fibrotic myocardium. **Diagnostic pearls:** Most commonly observed in the region of the cardiac apex. Filling defect on postcontrast scans indicative of thrombus formation. May calcify.	Usually occurs several weeks after transmural MI. Affected segments typically dys- or akinetic.
Inflammation		
Dilated cardiomyopathy (DCM) ▷ *Fig. 18.59*	Left ventricular dilation with systolic dysfunction with or without right ventricular dysfunction. **Diagnostic pearls:** Increased left ventricular diameter (> 3 cm/m^2 body surface), left ventricular ejection fraction < 45%, and contractile dysfunction.	Etiology includes genetics (familial DCM 2%), neuromuscular disorders, and myocardial ischemia. Medication is treatment of choice, followed by device therapy with ICD or cardiac transplantation. Echo/MRI is imaging modality of choice.
Hypertrophic cardiomyopathy (HCM)	Increased left ventricular mass due to asymmetric myocardial hypertrophy. **Diagnostic pearls:** Left ventricular wall thickness > 15 mm; asymmetric septal thickening (basal > apical); obstruction of left ventricular outflow tract (LVOT); normal cardiac shape.	Histologically, a genetic disease (autosomal dominant) of the cardiac sarcomer. No age or gender preference. Patients most often are asymptomatic. Echocardiogram/MRI is imaging modality of choice.
Restrictive cardiomyopathy (HCM)	Diastolic function is abnormal, whereas systolic function is preserved. **Diagnostic pearls:** Normal systolic function, normal wall thickness, and small left ventricular cavity; normal pericardium (< 3 mm) excludes constrictive pericarditis.	May be idiopathic without any known cause or secondary due to chemotherapy, radiation therapy, amyloidosis, hemochromatosis, glycogen storage disorders, or sarcoidosis. Echocardiogram/MRI is imaging modality of choice.
Myocarditis	Myocardial inflammation with subsequent necrosis with or without degeneration of myocytes. **Diagnostic pearls:** Delayed imaging may show late enhancement. Characterized by segmental myocardial dysfunction. Left ventricle (LV) or global dilation may be observed.	May be idiopathic, viral (Coxsackie B, Epstein–Barr virus, etc.), or due to autoimmune disorders (Takayasu arteritis, SLE, Wegener granulomatosis, etc.). May be fulminant, acute, chronic, or chronic persistent. Exclude ischemic causes on CT angiography. Echocardiogram/MRI is imaging modality of choice.

(continues on page 664)

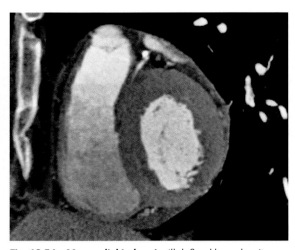

Fig. 18.54 Myocardial ischemia. Ill-defined hypodensity within subendocardial myocardium of AHA segment 4 and 5 due to > 75% stenosis of the left circumflex (LCX).

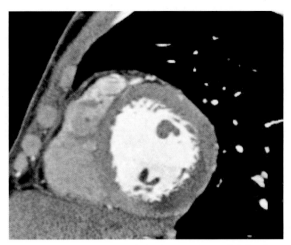

Fig. 18.55 Acute myocardial infarction (MI). Ill-defined transmural hypodensity in AHA segment 4 and 5 due to total occlusion of the LCX.

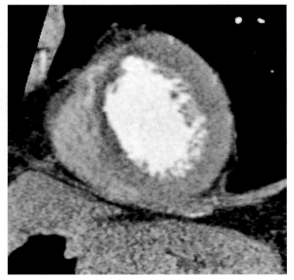

Fig. 18.56 Chronic MI. Thinning of the myocardium with diminished transmural perfusion and presence of fatty deposits in subendocardial myocardium in AHA segment 7 to 9 due to middle left anterior descending artery (LAD) total occlusion.

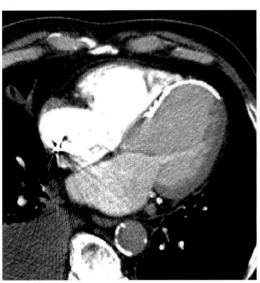

Fig. 18.57 Chronic MI. Septal thinning and calcification due to chronic MI.

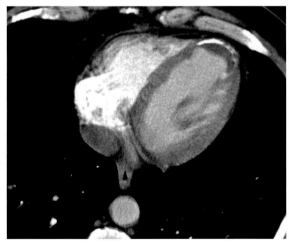

Fig. 18.58 Myocardial aneurysm. Partly calcified myocardial aneurysm of the cardiac apex with filling defect due to thrombus formation.

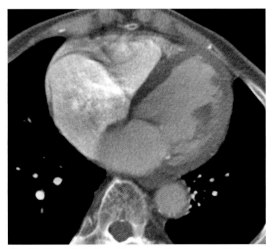

Fig. 18.59 Dilated cardiomyopathy. Increased left and right ventricular and atrial diameter.

Table 18.3   (Cont.) Heart

Disease	CT Findings	Comments
Pericardial effusion/ acute pericarditis ▷ *Fig. 18.60* ▷ *Fig. 18.61*	Fluid collection in the pericardial space. **Diagnostic pearls:** Well-defined water-density fluid collection between the myo- and pericardium along the contour of the heart; small effusions are usually found in the most dorsal part of the heart. Gas bubbles are indicative of an infection. CT density measurement is useful for assessing the underlying cause (chyle, blood, or serous fluid). Deformed ventricular contour with or without dilated IVC/SVC is indicative of pericardial tamponade.	Usually accidental finding. May be traumatic, postsurgical, neoplastic, infectious, inflammatory following acute MI, or due to collagenosis, uremia, or medication. **Pericardial tamponade** describes a situation of impaired diastolic ventricular filling with or without myocardial compression due to < 50 mL of fluid in the pericardial space. Pneumopericardium is usually posttraumatic.
Chronic pericarditis	Chronic pericardial effusion due to various causes. **Diagnostic pearls:** High-attenuation effusion (10–40 HU). Often associated with thickened, attenuating pericardium. Asymmetric accumulation suggests encapsulated effusion.	Typically due to chronic diseases, such as slow infections (e.g., TB), or irradiation.
Chronic constrictive pericarditis ▷ *Fig. 18.62*	Impaired ventricular filling due to abnormal pericardial thickening. **Diagnostic pearls:** Pericardial thickening (> 5 mm) with or without calcification. Pericardial enhancement indicates an active inflammatory process and can be used to distinguish effusion from thickened pericardium.	Any purulent and serofibrinous type of pericarditis may transform into chronic constrictive pericarditis. **Pericarditis calcarea** is a chronic constrictive pericarditis that is dominated by myocardial encasement due to a thinned but heavily calcified pericardium.
Takotsubo syndrome	"Broken heart" or stress-induced cardiomyopathy. **Diagnostic pearls:** Absence of relevant coronary artery stenosis; systolic ballooning of the left ventricular apex, and normal contraction of the base.	Diffuse coronary microvascular dysfunction is discussed as the underlying pathology. Typically observed in patients with physical or emotional stress. Usually resolves completely over time.
Congenital		
Coronary artery anomalies ▷ *Fig. 18.63*	Anomalous origin of coronary arteries. **Diagnostic pearls:** May affect left coronary artery (LCA), left circumflex (LCX), or right coronary artery (RCA). Anomalous LCA/LCX arises from right sinus of Valsalva, anomalous RCA from left sinus of Valsalva. Benign variants run either anteriorly to the pulmonary artery (PA) or posteriorly to the aorta. Malignant variants are encased between the aorta and PA.	Usually asymptomatic. No gender predilection. Primary congenital anomalies of the coronary arteries occur in 1% to 2% of the general population. LCX anomaly is the most common variant. In Bland–White–Garland syndrome, an anomalous LCA arises from the pulmonary artery. Typically observed in children who present with heart failure (> 90%), shortness of breath, angina with or without MI. Rare in adults.
Pericardial defect	Partial or complete absence of pericardial contour on CT scans. **Diagnostic pearls:** Most commonly (70%) affects the left side of the pericardium. Increased intrapulmonary protrusion of the left pulmonary artery (PA) and indentation of lung parenchyma between the ascending aorta and PA. Protrusion of fat or abdominal organs into the pericardium is indicative of a diaphragmatic pericardial defect (17%).	Rare anomaly. In 30% of cases, associated with other congenital abnormalities, including atrial septal defect, patent ductus arteriosus, bronchogenic cyst, pulmonary sequestration, mitral stenosis, and tetralogy of Fallot. In the absence of concomitant abnormalities, the patient is usually asymptomatic.
Pericardial cyst/diverticulum ▷ *Fig. 18.64*	Pericardial mass at the right anterior costophrenic angle. **Diagnostic pearls:** A pericardial cyst appears as a well-defined, thin-walled, round to oval mass with attenuation values between 0 and 20 HU. Calcification is rare. Diverticula communicate with the pericardium but are otherwise similar in CT appearance.	Rare lesions usually seen in asymptomatic patients. May mimic pulmonary/mediastinal mass on chest radiograph.

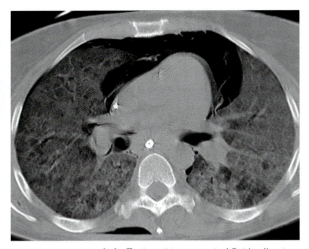

Fig. 18.60   Pericardial effusion. Discrete apical fluid collection in a bilateral pneumothorax in a patient suffering from a severe blunt accident.

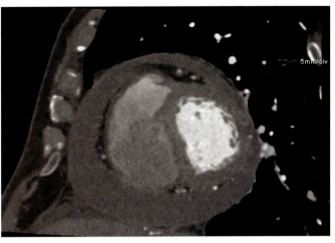

Fig. 18.61   Pericardial tamponade. Pericardial tamponade with marked fluid collection in the pericardial space and beginning of myocardial compression.

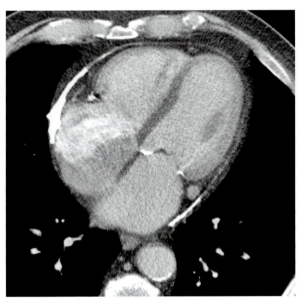

Fig. 18.62   Pericarditis calcarea. A thinned and heavily calcified pericardium. Concomitant pericardial enhancement indicates an active inflammatory process.

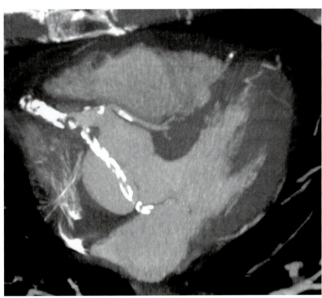

Fig. 18.63   Coronary artery anomalies. Common origin of LCA, LCX, and RCA from right sinus of Valsalva. The LCA is encased between the aorta and the pulmonary artery (malignant), whereas the LCX runs posteriorly to the aorta (benign).

Fig. 18.64   Pericardial cyst. Well-defined, waterlike, attenuating, thin-walled lobulated mass at the right anterior costophrenic angle.

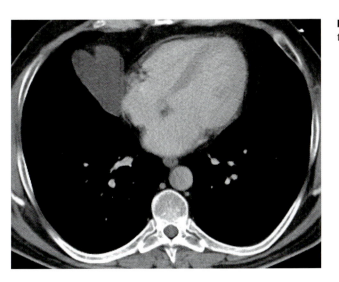

Table 18.3 (Cont.) Heart

Disease	CT Findings	Comments
Congenital heart disease ▷ *Fig. 18.65* ▷ *Fig. 18.66* ▷ *Fig. 18.67* ▷ *Fig. 18.68* ▷ *Fig. 18.69* ▷ *Fig. 18.70*	A variety of congenital heart anomalies with either right-left or left-right shunting. **Diagnostic pearls: Figure 18.65** lists the most common types, including endocardial cushion defects (atrial [ASDs] and ventricular septal defects [VSDs], common atrioventricular channel), persistent ductus arteriosus Botalli, pulmonary stenosis, tetralogy of Fallot, total anomalous pulmonary venous return, mitral or tricuspid atresia, Ebstein anomaly, coarctation, and transposition of large vessels.	Congenital heart disease is typically observed in newborns and, due to radiation issues, usually assessed with MRI. MRI allows precise noninvasive flow measurements and functional assessment. CT offers the benefit of significantly shorter examination times, making sedation typically obsolete. Recent introduction of low-dose dual-source technology allows image acquisition at < 1 ms.
Benign neoplasms		
Intracardiac thrombus ▷ *Fig. 18.58, p. 663*	Nonspecific intraluminal filling defect. **Diagnostic pearls:** Thrombus is hypodense (< 50 HU) in comparison to normal myocardium (70–90 HU). Left ventricular (LV) thrombus usually associated with aneurysm. Left atrial (LA) thrombus usually associated with LA dilation. Thrombus may calcify.	Underlying causes include deep vein thrombosis, left atrial fibrillation, presence of foreign material (pacemaker wires, etc.), previous heart surgery, and cardiomyopathy. LV thrombus most common, followed by LA thrombus. Right ventricular (RV) and right atrial (RA) thrombi are rare.
Cardiac myxoma ▷ *Fig. 18.71*	Most common primary neoplasm of the heart. **Diagnostic pearls:** Almost exclusively restricted to the atrium, 83% located in the LA, 12% in the RA; 5% in atypical location. Typically located at LA fossa ovalis. Nonattenuating intra-atrial filling defect seen on postcontrast scans. May contain cystic components.	Very slow-growing gelatinous neoplasm. May be sporadic or familial (Carney complex). Typically observed in middle-aged patients. Myxoma may obstruct the mitral valve. Surgical resection is treatment of choice in symptomatic patients.
Other benign neoplasms	**Diagnostic pearls:** Usually non- to slightly hyperattenuating intracardiac filling defects. Tumor localization is often indicative of tumor entity: fibroelastoma (valves); paraganglioma (LA); lipoma (RA/RV); fibroma (ventricular wall); lymphangioma (ubiquitous); rhabdomyoma (multilocular/intramyocardial).	Accidental finding on CT scans. MRI imaging is modality of choice. Combined T1- and T2- weighted MRI allows further differentiation between histologic subtypes.

(continues on page 668)

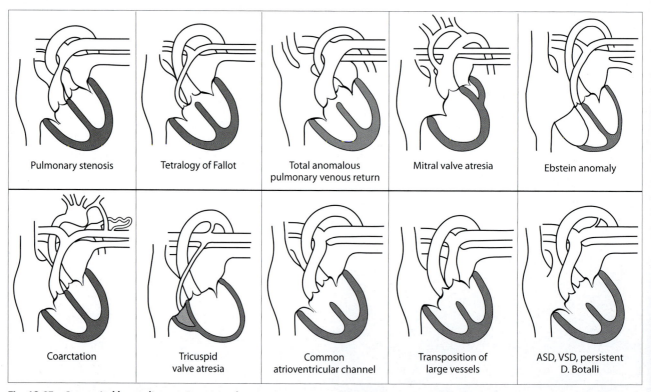

Pulmonary stenosis

Tetralogy of Fallot

Total anomalous pulmonary venous return

Mitral valve atresia

Ebstein anomaly

Coarctation

Tricuspid valve atresia

Common atrioventricular channel

Transposition of large vessels

ASD, VSD, persistent D. Botalli

Fig. 18.65 Congenital heart disease. Overview of most common types. (With kind permission from Springer Science+Business Media: Diagnostische und Interventionelle Radiologie, Kap. 21, Herz und Gefaesse, 2010, Vogl TJ, Reith W, Rummeny EJ. Figure 21.10.) ASD, atrial septal defect; VSD, ventricular septal defect; d. Botalli, ductus arteriosus Botelli.

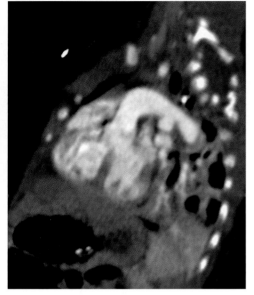

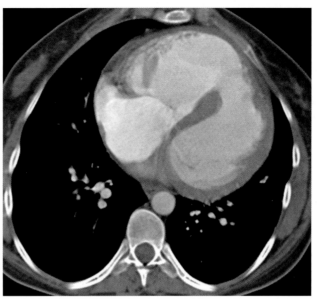

Fig. 18.66   Fallot tetralogy. Large ventricular septal defect (VSD) with overriding aorta, stenosis of pulmonary artery (on the left side of the aorta), and right ventricular hypertrophy.

Fig. 18.67   Large apical VSD.

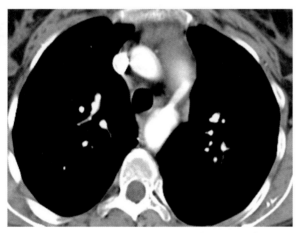

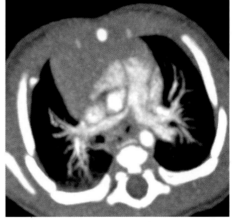

Fig. 18.68   Persistent ductus arteriosus (PDA) Botalli.

Fig. 18.69   Stenosis of the right pulmonary artery.

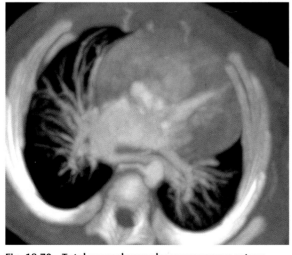

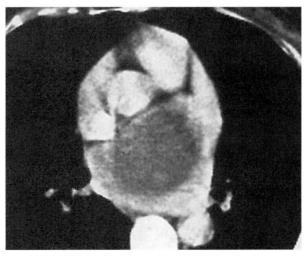

Fig. 18.70   Total anomalous pulmonary venous return. All four lung veins drain into the right atrium.

Fig. 18.71   Left atrial myxoma. Contrast-filling defect in an enlarged left atrium.

Table 18.3 (Cont.) Heart

Disease	CT Findings	Comments
Malignant neoplasms		
Intracardiac metastasis ▷ *Fig. 18.72*	**Diagnostic pearls:** Nonspecific intracardiac filling defect at any location.	Most common primaries are bronchial carcinoma, melanoma, and malignant lymphoma.
Other malignant neoplasms	**Diagnostic pearls:** Usually non- to slightly hyperattenuating intracardiac filling defects: lymphoma (RV); angiosarcoma (atrial septum); malignant fibrous histiocytoma (LA); rhabdomyosarcoma (ubiquitous/intramyocardial).	Primary cardiac sarcomas are rare. Accidental finding on CT scans. MRI is modality of choice. Combined T1- and T2-weighted MRI imaging allows further differentiation between histologic subtypes.
Valvular		
Aortic valve ▷ *Fig. 18.73a, b*	Regurgitation or stenosis of the aortic valve. **Diagnostic pearls:** *Aortic valve stenosis:* Typically associated with thickening, fusion with or without calcification of valve cusps or anulus, as well as with LV hypertrophy and poststenotic dilation of the aorta. *Aortic valve regurgitation:* Dilation of aortic roof, aortic valve anulus, and ascending aorta. Valve may also show vegetations.	Calcifications may be better depicted on CT scans. Amount of calcifications correlates with 5-y risk of LV failure. Functional parameters and valvular movement may be assessed on ECG-gated multiphasic CT scans. Echo/MRI is image modality of choice. Bicuspid aortic valve is the most common cardiovascular malformation, occurring in 2% of the population. Usually asymptomatic.
Mitral valve	Regurgitation or stenosis of the mitral valve. **Diagnostic pearls:** *Mitral valve stenosis:* Typically associated with narrowing, thickening, fusion with or without calcification of valve cusps or anulus. Often LA dilation and thrombi. *Mitral valve regurgitation:* LA and LV dilation in chronic regurgitation. Valve vegetation indicates rheumatic or infectious origin of disease.	Calcifications may be better depicted on CT scans. Functional parameters and valvular movement may be assessed on ECG-gated multiphasic CT scans but are usually better depicted by MRI and echo. Mitral valve prolapse describes midsystolic atrial bulging of thickened leaflets.
Pulmonary valve	Regurgitation or stenosis of the pulmonary valve. **Diagnostic pearls:** *Pulmonary valve stenosis:* Thickening, fusion with or without calcification of valve cusps or anulus; also, normal-sized heart and dilated pulmonary artery. *Aortic valve regurgitation:* Dilated pulmonary artery, RV, azygos vein, and IVC/SVC.	Pulmonary valve stenosis is usually congenital: in 80% solitary, in 20% associated with other congenital heart diseases. Aortic valve regurgitation is a rare condition. Echo/MRI is image modality of choice.
Tricuspid valve	Regurgitation or stenosis of the tricuspid valve. **Diagnostic pearls:** *Tricuspid valve stenosis:* Thickening, fusion with or without calcification of valve cusps; RA dilation (> 20 cm²). *Tricuspid valve regurgitation:* Valve often not directly visualized; dilated RA, RV, and IVC; systolic contrast reflux into dilated hepatic veins.	Tricuspid valve stenosis is most commonly due to rheumatic heart disease. Tricuspid valve regurgitation may be idiopathic, infectious, traumatic, or due to rheumatic heart disease. Carcinoid syndrome causes fibrous plaques on the tricuspid and pulmonary valve and is the second most common cause of tricuspid stenosis. Echo/MRI is the image modality of choice.

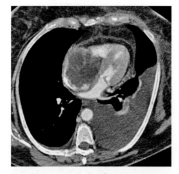

Fig. 18.72 Intracardiac metastasis of breast cancer. The cancer is seen nearly completely occluding the right atrium.

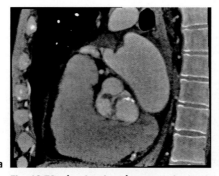

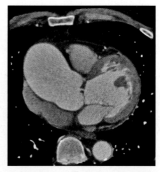

Fig. 18.73a, b Aortic valve stenosis. Aortic valve top view reconstruction shows thickening, fusion, and calcification of valve cusps (**a**). Left ventricular outflow tract (LVOT) MPR shows LV hypertrophy and poststenotic dilation of the aorta (**b**).

Table 18.4   Thoracic calcifications

Disease	CT Findings	Comments
Focal parenchymal calcifications		
Healed tuberculosis or fungal infection	Diffuse or laminated calcification of single or multiple nodules is characteristic. Calcified ipsilateral hilar lymph nodes in combination with a focal calcification in the lung parenchyma (the primary or Ghon lesion) are called the primary or Ranke complex (see also **Fig. 16.40, p. 613**).	Multiple pulmonary parenchymal lesions associated with splenic calcifications suggest histoplasmosis. Viable organisms may hibernate within calcified granulomas. Calcified pulmonary nodules due to previous infection with coccidioidomycosis are rare.
Broncholithiasis	Calcified endobronchial or peribronchial material that erodes, obstructs, or distorts the tracheobronchial tree. Distal mucous plugging and/or air trapping may be seen as a complication.	Uncommon disorder, most likely arising from previously infected (TB, histoplasmosis, etc.), calcified peribronchial lymph nodes that erode into and deform adjacent bronchi.
Hamartoma	Well-circumscribed, lobulated lesion measuring < 4 cm in diameter. Stippled or scattered calcifications are often seen on CT, although not evident in chest radiographs. Nodules may contain both fat and calcium. The frequency of calcification increases with tumor size.	Benign nodule composed of disorganized, mature mesenchymal and epithelial tissue. Commonly contains both cartilage and adipose tissue. Usually an incidental finding. Endobronchial hamartomas occur infrequently.
Bronchial carcinoid	Well-circumscribed tumor located within lobular, segmental, or large subsegmental bronchi. Calcification occurs in > 25% of cases and is observed slightly more often in centrally located tumors.	Stems from the amine precursor uptake decarboxylase (APUD) group of tumors, arising from the Kulchitsky cells of the respiratory endothelium.
Bronchogenic carcinoma	Eccentric calcification within a soft tissue pulmonary mass, usually bronchus associated.	Bronchogenic carcinoma does not primarily calcify but may engulf a preexisting granuloma. Rarely, dystrophic calcification may develop in areas of tumor necrosis.
Calcified metastases	Solitary or multiple calcified intrapulmonary nodules with a lymphatic (involvement of subpleural space) distribution pattern (see also **Fig. 16.88, p. 629**).	Pulmonary metastases of osteosarcoma are common but may not calcify when small. Other neoplasms that may produce calcified metastases are synovial cell sarcoma, chondrosarcoma, mucinous adenocarcinoma, and thyroid neoplasms.
Parasitic diseases (echinococcosis, paragonimiasis)	A pulmonary hydatid cyst presents as a solitary cystic mass with a right lower lobe predominance (adjacent to liver). In contrast to hepatic lesions, which commonly calcify, calcification of pulmonary hydatid cysts is rare. Thin-walled cysts, nodular and linear areas of increased opacity, focal air-space consolidation, and pleural effusions have been described in paragonimiasis. Calcification is a late phenomenon.	Echinococcosis is caused by two cestode species: *Echinococcus granulosus* and, less frequently, *Echinococcus multilocularis*. Lung involvement is observed in ~15% of cases. Pulmonary paragonimiasis is caused by the liver fluke *Paragonimus westermani*, which is usually ingested with raw crayfish or crabs. Pulmonary calcification due to other parasitic diseases is uncommon.
Bronchogenic cyst	Thin-walled cystic lesion with small curvilinear mural calcifications measuring up to a few centimeters in diameter. Predominantly found in central parts of the lung or within the mediastinum.	Rare cause of pulmonary or mediastinal calcification. Bronchogenic cysts usually do not calcify.
Pulmonary arteriovenous (AV) fistula	Lobulated, well-defined, enhancing lung lesion. Precontrast scans may be able to identify calcified phleboliths within the lesion.	Most AV fistulas do not calcify. Feeding vessels are often identifiable.
Diffuse parenchymal calcifications		
Healed histoplasmosis or varicella	Multiple micronodular pulmonary calcifications. Size and density of the nodules are best appreciated by using high-resolution CT.	If associated with both calcified mediastinal and calcified hepatic and splenic micronodules, histoplasmosis is the preferred diagnosis. Extrapulmonary calcified nodules are not a feature of healed varicella pneumonia.
Silicosis	Several small, randomly distributed nodules with a preference for middle and upper parts of both lungs. Central calcifications occur in 5% to 10% of cases and may be located subpleurally. Hilar and mediastinal lymphadenopathy is frequent. Occasionally, lymph nodes show circumferential calcifications (i.e., "eggshell" calcifications).	Silicosis-associated radiographic abnormalities occur after a latency period of up to 10 to 20 y after silica particle exposure. Complicated silicosis is characterized by development of progressive massive fibrosis (PMF) through coalescence of small nodules. PMF is commonly associated with local emphysema and may aggravate respiratory impairment.

(continues on page 670)

Table 18.4   (Cont.) Thoracic calcifications

Disease	CT Findings	Comments
Metastatic pulmonary calcification	Calcified alveolar septa, preferentially in the upper lung zones.	Numerous discrete septal calcium deposits due to combined hypercalcemia and hyperphosphatemia. Can occur with hyperparathyroidism, multiple myeloma, milk–alkali syndrome, hypervitaminosis D, sarcoidosis, and following iatrogenic calcium hyperinfusion.
Pulmonary alveolar microlithiasis	Diffuse ground-glass attenuation throughout both lungs. An increased number of calcifications can be found along bronchovascular bundles and within the subpleural space. Concomitant interstitial fibrosis and subpleural cysts are found in more advanced cases.	Rare condition of unknown etiology, resulting in calcification of the alveolar space. Patients are usually 20 to 40 y of age at the time of diagnosis, may initially be clinically asymptomatic, and show normal serum calcium and phosphorus levels. Late complications include respiratory failure and cor pulmonale.
Amyloidosis	**Tracheobronchial amyloidosis:** Characterized by multiple calcified nodules protruding into the trachea and bronchial wall, causing a bronchial obstruction. **Nodular pulmonary amyloidosis:** Characterized by multiple well-defined, round or oval areas of consolidation that calcify in ~50% of cases. **Diffuse parenchymal amyloidosis:** Nonspecific interstitial disease; does not calcify.	Extracellular deposition of insoluble fibrillar proteinaceous material. Approximately 10% of cases are primary or inherited. Most cases of amyloidosis occur concomitantly with other diseases, including multiple myeloma, other plasma cell dyscrasias, and inflammatory processes. The disease occurs in middle-aged and elderly patients. Respiratory involvement is observed in ~50% of patients.
Mitral stenosis	Two- to 8-mm noduli within alveolar spaces constituting mature bone. Predominance for lower lung zones. Comcomitant mitral valve calcification is common.	Associated with pulmonary venous hypertension and mitral valve disease.
Interstitial pulmonary ossification	**Dendriform type:** Diffusely branching areas of high attenuation, adjacent to the bronchovascular bundle. May be induced by scar formation or bronchiectasis. **Nodular type:** Multiple subpleural micronoduli of increased opacity.	Rare condition observed in association with diffuse lung injury, such as interstitial fibrosis, pulmonary edema, or recurrent bronchopneumonia. Dense areas in both subtypes are composed of mature bone. Presence of pulmonary ossifications has no prognostic significance.
Sarcoidosis	Speckled, amorphous, or popcorn-like calcifications of mediastinal lymph nodes. Circumferential or "eggshell" calcifications are uncommon; miliary pulmonary calcifications are extremely rare (see **Fig. 16.32, p. 609**).	Mediastinal lymph node calcifications occur in 3% to 10% of patients with sarcoidosis. Only diseased lymph nodes can calcify.
Hodgkin disease after therapy	Enlarged hilar and mediastinal lymph nodes with dense, coarse, or popcorn-like calcifications. Calcifications usually occur 1 to 9 y after radiation therapy, rarely after chemotherapy.	Superior mediastinal and hilar lymph nodes are the most commonly involved sites (> 95% of cases). Calcification in lymphoma before therapy is rare.
Pneumocystis carinii infection	Mediastinal nodal calcifications and calcified granulomas in parenchymal organs.	Has been reported in patients with acquired immunodeficiency syndrome (AIDS) who have *P. carinii* infection.
Pleural calcification		
Healed empyema	Unilateral thickening and fibrosis of the visceral pleura that may contain coarse calcifications. Usually a thick layer of soft tissue is found between calcified visceral pleura and the chest wall.	Typically observed in patients with a known history of chronic pleural inflammation. In the past, pleural injection of oil, an iatrogenic inflicted pneumothorax and thoracoplasty were used for treatment of TB, typically resulting in calcified pleural callosities.
Prior hemothorax	Unilateral thickening and fibrosis of the visceral pleura that may contain coarse calcifications. Soft tissue is seen between the chest wall and calcified pleura.	Known history of hemothorax must be present. Often posttraumatic rib changes are associated.
Asbestos exposure	Bilateral, sharply marginated linear thickenings and calcifications of the parietal pleura, most prominent along the diaphragmatic surfaces and in the lower half of the thorax (usually between the sixth and ninth ribs) (see **Figs. 17.6 [p. 632], 17.7 [p. 632], 18.5 [p. 641]**).	May occur 20 y or more after exposure to asbestos or talc. Progresses over time.
Localized fibrous tumor of pleura	Focal thickening of the pleura that may contain calcification.	No relation to asbestos exposure.

Table 18.4 (Cont.) Thoracic calcifications

Disease	CT Findings	Comments
Chest wall calcifications		
Costochondral calcification	Coarse calcification of the cartilaginous portions of the ribs.	Prevalence increases with age: affects 6% of individuals aged 20 to 29 y and ~50% of patients > 70 y of age.
Posttraumatic calcification	Focal calcification in the soft tissues of the chest wall; not associated with bone.	Occurs after direct soft tissue or muscle injury, with subsequent dystrophic mineral deposition.
Dermatomyositis	Calcifications within the subcutaneous tissue and occasionally in the interfascial muscular planes of the chest wall.	Peak occurrence in the first and sixth decades of life; characterized by symmetric proximal muscle weakness with associated cutaneous rash and vasculitis.
Bone tumor	Calcific or osseous mass adjacent to ribs, vertebral bodies, or sternum (see **Fig. 17.16, p. 635**).	Osteochondroma and chondrosarcoma are the most common calcified primary bone tumors affecting the chest wall. Fibrous dysplasia of the rib may be expansile and have a tumorlike appearance on CT.
Cardiovascular calcifications		
Arteriosclerosis	Intimal calcification of the aorta and/or anulus. The mitral valve anulus is often calcified as well. Coronary artery calcification is most commonly seen in the proximal LCX artery (see **Figs. 16.27a [p. 607], 18.35 [p. 653]**).	Increased diameter of the aorta is indicative of an aneurysm. Coronary artery calcifications are associated with coronary artery disease and may be semiquantified according to the method of Agatston by using ECG-triggered CT of the heart. Also, the amount of hydroxyapatite and the total plaque volume can be accurately measured.
Aortic valve disease	Stippled calcification of the aortic valve. If done without ECG triggering, streak artifacts due to cardiac motion are common (see **Figs. 16.27a [p. 607], 18.73a [p. 668]**).	Aortic valve calcification under the age of 50 is likely to be of rheumatic origin. Particularly if the aortic wall lacks calcifications, causes other than atherosclerosis are likely. Irrespective of the underlying pathology, the amount of calcification is directly associated with left heart insufficiency: patients with intense calcification of the leaflets and anulus bear a 75% risk within the next 5 y.
Rheumatoid mitral valve disease	Usually difficult to visualize on chest CT scans due to motion artifacts.	Aortic valve and anulus calcifications are usually concomitant. Left atrial wall may be calcified as well.
Myocardial infarction (MI)	Usually LV wall calcifications, most commonly observed near the apex with or without aneurysmal dilation (see **Fig. 18.57, p. 663**).	MI is the predominant cause. Calcified myocardial damage due to trauma, syphilis, myocarditis, rheumatic fever, or hyperparathyroidism is rare.
Pericarditis	Calcifications of the pericardium, most commonly observed near the atrioventricular groove (see **Fig. 16.62, p. 621**).	Common causes of pericarditis include TB, rheumatoid fever, bacterial pneumonia, MI, viral infection, syphilis, histoplasmosis, asbestosis, and trauma.
Left atrial myxoma or thrombus	Partly calcified LA soft tissue mass. Motion artifacts may mask atrial myxoma on normal chest CT scans.	A calcified left atrial appendage is highly indicative of a calcified thrombus.
Ductus arteriosus	Calcification and associated motion artifacts at the site of the ductus arteriosus Botalli.	May be difficult to differentiate from aortic calcification; typically represents an occluded ductus.

VI Abdomen and Pelvis

19 Liver

Christopher Herzog

With an average volume of 1400 to 1700 mL and a maximum craniocaudal expansion of 12 cm, the liver represents the largest parenchymatous organ of the body. Although liver size distinctly varies with body size and gender, a liver volume of ≥ 2000 mL and a craniocaudal stretch of ≥ 15 cm is equivalent to hepatomegaly. The normal proportion between the right and left liver lobe is 3:2. If there is gas in the biliary tree, it tends to be located centrally (see **Fig. 20.11, p. 707**), whereas gas in the portal branches (seen in intestinal ischemia) collects peripherally (see **Fig. 24.21, p. 753**). On computed tomography (CT) scans, gas usually is more prominent in the right than the left liver lobe (due to scanning in a supine position).

Overall density (attenuation) of normal adult liver on post-contrast CT scans amounts to 60 to 70 HU but may range between 38 and 80 HU on non–contrast-enhanced images. All lobes have approximately the same attenuation; thus, geographic variation of attenuation within an individual is usually < 10 HU. On non–contrast-enhanced scans, CT attenuation should be 8 to 10 HU greater than that of spleen or muscle. Portal as well as hepatic veins are seen as lower-attenuation branching structures within the parenchyma, whereas near-water-attenuating bile ducts are difficult to delineate. Abnormally decreased density usually is a sign of fatty infiltration (steatosis), but it may also be due to drug toxicity, infection (e.g., viral hepatitis), or diffuse tumor infiltration (e.g., lymphoma). In case of steatosis, CT attenuation decreases by ~15 HU per 10% increase in fat; > 15% fat infiltration on non–contrast-enhanced scans leads to masking of intrahepatic vessels (see **Fig. 19.33, p. 695**). Higher levels of fat infiltration cause an inversion of contrast, where liver vessels appear hyperdense as compared with liver parenchyma.

Abnormally increased liver density usually is observed in the presence of iron overload (hemochromatosis/hemosiderosis), but it may also be induced by other metals, such as copper (Wilson disease), iodine (amiodarone), gold (antirheumatic base treatment), and thallium. Rare causes are acute massive protein overload and glycogen storage diseases. CT attenuation increases proportionally with metal overload, but increase in attenuation strongly depends on effective beam energy and thus varies depending on tube voltage, type of scanner, and patient size. After proper intravenous contrast administration, the blood vessels are highly attenuating and help in delineating the lobular and segmental anatomy of the liver. The portal vein, formed by the confluence of the superior mesenteric vein and splenic vein, ascends through the hepatoduodenal ligament at the anterior margin of the inferior vena cava into the porta hepatis, where it bifurcates into the right and left portal vein. The hepatic artery lies anterior to the portal vein. The left portal vein extends over the anterior surface of the caudate lobe into the left lobe. The right portal vein bifurcates into anterior and posterior branches, which run through the central portions of the anterior and posterior segments. The segmental classification (S1–S8) of the liver is due to the anatomy of the portal vein branches (P1–P8), while hepatic vein anatomy is the landmark for the segmentation (**Fig. 19.1**).

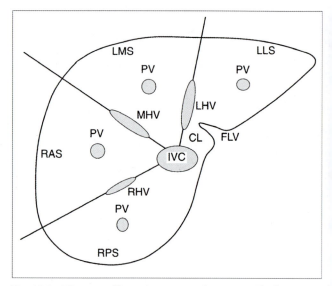

Fig. 19.1   Diagram of hepatic segmental anatomy. The hepatic venous anatomy provides landmarks for the fissures dividing the liver into lobes and segments.
CL   caudate lobe
FLV   fissure of the ligamentum venosum
IVC   inferior vena cava
LHV   left hepatic vein
LLS   lateral segment of the left lobe
LMS medial segment of the left lobe
MHV middle hepatic vein
PV   portal vein
RAS anterior segment of the right lobe
RHV right hepatic vein
RPS posterior segment of the right lobe
(Modified after Webb.)

At the higher level, the left hepatic vein and at the lower level, the left intersegmental fissure, which contains fat and the ligamentum teres, separate the medial and lateral segments of the left hepatic lobe. Similarly, the middle hepatic vein and interlobular fissure, which contains the gallbladder recess, separate the left and right hepatic lobes (**Fig. 19.2**). The right hepatic vein bisects the right lobe into the anterior and posterior segments, but the right intersegmental fissure cannot be visualized directly by CT. Sometimes an accessory right hepatic vein is present.

Some anatomical variants may resemble an abnormality. An unusually prominent lateral segment may extend laterally to the spleen (see **Fig. 19.13, p. 681**). The rare congenital absence of the right or left lobe results in hypertrophy of the contralateral lobe. Children who have received a left lateral segment liver transplant develop an unusually shaped liver for obvious reasons. The papillary process of the caudate lobe may sometimes appear separate from the liver and simulate an extrinsic mass. Scalloping of the diaphragm in the elderly may create an accessory fissure of the right hepatic lobe. This is a normal variant (**Fig. 19.3**).

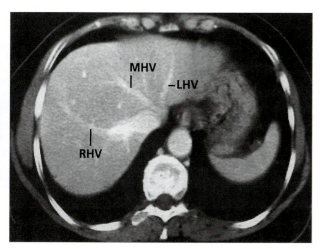

Fig. 19.2   Hepatic veins on contrast-enhanced CT.
LHV   left hepatic vein
MHV   middle hepatic vein
RHV   right hepatic vein

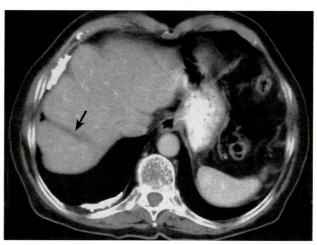

Fig. 19.3   Accessory "fissure" in an 83-year-old woman. Fissure caused by scalloping of the diaphragm is seen in the right lobe of the liver (arrow).

The bare area of the liver refers to the posterior surface of the liver, which is in direct contact with the diaphragm. It helps in differentiating pleural fluid collections, which are seen throughout the entire posterior aspect of the posterior perihepatic space, whereas peritoneal fluid stops medially at the bare area of the liver, except for patients with a liver transplant and consequently absent bare area (**Fig. 19.5, p. 677**).

CT images of the liver should be acquired in a helical scanning mode, with a slice collimation of at least 5 mm and a gantry rotation time ≤ 0.5s. On current multidetector-row CT scanners, slice collimation ranges from 1.2 to 0.6 mm and continuous volume data sets can be acquired within 2 to 8 seconds. These technical parameters give way for full liver coverage during one breath hold, as well as (near) isometric voxel size and thus artifact-free image reformation in any spatial orientation (coronal, sagittal, etc.). Best results for multiplanar image reformation can be obtained by reconstructing overlapping axial thin slices (≤ 3 mm) at 50% increment. Raw data should be acquired during inspiratory breath hold and with the patient lying in a supine position. The scan range usually extends from the lower parts of the lung to the lower margin of the liver. However, if liver imaging is performed in the course of an abdominal scan, scans may extend caudally to the symphysis. Optimal image contrast is achieved by applying window/level settings of 250/40 in native and delayed CT scans and 350/60 in postcontrast scans.

Proper timing of bolus injection of contrast material is key to sufficient liver visualization and thus requires adequate volume and rate of delivery. In patients with a normal body mass index (BMI), 100 to 120 mL of contrast material with an iodine concentration ≥ 320 mg I/mL are injected at a rate of 5 mL/s.

Four phases of liver parenchyma attenuation can be distinguished after contrast material injection (**Fig. 19.17, p. 683**): hepatic arterial phase (~18–25 s p.i.), portal venous phase (~30–40 s p.i.), parenchymal phase (~70–80 s p.i.), and delayed or equilibrium phase (2–5 min p.i.). The hepatic arterial phase (HAP) is suited for hepatic arterial angiography, the portal venous phase (PVP) for detection and characterization of hypervascular tumors. The parenchymal phase (PP) is a standard procedure in abdominal CT imaging, and the delayed phase (DP) may be added to further characterize hepatic masses (particularly useful for identification of cholangiocarcinomas and hemangiomas). A proper HAP shows densely opacified arteries, moderately enhanced portal veins, and only minimally enhanced liver parenchyma. During the PVP, portal and hepatic veins are densely opacified and hyperdense as compared with liver parenchyma, which also is maximally enhanced. In the PP, liver parenchyma, vessels, and most masses appear isodense. Nonenhanced CT scans of the liver can distinguish benign lesions such as fatty infiltration, calcifications, or cysts and thus may be used in the course of baseline scans in oncological staging but not for follow-up examinations.

Blood supply of normal liver parenchyma constitutes 75% of portal venous and 25% of arterial blood; that of liver tumors, 80% and 95%, respectively.

Highest diagnostic accuracy in detecting the number and determining the extent of liver lesions still is obtained by using CT arterial portography (CTAP). However, with the introduction of helical CT scanners and power injectors for continuous delivery of contrast material, this technique has largely been abandoned. Proper CTAP imaging requires injection of up to 150 mL of dilute iodine (150 mg I/mL) injected at a rate of 3 mL/s into a catheter placed in the superior mesenteric artery or splenic artery. Helical CT of the liver is then performed during the PVP and late venous phase. With this approach, lesions ≥ 1 cm are detected with up to 100% sensitivity and 91% specificity.

For multidetector-row CT, sensitivity and specificity range from 86% to 92% and 71% to 91%, respectively, depending not only on the type and vascularity of the lesion but also on the number of the contrast phase applied. Thus, for initial oncological staging, a triphasic protocol is recommended: scanning before contrast administration and during the late HAP and PVP. Any follow-up examination can be restricted to late arterial and venous scans in the presence of hypervascular lesions (hepatocellular carcinoma, metastases, carcinoids, etc.).

The differential diagnostic aspects of focal liver abnormalities as seen on CT are discussed in **Table 19.1. Table 19.2** discusses diffuse liver abnormalities.

Table 19.1   Focal liver lesions

Disease	CT Findings	Comments
Vascular		
Hepatic venous outflow obstruction (Budd–Chiari syndrome) ▷ *Fig. 19.4*	Segmental or global venous outflow obstruction. Often accompanied by large regenerative nodules. Hepatic veins usually not visualized or even clotted with thrombotic material (hypodense). **Scan recommendation:** Multiphasic CT (nonenhanced CT, portal venous phase [PVP], parenchymal phase [PP]). Nonenhanced CT: Typically, peripheral low attenuation of the liver parenchyma, with higher attenuation in central portions of the left lobe and the caudate lobe. PVP: Patchy enhancement on early contrast images. PP: Reverse of this pattern or persistent patchy central enhancement. **Diagnostic pearls:** Despite appropriate enhancement of the inferior vena cava (IVC), aorta, and hemiazygos vein, there is a lack of contrast in the hepatic veins. Characteristics include collateral gastric veins "flip-flop" pattern of central portions of the left liver lobe and caudate lobe on PVP (enhancement) and PP images (decreased enhancement).	Rare clinical entity of obstruction of hepatic venous outflow. Causing agents may be pregnancy, hypercoagulopathy states, oral contraceptives, invading tumors, and congenital webs. Occlusion may occur at the level of intrahepatic venules, hepatic veins, or the IVC. Associated findings include narrowing of the IVC and dilated collateral veins (azygos, hemiazygos, or subcutaneous), ascites, and portal thrombosis. Hepatomegaly, regional intrahepatic attenuation differences, and large regenerative nodules are characteristic.
Liver infarction ▷ *Fig. 19.5*	A wedge-shaped, low-attenuation lesion due to local vascular obstruction. Initially, infarcts are poorly marginated but become more discernible in a subacute/chronic situation. **Scan recommendation:** Biphasic CT (nonenhanced CT, PP). Nonenhanced CT: Wedge-shaped, low-attenuation lesion with poor delineation to surrounding liver tissue. The more subacute/chronic the infarction, the better demarcated the margins. PP: Distribution segmental or diffuse, non- or patchy heterogeneous enhancement, depending on degree and extent of occlusion. **Diagnostic pearls:** Wedge-shaped, low-attenuation lesions with segmental distribution on pre- and postcontrast scans.	Histologic feature of acute hepatic infarction is centrilobular necrosis with local hemorrhage. Chronic findings include focal atrophy of the involved segment and hypodense or cystic changes. The portal venous system accounts for 75% of the blood supply of the liver. Thus, hepatic infarction usually is caused by the superimposition of portal vein occlusion on preexisting hepatic artery stenosis. Etiology for hepatic artery stenosis includes atherosclerosis, embolism, thrombosis, vasculitis, and hypotension/shock. Portal vein occlusion/thrombosis may be (1) caused by pregnancy or oral contraceptives, (2) iatrogenic (during intra-abdominal surgery, surgery of thrombogenic organs (prostate, uterus, etc.), or (3) paraneoplastic (pancreas).
Infection		
Pyogenic abscess ▷ *Fig. 19.6*	Small abscesses are sharply defined lesions, often surrounded by a capsule and septated. They may aggregate into a single large cavity. **Scan recommendation:** Biphasic CT (nonenhanced CT, PP). Nonenhanced CT: Well-defined, round lesions, denser than water but less dense than liver. PP: Distinct enhancement of capsule and septa. No enhancement of central portion (necrosis). **Diagnostic pearls:** "Cluster of grapes" sign: cluster of multilocular collections of pus coalescing into larger centrally located septated cavities.	Destruction of hepatic parenchyma with localized collection of pus due to a bacterial infection. Twenty to 30% contain gas, but gas–fluid levels are rare. Immature abscesses may not be cystic. Usually occur in immunocompromised or older patients with predisposing conditions, such as biliary/pancreatic diseases, diverticulitis, colitis, appendicitis, trauma, and septicemia. Necrotic metastases (from sarcoma or ovarian carcinoma) may look alike and even become infected.
Opportunistic abscess ▷ *Fig. 19.7*	Multiple round hypodense hepatic lesions. Micronodular abscesses may even make liver appear almost normal or slightly heterogeneous. **Scan recommendation:** Biphasic CT (nonenhanced CT, PP). Nonenhanced CT: Multiple small hypodense lesions. PP: Lesions remain hypodense without any attenuation. **Diagnostic pearls:** Multiple ill-defined micronodular hypodense lesions seen on pre- and postcontrast scans.	Microabscesses typically are observed in immunocompromised patients and are caused by *Candida*, less commonly by *Aspergillus*, *Pneumocystis carinii*, or atypical mycobacteria. Because needle biopsy may be false-negative, open wedge biopsy is usually required for final diagnosis. Differential diagnosis: rule out biliary hamartomas, Caroli disease, and metastases. Typically, similar nodules are also found in the spleen and/or lung (septicemia).

(continues on page 678)

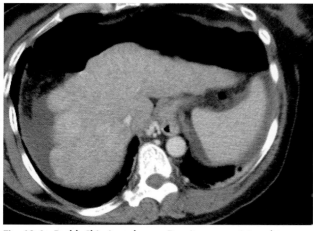

Fig. 19.4   Budd–Chiari syndrome. Despite appropriate enhancement of the inferior vena cava (IVC), aorta, and hemiazygos vein, there is a lack of contrast in the hepatic veins. Note the collateral gastric veins ventrally to the hemiazygos vein and medially to the cardia.

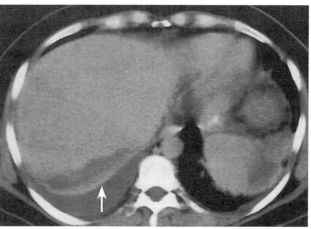

Fig. 19.5   Right liver lobe with decreased attenuation due to infarction after liver transplantation. The hyperdense stripe posterior to the right liver lobe represents the diaphragm (arrow). There is fluid on both sides of the diaphragm in the absence of a bare area.

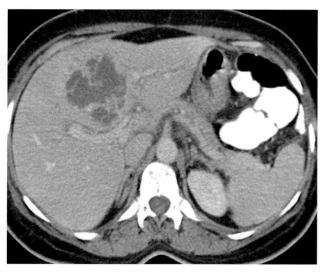

Fig. 19.6   Liver abscess with typical "cluster of grapes" sign. Cluster of multilocular pus collections coalesce into a larger centrally located septated cavity.

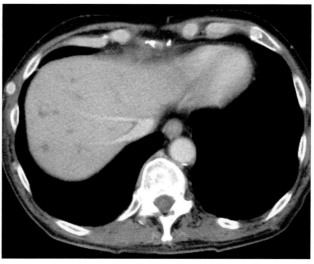

Fig. 19.7   Opportunistic abscesses. Multiple ill-defined, micronodular, hypodense lesions.

Table 19.1 (Cont.) Focal liver lesions

Disease	CT Findings	Comments
Amebic abscess ▷ *Fig. 19.8*	Peripherally located, well-defined, round, hypodense cystic lesion with enhancing capsule. **Scan recommendation:** Biphasic CT (nonenhanced CT, PP). Nonenhanced CT: Hypodense as compared with normal liver parenchyma. PP: Nonenhancing center, enhancing inner rim, and hypodense outer rim. **Diagnostic pearls:** Well-defined, round, targetlike lesions with preference for the right liver lobe.	Underlying infection is amebiasis of the cecum and ascending colon. In ~8% of cases, amebas invade liver through the portal venous system. Common in developing countries (~10% of the world population). May be complicated by rupture into the peritoneum, through the diaphragm, subphrenic abscess, biliary obstruction, or septic emboli. Do not touch lesions; antimicrobial therapy and cytotoxic drugs are treatment of choice. Differential diagnosis: rule out hepatic pyogenic abscess, hepatic hydatid cyst, and biliary cystadeno-carcinoma.
Echinococcal (hydatid) cyst ▷ *Fig. 19.9*	Large, well-defined, cystic liver mass surrounded by several peripheral satellite (daughter) cysts. **Scan recommendation:** Biphasic CT (nonenhanced CT, PP). Nonenhanced CT: Cysts appear hypodense to normal liver parenchyma. PP: Enhancement of cysts' walls and septations. **Diagnostic pearls:** Large well-defined, hypodense, cystic liver mass with intracystic septations, irregular wall calcifications surrounded by numerous (less hypodense) daughter cysts.	Caused by *Echinococcus granulosus* or *Echinococcus multilocularis:* parasitic eggs are ingested after contact with dogs or foxes/contaminated food or water. *E. granulosus* infiltrates liver within days, develops into typical hydatid cysts, and grows up to 3 cm per year in diameter. *E. multilocularis* effects a diffuse tissue infiltration, induces a granulomatous hepatic tissue reaction followed by necrosis, cavitation, and calcifications. Air–fluid levels typically represent cyst rupture and not infection. Rupture into the biliary tree is the most common complication, causing biliary dilation and cyst wall discontinuity. Clinical symptoms of biliary rupture are pain, fever, and jaundice. Treatment of choice is surgical resection; alternatively, percutaneous aspiration/injection and albendazole may be used.
Congenital		
Caroli disease ▷ *Fig. 19.10a, b*	Multiple low-attenuating cystic masses in the liver associated with a dilated biliary tree. **Scan recommendation**: Biphasic CT (nonenhanced CT, PVP, PP). Nonenhanced CT: Multiple round to saccular hypodense cysts. PP: Cysts may contain a hyperdense central "dot" representing enhancing portal radicles. **Diagnostic pearls:** Multiple well-delineated, round to saccular hypodense cysts with a hyperdense central "dot" during the PVP.	Rare condition characterized by multiple saccular dilations of the intrahepatic bile ducts throughout the liver. Medullary sponge kidney is associated in 80% of cases.
Trauma		
Biloma (bile pseudocyst) ▷ *Fig. 19.11*	Water-density, usually crescent or ovoid mass within or immediately adjacent to the liver. **Scan recommendation:** Biphasic CT (nonenhanced CT, PP). Nonenhanced CT: Near-water density. PP: No contrast enhancement of the wall or contents. **Diagnostic pearls:** Well-delineated, homogeneous, round, near-water-density lesions without enhancement after contrast application.	Intra- or extrahepatic collection of bile after traumatic rupture or surgery of the biliary tree.
Laceration ▷ *Fig. 19.12*	Irregular cleft or low-attenuation area that often extends to the periphery of the liver. A solitary (simple) or branching (stellate/radiating pattern may be seen. Often accompanied by intra- and perihepatic hemorrhage. **Scan recommendation:** Biphasic CT (nonenhanced CT, PP). Nonenhanced CT: Lacerations show near-water density. Hemorrhage may be acute (unclotted) or subacute (clotted). Unclotted blood (> 50 HU) and clotted blood (< 90 HU) typically are hyperdense to lacerations and liver parenchyma. PP: Active hemorrhage seen as contrast extravasation (Caveat: Injection rate must be ≥ 5 mL/s).	Small hyperdense blood clots may be detected within the laceration. Lacerations evolve from sharply marginated low-attenuation lesions into indistinguishable areas after several weeks.

(continues on page 680)

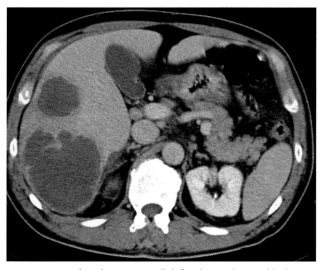

Fig. 19.8 Amebic abscesses. Well-defined, round, targetlike lesions with nonenhancing center, enhancing inner rim, and hypodense outer rim (edema).

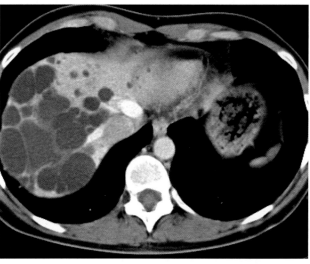

Fig. 19.9 Echinococcal (hydatid) cyst. Large well-defined cystic liver mass surrounded by several peripheral satellite (daughter) cysts.

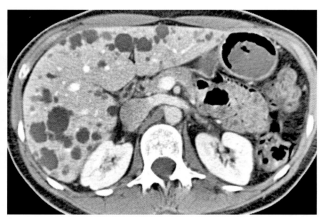

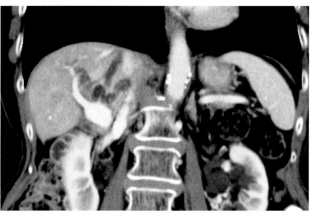

b

Fig. 19.10a, b Caroli disease. Multiple well-delineated round cysts. Hyperdense central dots (i.e., portal radicles) are not yet visible on the axial image during the hepatic arterial phase (HAP) (**a**), but they are seen on the coronal multiplanar reconstruction (MPR) during the portal venous phase (PVP) (**b**).

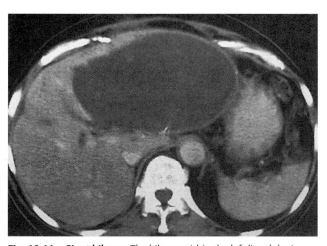

Fig. 19.11 Giant biloma. The biloma within the left liver lobe is secondary to biliary tree damage.

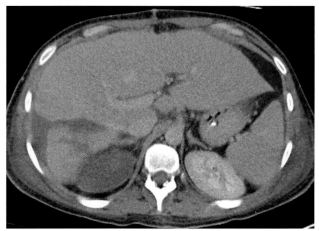

Fig. 19.12 Liver laceration due to blunt trauma. Hypodense irregular cleft is seen through the right liver lobe. Note the adjacent perihepatic fluid and nonattenuation of the right kidney.

Table 19.1 (Cont.) Focal liver lesions

Disease	CT Findings	Comments
Intrahepatic hematoma ▷ *Fig. 19.13a, b*	Round, oval, changing density patterns depending on acuteness of hemorrhage. **Scan recommendation:** Biphasic CT (nonenhanced CT, PP). Nonenhanced CT: Subacute hematoma usually hyperdense (< 90 HU), chronic hematoma (10–30 d after onset of bleeding) usually hypodense (20–25 HU). PP: Subacute hematoma may become isodense after CM. **Diagnostic pearls:** Hyperdense intrahepatic round, oval, or irregular lesions on nonenhanced CT scans.	Usually secondary to penetrating or blunt trauma, rarely due to adenoma, metastasis, or arteriovenous malformation (AVM). Differential diagnosis: bilioma: remains hypodense on all scans.
Subcapsular hematoma	Well-marginated, crescentic or lenticular fluid collection beneath the hepatic capsule. High-attenuation lesion in the beginning and diminishing gradually over several weeks to become a low-attenuation lesion. **Scan recommendation:** Biphasic CT (nonenhanced CT, PP). Nonenhanced CT: Subacute hematoma usually hyperdense (< 90 HU), chronic hematoma (10–30 d after onset of bleeding) usually hypodense (20–25 HU). PP: Subacute hematoma may appear isodense after CM. **Diagnostic pearls:** Well-marginated, crescentic fluid collection beneath the hepatic capsule.	May result from trauma, surgery, or percutaneous interventions (cholangiography, biopsy, portography, or biliary drainage procedures). Patients usually report right chest pain during breathing or pain radiating into the right shoulder. Pain usually diminishes within a few days, but it may continue. Keep patients on strong medication as needed.

Inflammation

Disease	CT Findings	Comments
Hepatic sarcoidosis ▷ *Fig. 19.14*	Presence of diffuse small noncaseating granulomas in the liver of patients with known Boeck disease (sarcoidosis). **Scan recommendation:** Biphasic CT (nonenhanced CT, PP). Nonenhanced CT/PVP: Multiple ill-defined, hypodense hepatic noduli or heterogeneous appearance of liver parenchyma, often accompanied by hepatosplenomegaly. PP: Hepatic noduli become isodense to normal liver parenchyma. **Diagnostic pearls:** Always consider in patients with lymphadenopathy and hepatosplenomegaly. Often also found in the spleen.	Histologically, noncaseating epithelioid granulomas with multinucleated giant cells of Langerhans type. Causing agent of granulomas unknown. Two thirds of patients are women 20 to 40 y old. Up to 80% of all patients with sarcoidosis present with involvement of abdominal organs, particularly of the liver and spleen. Treatment through corticosteroids, antiinflammatory agents, and cytotoxic drugs. May not be discernible from liver hamartoma, opportunistic abscesses, metastases.
Focal fatty infiltration ▷ *Fig. 19.15*	Varies from a small oval focus, typically adjacent to the intersegmental fissure, to segmental, lobar, or geographic distribution. No mass effect, contour change, or vascular displacement. **Scan recommendation:** Biphasic CT (nonenhanced CT, PP). Nonenhanced CT: Poor delineation to normal liver parenchyma (iso-/slightly hypodense). PP: Slightly hypodense as compared with normal liver parenchyma; noncompromised intralesional vessels. **Diagnostic pearls:** Poorly delineated lesion often adjacent to the intersegmental fissure slightly hypodense to normal liver parenchyma on all phases and noncompromising hepatic vessels.	Histologically regional reversible accumulation of triglycerides within hepatocytes that can simulate neoplasia. Typically associated with obesity, alcoholism, small bowel bypass surgery, diabetes, chemotherapy, hyperalimentation, blunt abdominal trauma, cystic fibrosis, congestive heart failure, Reye syndrome, steroid therapy, and Cushing syndrome. Lesion may occur and disappear within weeks.

(continues on page 682)

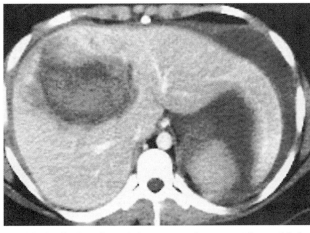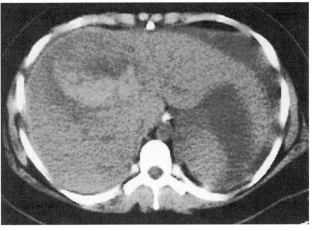

b

Fig. 19.13a, b   Intrahepatic hematoma. Precontrast image (**a**) shows a slightly hyperdense intrahepatic lesion surrounded by hypodense edema. Postcontrast image (**b**) shows normal attenuation of liver parenchyma but not hematoma. Note an unusually prominent lateral segment of the liver.

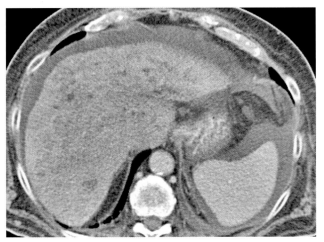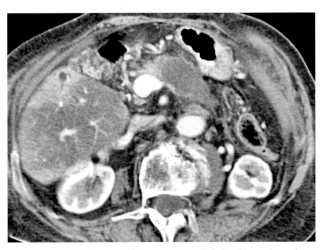

Fig. 19.14   Sarcoidosis of the liver. Multiple ill-defined, hypodense hepatic noduli. Signs of cirrhosis are evident in the nodular liver margin, marked ascites, and inhomogeneous parenchymal contrast, which is most likely also due to sarcoidosis. No involvement of the spleen is seen. Micrometastases or cystic liver hamartomas may have similar CT features.

Fig. 19.15   Focal fatty infiltration. Large ill-defined hypodense lesion in the right liver lobe, with noncompromising hepatic vessels.

Table 19.1 (Cont.) Focal liver lesions

Disease	CT Findings	Comments
Periportal edema ▷ *Fig. 19.16*	Nonenhancing low-density collection encasing the branches of the portal vein (see also **Fig. 24.3, p. 741**).	Common postoperative finding in liver transplants. Does not indicate rejection. May also occur in combination with significant edema of other abdominal organs.
Radiation hepatitis	Sharply defined band of diminished density in the liver corresponding to the radiation port.	May develop within days/months after radiation therapy (radiation dose ≥ 35 Gy). May show evidence of recovery.
Benign neoplasms		
Hepatic hemangioma ▷ *Fig. 19.17a–d*	Benign neoplasm of thin, fibrous stroma that surrounds multiple vascular channels lined by a single layer of endothelial cells. **Scan recommendation:** Multiphasic CT (nonenhanced CT, hepatic arterial phase [HAP], PP, delayed phase [DP]). Nonenhanced CT: Small hemangiomas are usually well-circumscribed masses isodense to blood. Large hemangiomas appear more heterogeneous and may contain central fibrotic cleft of low density. HAP: Early peripheral global or nodular enhancement. PP: Progressive centripetal filling usually isodense to blood. DP: Persistent global enhancement that stays isodense with blood. **Diagnostic pearls:** < 10 cm lesion commonly in subcapsular location (right > left liver lobe) with peripheral globular enhancements on HAP scans and progressive centripetal enhancement following contrast phases (flash filling). Hemangiomas usually are isodense to blood and thus show a similar enhancement pattern as the aorta.	The most common hepatic neoplasm, seen in 7% or more of the normal population. A significant proportion of hemangiomas does not present a characteristic pattern of contrast enhancement and may thus simulate metastasis. Metastases from breast carcinoma and gastrointestinal stromal tumor (GIST) may not be discernible from typical hemangiomas (see **Fig. 24.13, p. 747**). Hemangiomas grow slowly from childhood to adulthood, more rapidly during pregnancy. May spontaneously regress.

(continues on page 684)

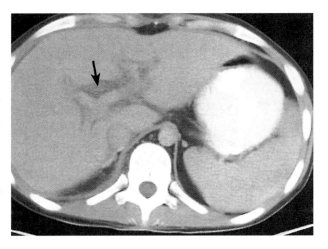

Fig. 19.16   Periportal edema. Low-density band (arrow) within the porta hepatis surrounding the branches of the portal vein.

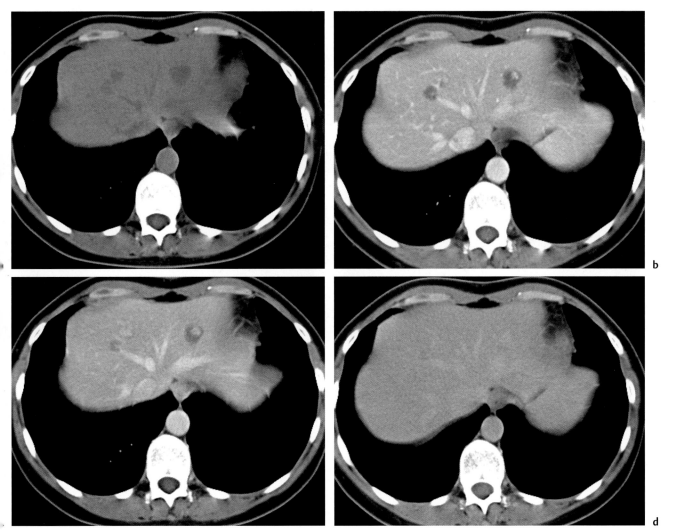

Fig. 19.17a–d   Hemangioma. Hypodense lesions in liver segments 2 and 8 on noncontrast scans (**a**). After contrast material injection, early peripheral nodular enhancement is seen during the HAP (**b**), progressive centripetal filling during the PP (**c**), and persistent global enhancement that stays isodense with blood during the DP (**d**).

Table 19.1   (Cont.) Focal liver lesions

Disease	CT Findings	Comments
Focal nodular hyperplasia (FNH) ▷ *Fig. 19.18a–c* ▷ *Fig. 19.19a, b*	Well-circumscribed benign hamartomatous liver lesion with subcapsular preference. Majority of FNH appear solitary and < 5 cm in diameter (80% of cases). **Scan recommendation:** Multiphasic CT (nonenhanced CT, HAP, PP, DP). Nonenhanced CT: Hypo- or isodense to normal liver parenchyma. Any central scar appears even more hypodense. HAP: Bright homogeneous enhancement. PP: Hypo-/isodense to normal liver parenchyma. DP: Isodense to normal liver parenchyma. If there is a scar, it is hyperdense. **Diagnostic pearls:** Well-differentiated mass with distinct homogeneous enhancement on HAP and continuously becoming isodense to liver parenchyma; on delayed images, often showing a hyperdense central scar. May resemble a cross section of a grapefruit.	Rare benign liver tumor most often seen in women between age 20 and 50 y. Histologically, a hyperplastic stroma response to local abnormal vasculature. Oral contraceptives have stimulating effect on FNH growth but are not responsible for existence per se. Usually incidentally detected, multiple in 7% to 20% of cases. Central scars are visible in ~70% of large and 30% of small FNHs. Central scar also seen in atypical HCCs, fibrolamellar hepatomas, hepatic adenomas, and giant hemangiomas. Absence of intratumoral calcifications, necrosis, and hemorrhage may help to differentiate from these lesions. Any definitive diagnosis requires hepatic biopsy.
Hepatic adenoma ▷ *Fig. 19.19a, b*	Heterogeneous subcapsular hypervascular lesion, on average 8 to 15 cm in diameter, with a preference for the right lobe of the liver and surrounded by a pseudocapsule. **Scan recommendation:** Multiphasic CT (nonenhanced CT, HAP, PVP, DP). Nonenhanced CT: Well-defined mass with intratumoral presence of hypodense (fat) and/or hyperdense (calcifications, hemorrhage) areas. HAP: Heterogeneous hyperdense enhancement. PVP: Hypo-/iso-/hyperdense to normal liver parenchyma. DP: Homogeneous isodense (to liver) enhancement. Pseudocapsule appears hyperdense as compared with normal liver parenchyma and adenoma. **Diagnostic pearls:** Well-defined, heterogeneous (intratumoral fat/hemorrhage), hypervascular lesion with pseudocapsule on DP images in a noncirrhotic liver.	Usually unilocular large lesions, typically in young women taking oral contraceptives. May also occur in men who use androgens or anabolic steroids. Multilocular adenomas (hepatic adenomatosis) seen in patients with glycogen storage disease or diabetes mellitus. Internal hemorrhage or necrosis is common (36%). Histologically, adenomas lack bile ducts and portal/central veins but contain hepatocytes that are arranged in cords/sheets. May contain malignant foci. Forming of a pseudocapsule due to compression of adjacent liver tissue. On CT scans, often indistinguishable from HCC, but presence of a pseudocapsule and absence of cirrhosis are suggestive.

(continues on page 686)

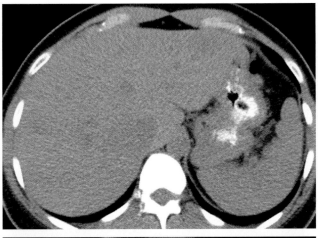
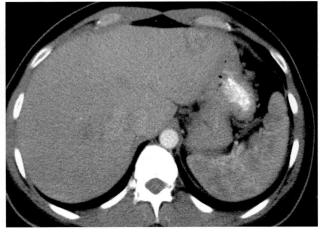
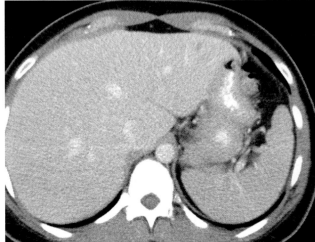

Fig. 19.18a–c   Focal nodular hyperplasia (FNH). On precontrast scans, a hypodense lesion (**a**) is visible ventrally in the left liver lobe (liver segment 2) with distinct homogeneous enhancement during the HAP (**b**) and becoming isodense to liver parenchyma during the PP (**c**). Note the hypodense central scar on all scans.

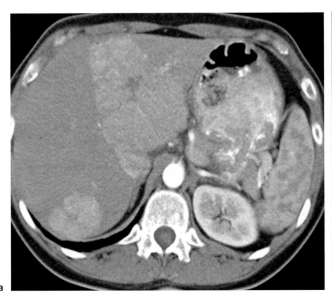
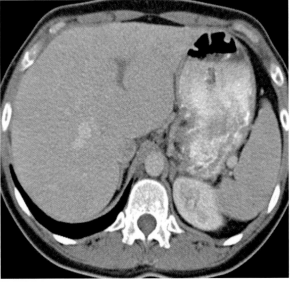

Fig. 19.19a, b   Hepatic adenoma. Large well-defined mass in the left liver lobe with a fatty center and hyperdense attenuation during the HAP (**a**). The lobe becomes isodense to normal liver parenchyma during the PP (**b**). Note also the small FNH in the right liver lobe (liver segment 6 dorsally) with similar attenuation features but a hypodense central scar that becomes slightly hyperdense during the PP.

Table 19.1   (Cont.) Focal liver lesions

Disease	CT Findings	Comments
Nodular regenerative hyperplasia ▷ *Fig. 19.20*	Either multiple micronodular or solitary macronodular, preferably hypervascular liver lesions. Size varies from < 1 mm (micronodular) to 4 cm (macronodular). **Scan recommendation:** Multiphasic CT (nonenhanced CT, HAP, PVP). Nonenhanced CT: Lesions isoattenuating to normal liver parenchyma. HAP/PVP: Homogeneously hyperdense lesions sometimes with hypodense peripheral "halo." **Diagnostic pearls:** Multiple micronodular liver lesions with hyperattenuation on both HAP and PVP images.	Histologically, regenerative nodules consist of hyperplastic hepatocytes surrounding dilated, atypically formed, large sinusoids. Peripheral halo, if present, evoked by enlarged surrounding sinuses (peliosis). May mimic metastases. Larger nodules may have central scar and thus be indistinguishable from FNH.
Mesenchymal (biliary) hamartoma ▷ *Fig. 19.14, p. 681*	Multiple micronodular (< 15 mm), low-density cystic or solid lesions. **Scan recommendation:** Multiphasic CT (nonenhanced CT, PVP, PP). Nonenhanced CT: Cystic lesions with near-water density. Solid lesions have low density compared with normal liver parenchyma. PVP: Cystic lesions isodense to water; solid lesions enhance strongly. PP: Cystic lesions remain isodense; solid lesions become isodense to normal liver parenchyma. **Diagnostic pearls:** Multiple small lesions with identical near-water attenuation on pre- and postcontrast scans.	Rare. Histologically, proliferated bile ducts embedded in mesenchymal tissue. May be associated with polycystic liver disease. Solid lesions may mimic hemangioma. Cystic lesions have similar CT features as sarcoidosis but without coexistent lesions in the spleen.
Hepatic cyst ▷ *Fig. 19.21*	Sharply delineated, round or oval lesion of near-water attenuation. **Scan recommendation:** Biphasic CT (nonenhanced CT, PP). Nonenhanced CT: Near-water density. PP: No contrast enhancement of the wall or contents. **Diagnostic pearls:** Well-delineated, homogeneous, round, near-water density lesions without enhancement after contrast application.	May be multiple. Incidence is ~2.5% in the Western population, higher in Asian women. Associated with von Hippel–Lindau disease, polycystic kidney disease, and autosomal dominant polycystic liver disease. In case of septations, irregular inner margins, intracystic components, and contrast attenuation rule out cystic neoplasm. Nonenhanced CT helps to distinguish intracystic hemorrhage (hyperdense) from neoplasm (hypodense).
Hepatic angiomyolipoma ▷ *Fig. 19.22a, b*	Sharply delineated hepatic mass of variable shape and diameter (0.5–30 cm) containing intralesional fat. **Scan recommendation:** Multiphasic CT (nonenhanced CT, PVP, PP). Nonenhanced CT: Heterogeneous attenuation depending on predominant tissue component. PVP: Strong attenuation (angioid components). PP: Delayed enhancement. **Diagnostic pearls:** Well-delineated hepatic mass with hyperattenuation on PVP scans and presence of intralesional fat and vessels.	Rare. Seen predominantly in patients with renal angiomyolipomas. Histologically, composed of fat, smooth muscle cells, and proliferating blood vessels.
Biliary cystadenoma	Cystic mass in the liver parenchyma with septated, multilocular appearance.	Rare lesion, primarily in middle-aged women. May recur and develop into a malignant cystadenocarcinoma. Distinction not important as surgical resection is treatment of choice for both. Differential diagnosis: liver abscess/hydatid cysts.
Hepatic lipoma	Distinct area of intrahepatic fat. Sometimes fine septa of soft tissue density are present. Identical low-attenuation values on pre- and postcontrast scans.	Rare. May be distinguished from focal steatosis (poorly discernible, blood vessels crossing through lesions) and metastases from liposarcoma (heterogeneous lesions with distinct attenuation on postcontrast scans).
Intrahepatic extension of a pancreatic pseudocyst	Round intrahepatic cystic mass or tubular lucencies simulating dilated bile ducts (see also **Fig. 20.11, p. 707**).	Complication of pancreatitis.

(continues on page 688)

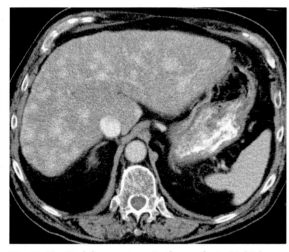

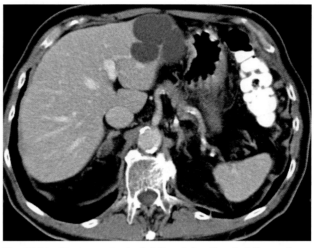

Fig. 19.20 Nodular regenerative hyperplasia. Multiple hepatic macronoduli with strong attenuation during the HAP are seen in a patient with underlying severe liver cirrhosis.

Fig. 19.21 Liver cysts in the left liver lobe. Sharply delineated, round or oval lesion of near-water attenuation without contrast enhancement of the cyst wall.

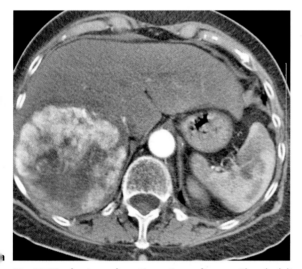

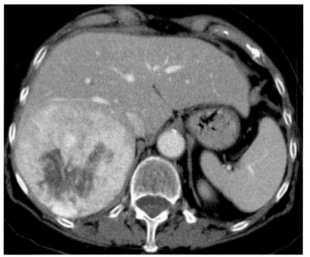

Fig. 19.22a, b Large hepatic angiomyolipoma. Sharply delineated hepatic mass with strong attenuation during the PVP (**a**) and delayed enhancement during the PP (**b**). Note intralesional vessels and fat.

Table 19.1   (Cont.) Focal liver lesions

Disease	CT Findings	Comments
Malignant neoplasms		
Hepatocellular carcinoma (HCC) ▷ *Fig. 19.23*	CT appearance is variable: focal, multinodular, or diffuse. May contain fatty tissue, necrosis, and, occasionally, calcifications. Portal vein invasion in 25% to 40%, hepatic vein invasion in up to 15%. **Scan recommendation:** Triphasic CT (nonenhanced CT, HAP, PVP). Nonenhanced CT: Hypodense mass with or without necrosis, calcification, fat. HAP: Heterogeneous wedge-shaped enhancement (perfusion abnormalities due to portal vein occlusion). PVP: Hypo isodense to liver parenchyma with local contrast accumulation. **Diagnostic pearls:** Large heterogeneous, hypervascular mass invading portal vein suspicious for HCC. Smaller HCC may mimic metastasis/hemangioma in cirrhotic liver.	The most common primary liver tumor. Predisposing conditions: cirrhosis due to ethanol or virus hepatitis, hemochromatosis, Wilson disease, Gaucher disease, glycogen storage disease (type 1), tyrosinosis, and biliary atresia. The total number and location of lesions are often difficult to estimate.
Fibrolamellar hepatocellular carcinoma (HCC) ▷ *Fig. 19.24*	Well-defined, large, solitary heterogeneous mass; often hypodense central scar and radial septa. Necrosis and calcification are common (30% of patients). **Scan recommendation:** Multiphasic CT (nonenhanced CT, HAP, PVP, DP). Nonenhanced CT: Well-defined hypodense mass. Necrosis and calcification are common. HAP: Hyperattenuating and heterogeneous. PVP: Hypo-/isodense to liver parenchyma. DP: Hyperdense scar/septa/capsule.	Rather uncommon form of HCC. Involves younger population and is unrelated to cirrhosis. Less malignant than standard HCC. Lymph node/lung metastases and biliary/vessel infiltration are signs of malignancy. May mimic FNH/HCC. Central scar on T2-weighted MRIs hyperintense in FNH versus hypointense in fibrolamellar HCC. HCC lacks scar and often comes with underlying cirrhosis.
Hepatic metastases ▷ *Fig. 19.25a–f*	Either hypo- (common) or hyperdense (less common) lesions with random distribution pattern within normal-enhancing liver tissue. Variable in size (few millimeters to several centimeters). **Scan recommendation:** Triphasic CT (nonenhanced CT, HAP, PP) necessary only for initial oncological staging. Nonenhanced CT: Iso-/hypoattenuating to normal liver parenchyma. HAP: Hypervascular metastases appear hyperdense. PP: Hypodense, sometimes hypodense center (central necrosis) with peripheral rim enhancement (viable tumor or compressed normal parenchyma). **Diagnostic pearls:** Hepatic cysts, hemangiomas, abscesses, sepsis, sarcoidosis, peliosis hepatis, and biliary hamartoma may mimic metastases. Vascular rim enhancement typical for epithelial metastases. Metastases of ovarian cystadenocarcinoma typically infiltrate liver from outside and thus may be found primarily in a subcapsular location. Breast cancer metastases may be indistinguishable from hemangiomas.	Most common liver malignancy (~20 times more common than all primary liver neoplasms combined). Common sites of origin are the colon, stomach, pancreas, breast, and lung. Usually multiple and involving both lobes. Right or left lobe involvement occurs in 20% and 3%, respectively. New appearance of a liver lesion in a patient with a known malignancy most indicative of a metastatic lesion. Pre- and early postcontrast scans are recommended to depict the maximum number of metastases. CT features lack histologic specificity except for vascularity. Pancreatic islet cell, carcinoid, renal cell carcinoma, sarcoma, pheochromocytoma, and germ cell tumors often are hypervascular. Cystadenocarcinoma and sarcoma (pancreas, GI, ovarian) often cystic (hypoattenuating). Mucinous carcinomas (colon, rectum, and stomach), treated breast, medullary thyroid, osteosarcoma, carcinoid, and leiomyosarcoma metastases frequently calcify.

(continues on page 690)

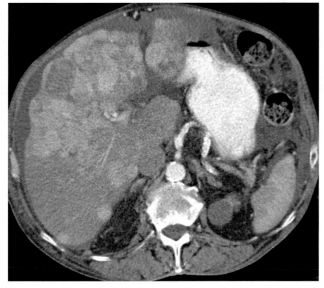

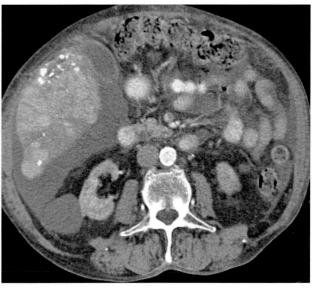

Fig. 19.23   Multifocal hepatocellular carcinoma (HCC). Visible is HCC with distinct enhancement during the HAP. Note also marked liver cirrhosis and perihepatic ascites.

Fig. 19.24   Fibrolamellar HCC. Large well-defined, heterogeneous mass with hypodense central scars, radiating septa, areas of necrosis, and calcifications.

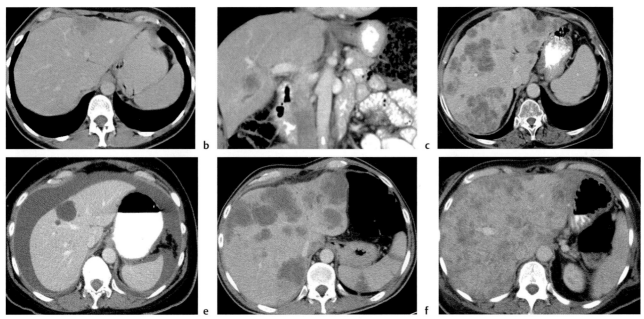

Fig. 19.25a–f   Hepatic metastases. Vessel infiltration (**a**) and local cholestasis (**b**) are typical signs of malignancy. CT appearance depends on primary neoplasm: vascular rim enhancement in colon carcinoma (**c**); subcapsular location in ovarian cystadenocarcinoma (**d**); mainly cystic in pancreatic cystadenocarcinoma (**e**); slightly hypervascular in pancreatic islet cell (i.e., neuroendocrine) tumor (**f**).

Table 19.1 (Cont.) Focal liver lesions

Disease	CT Findings	Comments
Hepatic lymphoma ▷ *Fig. 19.26*	Primary hepatic lymphomas (rare) or secondary involvement in Hodgkin disease or non–Hodgkin lymphoma. **Scan recommendation:** Biphasic CT (nonenhanced CT, PP). Nonenhanced CT necessary only for initial oncological staging. **Diagnostic pearls:** Primary liver lymphoma is a solitary mass with no distinguishing CT features. Secondary infiltrating lymphoma is usually impossible to differentiate from normal liver parenchyma. Nodular or mixed forms are often low attenuating and distinguishable on CT but less common.	Due to a high content of lymphatic tissue, lymphomas are often found in the periportal area. Primary lymphoma of the liver is rare, but secondary lymphomatous involvement is found in 60% of Hodgkin disease and in 50% of non–Hodgkin lymphomas. May complicate liver transplant.
Hepatic sarcomas (angiosarcoma, hemangiosarcoma, and hemangioendothelial sarcoma)	Hemorrhagic, hypervascular, heterogeneous tumor: multifocal or diffusely infiltrating. Size ranging from micronodular to large. Vascular channels within lesion may be capillary or cavernous. **Scan recommendation:** Triphasic CT (nonenhanced CT, PVP, DP) shows progressive enhancement over time. Nonenhanced CT: Single/multiple hypodense masses. Central hyperdensity represents fresh hemorrhage. PVP: Usually hypodense mass with heterogeneous nodular enhancement. Rarely peripheral nodular enhancement with centripetal progression. DP: Persistence of contrast material in central vessels. **Diagnostic pearls:** Multiphasic CT shows progression of contrast enhancement over time. Consider hemangiomas as differential diagnosis that usually enhance relative to blood vessels (aorta, vena cava).	Most common mesenchymal liver tumor (~2%) often associated with liver cirrhosis, hemochromatosis, or von Recklinghausen disease. Histologically, a malignant spindle cell tumor of endothelial origin, forming poorly organized vessels and growing along predefined vascular structures. Typically also involves skin, soft tissue, breast, liver, and spleen. Environmental carcinogens (such as thorotrast, polyvinyl chloride, etc.) and radiation exposure may trigger tumor growth.
Epithelioid hemangioendothelioma ▷ *Fig. 19.27a, b*	Well-defined, peripheral (often confluent), typically targetlike nodules. Calcifications rare. **Scan recommendation:** Multiphasic CT (nonenhanced CT, PVP, DP). Nonenhanced CT: Nodules of decreased attenuation as compared with normal liver. PVP/PP: Targetlike appearance: Hypodense center (myxoid stroma); hyperdense inner peripheral rim (highly vascularized); hypodense outer peripheral rim (edema). **Diagnostic pearls:** Targetlike appearance of peripherally located and partly coalescing lesions. Capsular retraction due to fibrosis and ischemia.	Low-malignant, slowly progressing, highly vascularized liver tumor of unknown etiology. Epithelioid cells stain positive for factor VIII–related antigen. Tumor affects women more than men (association with contraceptives?). Typical age group: 28 to 58 y. Eighty percent of patients survive 5 to 10 y after diagnosis. Nodule resection and liver transplantation are treatment of choice.
Peripheral (intrahepatic) cholangiocarcinoma (PCC) ▷ *Fig. 19.28a, b*	Heterogeneous large hepatic mass with dilated bile ducts and capsular retraction. Can be mass forming (well circumscribed), periductal infiltrating (i.e., branchlike growth along bile ducts with local obstruction of bile ducts), or intraductal growing (segmental/focal bile duct dilation). **Scan recommendation:** Multiphasic CT (nonenhanced CT, HAP, PP, DP). Nonenhanced CT: Well-defined, lobulated, hypodense mass often with punctuated calcifications and intrahepatic bile duct dilation. HAP: Rimlike enhancement. PP: Progressive centripetal filling usually not isodense to blood. DP: Distinct delayed enhancement (due to fibrotic stroma of tumors) **Diagnostic pearls:** Tumor often visible only on delayed images. Tumor margins often best depicted on DP/PP images.	PCC and intraductal growing cholangiocarcinoma often missed due to ill-defined margins and low attenuation. Five to 10 minutes after contrast injection is optimal for delayed imaging. Accounts for ~15% of liver cancers, but only 10% of all cholangiocarcinomas are intrahepatic. Associated with repeated cholangitis, hepatolithiasis, congenital cystic liver disease, and primary sclerosing cholangitis (PSC). Age peak: 50 to 60 y. Treatment of choice is surgical resection. Five-year survival rate is 30%.

(continues on page 692)

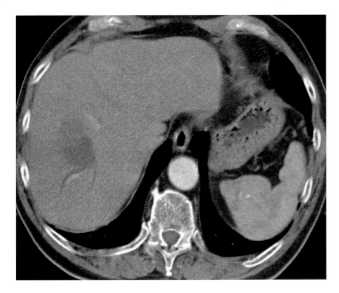

Fig. 19.26 Secondary hepatic and splenic involvement of a patient with non–Hodgkin lymphoma. Low-attenuating lesion in the liver and spleen. Local cholestasis in the liver is highly suspicious for a malignancy.

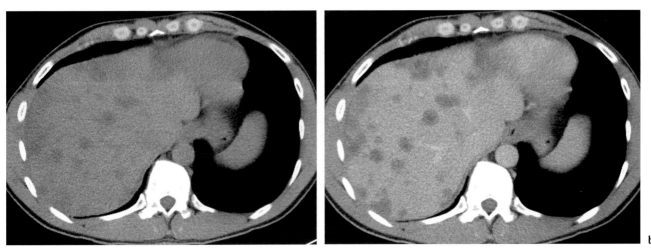

a ⁣ b

Fig. 19.27a, b Epithelioid hemangioendothelioma. Well-defined hypodense nodules on nonenhanced CT and targetlike appearance during the PVP.

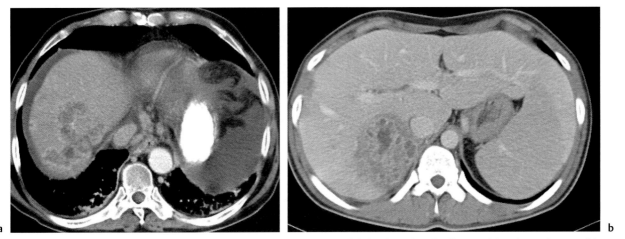

a ⁣ b

Fig. 19.28a, b Peripheral cholangiocarcinoma (PCC). Comparison of well-defined periductal-infiltrating (**a**) and mass-forming (**b**) type. Note the rimlike enhancement during the PVP.

Table 19.1 (Cont.) Focal liver lesions

Disease	CT Findings	Comments
Hepatoblastoma	Low-attenuation hepatic tumor with peripheral rim enhancement. **Scan recommendation:** Consider MRI instead of CT (radiation issues with children).	Most frequent hepatic malignancy in children, usually affecting the right lobe.
Embryonal sarcoma	Large liver tumor with numerous cystic regions. **Scan recommendation:** Consider MRI instead of CT (radiation issues with children).	Rare tumor found exclusively in pediatric patients; 75% occur in the right lobe.
Biliary cystadenocarcinoma ▷ *Fig. 19.29*	Large, well-defined, complex cystic mass with macroscopic nodules, septations, and, rarely, calcifications.	Eighty-five percent of tumors arise from intrahepatic bile ducts, 14% from extrahepatic bile ducts, and < 1% from the gallbladder. Distinction between (benign) cystadenoma and cystadenocarcinoma not important as surgical resection is treatment of choice for both.
Extrahepatic tumors	Tumors of adrenal, kidney, stomach, and gallbladder can invade or displace the liver and thus have an appearance similar to that of primary liver tumors.	Multiplanar reformations allow for better delineation of anatomical structures/pathology.

Table 19.2 Diffuse liver disease

Disease	CT Findings	Comments
Vascular		
Peliosis hepatis ▷ *Fig. 19.30*	Cystic dilation of the central vein of the hepatic lobule leading to blood filled endothelial-lined sinusoidal cavities. **Scan recommendation:** Multiphasic CT (nonenhanced CT, AP, PVP, DP). Nonenhanced CT: Depending on size of lesions liver may appear normal (lesions < 10 mm) or show multiple low-attenuation lesions. AP: Typically, ringlike high attenuation (although some lesions may show central attenuation). PVP: Centripetal contrast enhancement. DP: Lesions remain hyperdense as compared with normal liver parenchyma. **Diagnostic pearls:** Multiple hypodense nodular lesions on nonenhanced CT restricted to the liver with ringlike enhancement on early and late global enhancement on delayed postcontrast scans.	Two subtypes, histologically can be distinguished: parenchymal and phlebectatic. Only the phlebectatic type is lined by endothelium. Peliosis is a rare disorder of unknown etiology. There is an association with exposure to cytotoxic agents, long-term steroid use, chronic diseases (AIDS, TB, etc.), and immunosuppression. Differential diagnosis includes hypervascular metastases and hepatic hemangioma. Metastases appear hypodense on delayed images (wash-out phenomenon). Hemangiomas show similar centripetal progression of contrast attenuation, but enhancement pattern is more patchy/nodular.
Portal vein thrombosis ▷ *Fig. 19.31a, b*	Segmental to global hypoperfusion of the liver depending on extent and localization of the thrombus. Portal vein may be enlarged (acute) or normal (chronic) in size. **Scan recommendation:** Multiphasic CT (nonenhanced CT, PVP, DP). Nonenhanced CT: Segmental (wedge-shaped) or global hypodensity of liver parenchyma. PVP: Segmental to global hypoattenuation of the liver parenchyma. In acute thrombosis, walls of the portal vein may enhance, the thrombus not. In chronic thrombosis, usually enlarged collaterals termed *cavernous malformations*. DP: Necrotic areas hypodense; nonnecrotic areas hypo- to isodense to normal liver parenchyma. **Diagnostic pearls:** Clotted portal vein with segmental/global hepatic hypoperfusion on all scans.	May be caused by neoplasms, infections, cirrhosis, trauma, hypercoagulable states, or hepatic venous obstruction.

(continues on page 694)

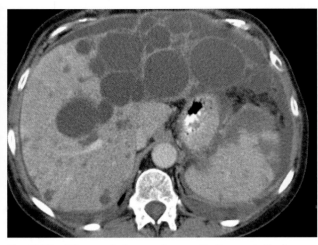

Fig. 19.29   Biliary cystadenocarcinoma. Cystic mass in the liver parenchyma with septated, multilocular appearance. Note the aggressive expansion of cysts.

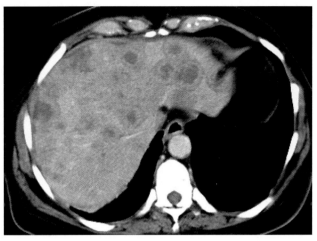

Fig. 19.30   Peliosis hepatis. Multiple hypodense nodular hepatic lesions with ringlike enhancement during PVP in a patient with acquired immunodeficiency syndrome (AIDS).

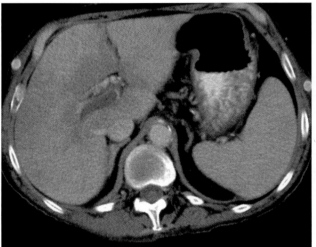

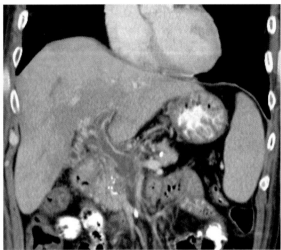

b

Fig. 19.31a, b   Portal vein thrombosis. Clotted portal vein with segmental hepatic hypoperfusion is clearly visible on axial (**a**) and coronal (**b**) images.

Table 19.2   (Cont.) Diffuse liver disease

Disease	CT Findings	Comments
Passive hepatic congestion ▷ *Fig. 19.32*	Backflow of venous blood into liver veins due to insufficient hepatic venous outflow. **Scan recommendation:** Contrast-enhanced CT. PVP/DP: Retrograde backflow of contrast into dilated IVC and hepatic veins. Often by formation of a contrast/noncontrast (blood) level in the IVC. Contrast in liver veins often higher than in the aorta. Often periportal hypodensity (due to perivascular lymphedema).	Typically caused by cardiac failure such as constrictive pericarditis, cardiomyopathy, right-side valvular disease, or congestive heart failure. Thus, typically accompanied by pericardial and pleural effusion, hepatomegaly, and ascites.
Inflammation		
Fatty liver (hepatic steatosis) ▷ *Fig. 19.33*	Fatty degeneration of hepatocytes due to a variety of infectious, toxic, and ischemic agents. **Scan recommendation:** Multiphasic CT (nonenhanced CT, PVP, DP). Nonenhanced CT: Diffuse/lobular/segmental hepatic hypoattenuation compared with spleen (normal liver parenchyma 10 HU > spleen). Inversion of contrast between vessel (hyperdense) and liver parenchyma (hypodense). PVP/DP: Often not visible on postcontrast scans. **Diagnostic pearls:** Liver hypodense compared with spleen. Contrast inversion between vessels and parenchyma on nonenhanced CT. Uncompromised course of hepatic vessels through fatty infiltrations.	Causative agents may be alcohol, cytotoxic drugs, obesity, diabetes mellitus, hepatitis, steroid treatment, hyperalimentation, or liver transplantation. Typically accompanied by hepatomegaly (75%). Hypodense lesions may be masked on noncontrast scans. May mimic diffuse hepatic infiltration from neoplasms or lymphoma. Contrast inversion between vessel and liver parenchyma indicates > 10% to 15% intrahepatic fat.
Cirrhosis ▷ *Fig. 19.34*	Nonreversible parenchymal destruction accompanied by fibrosis, nodular regeneration, and abnormal reconstruction of normal lobar architecture. **Scan recommendation:** Multiphasic CT (nonenhanced CT, PVP, DP). Nonenhanced CT: Nodular hyperdensity (> 70–140 HU) of liver parenchyma due to increased iron storage of regenerative nodules. PVP/PP: Nodular hyperdensity becomes isodense to liver parenchyma. DP: Late enhancement of fibrotic areas. **Diagnostic pearls:** Nodular liver contour with multiple hyperdense (> 70–140 HU) intrahepatic nodules on nonenhanced CT scans, accompanied by left lobular hypertrophy and right lobular atrophy.	Heterogeneous appearance of liver parenchyma with presence of regenerative nodules causing a nodular liver contour, enlargement of the caudate lobe and lateral segment of left lobe, and atrophy of the right lobe and medial segment of the left lobe. Three subtypes of cirrhosis depending on the type of nodular regeneration: micronodular (< 0.5 cm), due to alcohol abuse; macronodular (0.5 cm to several cm), due to viral hepatitis; mixed type, due to chronic bile duct obstruction. Splenomegaly, ascites, collateral veins, colonic interposition, and small bowel edema are associated findings.
Primary biliary cirrhosis (PBC)	Idiopathic liver cirrhosis of unknown etiology due to chronic destruction of intrahepatic bile ducts. **Scan recommendation:** Multiphasic CT (nonenhanced CT, PVP, DP). Nonenhanced CT: Nodular hyperdensity (> 70–140 HU) of liver parenchyma due to multiple regenerative nodules. PVP/PP: Regenerative nodules become isodense to liver parenchyma. DP: Late enhancement of fibrotic areas. **Diagnostic pearls:** nodular liver contour with multiple hyperdense intrahepatic nodules on nonenhanced CT scans, lobular hypertrophy, and atrophy.	PBC almost exclusively affects women between age 30 and 60 y. The etiology of the disease is unknown, but it is typically associated with other autoimmune diseases (scleroderma, Sjögren syndrome, and rheumatoid arthritis). Histologic features are damaged epithelial cells, necrotic bile ducts, and fibrosis of portal triads. Typical clinical symptoms include tiredness, pruritus (bilirubin), intermittent abdominal pain, and jaundice, but in 50% of cases, asymptomatic hepatomegaly is the first sign of PBC. Liver transplantation is the sole treatment option, but the risk of PBC recurrence in the transplant is slightly increased.

(continues on page 696)

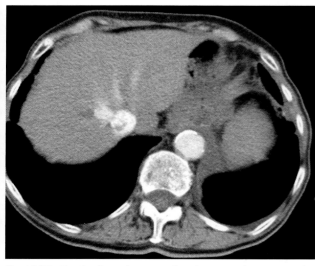

Fig. 19.32   Passive hepatic congestion. Presence of contrast in the dilated IVC and early high attenuation of large intrahepatic veins.

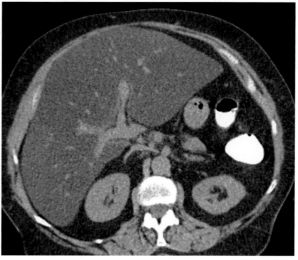

Fig. 19.33   Hepatic steatosis. Contrast inversion between vessels and parenchyma on nonenhanced CT.

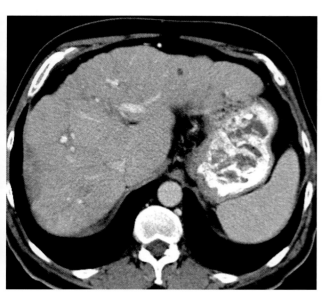

Fig. 19.34   Liver cirrhosis. Nodular liver contour with multiple hyperdense intrahepatic nodules, atrophy of the right liver lobe, and compensatory hypertrophy of the left liver lobe.

VI Abdomen and Pelvis

Table 19.2 (Cont.) Diffuse liver disease

Disease	CT Findings	Comments
Hemochromatosis ▷ *Fig. 19.35a, b*	Iron overload disorder with functional impairment of hepatocytes. **Scan recommendation:** Multiphasic CT (nonenhanced CT, PVP, DP). Nonenhanced CT: Homogeneous hyperattenuation (> 70–140 HU) of liver parenchyma due to increased iron storage. Hepatic and portal veins appear hypodense. PVP/PP: Difference in attenuation between liver parenchyma and vessels diminishes. **Diagnostic pearls:** Clear differentiation on nonenhanced CT between hyperdense liver parenchyma and hypodense vessels that diminishes on postcontrast scans.	Two subtypes of hemochromatosis: primary hemochromatosis, an autosomal recessive disorder of iron metabolism, with excessive deposition of iron in the liver, pancreas, myocardium, endocrine glands, joints, and skin; and secondary hemochromatosis, with iron deposition in the reticuloendothelial cells due to either increased iron intake (multiple transfusions, nutritive), or alcohol-induced toxic liver disease. Iron concentration directly proportional to the difference between actual and normal HU value (60 HU). Contrast only necessary to rule out/in HCC.
Wilson disease	Inflammatory periportal reaction followed by nodular liver cirrhosis due to sinusoidal and periportal copper deposition. **Scan recommendation:** Nonenhanced CT: Multiple hyperdense regenerating nodules and typical cirrhotic changes.	Autosomal recessive disease of copper metabolism usually diagnosed in childhood. Toxic levels of copper accumulate in the liver, brain, and cornea secondary to impaired biliary excretion.
Sarcoidosis	Nonspecific hepatosplenomegaly with diffuse small noncaseating granulomas in the liver of patients with known Boeck disease (sarcoidosis). **Scan recommendation:** Biphasic CT (nonenhanced CT, PP). Nonenhanced CT: Multiple hypodense hepatic noduli or simply heterogeneous appearance of liver parenchyma, often accompanied by hepatosplenomegaly. PVP/PP: Isodensity of hepatic noduli compared with normal liver parenchyma. **Diagnostic pearls:** Always consider in patients with lymphadenopathy and hepatosplenomegaly. Nodular pattern often seen in both liver and spleen.	Histologically, noncaseating epithelioid granulomas with multinucleated giant cells of Langerhans type. Granulomas usually more apparent in the portal triad regions than in the liver parenchyma. Causing agent unknown. Two thirds of patients are women between 20 and 40 y of age. Up to 80% of all patients with sarcoidosis present with involvement of abdominal organs, particularly of the liver and spleen. Treatment with corticosteroids, antiinflammatory agents, and cytotoxic drugs. Unusually concomitant involvement of the spleen and thus similar findings in **Fig. 21.10, p. 715.**
Amyloidosis	Nonspecific hepatomegaly and lymphadenopathy. **Scan recommendation:** Multiphasic CT (nonenhanced CT, PP, DP). Nonenhanced CT: Global or focal hypoattenuation of liver parenchyma. PP: Global or focal hypoattenuation of liver parenchyma. DP: Delayed contrast enhancement may be present. **Diagnostic pearls:** Global or focal hypoattenuation of liver parenchyma on pre- and postcontrast scans.	Deposition of fibrils of light-chain immunoglobulins in a perivascular location within the spaces of Disse.
Infection		
Tuberculosis (TB) ▷ *Fig. 21.12, p. 717*	Multiple round, hypodense hepatic lesions. **Scan recommendation:** Multiphasic CT (nonenhanced CT, PP). Nonenhanced CT: Multiple small, hypodense lesions. PP: Lesions remain hypodense—attenuation. **Diagnostic pearls:** Multiple micronodular hypodense lesions seen on pre- and post-contrast scans. In presence of miliar lesions, the liver may appear almost normal.	Occurs in patients after primary TB infection as a result of subsequent hematogenous spreading of the disease (miliary TB). Typically, also involves other parenchymatous organs, such as the kidneys, spleen, brain, and lung. Differential diagnosis: rule out biliary hamartomas, Caroli disease, and metastases. Concomitant involvement of the spleen as visible is typical.
Schistosomiasis	Multiple high-attenuating hepatic lesions ranging in size from a few millimeters to several centimeters. **Scan recommendation:** Multiphasic CT (nonenhanced CT, PP). Nonenhanced CT: Either a "tortoise shell" appearance of the liver with multiple hypodense, partly calcified lesions (*Schistosoma japonicum*) or low-density periportal changes combined with multiple hypodense, noncalcified lesions (*S. mansoni*). PP: Center of lesions hypodense, marked peripheral contrast enhancement.	Schistosomiasis is a parasitic disease caused by *Schistosoma japonicum* and *S. mansoni*. The disease is endemic in tropical countries (Africa, the Caribbean, eastern South America, southeast Asia, and the Middle East). Schistosomes live and mature in the portal veins, inciting a granulomatous reaction with central necrosis and eventually periportal fibrosis.

(continues on page 697)

Table 19.2 (Cont.) Diffuse liver disease

Disease	CT Findings	Comments
Neoplasms		
Diffuse hepatocellular carcinoma (HCC) ▷ *Fig. 19.23, p. 689*	Diffuse irregular, low-density changes, variable degree of contrast enhancement. **Scan recommendation:** Triphasic CT (nonenhanced CT, HAP, PVP). Nonenhanced CT: Hypodense mass with necrosis, calcification, fat. HAP: Heterogeneous enhancement (perfusion abnormalities due to portal vein occlusion). PVP: Hypo-/isodense to liver parenchyma with local contrast accumulation. **Diagnostic pearls:** Large heterogeneous, hypervascular mass invading the portal vein.	The most common primary liver tumor. Predisposing conditions: cirrhosis due to ethanol or virus hepatitis, hemochromatosis, Wilson disease, Gaucher disease, glycogen storage disease (type 1), tyrosinosis, and biliary atresia. The total number and location of lesions are often difficult to estimate. Treatment options include resection, chemoembolization, and liver transplantation depending on extent and cause of disease. Liver cirrhosis is often an overlying finding.
Diffuse metastatic disease ▷ *Fig. 19.25, p. 689*	Liver may be normal in size or show diffuse hepatomegaly due to multiple low-contrast lesions. Contrast enhancement usually shows subtle displacement of normal liver parenchyma with diffuse metastatic spreading. **Scan recommendation:** Triphasic CT (nonenhanced CT, HAP, PP) necessary only for initial oncological staging. Nonenhanced CT: Iso-/hypoattenuating to normal liver parenchyma. HAP: Hypervascular metastases appear hyperdense. PP: Hypodense, sometimes hypodense center (central necrosis) with peripheral rim enhancement (viable tumor or compressed normal parenchyma). **Diagnostic pearls:** Hepatic cysts, hemangiomas, abscesses, sepsis, sarcoidosis, peliosis hepatis, and biliary hamartoma may mimic metastases.	Most common liver malignancy. Common sites of origin are the colon, stomach, pancreas, breast, and lung. Usually involving both liver lobes. Pre- and early postcontrast scans are recommended to depict the maximum number of metastases. CT features lack histologic specificity except for vascularity. Pancreatic islet cell, carcinoid, renal cell carcinoma, sarcoma, pheochromocytoma, and germ cell tumors often are hypervascular. Cystadenocarcinoma and sarcoma (pancreas, GI, and ovarian) are often cystic (hypoattenuating). Mucinous carcinomas (colon, rectum, and stomach), treated breast, medullary thyroid, osteosarcoma, carcinoid, and leiomyosarcoma metastases frequently calcify.
Diffuse lymphoma	Multiple hypodense, poorly delineated lesions or diffuse infiltrating mass that is usually more clearly delineated on postcontrast scans. **Scan recommendation:** Biphasic CT (nonenhanced CT, PP): Nonenhanced CT only at initial oncological staging. PP: Micronoduli/diffuse mass remains hypodense as compared with normal liver parenchyma.	Commonly accompanied by lymphadenopathy and splenomegaly. Primary liver lymphoma is a solitary mass with no distinguishing features. Secondary infiltrating lymphoma is usually difficult to differentiate from normal liver parenchyma. Nodular or mixed forms are less common, low attenuating, and thus more distinguishable from normal liver parenchyma.

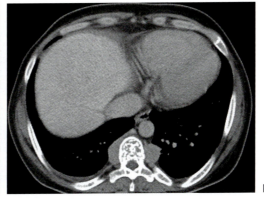

Fig. 19.35a, b   Hemochromatosis in a patient with thalassemia. On nonenhanced CT, clear differentiation between hyperdense liver parenchyma and hypodense vessels (**a**), which diminishes on postcontrast scans (**b**). Note the paravertebral soft tissue masses, which are pathognomonic for concomitant extramedullary hematopoiesis (see also **Fig. 18.33**).

VI Abdomen and Pelvis

20 Biliary System

Christopher Herzog

Diseases of the biliary system are usually diagnosed by using ultrasound, endoscopic retrograde cholangiography (ERCP), or percutaneous transhepatic cholangiography (PTC). Computed tomography (CT) typically comes into play for tumor staging in addition to ultrasound. However, most biliary abnormalities are found accidentally in the course of an abdominal CT scan.

Anatomically, the biliary system consists of intra- and extrahepatic bile ducts, as well as the gallbladder. Intrahepatic bile ducts parallel portal veins and hepatic arteries, empty into a right and left hepatic duct, measure < 1 mm in diameter, and thus are usually not visible on CT scans. Cholestasis describes continuous centripetal widening of the bile ducts due to a distal (near) occlusion. The differential diagnosis embraces hepatic and cholangioneoplasms, bile duct stones, and various forms of cholangitis (see **Fig. 20.9**).

The right and left hepatic ducts appear as ~3-mm-wide, near-water-dense linear structures on postcontrast images and join the common hepatic duct (CHD) (**Fig. 20.1**). The CHD is a thin-walled (< 1.5 mm) structure 3 to 4 mm in diameter located anterior to the portal vein and lateral to the hepatic artery (**Fig. 20.2**). A CHD with a diameter > 6 mm must be regarded as dilated. After joining the cystic duct, which drains the gallbladder, the CHD forms the common bile duct (CBD), or ductus choledochus, which measures up to 6 mm in diameter. Any diameter > 8 mm is indicative of biliary obstruction. However, after cholecystectomy, a diameter of up to 10 mm may still be normal. Typically, the CBD appears as a low-attenuating structure surrounded by enhancing pancreatic tissue. It has a low-attenuating wall, which is ≤ 1.5 mm in thickness. The CBD is distally confined by the sphincter of Boyden. After joining the main pancreatic duct (which also is confined by a separate sphincter), both ducts drain into the duodenum through the ampulla of Vater, which is confined by the sphincter of Oddi.

The gallbladder is an oval sac of near-water density located in the gallbladder fossa—a notch on the undersurface of the liver—with a wall thickness of 1 to 2 mm (**Fig. 20.3**). It may be anomalously located intrahepatically, suprahepatically, or even retrorenally. Intracystic septations occur in ~10% of patients and usually are not visible on CT scans. Duplication of the gallbladder or cystic duct is rare. Anatomically, the gallbladder is distinguished by the fundus, body, and neck. The distally located fundus usually is round and appears below the edge of the liver when filled. A common variation is the "phrygian cap," a partially septated fundus that is folded upon itself. The body is the midportion of the gallbladder and is usually adjacent to the hepatic flexure of the colon and the duodenum. The gallbladder drains via its proximally located neck into the cystic duct, which is usually 2 to 5 cm long, tortuous, and equipped with several spiral folds (valves of Heister).

On CT scans, usually the portal venous phase (PVP) and parenchymal phase (PP) (see Chapter 19) are best suited to distinguish intrahepatic bile ducts from liver parenchyma. Bile ducts and the gallbladder walls usually appear hypodense compared with surrounding parenchymal tissue. Thus, any increase in density after contrast application is indicative of an inflammation or additional local thickening of a neoplastic process.

The biliary tract wall and subtle calculi are best visualized by using multidetector-row spiral CT and thin-slice collimation (> 1.5 mm). Scanning with maximal kilovolt peak eases visualization of cholesterol gallstones. Dual-source CT scanners allow for dual-energy scans with 140 and 80 pkV and thus for optimized differentiation of stones without loss of overall image quality. Oral contrast is obsolete in patients with suspected stone disease due to potential masking of calculi near the ampulla of Vater.

After intravenous contrast, usually only 2% of iodine fluid is eliminated via the biliary system. Any presence of contrast in the gallbladder consequently is indicative of an impaired renal function. Intrahepatic bile ducts enhance only in case of a severely restricted renal clearance.

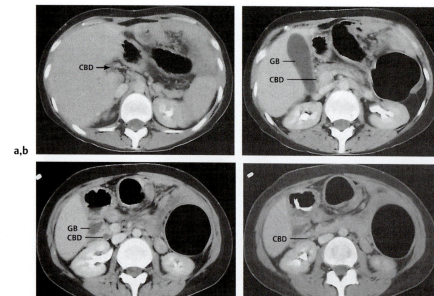

a,b

d,e

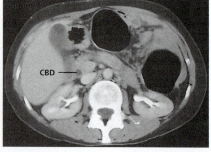

c

Fig. 20.1a–e   Anatomy of extrahepatic bile ducts. Common bile duct (CBD) formed by the junction of the left and right hepatic ducts (**a**). CBD and normal gallbladder (**b**). Intrapancreatic portion of the CBD (**c**). Junction of CBD and pancreatic duct (**d,e**). The latter appears as a thin, low-density structure joining the CBD. Typical narrowing of the CBD before entering the duodenum (**e**).

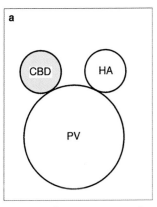 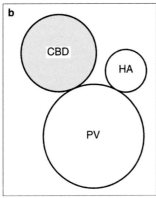

Fig. 20.2a, b Cross-sectional anatomy of the portal triad as visible on CT scans. Normal (**a**) versus dilated (**b**) CBD. (Modified after Webb.)

CBD common bile duct
HA hepatic artery
PV portal vein

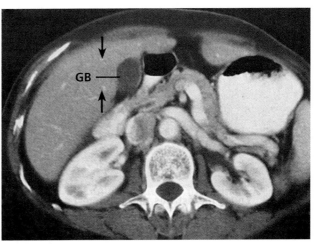

Fig. 20.3 Normal intrahepatic bile ducts. Usually, normal intrahepatic bile ducts are not seen clearly on CT, but they can be anticipated on good-quality images as low-density spots next to the enhanced portal branches (arrows). A normal, thin-walled gallbladder is also demonstrated.

A global gallbladder wall thickening and pericholecystic fluid are typical for cholecystitis. However, similar features are observed in a number of other conditions, such as liver failure, ascites, hypoalbuminemia, congestive heart disease, renal failure, and lymphatic obstruction (see **Fig. 20.6**). A gallbladder diameter > 5 cm is an indicator of biliary obstruction distal to the cystic duct. In most patients, the cystic duct cannot be identified as a structure separate from the gallbladder and the CHD. Gallstones within the cystic duct are a rare cause of proximal extrahepatic biliary obstruction and may cause cholangitis or obstructive jaundice (Mirizzi syndrome). Alternatively, after cholecystectomy, a long remnant may cause symptoms similar to cholecystolithiasis.

The characteristic CT appearance of distal biliary tract obstruction is shown in **Fig. 20.4 (p. 701)**. Abrupt interruption of the dilated CBD can easily be seen on CT scans and is a characteristic sign of malignancy. Patients with an unobstructed duct or benign stricture usually demonstrate a gradual tapering of the distal duct. It is important to differentiate benign choledochal cysts from physiologic bile duct dilation, such as choledochal cysts.

According to Todani, different types of choledochal cysts can be distinguished: solitary fusiform-extrahepatic (type I), extrahepatic supraduodenal diverticulum (type II), intraduodenal diverticulum/choledochocele (type III), fusiforme and intrahepatic cysts (type IVa), multiple extrahepatic cysts (type IVb), and multiple intrahepatic cysts (type V = Caroli disease) (see **Fig. 20.10**). The appearances of the cross section of the portal triad when the CBD is normal or dilated are presented in **Fig. 20.2**.

Gas in the biliary tree typically is observed after surgery, such as sphincterotomy and choledochoenterostomy. Less common causes include cholecystoduodenal gallstone fistula, choledochoduodenal fistula after perforated ulcer, choledochoenteric fistula due to carcinoma, and biliary tree damage after radiological interventions, such as Lipiodol (Ethiodol) embolization of liver metastases.

The differential diagnosis of biliary tract abnormalities is discussed in **Table 20.1**.

Table 20.1 Differential diagnosis of diseases of the biliary system

Disease	CT Findings	Comments
Inflammation		
Cholecystolithiasis ▷ *Fig. 20.4a–e*	Gallstones are composed of cholesterol, pigment (calcium bilirubinate), or a mixture of both. Stones are visible only if density is different than bile. Gaseous stones accrue by dehydration and excavation. Sludge consists of small cholesterol and pigment granules. **Scan recommendation:** Nonenhanced CT, although ultrasound is the imaging modality of choice. **Diagnostic pearls:** Typically, pure cholesterol stones are large and iso-/hypodense as compared with bile. Pigmented stones are hyperdense, numerous, and small. Mixed stones either are masked by bile or are peripherally calcified with a hypodense center. Gaseous stones show central hypodense air streaks. Sludge appears slightly more dense than bile and may effect an intracystic sludge/bile level.	Gallstones are usually accidental findings on CT scans. CT's sensitivity to detect gallstones amounts to 80% at maximum. Dual-energy CT is favorable, as cholesterol stones are nicely visualized at high-kilovolt peaks. Gallbladder folds may simulate (rimmed) gallstones. Consider the 5*F*'s (female, 40, fertile, fat, fair) as predisposing factors for cholecystolithiasis.
Choledocholithiasis ▷ *Fig. 20.5a, b*	Presence of gallstones in intra- or extrahepatic bile ducts with or without duct obstruction. The latter initially leads to extrahepatic cholestasis followed by intrahepatic cholestasis. **Scan recommendation:** Nonenhanced CT, although magnetic resonance cholangiopancreatography (MRCP) and endoscopic retrograde cholangiography (ERCP) are imaging modalities of choice. Cholesterol stones are visualized as hypodense filling defects. Pigmented stones usually appear hyperdense. **Diagnostic pearls:** Rule out dilation and truncation of CBD (normally < 6 mm) and cholestasis proximal to it. Twenty percent of stones are seen as homogeneous, high-attenuation structures within the water-attenuation bile or surrounded by soft tissue density of the duct. About 50% of stones are of soft tissue density and are recognized as target lesions surrounded by low-density bile or as a crescent sign.	Cholangiography is the examination of choice. Approximately 93% of all stones are secondary gallstones due to cholecystectomy, hyperalimentation, hemolytic anemias, metabolic syndrome, or ileocecal resection; ≤ 7% are primary duct stones due to bile duct sclerosis (recurrent cholangitis), congenital bile duct anomalies, motor disorder of the papilla of Vater, foreign bodies, or parasites. Typical clinical signs are acute abdominal pain. Persistent choledocholithiasis may lead to pruritus, jaundice, and pancreatitis. Whereas small stones may pass spontaneously or could be fragmented by mechanical lithotripsy, larger stones usually require endoscopic sphincterectomy or surgical removal. Thin collimation (≤ 1 mm) is necessary to display stones and ducts. Consider dual-source CT for better depiction of cholesterol stones.

(continues on page 702)

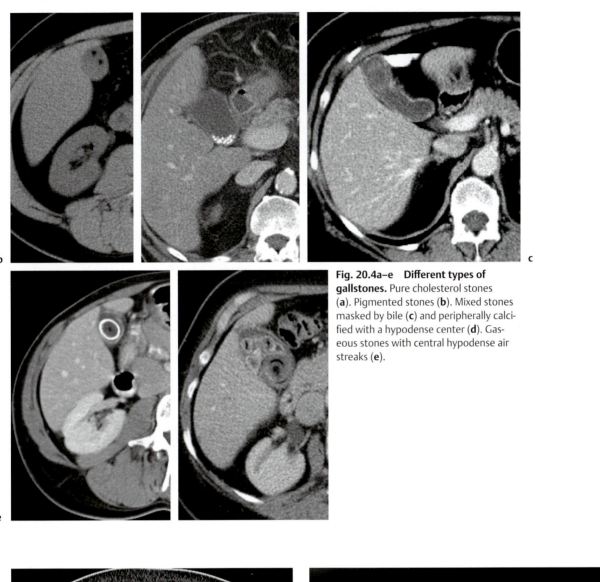

Fig. 20.4a–e   Different types of gallstones. Pure cholesterol stones (**a**). Pigmented stones (**b**). Mixed stones masked by bile (**c**) and peripherally calcified with a hypodense center (**d**). Gaseous stones with central hypodense air streaks (**e**).

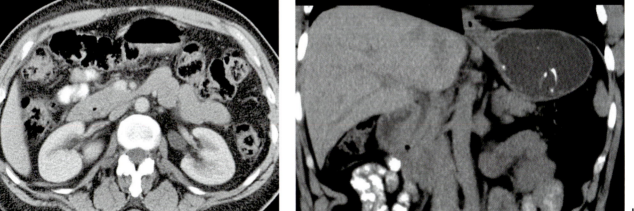

Fig. 20.5a, b   Choledocholithiasis. Obstruction of the distal CBD by a pure cholesterol stone, visible as a round hypodense nodule proximally to the sphincter of Oddi (**a**). Coronal multiplanar reconstruction (MPR) clarifies the location of the stone and shows intra- and extrahepatic cholestasis (**b**).

Table 20.1 (Cont.) Differential diagnosis of diseases of the biliary system

Disease	CT Findings	Comments
Cholecystitis ▷ *Fig. 20.6a–g*	Acute inflammation of gallbladder mainly (> 95%) due to cystic duct obstruction, to a lesser extent also due to secondary infection, inflammation, or ischemia. **Scan recommendation:** Multiphasic CT (nonenhanced CT, parenchymal phase [PP]). Nonenhanced CT: Regular thickening of gallbladder wall (> 3 mm) and stranding of pericholecystic fat, with or without gallstones. PP: Hyperattenuation of gallbladder wall, often showing three layers (hypodense wall edema within hyperdense inner and outer layer); also, pericholecystic fluid/stranding of fat. **Diagnostic pearls:** Thickened gallbladder wall and cholelithiasis are not suggestive of cholecystitis. Increased density of bile (> 20 HU), loss of clear demarcation of the gallbladder wall, and gallbladder lumen dilation (hydrops > 5 cm) are more specific findings.	Marked contrast enhancement of the gallbladder wall is typically seen in acute but not chronic cholecystitis. Irregular wall thickening with zones of low density and pericholecystic fluid collection are suggestive of complicated cholecystitis. Air within gallbladder lumen or wall is indicative of emphysematous cholecystitis (typically > 24 h after onset of symptoms). Focal interruption of gallbladder wall is a sign of rupture/necrosis. Irregular thickening of gallbladder wall, occasionally with calcifications and pericholecystic extension, typically is observed in the presence of xanthogranulomatous cholecystitis but also gallbladder carcinoma.
Adenomyomatosis	Nonspecific localized thickening of gallbladder wall and/or presence of intraluminal diverticula. **Scan recommendation:** Contrast-enhanced CT (DP): ~30 min after contrast administration (Biliscopin). **Diagnostic pearls:** Localized isodense, wall-adherent noduli surrounded by hyperattenuating bile fluid.	Hyperplastic mucosa, thickening of the muscularis, and expression of intramural diverticula (Rokitansky–Aschoff sinuses) are usually better depicted on MRCP or ultrasound. Predominantly found in the fundus of the gallbladder. Delayed scans after intravenous (IV) administration of Biliscopin are the only CT option to correctly visualize intraluminal diverticula.
"Porcelain" gallbladder ▷ *Fig. 20.7*	(Partly) calcified gallbladder wall. **Scan recommendation:** Biphasic CT (nonenhanced CT, PP): Mural calcifications visible on all scans. **Diagnostic pearls:** Calcification of the gallbladder wall.	Etiology unknown, most likely due to recurrent cholecystitis with accumulation of calcium carbonate in the wall of the gallbladder. Predisposing factor for gallbladder carcinoma.
Milk of calcium bile ▷ *Fig. 20.8*	Calcium carbonate collecting within gallbladder. **Scan recommendation:** Biphasic CT (nonenhanced CT, PP). Nonenhanced CT: High attenuating (> 140 HU) fluid within gallbladder. PP: Gallbladder wall may or may not enhance. **Diagnostic pearls:** Calcified liquid within the gallbladder.	Rare; incidence < 0.3% of CT scans. Typically due to gallbladder stasis. Occurs in middle-aged patients, more often in women than men.

(continues on page 704)

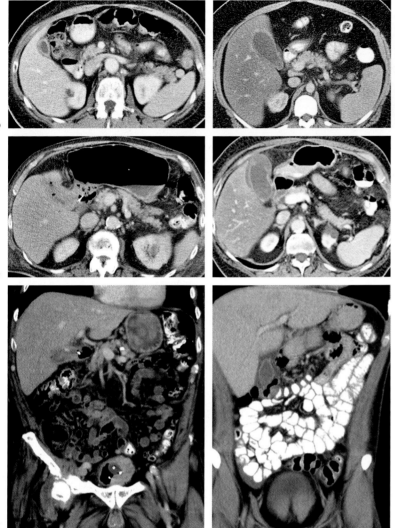

b

c

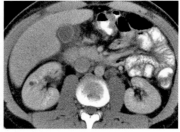

Fig. 20.6a–g CT features of cholecystitis. Acute cholecystitis (**a**). Chronic cholecystitis (**b**). Complicated cholecystitis with pericholecystic fluid (**c**). Emphysematous cholecystitis and rupture of the gallbladder wall and abscess formation within the abscess (**d**). Xanthogranulomatous cholecystitis with irregular thickening of the gallbladder wall (**e**). Coronal reformations clearly show if the liver is involved (**f**) or not (**g**).

e

f

g

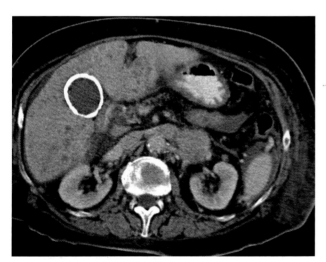

Fig. 20.7 "Porcelain" gallbladder. CT scan shows a porcelain gallbladder with a completely calcified gallbladder wall.

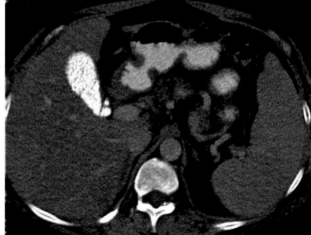

Fig. 20.8 Milk of calcium bile. The gallbladder is completely filled with calcified bile. Note a distinct hypodense line separating milk of calcium bile from liver parenchyma, which represents the gallbladder wall and thus excludes porcelain gallbladder as a possible differential diagnosis (see **Fig. 20.7**).

Table 20.1 (Cont.) Differential diagnosis of diseases of the biliary system

Disease	CT Findings	Comments
Primary sclerosing cholangitis (PSC) ▷ *Fig. 20.9a, b*	A chronic idiopathic inflammation of intra- and extrahepatic bile ducts. **Scan recommendation:** Multiphasic CT (nonenhanced CT, PP, delayed phase [DD]). Nonenhanced CT: Discontinuous dilation of bile ducts, which are partly filled with high-attenuating intraluminal calculi; in end stage, hypoattenuation of periportal region (fibrosis). PP: Slight enhancement of bile duct walls. DP: Late enhancement of periportal fibrosis. **Diagnostic pearls:** Cirrhotic liver with late-enhancing periportal fibrosis and discontinuous dilation of bile ducts, which are partly filled with high-attenuating calculi.	PSC typically affects young (< 50 y) male (> 70%) patients and is associated with other autoimmune diseases (e.g., Crohn disease, ulcerative colitis, and retroperitoneal fibrosis). Histologic features are bile duct destruction and severe periportal fibrosis. End stage of the disease is severe liver cirrhosis. Clinical symptoms are intermittent abdominal pain, obstructive jaundice, and elevated liver enzymes. Imaging modality of choice is MRI/MRCP, although diagnosis often is possible only with ERCP. Liver transplantation is the sole treatment option.
Congenital		
Choledochal cyst ▷ *Fig. 20.10a–c*	Segmental dilation of any portion of bile ducts, predominantly of the common duct. **Scan recommendation:** Biphasic CT (nonenhanced CT, PP). Nonenhanced CT: Well-demarcated, near-water density cyst within bile ducts, with or without dilation of the ductal system. PP: Slight enhancement of bile duct walls may be observed, but no enhancement of cysts. **Diagnostic pearls:** Nonenhancing intra- and extrahepatic cystic lesions with direct affiliation to the bile ducts. Thirty minutes after Biliscopin, choledochal cyst will fill with contrast media; any other cystic lesions will not.	A noncritical congenital malformation of large bile ducts, typically diagnosed during childhood and classified into five different types according to Todani (see introduction to this chapter). Clinical symptoms are intermittent abdominal pain, pruritus, and jaundice. Imaging modality of choice is MRI/MRCP. Complications (cholangitis/pancreatitis) may require surgical repair. Rule out other cystic lesions, including hepatic and pancreatic cysts, fluid collections, and enteric duplication cysts as differential diagnoses.
Caroli disease ▷ *Fig. 19.10a, b, p. 679*	Multifocal segmental saccular dilation of intrahepatic bile ducts (Todani cysts type V). **Scan recommendation:** Multiphasic CT (nonenhanced CT, PP). Nonenhanced CT: Multiple near-water-density, dilated intrahepatic bile ducts. PP: Very discrete central enhancement in cysts representing portal vein radicles. **Diagnostic pearls:** Multiple low-attenuation cystic lesions are seen throughout the liver associated with dilated intrahepatic bile ducts. Dilated bile ducts may surround the accompanying portal vein radicles in a pathognomonic fashion. Intrahepatic stone disease is often associated.	Rare congenital abnormality characterized by segmental dilation of intrahepatic bile ducts. Associated with cystic lesions of the kidneys. May simulate polycystic liver disease. Administration of biliary contrast agent (Biliscopin) 30 min prior to CT demonstrates contiguity of the cystic lesions with the biliary tree. Caroli syndrome is Caroli disease plus hepatic fibrosis. Clinical symptoms of CD are intermittent abdominal pain, pruritus, fever (cholangitis), and jaundice. Overall prognosis is poor. MRI/MRCP is imaging modality of choice.
Common bile duct (CBD) diverticulum	Diverticulum-like outpouchings of extrahepatic bile ducts in the presence of otherwise normal-sized bile ducts. **Scan recommendation:** Contrast-enhanced CT (DP): ~30 min after contrast administration (Biliscopin). **Diagnostic pearls:** Localized isodense and wall adherent diverticula are surrounded by hyperattenuating bile fluid.	Congenital diverticula of the CBD are uncommon. Diverticula in the intrahepatic ducts are rare. MRI/MRCP is imaging modality of choice.

(continues on page 706)

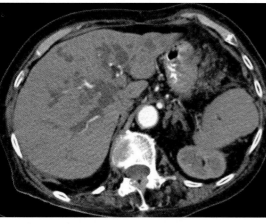
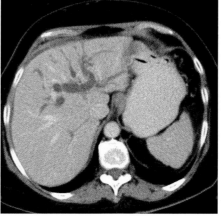

b

Fig. 20.9a, b   Primary sclerosing cholangitis (PSC) as compared with simple cholestasis. PSC (**a**) presents with discontinuous dilation of the bile ducts and a slightly irregular liver surface indicative of concomitant cirrhosis, whereas simple cholestasis (**b**) shows continuous centripetal widening of the bile ducts.

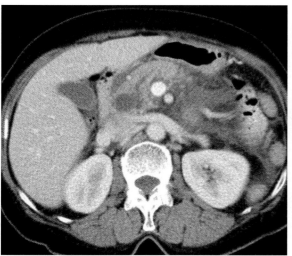
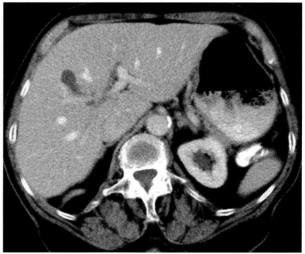

c

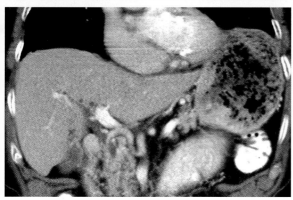

Fig. 20.10a–c   Choledochal cysts. A round lesion within the wall of the duodenum is seen in a patient with acute pancreatitis (type III, choledochocele) (**a**). Nonenhancing intrahepatic cystic lesion with direct affiliation to a slightly dilated bile duct (type IVa) (**b,c**).

Table 20.1 (Cont.) Differential diagnosis of diseases of the biliary system

Disease	CT Findings	Comments
Trauma		
Gallbladder trauma	Traumatic rupture of the gallbladder wall. **Scan recommendation:** Biphasic CT (nonenhanced CT, PP). Nonenhanced CT: Gallbladder often not discernible but distinct hypodense fluid in pericholecystic fat. High-attenuation of bile/high-attenuation of intra- or extracystic clots typically represents hemorrhage. PP: Gallbladder remains not discernible; blood and extracystic fluid remain isodense as on nonenhanced CT. **Diagnostic pearls:** Fluid collection in pericystic fat after trauma.	Often associated with laceration of the liver as well as the head/corpus of the pancreas. Typically observed in the wake of seat-belt injuries. Contrast material, milk of calcium bile, and gallstones should be excluded before making the diagnosis of hemobilia pericystic hemorrhage. Due to self-limitation of bleeding (intra-abdominal compartments), a no-touch treatment may often be favorable to laparotomy.
Postoperative fistula or cystic duct remnant	Postoperative leakage (fistula) after bile duct surgery or cystic duct remnant after cholecystectomy. **Scan recommendation:** Biphasic CT (nonenhanced CT, PP). Nonenhanced CT: Irregular cavity or tubular duct remnant isodense to CBD. PP: Slight enhancement in periphery of irregular cavity. Tubular duct remnant remains isodense to CBD. **Diagnostic pearls:** Irregular fluid collection with discrete peripheral contrast enhancement seen after bile duct surgery.	Patients with duct remnants often present symptoms similar to a cholecystitis. On the other hand, patients with fistulas may be symptom-free. If fistulas become secondary infection, typical symptoms are fever and abdominal pain. Caveat: Duct remnants may contain gallstones.
Infection		
Ascending (acute suppurative) cholangitis ▷ *Fig. 20.11*	Acute inflammation of intra- and extrahepatic bile ducts due to ascending infection. **Scan recommendation:** Biphasic CT (nonenhanced CT, PP). Nonenhanced CT: Dilated bile ducts appear either hypo- or hyperdense (pus), obstructing stones hypo-/iso-/hyperdense to bile. PP: Slightly hyperdense thickened bile duct wall. Demarcation of associated hepatic abscesses if present. **Diagnostic pearls:** Dilated bile ducts are seen filled with hyperattenuating material on precontrast scans and with distinct mural hyperattenuation on postcontrast scans.	Occurs typically due to acute bile duct obstructions (intraductal stones/iatrogenic/external lesions) after manipulation of bile ducts/pancreatic ducts during ERCP or after surgery (e.g., biliodigestive anastomosis/Whipple operation). Acute cholangitis usually caused by *Escherichia coli* infection. May quickly proceed to liver abscesses. Treatment of choice is antibiotic therapy and removal of obstructing agent.
Recurrent pyogenic cholangitis	Intra- and extrahepatic bile duct dilation (up to 3–4 cm in diameter) with associated biliary calculi and debris. **Scan recommendation:** Biphasic CT (nonenhanced CT, PP). Nonenhanced CT: The density of biliary stones is variable—usually either iso- or hyperdense as compared with normal liver parenchyma. PP: Markedly dilated, near-water-density extra- and intrahepatic bile ducts with slightly hyperdense, mildly thickened (2–3 mm) duct walls. **Diagnostic pearls:** Distinct cholestasis with numerous intra- and extrahepatic biliary stones but lacking gallbladder stones.	Endemic in Southeast Asia; also known as Asian cholangiohepatitis, intrahepatic pigment stone disease, and biliary obstruction disease. Parasites and bacteria are suspects as the cause. Typical clinical symptoms are recurrent fever, abdominal pain, and jaundice. Severe complications include liver abscess, biliary cirrhosis, and cholangiocarcinoma. Treatment of choice is long-term antibiotic therapy, surgical/interventional/endoscopic biliary drainage, and sphincterotomy. Differential diagnosis: cholangiocarcinoma (delayed enhancement on DP scans).
Worm infestation	Intraductal colonization of parasites/worms. **Scan recommendation:** Biphasic CT (nonenhanced CT, PP). Nonenhanced CT/PP: Soft tissue filling defects with or without obstruction of the bile ducts. **Diagnostic pearls:** Soft tissue filling defects with distinct cholestasis and lacking gallbladder stones.	*Ascaris* and liver flukes ascend from the duodenum into the bile ducts. Liver flukes (*Clonorchis sinensis* and *Fasciola hepatica*) are nematodes measuring 1 to 2 cm in length. They inhabit smaller bile ducts and form oval or linear filling defects. *Echinococcus* may cause partial obstruction due to cyst membranes, daughter cysts, or scolices discharged from a communicating hepatic cyst.

(continues on page 707)

Table 20.1   (Cont.) Differential diagnosis of diseases of the biliary system

Disease	CT Findings	Comments
Neoplasms		
Cholangiocarcinoma ▷*Fig. 20.12*	Intraductal neoplasm originating from epithelium of bile ducts. **Scan recommendation:** Multiphasic CT (nonenhanced CT, AP, PP). Nonenhanced CT: Often not discernible though hypodense lesion within dilated intra- or extrahepatic bile ducts. AP: Intrahepatic tumors often show an early peripheral enhancement subsequently followed by scattered central enhancement. PP: Distinct enhancement of bile duct walls. **Diagnostic pearls:** Mass at the level of bile duct bifurcation, hilar lymph nodes, distinct intrahepatic cholestasis, and biliary obstruction (Klatskin tumor).	Any obstruction between the level of confluence of hepatic ducts and the pancreatic portion of the common biliary duct is highly suspicious for cholangiocarcinoma. Cholangiocarcinoma usually arises in larger bile ducts and is identifiable on CT scans in 70%. Often associated with ulcerative colitis, sclerosing cholangitis, liver fluke disease, gallstones, and choledochal cysts. Treatment of choice is surgery or biliary stenting. Radiation therapy may be applied in a more palliative setting. Poor overall outcome (mean survival rate 6 months after diagnosis). Cholangiocarcinoma is typically accompanied by global intrahepatic bile duct dilation, whereas metastases or primary liver tumors usually cause either no or only segmental bile duct dilation.

(continues on page 708)

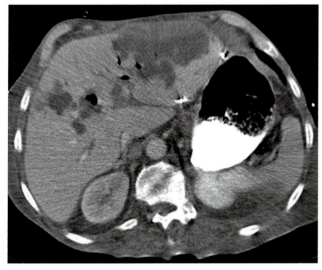

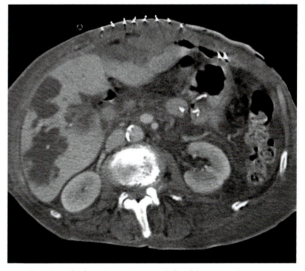

Fig. 20.11   Ascending cholangitis with aerobe after endoscopic retrograde cholangiography. In liver segment V, dilated bile ducts with distinct mural hyperattenuation during the parenchymal phase; in segments II/IV, abscess formation.

Fig. 20.12   Cholangiocarcinoma (Klatskin tumor). Mass at the level of bile duct bifurcation, local hilar lymph node, and marked intrahepatic cholestasis with clearly visible central dots representing portal radicles.

Table 20.1 (Cont.) Differential diagnosis of diseases of the biliary system

Disease	CT Findings	Comments
Ampullary carcinoma ▷ *Fig. 20.13*	Adenocarcinoma of the ampulla of Vater arising from epithelial cells of the CBD. **Scan recommendation:** Multiphasic CT (nonenhanced CT, acute phase [AP], PP). Nonenhanced CT: Soft tissue mass at papilla of Vater, cholestasis, and dilation of the pancreatic duct (double duct sign). AP: Ampullary mass hypodense as compared with pancreas. PP: Mass becomes isodense to pancreas. **Diagnostic pearls:** Mass at papilla of Vater with double duct sign and peripancreatic lymph nodes.	Often indistinguishable from primary pancreatic neoplasm; thus, scan parameters should allow parallel assessment of the pancreas: hydro-CT (100 mL of water orally 5 min prior to examination, 5 mL Buscopan IV); biphasic CT (AP/PP) thin-slice collimation and coronal MPR. Treatment of choice is surgery (Whipple operation). Overall prognosis is poor: 5-y survival rate < 40%.
Gallbladder carcinoma ▷ *Fig. 20.14*	Malignant neoplasm in > 90% of cases originating from epithelial cells of gallbladder wall. **Scan recommendation:** Biphasic CT (nonenhanced CT, PP). Nonenhanced CT: Eccentric thickening of the gallbladder wall/focal mass protruding into the gallbladder lumen, partly calcified. PP: The mass usually enhances well. **Diagnostic pearls:** Direct tumoral extension into the liver and portal vein is a frequent finding.	Gallbladder carcinoma associated with "porcelain" gallbladder and chronic inflammation due to gallstones. Affects mainly women (> 75%). Often simulates inflammatory gallbladder disease, especially in presence of gallstones or adjacent liver invasion. Cholecystectomy is treatment of choice.
Biliary intraductal papillary-mucinous neoplasm (IPMN)	IPMN of bile ducts. **Scan recommendation:** Biphasic CT (nonenhanced CT, PP). Nonenhanced CT: Segmental dilation of intra- and/or extrahepatic bile ducts. PP: Intraductal mass tends to attenuate after contrast but is usually not distinguishable from bile fluid. **Diagnostic pearls:** Segmental intrahepatic bile duct dilation without reasonable "downstream" obstruction.	Very rare disease, mainly affecting Southeast Asian populations. In presence of nodal-free disease, promising good prognosis after surgical resection of affected liver segments. Differential diagnosis: Klatskin tumor (usually leads to global intrahepatic cholestasis).
Pancreatic or metastatic carcinoma ▷ *Fig. 22.14, p. 727*	Abrupt bile duct interruption due to surrounding soft tissue mass. **Scan recommendation:** Biphasic CT (nonenhanced CT, PP). Nonenhanced CT: Global dilation of intra- and/or extrahepatic bile ducts. PP: Differentiation of retroperitoneal structures, lymph nodes, liver, and biliary system. **Diagnostic pearls:** Ill-defined mass in portal region leading to abrupt bile duct interruption and global intrahepatic bile duct dilation.	The most common causes are pancreatic carcinoma, lymphoma, and metastases to lymph nodes in the portal region. Direct invasion from other carcinoma of adjacent organs, such as stomach, kidney, and adrenal glands, is rare.

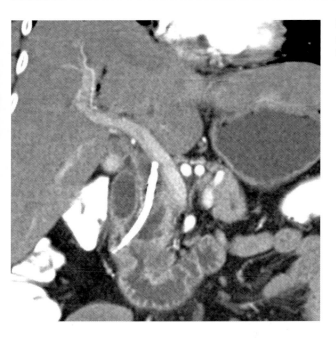

Fig. 20.13   Ampullary carcinoma. Inhomogeneous mass at papilla of Vater with dilated duct of Wirsung and stented CBD (double duct sign).

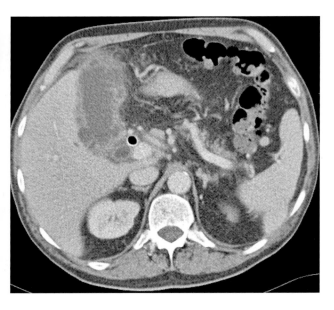

Fig. 20.14   Gallbladder carcinoma. Well-attenuating eccentric thickening of the gallbladder wall simulating inflammatory gallbladder disease and infiltrating into adjacent liver tissue.

21 Spleen

Christopher Herzog

Diseases of the spleen are primarily diagnosed by ultrasound. Computed tomography (CT) typically comes into play only if further evaluation is required. This includes posttrauma scans and staging in patients with lymphoma and other neoplastic diseases.

The spleen shows a marked variation in size and shape, but the typical size is 4 × 7 × 11 cm (thickness–width–length). Thickness corresponds to the distance from the inner to the outer border, width is the longest diameter on a transverse image, and length represents the maximal craniocaudal diameter. The length should not exceed 15 cm and the splenic volume or index (SI) not 480 mm³. Compared with body size, in children the spleen is relatively large. Common causes of splenomegaly include portal hypertension, lymphoma, acquired immunodeficiency syndrome (AIDS), intravenous (IV) drug abuse, chronic myelogenic leukemia, polycythemia vera, myelofibrosis, malaria, and infectious mononucleosis. The weight of the spleen can be estimated by SI × 0.55.

The spleen is embedded between the lateral abdominal wall, tail of the pancreas, left kidney, and stomach; thus, diseases of these organs may compromise its shape and anatomical localization. Physiologically, the lateral surface is confined by the abdominal wall and convex, whereas the medial surface usually is concave. A medial splenic bulge at this concave side represents a persistent fetal lobulation, but may easily be mistaken for a mass of the left adrenal, the tail of the pancreas, or the superior pole of the left kidney (**Fig. 21.1**). The diaphragmatic surface of the spleen often features a 2- to 3-cm-deep cleft with sharp, smooth margins, which must not be confused with splenic laceration, displaying predominantly fuzzy margins accompanied with perisplenic fluid (**Fig. 21.10, p. 715**).

Accessory spleens are found in 10% to 30% of individuals, usually appearing as isodense round nodules in the hilar region. They have no pathologic significance but may be mistaken for lymph nodes or other lesions. Contrast enhancement of accessory spleens is identical to that of the spleen itself. After splenectomy, accessory spleens may grow significantly in size and partly replace splenic function.

Peritoneal autotransplantation of splenic tissue after splenic trauma is called splenosis and must not be confused with peritoneal masses.

The splenic vessels enter the splenic hilum through the splenorenal ligament. The attachment of this ligament to the spleen creates an area 2 × 3 cm large on the medial surface of the spleen that is lacking in peritoneal covering. As the pancreatic tail transits the splenorenal ligament, this "bare area" may serve as an access route for pancreatic processes directly into the spleen. Additionally, although the spleen usually lies in a rather fixed intraperitoneal position, it may also be ectopic or mobile, with torsion of splenic vessels as a rare complication. Splenic encasement of the stomach is equally rare.

On precontrast scans, CT density of normal splenic tissue amounts to 40 to 60 HU, which is approximately 10 HU less than liver parenchyma. Increased values are observed in patients with thalassemia, sickle cell anemia, and hemochromatosis. However, changes in the density ratio most often are indicative of hepatic, not splenic, disease.

Diagnostic evaluation of the spleen should be performed preferentially during the parenchymal phase when there is homogeneous enhancement of the organ. During the arterial or portal venous phase, enhancement is patchy or striped (**Fig. 21.2**)—sometimes resembling a tiger skin—and thus may be misread as splenic infection, infarction, or even neoplastic lesions. The underlying cause for this enhancement pattern is delayed blood accumulation within the white matter (lymphatic follicles and reticuloendothelial tissue) of the spleen as compared with the red matter (vascular lakes). Precontrast scans of the spleen usually are suitable for identifying fresh hemorrhage. **Table 21.1** provides an overview of the differential diagnosis of diseases of the spleen.

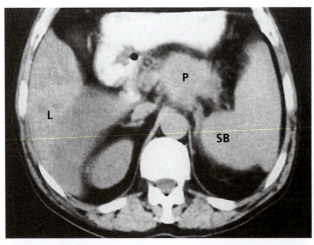

Fig. 21.1 Medial splenic bulge (SB) in a patient with pancreatic carcinoma (P) and liver metastases (L). Splenic bulge should not be confused with the upper pole of the left kidney, the pancreatic tail, or an adrenal mass.

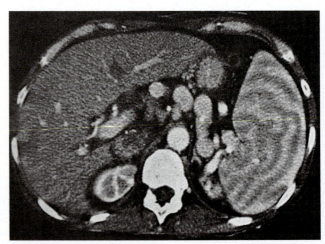

Fig. 21.2 "Zebra" spleen. Striped contrast enhancement of the spleen ("zebra" spleen), an unusual manifestation of the common inhomogeneous contrast enhancement of the splenic parenchyma during the first minute following contrast injection. The patient also has portal hypertension and splenomegaly with congestion of the portal and superior mesenteric veins.

Table 21.1 Differential diagnosis of diseases of the spleen

Disease	CT Findings	Comments
Vascular		
Portal hypertension ▷ *Fig. 21.3*	Splenomegaly associated with liver cirrhosis and ascites, as well as abdominal and/or retroperitoneal venous collaterals. **Scan recommendation:** Biphasic CT (portal venous phase [PVP], parenchymal phase [PP]). PVP: Optimal contrast of splenic and portal veins. PP: Optimal phase to assess venous collaterals. **Diagnostic pearls:** Splenomegaly, liver cirrhosis, ascites, enlarged portal vein, and numerous venous collaterals.	Common causes of portal hypertension include liver cirrhosis, pancreatic disease with portal obstruction, and portal vein thrombosis. Biphasic CT (especially PVP) important to assess portal vessels and venous collaterals.
Splenic infarct ▷ *Fig. 21.4*	Segmental to global ischemia of the spleen due to vascular occlusion. **Scan recommendation:** Biphasic CT (nonenhanced CT, PP). Nonenhanced CT: Nondiscernible from parenchyma. Calcifications may develop in chronic stages. PP: Wedge-shaped, nonattenuating peripheral parenchymal defect(s). Base typically abuts the splenic capsule, apex points toward the hilum. **Diagnostic pearls:** Wedge-shaped, nonattenuating peripheral parenchymal defect(s).	Acute infarction mainly caused by arterial emboli (atherosclerosis, atrial fibrillation, and aortic valve). Renal infarction often concomitant. Chronic infarction due to vascular (aneurysm, splenic vein thrombosis) and hematological (sickle cell anemia/leukemia, hypercoagulable states) reasons, splenic torsion, vessel infiltration (tumors, abscesses), as a complication of AIDS, chemotherapy, and chemoembolization (TACE) of the liver. Global infarction results in hypoattenuation of the spleen with or without hyperattenuating cortical rim (capsule).

(continues on page 712)

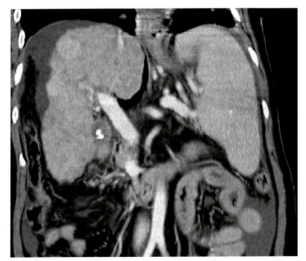

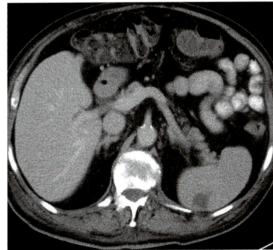

Fig. 21.3 Portal hypertension. Splenomegaly associated with liver cirrhosis, ascites, enlarged portal vein, and numerous venous collaterals.

Fig. 21.4 Splenic infarction. Wedge-shaped, nonattenuating peripheral parenchymal defect.

Table 21.1 (Cont.) Differential diagnosis of diseases of the spleen

Disease	CT Findings	Comments
Splenic vein thrombosis (SVT) ▷ *Fig. 21.5*	Nonspecific splenomegaly associated with nonenhancing (clotted) splenic vein. **Scan recommendation:** Multiphasic CT (nonenhanced CT, PVP, PP). Nonenhanced CT: Clotted vein usually not discernible from normal vessel. Calcifications in chronic stages. PVP: Nonattenuation of splenic vein. PP: Marked abdominal and retroperitoneal collaterals. **Diagnostic pearls:** Marked abdominal and retroperitoneal collaterals and nonenhancing (clotted) splenic vein.	Acute SVT may extend only up to the branching of the superior mesenteric vein, whereas chronic SVT usually is associated with portal vein thrombosis. On precontrast scans, fresh clot may appear hyperdense as compared with vessel walls.
Inflammation		
Sarcoidosis ▷ *Fig. 21.6*	Splenomegaly with multiple hypodense lesions. **Scan recommendation:** Biphasic CT (nonenhanced CT, PP). Nonenhanced CT: Hypodense parenchymal noduli of varying size (4 mm to 10 cm). PP: Sometimes discrete patchy enhancement of noduli, most often no enhancement. **Diagnostic pearls:** Enlarged periaortic and retrocrural lymph nodes and associated splenomegaly are seen with low-attenuation lesions on postcontrast scans.	Eleven to 42% of patients with sarcoidosis develop splenomegaly. Typically associated with abdominal, thoracal, and mediastinal lymphadenopathy. Patients with splenic sarcoidosis always also have pulmonary sarcoidosis. CT can only display (rare) focal lesions but not a (more common) diffuse splenic infiltration. Differential diagnosis: septicemia, tuberculosis (TB), micronodular metastases, Gaucher disease, and amyloidosis.
Congenital		
Polysplenia	Ectopic splenic tissue, predominantly in the hilus region of the spleen. **Scan recommendation:** Contrast-enhanced CT (PP), although ultrasound may suffice for diagnosis. **Diagnostic pearls:**Numerous small splenic, preferentially right-sided masses, bilateral distribution of usually left-sided visceral organs, and intrahepatic termination of the inferior vena cava (IVC) with continuation via the azygos vein.	Polysplenia in combination with left isomerism is called polysplenia syndrome. It is a rare anomaly, often associated with cardiovascular malformation, gastrointestinal (GI) malrotation, preduodenal portal vein, anomalous liver, and absence of a suprarenal vena cava. Asplenia and polysplenia syndrome may be pathogenetically related. Absence of a normal-sized spleen is a criterion to differ from patients with accessory spleens.
Accessory spleen (splenosis) ▷ *Fig. 21.7a, b*	Multiple, usually small spleens, predominantly left-sided, but often also bilateral. **Scan recommendation:** Contrast-enhanced CT (PP), although ultrasound may suffice for diagnosis. **Diagnostic pearls:** Small, round nodules near the splenic hilum with same texture and contrast enhancement as for a normally sized and located spleen.	Asymptomatic accidental finding in 10% to 30% of patients. May hypertrophy after splenectomy. Embryogenetically, a failure of splenic buds to unite within dorsal mesogastrium. Presence of a normal-sized spleen is a criterion to differ from patients with polysplenia (syndrome).
Congenital cyst ▷ *Fig. 21.8*	Unilocular, homogeneous, cystic lesion of the spleen. **Scan recommendation:** Biphasic CT (nonenhanced CT, PP). Nonenhanced CT: Water-density lesion with pencil-thin margins occasionally calcified. Hemorrhagic and protein-rich cysts may also be hyperdense as compared with normal spleen. PP: Usually nonenhancing. Contrast enhancement indicative of an infection. **Diagnostic pearls:** Well-defined, round cystic splenic lesion with water density.	Cysts may be congenital or acquired. Congenital cysts have a secreting inner (endothelial) lining. Differential diagnosis comprises abscesses (granulomatous, fungal, pyogenic, and parasitic), infarction, peliosis, hemangioma, lymphangioma, metastases (pancreatic, ovarian, and melanoma), and lymphoma.

(continues on page 714)

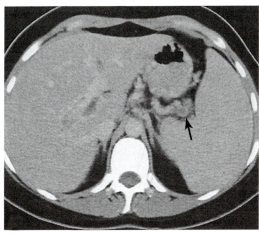

Fig. 21.5   Splenic vein thrombosis. Splenomegaly in a patient with idiopathic thrombocytosis. The splenic vein (arrow) is not opacified.

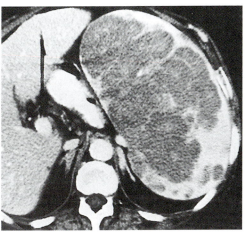

Fig. 21.6   Sarcoidosis. Splenomegaly with multiple low-attenuation lesions seen in a postcontrast scan.

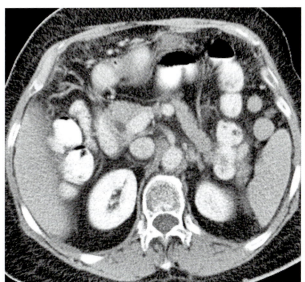

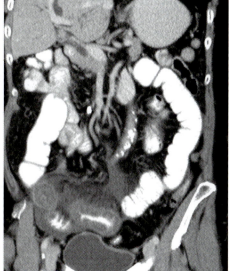

b

Fig. 21.7a, b   Splenosis. A patient with two accessory spleens (splenosis), located ventrally to the spleen (**a**). Lack of vascular anomalies excludes polysplenia syndrome (**b**).

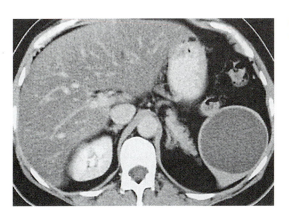

Fig. 21.8   Congenital splenic cyst. A water-density mass that is unilocular, homogeneous, nonenhancing, and sharply delineated is seen in the spleen.

Table 21.1 (Cont.) Differential diagnosis of diseases of the spleen

Disease	CT Findings	Comments
Trauma		
Subcapsular hematoma ▷ *Fig. 21.9*	Crescent or lenticular splenic lesion in subcapsular location that flattens or indents the surface of the spleen. Density depends on stage of hemorrhage. **Scan recommendation:** Biphasic CT (nonenhanced CT, PP). Nonenchanced CT: High- (acute) or low-density (subacute/chronic), sharply demarcated from adjacent normal splenic tissue. PP: Better delineation of extent of hematoma. **Diagnostic pearls:** In a patient with a history of trauma, characterized by hypo- to hyperdense, non-enhancing crescent lesion in subcapsular location.	Layered appearance of hematomas typically observed in subacute/chronic stages due to different maturation of blood products after sequential bleedings. Gas bubbles are a sign of secondary infection. Peri-/intrasplenic CM excretion indicative of traumatic vessel laceration. Chronic hematomas may calcify later. Subcapsular hematoma in combination with rupture of the splenic capsule may lead to life-threatening intra-abdominal bleeding.
Splenic laceration ▷ *Fig. 21.10*	Cleft defect through the spleen associated with perisplenic blood. **Scan recommendation:** Biphasic CT (nonenhanced CT, PP). Nonenhanced CT: Cleft defect as linear hypodensity partially or globally traversing the spleen. Concomitant hematoma may be high- (acute) or low-attenuating (subacute/chronic), depending on stage. PP: Cleft remains hypodense, but usually better delineation of extent of laceration is seen. **Diagnostic pearls:** Hypodense, nonenhancing cleft defect interrupting splenic margin(s), associated with perisplenic blood (hemoperitoneum).	Splenic laceration typically is associated with perisplenic blood (hemoperitoneum). If only the bare area of the spleen is involved, blood usually flows via the splenorenal ligament into the left anterior pararenal space and thus cannot be detected by peritoneal lavage. On postcontrast scans, hyperdense acute hematoma may be masked by hyperdense splenic parenchyma. An intraparenchymal hematoma may later develop into a pseudocyst. Treatment: usually "no touch" approach. Bleeding may compress itself.
Posttraumatic pseudocyst ▷ *Fig. 21.8, p. 713*	Typical late effect of an intraparenchymal hematoma. **Scan recommendation:** Biphasic CT (nonenhanced CT, PP). Nonenhanced CT: Clearly demarcated water-density (< 20 HU) lesion occasionally with a calcified rim. Intracystic blood clots may appear hyperdense. PP: Nonenhancing. **Diagnostic pearls:** Clearly defined, nonenhancing, water-density cystic splenic lesion with a calcified rim.	Effect of cystic degeneration of splenic hematoma. More common than congenital cysts. CT findings are identical to congenital cyst (**Fig. 21.8, p. 713**). Hemorrhagic cysts often calcify.
Infection		
Hydatid cysts	Large uni- or multilocular, well-defined, near-water-density cyst. **Scan recommendation:** Biphasic CT (nonenhanced CT, PP). Nonenhanced CT: Near-water-density lesion (10–45 HU), often with curvilinear, ringlike (hyperdense) calcifications. Daughter cyst may appear slightly hypodense as compared with mother cysts. PP: Enhancement of cyst wall and septations. **Diagnostic pearls:** Multilocular, clearly defined, water-density, enhancing cysts with ringlike, curvilinear calcifications.	The most common parasite of splenic hydatid cysts is *Echinococcus granulosus*. Usually the liver is involved. May appear multiloculated and may contain intracystic calcification. Search for concomitant parasitic cysts in the liver and peritoneal cavity. Differential diagnosis: Hydatid cysts typically show a strong rim enhancement on postcontrast scans.
Abscess ▷ *Fig. 21.11*	Unilocular (70%), sometimes multilocular (30%), liquefied pus collection within liver parenchyma. **Scan recommendation:** Biphasic CT (nonenhanced CT, PP). Nonenhanced CT: Hypodense, ill-defined parenchymal lesion. PP: No or peripheral rim enhancement. **Diagnostic pearls:** Enlarged spleen with singular or multiple ill-defined, hypodense, coalescing micronodular lesions. Look out for concomitant liver lesions.	Particularly observed in immunocompromised patients; otherwise rare. Common causative organisms are *Candida, Pneumocystis carinii,* and mycobacteria. May result from previous endocarditis. Often concomitant abscesses in the liver and kidneys. Gas bubbles are evidentiary but rare. Multilocular abscesses may show cluster sign similar to a hepatic abscess. Micronodular lesions are pathognomonic for fungal abscesses due to microvascular occlusions.

(continues on page 716)

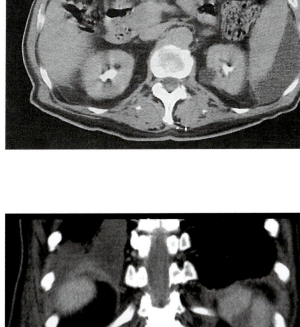

Fig. 21.9 **Splenic subcapsular hematoma.** The hematoma is seen laterally as a low-attenuation, sharply demarcated crescent mass. Cyst of the left kidney is an incidental finding.

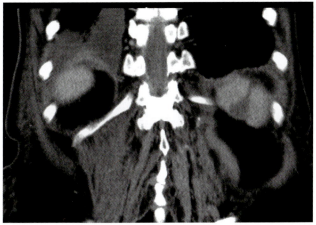

Fig. 21.10 **Splenic laceration.** Scan was taken weeks after trauma; thus, only a hypodense cleft defect in the central spleen is visible, but no perisplenic fluid (blood), as typically is the case in acute trauma.

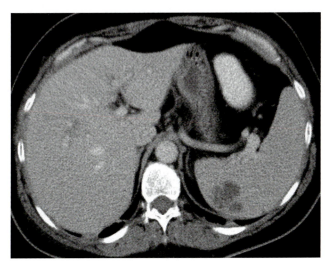

Fig. 21.11 **Splenic abscess.** The enlarged spleen exhibits a local area of partly coalescing micronodular lesions showing discrete rim attenuation.

Table 21.1 (Cont.) Differential diagnosis of diseases of the spleen

Disease	CT Findings	Comments
Splenitis	Poorly defined low-density mass in the spleen.	Rare complication of sepsis. May cause spontaneous splenic rupture.
Granulomatous infection ▷ *Fig. 21.12*	Splenomegaly with scattered punctate, low-attenuation lesions. **Scan recommendation:** Biphasic CT (nonenhanced CT, PP). Nonenhanced CT: Multiple hypoattenuating lesions. PP: Usually lesions are nonenhancing. **Diagnostic pearls:** Enlarged abdominal lymph nodes, ascites, and presence of multiple low-density lesions on pre- and postcontrast scans in the liver and spleen.	Typically associated with abdominal and thoracal lymphadenopathy. Splenomegaly is almost always present. Calcifications represent healed infection with TB, pneumocystic pneumonia, or histoplasmosis. Differential diagnoses: sarcoidosis, peliosis, micronodular metastases, and TB.

Neoplasms

Benign neoplasms

Disease	CT Findings	Comments
Hemangioma	Rare, but the most common primary benign neoplasm of the spleen. **Scan recommendation:** Multiphasic CT (nonenhanced CT, hepatic arterial phase [HAP], PVP, PP, delayed phase [DP]). Nonenhanced CT: Usually well-circumscribed masses isodense to blood. HAP: Early peripheral global or nodular enhancement. PP: Progressive centripetal filling usually isodense to blood. DP: Persistent global enhancement that stays isodense with blood. **Diagnostic pearls:** Peripheral globular enhancement on HAP scans and progressive centripetal filling in subsequent scans (flash filling).	Predominantly cystic lesions in the spleen that may contain speckled calcifications. No gender preference; peak age: 35 to 65 y. Hemangiomas usually are isodense to blood and thus show a similar enhancement pattern as the aorta. May be part of Klippel–Trenaunay syndrome, a generalized angiomatosis, including port wine–colored cutaneous hemangiomas, hemangiomas of the bowel and soft tissue, superficial venous varicosis, and unilateral bony hypertrophy of one extremity. Lesions may contain curvilinear calcifications.
Lymphangioma	Rare malformations consisting of multiple endothelium-lined cysts containing lymphatic fluid. **Scan recommendation:** Biphasic CT (nonenhanced CT, PP). Nonenhanced CT: Isodense to splenic parenchyma. PP: Discrete rim enhancement. **Diagnostic pearls:** Multiple low-density, low-enhancing, sharply marginated, thin-walled cysts, predominantly in a subcapsular location.	Lesions of childhood. The size of the lymphatic spaces varies from capillary to cavernous and cystic. Lesions may contain curvilinear calcifications. Rim enhancement is due to discrete enhancement of the lesion's wall. Differential diagnoses: histoplasmosis, TB, and micronodular hemangiomas.
Hamartoma ▷ *Fig. 21.13*	Usually single, spherical, predominantly solid mass lesions, but cysts may occur. **Scan recommendation:** Biphasic CT (nonenhanced CT, PP). Nonenhanced CT: Hypo- to isodense to spleen. PP: Variable from no attenuation to slight attenuation, but usually uniform. **Diagnostic pearls:** Imaging findings are nonspecific.	Rare. Hamartomas contain a mixture of normal and abnormal splenic tissue. Fatty components and amorphous calcifications are observed.

Malignant neoplasms

Disease	CT Findings	Comments
Angiosarcoma ▷ *Fig. 21.14*	An ill-defined, inhomogeneous, hypervascular mass composed of cystic and solid components. **Scan recommendation:** Biphasic CT (nonenhanced CT, PP). Nonenhanced CT: Variable density (cystic/solid components). PP: Variable enhancement. **Diagnostic pearls:** Several ill-defined, inhomogeneous, hypervascular, splenic and hepatic masses in patients with known exposition to Thorotrast.	Rare primary malignancy of the spleen, directly associated with Thorotrast exposure. Also occurs in liver, lung, brain, bones, and lymph nodes. First symptoms of disease often are fever, malaise, ascites, hepatosplenomegaly, anemia, leukopenia, and thrombocytopenia. Angiosarcomas grow rapidly and metastasize early. Poor prognosis: most patients die within 1 y after onset of symptoms.

(continues on page 718)

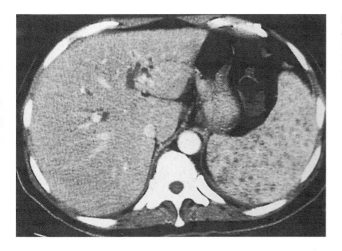

Fig. 21.12 *Mycobacterium avium intracellulare* **granulomas.** The granulomas are found in the spleen of a patient who is positive for human immunodeficiency virus (HIV). Also evident are micronodular, low-attenuation foci in the spleen and concomitant miliary hepatic involvement.

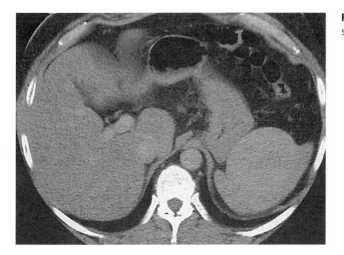

Fig. 21.13 **Splenic hamartoma.** After contrast administration, a slightly hyperdense spherical mass is visible in the splenic hilum.

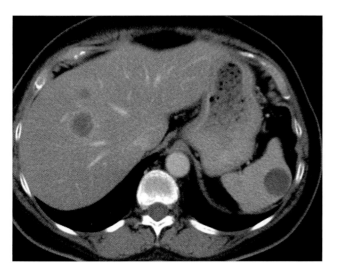

Fig. 21.14 **Angiosarcoma.** One of several similar ill-defined, cystic masses in the spleen with two of several concomitant liver metastases.

Table 21.1 (Cont.) Differential diagnosis of diseases of the spleen

Disease	CT Findings	Comments
Lymphoma ▷ *Fig. 21.15a, b*	Most common malignant neoplasia of the spleen. May be focal (lesions > 10 mm) or diffuse (typical). Always comes with a distinctly enlarged spleen. **Scan recommendation:** Biphasic CT (nonenhanced CT, PP). Nonenhanced CT: Focal lesions may sometimes be hypodense as compared with normal spleen parenchyma. Usually isodense (as in diffuse disease). PP: Iso-/hypodense to spleen. **Diagnostic pearls:** Splenomegaly with or without hypodense, nonenhancing lesions seen in patients with known lymphoma.	Splenic involvement observed in both Hodgkin disease and non–Hodgkin lymphoma. In Hodgkin disease, spleen considered as "nodal"; in non–Hodgkin lymphoma, as "extranodal" organ. Moderate splenomegaly is nondiagnostic of splenic involvement in Hodgkin disease. Even a normal-sized spleen may harbor lymphoma. AIDS-related lymphoma often presents as focal lesions.
Metastasis ▷ *Fig. 21.16*	Very unspecific: either solitary or multiple, cystic or solid. **Scan recommendation:** Biphasic CT (nonenhanced CT, PP). Nonenhanced CT: Solid metastases usually isodense; cystic metastases slightly hypodense as compared with normal spleen parenchyma. PP: Variable, central to peripheral to no enhancement. **Diagnostic pearls:** Unspecific but uniformly contrasting lesions with splenic and abdominal involvement in a patient with a known history of cancer.	Rare. The most common primaries (in decreasing frequency) are breast (20%), lung (21%), ovarian (9%), melanoma (7%), and prostate (5%). Typically, metastases are implanted in the spleen via hematogenous spread. The presence of calcifications almost excludes metastatic spread (exception: very rarely mucinous tumors of the stomach and colon). Cystic metastases observed particularly in ovarian carcinoma and sometimes melanoma. Biopsy is the method of choice for further diagnosis.
Leukemia	Spleen may be enlarged but usually has homogeneous, normal attenuation values (40–50 HU). **Scan recommendation:** Biphasic CT (nonenhanced CT, PP). Nonenhanced CT: Physiological attenuation of splenic parenchyma. Blood within vessels sometimes appears hypodense compared with vessel wall. **Diagnostic pearls:** Splenomegaly in a patient with known leukemia.	Spontaneous rupture of leukemic spleen occurs. A normal-sized spleen does not exclude splenic involvement. Different types of leukemia are not predictable from CT scans. Lymphadenopathy may be indicative, but otherwise absence does not exclude leukemia. Differential diagnoses: extramedullary hematopoiesis, other causes of splenomegaly.
Other		
Pancreatic pseudocyst ▷ *Fig. 21.16*	A pancreatic pseudocyst may be mistaken for a cystic mass of the spleen. **Scan recommendation:** Biphasic CT (nonenhanced CT, PP). Nonenhanced CT: Hypo- to isodense. PP: Marked abdominal and retroperitoneal collaterals.	History or imaging evidence of past acute pancreatitis may be obtainable.
Splenomegaly ▷ *Fig. 21.17*	Increased spleen volume (splenic index > 500 cm³). **Scan recommendation:** Biphasic CT (nonenhanced CT, PP). Nonenhanced CT: Variable. Density normal in congestive disease, extramedullary hematopoiesis and hemochromatosis. Low-attenuation in all other storage diseases. High attenuation in hemosiderosis. PP: Variable, depending on underlying cause. **Diagnostic pearls:** Enlarged spleen with convex medial border. Low attenuation typical for storage diseases, high attenuation for hemosiderosis.	CT appearance depending on underlying cause of splenomegaly: congestive disorders (e.g., portal vein occlusion, portal hypertension, and sickle cell anemia), extramedullary hematopoiesis; storage disorders (amyloidosis, primary hemochromatosis, and Gaucher disease), hemosiderosis, space-occupying lesions (cysts, neoplasms, and abscesses), and trauma (e.g., hematoma). Splenomegaly in combination with pancytopenia is termed *hypersplenism*.

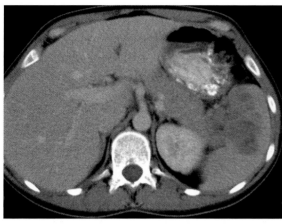 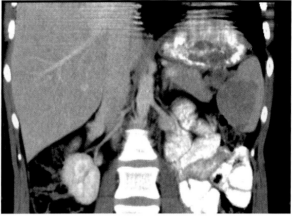

a   b

Fig. 21.15a, b   Non–Hodgkin lymphoma. Splenomegaly with low-attenuation, heterogeneous focal lesion on a postcontrast scan.

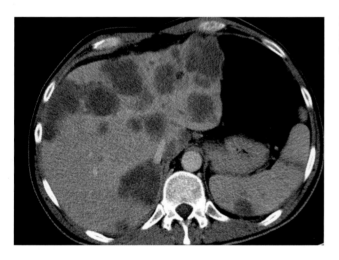

Fig. 21.16   Spleen metastases. Uniformly discrete, rim-enhancing liver and spleen lesions in a patient with a known history of pancreatic carcinoma.

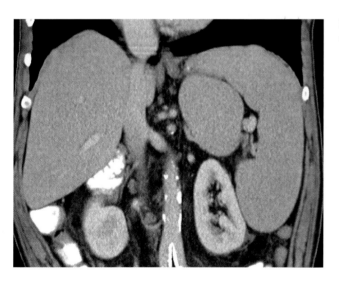

Fig. 21.17   Enlarged spleen. The enlarged spleen with convex medial borders is seen in a patient with pancytopenia (hypersplenism).

VI Abdomen and Pelvis

22 Pancreas

Christopher Herzog

A diagram of computed tomography (CT) landmarks of the pancreas and its surrounding organs is presented in **Fig. 22.1**. Size, shape, and retroperitoneal position of the pancreas show a marked variation in individuals. Usually the diameter of the pancreatic head does not exceed the transverse diameter of the adjacent vertebral body. In general, the pancreatic head-to-vertebra ratio is ~0.7 and pancreatic body-to-vertebra ratio ~0.3. Thus, the pancreas reduces harmonically from head to tail in sagittal diameter. Benchmark diameters are 3 cm for the head, 2.5 cm for the body, and 2 cm for the tail. There is gradual diminution of the pancreatic size with advancing age. The contour of the pancreas is smooth in ~80% of individuals (**Fig. 22.2**) and lobulated in ~20% (**Fig. 22.3**).

The main duct of the pancreas (duct of Wirsung) lies centrally in the longitudinal axis of the organ and does not exceed 3 to 4 mm in diameter; > 5 mm in diameter is regarded as pathological. The auxiliary pancreatic duct (duct of Santorini) and side branches of the main duct usually are not visible on CT scans.

Inhomogeneous fatty replacement (attenuation from −40 to −10 HU, **Fig. 22.4**) of pancreatic tissue is more common in the anterior aspect of the head of the pancreas, whereas the posterior aspect and the area around the common bile duct tend to be spared. It represents a common tissue abnormality of the pancreas and typically is associated with age and obesity, less frequently with cystic fibrosis, diabetes mellitus, and pancreatitis. The annular pancreas is a ring of pancreatic tissue surrounding and encasing the descending or transverse part of the duodenum. It is a congenital abnormality due to hypertrophy of the dorsal and ventral pancreatic duct or abnormal migration of the left ventral pancreatic bud to the right of the duodenum rather than to the left. Pancreas divisum is observed in patients with insufficient fusion of the dorsal and ventral bud of the pancreas. Although it may be a cause for otherwise inexplicable recurrent pancreatitis, it is often missed.

The portal vein is formed behind the neck of the pancreas by the confluence of the splenic and superior mesenteric veins. The uncinate process of the pancreas head extends between the superior mesenteric vein and the inferior vena cava. Occasionally, the tail or head is congenitally absent.

Differentiation from the adjacent duodenum is critical for sufficient evaluation of the pancreas. Patients should drink 1 l oz pure water (Hydro-CT) prior to the CT examination. This not only makes the duodenum appear hypodense in comparison to surrounding tissue, but also allows identification of hyperdense gallstones in the ampulla of Vater, which may otherwise be obscured by oral contrast medium. Differentiation may even be optimized by asking the patient to drink 300 mL water immediately before the exam and to subsequently rest on the right side for ~5 min before scanning is started. Additional administration of spasmolytic drugs (Buscopan) significantly decreases bowel motion and therefore has a direct impact on image quality. On precontrast scan, attenuation values of normal pancreatic tissue range from 30 to 50 HU.

Neoplasms usually are iso- to hypodense to normal pancreatic tissue and thus are masked on both precontrast and delayed postcontrast scans. Optimal visualization of malignancies is usually achieved on portal venous scans, when pancreatic tumors appear hypodense in contrast to typically strong enhancing pancreatic tissue. Endocrine-active tumors typically are enhancing—and thus discernible—only during the early arterial phase (AP).

In patients with acute pancreatitis, contrast enhancement helps to differentiate vital—and therefore attenuating—pancreatic tissue from nonenhancing necrotic tissue. Intravenous contrast administration is useful to distinguish pancreatic parenchyma from adjacent blood vessels, abdominal organs, or ligaments.

CT evaluation for neoplasms of the pancreas should be based on at least four contrast phases: noncontrast, or nonenhanced, CT; arterial phase (AP); portal venous phase (PVP); and parenchymal phase (PP). AP scans usually are acquired 25 to 30 seconds after the beginning of contrast injection, PVP immediately following this scan, and PP about 70 seconds after the beginning of contrast injection. For all other indications, three phases—nonenhanced, PVP, and PP—are sufficient. For follow-up examinations, usually only PVP and PP scans are necessary. Use of double-barrel power injectors,

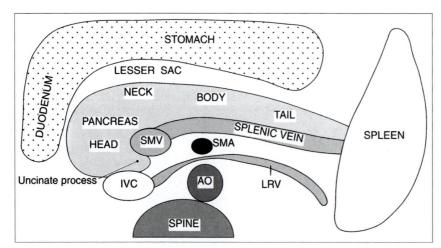

Fig. 22.1 Anatomy of the pancreas and its surroundings. (Modified after Webb.)
AO aorta
IVC inferior vena cava
LRV left renal vein
SMA superior mesenteric artery
SMV superior mesenteric vein

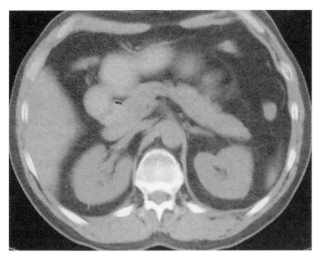

Fig. 22.2   Smoothly delineated normal pancreas. Parenchyma attenuation is isodense to many neighboring organs in this nonenhanced image.

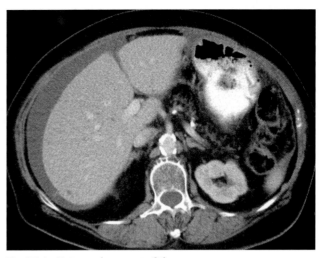

Fig. 22.4   Fatty replacement of the pancreas.

high-contrast flow ($\geq$ 3.5 mL/s), and application of bolus chaser technique with 50 mL saline following contrast media injection are critical to achieve optimal image contrast. It is also preferable to use contrast media concentrations of 350 mg I/mL or higher. The total amount of contrast media should not exceed 70 to 90 mL.

To identify even small pancreatic lesions and also be able to evaluate pancreatic ducts (ranging from 2.0 to 6.5 mm in diameter) on multidetector-row CT scanners, beam collimations < 1.5 mm and a slice thickness < 3 mm are required. The pancreatic duct is not always visible in all patients (**Fig. 22.5**). Optimal visualization of pancreatic ducts may often be achieved by using minimum intensity projection (MinIP) reformations.

The differential diagnoses of pancreatic abnormalities are discussed in **Table 22.1**.

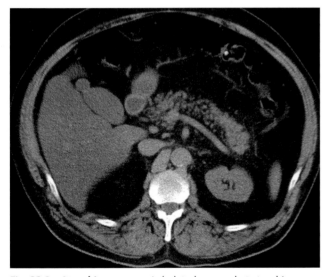

Fig. 22.3   Atrophic pancreas. Lobulated, somewhat atrophic pancreas with fat between lobules and fatty replacement of the pancreas body. Modest atrophy of pancreas is normal in the elderly.

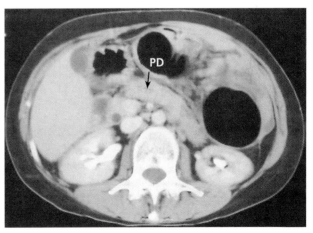

Fig. 22.5   A 10-mm slice through the body of the pancreas. The body, tail, and distal part of the head are visualized. The pancreatic duct (PD, arrow) is only barely visible within the body.

Table 22.1   Abnormal pancreas

Disease	CT Findings	Comments
Infection		
Pancreatic abscess ▷ *Fig. 22.6*	Well-defined cystic lesion in the pancreas. **Scan recommendation:** Biphasic CT (nonenhanced CT, parenchymal phase [PP]). Nonenhanced CT: Near-water fluid collection. Intracystic gas present in 30% to 50% of cases. PP: Slight rim enhancement. **Diagnostic pearls:** Well-defined cystic mass with intracystic gas in a patient with a known history of pancreatitis.	Rare, but severe complication of acute pancreatitis. In 30% of cases, there are multiple abscesses. Fistulous tracts are often responsible for intralesional gas collection. Without the presence of gas, abscesses often are indistinguishable from noninfected (pseudo-)cysts. Treatment: PAD, surgery (high mortality without).
Congenital		
Pancreas divisum ▷ *Fig. 22.7a, b*	Nonfusion of dorsal and ventral pancreatic buds. **Scan recommendation:** Biphasic CT (nonenhanced CT, PP). Nonenhanced CT: Large pancreatic head. Separation of ventral and dorsal pancreatic segment sometimes with a visible fatty cleft between both. Nonfusion of ducts visible on thin-slice minimum intensity projection (MinIP). PP: Hypoattenuation of necrotic areas (if present). **Diagnostic pearls:** Large pancreatic head with separate duodenal drainage of nonfused long (dorsal) and short (ventral) pancreatic duct in a patient with recurrent pancreatitis.	Failure of ventral pancreas in rotation during embryogenesis posteriorly to the duodenum to come (physiologically) into contact with the dorsal pancreas. Typical clinical symptoms are epigastric pain with or without vomiting in young patients due to recurrent episodes of idiopathic pancreatitis. Treatment (only in symptomatic patients): sphincteroplasty or surgery. Usually not diagnosed on CT scans. Magnetic resonance cholangiopancreatography (MRCP) modality of choice.
Annular pancreas ▷ *Fig. 22.8a, b*	Encasement of descending duodenum through ringlike pancreatic tissue. **Scan recommendation:** Biphasic CT (nonenhanced CT, PP). NECT: Obstructing band of pancreas tissue around descending duodenum with dilatation of stomach and proximal duodenum. PP: Better delineation of pancreatic tissue. Hypoattenuation of necrotic areas (if present).	Either due to hypertrophy of the dorsal and ventral pancreatic duct or to abnormal migration of the left ventral pancreatic bud to the right of the duodenum rather than to the left. Typically diagnosed during childhood. Clinical symptoms are epigastric pain with or without vomiting due to recurrent episodes of idiopathic pancreatitis, but pancreatitis is observed only in 20% to 30% of cases. Differential diagnosis: pancreatic or duodenal carcinoma.
Agenesis of dorsal pancreas	Congenital absence of tail, body, and neck of pancreas. **Scan recommendation:** Biphasic CT (nonenhanced CT, PP). Nonenhanced CT: Normal pancreatic head, absence of tail, and partial to complete absence of body. PP: No additional information. **Diagnostic pearls:** In cases with partial absence of the body, consider pancreatic atrophy.	Rare. Familial occurrence is indicative of potential hereditary mechanism. Agenesis is most likely a defect of the dorsal pancreatic bud. Typically asymptomatic, incidental finding. Symptomatic patients may present with recurrent abdominal pain and diabetes mellitus.
Trauma		
Pancreas laceration ▷ *Fig. 22.9a, b*	Traumatic laceration of the pancreas usually affecting either the neck or body. **Scan recommendation:** Biphasic CT (nonenhanced CT, PP). Nonenhanced CT: Hypodense cleft at side of laceration. Blood may appear hyperdense. PP: No additional information. **Diagnostic pearls:** (Hyperdense) peripancreatic fluid in a patient with seat-belt injury.	Typical complication in car accidents due to seat-belt injuries. Short-lasting but severe encasement between the spine dorsally and the compressed peritoneal cavity ventrally (through the seat belt) in combination with abrupt anteflexion of the body (due to abrupt braking) typically effects laceration within the body of the pancreas. Laceration is a severe posttraumatic injury that may easily be missed or misinterpreted on initial scans.

(continues on page 724)

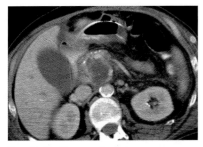

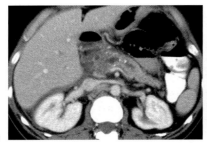

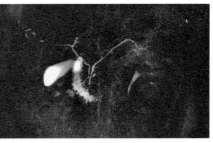

a

b

Fig. 22.6   Pancreatic abscess.
Well-defined cystic mass without intracystic gas in a patient with a known history of pancreatitis.

Fig. 22.7a, b   Chronic pancreatitis due to a pancreas divisum. Typical signs of chronic pancreatitis such as an irregularly dilated main pancreatic duct, glandular atrophy of the tail, pseudocysts in the head, and tissue calcifications in the body (**a**). Pancreas divisum is clearly shown on magnetic resonance cholangiopancreatography showing nonfusion of dorsal and ventral pancreatic buds (**b**). CT shows a large edematous pancreatic head—due to acute inflammation—with two separate orifices: the long duct dorsally, ill-defined due to edema, and the short duct ventrally, well-defined and round.

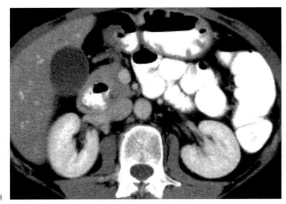

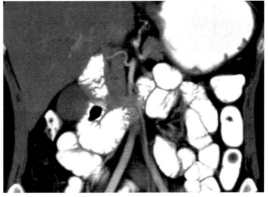

b

Fig. 22.8a, b   Annular pancreas. Encasement of the descending duodenum through ringlike pancreatic tissue on the axial scan (**a**), corresponding to the thin, linear soft tissue structure lateral to the descending duodenum on the coronal scan (**b**).

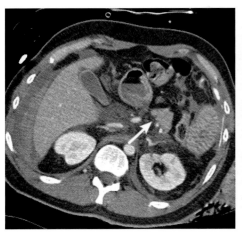

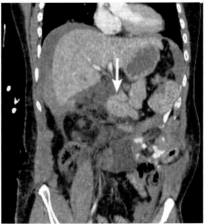

b

Fig. 22.9a, b   Traumatic laceration of the pancreas in a patient involved in a severe car accident.
There is marked hypodense fluid in the region of the pancreas head, which is completely destroyed and thus not visible. The pancreas body is displaced to the left and appears as a heart-shaped hyperattenuating structure ventrally to the left kidney (arrow) (**a**). Note the distinct exenteration of parts of the colon and small intestine to the left. The coronal multiplanar reconstruction reveals that the duodenum is cut proximally at the inferior part and displaced to the left (**b**). The displaced pancreas body is the triangular hyperattenuating structure cranial to it (arrow).

Table 22.1   (Cont.) Abnormal pancreas

Disease	CT Findings	Comments
Inflammation		
Acute pancreatitis ▷ *Fig. 22.10a–c*	Acute inflammation of the pancreas with various etiologies. **Scan recommendation:** Biphasic CT (nonenhanced CT, PP). Nonenhanced CT: Focal diffuse pancreas swelling (edema). Hypodense peripancreatic fluid/hyperdense stranding of peripancreatic fat. PP: Pancreatic tissue usually enhances homogeneously. Hypodense regions are indicative of necrosis. Rim attenuation is typical for abscess/phlegmon. **Diagnostic pearls:** Diffuse swelling of the pancreas, nonenhancing (necrotic) intrapancreatic regions, and peripancreatic fluid collection. May be accompanied by pleural effusions and fluid along the fascia of Gerota/within the pelvis (space of Douglas). *Renal halo sign* refers to inflammatory infiltration of the pararenal space with sparing of the perirenal space. Pancreatic hemorrhage can be seen as hyperdense peripancreatic fluid collection (> 60 HU).	Etiology includes alcohol abuse, trauma, cholelithiasis, penetrating peptic ulcer, hyperlipoproteinemia, hypercalcemia, and infection. Clinical severity and CT changes may not correlate. On CT scans, differentiation is possible between edematous (swelling of the pancreas and stranding of peripancreatic fat), exudative (peripancreating fluid collections), and necrotic (hypodense intrapancreatic regions within normal attenuating pancreatic tissue) pancreatitis. Phlegmonous extension is seen in ~20% of cases (mainly affecting patients with severe symptoms from the start). Any phlegmon may develop into a pseudocyst through progressive liquefaction of contents and development of a fibrous capsule. Hemorrhage/necrosis occurs in ~5% of cases, is associated with high mortality, and usually results from vessel erosion or occlusion. Pancreatic phlegmon usually extends into the lesser sac or to the left anterior pararenal space, less frequently to the transverse mesocolon and small bowel mesentery.
Chronic pancreatitis ▷ *Fig. 22.7, p. 723*	Irreversible glandular atrophy and dysfunction due to recurrent episodes of inflammation. **Scan recommendation:** Biphasic CT (nonenhanced CT, PP). Nonenhanced CT: Calcifications within atrophic pancreas (i.e., fatty degeneration). PP: Irregular dilation of the main pancreatic bile duct (best visible on thin-slice CT). May show hypodense thrombosis within otherwise hyperdense splenic vein or well-defined hypodense pancreas pseudocysts. **Diagnostic pearls:** Irregularly dilated main pancreatic duct, glandular atrophy, pseudocysts, and tissue calcifications.	Typically associated with alcohol abuse, but also observed in patients with recurrent cholelithiasis, pancreas divisum, or annular pancreas. Tissue calcifications arise from reaction and precipitation of pancreas enzymes with Ca^{++} (from pancreatic tissue). Often leads to glandular dysfunction with diabetes mellitus type II and fatty stool. Pancreatic duct dilation due to pancreatic carcinoma occurs in 80% of cases confined to the pancreas head or body and appears less irregular. Intraductal papillary mucinous neoplasm (IPMN) as another differential diagnosis may simulate chronic pancreatitis clinically and radiologically.
Pancreatic pseudocyst ▷ *Fig. 22.11*	Fibrous encapsulated fluid collection of inflammatory pancreatic exudate. **Scan recommendation:** Biphasic CT (nonenhanced CT, PP). Nonenhanced CT: Well-defined hypodense omental or retroperitoneal cystic lesion. Low-density intracystic gas bubbles seen in secondary infection. Cyst walls may calcify. PP: Rim attenuation of pseudocyst. **Diagnostic pearls:** Rim-enhancing, low-attenuating fluid collection in a patient with signs of chronic pancreatitis or following pancreas surgery/interventions.	Histologically, a collection of necrotic tissue, blood, and enzymatic pancreatic fluid, encapsulated by granulation tissue and later a fibrous wall. During maturation, the density of the contents may decrease as blood and debris liquefy. May remain within the pancreatic capsule, but is more common in extrapancreatic locations such as the peritoneal cavity, retroperitoneum, or even mediastinum. Observed in about 10% of patients with pancreatitis. Nearly 50% resolve spontaneously within 6 weeks; the rest require drainage. May simulate a necrotic or cystic tumor, pseudoaneurysm, or abscess.
Cystic fibrosis (CF)	Abnormal glandular function with lipomatous hypertrophy of the pancreas. **Scan recommendation:** Biphasic CT (nonenhanced CT, PP). Nonenhanced CT: Hypodense aspect of whole pancreas with or without several nodular cysts and calcifications. PP: Inhomogeneous, predominantly low-density attenuation (fatty infiltration) of the pancreas. **Diagnostic pearls:** Fatty degeneration of the pancreas with multiple nodular cyst and scattered calcifications.	CF is a recessively inherited multiorgan disease affecting particularly the lung, exocrine glands, and gut. Disorders of the pancreas are observed in > 80% of patients. CF is the major reason for an insufficient exocrine pancreatic function during childhood. Treatment through oral replacement of pancreas enzymes.

(continues on page 726)

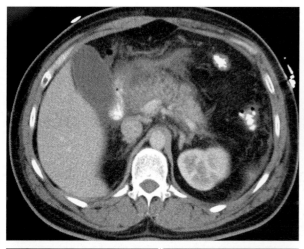
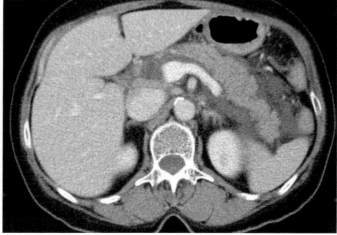

b

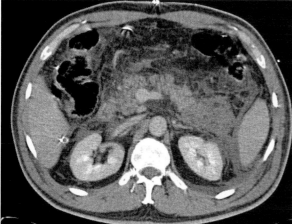

Fig. 22.10a–c   Three stages of acute pancreatitis. Edematous with diffuse swelling of the complete organ (**a**). Exudative with distinct peripancreatic fluid (**b**). Hypoattenuating tail on postcontrast scan indicative of focal necrosis (**c**). Note the thickened and collapsed inferior gastric wall anterior (**b**), both signs of concomitant mural inflammation.

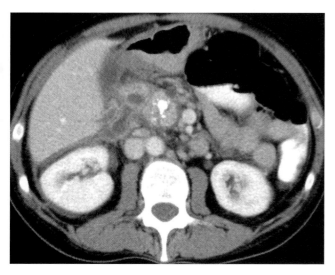

Fig. 22.11   Pancreatic pseudocyst. Fibrous, encapsulated, rim-enhancing, low-attenuating fluid collection between the pancreas head and the medial liver margin.

Table 22.1 (Cont.) Abnormal pancreas

Disease	CT Findings	Comments
Benign neoplasms		
Serous cystadenoma (or microcystic) tumor ▷ *Fig. 22.12a, b*	Cystic neoplasm, either macrocystic (cysts > 5 cm) or microcystic (cysts < 5 mm). **Scan recommendation:** Biphasic CT (nonenhanced CT, PP). Nonenhanced CT: Hypodense cysts. Calcifications may occur within a central scar. PP: Honeycomb pattern of microcystic adenoma with septal and capsular contrast enhancement. Macrocystic adenoma remains hypodense without enhancement. **Diagnostic pearls:** Well-defined, spongelike cystic mass in the head of the pancreas with distinct capsular/septal enhancement and normal width of main pancreatic duct (MPD).	Rare (~1% of pancreatic neoplasms). Histologically, a glycogen-rich mucinous tumor arising from centroacinar cells. Preferred location is the pancreas head, but it may occur in any part of the pancreas. Simple cysts of the pancreas may be multiple (e.g., von Hippel–Lindau disease, polycystic disease) but typically have no internal architecture. Differential diagnoses: IPMN, cystic islet cell tumor, and cystadenocarcinoma. Serous cystadenoma has no malignant potential, but differentiation from these other cystic neoplasms based on imaging alone is often impossible.
Pancreatic cyst	Usually congenital true cysts that are caused neither by neoplastic nor by inflammatory disease. **Scan recommendation:** Biphasic CT (nonenhanced CT, PP). Nonenhanced CT: Well-defined, round to oval, hypoattenuating cysts. PP: Lesions remain hypodense without enhancement.	Histologic true cysts with epithelial lining. Typically associated with cystic disease of the liver and other organs, such as autosomal dominant polycystic kidney disease (ADPKD) or von Hippel–Lindau disease. Solitary or multiple collection of near-water density is seen within the pancreas.
Malignant neoplasms		
Cystadenocarcinoma, mucinous cystic pancreatic tumor ▷ *Fig. 22.13*	Cystic neoplasm of varying size (3–10 cm) in the body or tail of the pancreas. **Scan recommendation:** Multiphasic CT (nonenhanced CT, portal venous phase [PVP], PP). Nonenhanced CT: Hypodense unilocular cystic mass with or without calcifications. PVP: Small tumors may be better delineated during an early contrast phase. PP: Distinct septal/capsular contrast enhancement. Macrocystic adenoma remains hypodense without enhancement. **Diagnostic pearls:** Unilocular cystic mass in the body or tail of the pancreas with hyperattenuation of thick, irregular wall on postcontrast scans.	Cystic malignant neoplasms represent < 10% of all malignant neoplasms. Cysts are typically located distal to the tumor, representing either pseudo- or retention cysts. As compared with simple cysts or pseudocysts, malignant neoplasms usually show higher central attenuation values and have irregular, thicker walls. Carcinomas may be masked in the presence of chronic inflammation. Ductal dilation often is the only abnormality on CT scans. In > 50% of patients, pancreatic duct (5–10 mm) and biliary tract dilation is observed. Stranding of peripancreatic fat is indicative of lymphangiosis and thus suspicious for extraglandular tumor growth. Mesenteric lymph nodes may be < 10 mm but still be infiltrated.
Ductal pancreas carcinoma ▷ *Fig. 22.14a, b*	Pancreas carcinoma arising from ductal epithelium of exocrine pancreas. **Scan recommendation:** Biphasic CT (nonenhanced CT, PP). Nonenhanced CT: Hypo-/isodense to normal pancreas tissue. PP: Heterogeneous, often poor enhancement. **Diagnostic pearls:** Heterogeneous, poorly enhancing irregular mass in the pancreas head with dilated common bile duct (CBD) and MPD (double duct sign).	Ductal pancreas carcinoma represents 95% of all pancreatic neoplasms. Histologically, presents as mainly mucinous adenocarcinomas. Sixty percent in the head, 20% in the body, 5% in the tail, and 15% diffuse. **Grading into three stages:** **I:** confined to pancreas **II:** stage I and regional lymph node metastases **III:** stage II and distant metastases

(continues on page 728)

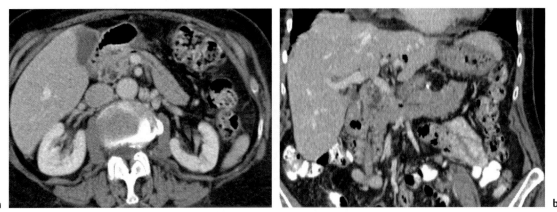

Fig. 22.12a, b   Serous cystadenoma (or microcystic) tumor. Well-defined, spongelike cystic mass in the head of the pancreas with distinct capsular/septal enhancement (**a**) and only slightly dilated, main pancreatic duct (**b**).

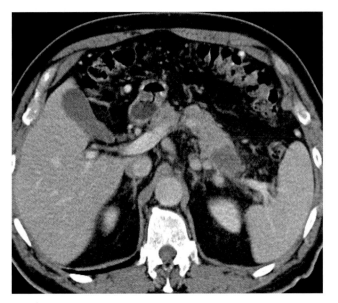

Fig. 22.13   Cystadenocarcinoma. Cystic mass in the body or tail of the pancreas with hyperattenuation of a thick, irregular wall on postcontrast scans.

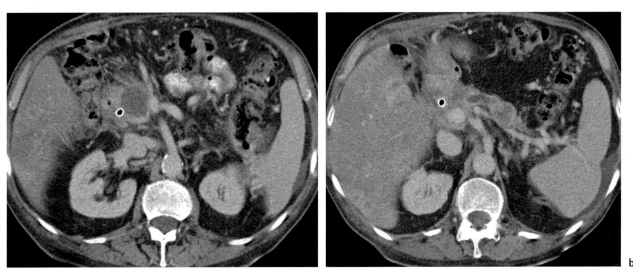

Fig. 22.14a, b   Ductal pancreas carcinoma. Heterogeneous, poorly enhancing irregular mass in the pancreas head with stent in the (previously dilated) common bile duct (CBD) and MPD (double duct sign).

Table 22.1 (Cont.) Abnormal pancreas

Disease	CT Findings	Comments
Islet cell tumor ▷ *Fig. 22.15a, b*	Neuroendocrine tumors arising from endocrine pancreatic cells (islet cells of Langerhans). **Scan recommendation:** Multiphasic CT (nonenhanced CT, arterial phase [AP], PVP). Nonenhanced CT: Small or large lesion, isodense to normal pancreatic tissue. Calcifications may be present. AP: Small islet cell tumors enhance usually strong and homogeneously. Large tumors may show ring enhancement with central necrotic low-density area. PVP: Tumors quickly become isodense (masked) to normal pancreas. **Diagnostic pearls:** A small hypervascular pancreatic mass with several liver lesions, showing a similar enhancement pattern.	Islet cell tumors are either secretory (functioning) or nonfunctioning. Secretory tumors are detected earlier due to clinical symptoms. Nonfunctioning tumors are usually large at the time of detection. Sixty to 75% of secretory islet cell tumors secrete insulin (insulinomas), and 20% are gastrin-secreting alpha-1 islet cell tumors (gastrinomas), causing Zollinger–Ellison syndrome. Rare islet cell tumors include those producing glucagon (alpha-2 cell), vasoactive intestinal peptide (VIPoma, non-beta cells), and somatostatin (somatostatinoma [delta cells]). Amine precursor uptake and decarboxylation cell tumors (APUDomas) are occasionally encountered in the pancreas. They produce adrenocorticotropic hormone (ACTH), antidiuretic hormone (ADH), and vasoactive intestinal polypeptide (VIP). Liver metastases are often detected before diagnosis of the primary islet cell tumor.
Papillary cystic carcinoma, solid and papillary tumor of the pancreas ▷ *Fig. 22.16*	Well-defined large (> 2 cm) heterogeneous mass in tail or body of the pancreas. **Scan recommendation:** Biphasic CT (nonenhanced CT, PVP). Nonenhanced CT: Well-defined, centrally hypodense mass, depending on hemorrhage/necrosis ratio. Calcifications may be present. PVP: Lesion remains centrally hypoattenuating with thick and strongly enhancing wall. **Diagnostic pearls:** Well-defined large (> 2–20 cm) tumor in the body or tail of the pancreas with coexistence of solid and cystic components.	Rare. Histologic solid and pseudopapillary structures surrounded by areas of necrosis and hemorrhage. Typically occurs in young (< 40 y) patients. Surgery is the treatment of choice. Rarely recurs after excision; thus, overall prognosis is good.
Intraductal papillary mucinous neoplasm (IPMN) ▷ *Fig. 22.17a, b*	Mucin-producing neoplasm arising from the epithelial lining of the MPD and/or branch pancreatic ducts (BPD type). **Scan recommendation:** Biphasic CT (nonenhanced CT, PVP). Nonenhanced CT: Dilated and tortuous main duct in MPD type. Rarely calcifications. Nonenhanced CT: Dilated and tortuous main duct in MPD type. Rarely calcifications. Grapelike cluster of multiple small hypodense cysts in BPD type. PVP: Subtle, irregular enhancement of cyst wall lining. **Diagnostic pearls:** Grapelike, hypoattenuating cluster of micronodular cysts within the uncinate process and emptying into a dilated MPD.	MPD IPMN usually located in body or tail, BPD type usually in the pancreatic head and uncinate process. Thirty percent of tumors transform into malignant variant. Usually diagnosed in patients older than 60 y. Symptomatic IPMN may cause pain, recurrent pancreatitis, diabetes mellitus, diarrhea, and weight loss. Treatment of choice is continuous monitoring in old and asymptomatic patients and surgical resection in young and symptomatic patients.
Pancreatic metastases	Pancreatic lesions without obstruction of the MPD. **Scan recommendation:** Biphasic CT (nonenhanced CT, PVP). Nonenhanced CT: Usually isodense to normal pancreas (melanoma: hyperdense). PVP: Variable; may resemble primary pancreas tumor. **Diagnostic pearls:** Intrapancreatic lesion(s) with concomitant intra-abdominal metastases (lymph nodes, adrenal glands, kidneys, liver).	Most often metastases are from melanoma, lung cancer, breast cancer, and ovarian cancer. Carcinoma of the stomach, gallbladder, and liver may directly invade pancreatic tissue. Lesions of the left adrenal gland and kidney initially displace the tail of the pancreas, subsequently invade peripancreatic fat, and may finally occlude the splenic vein.
Lymphoma ▷ *Fig. 22.18a, b*	Either a large, homogeneous, solid intraparenchymal mass or enlarged peripancreatic lymph nodes. **Scan recommendation:** Biphasic CT (nonenhanced CT, PVP). Nonenhanced CT: Diffuse pancreas enlargement with stranding of perihepatic fat, enlarged peripancreatic lymph nodes. PVP: Usually isoattenuating to pancreas; sometimes subtle enhancement of tumor. **Diagnostic pearls:** Enlarged peripancreatic lymph nodes or diffusely enlarged pancreas in a patient with known lymphoma.	Primary lymphoma represents < 1% of all pancreatic neoplasms. Secondary lymphomas are more common. Most common subtype is non–Hodgkin lymphoma. Treatment of choice usually is chemotherapy.

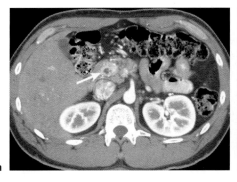
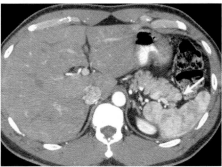

Fig. 22.15a, b   Islet cell tumors. Two hyperattenuating lesions on hepatic arterial phase (HAP) scans in the pancreas head (arrow) (with central necrosis) (**a**) and tail (small, round nodule) (arrow) (**b**).

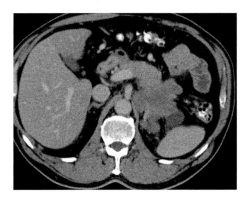

Fig. 22.16   Papillary cystic carcinoma. Irregular but well-defined large tumor in the tail of the pancreas with partly thickened hyperattenuating margins.

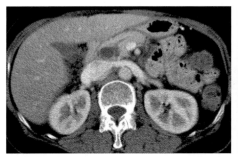
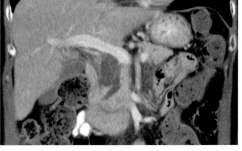

Fig. 22.17a, b   Intraductal papillary mucinous neoplasm (IPMN). Grapelike hypoattenuating cluster of micronodular cysts within the pancreas head with clear emptying into a dilated MPD (**a,b**).

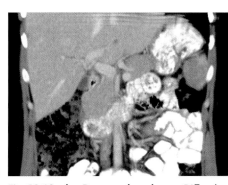
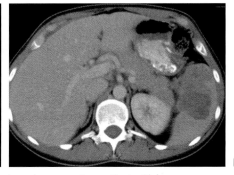

Fig. 22.18a, b   Pancreas lymphoma. Diffusely enlarged pancreas in a patient with known non–Hodgkin lymphoma (**a**). Note the concomitant involvement of the spleen (**b**).

23 Abdominal Wall

Christopher Herzog

The abdominal wall is composed of the following main layers: skin, subcutaneous tissue, muscles, transversalis fascia (which is a thin membrane), extraperitoneal fat, and peritoneum. The paired rectus abdominis muscles lie anteriorly and paramedian to the midline. The anterolateral or oblique muscle group is formed by the external oblique, internal oblique, and transversus abdominis muscles (**Fig. 23.1**). At the linea semilunaris, the aponeuroses of the oblique muscles extend medially to form the fibrous sheath of the rectus abdominis muscle. Above the arcuate line, the dorsal layer of the aponeuroses of both the internal oblique and transversus muscles pass posteriorly to the rectus muscle (**Fig. 23.1a**). Below the arcuate line, the aponeuroses of all three oblique muscles pass anterior to the rectus muscle (**Fig. 23.1b**). This transition zone forms a potential breaking point at the linea semilunaris and represents the site of so-called spigelian hernias. Both congenital and acquired defects (including trauma) of the abdominal wall can result in hernias. Typical subtypes are umbilical, paraumbilical, epigastric, hypogastric, incisional, and spigelian hernias (**Figs. 23.3 [p. 731], 23.4 [p. 733], 23.5 [p. 733], 23.6 [p. 733]**). Next to the inguinal canal, femoral and inguinal hernias are observed (**Figs. 23.7 [p. 733], 23.8 [p. 733]**), the latter being further subdivided into direct and indirect hernias. Direct or medial hernias protrude via the Hesselbach triangle and usually extend either into the scrotum or the labium majus. Indirect or lateral hernias pass via the internal inguinal ring along the inguinal canal and protrude through the external inguinal ring. Less common entities are obturator and lumbar hernias.

The posterior muscle group of the abdominal wall includes the latissimus dorsi, quadratus lumborum, and paraspinal muscles.

Primary tumors of the abdominal wall are rare; thus, most neoplasms either originate from abdominal organs and contiguously extend into the abdominal wall or represent metastases. Inflammatory and infectious conditions are observed more often, but typically they affect the abdominal wall only secondarily. However, characteristic structural changes in the subcutaneous tissue and muscles in most cases are visible on computed tomography (CT) scans.

Classic CT findings of pathologies of the abdominal wall are given in **Table 23.1**. Secondary changes in the abdominal wall, which are caused by intra-abdominal pathology, are discussed in subsequent chapters and thus are mentioned only in passing in **Table 23.1**.

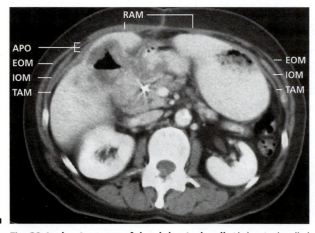 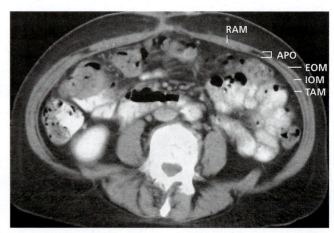

Fig. 23.1a, b Anatomy of the abdominal wall. Abdominal wall above (**a**) and below (**b**) the arcuate line. Superior to the arcuate line, the aponeuroses of the internal oblique and transversus muscles pass posterior to the rectus muscle. Inferior to the arcuate line, all pass anterior to the rectus muscle.
APO aponeuroses of the abdominal muscles
EOM external oblique muscle
IOM internal oblique muscle
RAM rectus abdominis muscle
TAM transversus abdominis muscle

Abnormalities of the Abdominal Wall **731**

Table 23.1 Abnormalities of the abdominal wall

Disease	CT Findings	Comments
Vascular		
Varices ▷ *Fig. 23.2a, b*	Increased number and size of venous vessels in the subcutaneous fatty tissue. **Scan recommendation:** Biphasic CT (nonenhanced CT, portal venous phase [PVP], parenchymal phase [PP]). Nonenhanced CT: Subcutaneous vasculature, isodense to other vessels. PVP: Portal venous hypertension with recanalization of the umbilical vein and dilated paraumbilical veins (caput medusae). PP: Typical venous enhancement.	Main cause of abdominal wall varices is an occlusion of the central venous system in the abdomen, pelvis, or chest. Location of collateral vessels indicative of the most likely site of the obstruction.
Hernias		
Paraumbilical hernia ▷ *Fig. 23.3*	Ventral hernia near the umbilicus, filled with mesenteric fat with or without loops of bowel. **Scan recommendation:** Biphasic CT (nonenhanced CT, PP). Nonenhanced CT: Control scan for PP (calcifications, etc.). PP: Best visualization of mesenteric vessels. **Diagnostic pearls:** Oral and rectal contrast is important to better differentiate bowel lumen. In children, preferably nonenhanced CT (radiation/contrast medium).	Acquired hernia in adults due to separation of the rectus abdominis muscle. Secondary to obesity, multiple pregnancies, or other causes of increased abdominal pressure. Differential diagnosis: umbilical hernia.

(continues on page 732)

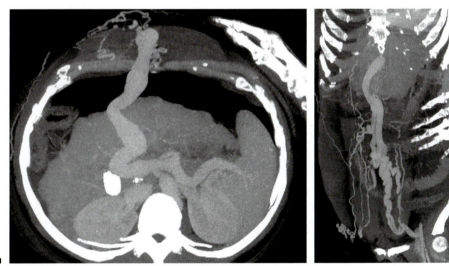

a   **b**

Fig. 23.2a, b Abdominal wall varices. Signs of liver cirrhosis—small liver, nodular margin, and marked ascites (**a**)—with recanalization of the umbilical vein and dilated paraumbilical veins (caput medusae) due to portal venous hypertension (**b**).

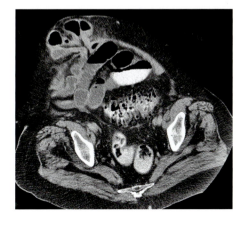

Fig. 23.3 Paraumbilical hernia. Incarcerated hernia filled with ileal bowel loops, leading to an ileus with marked dilation of the upstream small intestine.

VI Abdomen and Pelvis

Table 23.1 (Cont.) Abnormalities of the abdominal wall

Disease	CT Findings	Comments
Umbilical hernia ▷ *Fig. 23.4*	Ventral hernia straight through the umbilicus, filled with mesenteric fat with or without loops of bowel. **Scan recommendation:** Biphasic CT (nonenhanced CT, PP). Nonenhanced CT: Only necessary as a control for hyperattenuating findings on PP scans (calcifications, etc.). PP: Best phase for visualization of mesenteric vessels. **Diagnostic pearls:** Oral and rectal contrast is important to better differentiate bowel lumen. In children, preferably nonenhanced CT (radiation/contrast medium).	Acquired hernia in infants. Herniation through a weak umbilical scar. Usually resolves during childhood.
Epigastric/hypogastric hernia	Midline hernia, either between the umbilicus and the xiphoid process (epigastric) or below the umbilicus (hypogastric), filled with mesenteric fat with or without loops of bowel. **Scan recommendation:** Biphasic CT (nonenhanced CT, PP). Nonenhanced CT: Only necessary as a control for hyperattenuating findings on PP scans (calcifications, etc.). PP: Best phase for visualization of mesenteric vessels. **Diagnostic pearls:** Oral and rectal contrast important to better differentiate bowel lumen. In children, preferably nonenhanced CT (radiation/control medium).	Acquired hernia in adults due to separation of the rectus abdominis muscle. Secondary to obesity, multiple pregnancies, or other causes of increased abdominal pressure.
Incisional hernia ▷ *Fig. 23.5*	Ventral hernia following abdominal wall incision and filled with mesenteric fat with or without loops of bowel. **Scan recommendation:** Biphasic CT (nonenhanced CT, PP). Nonenhanced CT: Only necessary as a control for hyperattenuating findings on PP scans (calcifications, etc.). PP: Best phase for visualization of mesenteric vessels. **Diagnostic pearls:** Oral and rectal contrast is important to better differentiate bowel lumen. In children, preferably nonenhanced CT (radiation/contrast medium).	Delayed complication in ~4% of abdominal operations. Usually occurs within first 16 weeks after surgery.
Spigelian hernia ▷ *Fig. 23.6*	Paramedian infraumbilical herniation of mesenteric fat with or without loops of bowel between the internal and external oblique muscles. **Scan recommendation:** Biphasic CT (nonenhanced CT, PP). Nonenhanced CT: Only necessary as a control for hyperattenuating findings on PP scans (calcifications, etc.). PP: Best phase for visualization of mesenteric vessels. **Diagnostic pearls:** Herniation of bowel loops between the internal and external oblique muscles below the navel with a narrow hernia neck with or without signs of an abdominal ileus (incarceration).	Spigelian hernias occur spontaneously or postoperatively. They represent < 2% of ventral abdominal hernias. Herniation occurs through the fascia below the level of the navel, lateral to the junction of the linea semilunaris (i.e., lateral margin of the rectus muscle sheath) and the arcuate line. The contents of the hernia characteristically lie between the internal and external oblique muscles. The hernia neck may be narrow, and incarceration of bowel loops is not uncommon.
Inguinal hernia ▷ *Fig. 23.7*	Herniation of mesenteric fat with or without loops of bowel into the inguinal canal. **Scan recommendation:** Biphasic CT (nonenhanced CT, PP). Nonenhanced CT: Only necessary as a control for hyperattenuating findings on PP scans (calcifications, etc.). PP: Best phase for visualization of mesenteric vessels. **Diagnostic pearls:** The neck of a direct hernia lies medially and the neck of an indirect hernia lies laterally to the inferior epigastric vessels.	Inguinal hernias may be either direct or indirect. Direct hernias protrude via the Hesselbach triangle and usually extend into the scrotum or the labium majus. Indirect hernias pass via the internal inguinal ring along the inguinal canal and protrude through the external inguinal ring. Complete hernias may extend into the scrotum (along spermatic cord) or labium majus.
Femoral hernia ▷ *Fig. 23.8*	Herniation of mesenteric fat with or without loops of bowel medially to the inguinal canal. **Scan recommendation:** Biphasic CT (nonenhanced CT, PP). Nonenhanced CT: Only necessary as a control for hyperattenuating findings on PP scans (calcifications, etc.). PP: Best phase for visualization of mesenteric vessels. **Diagnostic pearls:** The neck of a direct hernia lies medially and the neck of an indirect hernia lies laterally to the inferior epigastric vessels.	Femoral hernias protrude medially to femoral vessels, anteriorly to the pubic ramus, and posteriorly to the inguinal ligament. They occur predominantly in women (~70%) and are significantly more prone to bowel strangulation than inguinal hernias. The Richter hernia is a subentity, containing only a small portion of antimesenteric bowel circumference.

(continues on page 734)

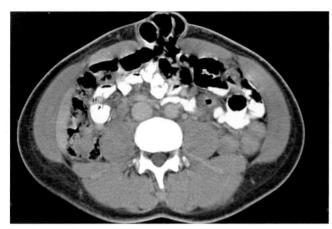

Fig. 23.4   Umbilical hernia. Ventral hernia straight through the umbilicus, filled with small bowel loops but no signs of an ileus.

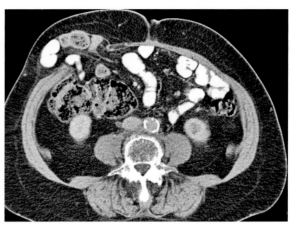

Fig. 23.5   Incisional hernia on the right lateral wall, filled with small intestine bowel loops. There are no signs of an incarceration. Note the clear separation between the rectus abdominis and obliquus internus/externus muscles, which is proof of an incisional hernia.

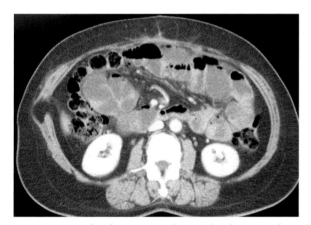

Fig. 23.6   Spigelian hernia. Note the spigelian hernia on the right side with presence of abdominal fat between the internal and external oblique muscles.

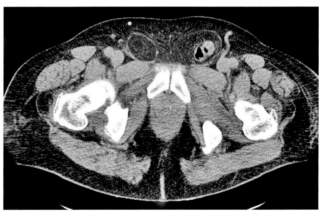

Fig. 23.7   Bilateral inguinal hernia. On the right side, the inguinal canal contains solely abdominal fat; on the left, it contains soft tissue, representing herniated bowel. Note the inguinal ligament, a thin soft tissue–equivalent linear structure dorsal to the hernia.

Fig. 23.8   Femoral hernia. A femoral hernia is seen on the left side protruding medially to the femoral vessels, anteriorly to the pubic ramus, and posteriorly to the inguinal ligament.

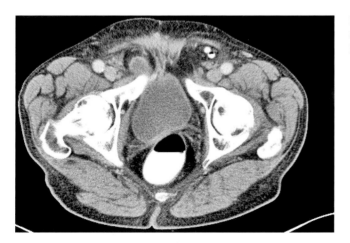

Table 23.1 (Cont.) Abnormalities of the abdominal wall

Disease	CT Findings	Comments
Obturator hernia	Herniation of bowel loops between obturator and pectineus muscles. **Scan recommendation:** Biphasic CT (nonenhanced CT, PP). Nonenhanced CT: Only necessary as a control for hyperattenuating findings on PP scans (calcifications, etc.). PP: Best phase for visualization of mesenteric vessels. **Diagnostic pearls:** Bowel loop interposed between obturator (posteriorly) and pectineus (anteriorly) muscle.	Typically occurs in elderly women due to a laxity in or defect of the pelvic floor. Obturator hernias have a right-sided preference, thus predominantly contain small bowel loop, such as the ileum.
Lumbar hernia	Dorsolateral herniation of mesenteric fat, bowel loop with or without kidneys. **Scan recommendation:** Biphasic CT (nonenhanced CT, PP). **Diagnostic pearls:** Superior lumbar herniation (SLH) through the lumbar triangle of Grynfeltt–Lesshaft, inferior lumbar herniation (ILH) through the triangle of Petit.	Rare acquired hernia in the flank region, usually between ages 50 and 70 y. SLH occurs through the lumbar triangle of Grynfeltt–Lesshaft, which is bordered by the 12th rib, internal oblique muscle, and paraspinous muscles. ILH occurs through the lumbar triangle of Petit, which is bordered by the iliac crest, external oblique muscle, and latissimus dorsi muscle.

Infection/inflammation

Disease	CT Findings	Comments
Abscess ▷ **Fig. 23.9**	Sharply defined near-water-density fluid collections, often surrounded by a capsule. **Scan recommendation:** Multiphasic CT (nonenhanced CT, PP). Nonenhanced CT: Well-defined, round lesions, denser than subcutaneous fatty tissue, but less dense than abdominal wall musculature. PP: Distinct enhancement of capsule and septa. No enhancement of central portion (necrosis).	Gas or gas–fluid level is seen in only 30% of abdominal wall abscesses. Over time smaller lesions may aggregate into a single large cavity. May result from a direct route of an intra-abdominal process such as Crohn disease, diverticulitis, appendicitis, and perforated neoplasms. Typical postoperative complication. PAD is the usual treatment of choice, followed by surgical excision.
Cellulitis/phlegmon ▷ **Fig. 23.10**	Diffuse but localized inflammation of the subcutaneous fatty tissue with or without involvement of muscle sheets and/or peritoneal fascia. **Scan recommendation:** Biphasic CT (nonenhanced CT, PP). Nonenhanced CT: Ill-defined hyperdensity of the subcutaneous fatty tissue with or without involvement of underlying muscles/fascia. **Diagnostic pearls:** Ill-defined localized hyperdensity of the subcutaneous fatty tissue in patients after surgery or skin injury.	Most commonly resulting from a postsurgical, posttraumatic wound infection. By definition, lacking gas or fluid. Treatment often protracted: intravenous (IV) antibiotics with or without surgical exposure.
Necrotizing fasciitis	Extensive necrosis of subcutaneous tissues and fascia. **Scan recommendation:** Multiphasic CT (nonenhanced CT, PP). Nonenhanced CT: Loss of conspicuity of fascial layers and increased density of fatty tissue. PP: Distinct enhancement of fatty tissue and fascial layers. **Diagnostic pearls:** Diffusely increased density of fatty tissue and subtle subcutaneous gas collections (lung window).	Characteristic complication of necrotizing pancreatitis. Subcutaneous gas collections are common.
Edema ▷ **Fig. 23.11**	Streaky opacities of fluid density in the subcutaneous tissue. **Scan recommendation:** Biphasic CT (nonenhanced CT, PP). Nonenhanced CT: Symmetrical but diffuse fluid-density congestion of subcutaneous fatty tissue with or without underlying muscles/fascia.	Causes for subcutaneous edema include heart failure, hypoproteinemia, and various other systemic diseases.

(continues on page 736)

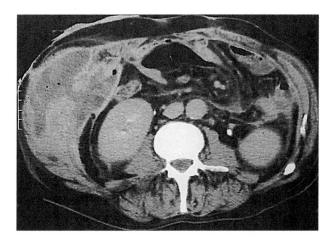

Fig. 23.9   Abdominal wall abscess. The muscular layers of the abdominal wall are separated by low-attenuation pus with discrete nodular gas collections.

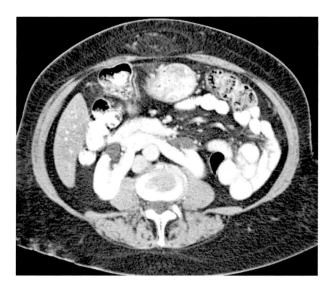

Fig. 23.10   Abdominal wall cellulitis. Ill-defined localized stranding of ventral subcutaneous fatty tissue in a patient a few days after laparoscopic appendectomy. The patient also has a horseshoe kidney.

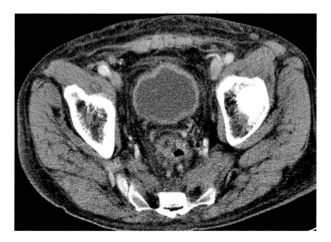

Fig. 23.11   Abdominal wall edema. Streaky opacities of fluid density in the subcutaneous tissue.

Table 23.1   (Cont.) Abnormalities of the abdominal wall

Disease	CT Findings	Comments
Congenital		
Muscular atrophy ▷ *Fig. 23.12*	Diffuse muscular atrophy affects several muscle groups on both sides of the midline. Focal atrophy usually is unilateral and restricted to a single muscle group. **Scan recommendation:** Biphasic CT (nonenhanced CT, PP). Nonenhanced CT: Atrophic muscles decreased in size and density (due to an increased fat content). PP: Atrophic muscles appear hypodense compared with normal musculature.	Diffuse muscular atrophy usually is associated with congenital or acquired neuromuscular disease. Focal atrophy typically is a delayed complication of transverse or subcostal abdominal incision, probably due to a denervation injury. Focal and diffuse atrophy may both cause disappearance of whole muscle layers on CT scans.
Trauma		
Hematoma	Round or spindle-shaped mass, usually in the rectus sheath or subcutaneous tissue. **Scan recommendation:** Biphasic CT (nonenhanced CT, PP). Nonenhanced CT: Iso- to hyperdense to muscles, depending on stage. PP: No additional information. **Diagnostic pearls:** A nonenhancing, hyperdense mass on precontrast scans. Density of the lesion decreases and approaches that of plain serum after 2 to 4 weeks.	May occur spontaneously due to muscle strain or secondary to trauma, surgery, or anticoagulation. Seat-belt injuries may lead to abdominal wall disruption, resulting in a transverse tear of the rectus muscle. Associated hemorrhage thus is not confined to the rectus sheath. Chronic hematoma often shows sedimentation of hyperdense iron particles. Hematoma may cross the midline below but not above the arcuate line.
Trapped air	Gas bubbles within subcutaneous fatty tissue, muscles, or fascial layers. **Scan recommendation:** Biphasic CT (nonenhanced CT, PP). Nonenhanced CT: Small, low-attenuating gas bubbles. PP: No additional information.	May result from penetrating injury of the abdominal wall, thoracic injuries, forced ventilation, or aerogenous germs.
Rhabdomyolysis	Excessive release of myoglobin from traumatic, ischemic, or toxic damaged muscle. **Scan recommendation:** Biphasic CT (nonenhanced CT, PP). Nonenhanced CT: Sometimes focal hypodense areas within affected muscle. PP: Affected areas remain hypodense.	Typical causes include severe soft tissue injury, surgical interventions, and compartment syndrome. Other causes are medications (neuroleptica, statins, cocaine, and propofol), malignant hyperthermia, alcohol intoxication, autoimmune reactions, inflammation, and muscle infection. Rhabdomyolysis often causes renal failure (crush syndrome).
Benign neoplasms		
Lipoma	Smooth encapsulated fatty mass within subcutaneous fatty tissue, abdominal muscles, or adjacent tendon sheaths. **Scan recommendation:** Multiphasic CT (nonenhanced CT, PP). Nonenhanced CT: Isodense to subcutaneous fat. PP: No enhancement. **Diagnostic pearls:** Easy to diagnose in nonfatty tissue. Often invisible in subcutaneous fat.	A fat-containing spigelian hernia may mimic lipoma of the abdominal wall. It is often possible to indirectly visualize lipomas within the subcutaneous fatty tissue by considering the space-occupying effect of the lesions in the form of side differences in the outer shape of the abdominal wall.

(continues on page 737)

Table 23.1   (Cont.) Abnormalities of the abdominal wall

Disease	CT Findings	Comments
Hemangioma	Well-enhancing vascular mass in the subcutaneous or muscular tissue. **Scan recommendation:** Multiphasic CT (nonenhanced CT, arterial phase [HAP], PP, delayed phase [DP]). Nonenhanced CT: Usually well-circumscribed masses isodense to blood. AP: Early peripheral global or nodular enhancement. PP: Progressive centripetal filling isodense to blood. DP: Persistent global enhancement that stays isodense with blood. **Diagnostic pearls:** Peripheral globular enhancements on AP scans and progressive enhancement during following contrast phases. Hemangiomas usually show a similar enhancement pattern as the aorta.	Histologically, a benign neoplasm of thin, fibrous stroma that surrounds multiple vascular channels lined by a single layer of endothelial cells. Large hemangiomas appear heterogeneous and may contain a central fibrotic cleft of low density. May contain calcified phleboliths.
Neurofibroma	Usually multiple round soft tissue masses in the subcutaneous tissue of the abdominal wall. **Scan recommendation:** Biphasic CT (nonenhanced CT, PP). Nonenhanced CT: Isodense to abdominal wall musculature. PP: Iso- to hyperdense compared with muscles. **Diagnostic pearls:** Peripheral globular enhancements on AP scans and progressive enhancement during following contrast phases. Hemangiomas usually show a similar enhancement pattern as the aorta.	Neurofibromas mainly lie within the subcutaneous fatty tissue of patients with neurofibromatosis. In some patients, they may be found within the musculature. Spinal involvement or long plexiform neurofibromas of peripheral nerves may also be apparent on CT. CT usually is performed for staging.
Sebaceous cyst	Well-defined, fluid-density mass in the subcutaneous tissues. **Scan recommendation:** Biphasic CT (nonenhanced CT, PP). Nonenhanced CT: Hypo- to isodense to abdominal wall musculature. PP: No enhancement.	Slow-growing benign mass, usually asymptomatic.

(continues on page 738)

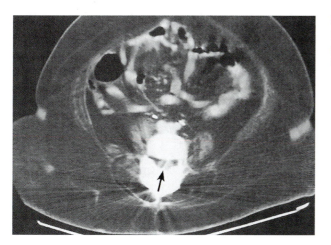

Fig. 23.12 Diffuse muscular atrophy. Abdominal wall musculature and spinal muscles are atrophic and hardly identifiable due to fatty replacement. The patient shows significant spinal stenosis (arrow), which may have caused muscular atrophy of the trunk.

VI Abdomen and Pelvis

Table 23.1 (Cont.) Abnormalities of the abdominal wall

Disease	CT Findings	Comments
Tumoral ossification ▷ *Fig. 23.13*	Well-defined, calcified conglomerates within soft tissue. **Scan recommendation:** Biphasic CT (nonenhanced CT, PP). Nonenhanced CT: Hyperdense (calcified) compared with all other tissues of the abdominal wall. PP: No enhancement.	May occur anywhere in the body. A rare occurrence in the abdominal wall.
Malignant neoplasms		
Soft tissue sarcoma ▷ *Fig. 23.14*	Ill-defined, inhomogeneous mass, often containing areas of hemorrhage or necrosis. **Scan recommendation:** Biphasic CT (nonenhanced CT, PP). Nonenhanced CT: Ill-defined, inhomogeneous mass. PP: Only nonnecrotic areas enhance after contrast injection. **Diagnostic pearls:** Ill-defined heterogeneous mass with inhomogeneous contrast enhancement.	Rare in the abdominal wall. Local recurrence and distant metastases following surgical resection are common. Diameter of metastases characteristically already measures several centimeters at the time of diagnosis.
Lymphoma ▷ *Fig. 23.15*	Diffuse, relatively low-attenuating infiltration of abdominal wall musculature. **Scan recommendation:** Biphasic CT (nonenhanced CT, PP). Nonenhanced CT: Isodense to abdominal wall musculature. PP: Slightly hyperdense compared with muscle.	Primary lymphoma of the abdominal wall is very rare; direct infiltration from an intra-abdominal origin is more common.
Desmoid tumor	Characteristically unilateral, well-defined, round or oval soft tissue mass. **Scan recommendation:** Biphasic CT (nonenhanced CT, PP). Nonenhanced CT: Isodense to abdominal wall musculature. PP: Enhances strongly. **Diagnostic pearls:** Well-defined, round, strongly enhancing soft tissue mass, restricted to one side of the abdomen.	Rare, locally invasive fibroblastic proliferation arising from the aponeurosis of abdominal muscles (i.e., aggressive fibromatosis). Desmoid tumors measure between 5 and 15 cm in diameter, are restricted to one side of the body, are more common in women, do not metastasize, and frequently recur. The typical age peak is 23 to 40 y. Twenty-nine percent of patients with Gardner syndrome develop desmoid tumors of the abdominal wall.
Metastases	Well-defined nodules in the subcutaneous tissue, skin, or muscles. **Scan recommendation:** Biphasic CT (nonenhanced CT, PP). Nonenhanced CT: Iso- to hyperdense to muscles. Malignant melanoma metastases appear slightly inhomogeneous in texture. PP: Iso- to hyperdense compared with muscles. **Diagnostic pearls:** If malignant melanoma is suspected primary, check mesentery (originates from ectoderm) for further metastases.	Exclusively hematogenous metastases. Characteristic locus for metastases of malignant melanoma, but primary tumor itself may also look alike. Other types are lung, breast, ovarian (endometriosis), and renal cell carcinoma. May also be iatrogenic due to previous surgery.
Tumor extension per continuitatem	Contiguous infiltration of abdominal muscles and adjacent soft tissue. **Scan recommendation:** Biphasic CT (nonenhanced CT, PP). Nonenhanced CT: Isodense to abdominal wall musculature. PP: Iso- to hyperdense compared with muscles.	Neoplasms originating from superficial abdominal organs are prone to extend into the abdominal wall. Likely primaries include malignancies of the transverse colon, gallbladder, urinary bladder, liver, and omentum. May also develop within a scar due to previous surgery.

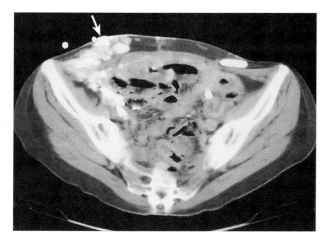

Fig. 23.13 Calcifications. Tumorlike calcifications within the subcutaneous tissue of the right abdominal wall (arrow).

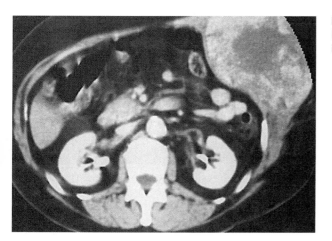

Fig. 23.14 Soft tissue sarcoma of the abdominal wall. A large inhomogeneously attenuating mass bulges the peritoneal cavity without infiltrating.

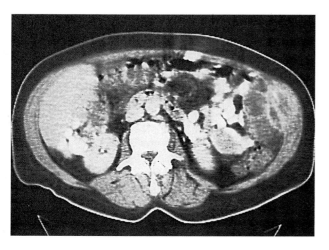

Fig. 23.15 Non–Hodgkin lymphoma. The main part of the tumor lies within the abdominal cavity, but it also infiltrates muscle layers of the left abdominal wall. The tumor consists of enhancing and necrotic components.

24 Gastrointestinal Tract

Christopher Herzog

Together with abdominal magnetic resonance imaging (MRI), computed tomography (CT) has become the chief imaging modality for the assessment of abdominal pain. Whereas MRI has its strengths in organ-based diagnostics, CT is a superb modality for any kind of staging examination.

Multidetector CT scanners allow for subsecond image acquisition and overall scan times < 10 seconds, making motion and breathing artifacts a negligible issue in assessing parenchymatous abdominal organs on CT scans. However, instruction and preparation play an important role in properly displaying the intestine. The stomach and duodenum should therefore be assessed by applying the hydro-CT technique, the distal parts of the small intestine by proper administration of oral contrast material, and the colon by rectal filling with oral contrast. Optimal opacification of the stomach and small intestine is achieved by slowly and continuously drinking 1500 mL of either a 2% mixture of Gastrografin or a 1% mixture of barium sulfate suspension (contraindication is suspected perforation due to a high risk of barium-induced peritonitis) over a period of 60 minutes prior to the examination. Optimal colonic opacification is achieved by rectal instillation of 300 mL of 2% water-soluble contrast medium. Virtual colonography (see **Figs. 24.36 [p. 763], 24.37 [p. 763], 24.40 [p. 764]**) requires bowel cleansing and stool tagging with oral contrast 24 hours prior to the examination, as well as transrectal insufflation of air or carbon dioxide—depending on availability—immediately prior to the examination. Although the method offers high diagnostic accuracy in experienced hands, its clinical relevance is usually still restricted to assessment of patients in whom conventional colonoscopy is either not possible (see **Fig. 24.40 [p. 764]**) or not desired.

Intravenous (IV) contrast medium (≥ 300 mg I/mL administered with a flow rate of > 3.5 mL/s) is required for all abdominal scans. Usually scanning during the parenchymal phase (PP; ~70–80 seconds after starting contrast injection) suffices. However, when assessing arterial or portal venous abdominal vessels, higher flow rates (5 mL/s) and proper timing of contrast injection are critical; use of the bolus-triggering technique is therefore highly recommended. The bolus triggering scout may be placed in the aorta at the level of the celiac trunk, and scanning is started either immediately after a mean aortic density of 160 HU is reached (arterial phase [AP]) or with a delay of 10 seconds (portal venous phase [PVP]).

CT may be used to assess the stomach. However, in experienced hands, barium studies still have a higher diagnostic accuracy in identifying relevant pathology and may even be better than endoscopy in detecting scirrhous carcinoma. The thickness of the well-distended stomach wall ranges from 2 to 5 mm, as measured at the depth of a rugal fold. Any measurement > 1 cm is considered abnormal. Rugal thickness varies (**Figs. 24.1, 24.2**). The gastroesophageal junction often appears as a focal thickening on CT and may be confused with a lesion, particularly if the stomach is not fully distended. Viscous stomach contents may simulate nonexistent wall thickening (**Fig. 24.3**). Because the diagnostic accuracy of CT in detecting abnormalities of the stomach is rather low, it may be better to use it for adjuvant abdominal staging and assessment of perigastric tissue.

The small bowel and its mesentery typically lie in the central abdominal cavity and may be found on CT scans between the level of the renal hilum and the aortic bifurcation. The wall of normally distended contrast-filled small bowel loops measures < 3 mm in thickness. Jejunal and ileal folds may be visible but usually measure at most 2 to 3 mm in thickness (**Fig. 24.4**). Healthy bowel loops usually show a well-defined, homogeneous, hyperattenuating wall on postcontrast scans and no visible locoregional lymph nodes or stranding of surrounding mesenteric fat. The latter is always suspicious of an inflammatory/infectious/neoplastic process. A general thickening of small bowel folds may be due to hypoproteinemia, radiation enteritis, ischemia, or an adjacent inflammatory process and thus be nonspecific. However, infectious diseases, such as tuberculosis, cryptosporidiosis, and cytomegalovirus infections, may also cause thickening of small intestine and colonic mucosa. These diseases particularly occur in immunocompromised patients.

The wall of normally distended colon measures ≤ 3 mm in thickness (**Fig. 24.5**). Any wall thickness > 4 mm is considered

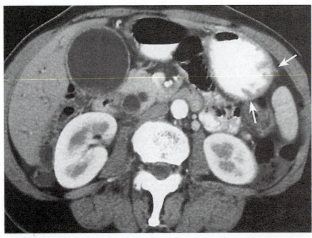

Fig. 24.1 Rugal folds. Normal-sized rugal folds in the contrast-filled stomach (arrows) of a patient with a biliary obstruction.

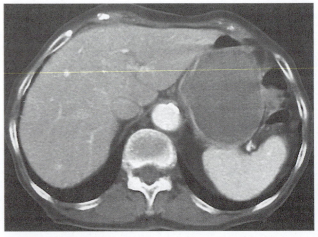

Fig. 24.2 Rugal folds. Well-distended stomach with flattening of the rugal folds.

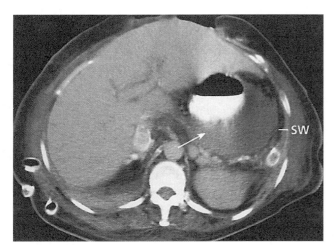

Fig. 24.3   Liver transplant patient with periportal edema. Viscous contents of the stomach create a false-positive thickened stomach wall (SW). Note the streaks of contrast media slowly penetrating into the viscous contents (arrow).

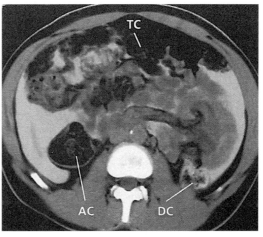

Fig. 24.5   Topographic relations of the colon in the upper abdomen. Contrast medium in the ascitic fluid eases the retroperitoneal location of the ascending (AC) and descending (DC) colon. The ascending colon is distended with gas, and its wall appears very thin. The descending colon is collapsed—which is common—and therefore has a thicker wall. The transverse colon (TC) floats behind the anterior abdominal wall and contains gas.

suspicious. A wall thickness > 6 mm is definitely not normal. The colon is sharply outlined by surrounding pericolonic fat; thus, stranding of pericolonic fat is indicative of a pathologic process. Local mural thickening may be caused by surgical anastomosis, but apart from this is always highly suspicious of a malignancy.

The jejunum, ileum, cecum, transverse colon, and sigmoid are intraperitoneal structures; the distal duodenum and ascending and descending colon lie in the retroperitoneal space (**Fig. 24.5**). The ascending colon is located in the far right lateral abdomen, reaching from the cecum up to the right hepatic flexure just below the liver. The descending colon lies in the far left lateral abdomen and stretches from the splenic flexure to the pelvic brim. It is usually collapsed. The position and length of the transverse colon and sigmoid vary, depending on the extent of the mesocolon and sigmoid mesentery, respectively. Thus, a diverticulitis in the presence of an elongated sigmoid may project the maximum pain into the right lower abdomen. Anterior and lateral surfaces of the proximal rectum are covered by peritoneum, whereas the distal rectum is completely extraperitoneal.

Congenital malrotation of the bowel usually is an incidental finding and may include transposition of the superior mesenteric artery.

A malrotated distal duodenum is usually found in the right abdomen, with the cecum and large bowel lying in the left abdomen.

A retrogastric colon is observed in 0.2% of patients: in these patients, the transverse colon and splenic flexure are positioned posterior to the stomach (types I and II), and sometimes posterior to the spleen and anterior to the pancreas (type III). Although it is usually an isolated finding, this anomaly may be associated with small bowel malrotation.

Interposition of the colon between the right hemidiaphragm and the liver may take place anteriorly or posteriorly but is of no pathologic significance. Anterior colonic interposition is common in patients treated with neuroleptic medication and may be confused with pneumoperitoneum. Chilaiditi syndrome describes a symptomatic clinical presentation with abdominal pain that worsens during deep inspiration (**Fig. 24.6**). Posterior colonic

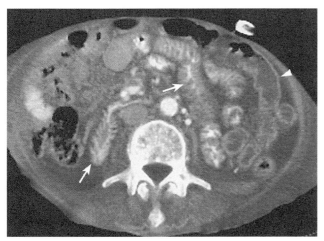

Fig. 24.4   Small bowel folds. Normal small bowel folds (arrows) as visualized after administration of water-soluble contrast material. Note the absence of folds in the colon (arrowhead).

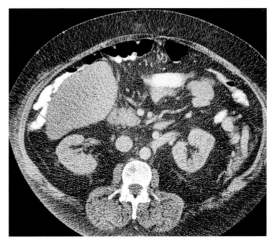

Fig. 24.6   Chilaiditi syndrome. Anterior interposition of the right transverse colon between the right hemidiaphragm and the liver in a patient with recurrent inspiratory pain (Chilaiditi syndrome).

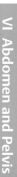

VI Abdomen and Pelvis

interposition is usually associated with right renal agenesis, ectopia, or nephrectomy.

Mobile portions of the bowel are more often injured than retroperitoneally located portions. CT is usually performed to assess the intra-abdominal extent of injury. Findings may include bowel wall hematoma, laceration, perforation, and herniation. Pneumoperitoneum, pneumoretroperitoneum, and pneumomediastinum may be concomitant after perforation of the colon. Small gas collections may be missed on soft tissue CT images; thus, additional provision of lung window

CT images is highly recommended in patients with acute abdominal pain. Free intra-abdominal or intrapelvic fluid may be the only sign of bowel perforation. Hematoma and laceration of the bowel walls appear as focal mural thickening and edema. Rupture of the diaphragm may result in bowel herniation into the thoracic cavity. It is better seen on the left side, as the diaphragm is concealed by the liver on the right side.

Differential diagnoses of gastrointestinal abnormalities are discussed in **Tables 24.1, 24.2,** and **24.3.**

Table 24.1 Abnormal stomach

Disease	CT Findings	Comments
Vascular		
Gastric varices	Pathologic enlargement of intramural and/or submucous gastric veins. **Diagnostic pearls:** Well-defined clusters of round or tubular structures running along the circumference of the gastric fundus/posteromedial gastric wall that enhance with contrast and are inseparable from the wall (see **Fig. 16.4, p. 594**).	Reopening of venous collaterals typically in the wake of splenic vein thrombosis or portal hypertension. Retroperitoneal and umbilical varices are optimally visualized on CT scans. Peripancreatic varices and cavernous transformation of the splenic vein are equally well visualized by angiography.
Inflammation		
Gastritis	Multifactorial inflammation of the gastric mucosa. **Diagnostic pearls:** Three-layered appearance of gastric wall—hyperattenuating mucosa and serosa, as well as hypoattenuating submucosa; also, partly thickened hyperdense gastric folds.	Atrophic gastritis: Tubular stomach with thin, smooth mucosa. Erosive gastritis: Areas of edematous/ulcerated mucosa. Multifactorial etiology: Drugs, radiation, stress, lymphoma, caustic ingestion, infectious (*Helicobacter pylori*, human immunodeficiency virus [HIV], tuberculosis [TB]; Crohn disease).
Emphysematous gastritis ▷ *Fig. 24.7*	Gastritis with concomitant intramural gas collections. **Diagnostic pearls:** Thickened gastric wall with streaklike or mottled intramural gas bubbles associated with large amounts of secretions and debris.	Particularly due to infections with *Escherichia coli, Clostridium perfringens,* and *Staphylococcus aureus.* Poor prognosis (up to 80% mortality). Use water-soluble contrast media to avoid perforation-associated peritoneal complications.
Gastric ulcer	Craterlike mucosal lesion of the stomach. **Diagnostic pearls:** Rarely visualized as irregularity or contrast medium collection protruding into the gastric wall. Usually hyperattenuation of gastric wall. CT helps to rule out perforation: Stranding of perigastric fat with or without free air in lesser sac/abdomen.	Difficult to distinguish malignant (more often on the greater curvature) from benign gastric ulcers (typically on lesser curvature and posterior wall). Use water-soluble contrast media (risk of perforation). Double-contrast barium fluoroscopy is imaging modality of choice. *H. pylori* irradiation and H2-receptor antagonists are therapies of choice. Consider surgery only in case of recurrence or complications.
Ménétrier disease ▷ *Fig. 24.8a, b*	Hyperplastic gastropathy characterized by prominent rugae along the greater curvature and sparing of the antrum. **Scan recommendation:** Biphasic CT (nonenhanced CT, parenchymal phase [PP]). Nonenhanced CT: Markedly thickened gastric folds. PP: Three-layered appearance of stomach fold with submucous edema and high-attenuation mucosa and serosa. **Diagnostic pearls:** Elongation and thickening of the rugal folds are seen in the presence of otherwise normal gastric wall.	Condition characterized by hyperrugosity, mucosal hypertrophy, and hyposecretion of acid. Rarely seen on CT scans. Fluoroscopy is imaging modality of choice. Medical therapy (anticholinergic antibiotics) is preferable and thus done prior to surgery (gastrectomy with or without vagotomy). CT is not an indication in this disease, but may still present with typical features.

Table 24.1   (Cont.) Abnormal stomach

Disease	CT Findings	Comments
Zollinger–Ellison syndrome	Severe peptic ulcer disease due to pancreatic gastrinoma. **Scan recommendation:** Triphasic CT (nonenhanced CT, arterial phase [AP], portal venous phase [PVP]). Nonenhanced CT: Thickened gastric walls, hypodense (liver) metastases. AP: Hyperattenuation of primary lesion with or without metastases. PVP: Hyperattenuation of gastric folds (gastritis), vessel invasions, general overview of abdomen. **Diagnostic pearls:** Thickened rugal folds, normal gastric wall thickness, multiple peptic ulcers, liver metastases, and hypervascular pancreatic mass.	Pancreatic gastrinomas are non-beta-cell islet cell tumors of the pancreas causing overproduction of gastric acid secretion and in the wake of it severe ulcerations in the upper gastrointestinal (GI) tract. CT is particularly helpful to detect perforation. Treatment of choice is medical therapy with H1/H2-receptor antagonist. Surgery is useful to remove the primary tumor, as well as stomach or liver metastases.
Pancreatitis ▷ *Fig. 22.10, p. 725*	Thickening of the inferior gastric wall associated with signs of acute pancreatitis.	Common cause of gastric wall thickening. Rarely associated with a pseudocyst of the gastric wall.

(continues on page 744)

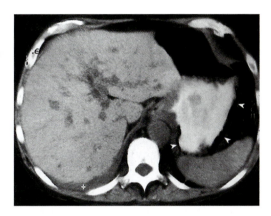

Fig. 24.7   Emphysematous gastritis. The thickened gastric wall is atonic and contains gas (arrows). (Reprinted from Krestin GB. Radiology of the Acute Abdomen. Stuttgart: Thieme; 1994, with permission.)

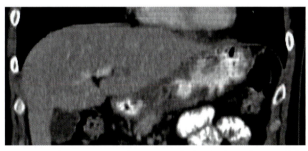 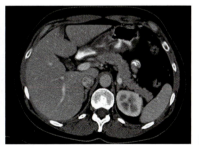

Fig. 24.8a, b   Ménétrier disease. Markedly thickened gastric folds (**a**) with submucous edema and high-attenuation mucosa and serosa (**b**).

Table 24.1 (Cont.) Abnormal stomach

Disease	CT Findings	Comments
Congenital		
Gastric duplication	Rounded left upper quadrant cystic mass adjacent to the stomach. **Diagnostic pearls:** Cystic lesions attached to the greater curvature but without communication to the stomach. May show calcifications.	Rare malformation of the GI tract, usually presenting as gastric outlet obstruction. Distinction from pancreatic, omental, splenic, or mesenteric cyst may not be possible.
Gastric diverticulum	A sac opening from the stomach. **Diagnostic pearls:** A thin-walled, cystic-appearing mass lying adjacent to the fascia of Gerota and the left adrenal gland.	Typically congenital but may also be acquired. Can be confused with an adrenal mass, pancreatic cyst, renal cyst, duplication cyst, or bowel diverticulum. Rare complications are ulceration, malignant transformation, and bleeding. Usually no treatment is necessary.
Trauma		
Hiatal hernia ▷ *Fig. 24.9a–f*	Protrusion of (part) of the stomach through the esophageal hiatus of the diaphragm. **Diagnostic pearls:** Axial hernias often resemble esophageal masses. A second contrast-filled lumen lateral to the distal esophagus is always conspicuous for paraesophageal hernia. Best visualized on coronal reformations. Rule out other cystic mediastinal masses.	Differentiation between axial (sliding) hernias and paraesophageal hernias. In axial hernias, the gastroesophageal (GE) junction and the cardia are displaced intrathoracically. In paraesophageal hernias, the fundus with or without the GE junction is displaced intrathoracically. A complete intrathoracic herniation of the entire stomach is called upside-down stomach.
Benign neoplasms		
Eosinophilic granuloma	Gastric wall thickening in the wake of an eosinophilic gastritis, which can simulate malignancy. **Diagnostic pearls:** Thickened gastric folds in the body of the stomach with antral rigidity and stenosis.	Local gastric wall thickening simulating malignancy may also be caused by syphilis, pseudolymphoma, TB, Crohn disease, and radiation. In patients with acquired immunodeficiency syndrome (AIDS), similar changes may be caused by cytomegalovirus (CMV) or cryptosporidiosis infection.
Adenomatous polyp	Pedunculated mass projecting into the gastric lumen. **Diagnostic pearls:** Oval or round mass protruding into the gastric lumen and thickening of the adjacent gastric wall.	The most common benign neoplasm of the stomach. Differential diagnoses include lipoma; leiomyoma; neurogenic, fibrous, vascular, glomus, or granular cell tumor; myoblastoma; and hemangiopericytoma.
Benign intramural gastric tumors ▷ *Fig. 24.10a, b*	Homogeneous, well-defined submucosal masses with smooth surface. **Diagnostic pearls:** Fatty tissue between tumor and adjacent organs is preserved. Lipomas usually are hypoattenuating (−60 to −130 HU); leiomyomas are strong enhancing, may show intratumoral calcifications and ulcerations within the inner margin; neurofibromas and schwannomas typically occur as multilocular nodular lesions.	Benign gastric tumors of different histologic origin, usually leiomyomas, lipomas, neurofibromas, schwannomas, hemangiomas, or lymphangiomas. Typically located in the antrum and body of the stomach. Differentiation from malignant gastric tumors usually not possible on CT scans. Barium contrast fluoroscopy is the imaging method of choice.
Ectopic pancreas	**Diagnostic pearls:** Smooth submucosal mass with central umbilication, most commonly on the greater curvature of the distal antrum close to the pylorus.	Central umbilication represents the orifice of the aberrant pancreatic duct rather than ulceration.

(continues on page 746)

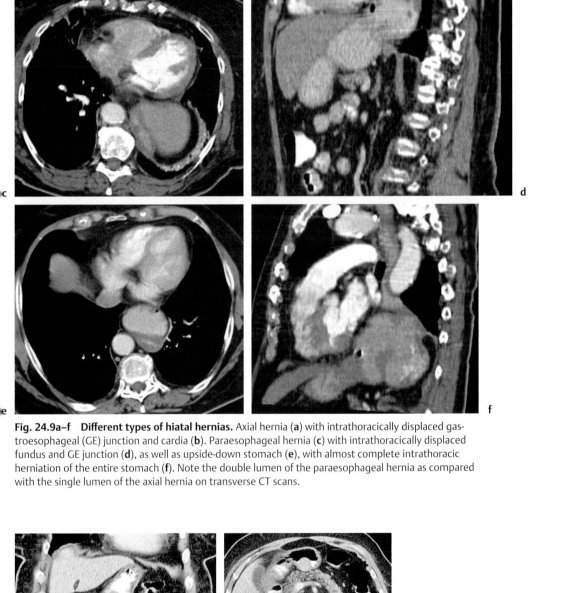

Fig. 24.9a–f   Different types of hiatal hernias. Axial hernia (**a**) with intrathoracically displaced gastroesophageal (GE) junction and cardia (**b**). Paraesophageal hernia (**c**) with intrathoracically displaced fundus and GE junction (**d**), as well as upside-down stomach (**e**), with almost complete intrathoracic herniation of the entire stomach (**f**). Note the double lumen of the paraesophageal hernia as compared with the single lumen of the axial hernia on transverse CT scans.

Fig. 24.10a, b   Submucosal gastric leiomyoma. Homogeneous, well-defined, strong enhancing submucosal mass with smooth surface.

Table 24.1 (Cont.) Abnormal stomach

Disease	CT Findings	Comments
Malignant neoplasms		
Gastric carcinoma ▷ *Fig. 24.11a–d*	Mucosal tumor of the stomach, either locally infiltrating polypoid or diffuse infiltrating circumferential mass. **Diagnostic pearls:** Focal mucosal thickening with or without ulceration. Stranding of perigastric fatty tissue is indicative of extragastric growth. Scirrhous carcinomas typically induce distinct global thickening of the whole stomach. Mucinous carcinomas appear hypoattenuating (mucin) as compared with normal gastric wall with presence of intratumoral calcifications.	Histologically, papillary, tubular, or mucinous adenocarcinoma, "signet ring" cell carcinoma. Carcinoma in situ without infiltration of the lamina propria; early carcinoma restricted to mucosa and submucosa; advanced carcinoma with infiltration of the muscularis propria and serosa. **CT staging:** Stage I: Intraluminal mass without gastric wall thickening Stage II: Intraluminal mass with wall thickness > 10 mm Stage III: Extension into adjacent organs and presence of perigastric lymph nodes Stage IV: Distant metastases CT less accurate in staging; tendency to under- rather than overstage.
Teratoma	**Diagnostic pearls:** Large, well-marginated intramural mass with one or more cystic components. Fat and calcification are common.	Rare tumor, mainly seen in children. Usually contains skin appendages, cartilage, bone, and adipose tissue.
Lymphoma ▷ *Fig. 24.12*	Involvement of stomach may be primary or secondary. **Diagnostic pearls:** Typically manifests with > 1-cm thickening of a large area of the stomach, if not the entire stomach wall. Wall thickening may ≤ 3 cm. Outer contour of lymphoma usually smooth or lobulated. Surrounding fat planes are preserved. Gastric folds may be thickened but typically are sustained.	Up to 5% of all malignant gastric tumors are lymphomas, either secondary as part of generalized lymphoma or (in 10%) as isolated GI lymphomas. Primary lesions are either high-grade non–Hodgkin (B-cell) or low-grade mucosa-associated lymphoid tissue (MALT) lymphomas. It is often difficult to distinguish gastric lymphomas from adenocarcinomas or severe peptic gastritis (Ménétrier disease).
Leiomyosarcoma	Large (usually > 10 cm in diameter), mainly extraluminal mass. **Diagnostic pearls:** Central necrosis and calcifications are common. Early settlement of liver metastases (often with central necrosis).	Leiomyosarcomas make up only 0.5% of gastric neoplasms; 60% of GI leiomyosarcomas occur in the stomach.
Gastrointestinal stromal tumor (GIST) ▷ *Fig. 24.13a–c*	Well-defined, exophytic gastric mass often with central ulceration. **Diagnostic pearls:** May be hypo- or hyperattenuating on postcontrast scans. Calcified in 30% of cases. Metastases occur in the lung, peritoneal cavity, and liver.	Most common mesenchymal tumor of the GI tract; > 60% occur in stomach, followed by small bowel. Surgical resection is treatment of choice. Chemotherapy (Gleevec) should be considered only in case of metastases. Prognosis is dependent on completeness of surgical resection (5-y survival 15%–67%).
Metastases	Most commonly hematogenous spread and direct invasion. Rarely lymphatic spread. **Diagnostic pearls:** Hydro-CT is more sensitive for detecting intramural lesions. Enhancement pattern is similar to primary tumor. Look out for metastases in surrounding organs. Metastases of malignant melanoma typically appear hypodense compared with gastric wall.	Malignant melanoma and lung and breast carcinoma are the most common primary tumors with a hematogenous spread to the stomach. Hepatocellular, pancreas, and colon carcinomas are the predominant primary neoplasms leading to direct invasion of metastases. Lymphatic spread is mainly through colon and esophageal carcinoma. It is often difficult to distinguish metastases from primary gastric tumors.

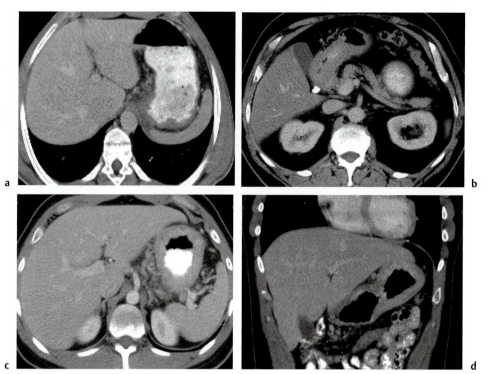

Fig. 24.11a-d   Adenocarcinoma of the stomach. Adenocarcinoma may present as a subtle intraluminal mass such as in the scan of the posterior wall (**a**) or as focal circular thickening in the gastric antrum (**b**). Distinct global thickening of the whole stomach is typical for scirrhous carcinomas (**c,d**). Note the increased perigastric lymph nodes (**a,c**).

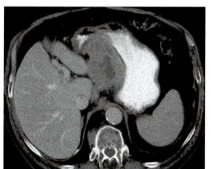

Fig. 24.12   Primary gastric lymphoma. Smooth, marginated, large submucous lesion of the lesser curvature with central necrosis and marked bulging into the gastric lumen.

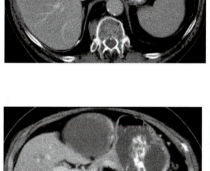

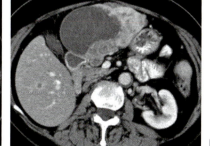

Fig. 24.13a–c   Gastrointestinal stromal tumor (GIST). Hypodense intragastric mass (**a**) with metastases to the small intestine and liver (**b**), showing a hemangioma-like attenuation pattern of liver metastases (**c**).

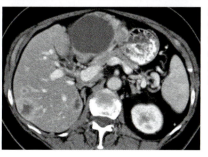

Table 24.2 Abnormal small intestine

Disease	CT Findings	Comments
Vascular		
Ischemia ▷ *Fig. 24.14a, b*	Insufficient blood supply due to arterial or venous occlusion (ischemic enteritis). **Diagnostic pearls:** Lack of mucosal enhancement typical for superior mesenteric artery (SMA) occlusion (clots in SMA?) due to compromised arterial blood flow. "Target" sign appearance of bowel wall (low-attenuating edematous submucosa framed by hyperdense mucosa and serosa) typical for shock bowel (i.e., reperfusion following hypotension). Rarely pneumatosis intestinalis.	Arterial occlusion is predominant cause (90%); venous occlusion accounts for < 10%. Clinical symptoms are sudden onset of abdominal pain, diarrhea, and vomiting. Emergency surgery is usually the treatment of choice. Prognosis depends on the speed of treatment and the amount of small bowel affected. If SMA clot is ruled out, check superior mesenteric vein (SMV) for occlusion (i.e., outflow obstruction), typically accompanied by mesenteric fat stranding.
Pneumatosis intestinalis ▷ *Fig. 24.15*	Submucosal/subserosal gas collection. **Diagnostic pearls:** Beadlike intramural gas with or without portal venous, mesenteric, and biliary gas collections.	May affect colon with or without small bowel. Intraluminal gas with increased intramural pressure or mucosal damage by enteric organism may result in gas permeation into the bowel wall. Etiologic agents are ischemia, bowel disruption, bacterial infection, and autoimmune diseases.
Vasculitis ▷ *Fig. 24.14a, b*	Concomitant inflammation of intramural blood vessels in the wake of systemic diseases. **Diagnostic pearls:** Thickened hypoattenuating bowel wall with distinct stranding of mesenteric fat. In an acute setting, vasculitis is indistinguishable from shock bowel.	Usually affects the entire small intestine. Multifactorial agents: autoimmune diseases, drug-related, infection-triggered, paraneoplastic, and arthritis induced. Radiation vasculitis is typically confined to the treatment portal. Usually indistinguishable from ischemic enteritis (check patient history).
Graft versus host reaction ▷ *Fig. 24.16*	Rare concomitant bowel affliction in patients who have undergone bone marrow transplantation. **Diagnostic pearls:** Diffuse, nonspecific mural thickening involving entire intestine from stomach to colon as well as stranding of mesenteric fat and lymphadenopathy.	The most common GI complication after bone marrow transplantation. Clinical symptoms are profuse secretory diarrhea, cramping, and malabsorption caused by immunocompetent T cells of the donor reacting against host tissues.
Inflammation		
Crohn disease ▷ *Fig. 24.17a, b*	Discontinuous, chronic, recurrent transmural inflammation. **Diagnostic pearls:** Discontinuous segmental thickening and target appearance of bowel wall seen in the acute phase, with mesenteric stranding, fistulas, abscess formation, and lymphadenopathy. Also characterized by long-segment narrowing with discontinuous segmental stenosis and homogeneous late enhancement of thickened bowel wall (transmural fibrosis) during delayed phase (DP) CT in chronic stage.	Histologically, lymphoid aggregates, coalescing into noncaseating granulomas. Typically affects the distal ileum, but skip lesions may be found everywhere in the intestine. Fistulas may be better seen on precontrast scans (hyperattenuating oral contrast material within the mesentery), but hydro-CT is better at identifying mural contrast attenuation.
Hypoproteinemia	Thickened bowel folds associated with distinct stranding of mesenteric fat and poor delineation of segmental mesenteric veins; relative sparing of retroperitoneal fat.	Hypoalbuminemia most often due to cirrhosis, nephrosis, intestinal lymphangiectasia, or SMV thrombosis. Exclude wall edema due to focal lesions occluding mesenteric veins.
Whipple disease	Bacterial infection leading to malabsorption and chronic diarrhea. **Diagnostic pearls:** Micronodular irregularities on thickened folds in the proximal small intestine, distinct submucosal edema, and near-fat-density mesenteric lymph nodes.	Rare disease. Caused by *Tropheryma whippelii* bacteria. Micronodular irregularities represent bacteria-laden macrophages within the lamina propria. Submucosal edema is due to malabsorption leading to hypoalbuminemia.

(continues on page 750)

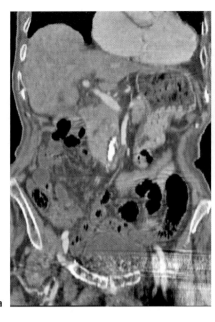

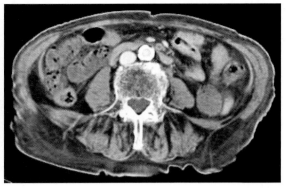

Fig. 24.14a, b CT features of small bowel ischemia. Superior mesenteric artery (SMA) occlusion with a clearly visible clot, dilated small bowel loops in the left, and segmental wall thickening in the right abdominal cavity (**a**). Wall edema of the small intestine in the ileocecal region with patchy "target sign" appearance. (**b**). The target appearance is also typical for patients with vasculitis.

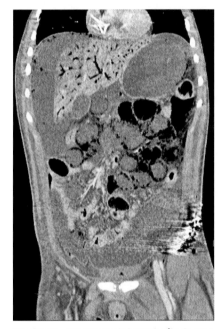

Fig. 24.15 Pneumatosis intestinalis. Severe pneumatosis intestinalis presenting with beadlike intramural and biliary gas collections.

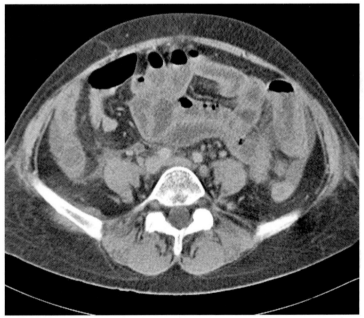

Fig. 24.16 Graft versus host reaction. Diffuse nonspecific mural thickening involving the entire intestine from the stomach to the colon. Stranding of mesenteric fat and lymphadenopathy can be seen in the mesenteric root.

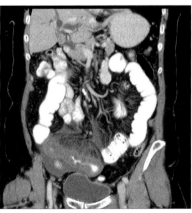

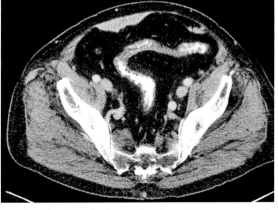

Fig. 24.17a, b Crohn disease. Mesenteric stranding, local lymphadenopathy, discontinuous segmental thickening, and target appearance of terminal ileum during the acute phase (**a**). The cecum is also involved. Long-segment narrowing with discontinuous segmental stenosis in the chronic phase (**b**).

Table 24.2 (Cont.) Abnormal small intestine

Disease	CT Findings	Comments
Sprue (nontropical or tropical)	Malabsorption due to an intolerance to gluten (nontropical) or observed in inhabitants of tropical countries. **Diagnostic pearls:** Distended fluid-filled small bowel loops with prominent folds in the distal jejunum and ileum, as well as mesenteric lymph nodes.	Common cause of malabsorption. Typically diagnosed in children. Second peak between age 20 and 40 y. Fluoroscopy is imaging modality of choice. CT findings often not typical. Gluten-free diet (nontropic) and antibiotics are therapies of choice.
Congenital		
Malrotation	Insufficient or nonrotation of the small intestine during embryogenesis. **Diagnostic pearls:** Colon located left and small bowel right in the abdominal cavity. SMV on the left side of SMA. Often hypoplasia of pancreas/aplasia of uncinate process is seen.	Three grades of malrotation: Reversed rotation, incomplete rotation, and nonrotation. May cause a volvulus. Usually diagnosed in children (80% < 1 y). Treatment of choice is surgical repair after Ladd.
Meckel diverticulum ▷ *Fig. 24.18a, b*	Persistent congenital omphalomesenteric duct forming an ileal diverticulum. **Diagnostic pearls:** Blind-ending saccular outpouching usually located 40 to 70 cm proximal of ileocecal valve.	Histologically, incomplete occlusion of ileal anastomosis of vitelline duct during embryogenesis. Clinical symptoms (if symptomatic) are bleeding, perforation, inflammation, and abscess formation. May contain ectopic gastric or pancreatic tissue.
Duplication cyst	Bowel-like tubular structures that are not connected with the bowel lumen. **Diagnostic pearls:** Cystic nonenhancing mass contiguous to a segment of normal small bowel.	Most common in the small bowel and esophagus. Spinal anomalies are often associated. CT-guided aspiration biopsy and injection of contrast material into the cystic cavity are diagnostic.
Trauma		
Blunt trauma ▷ *Fig. 22.9a, b, p. 723*	Typically due to seat-belt injuries, but any other abdominal trauma (e.g., falls and assaults) may be causative. **Diagnostic pearls:** Extraluminal oral contrast specific for bowel perforation. A dense mesenterial clot (sentinel clot) indicates a likely location of bleeding. Extraluminal/intra-abdominal gas not specific for bowel perforation (alternative causes may be barotraumas and mechanical ventilation). Use lung and abdominal window/level settings for image assessment.	Due to its rather fixed position, the duodenum is the most frequently injured segment of small bowel. Retroperitoneal rupture of the duodenum is usually evident on CT but not on plain films. Very often intramural hematoma is the cause of obstruction. Gas and fluid in the anterior pararenal space indicate retroperitoneal duodenal rupture.
Hematoma ▷ *Fig. 24.19*	Locoregional thickening of the small bowel wall and valvulae. **Diagnostic pearls:** Hyperattenuating (52–80 HU) solid intramural mass is seen on noncontrast scans. A partially cystic mass with fluid layers may be observed in cases of anticoagulation-induced bleeding.	Intramural hematoma of the small bowel is most commonly due to blunt abdominal trauma (50%), anticoagulation treatment (10%), pancreatic disease (10%), and collagenosis. Any isodense mural mass is unlikely to be a hematoma. Rule out tumors such as lymphoma, melanoma, or an inflammatory condition.
Infection		
Tuberculosis (TB) (cytomegalovirus [CMV], cryptosporidiosis)	Thickened mucosal folds and wall particularly affecting the ileocecal region. Stierlin sign: Narrowing of ileocecal area. Fleisher sign: Hypertrophy of ileocecal valve. **Diagnostic pearls:** Lymphadenopathy with hypoattenuating center (necrosis), nodular omental and mesenteric thickening (typically for miliary TB), high-attenuating ascites, nodules in the liver and spleen, and hepatosplenomegaly.	May result from a secondary reaction of pulmonary TB (miliary TB). Often also a *Mycobacterium avium intracellulare* infection in patients with AIDS. **Differential diagnosis:** CMV: Often with severe ulcerations, causing mesenteric stranding. Cryptosporidiosis: Mural thickening and usually nonnecrotic lymphadenopathy.

Table 24.2   (Cont.) Abnormal small intestine

Disease	CT Findings	Comments
Benign neoplasms		
Leiomyoma ▷ *Fig. 24.20*	Smooth, round intramural lesion with intraluminal protrusion. **Diagnostic pearls:** A large, homogeneous, intra- or extraluminal mass. Low-attenuation center indicative for necrosis; may calcify.	The most common benign neoplasm of the small bowel; 50% > 5 cm in diameter.
Lipoma	**Diagnostic pearls:** Solitary small, fat-density-like mass located intramurally or intraluminally.	Characteristically changes shape when compressed.

(continues on page 752)

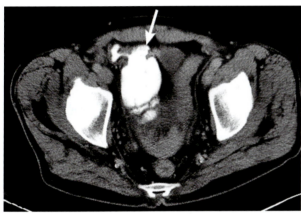
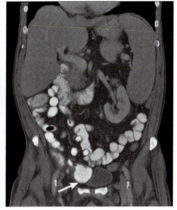

a   b

Fig. 24.18a, b   Meckel diverticulum. Well-distended, blind-ending saccular outpouching in the lower right abdomen between the right acetabulum and bladder (arrows).

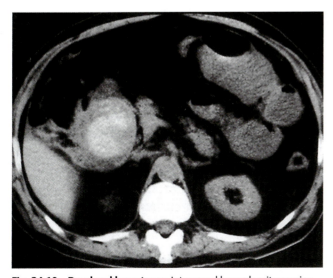
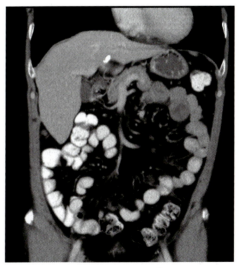

Fig. 24.19   Duodenal hematoma. Intramural hyperdensity causing widening of the circumference of the duodenum and effacement of the valvulae conniventes in a hemophiliac. (Reprinted from Krestin GB. Radiology of the Acute Abdomen. Stuttgart: Thieme; 1994, with permission.)

Fig. 24.20   Leiomyoma. A smooth, homogeneous, extraluminal mass adhering to the proximal jejunum. Note the homogeneous but discrete contrast enhancement and central necrosis. The leiomyoma is not distinguishable from a leiomyosarcoma.

VI Abdomen and Pelvis

Table 24.2   (Cont.) Abnormal small intestine

Disease	CT Findings	Comments
Pseudotumor ▷ *Fig. 24.21a, b*	Unopacified small bowel. May simulate a mass. **Diagnostic pearls:** Use multiplanar reconstruction (MPR) for further assessment or rescan after additional oral contrast.	Loops of bowel that have altered motility (e.g., following a Whipple or Billroth II procedure) may mimic a pseudotumor of the small bowel. Also, unopacified small bowel diverticula or malrotation of the small bowel may simulate pancreatic, intra-abdominal, or even pelvic masses.
Polyp (adenomatous or hamartomatous)	May be hereditary or nonhereditary, with or without other associated lesions. **Diagnostic pearls:** Small, often multiple, intraluminal filling defects. Polyps are more common in the colon. If multiple, polyps usually < 5 mm in diameter.	May be associated with polyposis syndromes including Peutz–Jeghers syndrome, Rendu–Osler–Weber syndrome, Cowden syndrome, Cronkhite-Canada syndrome, Gardner syndrome, and familial polyposis.
Malignant neoplasms		
Adenocarcinoma	Rare primary neoplasm of the small intestine. **Diagnostic pearls:** Annular solid enhancing mass of soft tissue density found on the bowel wall. May be ulcerated.	Often associated with small bowel obstruction or GI bleeding. Most common in the jejunum.
Leiomyosarcoma	Large, well-defined, strongly enhancing inhomogeneous mass with or without necrosis and calcifications. **Diagnostic pearls:** CT-based differentiation between leiomyoma and leiomyosarcoma is not possible (see **Fig. 24.20, p. 751**).	Approximately 50% of small bowel smooth muscle tumors are malignant. The remainder are benign leiomyomas.
Lymphoma ▷ *Fig. 24.22a, b*	Typically malignant neoplasm from B lymphocytes. **Diagnostic pearls:** Either diffuse bowel wall thickening or segmental annular mass with ulcerations with or without mesenteric lymphadenopathy.	Most common manifestation of non–Hodgkin lymphoma. Intussusception is frequent.
Neurogenic tumor	Single or multiple, sessile or pedunculated masses of soft tissue density that enhance with contrast and may contain ulcerations.	Associated with neurofibromatosis.
Carcinoid tumor	Neuroendocrine active primary malignant neoplasm of small bowel. **Diagnostic pearls:** Mesenteric mass of soft tissue density with spiculated margins; retraction of the bowel loops toward itself is characteristic.	Hepatic or lymph node metastases may be present. Tumors arise from enterochromaffin cells of Kulchitsky. After liver metastasis, typical clinical signs include flush, diarrhea, and cardia-related symptoms.
Metastases ▷ *Fig. 24.23*	Spread may be contiguous, hematogenous, or intraperitoneal. **Diagnostic pearls:** Heterogeneous appearance—soft tissue nodules, scirrhous lesions, intramural deposits, or polypoid intraluminal masses. Greatest portion of metastatic deposits is usually located in the mesentery adjacent to the wall of the small bowel.	Most common primary tumors include carcinomas of the lung, breast, colon, pancreas, kidney, uterus, and skin.
Gastrointestinal stromal tumor (GIST) ▷ *Fig. 24.13, p. 747*	Well-defined, exophytic gastric mass often with central ulceration. **Diagnostic pearls:** May be hypo- or hyperattenuating on postcontrast scans; calcified in 30% of cases. Metastasizes to the lung, peritoneal cavity, and liver.	Most common mesenchymal tumor of the GI tract; > 60% occur in stomach, followed by small bowel. Surgical resection is treatment of choice. Consider chemotherapy (Gleevec) only in case of metastases. Prognosis depends on the completeness of surgical resection (5-y survival 15%–67%).

(continues on page 754)

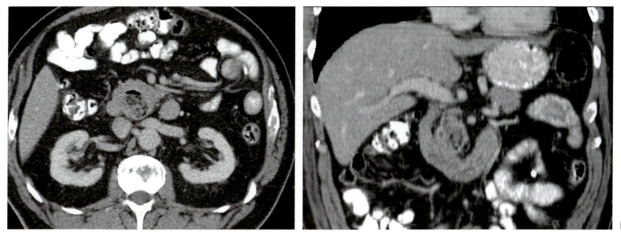

a · b

Fig. 24.21a, b   Pseudotumor of the duodenum. Lesion with central necrosis in the horizontal portion of the duodenum on axial scan (**a**), which proved to be a mucus-filled duodenal diverticulum on multiplanar reconstruction (MPR) (**b**).

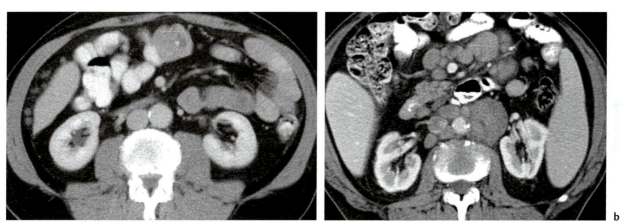

a · b

Fig. 24.22a, b   CT appearance of small bowel lymphoma. Segmental annular lesion at the level of the navel with mucosal ulceration (central hyperdensity) but without lymphadenopathy (**a**). Diffuse thickening of the horizontal portion of the duodenum associated with bulky mesenteric and retroperitoneal lymphadenopathy (**b**).

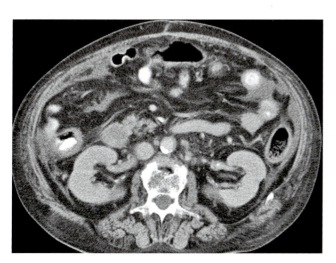

Fig. 24.23   Metastasis in the small bowel. Small bowel metastasis of pancreas carcinoma (hypodense mural nodule) infiltrating the horizontal portion of the duodenum. Ascites and mesenteric stranding are signs of peritoneal carcinosis.

Table 24.2 (Cont.) Abnormal small intestine

Disease	CT Findings	Comments
Others		
Volvulus ▷ *Fig. 24.24a–c*	Twisting of small bowel around its mesenteric axis. **Diagnostic pearls:** "Whirl" sign: Small bowel loops and their mesenteric attachment converge centrally at the point of torsion. Typically, SMV winds around SMA. "Coffee bean" sign: U-shaped configuration of bowel loops.	Acute onset of abdominal pain. Markedly dilated bowel loops seen on plain abdominal radiographs. May lead to ischemia and necrosis of bowel due to vessel strangulation. Treatment of choice usually is surgery.
Intussusception ▷ *Fig. 24.25a, b*	Bowel trapped within bowel. **Diagnostic pearls:** Cockade sign: Three concentric layers forming a soft tissue mass (inner layer representing the lumen of the intussuscepted bowel; the middle layer, mesenteric fat; and the outer layer, the intussuscipiens). May appear sausagelike if cut longitudinally (use MPR). Also seen: Proximal bowel distention and distal tiny, non-contrast-filled (i.e., "hungry") bowel loops.	Typically painful, short-segment, palpable intra-abdominal mass; often transient. Equally affects men and women of all age groups. A typical postoperative complication (disturbed bowel motility and adhesions). Etiology is often obscure. Always rule out inflammation, tumors (benign and malignant), and diverticula (Meckel diverticulum).
Gallstone ileus	Mechanical obstruction of the small bowel through intraintestinal impaction of gallstones. **Diagnostic pearls:** Rigler's triad: Multiple dilated small bowel loops with fluid and gas, a calcified stone in the lower abdomen, and gas in the biliary tree or gallbladder.	Typical complication of chronic cholecystitis. Erosion of gallbladder wall and transmural passage into small intestine. May also occur after repeated endoscopic retrograde cholangiography (ERCP) or sphincterectomy.
Small bowel obstruction ▷ *Fig. 24.26*	Primary or secondary obstruction of the small intestine. **Diagnostic pearls:** *Simple obstruction:* Dilated fluid-filled, thin-walled loops of small intestine with or without air–fluid levels. *Closed loop obstruction:* Obstruction at two ends. One or several grossly distended, fluid-filled U-shaped loops with two adjacent limbs showing a zone of abrupt transition (i.e., incarceration). *Strangulating obstruction:* Slight circumferential wall thickening and enhancement (target sign) and engorgement of mesenteric vessels indicate mild ischemia. Increased bowel wall attenuation, mesenteric hemorrhage, and pneumatosis indicate severe ischemia and infarction.	May be mechanical (i.e., intrinsic or extrinsic) or nonmechanical. Typical extrinsic causes are diverticulitis, appendicitis, hernias, adhesions, and peritoneal carcinomatosis. Typical intrinsic causes are intraluminal lesions, neoplasms, inflammations (e.g., Crohn disease), and infections. Nonmechanical bowel obstruction is mainly due to neuromuscular disturbances.
Diverticular disease ▷ *Fig. 24.27a, b*	Antimesenteric outpouching of small intestine wall. **Diagnostic pearls:** Small bowel diverticula, segmental mural thickening, and luminal narrowing in combination with mesenteric stranding are highly suspicious for small bowel diverticulitis. Locoregional mesenteric gas is indicative of abscess formation. Free intra-abdominal gas is indicative of free perforation. Use lung and abdominal window/level settings for assessment.	Rare. May mimic Crohn disease and appendicitis.

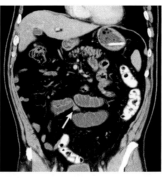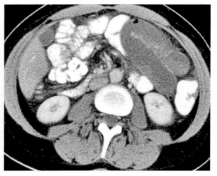

Fig. 24.24a–c   Small bowel dilation. Volvulus with "whirl" sign due to twisting of the small bowel around its mesenteric axis (**a**). MPR clearly reveals the point of twisting with dilated bowel loops proximally and nondilated bowel loops distally to it (arrow) (**b**). Another patient showing a typical "coffee bean" sign of dilated small bowel loops (**c**).

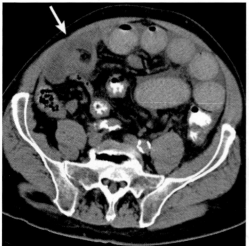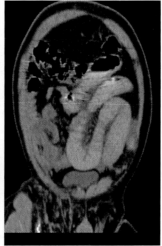

Fig. 24.25 a, b   Intussusception of ileal bowel loops. Axial scan shows typical cockade sign in the right lower abdomen (arrow), as well as proximal bowel distention and distal "hungry" bowel loops (**a**). On MPR, the intussusception appears sausagelike (**b**). Note the normal-sized, well-opacified distal ileum and colon.

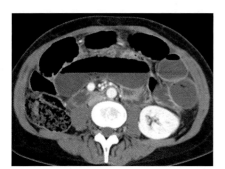

Fig. 24.26   Small bowel obstruction due to transmesenteric postoperative hernia. Dilated small bowel with no overlying omental fat displacing both hepatic flexures inferiorly and posteriorly and the main mesenteric trunk to the right. The right hepatic flexure is stool-filled; the left hepatic flexure contrast, media-filled.

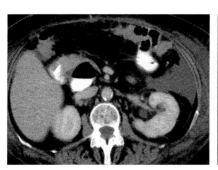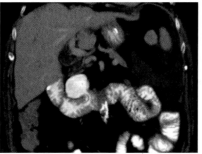

Fig. 24.27a, b   Duodenal diverticula in typical location. Antimesenteric outpouching with air/contrast level on axial scan (**a**) and coronal MPR (**b**).

Table 24.3   Abnormal colon

Disease	CT Findings	Comments
Vascular		
Ischemia/infarction ▷*Fig. 24.28a–c*	Insufficient blood supply due to arterial or venous occlusion. **Diagnostic pearls:** Markedly dilated small bowel loops and segmental wall thickening; clots in internal mammary artery and vein; three-layered appearance of bowel on postcontrast scans (target sign): low-attenuating edematous submucosa framed by hyperdense mucosa and serosa (i.e., shock bowel); stranding of mesenteric fat. Pneumatosis intestinalis and mesenteric or portal venous gas are usually visible earlier on CT than on plain films.	Typical symptoms are acute abdominal pain and rectal bleeding. Precipitating factors include bowel obstruction, vascular thrombosis, and recent surgery. Ischemic colitis is a predominantly left-sided, segmental, or diffuse disease and may mimic pseudomembranous colitis. Arterial occlusion predominant cause (90%); venous occlusion accounts for < 10%. Prognosis depends on the speed of treatment and the amount of small bowel affected.
Epiploic appendagitis ▷*Fig. 24.29*	Acute infarction/inflammation of epiploic appendages. **Diagnostic pearls:** Oval to round pericolonic fatty mass with hyperattenuating ring, surrounded by stranding of mesenteric fatty tissue.	Torsion of epiploic appendages leads to thrombosis and thus infarction of small veins. Important differential diagnosis to diverticulitis and appendicitis. CT pattern is pathognomonic. Treatment primarily with analgetics. Surgery only required in cases with larger infarctions.
Infection		
Typhlitis ▷*Fig. 24.30a, b*	Transmural inflammatory and sometimes necrotizing process. **Diagnostic pearls:** Inhomogeneous wall thickening of the cecum and ascending colon; occasionally, spreading to the distal ileum and/or appendix. Pneumatosis and pericolic inflammatory changes are common. Perforation and pericolic abscess formation may occur.	Histologically, an inflammatory process of the mucosa with deep ulcerations and necrosis due to local ischemia. Particularly observed in neutropenic patients, including leukanemia, HIV, chemotherapy, aplastic anemia, bone/organ transplants, and lymphoma. Treatment of choice is antibiotics/antiinflammatory drugs. In severe cases, surgical resection is needed.
Pseudomembranous colitis ▷*Fig. 24.31a, b*	*Clostridium difficile*–induced acute inflammation of the colonic mucosa with or without submucosa. **Diagnostic pearls:** Pancolitis with nodular circumferential wall thickening (≤ 15 mm). Oral contrast between the thickened folds may create an "accordion" sign. "Targetlike" appearance of colon wall: Hypodense (i.e., edematous) submucosa embedded between hyperintense mucosa and serosa. Usually most prominent in the ascending and transverse colon.	Usually a complication of antibiotic therapy with copious nonbloody diarrhea, abdominal cramps, and tenderness. Secondary to cytotoxin produced by *C. difficile*. CMV colitis causes wall thickening of the right colon and the terminal ileum only, without lymphadenopathy, and is usually seen in patients with AIDS.

(continues on page 758)

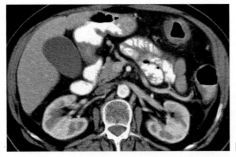 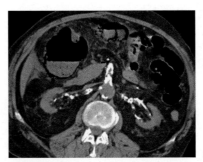 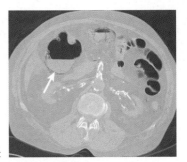

a   b   c

Fig. 24.28a–c   CT findings in ischemic colon. Dilation of the descending colon and segmental wall thickening with "target" sign (**a**). Restriction of changes to the left-sided colon is indicative of ischemic origin (**b**). Pneumatosis intestinalis (arrow) in another patient is particularly visible when using lung window CT scans (**c**).

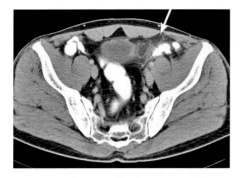

Fig. 24.29   Epiploic appendagitis. Oval to round pericolonic fatty mass (arrow) in the left lower abdomen with hyperattenuating ring, surrounded by stranding of mesenteric fatty tissue.

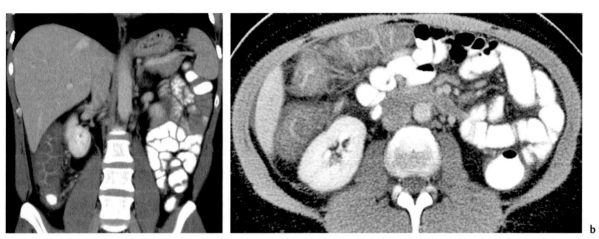

Fig. 24.30a, b   Typhlitis. Marked wall thickening of the cecum and ascending colon (**a**). Axial scan shows no involvement of descending and transverse colon (**b**).

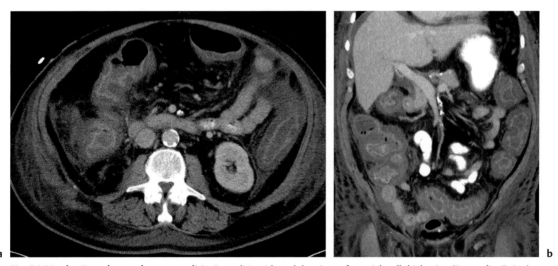

Fig. 24.31a, b   Pseudomembranous colitis. Pancolitis with nodular circumferential wall thickening ("accordion" sign) (**a**) and targetlike appearance of colonic wall (**b**).

Table 24.3 (Cont.) Abnormal colon

Disease	CT Findings	Comments
Infectious colitis	Diffuse or segmental wall thickening with or without mucosal ulcerations. **Diagnostic pearls:** *Actinomycosis:* Predominantly in the ileocecal and rectosigmoid colon. Cecum may appear shrunken (differential diagnosis: TB) but lack of mass or fistulous tracts. *Amebiasis:* Irregular thickening of the colonic wall sometimes masslike. Often skip lesions. Cecum is involved in 90% of cases. Ileum is spared. *Campylobacter:* Concomitant wall thickening of small intestine and colon. *CMV:* Nodular wall thickening involving cecum and proximal colon. May also affect the terminal ileum. *E. coli:* May primarily affect the transverse colon but often the whole colon. *Herpesvirus/chlamydia/gonorrhea:* Typically found in the rectosigmoid colon. *Histoplasmosis:* Usually affects ileocecal region. *Salmonellosis/yersiniosis:* Predominantly ileum, but may also spread to cecum and right colon. *Schistosomiasis:* Multiple polypoid filling defects in the sigmoid colon or rectum. Larger lesions may mimic carcinoma. *Shigellosis:* Nodular mucosal thickening affecting mainly the left-sided colon. *TB:* Thick-walled, shrunken cecum, narrowed terminal ileum, and thickened ileocecal valve (Fleischner sign). *Worm infestation (Ascaris and Trichuris):* Bolus of ascariasis may cause a solitary filling defect. Trichuriasis may induce excessive mucus production and numerous irregular filling defects.	*Actinomycosis:* Typically in the wake of appendicitis or after insertion of intrauterine device (IUD). *Amebic colitis:* Often cannot be morphologically differentiated from primary adenocarcinoma or paracolic mass in the wake of diverticulitis. *CMV:* Without biopsy, difficult to differentiate from Crohn disease diagnosis. *Herpesvirus/chlamydia/gonorrhea:* Usually sexually transmitted. *Histoplasmosis:* May mimic appendicitis. *Salmonellosis/yersiniosis:* Both always involve the ileum. Marked thickening of wall and folds. *Schistosomiasis:* Filling defects (granulomas) are a late manifestation of heavy infestation and chronic exposure to *Schistosoma.* *TB:* Colonic TB is almost exclusively limited to the cecum. May lead to neoplasmlike colonic stenoses. *Worm infestation: Trichuris trichiura* is a relatively common inhabitant in the cecum and appendix. Symptomatic infections occur commonly in the tropics and subtropics.
Appendicitis ▷*Fig. 24.32a–d*	Inflammation and subsequent infection of the appendix due to an acute luminal obstruction. **Diagnostic pearls:** Dilated appendix (> 6 mm), hyperattenuation and thickening of appendicular (and sometimes also cecal) wall, and periappendicular fat stranding. Calcification represents a fecalith.	An appendicular abscess appears as a well-demarcated fluid collection in the right lower quadrant of the pelvis. High diagnostic accuracy (> 97%) for CT as compared with all other diagnostic methods. Differential diagnoses: diverticulitis and epiploic appendagitis.
Diverticulosis	Small, flask-shaped, air-containing diverticula in the colonic wall. Usually incidental finding.	Occurs in 6% to 8% of the Western population, increasing with age. Highest incidence in the sigmoid.
Diverticulitis ▷*Fig. 24.33a–c*	Inflammation with or without perforation of saccular outpouchings in the antimesenteric colon wall. **Diagnostic pearls:** Diverticula, segmental mural thickening, and luminal narrowing in combination with mesenteric fat stranding are highly suspicious for diverticulitis (stage I/IIA). Locoregional mesenteric gas points to abscess formation (stage IIB). Free intra-abdominal gas is indicative of free perforation (stage IIC). Use lung and abdominal window/level settings for assessment.	Occurs in 10% to 25% of patients with diverticulosis due to obstruction of the diverticular neck and subsequent diverticular distention and perforation. **Staging and management per Hansen and Stock:** Stage 0: Asymptomatic diverticulosis Stage I: Inflammation restricted to bowel wall (i.e., no wall thickening) Stage IIA: Phlegmonous Stage IIB: Abscess-forming Stage IIC: Free perforated Stage III: Chronically relapsing Stages I and IIA are usually managed conservatively, stages IIB and III, surgically.

(continues on page 760)

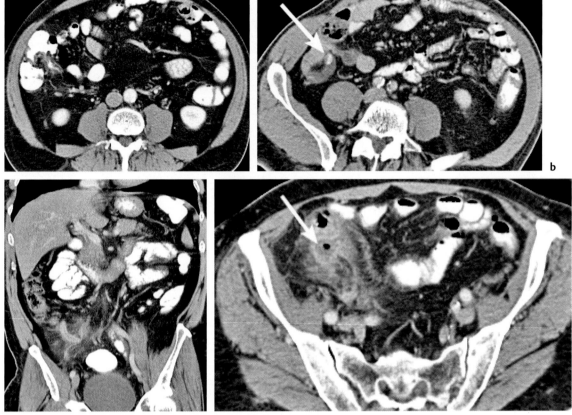

Fig. 24.32a–d   CT appearance of appendicitis. Simple appendicitis with discrete periappendicular fat stranding (**a**). Clearly visible fecalith within normal appendix (arrow) (**b**). Acute periappendicular inflammation and exudation (**c**). Appendicular abscess with central air bubble (arrow) (**d**).

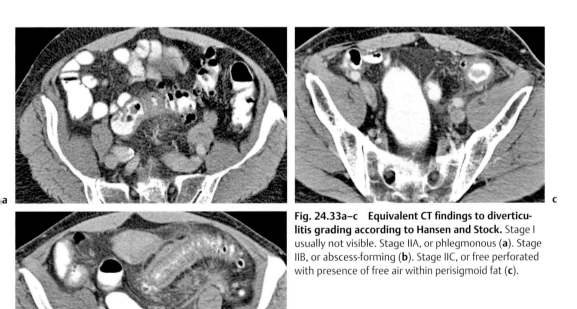

Fig. 24.33a–c   Equivalent CT findings to diverticulitis grading according to Hansen and Stock. Stage I usually not visible. Stage IIA, or phlegmonous (**a**). Stage IIB, or abscess-forming (**b**). Stage IIC, or free perforated with presence of free air within perisigmoid fat (**c**).

Table 24.3   (Cont.) Abnormal colon

Disease	CT Findings	Comments
Trauma		
Hematoma/laceration ▷*Fig. 24.34*	Focal thickening of the bowel wall. **Diagnostic pearls:** Hyperattenuating (52–80 HU) solid intramural mass on noncontrast scans. A partially cystic mass with fluid layers may be observed in cases of anticoagulation-induced bleeding.	Intra-abdominal or retroperitoneal hemorrhage may be associated.
Perforation	Pneumoperitoneum or pneumoretroperitoneum. **Diagnostic pearls:** Extraluminal oral contrast specific for colon perforation. Extraluminal/intra-abdominal gas not specific for colon perforation (alternative causes may be barotraumas and mechanical ventilation).	Use lung and abdominal window/level settings for image assessment.
Inflammation		
Crohn colitis ▷*Fig. 24.17, p. 749*	Discontinuous chronic recurrent transmural inflammation. **Diagnostic pearls:** Thickening of the bowel wall and "sandwich" sign of bowel wall (edematous submucosa between hyperattenuating mucosa and serosa). Abscesses, fistulas, and regional adenopathy may be present.	Terminal ileum involved in 80%, ascending colon in 20% to 55%. Rectum and sigmoid are usually spared. Initial inflammation is confined to the mucosa; thus, barium study and endoscopy are more sensitive for detecting these changes.
Ulcerative colitis	Idiopathic chronic inflammation affecting primarily the colorectal mucosa and submucosa. **Diagnostic pearls:** Pancolitis with thickened target-like colonic wall (< 10 mm), luminal narrowing, stranding of pericolonic fat, and fibrofatty perirectal proliferation (presacral space > 2 cm). Changes may be only subtle and constricted to the rectum. Extraluminal extension of the disease is uncommon, unlike in Crohn disease.	Chronic inflammation confined to the mucosa and exclusively progressing retrograde and continuous from the rectum to the cecum. Within the first 10 y, the risk of colonic cancer increases by 2% annually. Barium enema and colonoscopy are much more sensitive than CT in the diagnosis of initial inflammation.
Radiation enteritis	Iatrogenic-induced damage to the bowel wall due to therapeutic abdominal irradiation. **Diagnostic pearls:** *Acute changes:* Nonspecific wall thickening, target sign *Chronic changes:* Bowel wall thickening, fibrosis, and luminal narrowing Perirectal fat proliferation (> 10 mm) with accompanying pararectal fibrosis (halo sign).	Complication after radiation therapy with > 40 to 50 Gy. Affects ~10% of treated patients. Radiation enteritis may occur up to 20 y after treatment, radiation colitis within 2 y after radiation. Typically confined to the rectum (pelvic irradiation is very common).
Graft versus host reaction ▷*Fig. 24.16, p. 749*	Rare concomitant bowel affection in patients who underwent bone marrow transplantation. Diagnostic pearls: Diffuse nonspecific mural thickening involving the entire intestine from the stomach to the colon, as well as stranding of mesenteric fat and lymphadenopathy.	The most common GI complication after bone marrow transplantation. Clinical symptoms are profuse secretory diarrhea, cramping, and malabsorption caused by immunocompetent T cells of the donor reacting against host tissues.
Colitis cystica profunda	Rectosigmoid wall thickening due to multiple submucosal cysts. **Diagnostic pearls:** Multiple, up to 2-cm submucosal low-density cystic lesions in the rectum with or without sigmoid.	Unknown etiology (inflammatory or traumatic). The cysts are filled with thick mucinous material and lined by a cuboidal flattened epithelium. Presents clinically with bright rectal bleeding, mucus discharge, and diarrhea. Commonly associated with solitary ulcer syndrome and rectal prolapse.
Amyloidosis	Submucosal deposition of fibrils of light-chain immunoglobulins. **Diagnostic pearls:** Normal or thickened rectal wall with small hypoattenuating polypoid lesions. On venous phase images, delayed contrast enhancement may be present.	May be primary or secondary. Preferentially involves the rectal submucosa, which thus represents a preferred site for diagnostic biopsy (even in the absence of CT findings).

Table 24.3   (Cont.) Abnormal colon

Disease	CT Findings	Comments
Pneumatosis cystoides coli ▷*Fig. 24.35a, b*	Cystic/linear gas collection in submucosal/subserosal layers of the GI tract. **Diagnostic pearls:** Intramural gas collection within normal-sized colonic wall. Findings may be completely missed on soft tissue CT images (lung window is the key).	May be idiopathic, associated with chronic obstructive pulmonary disease, or secondary to surgery or ischemia. Lack of intravascular or biliary air (liver) indicates idiopathic origin.
Benign neoplasms		
Lipoma	**Diagnostic pearls:** Submucosal mass with fatlike density and smooth margins.	The most common submucosal tumor in the colon. Typically occurs in the cecum and ascending colon.
Leiomyoma	**Diagnostic pearls:** Large, strongly enhancing soft tissue mass in the bowel wall that may contain necrosis and ulceration.	Rare in the colon, more common in the upper GI tract.
Schwannoma	**Diagnostic pearls:** Multiple strongly attenuating tumors characteristically located on the mesenteric side of the colon. May show central necrosis.	Associated with neurofibromatosis type 1 (Recklinghausen disease).

(continues on page 762)

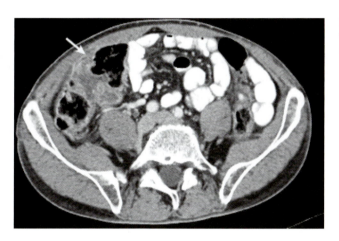

Fig. 24.34   Colonic wall hematoma. Colonic wall hematoma due to anticoagulation therapy appears as partially cystic submucous mass with fluid layers (arrow).

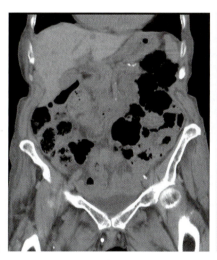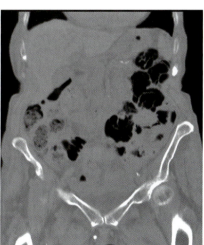

Fig. 24.35a, b   Idiopathic pneumatosis cystoides coli. Soft tissue MPR shows normal-looking distended colon loops (**a**) and thus completely misses marked submucosal gas collection within the entire left colon (**b**).

a

b

Table 24.3   (Cont.) Abnormal colon

Disease	CT Findings	Comments
Malignant neoplasms		
Adenomatous polyp ▷*Fig. 24.36a,b*	Sessile or broad-based polypoid mass in the luminal side of the colonic wall. **Diagnostic pearls:** Incidental finding on axial CT scans. Polyps usually enhance after contrast. Apply CT virtual colonoscopy. Use prone and supine scans (to differentiate from stool).	Adenomatous polyps account for $>$ 50% of all polyps; $>$ 2 cm considered malignant. Multiple polyps may be associated with a polyposis syndrome. CT colonoscopy allows detection of polyps $\geq$ 10 mm with $>$ 95% accuracy. CT colonoscopy requires adequate patient preparation (bowel cleansing, stool tagging, and CO_2 insufflation).
Villous adenoma	Adenomatous polyp containing predominantly villous elements. **Diagnostic pearls:** Low-attenuating ($<$ 10 HU), irregular polypoid mass, usually located in the rectum or sigmoid colon. May occupy $>$ 50% of the lumen.	Characteristic CT appearance of villous adenomas is based on high mucus content. When using CT to evaluate a suspected villous adenoma, oral and rectal contrast material should not be used.
Giant anorectal condyloma acuminatum	Sexually transmitted wart in the rectoanal region. **Diagnostic pearls:** Attenuating infiltrating mass with a cauliflower-like surface appearance and subcutaneous tissue/perirectal fat infiltration.	Associated with human papillomavirus. Also called Buschke–Löwenstein tumor. May show different histologic patterns and even malignant transformation. CT cannot distinguish histologic subtypes.
Carcinoid	Neuroendocrine tumors arising from endocrine cells. **Diagnostic pearls:** Polypoid soft tissue mass is found in the appendix or right colon, less commonly in the rectum. Strong enhancement is seen during the arterial phase.	Small appendicular carcinoids are usually benign. Large, broad-based intraluminal tumors in elderly patients suggest a less common malignant carcinoid. Flush symptom occurs after hepatic spread.
Adenocarcinoma ▷*Fig. 24.37a–c* ▷*Fig. 24.38, p. 764*	Segmental wall thickening and luminal narrowing. **Diagnostic pearls:** Intraluminal or intramural mass, often no or only distinct attenuation; extracolonic growth, necrosis, and perforation. Stranding of pericolonic fat indicates transmural growth. Low-attenuation and subtle calcifications are typical for mucinous adenocarcinoma.	Adenocarcinomas represent 95% of all colon cancers. Histologic subtypes are mucinous (signet ring cells), mucin-producing, and colloid. Most common tumor of the GI tract. Lymphatic spread and size of lymph nodes do not correlate. **Modified Dukes staging:** Stage A (T1N0M0): Restricted to (sub)mucosa Stage B (T2or3N0M0): Limited to serosa/pericolonic tissue Stage C (T2or3N1M0): Lymphatic spread Stage D (any T, any N, M1): Distant metastases
Metastatic disease ▷*Fig. 24.38, p. 764*	Segmental or multifocal wall thickening with or without luminal narrowing. **Diagnostic pearls:** Features usually are indistinguishable from those of primary colonic cancer.	Primary tumors of the uterus, ovary, prostate, bladder, pancreas, kidney, and stomach may directly invade nearby colonic segments or induce distant seeding through ascites.
Lymphoma ▷*Fig. 24.39, p. 764* ▷*Fig. 24.40a, b, p. 764*	Segmental wall thickening with mucosal ulcerations. **Diagnostic pearls:** Most common in the cecum. Associated with massive mesenteric/retroperitoneal lymphadenopathy.	Rare; represents only 1.5% of all abdominal lymphoma. Usually non–Hodgkin lymphoma.
Other		
Mechanical bowel obstruction	Primary or secondary obstruction of the small intestine. **Diagnostic pearls:** *Simple obstruction:* Dilated fluid-filled, thin-walled loops of small intestine with or without air–fluid levels. *Closed loop obstruction:* Obstruction at two ends. One or several grossly distended fluid-filled U-shaped loops with two adjacent limbs showing a zone of abrupt transition (i.e., incarceration). *Strangulating obstruction:* Slight circumferential wall thickening and enhancement (target sign), as well as engorgement of mesenteric vessels, indicate mild ischemia.	Causes may be intrinsic or extrinsic. Typical extrinsic causes are diverticulitis, appendicitis, hernias, adhesions, and peritoneal carcinomatosis. Typical intrinsic causes are intraluminal lesions, neoplasms, inflammations, and infections.
Colonic pseudo-obstruction	Dilated colonic loops containing gas, stool, and possibly contrast medium. **Diagnostic pearls:** Often concomitant dilation of small bowel loops. CT findings in general are nonspecific.	Pseudo-obstruction may be induced by ischemia, inflammation (toxic megacolon), impaired neuromuscular function (diabetic neuropathy, uremia, and hypokalemia), postoperative paralytic ileus, and iatrogenic causes (vagotomy and irradiation).

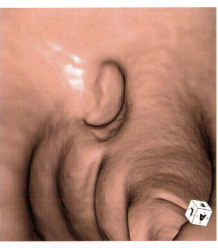

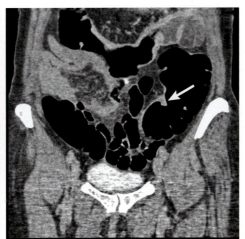

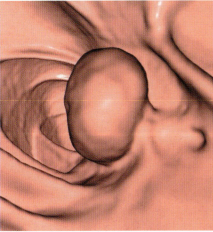

Fig. 24.36a–c   Adenomatous polyps. CT appearance of a sessile polyp (arrow) in the distal part of the descending colon (virtual colonography [**a**] and MPR [**b**]) as well as of a broad based polyp (arrow) in the ascending colon (virtual colonography [**c**]).

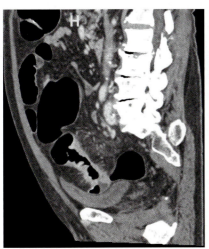

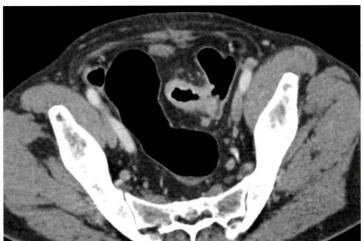

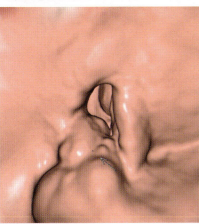

Fig. 24.37a–c   Sigmoid adenocarcinoma. Luminal narrowing and wall thickening on MPR would correspond to Dukes A classification (**a**). However, perisigmoidal fat stranding on axial scan indicates stadium Dukes B (**b**), but local lymphadenopathy led to a final stage Dukes C. Note significant luminal narrowing in virtual colonography (**c**).

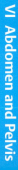

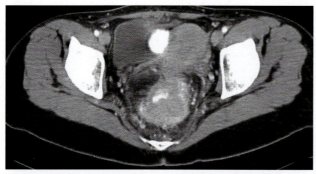

Fig. 24.38   Rectal adenocarcinoma. The tumor is limited to the serosa, and there is no evidence of local lymphadenopathy, thus corresponding to a stage Dukes B or T2N0M0.

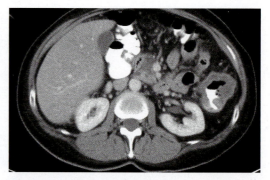

Fig. 24.39   Metastatic disease. Segmental wall thickening and luminal narrowing in the descending colon due to a metastasis from adenocarcinoma of the pancreas head, which is also visible.

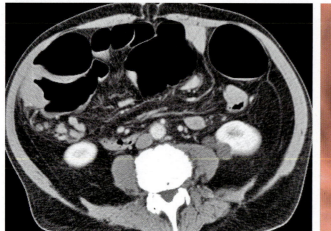

a

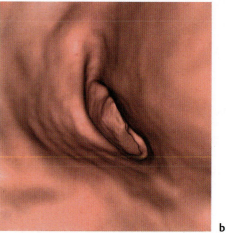

b

Fig. 24.40a, b   Primary colonic lymphoma. Segmental wall thickening lateral in the ascending colon (**a**). Incidental finding during preoperative virtual colonography (**b**) in a patient with a nonpassable sigmoid cancer (same patient as in **Fig. 24.37**).

25 Peritoneum and Mesentery

Christopher Herzog

The peritoneal space is an anatomically complex cavity and under normal physiological conditions nonvisible on computed tomography (CT) scans. However, **Fig 25.1** displays CT scans of a patient with heavy ascites, which has been made even more attenuating through intraperitoneal contrast application. In combination with **Fig. 25.2**, it thus allows for an identification of all relevant peritoneal structures and spaces.

The peritoneal cavity is subdivided by peritoneal plicas into several different compartments and recesses (**Fig. 25.2**), which are anatomically interconnected.

The *transverse mesocolon,* which affixes the transverse colon to the retroperitoneum, is a major barrier dividing the abdominal cavity into supramesocolic and inframesocolic compartments. The *inframesocolic compartment* or space is further subdivided by the small bowel mesentery into the right and left inframesocolic space.

The *right inframesocolic space* is laterally defined by the peritoneal attachment of the ascending colon, as well as medially and caudally by the mesenteric root.

The *left inframesocolic space* is laterally and caudally to the left delineated by the peritoneal attachments of the descending colon and the sigmoid. On the right side, it opens caudally into the *right paracolic gutter,* which lies lateral to the mesenteric attachment of the ascending colon. The *left paracolic gutter* lies lateral to the peritoneal attachments of the descending colon and the sigmoid. These four inframesocolic spaces and barriers are better visualized on cross-sectional CT scans than the transverse mesocolon.

The supramesocolic space is subdivided into the right and left subphrenic spaces, the subhepatic space, the Morison pouch, and the lesser sac. On the right side, the right paracolic gutter extends cranially into the posterior subhepatic space and the Morison pouch, which represents the most dependent portion of the peritoneal cavity in the right upper quadrant. It also is a frequent site of intraperitoneal fluid collections, which may extend even to the right subphrenic space (supramesocolic space) if the fluid volume suffices. Both paracolic gutters connect the inframesocolic space with the pelvis, where the pouch of Douglas and two lateral paravesical recesses are the most dependent parts and thus frequent sites of intraperitoneal fluid collections.

Because the left coronary ligament lies more anteriorly as compared with the right, the left subphrenic space extends less posteriorly than the right. The lesser sac lies dorsally to the lesser omentum, the stomach, the duodenum, and the gastrocolic ligament but ventrally to the body of the pancreas and the spleen. It is connected with the peritoneal space through the foramen of Winslow, or foramen epiploicum—which hides behind and below the porta hepatis. The lesser sac may extend downward between the anterior and posterior plicas of the greater omentum. The superior recess of the lesser sac usually extends upward to the diaphragm surrounding the caudate lobe of the liver (**Fig. 25.1a**).

The mesentery of both the small and large bowel and various ligaments provide a barrier not only for the free movement of fluid, cells, and germs but also for the direct spread of diseases within the abdominal cavity. However, in the absence of ascites, identification of individual ligaments may be difficult, as mesentery and intraperitoneal fatty tissue show similar Hounsfield unit (HU) values. Mesentery and ligaments contain blood vessels and therefore may be better identified on postcontrast CT-scans. Mesenteric lymph nodes usually are not discernible due to their predominant fat content. Only reactive nodes appear as well-defined oval or round soft tissue densities.

Nevertheless, several ligaments of the supramesocolic cavity usually can be identified on CT scans.

The *right triangular ligament* forms from the coalescence of the superior and inferior plica of the right coronary ligament and separates the right subphrenic space from the Morison pouch. The *left triangular ligament* forms from the superior and inferior plica of the left coronary ligament and is located along the superior aspect of the left hepatic lobe.

The *gastrophrenic ligament* runs from the dome of the left diaphragm to the stomach and is easily missed on CT.

The *gastropancreatic plica* (**Fig. 25.1b**) forms around the proximal left gastric artery as it courses superiorly. It attaches the gastric fundus to the retroperitoneum and partially separates the superior recess of the lesser sac from the splenic recess.

The *falciform ligament* (**Fig. 25.1c**) is a remnant of the ventral mesogastrium, which contains the *ligamentum teres* and the obliterated umbilical vein. This vein may be recanalized in situations with decreased venous hepatic outflow.

The *gastrosplenic ligament* (**Fig. 25.1d**) is a remnant of the dorsal mesogastrium, connecting the greater curvature of the stomach with the splenic hilum. It contains short gastric arteries (rami gastrici breves), forms the lateral border of the lesser sac, and may be affected by processes of the stomach or pancreatic tail.

The *phrenicocolic ligament* is fixed to the spleen and attaches the proximal part of the descending colon to the left hemidiaphragm. By separating the left subphrenic space from the remainder of the peritoneal cavity, it inhibits free flow from the left paracolic gutter to the left subphrenic space. Pancreatic processes can spread via this ligament and involve the splenic flexure of the colon.

The *gastrocolic ligament* connects the greater curvature of the stomach with the superior aspect of the transverse colon. It contains gastroepiploic vessels and forms a portion of the greater omentum.

The *gastrohepatic ligament* is part of the lesser omentum and connects the medial aspect of the liver with the lesser curvature of the stomach. It contains the left gastric artery, coronary vein, and small lymph nodes. It is a common site of varices, pancreatic phlegmon, and metastases from malignant esophageal, gastric, or biliary neoplasms.

The *hepatoduodenal ligament* represents the inferior edge of the gastrohepatic ligament and delineates the foramen of Winslow.

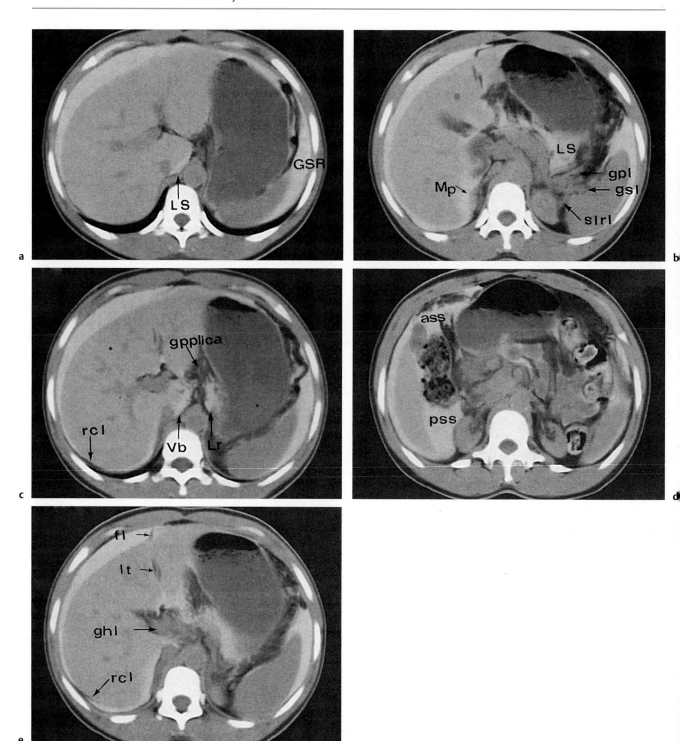

Fig. 25.1a–e   CT anatomy of the peritoneal space and ligaments in the upper abdomen, as seen on five different levels. The patient has ascites; a water-soluble contrast medium has been administered, which helps to visualize the peritoneal space.

ass	anterior subhepatic space
fl	falciform ligament
ghl	gastrohepatic ligament
gpl	gastropancreatic ligament
gpplica	gastropancreatic plica
gsl	gastrosplenic ligament
GSR	gastrosplenic recess
Lr	lateral recess of the lesser sac
LS	lesser sac
lt	ligamentum teres
Mp	Morison pouch
pss	posterior subhepatic space
rcl	right coronary ligament
slrl	splenorenal ligament
Vb	vestibulum

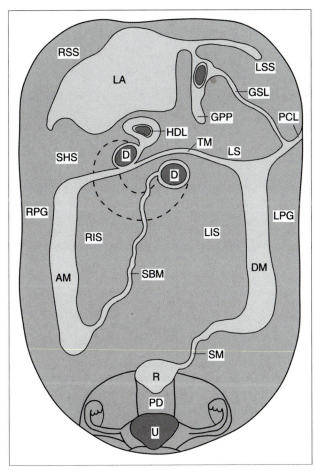

Fig. 25.2   Topography of the posterior abdominal wall. Supramesocolic compartment. (Modified from Wegener.)

D   duodenum
GPP gastropancreatic plica
GSL gastrosplenic ligament
HDL hepatoduodenal ligament with portal vein
LA   liver attachment
LS   lesser sac
LSS left supramesocolic space
PCL phrenicocolic ligament
RSS right supramesocolic space
SHS subhepatic space
TM   transverse mesocolon

Inframesocolic compartment.

AM   attachment of ascending mesocolon
DM   attachment of descending mesocolon
LIS left infracolic space
LPG left paracolic gutter
PD   pouch of Douglas
R   rectum
RIS right infracolic space
RPG right paracolic gutter
SM   root of the mesentery
U   uterus and adnexa

It extends from the proximal duodenum to the porta hepatis and contains the common hepatic duct, common bile duct, hepatic artery, and portal vein. It is a common route for spreading of carcinomas of the gallbladder and the biliary system.

The *transverse mesocolon* lies in the inframesocolic abdomen, contains middle colic vessels, and is a common site for spreading of pancreatic or colic processes.

The *greater omentum* is located anterior to the small bowel and represents the inferior continuation of the gastrocolic ligament.

It is formed by a double reflection of the dorsal mesogastrium and has four layers of peritoneum.

The *small bowel mesentery* extends from the ligamentum of Treitz in the left upper quadrant down to the ileocecal valve, totaling a distance of ~15 cm. It contains superior mesenteric vessels.

The *sigmoid mesocolon* contains sigmoid and hemorrhoidal vessels and forms a pathway from the pelvis to the abdomen as it coalesces with the *broad ligament* in women. Infections and neoplasms of the sigmoid can spread not only to the pelvis, but also vice versa, with ovarian processes involving the sigmoid colon.

The *broad* and *round ligaments* serve as anterior suspenders of the uterus. The broad ligament contains uterine vessels branching from the internal iliac vessels, as well as lymph vessels and nerves. The ureters course distally through the base of the broad ligament. The lowermost portion of the broad ligament is called the cardinal ligament, which is the main supporter of the cervix and upper vagina. The round ligaments extend into the inguinal canal and farther down to the labia majora.

The *medial umbilical ligament* and the *lateral umbilical folds* are two ligament-like structures within the anterior wall of the abdomen. The latter contain hypogastric vessels.

Free intraperitoneal fluid can be seen on CT scans only in the presence of volumes > 50 mL. In the supramesocolic compartment, it initially collects within the Morison pouch and extends from there via the paravesical fossae into the paracolic gutters. In the inframesocolic compartment, fluid preferentially collects in the fossa of Douglas. In the presence of large amounts of ascites, bowel loops typically are centrally positioned, and the mesentery can be clearly delineated.

Loculated (encapsulated) ascites indicates adhesions, whether benign or malignant. Thus, bowel loops do not float free within the central abdomen, but are displaced by loculated fluid. Unfortunately, CT attenuation of benign and malignant ascites is similar, thus rendering any CT-based differentiation impossible. Instead, distribution patterns may be suggestive. Unlike benign ascites, the amount of malignant ascites in the lesser sac typically matches the amount observed within the peritoneal cavity. Fluid predominantly confined to the lesser sac is more typically characteristic of diseases of the pancreas or abscesses of the lesser sac. Abscesses are loculated fluid collections with mass effect. CT attenuation usually is between 15 and 35 HU. The most sensitive CT feature is the presence of extraluminal gas, which is seen in only ~30% of all abscesses. (Loculated gas within any abdominal mass is always indicative of an abscess or necrosis formation.) A well-defined, hyperattenuating wall is a classic feature of a mature abscess.

CT is superior to plain film radiographs in detecting free intraperitoneal air, which usually collects ventrally in the midabdomen, beneath the abdominal musculature. Following surgical interventions, small amounts of free air may be detected up to 7 days on CT scans.

Relevant peritoneal and mesenteric processes can usually be identified on nonenhanced CT scans. Postcontrast scans are often useful to better delineate vessels and differentiate between solid and necrotic and cystic lesions. Irrespective of the scan technique, mesenteric abnormalities are detected much easier if the intestines are well opacified and thus in patients who previously received sufficient oral contrast. Usually patients should drink 1.5 L over a period of 60 to 90 minutes prior to the scan. On the CT table, rectal infusion of contrast media may further increase diagnostic accuracy. **Table 25.1** lists the most relevant differential diagnoses of the peritoneum and mesentery.

Table 25.1 Peritoneal, mesenteric, and omental collections and masses

Disease	CT Findings	Comments
Vascular		
Omental infarction	Wedge-shaped to ovoid omental mass with hyperattenuated streaks. **Scan recommendation:** Biphasic CT (nonenhanced CT, delayed phase [DP]). Nonenhanced CT: Ill-defined, heterogeneous stranding of omental fatty tissue. Sometimes hyperdense free fluid collection. DP: No enhancement. **Diagnostic pearls:** Ill-defined mass with hyperdense stranding of omental fatty tissue in the right lower quadrant.	Typically located between the anterior abdominal wall and colon. Congestion of omental fatty tissue due to a segmental infarction/ischemia. Additional findings may be a focal inflammation with or without thickening of colonic and abdominal wall. Treatment: conservative or surgical excision (laparoscopy), depending on clinical presentation. Differential diagnosis: Acute appendicitis, epiploic appendagitis.
Infection		
Peritonitis ▷ *Fig. 25.3a, b*	Infectious, sometimes inflammatory affection of the peritoneum with or without the peritoneal cavity. **Scan recommendation:** Biphasic CT (nonenhanced CT, DP). Nonenhanced CT: Hypodense intraperitoneal fluid collection. Hyperdense stranding and thickening of peritoneal fat. DP: Slight hyperattenuation of soft tissue stranding and peritoneum. **Diagnostic pearls:** Slight hyperattenuation of thickened peritoneum on postcontrast scans.	Arises from a posttraumatic or iatrogenic infection of the abdominal cavity. Acute peritonitis: Intraperitoneal fluid, dilated mesenteric vessels, stranding of mesenteric fat, and enhancement of peritoneal membranes. Chronic peritonitis: Extensive thickening of the peritoneum and adhesions (e.g., tuberculous peritonitis). Symptoms: Abdominal pain, fever. May lead to sepsis; thus, fast treatment is required: antibiotics, surgery.
Intraperitoneal abscess ▷ *Fig. 25.4a, b*	Intraperitoneal fluid collections with mass effect. **Scan recommendation:** Biphasic CT (nonenhanced CT, DP). Nonenhanced CT: Low-attenuation (10–40 HU) fluid collection often with gas bubbles. DP: Strong rim enhancement. **Diagnostic pearls:** Low-attenuation intraperitoneal fluid collection with rim enhancement and gas bubbles. The surrounding peritoneal membrane becomes thicker and enhancing when the abscess matures.	Infected local peritonitis typically after perforation (ulcer, diverticulum), surgery, or inflammation (pancreatitis, pericholecystitis). Commonly found in the right subphrenic space, the subhepatic space, and the pouch of Douglas. Oral contrast, important to differentiate from fluid-containing bowel loops. Gas bubbles are pathognomonic but occur in 30% of cases. Air–fluid levels may indicate a fistula to bowel loops. Treatment: Percutaneous abscess drainage (PAD) and antibiotics. Surgery is secondary treatment.
Tuberculosis (TB) ▷ *Fig. 25.4a, b*	Mesenteric and omental masses and adenopathy. **Scan recommendation:** Biphasic CT (nonenhanced CT, DP). Nonenhanced CT: Relatively high-density (15–30 HU), well-defined ascites. DP: Hyperattenuation of thickened peritoneum. **Diagnostic pearls:** Enlarged lymph may show rim enhancement.	Hematogenous disseminated TB from a distant focus (primary complex), usually from the lung. Rare, but often seen in immunocompromised patients.
Mesenteric lymphadenitis	Localized moderate enlargement of mesenteric lymph nodes associated with thickening of the wall of the distal ileum and cecum. **Scan recommendation:** Biphasic CT (nonenhanced CT, DP). Nonenhanced CT: No additional information. DP: Enhancement of lymph nodes and thickened bowel wall.	Usually caused by *Yersinia enterocolitica*, *Campylobacter jejuni*, or nontyphoid *Salmonella* species. Clinically, an important differential diagnosis of appendicitis and Crohn disease.

(continues on page 770)

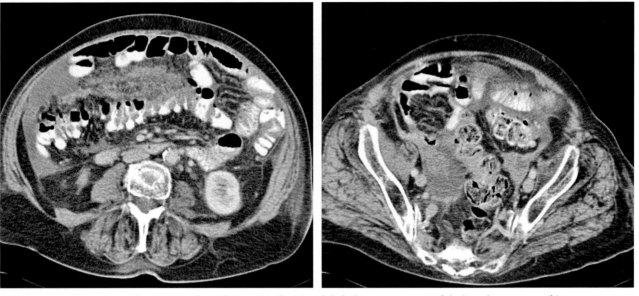

a b

Fig. 25.3a, b   Peritonitis. Soft tissue stranding of mesentery fat (**a**) and slight hyperattenuation of thickened peritoneum (**b**) on postcontrast CT scans.

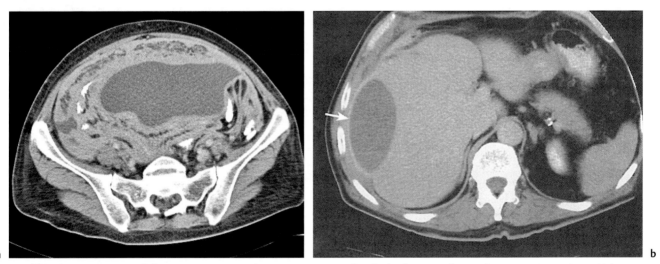

a b

Fig. 25.4a, b   Intraperitoneal abscesses. Mesenteric abscess presenting as a low-fluid collection with rim-enhancement in a patient with known tuberculosis (**a**). Subphrenic abscess (**b**). A lesion with similar CT appearance is located between the liver and right hemidiaphragm (arrow).

Table 25.1 (Cont.) Peritoneal, mesenteric, and omental collections and masses

Disease	CT Findings	Comments
Internal hernias		
Paraduodenal hernia (PDH) ▷ *Fig. 25.5*	Cluster of dilated bowel loops with distorted mesenteric vessels. **Scan recommendation:** Biphasic CT (nonenhanced CT, DP). Nonenhanced CT: Usually suffices for diagnosis. Oral contrast more important. DP: Better delineation of distorted mesenteric vessels. **Diagnostic pearls:** Cluster of dilated small bowel loops lateral to the ascending or descending duodenum.	Rare herniation of bowel loops through an acquired or congenital defect of the mesentery. Right PDH (25%): Herniation through abnormal mesentericoparietal fossa of Waldeyer (lateral to ascending part of the duodenum). Left PDH (75%): Herniation through abnormal paraduodenal mesenteric fossa of Landzert (next to the ligament of Treitz).
Transmesenteric hernia ▷ *Fig. 24.26, p. 755*	Cluster of dilated bowel loops with distorted mesenteric vessels. **Scan recommendation:** Biphasic CT (nonenhanced CT, DP). Nonenhanced CT: Usually suffices for diagnosis. Oral contrast more important. DP: Better delineation of distorted mesenteric vessels. **Diagnostic pearls:** Dilated small bowel volvulus with twisted mesenteric vessels ("swirl" sign). Displacement of main mesenteric trunk to the left or right. Displacement of hepatic flexure inferiorly and posteriorly (common) or medial displacement of ascending/descending colon.	Typical postoperative complication after bowel surgery (Roux-Y, Whipple, etc.). In most cases, herniation of small bowel loops through artificial opening in mesentery of colon or small bowel (> 75% of cases through transverse mesocolon).
Trauma		
Hematoma ▷ *Fig. 25.6*	Local intraperitoneal or mesenteric fluid collection that otherwise mimics ascites. **Scan recommendation:** Multiphasic CT (nonenhanced CT, DP). Nonenhanced CT: High-attenuating (30–80 HU). DP: No enhancement. **Diagnostic pearls:** Nonenhanced CT is important to avoid false-positive interpretation of high-attenuating blood as contrast media uptake. Attenuation may appear inhomogeneous due to incomplete coagulation.	Usually resulting from blunt trauma (particularly of the spleen and liver), bowel perforation with vascular erosion, spontaneous rupture of vascularized tumors (hepatoma, cavernous hemangioma, hepatic adenoma, angiosarcoma), extrauterine pregnancy, bleeding disorders, or excessive anticoagulation. In chronic hematoma (> 1–2 weeks) attenuation drops to 0 to 20 HU. Treatment only in symptomatic patients (e.g., secondary infection, abscess formation, or bowel obstruction). PAD is treatment of choice.
Inflammation		
Ascites ▷ *Fig. 25.7*	Intraperitoneal fluid collection. **Scan recommendation:** Biphasic CT (nonenhanced CT, DP). Nonenhanced CT: Low-attenuation fluid collection (< 30 HU). Density increases with protein content. Typical ascites: bile < 20 HU; urine ~10 to 15 HU; chylous fluid < 0 HU. DP: Rim enhancement indicates concomitant peritoneal inflammation and abscess formation. **Diagnostic pearls:** Loculation (nonuniform distribution) of ascites indicates postoperative, inflammatory, or neoplastic adhesions. Dense (> 30 HU) ascites suggests intraperitoneal hemorrhage or TB. The lesser sac usually is only moderately filled. Large amount of ascites in the lesser sac, small nodules on the smooth surfaces of the liver and spleen, and mesenteric lymph nodes are characteristic of peritoneal carcinomatosis.	Ascites may develop from right heart failure, abdominal vein occlusion, constrictive pericarditis, hypoalbuminemia, liver failure, myxedema, peritonitis, pancreatitis, intestinal perforation, glomerulonephritis, peritoneal carcinomatosis, and malignant lymphomas (blockage of lymph flow). The combination of fibrous ovarian tumors, hydrothorax, and benign ascites is called Meigs syndrome. Discrete ascites appears either as a hypodense rim around intraperitoneal organs (particularly the right liver lobe and the spleen) or small fluid collections in the Morison pouch, perihepatic, or Douglas space. Larger amounts of ascites lead to fluid collection in paracolic gutters and centralization of small bowel loops in the uppermost part of the peritoneal cavity.
Biliary ascites, biloma	Well-defined, low-density fluid collection in the left or right supramesocolic space. **Scan recommendation:** Multiphasic CT (nonenhanced CT, hepatic arterial phase [HAP], portal venous phase [PVP], DP). Nonenhanced CT: Low-density fluid collection (~20 HU) DP: Rim enhancement indicative of infection/inflammation.	Usually iatrogenic or posttraumatic, rarely spontaneous rupture of the gallbladder. Bile causes local inflammation, sealing the fluid collection near the porta hepatis (i.e., biloma).

(continues on page 772)

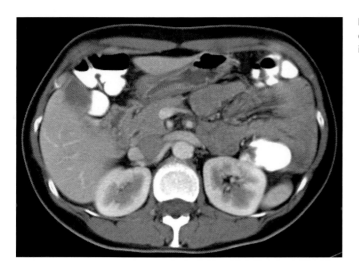

Fig. 25.5 Paraduodenal hernia to the left. Cluster of poorly opacified small bowel loops lateral to the well-opacified descending duodenum.

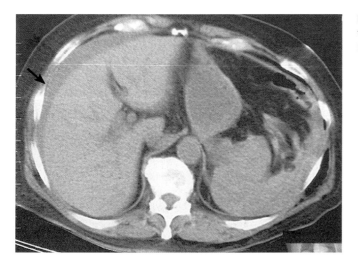

Fig. 25.6 Intraperitoneal hematoma due to hepatic laceration. A hyperdense crescent perihepatic lesion is visible on noncontrast scan.

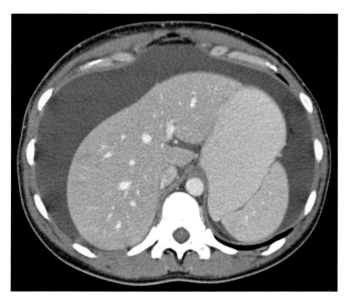

Fig. 25.7 Ascites. Near-water density surrounding the liver, stomach, and spleen.

Table 25.1 (Cont.) Peritoneal, mesenteric, and omental collections and masses

Disease	CT Findings	Comments
Pancreatic ascites ▷ *Fig. 22.10a–c, p. 725*	Diffuse, low-density fluid collection in peripancreatic fatty tissue, lesser sac, and anterior pararenal space (i.e., ventral to fascia of Gerota). **Scan recommendation:** Multiphasic CT (nonenhanced CT, HAP, PVP, DP). Nonenhanced CT: Sufficient for visualization of ascites. DP: Additional information of pancreatic perfusion (necrosis).	Typically observed in patients with pancreatitis, after seat-belt injury (disruption of pancreas corpus [spine as hypomochlion, or center of rotation]), or following pancreas surgery.
Fibrosing mesenteritis (retractile mesenteritis, mesenteric panniculitis, mesenteric lipodystrophy) ▷ *Fig. 25.8*	Separation of bowel loops with kinking and angulation, mesenteric thickening with fine stellate pattern. **Scan recommendation:** Biphasic CT (nonenhanced CT, DP). Nonenhanced CT: May contain calcified or enlarged mesenteric lymph nodes and central necrotic cysts. DP: Visualization of encased mesenteric vessels. May show slightly enhancing pseudocapsule. **Diagnostic pearls:** Mesenteric stellate mass encasing mesenteric vessels with a preserved hypodense (fat) perivascular halo.	Inflammation, fibrosis, and fatty infiltration of the mesentery. Usually located in the root of small bowel mesentery, less often in mesentery root of the colon, the omentum, or within the retroperitoneum (peripancreatic tissue). Associated with Gardner syndrome and fibrosing mediastinitis. Multiple mesenteric soft tissue masses represent fibromas. Panniculitis is regarded as an early stage of fibrosing mesenteritis. Typically appears as ill-defined soft tissue stranding of mesenteric fat.

Benign neoplasms

Disease	CT Findings	Comments
Pancreatic pseudocyst	Well-defined, near-water-density (retro-) peritoneal or mesenteric mass. **Scan recommendation:** Biphasic CT (nonenhanced CT, DP). Nonenhanced CT: Circumscript near-water-density (< 15 HU) mass. DP: Often distinct rim enhancement. See also **Fig. 22.11, p. 725.**	The most common lesion of the lesser sac. May invade the mesentery. Likely only in patients with an acute or chronic pancreatitis. Treatment of choice in symptomatic patients is transgastral/percutaneous drainage.
Mesenteric cyst (omental cyst, duplication cyst, lymphangioma) ▷ *Fig. 25.9*	Usually near-water-density, single or multilocular cysts up to several centimeters in size. **Scan recommendation:** Multiphasic CT (nonenhanced CT, DP). Nonenhanced CT: Attenuation between chylous (< 0 HU) and blood (> 40 HU), depending on main cyst content. In chronic cases, rim calcifications. DP: Sometimes discrete rim enhancement. **Diagnostic pearls:** Low-attenuation, fluid-filled intra-abdominal cyst with thin rim and subtle internal septa.	Hamartomatous lesions lined by mesothelial cells with chylous, serous, or occasionally hemorrhagic fluid contents. Usually asymptomatic. Omental cysts may be pedunculated. In some cases, a water–fat level is present. Differential diagnoses include pancreatic (pseudo-) cyst, cystic mesothelioma, and cystic teratoma.
Fibromatosis (desmoid tumor)	Well-defined, usually large encapsulated homogeneous mass of variable attenuation and enhancement. **Scan recommendation:** Biphasic CT (nonenhanced CT, PVP). Nonenhanced CT: Isodense to muscle. PVP: Usually discrete enhancement. Optimal for visualization of encased mesenteric vessels.	Histologically, an aggressive tumor composed of fibroblastic tissue. Fibromatosis is the most common primary tumor of the mesentery. Known association with local trauma, Gardner syndrome, estrogen therapy, and surgery. Typically involves small bowel mesentery and leads to displacement and obstruction of bowel loops. Infiltration into adjacent organs/muscles is observed.
Lipoma	Well-defined, marginated, nonenhancing, fat-density mass. **Scan recommendation:** Multiphasic CT (nonenhanced CT, DP). Nonenhanced CT: Low attenuation (~10–15 HU with minimal values below 0 HU). DP: No enhancement. **Diagnostic pearls:** Low-attenuation framed lesion without internal septations.	The second most common primary benign solid tumor of the mesentery.

Table 25.1   (Cont.) Peritoneal, mesenteric, and omental collections and masses

Disease	CT Findings	Comments
Neurofibroma	Well-defined, low-density mesenteric mass. **Scan recommendation:** Biphasic CT (nonenhanced CT, DP). Nonenhanced CT: Well-defined hypoattenuating mass. DP: Homogeneous enhancement.	Histologically, lesions are built of endoneural myxoid matrix. May arise as isolated lesions or be part of a clinically proven neurofibromatosis.
Splenosis ▷ *Fig. 21.7a, b, p. 713*	Single or multilocular intra-abdominal soft tissue masses. **Scan recommendation:** Biphasic CT (nonenhanced CT, DP). Nonenhanced CT: Well-defined spleenlike attenuation. DP: Homogeneous spleenlike attenuation. **Diagnostic pearls:** Single or multilocular nodules on the serosal surface of the small bowel, greater omentum, or parietal peritoneum with spleenlike attenuation.	Autotransplantation of splenic tissue after splenic trauma or splenectomy. Usually asymptomatic, but may cause abdominal pain or gastrointestinal hemorrhage.
Castleman disease (angiomatous lymphoid hamartoma)	Large homogeneous, well-defined mass. **Scan recommendation:** Multiphasic CT (nonenhanced CT, HAP, PVP, DP). Nonenhanced CT: Well-defined, isodense to muscle. DP: Moderate contrast enhancement.	Two histologic subtypes: Hyaline-vascular (90%) and plasma cell type (10%). Benign massive enlargement of lymph nodes. Most (70%) occur in the mediastinum of young healthy people, but also in the mesentery and omentum.

(continues on page 774)

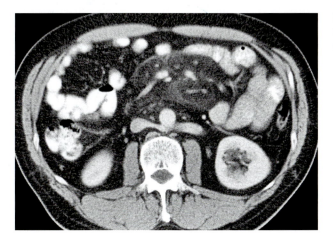

Fig. 25.8   Panniculitis. Discrete localized soft tissue stranding within the mesenteric root simulating a slightly enhancing pseudocapsule and encasement of mesenteric vessels.

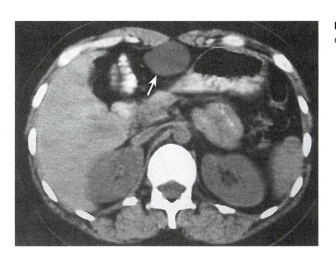

Fig. 25.9   Mesenteric cyst. Smooth, thin-walled, near-water-density collection between the greater curvature and abdominal wall (arrow).

Table 25.1   (Cont.) Peritoneal, mesenteric, and omental collections and masses

Disease	CT Findings	Comments
Malignant neoplasms		
Pseudomyxoma peritonei ▷ *Fig. 25.10a,b*	Diffuse, multiseptated fluid collection with loculations. **Scan recommendation:** Multiphasic CT (nonenhanced CT, DP). Nonenhanced CT: Multiple grapelike, hypodense (15–30 HU) intra-abdominal cysts. Cyst walls partly calcified. DP: Hyperattenuating, thickened peritoneal and omental surface. **Diagnostic pearls:** Multiple grapelike hypodense cysts with rim enhancement, scalloping of liver/spleen surface, and displacement of intestinal structures and mesentery. See also **Fig. 29.62, p.832.**	Rare disease. Histologically, an intraperitoneal accumulation of gelatinous, mucinous material, which usually derives from the spread of ovarian mucinous cystadenocarcinoma. Malignant degeneration of an appendicular mucocele is a less common cause. Other (rare) origins include stomach, colon, uterus, bile ducts, and pancreas. Contrast media enhances solid components and improves the visibility of the septations. Mucinous components remain hypoattenuating.
Lymphoma ▷ *Fig. 24.22a, b, p. 753*	Well-defined soft tissue density masses > 10 mm in size. **Scan recommendation:** Multiphasic CT (nonenhanced CT, DP). Nonenhanced CT: Isodense to muscle. DP: Homogeneous enhancement. **Diagnostic pearls:** Well-defined, partly coalescing homogeneous enhancing masses.	The most common neoplastic mesenteric mass. Predominantly non–Hodgkin lymphomas (61%), Hodgkin disease involves the mesentery in only 5% of cases. Lymphomas typically encase instead of invade mesenteric vessels, which may result in a "sandwich sign."
Peritoneal carcinomatosis (PC) ▷ *Fig. 25.11a–c*	Any combination of ascites, nodular omental thickening, mesenteric stranding, scalloping of parenchymal organ's contours, and enlarged mesenteric lymph nodes. **Scan recommendation:** Biphasic CT (nonenhanced CT, DP). Nonenhanced CT: Lymph nodes, ascites, and omentum hypoattenuating. DP: Enhancement of peritoneal/omental nodularities. **Diagnostic pearls**: Omental caking, bowel obstruction (subileus), and enlarged mesenteric lymph nodes.	Appearance of PC ranges from a thickened nodular peritoneal surface to a cakelike omental mass. Peritoneal metastases most commonly derive from ovarian, colonic, or gastric cancer. Calcification and cystic lesions on liver/spleen contour or peritoneal surface suggests ovarian cystadenocarcinoma. Ascites presents in > 70% and may be loculated. Omental fat is involved in > 70% and appears normal, permeated with multiple discrete enhancing nodules, or as diffuse caking (omental caking). Mesenteric involvement is present in > 60% mainly as diffuse or stellate soft tissue stranding. Diagnostic accuracy of CT in the diagnosis of PC is low.
Malignant mesothelioma (MM)	Peritoneal associated with calcified pleural plaques. **Scan recommendation:** Biphasic CT (nonenhanced CT, DP). Nonenhanced CT: Subtle to distinct calcified plaques. DP: Homogeneous enhancement. **Diagnostic pearls:** Stellate peritoneal mass or omental caking, infiltrating vessels and adjacent viscera. Calcifications are present in the majority of cases. Disproportionately little ascites in 90%.	MM is associated with excessive exposure to asbestos (~20–40-y latent period). Twenty-five percent of MM cases arise from the peritoneum. Three histologic subtypes: 1. Carcinomatous type (most common): Diffuse thickening of the peritoneum, multiple mesenteric and peritoneal nodules, and fixation of the small bowel 2. Sarcomatous type (20%): Large encapsulated mass with local invasion 3. Mixed type
Liposarcoma ▷ *Fig. 25.12*	Nodular myxoid mass with regions of hemorrhage and necrosis. **Scan recommendation:** Biphasic CT (nonenhanced CT, DP). Nonenhanced CT/DP: Appearance variable, depending on main tissue component. Often multiple heavily calcified lesions.	Most common in the retroperitoneum, rare in the omentum or mesentery. Five histologic subtypes: pleomorphic, round cell, myxoid, sclerosing, and lipomalike. Often indistinguishable from lipoma.
Spindle cell tumors **(leiomyoma, leiomyosarcoma)**	Large heterogeneous, solid mass typically with cystic spaces representing necrosis. **Scan recommendation:** Multiphasic CT (nonenhanced CT, HAP, PVP, DP). Nonenhanced CT: Appearance variable, depending on main tissue component. DP: Intense contrast enhancement of the solid components.	The most common primary omental tumor. Leiomyosarcoma is more common than leiomyoma.

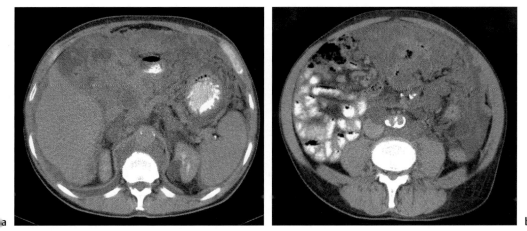

Fig. 25.10a, b Pseudomyxoma peritonei. Diffuse, multiseptated intra-abdominal fluid collection with loculations.

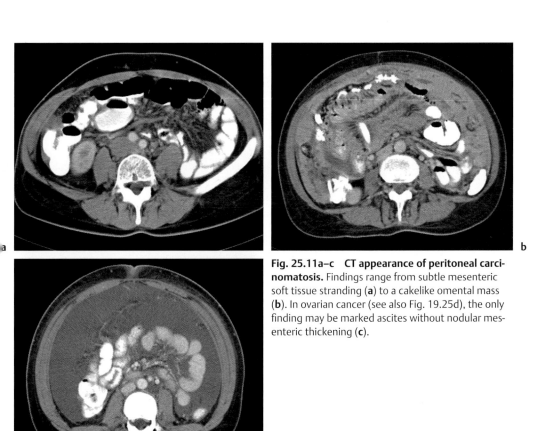

Fig. 25.11a–c CT appearance of peritoneal carcinomatosis. Findings range from subtle mesenteric soft tissue stranding (**a**) to a cakelike omental mass (**b**). In ovarian cancer (see also Fig. 19.25d), the only finding may be marked ascites without nodular mesenteric thickening (**c**).

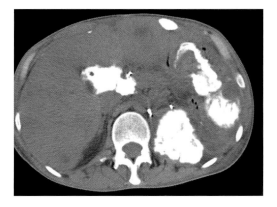

Fig. 25.12 Peritoneal liposarcoma presenting with multiple heavily calcified lesions.

26 Retroperitoneum

Christopher Herzog

The retroperitoneal space is defined by several fascial planes. The inner and anterior border of the retroperitoneum is formed by the posterior peritoneum. The transversalis fascia forms the outer or posterior border. Anterior and posterior renal fasciae fuse behind the colon and form a single lateroconal fascia. These fascial boundaries form three extraperitoneal compartments (**Fig. 26.1**).

1. *The anterior pararenal space* extending from the posterior parietal peritoneum to the anterior renal fascia and confined laterally by the lateroconal fascia. It contains the ascending and descending colon, the duodenal loop, and the pancreas. Fluid collections in the anterior pararenal space, unless intrapancreatic, are usually confined to the site of origin but may sometimes extend into the small-bowel mesentery and the transverse mesocolon, respectively.
2. *The two perirenal spaces* encompass each one kidney, adrenal gland, and perirenal fat. Both spaces do not communicate across the midline, although the anterior renal fascia below the level of the renal hila occasionally appears non-interrupted

across the midline. Normal thickness of the renal fascia ranges from 1 to 2 mm. The posterior renal fascia is usually better depicted than the anterior. An abnormally thick (> 2–3 mm) renal fascia may be caused by edema, hyperemia, fibrosis, lipolysis, inflammation, malignancy, or trauma.
3. *The posterior pararenal space* extending from the posterior renal fascia to the transversalis fascia. This relatively thin layer of fat continues uninterruptedly as the properitoneal fat of the abdominal wall, external to the lateroconal fascia. It is medially confined by the psoas muscle and contains no organs.

Normal retroperitoneal *lymph nodes* appear on CT scans as small soft-tissue densities in the vicinity of abdominal and pelvic blood vessels and may range from 3 to 10 mm in size. Pancreatic, celiac, and superior mesenteric lymph nodes are usually not visible unless they are enlarged. Whereas in the abdomen and pelvis, only lymph nodes > 1.5 cm in diameter are considered abnormal, retroperitoneal lymph nodes > 6 mm in diameter are suspicious. Also, a solitary pelvic or abdominal lymph node > 10 mm in diameter or a cluster of multiple small nodes are conspicuous. Appropriate bowel loops opacification with oral contrast medium is important to allow differentiation from adenopathy. Intravenous contrast material helps to distinguish strongly enhancing vascular cross sections from lymph nodes, which usually enhance less strongly.

The *abdominal aorta* measures < 3 cm in diameter and tapers gradually in caliber before bifurcating into the common iliac arteries at the level of L3–L4. Abnormalities of the aorta and its branches such as aneurysms, atherosclerosis, thrombus formation, or dissection are best evaluated using contrast-enhanced scans acquired during the arterial phase. Optimal vessel opacification is achieved when applying bolus triggering technique (with the monitor scan placed on the aorta at the level of the celiac trunk) and contrast media flow rates of 4 to 5 mL/s. In addition, the iodine concentration of the contrast medium should be at least 350 mg I/mL. Thin collimation multidetector CT technology allows multiplanar reconstruction of equal quality due to an isotropic voxel size.

The *inferior vena cava* (IVC) is formed by the junction of the right and left common iliac veins just caudal to the aortic bifurcation and parallels the abdominal aorta on the right side. The cross-sectional diameter of the IVC usually amounts to 2 to 3 cm, and its shape may vary from slitlike to rounded. A collapsed IVC at multiple levels can be observed in patients with severe hypovolemia. A round and widened IVC may be indicative of heart failure. Forced inspiration and expiration usually provoke changes in the vascular diameter of the IVC. The differential diagnosis of various retroperitoneal abnormalities is given in **Table 26.1**.

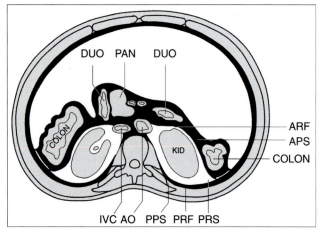

Fig. 26.1 Retroperitoneal compartments. Darkened areas: anterior and posterior pararenal space; white areas: perirenal space. (Modified from Krestin.)

AO aorta
APS anterior pararenal space
ARF anterior renal fascia
DUO duodenum
IVC inferior vena cava
KID kidney
PAN pancreas
PPS posterior pararenal space
PRF posterior renal fascia
PRS perirenal space

Table 26.1   Retroperitoneal abnormalities

Disease	CT Findings	Comments
Vascular		
Atherosclerosis ▷ *Fig. 18.35a, b, p. 653*	Fatty deposits (atheromas) inside the arterial walls leading to stenosis and calcification of the arteries. **Diagnostic pearls:** Vessel tortuosity, intimal calcification, noncalcified atheromatous plaques, and sometimes thrombus formation.	Atherosclerotic risk factors (see Framingham risk factors) initiate vascular stress with subsequent local vascular inflammation, progressive intimal thickening, and finally stenosis. May also lead to formation of an intravasal thrombus or an aneurysm. Plaques may be calcified (stable) or noncalcified (more prone to rupture) (e.g., atheromas). Eccentric array of calcifications is an important differentiator to aortic dissection (centrally displaced intima).
Aortic aneurysm ▷ *Fig. 26.2a–c*	Segmental to total saccular or fusiform aortic dilation > 3 cm in diameter. **Diagnostic pearls:** Thickened, often calcified, aortic wall; calcifications found on outer wall of dilated aorta; presence of noncalcified plaques/thrombus. Perianeurysmal fat stranding indicates inflammatory fibrosis. Discontinuity of the aneurysm wall and periaortic hematoma are indicative of rupture.	Observed in 1% to 3% of the Western population, mainly due to atherosclerosis. **Crawford classification for staging:** Type 1: Aneurysm from left subclavian artery to renal arteries. Type 2: Aneurysm from left subclavian artery to aortic bifurcation. Type 3: Aneurysm from middescending aorta to aortic bifurcation. Type 4: Aneurysm from upper abdominal aorta and all or none of the infrarenal aorta. The risk of rupture increases with aneurysm diameter. Surgical/interventional repair required for > 1 cm/y diameter growth rate or an aneurysm size > 5 cm. Differential diagnosis: Intramural hematoma (IMH)/ aortic dissection.

(continues on page 778)

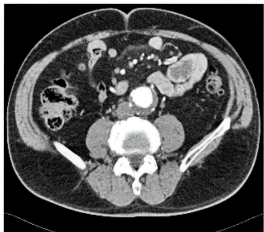

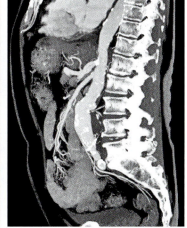

a

b

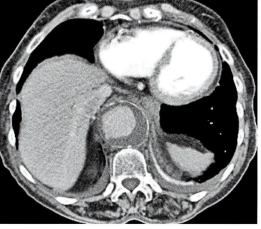

c

Fig. 26.2a–c   Abdominal aorta aneurysms, Crawford type IV. Subrenal segmental aortic dilation > 3 cm in diameter (**a,b**). Suprarenal aortic dilation > 5 cm with perianeurysmal inflammatory fibrosis and discontinuity of the right laterodorsal aneurysm wall requiring immediate surgery due to high risk of rupture (**c**).

VI Abdomen and Pelvis

Table 26.1   (Cont.) Retroperitoneal abnormalities

Disease	CT Findings	Comments
Aortic dissection ▷ *Fig. 18.40a–c, p. 655*	Spontaneous intimal tear with continuous mucosal wall separation. **Diagnostic pearls:** On nonenhanced CT, calcified intima are displaced centrally. On contrast-enhanced CT (arterial phase), contrast-filled double (true and false lumen) channel with an intervening intimal flap spirals down the aorta. *Indicators of the false lumen:* • Usually the larger lumen with delayed contrast • A "beak" sign: An acute angle between the dissected flap and the outer wall • Presence of cobwebs: Thin mucosal strands crossing the false lumen • Intraluminal thrombus with centrally displaced intima (calcifications). In general, eccentric array of calcifications is an important differentiator to aortic dissection (centrally displaced intima). Characterized by a contrast-filled double channel with an intervening intimal flap. True and false lumen usually opacify at different paces, the true lumen first. Intraluminal thrombosis, dilation of the aorta with compression of the true lumen, and irregular contour of the contrast-filled part of the aorta are other common findings.	Histologically, a cystic media necrosis from either atherosclerosis or congenital disorders. May be due to collagen disorders (Ehlers–Danlos syndrome, Marfan syndrome, Turner syndrome, osteogenesis imperfecta, etc.), trauma, hypertension, or pregnancy (> 50% of dissections in women). **Stanford classification of dissections:** **Type A:** Entry of dissection in ascending aorta (70%) **Type B:** Entry of distal to left subclavian artery (30%) Intimo-intimo intussusception is observed in cases of complete circumferential dissection. Typical complications include occlusion of the aortic side branches and continuation into the iliac arteries. Multiplanar reconstruction (MPR) is useful for assessment of exact dimension of dissection. Look out for distal re-entry. Typical pitfalls are streak (i.e., motion artifacts in the ascending aorta). When in doubt, perform electrocardiogram (ECG)-triggered CT.
Aortic surgery ▷ *Fig. 26.3a, b*	History of previous interventional stent or surgical graft placement. **Diagnostic pearls:** Any high-attenuating homogeneous perigraft mass with decreasing HU values > 2 weeks after surgery suggests hematoma. Fluid–fluid levels indicate sedation of hemoglobin. Irregular, septated periaortic fluid or gas collection is indicative of an infected graft. Irregular, periaortic fat stranding on nonenhanced CT and moderate attenuation on postcontrast scans is typical of stent/graft infection. Septated periaortic fluid or gas collection is highly suspicious of abscess formation. The lack of luminal contrast enhancement is observed in thrombosis. A blood-equivalent mass lesion with rim enhancement and with or without septations may represent a pseudoaneurysm.	Aortic graft may be end-to-side, end-to-end, or intra-aneurysmal. Grafts may extend into the iliac arteries (Y graft). Ventral collections of perigraft gas and fluid shortly after surgery may be a normal postoperative finding. Differential diagnoses: seroma and lymphocele. A common complication of endovascular aneurysm repair (EVAR) represent endoleaks, which may continue to perfuse and pressurize the aneurysm sac, thereby conferring an ongoing risk of aneurysm enlargement and/or rupture. **Endoleaks** are classified by the source of blood flow and organized into five categories: **I:** Attachment site leaks **II:** Collateral vessel leaks **III:** Graft failure (i.e., midgraft hole, junctional leak, or disconnect) **IV:** Graft wall porosity **V:** Endotension (with or without endoleak)
Circumaortic left renal vein	Congenital anomaly of the left renal vein. **Diagnostic pearls:** One of two left renal veins crosses the aorta anteriorly and posteriorly to join the IVC.	Incidence: 1.5% to 8.7%.
Retroaortic left renal vein	**Diagnostic pearls:** One left renal vein crosses the aorta posteriorly.	Incidence: 2% to 2.5%. In 0.1% of cases, a concomitant retrocaval ureter is seen.
Caval transposition/left inferior vena cava (IVC) ▷ *Fig. 26.4*	Congenital anomaly of the IVC inferior to renal veins. **Diagnostic pearls:** On caudal sections, the IVC parallels the aorta to the left and ends at the level of the left renal vein, which crosses the aorta either anteriorly or posteriorly to form a normal right suprarenal IVC.	Incidence: 0.2% to 0.5%.
Duplication of the inferior vena cava (IVC)	Persistence of both supracardinal veins. **Diagnostic pearls:** Left and right IVC inferior to the renal vein. Left IVC drains into the left renal vein, which crosses the aorta in normal fashion and joins the IVC. May be combined with an azygos/hemiazygos continuation of the IVC.	Incidence: 0.2% to 3.0%. A duplicated IVC may mimic a prominent left gonadal vein. The latter can be traced to the level of the inguinal canal or ovary, whereas a duplicated IVC ends at the level of the left common iliac vein.
Azygos continuation of the inferior vena cava (IVC)	Failure to form right subcardinal-hepatic anastomosis, resulting in atrophy of the right subcardinal vein. **Diagnostic pearls:** Intrahepatic vena cava is absent, and the IVC passes the diaphragm posteriorly as the azygos vein, which joins the superior vena cava (SVC) at the physiological location in the right peribronchial location.	Incidence: 0.2% to 4.3%. It is associated in 85% of cases with congenital heart disease; left pulmonary isomerism, polysplenia, dextrocardia, and intracardiac defects. Transposed abdominal viscera are also commonly associated.

Table 26.1   (Cont.) Retroperitoneal abnormalities

Disease	CT Findings	Comments
Thrombosis of the inferior vena cava (IVC) ▷ *Fig. 26.5a, b*	**Diagnostic pearls:** A low-density intraluminal filling defect in a focal enlarged IVC, often surrounded by a rim of high density representing the vessel wall. The presence of gas bubbles within the caval filling defect indicates septic thrombosis.	May result from bland or septic thrombosis, but is more commonly secondary to direct tumor invasion from the kidney, adrenals, or liver.

(continues on page 780)

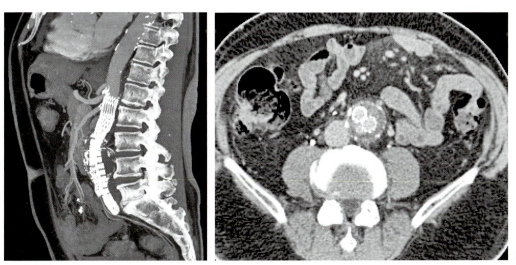

a   b

Fig. 26.3a, b   Follow-up after interventional stent placement (same patient as Fig. 26.2a,b). Stent fully covers the previous aneurysm (**a**) but shows type I endoleak at the attachment side of the iliac legs (**b**).

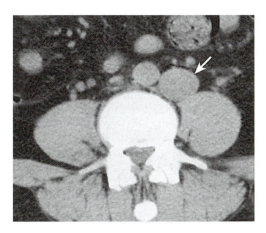

Fig. 26.4   Caval transposition. The IVC (arrow) parallels the aorta on the left.

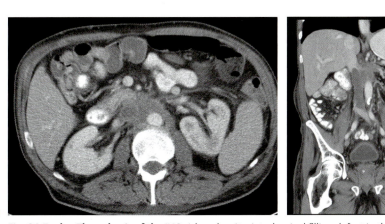

a   b

Fig. 26.5a, b   Thrombosis of the IVC. A low-density, intraluminal filling defect in the infrarenal IVC by a rim of high density representing the vessel wall. Axial scan identifies infiltrating retroperitoneal lymphoma as the underlying cause.

Table 26.1 (Cont.) Retroperitoneal abnormalities

Disease	CT Findings	Comments
Inflammation		
Retroperitoneal fibrosis ▷ *Fig. 26.6*	Thick, fibrous soft tissue encasing retroperitoneal vessels. **Diagnostic pearls:** A distinctly enhancing, fibrous sheet/bulky mass extending from the kidneys to the sacrum. Also seen: encasing of the aorta, IVC, iliac vessels, and ureters. Retroperitoneal fibrosis usually displaces the ureters medially, unlike retroperitoneal lymphadenopathy, which tends to displace them laterally.	Proliferation of fibrous and inflammatory tissue in the retroperitoneum. Seventy percent of cases are idiopathic; 30% are secondary to either drugs (methysergide or ergotamine) or malignant tumors, which cause a desmoplastic reaction that is morphologically indistinguishable from retroperitoneal fibrosis.
Sarcoidosis	Lymphadenopathy associated with hepatosplenomegaly in the absence of signs of portal hypertension. **Diagnostic pearls:** Discrete lymph node swelling, unlike in malignant lymphoma.	Histologically, well-defined granulomas with a rim consisting of fibroblasts and lymphocytes. Usually associated with chronic pulmonary sarcoidosis (75%). Differentiation from lymphoma may be difficult without biopsy.
Amyloidosis	Lymphoma-like lymph node enlargement. **Diagnostic pearls:** Nonspecific hepatomegaly and lymphadenopathy. Mural involvement of gastrointestinal (GI) organs is more common.	Deposition of protein-polysaccharide material in various organs. Can be either primary or secondary to advanced age, rheumatoid arthritis, multiple myeloma, lymphoreticular malignancy, or chronic infections.
Whipple disease	Bacterial infection leading to malabsorption and chronic diarrhea. **Diagnostic pearls:** Lymphadenopathy with central areas of low density, caused by deposition of fat and fatty acids.	Characteristic of Whipple disease but may also occur in Crohn disease, treated lymphoma, and metastases.
Castleman disease	Rare benign lymphoproliferative hyperplasia of the lymph nodes. **Diagnostic pearls:** Well-defined muscle density mass with a thin, enhancing rim that may contain spotty central calcifications.	Histologically, hyaline vascular (90%), plasma cell (9%), or mixed types. Observed in middle-aged adults without any gender preponderance. Castleman disease is indistinguishable from lymphoma. Seventy percent of the lesions occur in the middle or posterior mediastinum, rarely in the retroperitoneum.
Benign lymphadenopathy ▷ *Fig. 26.7*	**Diagnostic pearls:** Reactively enlarged lymph nodes up to 2 cm, especially in immunosuppressed patients.	Relatively rare. In immunocompromised patients, it is impossible to distinguish between lymphomas and metastases of Kaposi sarcoma.
Congenital		
Undescended testes	**Diagnostic pearls:** Small retroperitoneal focus of soft tissue anywhere along the course of the gonadal vein from the inguinal region to the renal vein. Growth indicates malignancy.	Eighty percent of maldescended testes are located distal to the inguinal ring, 20% are above and usually adjacent to the iliac vessels. Congenital absence of testes occurs.
Trauma		
Hematoma	Irregular soft tissue mass that obscures, compresses, or distorts normal retroperitoneal structures. **Diagnostic pearls:** During acute stage, hematomas are high-attenuating. Subacute hematomas appear heterogeneous with higher density centrally and a more lucent periphery (due to liquefaction). Chronic hematomas may develop a thick calcified capsule.	Either spontaneous or secondary to trauma, vascular tumors, aneurysm rupture, blood dyscrasias, anticoagulation therapy, or long-term hemodialysis. Usually contained within well-defined muscle groups and spontaneously resolving.
Infection		
Tuberculosis (TB)	**Diagnostic pearls:** Lymphadenopathy in mesenteric and peripancreatic lymph nodes. Central areas of low attenuation and inflammatory rim enhancement following intravenous (IV) contrast administration are typical, but they may also be seen in metastatic nodes.	Complicates pulmonary disease in 6% to 38% of immunocompromised patients. May be due to *Mycobacterium tuberculosis* or *M. avium intracellulare* (MAI). The latter typically shows lymph nodes with distinct central necrosis.
Abscess ▷ *Fig. 26.8a, b*	**Diagnostic pearls:** Well-defined mass of fluid density with or without gas bubbles. Usually strong rim enhancement.	The most common causes are colonic perforation, pancreatic abscess, duodenal perforation, and surgical contamination. Very common in immunocompromised patients.

(continues on page 782)

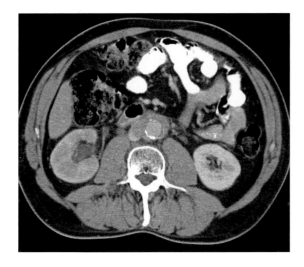

Fig. 26.6   Retroperitoneal fibrosis. Proliferation of retroperitoneal fibrous tissue encasing the aorta, right ureter, and IVC. The left ureter is not visible and may also be encased.

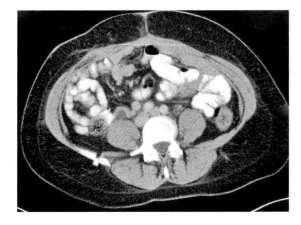

Fig. 26.7   Benign lymphadenopathy in acquired immunodeficiency syndrome (AIDS). Reactively enlarged lymph nodes ventral to the IVC and between the common iliac arteries.

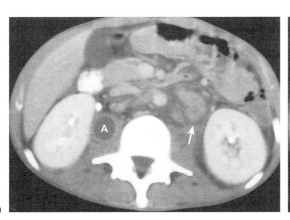

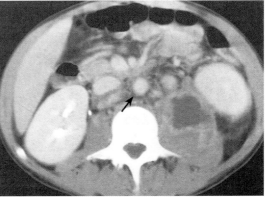

a   b

Fig. 26.8a, b   Benign lymphadenopathy and psoas abscesses in AIDS. Right-sided psoas abscess (A) and para-aortic lymphadenopathy (arrow) in a 21-y-old man (**a**). Ten months later, a new psoas abscess on the left displaces the left kidney (**b**). Lymphadenopathy now is less extensive, but fibrotic changes have appeared in the periaortic fat (arrow).

Table 26.1   (Cont.) Retroperitoneal abnormalities

Disease	CT Findings	Comments
Benign neoplasms		
Lymphocele	Homogeneous, low-attenuating fluid collection due to iatrogenic disruption of lymphatics. **Diagnostic pearls:** Smoothly marginated (very thin), waterlike, hypodense lesion. Secondary infection may result in higher attenuation values.	Typically occurs several weeks after retroperitoneal surgery or intervention.
Urinoma (perirenal pseudocyst)	Water-dense mass that partially or completely occludes the perirenal compartment. **Diagnostic pearls:** In acute stages, leakage of contrast material into the urinoma may be visible. Chronic urinoma may extend down to the pelvic inlet.	Ill-definition from adjacent structures or attenuation values > 30 HU is suspicious of an infection. A thick, enhancing rim is typically observed in abscess formation.
Seroma	**Diagnostic pearls:** Collection of near-water-density fluid, usually in a postoperative patient at or near the site of operation.	May become infected and develop into an abscess.
Cystic lymphangioma	**Diagnostic pearls:** Solitary or multilocular cystic mass with slightly enhancing, thin walls.	Neoplasms that almost exclusively occur in the neck or groin. Very rarely found in the retroperitoneum.
Pancreatic pseudocyst ▷ *Fig. 22.11, p. 725*	Fibrous encapsulated fluid collection of inflammatory pancreatic exudate. **Diagnostic pearls:** Near-water-density mass with enhancing walls.	May invade the retroperitoneal space but usually stays outside Gerota fascia.
Malignant neoplasms		
Lymphoma ▷ *Fig. 26.9a, b* ▷ *Fig. 26.10*	**Diagnostic pearls:** Well-defined enlarged lymph nodes that may coalesce into large conglomerates. Typically results in arterial displacement of vessels and ureters. Attenuation of enlarged lymph nodes is similar to that of muscle tissue (40–60 HU).	CT does not provide any information concerning the type of lymphoma. It can only detect enlarged lymph nodes. **Staging according to Ann Arbor classification (I–IV):** Involvement of only one (stage I) or two (stage II) nodal regions on one side of the diaphragm has a better prognosis than involvement of nodal regions on both sides of the diaphragm with or without involvement of extralymphatic organs (stages III and IV).
Testicular neoplasm ▷ *Fig. 26.11*	The most common malignancy in men age 20 to 34 y. **Diagnostic pearls:** Enlarged, low-attenuation, para-aortic lymph nodes near the renal hilum.	About 95% of neoplasms are germ cell tumors, including seminoma, embryonal cell tumor, teratocarcinoma, choriocarcinoma, and mixed-element tumors.
Other metastatic tumors ▷ *Fig. 26.12*	Enlarged retroperitoneal lymph nodes in the pelvic and abdominal regions. **Diagnostic pearls:** Any round lymph node > 1 cm and without central fat hilus is suspect. Metastatic lymph node enlargement is less pronounced than in malignant lymphoma. Metastatic nodes may not be enlarged.	Cervical, prostatic, bladder, uterine, renal, and ovarian carcinomas frequently metastasize to retroperitoneal lymph nodes. Other primaries include lung and GI carcinomas. Modest lymph node enlargement in renal cell carcinoma patients may be reactive, not metastatic.

(continues on page 784)

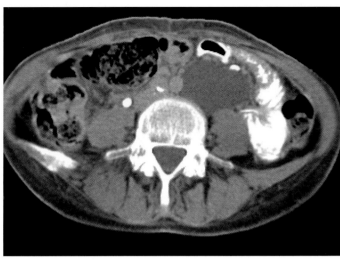
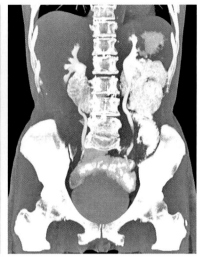

a **b**

Fig. 26.9a, b   Large left-sided retroperitoneal lymphoma. CT urography shows medial displacement of the left ureter on axial scan (**a**) and coronal multiplanar reconstruction (MPR) (**b**).

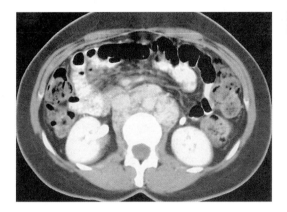

Fig. 26.10   Hair cell leukemia. Densely packed para-aortic mass of distinctly but inhomogeneously enhancing enlarged lymph nodes.

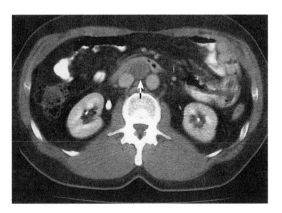

Fig. 26.11   Metastatic testicular seminoma. Low-attenuation enlarged lymph node (arrow) is seen between the aorta and the IVC at the level of the renal hilum.

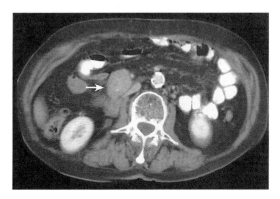

Fig. 26.12   Carcinoid tumor metastatic to retroperitoneal lymph nodes. The strongly enhancing mass compresses the IVC (arrow).

Table 26.1 (Cont.) Retroperitoneal abnormalities

Disease	CT Findings	Comments
Mesodermal tumors ▷ *Fig. 26.13* ▷ *Fig. 26.14* ▷ *Fig. 26.15*	Large mass that may be solid (soft tissue density), mixed, or pseudocystic (water-like density). **Diagnostic pearls:** CT attenuation depends on the main soft tissue component. A leiomyosarcoma is strongly enhancing with a central necrosis. A liposarcoma has higher attenuation than normal retroperitoneal fat and shows large soft tissue components. The lack of soft tissue suggests a benign lipoma.	Fifty percent of all mesodermal tumors are primary retroperitoneal neoplasms, of which 85% are malignant. Liposarcoma is the most common type. Even a subtle area of negative CT values in a solid retroperitoneal mass is highly suspicious of liposarcoma. Other tumor entities are leiomyosarcoma, malignant fibrous histiocytoma, fibrosarcoma, malignant hemangiopericytoma, and malignant mesenchymoma.
Neurogenic tumors ▷ *Fig. 26.16*	Small, well-defined, round to oval retroperitoneal mass. **Diagnostic pearls:** Hypodense masses near the course of a nerve.	Neurogenic tumors represent 30% of primary retroperitoneal tumors. Usually occur in patients younger than 30 y. Ganglioneuroma, pheochromocytoma, and neurofibroma are the most common benign tumors. Neuroblastoma is a common malignancy in children younger than 6 y. Patients with von Hippel–Lindau syndrome, tuberous sclerosis, or neurofibromatosis have a genetic predisposition for neurogenic tumors.

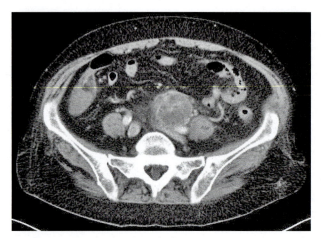

Fig. 26.13 Leiomyosarcoma. The leiomyosarcoma presents with central necrotic components and a strongly enhancing rim.

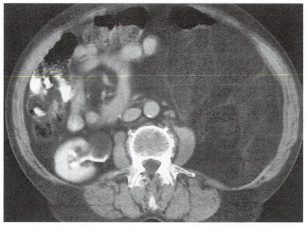

Fig. 26.14 Retroperitoneal liposarcoma. A huge fatty mass on the left displaces the bowel anteriorly and medially.

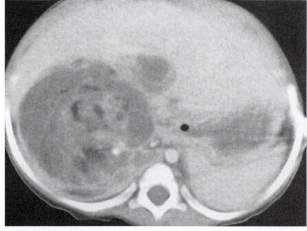

Fig. 26.15 Retroperitoneal teratoma in a 1-y-old girl. A large hypodense, inhomogeneous mass displaces the liver. It contains fat, fibrous components, and calcifications.

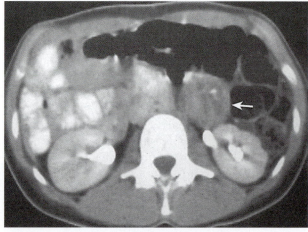

Fig. 26.16 Retroperitoneal neurilemoma. A round, inhomogeneously enhancing, partly calcified mass (arrow) near the left psoas muscle.

27 Kidneys

Francis A. Burgener

The kidneys are surrounded by perinephric fat, resulting in excellent delineation of their margins. The renal parenchyma has a relatively uniform density of 30 to 50 HU on precontrast computed tomography (CT) scans, which does not permit differentiation between the renal cortex and medulla. The attenuation of urine in the collecting system is similar to water.

Renal arteries arise posterior to the corresponding *renal veins*, which are usually somewhat larger. The right renal artery crosses posterior to the inferior vena cava, whereas the left renal vein crosses anterior to the aorta.

After an intravenous (IV) contrast material bolus, the attenuation in the renal cortex increases more rapidly than in the medulla, permitting differentiation between these two compartments within the first minute. After that time the density of the renal parenchyma becomes uniform again, as the renal medulla enhances more slowly than the cortex, which already depicts early contrast washout. Following an IV contrast material infusion, the renal parenchymal density increases uniformly, and differentiation between the cortex and medulla is not feasible.

The renal parenchyma is tightly invested by a rigid *renal capsule* composed predominantly of fibrous tissue. The capsule is rarely, if ever, visualized by CT. Because of the rigidity of the renal capsule, a subcapsular process such as a hematoma compresses primarily the adjacent renal parenchyma, which becomes flattened by the pathologic fluid collection and often assumes a lenticular shape.

Between the renal capsule and the *renal fascia* (perirenal fascia, Gerota fascia anteriorly, and Zuckerkandl fascia posteriorly), which is commonly seen on CT scans, lies the *perirenal space,* composed largely of fatty tissue. Bridging connective tissue septa connecting the renal capsule with the renal fascia may divide this space into smaller subunits. A fascia measuring ≥ 3 mm in width is an abnormal but totally nonspecific finding. It has been reported in a variety of conditions, including inflammatory, malignant, and traumatic processes, or may be caused by edema and fibrosis. The pararenal compartment is located outside the renal fascia. An *anterior pararenal compartment* containing the pancreas, duodenum (with the exception of the bulb), and both the ascending and descending colon is distinguished from the *posterior pararenal compartment,* which contains no major organs. Although these retroperitoneal compartments are anatomically well defined, an infectious or tumorous process can easily spread from one space to the other. Furthermore, pelvic disease, especially involving the rectosigmoid, may spread cephalad into the perirenal and pararenal compartments (**Fig. 27.1**).

CT is valuable in the detection, localization, and characterization of focal renal mass lesions. The most common renal mass in the adult is a benign cyst. *Cysts* may be solitary or multiple and are usually round and located in the cortex. Characteristic CT features include a homogeneous density close to water (0–20 HU), a smooth margin with sharp demarcation from the adjacent renal parenchyma, no detectable wall when projecting beyond the renal outline, and no enhancement after IV contrast material administration (**Fig. 27.2**). A cyst smaller than

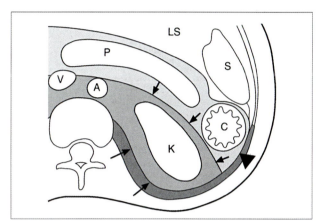

Fig. 27.1 Extraperitoneal anatomy of the left flank. Light gray area: anterior pararenal space; medium gray area: perirenal space; dark gray area: posterior pararenal space; short arrows: anterior renal fascia; long arrows; posterior renal fascia; arrowhead: lateroconal fascia.

A aorta
C colon
K kidney
LS lesser sac
P pancreas
S spleen
V inferior vena cava

the image slice thickness may be volume-averaged, resulting in falsely high attenuation values before and particularly after contrast enhancement. Truly high-density cysts occur and are caused by proteinaceous material or "milk of calcium" in the cystic fluid, infection, or hemorrhage into the cyst (**Fig. 27.3**). Milk of calcium may also be found in a calyceal diverticulum (**Fig. 27.4**). Thin intracystic septation occasionally occurs in benign renal cysts, but other entities, such as multilocular renal nephromas, Wilms tumors, and abscesses, must be considered. The Bosniak classification is commonly used to assess cystic renal lesions (**Table 27.1**).

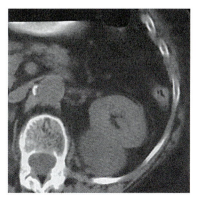

Fig. 27.2 Renal cyst. A renal mass of homogeneous density close to water displacing the left kidney anteriorly is seen on this nonenhanced scan.

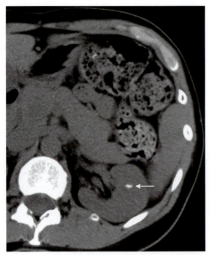
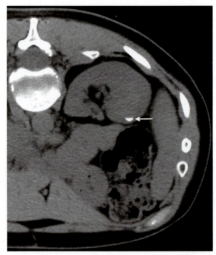
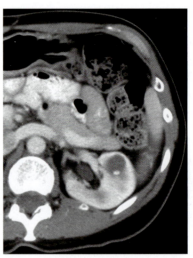

a   b   c

Fig. 27.3a–c   High-density renal cyst with tiny intracystic calcification. Supine view (**a**). An isodense anterolateral enlargement of the left kidney containing a tiny calcification (arrow) is seen on this nonenhanced scan. Prone view (**b**). In this position, the tiny calcification (arrow) is moving to the most dependent portion of the kidney. Supine postcontrast enhancement (**c**). A well-demarcated cyst without enhancement can be differentiated from the enhanced normal renal parenchyma. The tiny intracystic calcification is located at the most dependent portion of the renal cyst.

Solid renal mass lesions are usually irregularly shaped with poor demarcation from the normal renal parenchyma (**Fig. 27.5**). Characteristic CT features include an inhomogeneous density that is close to the renal parenchyma (30–50 HU) and increases after IV contrast administration. Compared with the surrounding renal parenchyma, solid renal mass lesions are frequently slightly hypodense, but because of small differences in attenuation on precontrast scan, these lesions may be appreciated only after IV contrast administration, as they usually enhance considerably less than normal renal parenchyma. A solid renal mass lesion must be considered malignant until proven otherwise and requires prompt clinical workup, including surgical exploration.

Renal lesions that do not unequivocally display CT criteria of either a benign cyst or a solid tumor represent *indeterminate masses*. They account for about 10% of all focal renal lesions. The renal mass may be indeterminate for technical reasons, such as breathing artifacts and volume-averaging effects. Cystlike renal masses may be considered indeterminate if they demonstrate a thick wall, calcifications, multiple septa, indistinct interface with the renal parenchyma, high attenuation of the cyst content (≥ 25 HU), and/or some contrast enhancement. Complicated (hemorrhagic) cysts, abscesses, and benign and malignant cystic or necrotic tumors may all represent as indeterminate masses by CT criteria (**Fig. 27.6**). They correspond to types 3 and 4 in the Bosniak classification of cystic renal lesions and usually require prompt clinical workup, including percutaneous biopsy or surgical exploration.

Calcifications in a focal renal lesion occur in both benign and malignant conditions (**Fig. 27.7**). Peripheral curvilinear

Fig. 27.4   "Milk of calcium." Calcium–fluid level is visible in a calyceal diverticulum.

Table 27.1   Bosniak classification of cystic renal lesions

1   Simple cyst
    Well-defined round mass of water attenuation
    Hairline-thin imperceptible wall
    No enhancement

2   Minimally complicated cyst
    Cluster of cysts/septated cyst
    Minimal curvilinear calcification
    Minimally irregular wall
    High-density content (> 25 HU)

2F Follow-up cyst
    Hairline-thin septum
    Wall with perceived enhancement
    Intrarenal lesion > 3 cm with high density content

3   Complicated (surgical) cyst
    Irregular, thickened septa
    Measurable enhancement
    Coarse, irregular calcifications
    Irregular margin
    Multiloculated lesion
    Uniform wall thickening
    Nonenhancing nodular mass

4   Malignant cyst
    Irregular wall thickening
    Solid enhancing elements
    Large cystic/necrotic component

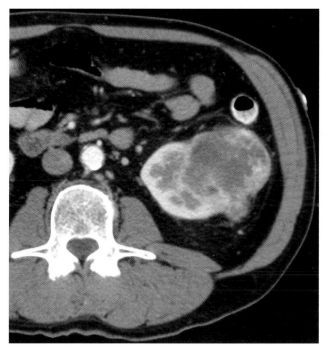

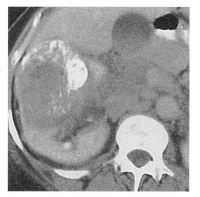

Fig. 27.7   Calcification in renal cell carcinoma. A large mass with irregular calcifications is seen in the right kidney.

Fig. 27.5   Renal cell carcinoma. A poorly defined lesion with less contrast enhancement than the adjacent normal renal parenchyma is seen in the lateral aspect of the kidney.

calcifications in a cystlike lesion with homogeneous, near-water-density fluid content and the absence of both a soft tissue mass and thickened (focal or uniform) wall is likely to be benign. In addition to calcified renal cysts, aneurysms and arteriovenous malformation must be considered. In hydatid (echinococcal) disease, a larger partially calcified cyst with a thin or thick wall containing daughter cysts is diagnostic. Amorphous or punctate calcifications associated with a solid or partially cystic mass are found in a variety of benign (e.g., oncocytoma) or malignant tumors (e.g., renal cell carcinomas, Wilms tumor, and metastases), tuberculosis (TB) and other granulomatous diseases, and old abscesses and hematomas (**Fig. 27.8**).

Diffuse renal parenchymal calcifications (*nephrocalcinosis*) occur most often in the renal medulla, especially in the renal papilla,

where the largest urine concentration is attained (**Fig. 27.9**). *Medullary nephrocalcinosis* is found with medullary sponge kidney, hyperoxaluria, and conditions associated with hypercalcemia and hypercalcinuria (e.g., hyperparathyroidism, renal tubular acidosis, milk–alkali syndrome, Cushing syndrome, vitamin D intoxication, sarcoidosis, bone metastases, multiple myeloma, and osteoporosis). *Papillary calcifications* are also encountered with papillary necrosis and TB.

Cortical nephrocalcinosis is rare and limited to diseases primarily involving the renal cortex (e.g., acute cortical necrosis and occasionally glomerulonephritis).

Renal calculi are readily detected by CT even if they are not calcified. Nonopaque calculi account for approximately 10% of all renal calculi and consist of uric acid, xanthine, or matrix (mucoprotein/mucopolysaccharide). Urographic differentiation from tumors and blood clots is often not possible. CT can, however, readily distinguish calculi from other nonopaque filling defects because of a difference in density. Nonopaque calculi have a CT density exceeding 50 HU, whereas tumors of all types have soft tissue attenuation values of less than 50 HU.

Perinephric fluid collections complicating a renal transplant are caused by lymphocele, urinoma, hematoma, and abscess formation. Lymphoceles are the most common peritransplant fluid collections, characteristically occurring within 2 to 3 weeks after transplantation. They tend to be large, may be septated, and are usually located

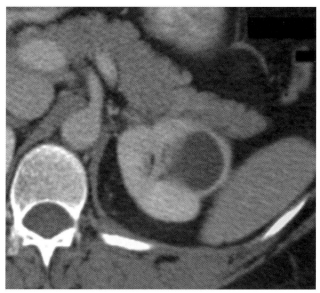

Fig. 27.6   Cystic renal cell carcinoma. A well-demarcated, hypodense lesion mimicking a cyst is apparent in the lateral aspect of the left kidney on this contrast-enhanced scan.

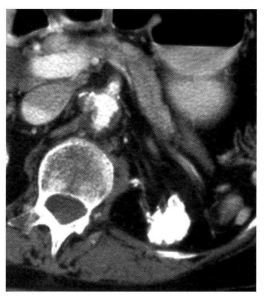

Fig. 27.8   Tuberculous autonephrectomy. A small, shrunken, scarred, nonfunctioning calcified left kidney is seen.

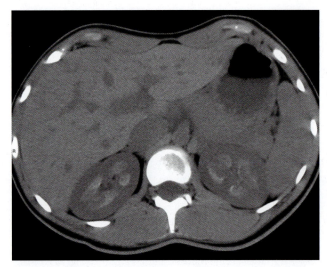

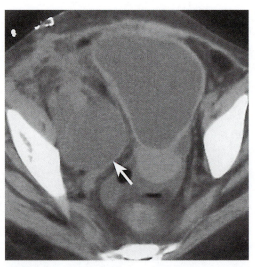

Fig. 27.9   Medullary nephrocalcinosis. Diffuse medullary calcifications are evident in both kidneys.

Fig. 27.10   Lymphocele in renal transplant. A large fluid collection (arrow) is visible in the right hemipelvis after renal transplantation. The density of the lymph in the lymphocele is similar to the urine in the adjacent distended bladder.

medial and inferior to the lower pole of the transplant (**Fig. 27.10**). Urinomas can occur at any time after transplantation and are caused by an anastomotic leak or are secondary to a vascular injury causing a focal necrosis with subsequent leak in the urinary system. Hematomas can be differentiated in the acute stage by their higher CT density. Abscesses can be unequivocally diagnosed only if they contain gas. Transplant failure caused by rejection, acute tubular necrosis, and cyclosporine-induced nephrotoxicity cannot be reliably differentiated by CT. Nevertheless, a rapid increase in the size of a failing transplant suggests acute rejection.

The differentiation of focal lesions in the kidney and perinephric space is discussed in **Tables 27.2** and **27.3**, respectively.

Table 27.2   Focal renal lesions

Disease	CT Findings	Comments
Renal ectopy ▷ *Fig. 27.11* ▷ *Fig. 27.12* ▷ *Fig. 27.13a, b* ▷ *Fig. 27.14*	Malpositioned kidneys are readily located and identified as functioning renal parenchyma after contrast enhancement. In **horseshoe kidneys,** the lower poles of both kidneys are fused by a parenchymal or fibrous isthmus across the midline at L4–L5 between the aorta and inferior mesenteric artery. The long renal axis is medially oriented, and renal pelvises and ureters are situated anteriorly. Upper pole fusion is rare (10%). Complications include hydronephrosis secondary to ureteral pelvic junction (UPJ) obstruction, renal calculi, infection, and vesicoureteral reflux.	In **longitudinal ectopy,** the kidney is malpositioned in any location from the thorax to the sacrum. Pelvic kidney is the most common location and frequently associated with vesicoureteral reflux, hydronephrosis, hypospadia, and contralateral renal agenesis. In **crossed ectopy,** the malpositioned kidney is commonly fused with the contralateral kidney. A large kidney with usual outline and two collecting systems on one side and an absent kidney on the contralateral side are diagnostic. In **renal fusion,** the fused kidneys are located in the midline and may assume the shape of a horseshoe, disk, or pancake. Ureteral obstruction by aberrant arteries is frequently associated. In **renal malrotation,** the collecting system is usually positioned anteriorly. Differential diagnosis: A malpositioned kidney may also be caused by a large adjacent mass.
Renal duplication ▷ *Fig. 27.15*	Two separate renal sinuses and pelvises are seen, separated by a parenchymal bridge. Upper pole moiety is subject to obstruction and may simulate an upper pole mass on excretory urography when completely obstructed. Hydronephrosis and hydroureter of the obstructed upper collecting system is readily diagnosed by CT. Lower pole moiety is subject to vesicoureteral reflux.	In complete renal and ureteral duplication, the ureter draining the upper system inserts ectopically medial and below the orthotopic ureter into the bladder trigonum or urethra and may be associated with an **ectopic ureterocele.** Other congenital renal anomalies are partial duplication, supernumerary kidney, and renal hypoplasia or agenesis.

(continues on page 790)

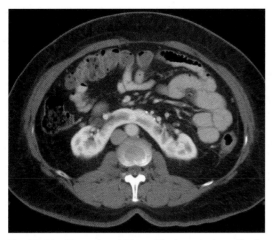

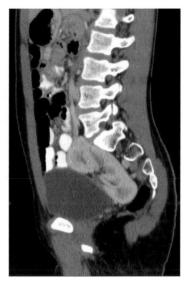

Fig. 27.12 Pelvic kidney. The enlarged kidney is located between the sacrum and urinary bladder.

Fig. 27.11 Horseshoe kidney. The lower poles of both kidneys are fused by a parenchymal isthmus, with the renal pelves and ureters being situated anteriorly.

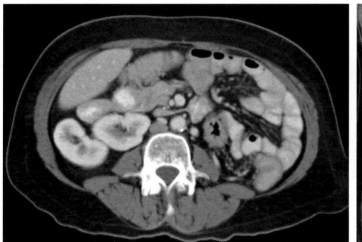

a

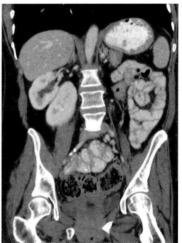

b

Fig. 27.13a, b Crossed renal ectopy. Axial (**a**) and coronal (**b**) views showing a malpositioned left kidney located on the right side that is partially fused with the right kidney.

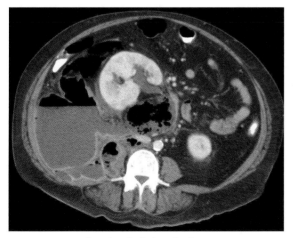

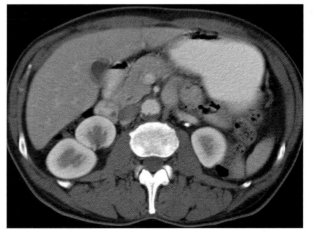

Fig. 27.14 Displaced right kidney by large retroperitoneal abscess. The right kidney is rotated and displaced medially by a large right retroperitoneal abscess containing a long air–fluid level.

Fig. 27.15 Supernumerary kidney. Two kidneys are seen on the right side, one on the left side. All three kidneys are functioning normally. Differential diagnosis: renal duplication where either the upper or lower pole moiety is malfunctioning.

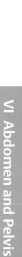

Table 27.2 (Cont.) Focal renal lesions

Disease	CT Findings	Comments
Renal sinus lipomatosis/ fibrolipomatosis ▷ *Fig. 27.16*	Extensive proliferation of fat in the renal sinus associated with loss of renal parenchyma is characteristic. It may result in concentric encroachment of the renal collecting system (trumpetlike pelvocaliceal system on urography), but without obstruction.	Etiology: (1) normal increase of sinus fat with aging and in obesity; (2) vicarious proliferation of sinus fat with renal atrophy of any cause; (3) fibrolipomatosis induced by extravasation of urine into the renal sinus (e.g., in chronic prostatism).
Hydronephrosis ▷ *Fig. 27.17a, b* ▷ *Fig. 27.18*	Dilated collecting system evident as water-density structure within normal or enlarged kidney on nonenhanced images. High-density urine in obstructed system suggests pyonephrosis. After enhancement, a persistent nephrogram and delayed and decreased contrast medium excretion are characteristic. In long-standing obstruction, the kidney appears as a fluid-filled cyst with a thin rim of solid renal tissue draped around it.	Early hydronephrosis can be differentiated from an extrarenal pelvis and postobstructive uropathy by the persistent nephrogram and delayed urinary contrast material excretion after contrast enhancement. Level of obstruction can easily be identified with CT by following the dilated collecting system and ureter to the point of obstruction. Nonopaque calculi have a CT density of at least 50 HU and can therefore be differentiated from soft tissue lesions that have a lower density. Freely mobile filling defects in the collecting system other than renal calculi include blood clots and fungus balls.
Renal cyst ▷ *Fig. 27.19* ▷ *Fig. 27.20* ▷ *Fig. 27.21*	Solitary or multiple sharply delineated, homogeneous lesions of near-water density (0–20 HU). Wall either very thin or not detectable when projecting beyond the renal outline. No contrast enhancement. Hemorrhagic cysts may demonstrate a fluid–fluid level or hematocrit effect due to settling of red blood cells. The Bosniak classification is commonly used for the CT assessment of cystic renal lesions (see **Table 27.1**).	Most common renal mass in adults. Higher than water attenuation values in a renal cyst are found with hemorrhage into the cyst, contrast material leakage into the cyst (caused by either communication with the collecting system or diffusion), calcification of the cyst wall or the cyst content (milk of calcium or calcium carbonate), high protein content of cyst fluid, and infection. Partial volume averaging with normal adjacent renal parenchyma (e.g., in cysts smaller in diameter than the CT slice thickness) also results in a higher displayed attenuation value of the cyst.
Parapelvic cyst (renal sinus cyst)	Features of a benign renal cyst, but located adjacent to the renal sinus. Differentiation from an ectatic renal pelvis may require IV contrast administration demonstrating lack of enhancement of the cyst.	Occurs frequently in the fifth and sixth decade of life and is almost always asymptomatic. Very rare complications may include obstructive caliectasis and renal vascular hypertension due to compression of renal arteries.
Autosomal dominant polycystic kidney disease (ADPKD) ▷ *Fig. 27.22* ▷ *Fig. 27.23*	Bilateral, often markedly enlarged kidneys with lobulated contours but often not symmetrically involved. Multiple cysts of different sizes cause splaying and distorting of the collecting system and may demonstrate varying densities due to blood products of different ages. Unilateral involvement is exceedingly rare.	Also referred to as adult polycystic kidney disease. Cysts are often also present in the pancreas, spleen, and lungs. Progressive renal failure and hypertension are usually evident in the fourth decade but occasionally as early as childhood or young adulthood.
Autosomal recessive polycystic kidney disease (ARPKD)	Symmetric, slightly enlarged kidneys with numerous tiny cysts (usually 1–2 mm, occasionally larger but always < 1 cm). They represent abnormally proliferated and dilated collecting tubules and do not produce calyceal or renal pelvis distortion. After IV contrast material administration, a prolonged and increasingly hyperintense, heterogeneous nephrogram is seen with delayed and decreased urinary contrast medium excretion.	Also referred to as infantile polycystic kidney disease. Occurs in neonates and children younger than 5 y. Associated with dilated bile ducts, periportal fibrosis, and pancreatic fibrosis. Neonatal death occurs in up to 50% of cases from pulmonary hypoplasia with long–term survival improving substantially after the newborn period.

(continues on page 792)

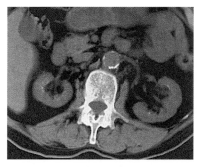

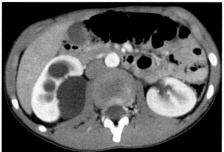

Fig. 27.16   Renal sinus lipomatosis. Enlarged fatty areas are seen in both renal hila, especially on the left side. Note tiny punctate calcifications bilaterally in the area of the renal papillae due to hyperparathyroidism.

Fig. 27.17a, b   Hydronephrosis (two cases). A large cystic area is evident in the right renal hilum caused by a ureteral pelvic junction (UPJ) obstruction (**a**). A dilated collecting system (arrow) of the left kidney with persistent dense nephrogram and delayed contrast excretion is characteristic (**b**). The hydronephrosis is caused by a large and partially thrombosed abdominal aortic aneurysm projecting anterior to the lumbar vertebra.

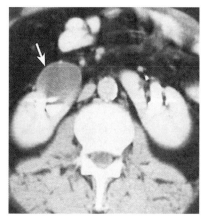

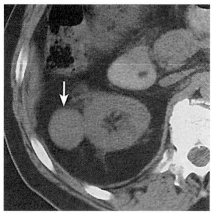

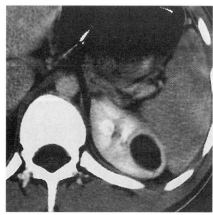

Fig. 27.18   Hydronephrosis in horseshoe kidney. A hydronephrosis (arrow) is seen on the right side of a horseshoe kidney evident by the medially oriented long renal axis and the anteriorly located renal pelvis.

Fig. 27.19   Renal cyst. A renal cyst (arrow) with a precontrast density similar to the adjacent renal parenchyma is seen.

Fig. 27.20   Renal cyst. A sharply delineated, homogeneous lesion of near-water density is seen within the left kidney following intravenous contrast material administration.

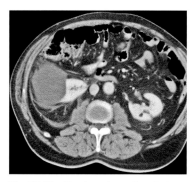

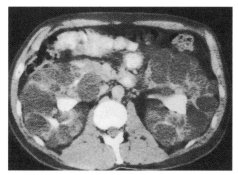

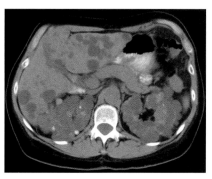

Fig. 27.21   Ruptured renal cyst. A large right renal cyst with poor definition on its superolateral border and obliteration of the adipose tissue in the adjacent perirenal space is seen.

Fig. 27.22   Adult polycystic kidney disease. Bilateral enlarged kidneys with multiple cysts are seen.

Fig. 27.23   Adult polycystic kidney disease. Bilateral enlarged kidneys with multiple cysts are seen. Note multiple hepatic cysts and a suggestion of small pancreatic cysts.

Table 27.2 (Cont.) Focal renal lesions

Disease	CT Findings	Comments
Multicystic dysplastic kidney ▷*Fig. 27.24*	Unilateral involvement consisting of a small or large single-chamber or multiloculated cystic mass, often with central or peripheral calcifications. No functional renal parenchyma is detectable after contrast administration (unlike multilocular cystic nephroma and unilateral polycystic kidney disease).	Frequent cause of palpable abdominal mass in an otherwise healthy infant or child resulting from failed fusion of the metanephros and ureteric bud. Compensatory hypertrophy of the contralateral kidney is usually present, often with an element of ureteropelvic obstruction.
Multilocular cystic nephroma (multilocular cystic renal tumor) ▷*Fig. 27.25* ▷*Fig. 27.26*	Single or multiple fluid-filled cysts measuring up to 10 cm, often replacing an entire renal pole (usually lower pole). Cysts are often separated by thick septa and sharply demarcated from the normal renal parenchyma. Peripheral and central calcifications of circular, stellate, flocculent, or granular nature in up to 50% of cases. Cyst wall and septations enhance after contrast administration.	Occurs in children younger than 5 y (M:F = 3:1) and in 40- to 70-y-old adults with strong female predominance. On ultrasound, multiple cystic masses separated by highly echogenic septa are evident. Cystic Wilms tumor and cystic renal cell carcinoma must be differentiated. Nodular thickening of the cyst wall and/or septa may be the clue for a malignancy.
Medullary cystic disease ▷*Fig. 27.27*	Bilateral small kidneys with multiple small medullary cysts that do not extend to the renal margins are characteristic.	Rare, in the majority of cases inherited, disorder manifesting itself in adolescents and young adults with progressive renal failure.
Medullary sponge kidney	Bilateral, unilateral, or segmental ectasia of the tubules in often enlarged papilla presenting after IV contrast material administration as tubular structures radiating from the calyx into the papilla. In approximately half of the cases, small calculi measuring up to 5 mm are clustered in the ectatic tubules of the papilla.	Usually an incidental finding in asymptomatic young to middle-aged adults. Differential diagnoses include medullary nephrocalcinosis (no ectatic tubules, calcifications beyond pyramids), renal TB (calcifications larger and more irregular), and papillary necrosis (partial or total papillary slough).
Acquired cystic disease of dialysis ▷*Fig. 27.28*	Small kidneys with largely preserved contours, as the cysts varying from 0.5 to 2 cm in diameter are mostly intrarenal. Complications include hemorrhage and development of renal adenomas and carcinomas.	Up to 50% of patients on chronic dialysis. Incidence increases with time, particularly after the third year. Cystic disease may regress after renal transplantation. Renal carcinomas are associated in 7% of patients.
Von Hippel–Lindau disease ▷*Fig. 27.29a, b*	Combination of multiple renal cysts and solid tumors (carcinomas, adenomas, and hemangiomas) characteristic. Renal carcinomas are often small, < 2 cm in size, and may occur within the cysts themselves. Involvement usually bilateral and multicentric.	Inherited (autosomal dominant) neurocutaneous dysplasia complex with onset in the second to third decade. Retinal angiomatosis, cerebellar and spinal hemangioblastomas, pheochromocytomas, pancreatic tumors and cysts, hepatic adenomas, and hemangiomas may be associated.

(continues on page 794)

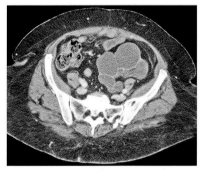

Fig. 27.24   Multicystic dysplastic kidney. A multiloculated cystic mass without functional renal parenchyma is apparent in the pelvis.

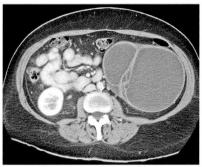

Fig. 27.25   Multilocular cystic nephroma. A large multiloculated mass is evident in the inferior pole of the left kidney.

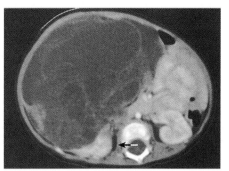

Fig. 27.26   Multilocular cystic nephroma. Large septated cystic mass originating from the right kidney (arrow) occupies over half of the abdominal cavity at this level.

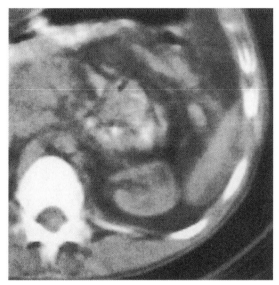

Fig. 27.27   Medullary cystic disease. Shrunken kidney with small cysts is seen. Findings were identical on the contralateral side.

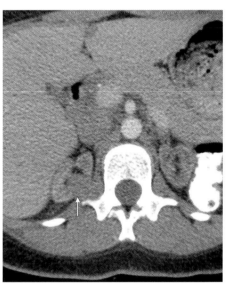

Fig. 27.28   Acquired cystic disease of dialysis. Bilateral small kidneys with tiny cysts and a small renal cell carcinoma (arrow) in the posterior aspect of the right kidney are evident.

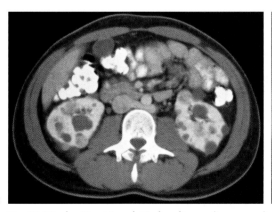

a

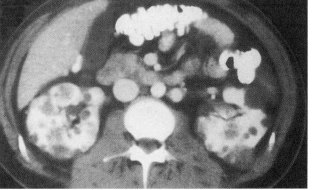

b

Fig. 27.29a, b   Von Hippel–Lindau disease (two cases). Multiple bilateral cystic and solid mass lesions in slightly enlarged bilateral kidneys are seen in both patients.

VI Abdomen and Pelvis

Table 27.2 (Cont.) Focal renal lesions

Disease	CT Findings	Comments
Renal pseudotumor ▷ *Fig. 27.30*	Focal enlargement of normal renal parenchyma simulating a tumor on other imaging studies. On CT, the mass has all the characteristics of normal renal tissue, including enhancement after IV contrast medium administration.	These anomalies include: **Fetal lobulations:** cortical bulges centered over corresponding calyces **Dromedary hump:** in the midportion of the left kidney due to prolonged pressure by the spleen during fetal development **Column of Bertin:** focal hypertrophy of the septal cortex in the midportion of the kidney causing deformation of the adjacent calyces and infundibula **Hilar lip:** supra- and infrahilar cortical bulge above and below the renal sinus **Nodular compensatory hypertrophy:** hypertrophied normal renal tissue secondary to focal renal scarring
Renal adenoma ▷ *Fig. 27.31*	Solitary or, less commonly, multiple cortical nodules measuring by definition < 3 cm in diameter. CT appearance is similar to renal cell carcinoma of the same size, that is, homogeneous and minimally hypodense to isodense on the precontrast and markedly hypodense on the postcontrast examination.	Most common cortical lesion at autopsy. May be a precursor of a renal cell carcinoma. **Metanephric adenoma** typically presents as a slightly hypoattenuating mass with little enhancement and occasionally small calcifications. **Juxtaglomerular tumor (reninoma)** is indistinguishable on CT from a renal adenoma but presents clinically with marked hypertension.
Oncocytoma ▷ *Fig. 27.32*	Solid 1- to 14-cm mass that is sharply separated from the cortex, does not invade the collecting system, and is rarely calcified. A central stellate, nonenhancing scar of lower density secondary to infarction and hemorrhage is characteristic but seen only in larger lesions (33%). After contrast administration, a homogeneous contrast enhancement that is only slightly less dense than the renal parenchyma is common, but occasionally poor tumor enhancement is found.	Seen in middle-aged patients, with a slight male predominance. Histologically, this benign tumor may be mistaken for a well-differentiated renal cell carcinoma with oncocytic features.
Angiomyolipoma (renal hamartoma) ▷ *Fig. 27.33* ▷ *Fig. 27.34* ▷ *Fig. 27.35* ▷ *Fig. 27.36*	Single or multiple renal masses ranging from 1 to 8 cm in diameter with attenuation values ranging from −100 HU (fat) to +150 HU (calcifications). Scattered punctate calcifications are rare (6%). Demonstration of intratumoral fat (≤ 20 HU) is characteristic, even if the tumor is composed mainly of vascular tissue, muscle, and hemorrhage, resulting in CT values > 20 HU in most parts of the lesion. After contrast administration, inhomogeneous tumor enhancement sparing only the fatty tissue and areas of necrosis is characteristic.	Occurs as an isolated lesion in middle-aged women (4:1 female predominance) or as renal manifestation in tuberous sclerosis (▷ *Figs. 27.37, 27.38*), where tumors are commonly multiple and bilateral. Although the CT diagnosis of angiomyolipomas is highly suggestive by the demonstration of fatty tissue, occasionally rare tumors such as renal lipomas, liposarcomas, and Wilms tumor containing small amounts of fatty tissue cannot be absolutely excluded. Renal cell carcinomas may occasionally also contain fatty tissue and calcifications.

(continues on page 796)

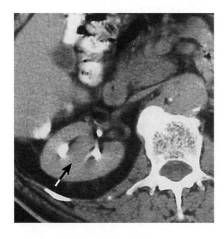

Fig. 27.30 Renal pseudotumor (column of Bertin). Hypertrophy of the septal cortex (arrow) simulates an intrarenal mass lesion on urography by causing an extrinsic filling defect on the collecting system.

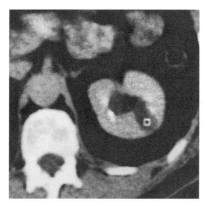

Fig. 27.31   Renal adenoma. A small hypodense lesion is seen in the renal cortex after contrast enhancement. On the precontrast scan, the lesion was isodense with the adjacent renal parenchyma and therefore not appreciated.

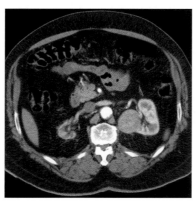

Fig. 27.32   Oncocytoma. A large solid mass with less enhancement than the adjacent renal parenchyma is seen originating from the medial aspect of the left kidney.

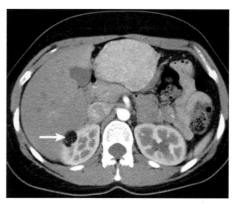

Fig. 27.33   Angiomyolipoma. A small, fatty lesion (arrow) is seen in the lateral aspect of the right kidney.

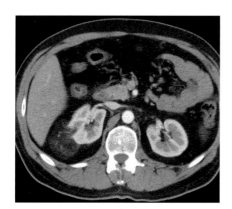

Fig. 27.34   Angiomyolipoma. A large, predominantly fatty lesion with mild enhancement of the nonfatty components is seen on the posterolateral aspect of the right kidney.

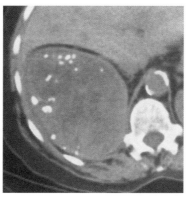

Fig. 27.35   Angiomyolipoma. A large, well-defined mass containing fatty foci and scattered calcifications are seen. Calcifications are rare in this condition (only 6% of cases).

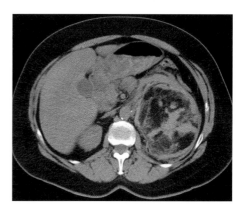

Fig. 27.36   Hemorrhagic angiomyolipoma. Spontaneous rupture of an angiomyolipoma is a frequent complication resulting in a large complex renal mass with extension into the perirenal and pararenal space, as seen here on the left side.

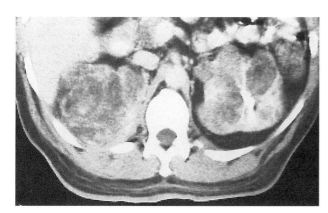

Fig. 27.37   Tuberous sclerosis. Bilaterally enlarged and deformed kidneys containing large inhomogeneous tumor masses (angiomyolipomas) with fatty components are characteristic.

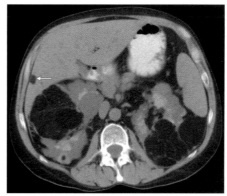

Fig. 27.38   Tuberous sclerosis. Bilateral large and deformed kidneys containing huge angiomyolipomas with considerable fatty components are seen. Note the small hamartoma in the liver (arrow).

Table 27.2 (Cont.) Focal renal lesions

Disease	CT Findings	Comments
Renal cell carcinoma ▷ *Fig. 27.39* ▷ *Fig. 27.40* ▷ *Fig. 27.41* ▷ *Fig. 27.42*	Homogeneous or heterogeneous, irregularly shaped, and poorly demarcated mass producing an irregular or lobulated renal contour and distortion of the collecting system. The attenuation is slightly less than that of normal renal parenchyma. Less commonly, the tumor is isodense or hyperdense (e.g., after recent intratumoral hemorrhage and tumor calcifications) on precontrast scans. Rarely, renal cell carcinomas are largely to completely cystic. Calcifications occur in 20% of patients and usually are central and amorphous or peripheral and curvilinear in cystic renal cell carcinomas. Intratumoral metaplasia into fatty marrow occurs occasionally in larger lesions. After contrast administration, the nonnecrotic parts of the tumor demonstrate an unequivocal increase in density, that is, less than the surrounding normal renal parenchyma, making the tumor more apparent on contrast-enhanced scans. Tumor spread to the perinephric fat, local lymph nodes and vessels, and adjacent organs can also be depicted in more advanced stages.	Most common malignant renal tumor, accounting for > 80% of all renal primaries. Twice as frequent in men as women and rare in patients younger than 40 y (peak age 55 y). Gross hematuria (60%) and flank pain (50%) are the most common clinical presentation. Bilateral involvement in 2% of cases. CT is most valuable for both diagnosing and staging. **Robson staging system:** **Stage I:** tumor confined to kidney **Stage II:** tumor spread to perinephric fat **Stage IIIA:** tumor spread to renal vein or inferior vena cava (IVC) **Stage IIIB:** tumor spread to local lymph nodes **Stage IIIC:** tumor spread to both local vessels and lymph nodes **Stage IVA:** tumor spread to adjacent organs (except ipsilateral adrenal) **Stage IVB:** distant metastases
Medullary renal tumor	Large, ill-defined mass centered in the renal medulla with extension into the renal sinus and cortex. Contrast enhancement may be heterogeneous due to varying amounts of hemorrhage and necrosis. Renal medullary carcinoma and collecting duct carcinoma are differentiated.	**Renal medullary carcinoma** (▷ *Fig. 27.43*): Highly aggressive malignant tumor of epithelial origin occurring almost exclusively in adolescent and young adult blacks with sickle cell trait (not with hemoglobin SS sickle cell disease), with mean survival rate of 15 weeks from diagnosis. Presents as large, ill-defined, heterogeneous mass centered in the renal medulla with extension into the renal sinus and cortex and nonuniform contrast enhancement. **Collecting duct carcinoma (Bellini)** (▷ *Fig. 27.44*): High-grade, infiltrative neoplasm centered in the renal medulla with renal sinus invasion, cortical extension, and metastases in 40% at presentation. Mean age 55 y (range 13–80 y).
Renal transitional cell carcinoma ▷ *Fig. 27.45* ▷ *Fig. 27.46*	Small tumors are often not detectable on precontrast scans but present as a smooth or irregular (frondlike) filling defect in the opacified renal pelvis. Contrast enhancement of the tumor itself is only subtle (8–40 HU precontrast, up to 55 HU postcontrast). Larger tumors cause hydronephrosis, obliterate the peripelvic fat, and invade the renal parenchyma and vessels, but they do not affect renal contour. Tumor calcifications are very rare.	Most common uroepithelial tumor (85%), multiple in one third of the cases. Majority (70%) of patients are men older than 60 y. Hematuria occasionally associated with flank pain is the most common clinical presentation. **Squamous cell carcinoma** (15%) is frequently associated with chronic leukoplakia. Renal calculi are present in 50% of patients, and tumor calcification occurs in 10%. The prognosis is very poor, as the tumor is usually well advanced at the time of diagnosis. **Nephrogenic adenoma** is an uncommon benign metaplastic response to a urothelial injury or prolonged irritation presenting as a papillary or polypoid filling defect in the renal pelvis. Malignant transformation is rare.

(continues on page 798)

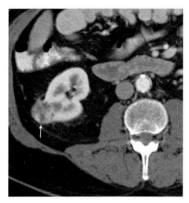

Fig. 27.39 Renal cell carcinoma. An inhomogeneously enhancing mass is seen in the posterolateral aspect of the right kidney (arrow).

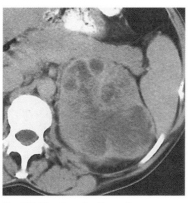

Fig. 27.40 Renal cell carcinoma. Large renal mass with hypodense areas due to tumor necrosis is evident.

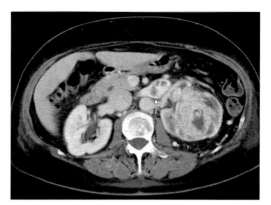

Fig. 27.41 Renal cell carcinoma. A large mass with inhomogeneous enhancement is seen in the left kidney. The tumor extends into the left renal vein (arrow), which is focally enlarged and depicts filling defects.

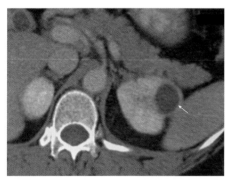

Fig. 27.42 Renal cell carcinoma. A well-defined homogeneous lesion with minimal enhancement is seen in the lateral aspect of the left kidney, mimicking a renal cyst.

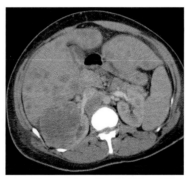

Fig. 27.43 Renal medullary carcinoma. A large right renal mass with multiple liver metastases is seen.

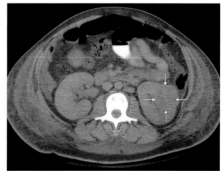

Fig. 27.44 Collecting duct carcinoma (Bellini). A renal mass (arrows) originating in the renal medulla and isodense to the normal renal parenchyma on this precontrast scan is seen in the left kidney.

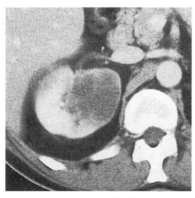

Fig. 27.45 Transitional cell carcinoma. A large, hypodense mass is shown in the area of the renal hilum.

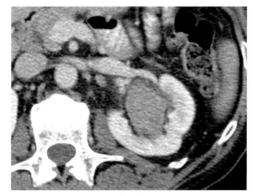

Fig. 27.46 Transitional cell carcinoma. A large, poorly enhancing mass lesion is seen in the left renal hilum.

VI Abdomen and Pelvis

Table 27.2 (Cont.) Focal renal lesions

Disease	CT Findings	Comments
Wilms tumor (nephroblastoma) ▷ *Fig. 27.47* ▷ *Fig. 27.48*	Large, inhomogeneous mass often with central hypodense areas representing cysts, necrosis, and/or hemorrhage. Calcifications are unusual. An enhanced rim of compressed renal parenchyma (pseudocapsule) is frequently present. Rarely, a large cyst with irregularly thickened wall and septa is the dominant feature. Tumor invasion into the renal vein occurs in one third of cases. In adults, the tumor is virtually indistinguishable from a renal cell carcinoma, except for a large central necrosis, which is more typical for the latter. **Staging:** 1. Tumor limited to kidney 2. Local extension into perirenal tissue, renal vein, and/or para-aortic lymph nodes 3. Not totally resectable (peritoneal implants, distant lymph node metastases in abdomen and pelvis) 4. Hematogenous metastases and/or lymph node metastases above diaphragm 5. Bilateral renal involvement	Most often in children between 1 and 5 y of age presenting usually with an asymptomatic abdominal mass. Hypertension, hematuria, aniridia, and hemihypertrophy (Beckwith–Wiedemann syndrome) may be associated. Metastases to lungs are frequent, less common to liver and lymph nodes. In contrast to neuroblastomas, bone metastases and tumor calcifications are rare. **Mesoblastic nephroma (▷ *Fig. 27.49*):** Benign intrarenal mass in neonates with CT appearance similar to Wilms tumor, but without venous extension. **Nephroblastomatosis:** Multiple nodules of primitive metanephric tissue. Benign condition with unilateral or bilateral renal involvement predisposing to the development of a Wilms tumor.
Rhabdoid tumor of the kidney	Centrally located, heterogeneous renal mass with indistinct borders and frequent central necrosis. Tumor lobules may be outlined by linear calcifications. Subcapsular crescent-shaped hematoma is associated in half of the cases.	Most aggressive renal neoplasm in childhood, typically occurring before the age of 2. May be associated with primary brain tumor of neuroectodermal origin (e.g., medulloblastoma, primitive neuroectodermal tumor [PNET]).
Renal lymphoma ▷ *Fig. 27.50* ▷ *Fig. 27.51* ▷ *Fig. 27.52*	Homogeneous infiltrate or mass, slightly hypodense on pre-contrast and markedly hypodense on postcontrast scans. Bilateral involvement common. Manifestations: 1. Renal enlargement caused by diffuse infiltration with maintenance of the normal renal contour 2. Multiple nodules 3. Solitary intrarenal mass 4. Retroperitoneal disease extending into the renal pelvis 5. Compression of the collecting system or vascular structures causing hydronephrosis or a nonfunctioning kidney After contrast enhancement, the lymphomatous tissue increases only slightly in attenuation.	Late manifestation of the disease, caused by hematogenous spread or direct extension from adjacent pararenal lymphoma. Absence of clinical symptoms in > 50% of patients. Leukemia can also produce bilateral renal enlargement and intrarenal masses (▷ *Fig. 27.53*).
Renal metastases ▷ *Fig. 27.54* ▷ *Fig. 27.55* ▷ *Fig. 27.56*	Solitary renal mass or, more commonly, multiple nodules of varying sizes. Metastases are usually small and do not distort the renal contour or the collecting system.	Most common renal malignancy at autopsy, but infrequently diagnosed antemortem. Lung and breast carcinomas are the most common primaries, but stomach, colon, pancreas, cervix, and gonads are other sites of origin.

(continues on page 800)

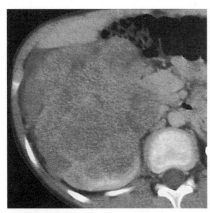

Fig. 27.47 Wilms tumor. A large, inhomogeneous mass originating from the right kidney is seen.

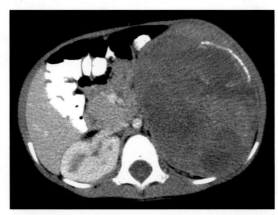

Fig. 27.48 Wilms tumor. A large, slightly inhomogeneous, hypodense left renal mass with peripheral calcification is seen.

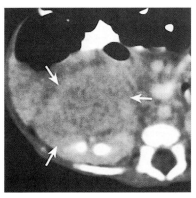

Fig. 27.49 Mesoblastic nephroma. The soft tissue mass (arrows) in a neonate originates from the posteriorly displaced right kidney, with the contrasted collecting system seen as two white dots just anterior to the visualized right rib.

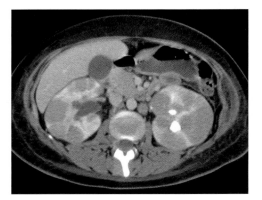

Fig. 27.50 Renal lymphoma. Bilateral enlarged kidneys with multiple hypodense lesions are evident in this postcontrast scan. Enlarged retroperitoneal lymph nodes are also seen.

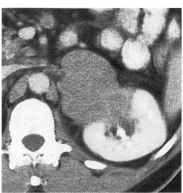

Fig. 27.51 Non–Hodgkin lymphoma. A large, hypodense, homogeneous mass is seen in the retroperitoneum extending into the renal hilum.

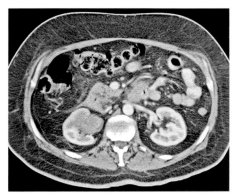

Fig. 27.52 Burkitt lymphoma. A large right central renal mass that is poorly demarcated against the normal renal parenchyma is seen on this postcontrast examination.

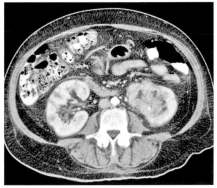

Fig. 27.53 Leukemia. A poorly defined mass in the left kidney and small peripheral nodules in the cortex of the right kidney, giving it a somewhat striated appearance, are leukemic renal manifestations.

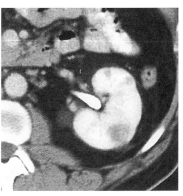

Fig. 27.54 Renal metastases. Three poorly defined, hypodense nodules are seen in the renal cortex (metastases from bronchogenic carcinoma).

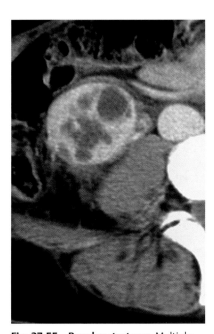

Fig. 27.55 Renal metastases. Multiple hypodense lesions of different sizes are shown in the right kidney on this postcontrast scan (melanoma metastases).

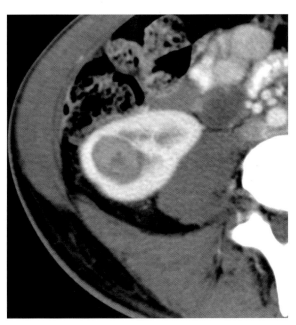

Fig. 27.56 Renal metastasis. A solitary hypodense lesion is seen in the lateral aspect of the right kidney on this postcontrast scan (metastasis from a squamous cell carcinoma originating in the hypopharynx).

Table 27.2 (Cont.) Focal renal lesions

Disease	CT Findings	Comments
Mesenchymal renal tumors (benign or malignant) ▷ *Fig. 27.57* ▷ *Fig. 27.58*	No characteristic features except for the demonstration of fatty tissue in lipomas and liposarcomas (see also angiomyolipoma) and the irregular peripheral contrast enhancement proceeding centrally in hemangiomas.	Very rare. **Ossifying renal tumor of infancy** presents as benign calcified (80%) filling defect in the renal pelvis with poor enhancement on CT.
Renal abscess ▷ *Fig. 27.59*	Cavitating mass with thick, irregular wall and liquefied center of decreased density simulating a necrotic neoplasm. After contrast administration, the wall of the abscess enhances, whereas the liquefied central part of the abscess does not. Perinephric extension and thickening of the renal fascia are common. Demonstration of gas bubbles or a gas–fluid level within the mass is virtually diagnostic but only rarely present.	The CT appearance of a renal abscess may be difficult to differentiate from a necrotic renal cell carcinoma.
Pyelonephritis, acute ▷ *Fig. 27.60* ▷ *Fig. 27.61* ▷ *Fig. 27.62* ▷ *Fig. 27.63*	Renal involvement may be unilateral or bilateral, diffuse or, more commonly, focal. Findings depend on the severity of the infection. Size of the involved kidney is normal to diffusely enlarged. On the precontrast scan, the affected renal area is isodense to slightly hypodense and poorly marginated. Occasionally, inflammatory (edematous) changes in the perinephric fat and mild thickening of both the renal fascia and the walls of the renal pelvis and calyces can be appreciated. Slight dilation of the renal pelvis and ureter is frequently also present. After contrast enhancement, a patchy inhomogeneous enhancement is evident that is, however, less than in the nonaffected part of the kidney. These hypoattenuating zones extending from the papilla into the cortex are typically wedge-shaped in the nephrographic phase. Other findings include poor corticomedullary differentiation after an intravenous material bolus and a striated nephrogram that may persist for an extended period of time.	Most commonly an ascending *Escherichia coli* infection presenting with fever, chills, and flank pain. Patients with altered host resistance (e.g., diabetes, immunosuppression), mechanical or functional ureteral or bladder outlet obstruction, including stones, and chronic catheterization are predisposed. Hematogenous route of infection accounts for 15% of cases. May occur at any age, with marked female prevalence. Acute focal pyelonephritis is also referred to as renal phlegmon. **Emphysematous pyelonephritis** *(▷ Fig. 27.64)* is a life-threatening necrotizing infection usually in diabetics. Mottled areas of gas extending radially along the pyramids are diagnostic. Gas may also be found in the perinephric and retroperitoneal space and occasionally the renal veins. **Chronic atrophic pyelonephritis** is usually associated with vesicoureteral reflux. Calyceal dilation with overlying cortical scarring, preferentially located in the polar regions, is characteristic.
Xanthogranulomatous pyelonephritis ▷ *Fig. 27.65*	Diffuse or, much less commonly, focal renal enlargement with poor or no contrast excretion (global or focal). Solitary or multiple nonenhancing masses with lobulated contours and frequent extension into the perinephric space and occasionally adjacent organs are a typical presentation. A large central calculus and a pyonephrotic collecting system that may be distorted or partially replaced by the inflammatory masses are characteristically present.	Chronic suppurative granulomatous infection in a chronically obstructed kidney (usually due to nephrourolithiasis), occasionally by stricture or tumor. Most cases are associated with *Proteus* infections. All ages are affected (peak: fourth to fifth decade), with a 3:1 female predominance. Involvement may be diffuse (90%) or focal (tumefactive form).

(continues on page 802)

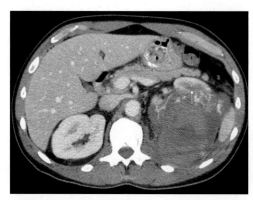

Fig. 27.57 Renal angiosarcoma. A huge hypodense renal mass is seen in the left kidney displacing its noninvolved small anterior portion (arrow) anteriorly.

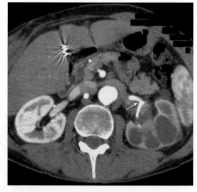

Fig. 27.58 Renal rhabdomyosarcoma. An infiltrating hypodense mass causing enlargement of the left kidney encircles and angulates the left renal artery (arrow).

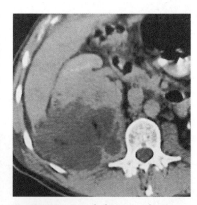

Fig. 27.59 Renal abscess. A large renal abscess in the posterior aspect of the right kidney is seen as a hypodense lesion extending into the perirenal and pararenal spaces and psoas muscle.

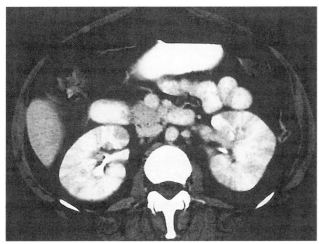

Fig. 27.60 Acute pyelonephritis. After contrast enhancement, linear, radially oriented, low-density areas are seen in the renal parenchyma bilaterally.

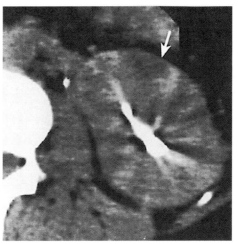

Fig. 27.61 Focal nephritis. A larger, poorly defined, hypodense area (arrow) is evident after contrast enhancement. The patchy, inhomogeneous enhancement of the enlarged remaining kidney indicates a more widespread pyelonephritic involvement.

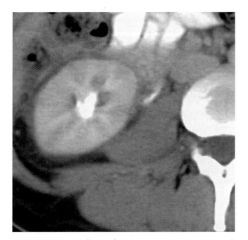

Fig. 27.62 Pyelonephritis. A persistent striated nephrogram is seen in the enlarged right kidney.

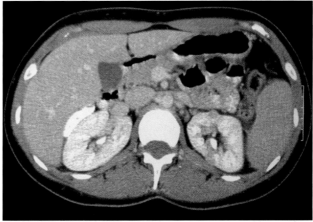

Fig. 27.63 Pyelonephritis. Bilateral enlarged kidneys with a patchy to striated nephrogram are shown.

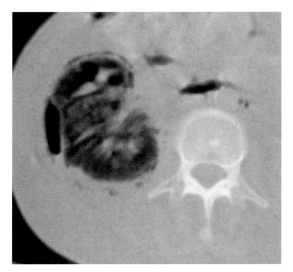

Fig. 27.64 Emphysematous pyelonephritis. An enlarged right kidney depicting extensive streaky to mottled gas collections throughout the renal parenchyma with extension into the perirenal space is seen.

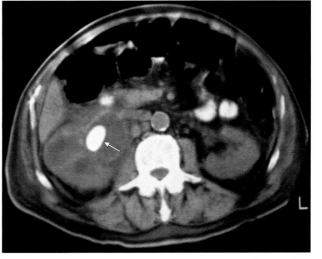

Fig. 27.65 Xanthogranulomatous pyelonephritis. Diffuse renal enlargement with several hypodense masses and a large calculus (arrow) in the renal pelvis is seen.

Table 27.2   (Cont.) Focal renal lesions

Disease	CT Findings	Comments
Renal trauma ▷ *Fig. 27.66* ▷ *Fig. 27.67* ▷ *Fig. 27.68*	**Intrarenal (renal contusion):** Focal area of decreased nephrogram with poor opacification of corresponding calyces. **Subcapsular:** Lenticular defect with flattening of the adjacent renal parenchyma. On precontrast scan, the hematoma is usually hypodense, but immediately after injury, occasionally a higher density than the surrounding kidney may be found. After contrast administration, the density of the nonenhancing hematoma is always markedly decreased compared with the normal renal parenchyma.	Renal biopsies, extracorporeal shock-wave lithotripsy, and trauma are common causes. Spontaneous hematomas in the absence of bleeding diathesis should raise suspicion of an underlying malignancy or an angiomyolipoma. **Classification of renal trauma:** 1. Limited to renal parenchyma: renal contusion or subcapsular hematoma without disruption of calyceal system and renal capsule. 2. Complete laceration or renal fracture with involvement of renal capsule and/or calyceal system. 3. Shattered kidney (multiple separate renal fragments) or injury to the renal vascular pedicle.
Renal infarction ▷ *Fig. 27.69* ▷ *Fig. 27.70*	**Regional:** Peripheral wedge-shaped areas of decreased density, typically between calyces and most obvious after contrast administration. **Total (renal artery occlusion):** After contrast enhancement, a thin subcapsular rim of high density caused by capsular collaterals to the outer cortex surrounds a central zone of diminished density.	Caused by trauma (avulsion of the renal artery), embolism, thrombosis, and renal vein thrombosis. The latter is diagnosed by an enlarged renal vein containing a filling defect on enhanced CT scans. An exaggerated and prolonged corticomedullary differentiation may be evident in the acute stage.
Arteriovenous malformation (AVM) ▷ *Fig. 27.71*	Well-defined intrarenal mass lesion with attenuation values similar to the aorta or IVC before and after contrast administration. Large feeding and draining vessels are also characteristic. Curvilinear calcifications are rare.	Congenital or acquired (trauma, biopsy, spontaneous rupture of an aneurysm, very vascular malignant neoplasm). Intrarenal aneurysm or pseudoaneurysm of the renal artery may present similarly except for the absent feeding and draining vessels.

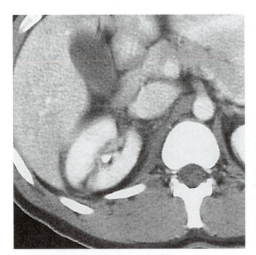

Fig. 27.66   Renal fracture. Complete transection of the right kidney is seen.

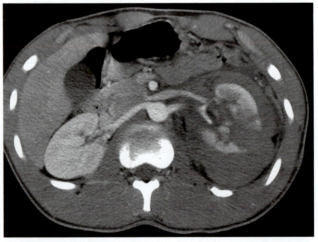

Fig. 27.67   Renal trauma. Shown here is a shattered left kidney with a large surrounding hematoma extending into the perirenal and pararenal space.

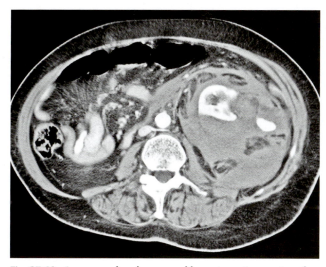

Fig. 27.68   Large renal and pararenal hematoma in a ruptured angiomyolipoma. A ruptured kidney with a huge surrounding hematoma is seen. The angiomyolipoma is not appreciated on this image.

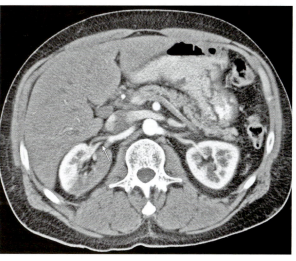

Fig. 27.69   Renal infarction. Nonperfusion of the lower half of the right kidney. A thrombus (arrow) in the enlarged nonopacified right renal artery is also evident.

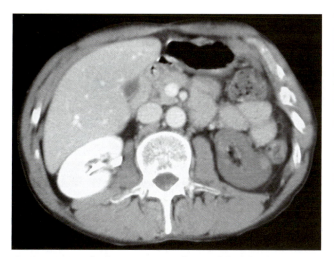

Fig. 27.70   Renal infarction. Nonperfusion of the left infarcted kidney is seen.

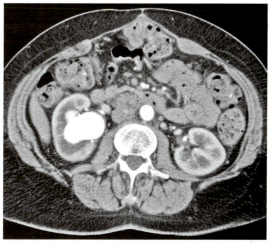

Fig. 27.71   Renal artery aneurysm. A large right central renal mass enhancing immediately with the same intensity as the abdominal aorta is characteristic.

Table 27.3 Focal lesions in the perinephric space

Disease	CT Findings	Comments
Urinoma ▷ *Fig. 27.72*	Localized or diffuse cystic lesion of low density with attenuation values ranging from −10 to +20 HU. Contrast extravasation into the fluid collection may be evident on late enhanced images. Long-standing urinomas may have well-defined walls. Large urinomas may dissect along tissue planes into the pelvis.	Usually associated with urinary tract obstruction, renal trauma, or iatrogenic interventions, although nonobstructive infectious and spontaneous urinomas occur.
Lymphocele	Homogeneous cystic, occasionally septated lesion with CT appearance similar to urinoma.	Develops usually 2 weeks or more after lymph node dissection or renal surgery.
Lipoma and fibroma	Small, homogeneous, well-circumscribed mass lesions originating from the renal capsule or fascia or perinephric fat.	Usually incidental findings. Benign mesenchymal tumors are even rarer than their malignant counterparts.
Liposarcoma	Variable appearance ranging from a soft tissue mass with only little adipose tissue (poorly differentiated liposarcoma) to a predominantly fatty, somewhat heterogeneous mass with irregularly thickened linear or nodular septa (well-differentiated liposarcoma) or a cystic lesion (myxoid liposarcoma). Larger tumors tend to displace rather than invade the renal parenchyma and have a smooth interface. Contrast enhancement is variable but tends to be poor.	Most common mesenchymal sarcoma originating from the perinephric fat or renal capsule and fascia. Other rare primary perinephric malignancies are malignant fibrous histiocytomas, leiomyosarcoma, and angiosarcoma.
Metastases and lymphoma ▷ *Fig. 27.73*	Findings depend on histology of the primary lesion and mode of tumor spread.	Direct extension or local metastases from primary renal, adrenal, and retroperitoneal malignancies. Rarely hematogenous or lymphangitic spread from more distant organs.
Abscess ▷ *Fig. 27.74* ▷ *Fig. 27.75* ▷ *Fig. 27.76*	Low-density mass, often with thick, irregular walls, that may enhance. Inflammatory (edematous) changes surrounding the lesion are common. Thickened renal fascia and perinephric strands may also be associated. Gas presenting as bubbles or air–fluid levels within the lesion is virtually diagnostic but only rarely present.	Usually an extension of underlying renal disease, especially a concomitant renal abscess. Diabetes mellitus and uronephrolithiasis are common predisposing factors. Other inflammatory conditions, such as pancreatitis, diverticulitis, and appendicitis, may spread into the perinephric space.
Hematoma ▷ *Fig. 27.77* ▷ *Fig. 27.78*	Well- (hemorrhagic cyst) to poorly defined, often inhomogeneous mass lesion that may displace the adjacent kidney. CT densities range from 80 HU (acute) to 20 HU (chronic). Rarely, a fluid–fluid level is evident, caused by the settling of cellular elements within the hematoma (hematocrit effect). No enhancement on the postcontrast scan unless acutely bleeding.	Traumatic etiologies include blunt or penetrating trauma, renal biopsy, percutaneous nephrostomy and nephrolithotomy, and extracorporeal shock-wave lithotripsy. Spontaneous (nontraumatic) etiologies include nephritis, arthritis, lupus, polyarteritis nodosa, acquired cystic disease of dialysis, renal tumors, blood dyscrasia, anticoagulation therapy, and aneurysms of the renal artery and abdominal aorta.

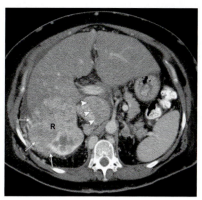

Fig. 27.72 Urinoma. A large, homogeneous fluid collection is seen extending from the ruptured right kidney into the perirenal and pararenal space.

Fig. 27.73 Renal cell carcinoma with local extension. A right renal cell carcinoma (R) with extension into the pararenal space (arrows), liver, and inferior vena cava (arrowheads) is seen.

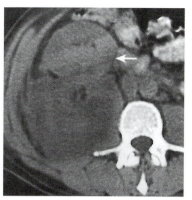

Fig. 27.74 Posterior perirenal and pararenal abscess. A hypodense mass is shown in the posterior renal fossa displacing the right kidney (arrow) anteriorly.

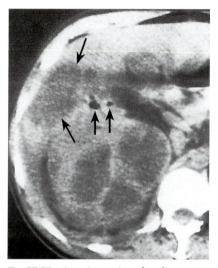

Fig. 27.75 Anterior perirenal and pararenal abscess. A hypodense area (long arrows) is seen anterolateral to the enlarged kidney affected by xanthogranulomatous pyelonephritis. The abscess extends into the duodenum, resulting in a renoduodenal fistula containing small air bubbles (short arrows).

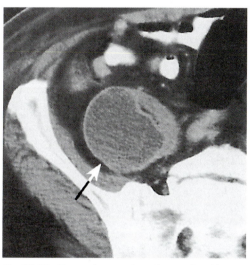

Fig. 27.76 Psoas abscess. A cystic mass is evident in the right psoas muscle.

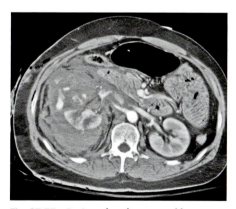

Fig. 27.77 Perirenal and pararenal hematoma. A ruptured (shattered) right kidney with large surrounding hematoma extending into the perirenal and pararenal space is seen.

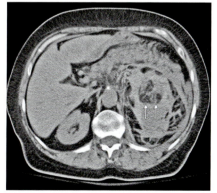

Fig. 27.78 Renal hematoma with perirenal and pararenal extension. A large intrarenal hematoma with hematocrit fluid level (arrows) secondary to a ruptured angiomyolipoma evident by its fatty components is seen. The soft tissue stranding in the perirenal and pararenal fat indicates extension of the hematoma into these spaces.

28 Adrenal Glands

Francis A. Burgener

The adrenal glands are small retroperitoneal structures readily identified by computed tomography (CT). They are located lateral to the spine at the level of the eleventh and twelfth rib and embedded in the perinephric fat that separates the kidney from the anterior (Gerota) and posterior (Zuckerkandl) renal fascia. On CT, normal adrenals extend 2 to 4 cm in a caudocranial direction and display a variety of shapes. The limbs of the adrenal glands have a uniform thickness of 5 to 8 mm with straight or concave margins. A limb thickness exceeding 10 mm is highly suggestive of adrenal disease with the exception of sites where two limbs converge.

On axial images, the right adrenal gland usually has an oblique linear configuration, paralleling the crus of the diaphragm, and rarely an inverted V, an inverted Y, an X, H, or triangular shape (**Fig. 28.1**). The right adrenal usually lies 1 to 2 cm superior to the upper pole of the right kidney and immediately posterior to the inferior vena cava. The right adrenal gland is also sandwiched between the right crus of the diaphragm medially and the right lobe of the liver laterally.

The left adrenal most often has an inverted V or an inverted Y shape and occasionally assumes a triangular shape on axial images (see **Fig. 28.1**). The left adrenal lies lateral to the crus of the left diaphragm and posterior and slightly medial to the tail of the pancreas and the stomach. The lower portion of the left adrenal may be in contact with the anteromedial aspect of the upper pole of the left kidney. The left adrenal is generally slightly caudal to the right adrenal.

Differentiating between a *benign adrenal adenoma,* an incidental finding in 2% of the general population and an *adrenal metastasis,* the overall fourth most common metastatic site in the body, is a great challenge in the staging of a tumor patient.

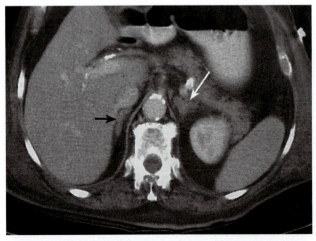

Fig. 28.1   Normal anatomy. The right adrenal (short arrow) has an oblique linear configuration paralleling the crus of the diaphragm. The left adrenal (long arrow) has a triangular shape.

Adrenocortical adenomas typically measure less than 4 cm in diameter (average size about 2 cm), enhance only mildly but uniformly after contrast material administration, and depict a relatively rapid contrast washout on delayed scans (**Fig. 28.2**). Adrenal metastases frequently measure often more than 3 cm in diameter, may be inhomogeneous, particularly when larger, tend to enhance more and less uniformly than adenomas, and demonstrate a relatively slow contrast washout. A contrast washout of 50% at 10 minutes after injection is suggestive of a benign adenoma. However, because of the substantial variability in the vascularity of metastases ranging from hypovascular to hypervascular, benign and malignant lesions cannot reliably be differentiated based on their difference in contrast enhancement and washout rates. Adrenal adenomas contain intracytoplasmic lipids (steroids) to a varying degree. Depending on the amount of these lipids, the density of these lesions is accordingly decreased when compared with soft tissue masses not containing any fat. Therefore, on a nonenhanced scan, a uniform CT density of less than 20 HU in a solid lesion strongly suggests a benign adenoma. Fat suppression techniques in magnetic resonance imaging (MRI) appear even more useful for the differentiation between benign adrenal adenomas and metastases. The approach that appears most promising is the combined use of an in-phase/out-of-phase gradient echo technique. This chemical shift-imaging method allows assessment of the intracellular fat content. Benign adenomas containing intracytoplasmic lipids lose signal intensity on out-of-phase images, whereas metastases do not. However, adenomas that do not contain lipids in sufficient quantities and other benign masses cannot be differentiated from metastases with this technique. More recently, positron emission tomography (PET) scan has been shown to more accurately identify adrenal metastases when the primary tumor takes up F 18 fluorodeoxyglucose.

Adrenal calcifications are associated with tumors, hemorrhage, and infections. Tumor calcifications (**Fig. 28.3**) are very common in neuroblastomas (80%); not unusual in myelolipomas, pheochromocytomas, and adrenal carcinomas (about 20% each); and rare in cortical adenomas. Calcifications in adrenal hemorrhage (**Fig. 28.4**) and infections are late sequelae of the disease occurring usually 1 y or later after the insult. Adrenal hemorrhage may be traumatic or nontraumatic (e.g., neonatal stress, surgery, burns, hypotension with shock, pregnancy, hemorrhagic diathesis, coagulopathy, and anticoagulation therapy). Calcification in a hemorrhagic pseudocyst characteristically is curvilinear ("eggshell" calcification). Infections commonly associated with adrenal calcifications include tuberculosis, histoplasmosis, and Waterhouse–Friderichsen syndrome (fulminant meningococcemia). Bilateral adrenal hemorrhage and infections with destruction of more than 90% of the adrenal cortex result in adrenal insufficiency (Addison disease).

The differential diagnoses of focal or diffuse adrenal enlargement are discussed in **Table 28.1.**

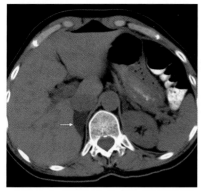 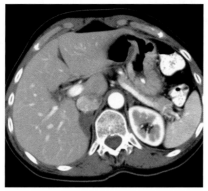 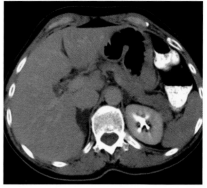

a   b   c

Fig. 28.2a–c   Contrast material washout of a benign adrenal cortical adenoma. (a) Precontrast. An enlarged, uniformly hypodense right adrenal (arrow) is seen bordered by the inferior vena cava anteriorly, the liver laterally, and the right crus of the diaphragm medially. **(b)** Postcontrast (30 s after intravenous (IV) contrast material injection). Mild homogeneous enhancement of the enlarged right adrenal is seen. **(c)** Postcontrast (10 min after IV contrast material injection). Contrast material washout from the enlarged right adrenal is virtually complete.

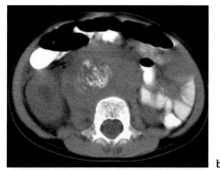 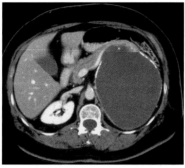 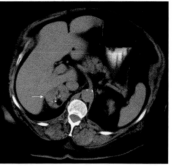

a   b   c

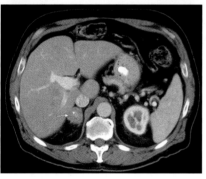

Fig. 28.3a–d   Adrenal tumor calcifications. Neuroblastoma (**a**). A large mass with irregular speckled central calcification is seen. Pheochromocytoma (**b**). A huge nonenhancing, low-density lesion with curvilinear calcifications is seen in the left abdomen. Myolipoma (**c**). A soft tissue mass (arrow) with foci of fat and tiny calcifications is seen. Adrenal cortical adenoma (**d**). A small soft tissue lesion (arrow) with a tiny calcification is seen.

d

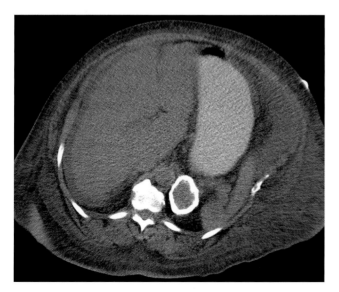

Fig. 28.4   Calcified adrenal hematoma. Extensive rim calcification in an enlarged left adrenal is evident.

VI Abdomen and Pelvis

Table 28.1 Focal or diffuse adrenal enlargement

Disease	CT Findings	Comments
Adrenal pseudotumors	Both normal anatomical and pathologic structures can simulate an adrenal mass, especially on the left side. Such structures include medial lobulation of the spleen, accessory spleen, outpouchings of adjacent stomach or small bowel, colonic interposition between the kidneys and liver, tortuous renal vessels, tortuous splenic artery, portosystemic venous collaterals in portal hypertension (e.g., spontaneous splenorenal shunt), and masses arising from the kidneys, liver, pancreas, or retroperitoneum.	Most of these pseudotumors can be differentiated from a true adrenal lesion with proper administration of intravenous (IV) and oral contrast material. Furthermore, a normal adrenal gland is present in these conditions.
Adrenal cyst and pseudocyst	Small to very large, usually unilateral, round, low-density mass with a smooth, well-defined contour. Rim calcification is rare except in echinococcal cysts and hemorrhagic pseudocysts.	Rare. True cysts are endothelial (e.g., lymphangiomatous or angiomatous), epithelial, or parasitic in origin. Pseudocysts are more common and result from hemorrhage and necrosis.
Adrenal cortical hyperplasia ▷ *Fig. 28.5*	Diffuse bilateral adrenal enlargement with preservation of the normal glandular shape. Hyperplastic glands usually have smooth outlines. Less commonly, the enlarged adrenals may have a nodular or lumpy appearance, with nodules measuring up to 2 cm in diameter (macronodular hyperplasia).	**Cushing syndrome** (hypercortisolism) is caused in 80% of cases by bilateral adrenal cortical hyperplasia, but in one third of the patients, the adrenals are normal by CT criteria. The syndrome is 4 times more common in women, with the highest incidence between 20 and 40 y of age. **Conn syndrome** (primary aldosteronism) presents in 20% of cases with bilateral nodular adrenal hyperplasia and is characterized by mild hypertension, hypokalemia, sodium retention, and reduced plasma renin levels. **Congenital adrenal cortical hyperplasia** (inborn block of adrenal cortical steroid production) causes in utero virilization of female offsprings and precocious puberty in male offsprings.
Adrenal cortical adenoma ▷ *Fig. 28.3a–d, p. 807* ▷ *Fig. 28.6* ▷ *Fig. 28.7*	Unilateral, well-defined, homogeneous mass measuring 2 to 4 cm in diameter. Depending on the lipid content, density ranges from soft tissue to near water. In the latter case, ultrasound may confirm the solid nature. Calcification is rare. IV contrast enhancement typically is mild, and the contrast washout is rapid. Differentiation from metastases is discussed in greater detail in the introductory text to this chapter.	Most common adrenal mass and most frequently nonhyperfunctioning and incidentally diagnosed. Increased occurrence in elderly, obese, or hypertensive patients or with carcinomas of the bladder, kidney, or endometrium. Hyperfunctioning adrenal adenomas are responsible for 15% of cases with Cushing syndrome. **Aldosteronomas** are responsible for 80% of Conn syndrome. The tumor averages less than 2 cm in diameter (range 0.5–3.5 cm) and is located twice as frequently on the left than the right side. On MRI, its signal intensity is typically increased on T2-weighted imaging when compared with nonhyperfunctioning adenomas.
Pheochromocytoma ▷ *Fig. 28.8* ▷ *Fig. 28.9* ▷ *Fig. 28.10*	Usually unilateral, large soft tissue mass measuring 3 to 12 cm in diameter. Smaller tumors may be entirely solid. Hemorrhage and necrosis are commonly present in larger tumors, producing central regions of low density to an almost completely cystic appearance that may be difficult to differentiate from a true cyst or pseudocyst. Calcifications are present in up to 20% of cases. After IV contrast administration, a marked enhancement with slow washout is present in nonnecrotic areas.	Secretion of high amounts of catecholamines results in paroxysmal attacks characterized by hypertension, diaphoresis, tachycardia, and anxiety. Elevated urinary metanephrine and vanillylmandelic acid levels are characteristic. Approximately 10% are bilateral, 10% malignant, 10% extra-adrenal (organ of Zuckerkandl at origin of inferior mesenteric artery, para-aortic sympathetic chain, gonads, urinary bladder, and mediastinum), 10% familial (associated with Sipple or multiple endocrine neoplasia [MEN II] syndrome, mucosal neuroma or MEN III syndrome, von Hippel–Lindau syndrome, or neurofibromatosis).

(continues on page 810)

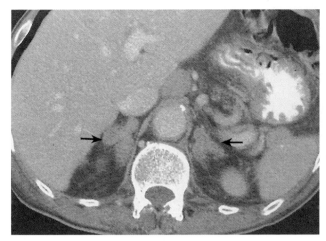

Fig. 28.5　Cortical hyperplasia. Diffuse bilateral adrenal enlargement with nodular appearance (arrows) is seen.

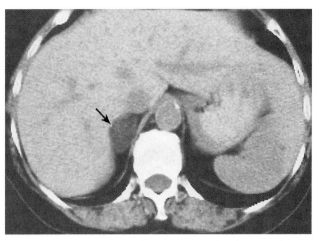

Fig. 28.6　Adrenal cortical adenoma. A well-defined, homogeneous, low-density mass (arrow) is seen.

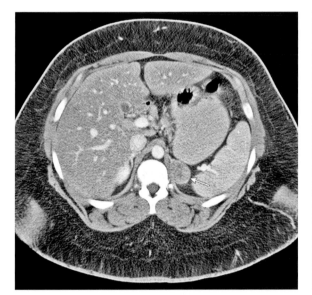

Fig. 28.7　Adrenal cortical adenoma. An enlarged left adrenal (arrow) with little contrast enhancement is seen.

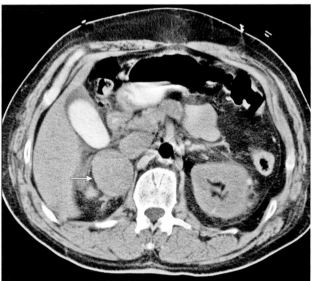

Fig. 28.8　Pheochromocytoma. A round, well-defined, homogeneous soft tissue mass (arrow) originating in the right adrenal is seen. Note also the milk of calcium bile (lime bile syndrome).

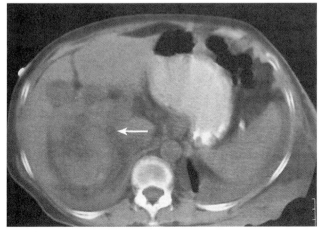

Fig. 28.9　Pheochromocytoma. A large mass (arrow) is seen with central regions of low density due to necrosis. Increased density of the perirenal fat is caused by hemorrhage from the pheochromocytoma.

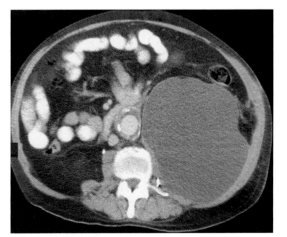

Fig. 28.10　Pheochromocytoma. A large cystlike lesion without enhancement is seen in the left abdomen. The finding is the sequela of extensive necrosis and hemorrhage within the original tumor.

Table 28.1   (Cont.) Focal or diffuse adrenal enlargement

Disease	CT Findings	Comments
Myelolipoma ▷ *Fig. 28.11* ▷ *Fig. 28.12* ▷ *Fig. 28.13*	Unilateral, usually small, well-defined mass, but occasionally measuring up to 12 cm in diameter. The lesion consists primarily of fatty tissue that may contain foci of calcifications in 20%. Less commonly, the tumor is of soft tissue density with small regions of fatty tissue.	Rare benign asymptomatic tumor consisting of myeloid (megakaryocytes) and erythroid elements and mature fat cells. Flank or abdominal pain may develop secondary to hemorrhage or necrosis.
Mesenchymal adrenal tumors	CT features are not characteristic except in cavernous hemangiomas that present as low-density masses with central and/or peripheral calcifications (phleboliths) and a distinctive enhancement pattern (peripheral discontinuous ring of nodules) seen immediately after IV contrast material administration.	Extremely rare. Besides hemangiomas, other lesions such as lymphangiomas, fibromas, neurofibromas, myomas, and hamartomas, as well as their malignant counterparts, occur.
Neuroblastoma ▷ *Fig. 28.14* ▷ *Fig. 28.15* ▷ *Fig. 28.16* ▷ *Fig. 28.17*	Irregular, usually unilateral soft tissue mass frequently containing low-density areas due to hemorrhage and necrosis and punctate to coarse calcifications. Considerable inhomogeneous enhancement is typically evident after IV contrast material administration. Invasion of the kidney and retroperitoneal lymph nodes with extension across the midline and encasement of the inferior vena cava, aorta, and its major vessels is characteristic in the advanced stage.	Approximately 80% occur in children younger than 3 y. Vanillylmandelic acid and homovanillic acid in urine are characteristic. Metastases (bone 60%, lymph nodes 40%, liver 15%, intracranial 14%, and lungs 10%) are already present in the majority of children at the time of diagnosis. Histologic spectrum ranges from the highly malignant **sympathicogonioma** to the relatively benign **ganglioneuroma** Adult neuroblastomas are rare and extra-adrenal sites are more frequent (e.g., mediastinum, retroperitoneum, and pelvis), and calcifications are uncommon.
Adrenal cortical carcinoma ▷ *Fig. 28.18* ▷ *Fig. 28.19*	Unilateral, inhomogeneous soft tissue mass usually measuring more than 4 cm at the time of diagnosis. Tumor diameters in excess of 10 cm are not unusual. They commonly contain low-density areas due to necrosis. Contrast enhancement is inhomogeneous, and the washout is delayed. Dystrophic calcifications are more common than in adenomas. Frequent complications, especially in larger lesions, include tumoral hemorrhage and central necrosis.	Occurs at any age and presents commonly with abdominal pain and palpable mass. Fifty percent of adrenal cortical carcinomas are hormonally active (twice as common in women), and patients may develop Cushing syndrome.

(continues on page 812)

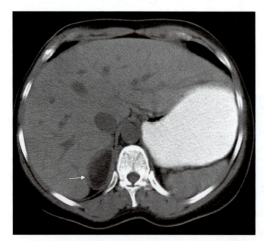

Fig. 28.11   Myelolipoma. An ovoid predominantly fatty lesion (arrow) is seen originating in the right adrenal.

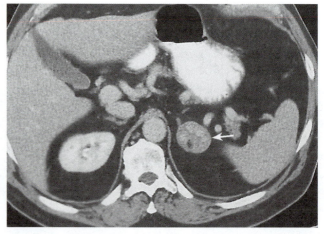

Fig. 28.12   Myelolipoma. A well-defined soft tissue mass (arrow) is seen containing a small focus of fatty tissue.

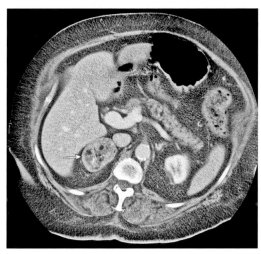

Fig. 28.13 **Myelolipoma.** A soft tissue lesion (arrow) containing several foci of fatty tissue and tiny calcifications is seen.

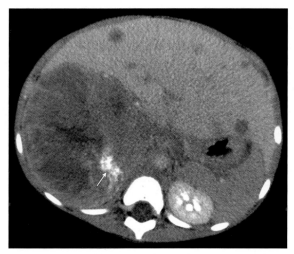

Fig. 28.14 **Neuroblastoma.** A large inhomogeneous soft tissue mass with calcifications (arrow) is seen in the right sub-hepatic region with extension into the retroperitoneum. Note also the peripheral low-density lesion in the liver representing metastases.

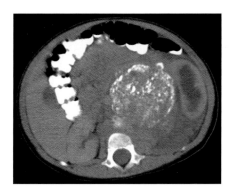

Fig. 28.15 **Neuroblastoma.** A large mass with extensive speckled calcifications is seen.

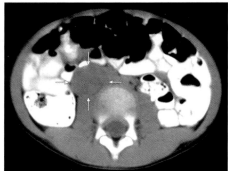

Fig. 28.16 **Ganglioneuroma.** A homogeneous round lesion (arrows) with similar to slightly less density than the surrounding muscle is seen.

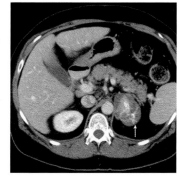

Fig. 28.17 **Ganglioneuroma.** An ovoid mass (arrow) with patchy enhancement is seen originating from the left adrenal.

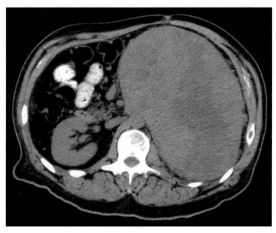

Fig. 28.18 **Adrenal cortical carcinoma.** A huge soft tissue mass with multiple hypodense areas caused by tumor necrosis is evident in the left abdomen.

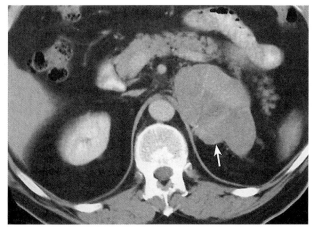

Fig. 28.19 **Adrenal cortical carcinoma.** A large mass (arrow) with slightly hypodense central regions is seen.

Table 28.1   (Cont.) Focal or diffuse adrenal enlargement

Disease	CT Findings	Comments
Adrenal metastases ▷ *Fig. 28.20* ▷ *Fig. 28.21* ▷ *Fig. 28.22*	Unilateral or bilateral. Usually relatively small lesions, but may attain any size. The density of the metastases is similar to the primary tumor or other metastatic deposits, provided they are comparable in size. Small metastases tend to be homogeneous, but with increase in size, intratumoral hemorrhage and necrosis occur more frequently. Marked contrast enhancement with delayed washout is typical after IV contrast material administration. Direct extension occurs from renal and pancreatic carcinomas. Differentiation of small adrenal metastases from adrenal adenomas is discussed in greater detail in the introductory text of this chapter.	Hematogenous adrenal metastases originate in order of decreasing frequency from carcinomas of the lung, breast, gastrointestinal tract, or thyroid, and melanomas. A small adrenal mass in a patient with a known tumor is, however, more likely a cortical adenoma than a metastatic deposit. **Primary adrenal lymphoma** is exceedingly rare and of the non-Hodgkin variety. In secondary lymphoma, retroperitoneal lymphadenopathy is usually present.
Adrenal granuloma ▷ *Fig. 28.23* ▷ *Fig. 28.24*	Unilateral or, more commonly, bilateral adrenal enlargement, often with hypodense regions representing necrosis. Calcification may subsequently develop which can become quite dense. Such calcifications in the absence of a soft- tissue mass strongly suggest chronic granulomatous disease rather than tumor. Contrast enhancement is usually modest.	Tuberculosis, histoplasmosis, and blastomycosis are the most frequent infectious sources. **Adrenal abscesses** are rare in adults but occur more frequently in neonates secondary to meningococcal infections (Waterhouse–Friderichsen syndrome). **Addison disease** (adrenal insufficiency) may be a late sequela of granulomatous disease, especially histoplasmosis. Autoimmune disease (idiopathic) and pituitary insufficiency are more common causes.
Adrenal hemorrhage ▷ *Fig. 28.25* ▷ *Fig. 28.26*	Unilateral or bilateral homogeneous adrenal masses measuring up to 3 cm. Lesions are either hyperdense or of soft tissue density. Progressive decrease in size and density of the adrenal masses on follow-up examinations. Calcifications may develop as late sequelae. Development of a hemorrhagic pseudo-cyst, often with curvilinear (eggshell) calcification, is another late presentation.	Anticoagulation therapy is the most common cause. Bleeding diathesis, sepsis, shock, trauma, major surgery, and pregnancy are other predisposing factors. Bilateral involvement may result in acute adrenal insufficiency that is potentially fatal. If not fatal, **Addison disease** may be a late sequela. Posttraumatic adrenal hemorrhage is limited in 85% to the right side. Right adrenal hemorrhage is also a complication of liver transplantation. In the neonate, adrenal hemorrhage may be associated with birth trauma, hypoxia (prematurity), septicemia, and bleeding disorders.

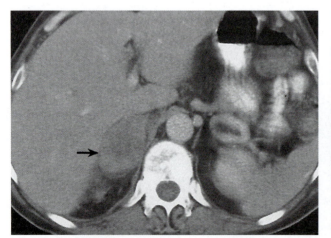

Fig. 28.20   Adrenal metastasis. A right adrenal metastasis (arrow) originating from a bronchogenic carcinoma is seen.

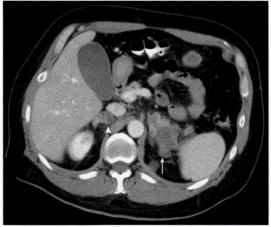

Fig. 28.21   Adrenal metastases. An enlarged and deformed left adrenal (arrow) with multiple hypodense nodules is seen. A small hypodense metastasis (arrowhead) is also seen in the nonenlarged right adrenal. The primary tumor was a bronchogenic carcinoma.

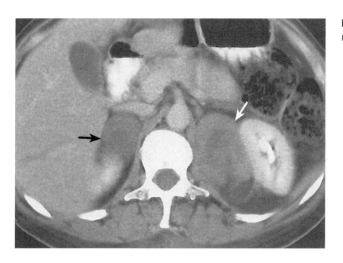

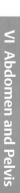

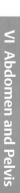

Fig. 28.22 Bilateral adrenal metastases. Large bilateral adrenal metastases (arrows) are seen originating from a liposarcoma.

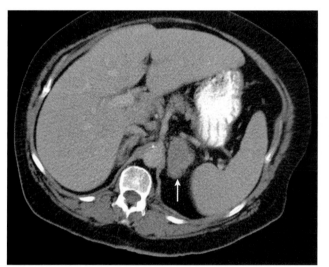

Fig. 28.23 Adrenal histoplasmoma. An enlarged, triangular, left adrenal (arrow) is seen with slightly reduced attenuation centrally when compared to its periphery.

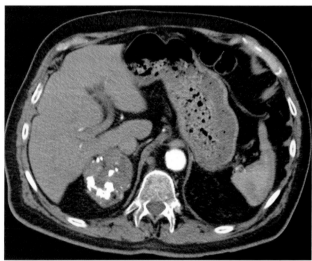

Fig. 28.24 Adrenal tuberculoma. An enlarged right adrenal with scattered irregular dense calcifications and small hypodense foci is seen.

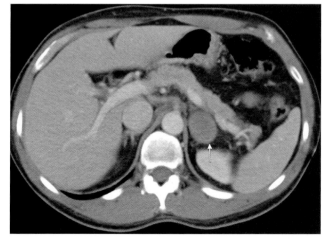

Fig. 28.25 Adrenal hematoma (subacute). An enlarged left adrenal (arrow) without enhancement is seen.

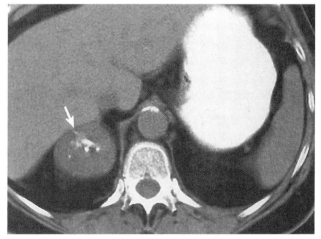

Fig. 28.26 Calcified adrenal hematoma. An enlarged right adrenal gland (arrow) with irregular central calcifications is seen.

29 Pelvis

Grégory Dieudonné and Francis A. Burgener

An understanding of soft tissue and bony pelvic anatomy on computed tomography (CT) aids in the detection of pelvic diseases and recognition of their patterns of spread. Nearly all major organ systems are represented in the pelvis, including the gastrointestinal (GI), genitourinary, central and peripheral nervous, angiolymphatic, and musculoskeletal systems. The limits of the pelvis are defined by the innominate bones, sacrum, and coccyx. The internal and external pelvic muscular and bony frameworks are relevant, as disease processes arising in these structures sometimes manifest within the pelvic cavity (**Figs. 29.1, 29.2**).

The *pelvic peritoneal reflections* delineate significant but not insurmountable boundaries between extraperitoneal structures and the peritoneal cavity. The peritoneal reflections over the pelvic organs, vessels, and ligaments define several peritoneal pelvic cavity recesses, the largest and most gravity-dependent of which is the rectovesicle pouch. The rectovesicle pouch, along with the pelvic portion of the greater omentum, is one of the most common sites of tumor implants in peritoneal carcinomatosis.

Pelvic peritoneal reflections often form anatomical landmarks recognizable on CT images where they envelop organs and the associated vascular and lymphatic systems. The peritoneal reflection forming the sigmoid mesocolon encompasses a portion of the proximal rectum and sigmoid colon, along with their associated angiolymphatic structures. The sigmoid mesocolon is more easily seen in the presence of ascites (**Fig. 29.3**). In addition, the small bowel and its mesentery, as well as their associated pathologic processes, often extend into the pelvis (**Fig. 29. 4**).

In women, the broad ligament is that part of the peritoneal reflection surrounding the margins of the uterus, fallopian tubes, and proximal round ligaments extending to the pelvic sidewall. The ovary is attached to the posterior broad ligament by the mesovarium. The peripheral broad ligament from the ovary to the pelvic sidewall that contains the ovarian vessels is referred to as the *suspensory ligament of the ovary*. The uterus divides the rectovesical pouch into the anterior vesicouterine pouch and the posterior rectouterine pouch, also known as the *cul-de-sac* or *pouch of Douglas.*

Although the remaining pelvic structures, such as the rectum, anus, distal ureters, bladder, cervix, vagina, seminal vesicles, prostate, and sidewall structures, do not readily protrude into the pelvic peritoneal cavity, they are often associated with fascial planes that frequently confine pathologic processes. These boundaries localize lesions to their site of origin, guiding the differential diagnosis of a pelvic mass.

Ectopic organs, such as pelvic kidneys (**Fig. 29.5**), are readily identified on CT. Pelvic testicles present as elliptical foci along the course of the testicles' descent, frequently within the inguinal canal (**Fig. 29.6**).

Some surgical procedures may result in *pseudolesions* due to the displacement of normal pelvic structures. In particular, abdominoperineal resection of the rectum can result in a posterior presacral position of the uterus in women or the prostate and seminal vesicles in men (**Fig. 29.7**). These normal presacral masses must be distinguished from presacral recurrent tumor and postoperative fibrosis. If a suspicious mass is encountered, biopsy is warranted. If there is question that a presacral mass is a displaced normal structure such as the seminal vesicles or uterus, magnetic resonance imaging (MRI) is often helpful.

Midline or lateral surgical transposition of the ovaries in women can also be problematic if the history of this procedure is not elicited, especially if there is a superimposed functional cyst. Lateral surgical ovarian transposition procedures are sometimes performed to preserve ovarian function in young women with cervical carcinoma who will receive radiation therapy. The ovaries are placed in the iliac fossae or high in the lateral abdomen (**Fig. 29.8**). Midline ovarian transposition may be performed in young women who will receive pelvic nodal radiation for lymphoma.

Other iatrogenic "pseudolesions" are intestinal urinary reservoirs in patients with urinary diversions, tissue expanders to displace bowel from radiation ports prior to radiation therapy (**Fig. 29.9**), and implanted reservoirs for penile prostheses and artificial sphincters.

Renal and pancreatic transplants are usually placed within the pelvis (**Fig. 29.10**). Although they are typically imaged with ultrasound, CT is occasionally performed. The pancreatic transplant is often connected to the bladder by a segment of bowel to allow drainage of exocrine fluids. Care must be taken to avoid confusing this with an abnormal collection. Renal and pancreatic peritransplant collections, such as hematomas, seromas, abscesses, urinomas, lymphoceles, and pancreatic pseudocysts, are readily detected with CT.

The accompanying tables of differential diagnoses of pelvic pathologic processes are predominantly organized by organ of origin. However, because the exact site of origin is not always evident, tables relating to a variety of lesions disseminating within the peritoneal cavity and originating from the pelvic cavity walls are also included. **Table 29.1** discusses pelvic GI lesions, **Table 29.2** lesions of the female and male pelvis, **Table 29.3** urinary bladder lesions, and **Table 29.4** peritoneal and extraperitoneal lesions.

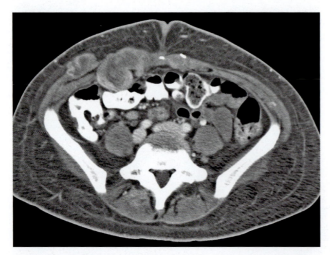

Fig. 29.1 Abdominal wall desmoid. Heterogeneously enhancing soft tissue mass in the anterior abdominal wall with impression onto the colon.

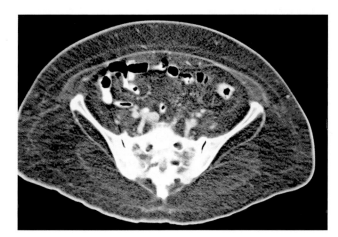

Fig. 29.2 Muscular dystrophy. Diffuse fatty replacement of muscles.

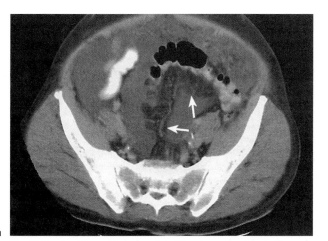

a

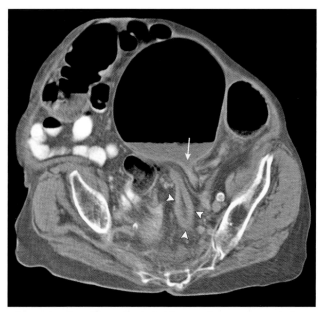

b

Fig. 29.3a, b Sigmoid mesocolon. The sigmoid colon and its mesentery (arrows), referred to as the sigmoid mesocolon, are suspended by pelvic ascites in this patient with carcinomatosis (**a**). Distended air–fluid-filled sigmoid tapering to a beak (arrow) without perceived wall thickening/mass. Note the collapsed twisted segment (arrowheads) of the distal sigmoid (sigmoid volvulus: twisting of the mesocolon about its mesenteric axis) (**b**).

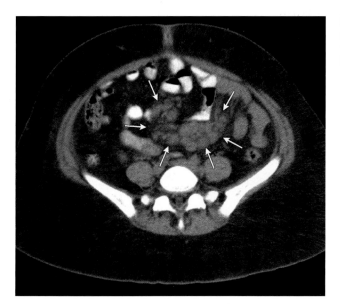

Fig. 29.4 Mesenteric adenopathy. Multiple soft tissue attenuation nodes distributed within the small bowel mesentery (arrows); contrast this with the nonopacified bowel segments within the left anterior hemipelvis.

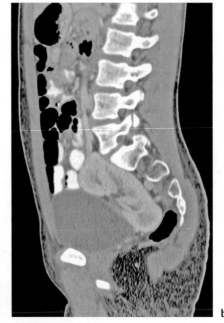

Fig. 29.5a, b **Congenital pelvic kidney.** Axial (**a**) and parasagittal (**b**) views showing the ectopic location of the left kidney within the pelvis.

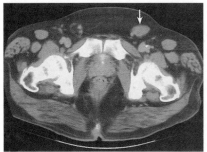

Fig. 29.6 **Undescended testis.** The undescended testicle (arrow) in this patient is within the left inguinal canal.

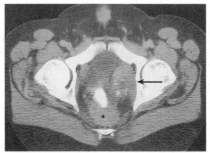

Fig. 29.7 **Pelvis following abdominoperineal resection for rectal carcinoma.** Normal presacral prostate position (star) following abdominoperineal resection. There is also partially calcified left obturator adenopathy (arrow) due to recurrent tumor.

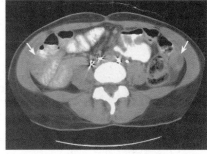

Fig. 29.8 **Ovarian transposition.** The ovaries (arrows) were surgically placed in the lateral abdomen in this patient undergoing pelvic radiation for cervical carcinoma.

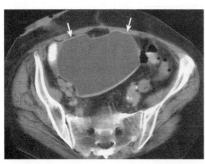

Fig. 29.9 **Tissue expander.** Surgically placed expandable device (arrows) that is used to displace the bowel from the area of a radiation port.

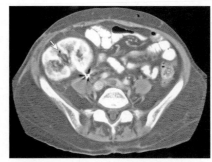

Fig. 29.10 **Renal transplant.** Kidney within the anterior right hemipelvis. Note the surgical clips, focus of calyceal gas (arrow). This patient has a filling defect (thrombus) within the left common iliac vein.

Table 29.1   Pelvic gastrointestinal lesions

Disease	CT Findings	Comments
Carcinoma ▷ *Fig. 29.11* ▷ *Fig. 29.12*	Segmental wall thickening or polypoid luminal masses. Search for lymph nodes, hepatic metastases, and peritoneal or omental tumor implants.	Often difficult to distinguish bowel contractions and luminal fecal material from focal lesion. Rescan area of concern or barium enema versus small bowel follow-through may be necessary to confirm in the absence of associated secondary signs of tumor (e.g., perienteric fat infiltration).
Lymphoma ▷ *Fig. 29.13*	Segmental or diffuse, irregular or smooth bowel wall thickening, sometimes associated with luminal expansion. May occur with or without adenopathy.	These are typically non–Hodgkin lymphomas. Gastrointestinal (GI) lymphoma may also be encountered in patients positive for human immunodeficiency virus (HIV) and in posttransplant lymphoproliferative disorder.
Mesenchymal neoplasms ▷ *Fig. 29.14*	Polypoid luminal or exophytic intermediate-attenuation mass causing luminal narrowing. The presence of calcifications would favor this diagnosis. Lipomas (see also **Fig. 29.25**) typically are polypoid and usually have uniform fat attenuation.	Other types of mesenchymal neoplasms are leiomyomas, leiomyosarcomas, and carcinoid tumors. Cystic necrosis is often seen in leiomyosarcomas. Carcinoid tumors may have associated mesenteric fibrotic response, which can lead to intestinal ischemia.
Metastases ▷ *Fig. 29.15a, b*	Soft tissue nodules, adjacent to or impinging on the small bowel lumen. Scirrhous lesions, intramural deposits, or polypoid intraluminal masses may be present. The greatest portion of the metastatic deposit is located in the mesentery adjacent to the wall of the small bowel. An omental "cake" may be recognized as an extensive soft tissue mass separating the colon or small bowel from the anterior abdominal wall.	Most common primary tumors are carcinomas of lung, breast, colon, pancreas, kidney, uterus, and skin.

(continues on page 818)

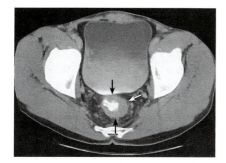

Fig. 29.11   Rectal carcinoma. Nearly completely circumferential rectal tumor (arrows) with associated perirectal lymph nodes.

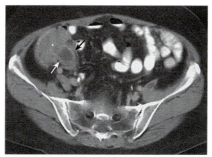

Fig. 29.12   Cecal carcinoma. The tumor (star) also obstructs the appendix (arrows).

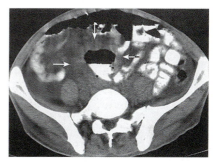

Fig. 29.13   Small bowel lymphoma. Extraluminal contrast and air fill a necrotic lymphomatous mass (arrows) in this patient positive for human immunodeficiency virus (HIV).

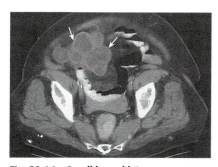

Fig. 29.14   Small bowel leiomyosarcoma. Cystic exophytic distal ileal tumor (arrows).

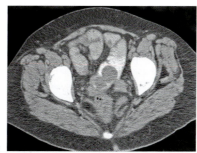
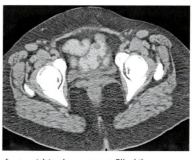

Fig 29.15a, b   Melanoma. Polypoid filling defects within the contrast-filled ileum.

VI Abdomen and Pelvis

Table 29.1 (Cont.) Pelvic gastrointestinal lesions

Disease	CT Findings	Comments
Diverticulitis ▷ *Fig. 29.16*	Segmental wall thickening with or without pericolonic infiltrative changes, fistulas, and/or abscesses. Usually occurs in patients with visible diverticula.	Majority of cases involve sigmoid colon, rarely other colonic sites or small bowel diverticula.
Inflammatory bowel disease ▷ *Fig. 29.17* ▷ *Fig. 29.18* ▷ *Fig. 29.19*	Segmental or diffuse, irregular or smooth bowel wall thickening, with or without perienteric infiltration.	Examples include Crohn disease, which may involve several bowel segments, with or without fistulas; typically spares rectum. May also observe associated mesenteric fibrofatty proliferation. Graft versus host disease can lead to fold and wall thickening and can be associated with pneumatosis intestinalis. Radiation enteritis can be acute and present within a few weeks of therapy, or chronic, manifesting a few months or more after therapy. Acute effects are due to direct cellular toxicity and chronic effects from a radiation-induced vasculitis.
Infectious enterocolitis ▷ *Fig. 29.20*	Segmental or diffuse, irregular or smooth bowel wall thickening. Nonneoplastic bowel wall thickening will often result in a low- (near-water) attenuation value at the sites of involvement.	Examples include pseudomembranous colitis, which may produce marked wall thickening, and other microbial agents, such as cytomegalovirus, which is a common HIV-related infection.
Ischemia ▷ *Fig. 29.21* ▷ *Fig. 29.22* ▷ *Fig. 29.23a–c*	Segmental or diffuse, irregular or smooth bowel wall thickening with or without pneumatosis intestinalis.	Survey mesenteric arteries and veins for the presence of thrombi and/or gas. Ischemia typically spares the rectum because of its dual blood supply.

(continues on page 820)

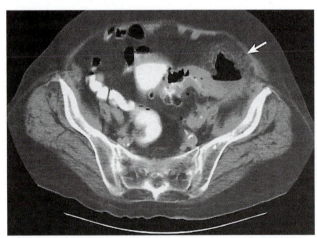

Fig. 29.16 Diverticulitis with abscess. Localized perforation (arrow) has led to abscess formation in this patient with diverticulitis.

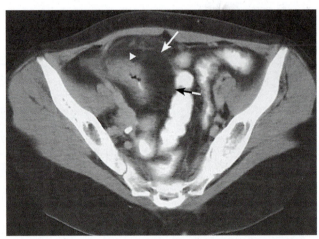

Fig. 29.17 Crohn disease. Terminal ileum with wall thickening (arrowhead) and associated fibrofatty mesenteric proliferation (arrows).

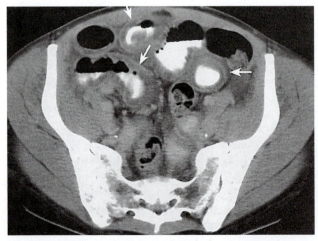

Fig. 29.18 Graft versus host disease. Small bowel graft versus host disease with wall thickening (arrows) following bone marrow transplant for lymphoma.

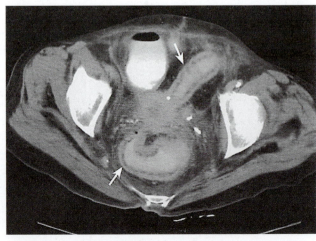

Fig. 29.19 Radiation enteritis. Rectosigmoid wall thickening (arrows) due to chronic radiation enteritis several years following treatment of a gynecological malignancy.

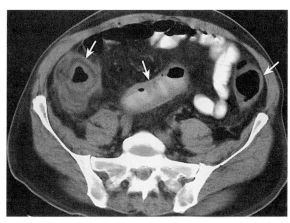

Fig. 29.20 Pseudomembranous colitis. Patient who had previously received antibiotics returned 2 weeks after appendectomy with abdominal pain. Note the typical pattern and appearance of the colonic wall (arrows) in this condition.

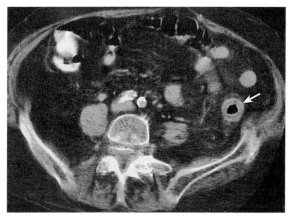

Fig. 29.21 Left colon ischemia. Patient with abdominal pain and hematochezia has a thickened descending colon wall (arrow).

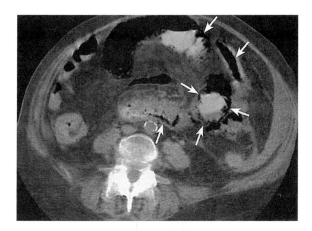

Fig. 29.22 Ischemic small bowel with pneumatosis. Typical pattern of pneumatosis and wall thickening (arrows) in the setting of ischemic/infarcted bowel. Note the pneumatosis encircling luminal contents when the bowel is seen in transverse section.

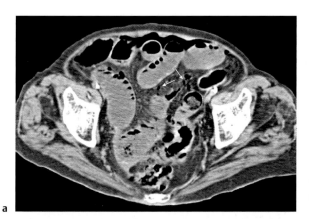

a

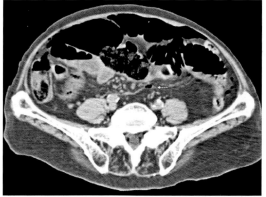

b

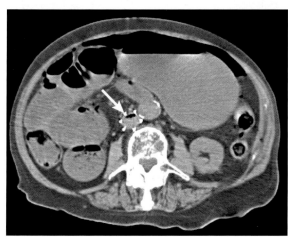

c

Fig 29.23a–c Infarcted bowel. Venous gas (short arrows) (a,b). Inferior vena cava (IVC) gas (long arrow) and pneumoperitoneum (**c**).

Table 29.1   (Cont.) Pelvic gastrointestinal lesions

Disease	CT Findings	Comments
Endometriosis	Mixed or uniform intermediate- to high-attenuation focal or diffuse mural masses.	High-attenuation adnexal masses with fluid–fluid levels on nonenhanced scans may be an associated finding. Often indistinguishable from neoplasia by CT alone.
Intussusception ▷ *Fig. 29.24* ▷ *Fig. 29.25a–d*	Short-axis section of bowel produces target appearance, and long-axis section of bowel produces ribbon appearance of involved segment with or without associated high-attenuation oral contrast and low-attenuation mesenteric fat.	Often idiopathic in children. Identifiable causes are more common in adults and include polypoid neoplasms and Meckel diverticula.
Congenital lesions	Cystic or tubular masses in or adjacent to the bowel wall.	Duplication cysts may communicate with the bowel or be associated with rectogenitourinary fistulas, duplications of genital structures, or skeletal abnormalities.
Appendicitis/mucocele ▷ *Fig. 29.26*	Thick-walled or distended appendix with or without appendicolith or periappendiceal abscess/infiltrative changes.	In middle-aged or older patients with appendicitis or mucocele, rule out underlying cecal malignancy (see also **Fig. 29.12, p. 817**).
Pneumatosis intestinalis	Intramural air may be difficult to recognize on standard soft tissue windows and levels. Viewing images at settings for lung detail can facilitate detection (see **Fig. 29.22, p. 819**).	Differential diagnosis includes ischemia/infarction and less ominous etiologies, such as scleroderma. Clinical correlation is frequently the best predictor of its significance.

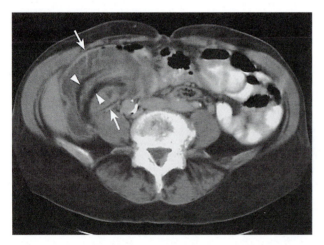

Fig. 29.24   Intussusception. Idiopathic ileocolonic intussusception (arrows) in an adult. Note the ribbon appearance (arrowheads) of the intussuscepted small bowel mesenteric fat.

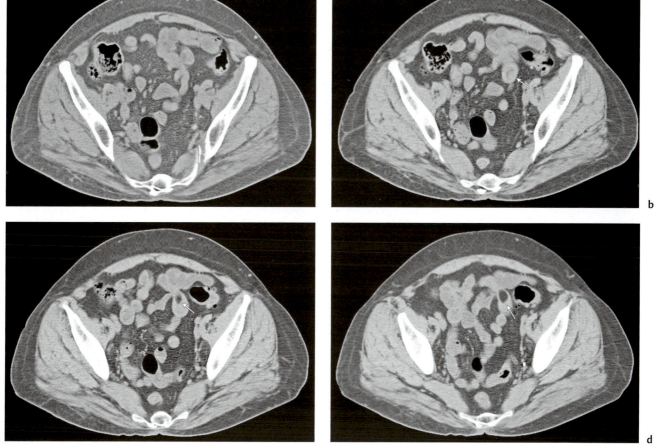

Fig. 29.25a–d   Small bowel lipoma (intussusception). Intraluminal fat attenuation mass (arrow) serving as the lead point.

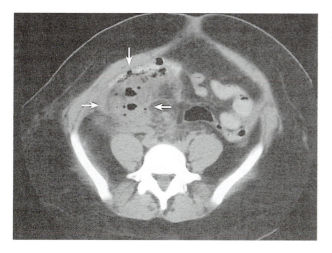

Fig. 29.26   Perforated appendicitis. Localized right lower quadrant mesenteric air and fluid (arrows) following appendiceal perforation.

Table 29.2   Reproductive system lesions

Disease	CT Findings	Comments
Female		
Ovary and tubes		
Carcinoma ▷ *Fig. 29.27* ▷ *Fig. 29.28*	Cystic and/or solid masses with or without ascites and omental or peritoneal surface tumor implants. Debris and septations within cysts are sometimes difficult to recognize on CT.	Isolated cystic masses < 5 cm in women of childbearing age are most often benign functional cysts, but if > 2.5 cm, masses require short-interval follow-up by clinical exam or ultrasound to ensure resolution.
Benign neoplasms	Cystic and/or solid masses. In the absence of obvious metastases, benign neoplasms cannot be reliably distinguished from malignant neoplasms on CT.	Includes adenomas, fibromas, serous or mucinous cystadenomas, and dermoids/teratomas. Meigs syndrome is the association of ovarian fibroma, hydrothorax (usually right-sided), and ascites.
Dermoid/teratoma ▷ *Fig. 29.29* ▷ *Fig. 29.30a, b* ▷ *Fig. 29.31*	Frequently contains fat and/or calcifications/ossifications. May have cystic or soft tissue components.	Other fat-containing adnexal masses, such as lipomas and lipoleiomyomas, are rare.
Metastases ▷ *Fig. 29.32* ▷ *Fig. 29.33*	Usually solid-appearing; not commonly recognized on CT.	Common sites of origin include bowel and breast.
Functional cysts ▷ *Fig. 29.34a, b*	May appear cystic or solid, depending on the amount of associated internal debris/hemorrhage. Polycystic ovaries (Stein–Leventhal syndrome) often manifest as bilateral ovarian enlargement, but the cysts are small (usually < 1.5 cm).	Often a consideration in women of childbearing age (see comments on carcinoma). Small cystic adnexal lesions in postmenopausal women on CT are not uncommon. If the cysts lack septations or enhancing components and are of water attenuation, they can represent "retained" functional cysts; if < 3 cm, they sometimes can be followed. Caution must be exercised in the setting of family history of ovarian carcinoma and for the larger cystic lesions. Congenital cysts are rare.
Endometriosis ▷ *Fig. 29.35*	Complex masses most commonly involving adnexal regions. May contain fluid or higher attenuation material (blood), fluid–fluid levels.	May secondarily involve abdominal wall, bowel, or ureters, causing hydronephrosis.
Tubo-ovarian abscess (TOA) ▷ *Fig. 29.36*	Typically a multiloculated appearance. May be unilateral or bilateral.	
Hydrosalpinx	Serpentine fluid-filled tube ending in bulbous cystic mass(es).	In the setting of fever, consider pyosalpinx.

(continues on page 824)

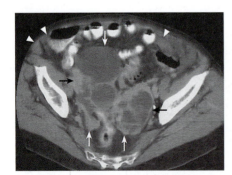

Fig. 29.27   Ovarian carcinoma. Typical appearance of a cystic and solid carcinoma (arrows) involving both adnexa. Ascites and omental tumor implants (arrowheads) are also present.

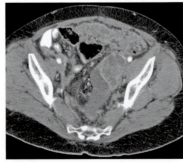

Fig. 29.28   Ovarian carcinoma with peritoneal implants. Cystic left ovarian mass with ascites and omental "caking."

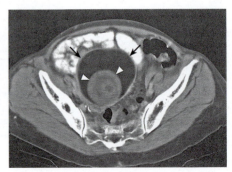

Fig. 29.29   Ovarian dermoid. Large fat-containing dermoid (arrows) with a Rokitansky nodule (arrowheads).

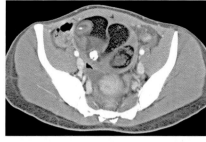
a

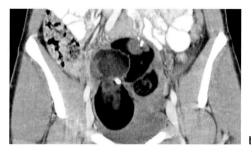
b

Fig. 29.30a, b   Dermoid. Axial (**a**) and coronal (**b**) views of a heterogeneous complex mass comprised of fat, soft tissue, and calcific attenuation.

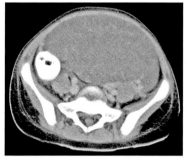

Fig. 29.31   Mixed germ cell tumor. Large solid, mildly heterogenously enhancing mass filling the pelvic cavity.

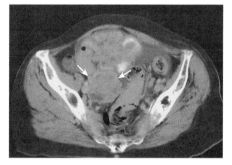

Fig. 29.32   Metastatic breast carcinoma. Patient with widely metastatic tumor also involving the right adnexa (arrows).

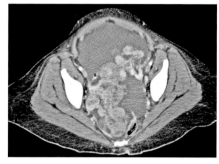

Fig. 29.33   Krukenberg tumors. Enhancing masses deposited about the adnexa.

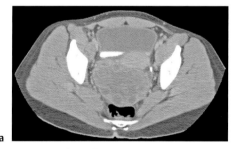
a

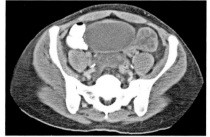
b

Fig. 29.34a, b   Polycystic ovaries (ovarian hyperstimulation). Markedly enlarged right ovary in pouch of Douglas (**a**) and less enlarged left ovary (**b**), both with peripherally distributed follicular cysts.

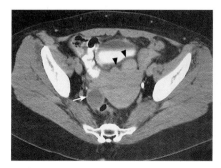

Fig. 29.35   Endometriosis. Typical pattern of an adnexal endometrioma (arrow) with a "hematocrit effect." This is not pathognomonic of endometrioma, however, and other cystic adnexal lesions should also be considered. This patient also has uterine fibroids (arrowheads).

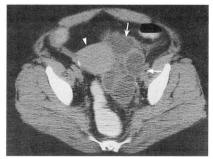

Fig. 29.36   Tubo-ovarian abscess (TOA). Typical appearance of TOA (arrows) with a pattern of multiple compartments that is often a manifestation of a dilated, tortuous fallopian tube (pyosalpinx), in addition to discrete abscesses. The uterus (arrowhead) is displaced to the right.

Table 29.2 (Cont.) Reproductive system lesions

Disease	CT Findings	Comments
Ectopic pregnancy	Indistinguishable from tumors or functional cysts.	Must consider this possibility in women of childbearing age. Pregnancy testing required if pregnancy a possibility.
Uterus and cervix		
Carcinoma ▷ *Fig. 29.37* ▷ *Fig. 29.38*	Focal or diffuse mass, often lower attenuation than myometrium following intravenous (IV) contrast. Often originates centrally; if associated with obstruction, nonenhancing hydrometrium/hematometrium may be visible.	Actual neoplastic focus can be inapparent, and frequently the only CT manifestation is an obstructed, fluid-filled uterus. Often impossible to distinguish benign cervical stenosis obstructing the uterus from malignant obstruction.
Gestational trophoblastic disease	All forms have a central, predominantly low-attenuation mass with areas of enhancement after contrast administration. The uterus may be enlarged. Choriocarcinoma and invasive mole may have myometrial invasion. Choriocarcinoma may metastasize, typically to lungs, vagina, brain, liver, kidney, and bones.	Spectrum of proliferative pregnancy-related trophoblastic tissue includes the hydatidiform mole, invasive mole, and choriocarcinoma. They are typically diagnosed with β-human chorionic gonadotropin (HCG) levels and ultrasound. There may be associated enlarged ovaries due to thecal-luteal cysts.
Sarcoma ▷ *Fig. 29.39*	Enlarged uterus with low- or isoattenuating masses often indistinguishable from other malignancies. The tumor may occupy and enlarge the central uterine cavity or be eccentric and focal with endoexophytic appearance.	Large tumors are often associated with "necrotic" appearance. Malignant change in a leiomyoma is rare, and by radiologic means alone, it is difficult to distinguish a focal leiomyoma from leiomyosarcoma. Rapid changes in size of a known lesion should be considered suspicious.
Lymphoma	Diffuse uterine and/or cervical enlargement or lobular contours mimicking fibroids.	Secondary involvement of female genitourinary (GU) tract is not uncommon in advanced non–Hodgkin lymphoma; primary lymphoma is rare.
Leiomyomas ▷ *Fig. 29.40*	Low- or isoattenuating masses, often more conspicuous after contrast. May be pedunculated, with or without calcifications. Uncommonly associated with areas of fatty change.	The most common uterine mass affecting 25% of women of reproductive age; often present in patients with other types of uterine or adnexal pathology.
Adenomyosis	Diffuse uterine enlargement or lobular wall thickening.	
Benign endometrial proliferative conditions	Central uterine low attenuation following IV contrast; may be indistinguishable from retained fluid.	Types include endometrial hyperplasia and polyps. In postmenopausal women, hormone replacement therapy may stimulate the endometrium. In premenopausal women, the endometrium is most prominent in the secretory (luteal) phase (usually < 1.5 cm thickness). Gestational sacs and decidual reactions (casts) in ectopic pregnancy should be considered, but they are unlikely possibilities because of routine pre-CT screening of women of childbearing age.
Nabothian cysts	Single or multiple typically round, low-attenuation cervical foci.	Form secondary to stenosis of the cervical glands. Differential diagnosis is with small cervical fibroids.
Congenital anomalies ▷ *Fig. 29.41a–c*	Unicornuate and duplex (bicornuate, uterine didelphys, septate) uteri may have unusual contours mimicking masses.	Observe for associated anomalies (e.g., undilated renal agenesis with unicornuate uterus).
Infection ▷ *Fig. 29.42*	Central fluid and/or gas.	In premenopausal women, uterine infection is usually associated with pelvic inflammatory disease or prior surgery. In postmenopausal women, there is often an associated malignancy. Postpartum uterine cavity air may be seen normally in the immediate period following uncomplicated cesarean sections and vaginal deliveries and is therefore not absolutely pathognomonic of infection in this setting.

(continues on page 826)

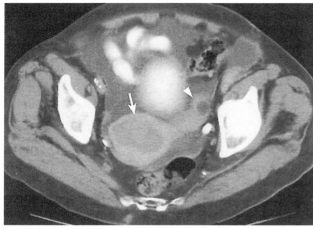

Fig. 29.37 Endometrial carcinoma. Typical pattern of enhancing central uterine mass due to carcinoma (arrow). This patient also has a synchronous cystic and solid ovarian malignancy (arrowhead).

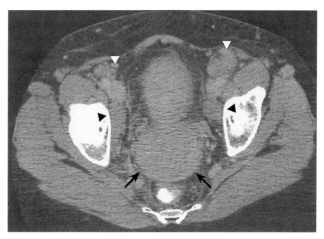

Fig. 29.38 Cervical carcinoma. Large cervical tumor (arrows) with several enlarged metastatic lymph nodes (arrowheads).

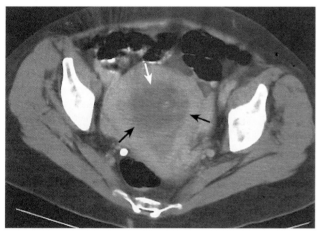

Fig. 29.39 Uterine sarcoma. Sarcomas (arrows) often present with larger masses than the more common endometrial malignancy.

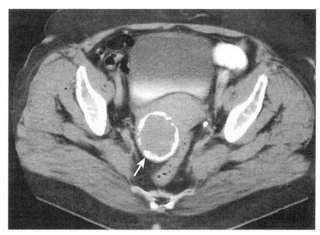

Fig. 29.40 Leiomyoma. Rim-calcified uterine leiomyoma (arrow) in this postmenopausal woman.

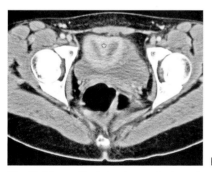
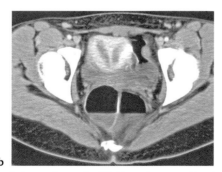
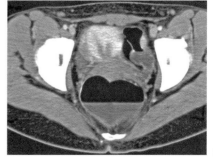

a   b   c

Fig. 29.41a–c Septate uterus. Septum through the uterine cavity (*). Note the normal fundus (in contradistinction to bicornuate uterus).

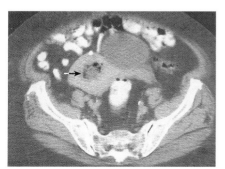

Fig. 29.42 Clostridial uterine infection. A postmenopausal woman's uterine infection (arrow) with this gas-forming organism was secondary to an underlying endometrial carcinoma.

Table 29.2   (Cont.) Reproductive system lesions

Disease	CT Findings	Comments
Vagina and vulva		
Carcinoma	For primary malignant tumors, a locally invasive mass may be evident on CT. In vulvar carcinoma, early metastatic nodal involvement of inguinal and subsequently pelvic nodes occurs. Tumors involving the proximal two thirds of the vagina first metastasize to deep pelvic nodes and tumors of the distal one third to inguinal nodes.	Vaginal and vulvar carcinomas are most frequently squamous cell carcinomas (85%–95%). Clear cell vaginal adenocarcinoma is associated with in utero exposure to diethylstilbestrol (DES). Direct vaginal invasion by cervical or uterine malignancies and metastatic vaginal lesions are additional considerations when encountering vaginal masses. Nonmalignant lesions, including endometriosis, can occur in the vagina and mimic malignancies.
Embryonal rhabdomyosarcoma ▷ *Fig. 29.43*	Vaginal mass with local invasion.	Usually in children younger than 5 y.
Congenital ▷ *Fig. 29.44*	Various malformations, including vaginal absence, atresia, septations, and duplications. Hydro- or hematocolpos (with or without uterine obstruction) may present as a low-attenuation central mass. Cystic peripheral vaginal area lesions may be due to Gartner duct cysts (wolffian duct remnants) or ectopic ureters.	Acquired vaginal obstructions are extremely rare.
Bartholin cyst ▷ *Fig. 29.45*	Up to 5 cm in size, these vulvovaginal gland cysts are not uncommon and occur at all ages.	May be involved in acute gonorrheal infections or result from stenosis of the orifice from prior infection. May fluctuate in size with repeated inflammation.
Male		
Prostate		
Carcinoma ▷ *Fig. 29.46* ▷ *Fig. 29.47*	Variable attenuation, frequently unrecognizable on CT in the absence of gross extraprostatic extension of disease. Often superimposed on benign prostatic hypertrophy (BPH) and biopsy changes.	Associated signs of advanced disease include seminal vesicle enlargement due to invasion (vs obstruction), adenopathy, and blastic pelvic bone metastases (vs bone islands).
Benign prostatic hypertrophy (BPH)	Diffuse, usually symmetric homogeneous or heterogeneous gland. Associated secondary signs of outlet obstruction may be present (thick wall bladder, bladder diverticula, and hydronephrosis).	Weight can be estimated from volume assuming a specific gravity for prostate tissue of 1.05 using the formula weight $= 0.55 \times$ length $\times$ AP $\times$ transverse extent. Normal prostates are usually < 30 g in adults.
Infection	Generalized enlargement, sometimes with focal fluid collections.	
Cystic foci	Focal low-attenuation lesions. If transurethral resection of the prostate (TURP) defect at bladder base, may fill with bladder contrast.	Nonsurgical midline foci are typically congenital, such as utricle and müllerian duct cysts. Eccentric foci often represent acquired processes, such as retention cysts, cystic degeneration in BPH, and abscesses. Ectopic ureters may open into the urethra or genital tract, and the most distal ureter is often dilated.
Seminal vesicle		
Neoplasm ▷ *Fig. 29.46*	Usually unilateral, homogeneous or inhomogeneous mass.	Primary benign and malignant seminal vesicle tumors are uncommon; secondary involvement from prostate, bladder, or rectal carcinomas occurs more frequently. May be difficult to distinguish from non-neoplastic cystic seminal vesicles.
Cystic seminal vesicles ▷ *Fig. 29.48*	Low-attenuation mass, unilateral or bilateral; look for associated urinary tract abnormalities (including cryptorchidism).	**Congenital:** Often associated with renal and/or collecting system anomalies (e.g., agenesis, duplication, and ectopic ureters). **Acquired:** As a result of obstruction, (e.g., due to prostate carcinoma). An association between bilateral cystic seminal vesicle changes and polycystic kidneys has been described.
Infection and hemorrhage	Often indistinguishable from and sometimes superimposed on seminal vesical neoplasms or obstructive processes. On unenhanced CT scan, acute hemorrhage (e.g., from prostate biopsies) may be of high attenuation compared with adjacent tissue.	

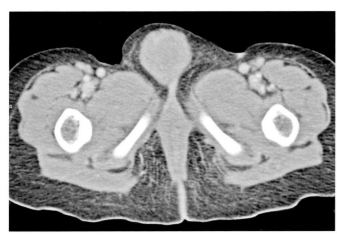

Fig. 29.43   Vulvar rhabdomyosarcoma. Solid enhancing mass bulging the upper right major labium and mons pubis.

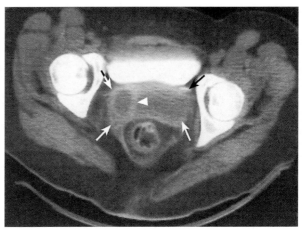

Fig. 29.44   Congenital vaginal obstruction with septum. Congenital hydrocolpos (arrows) with sagittal septum (arrowhead).

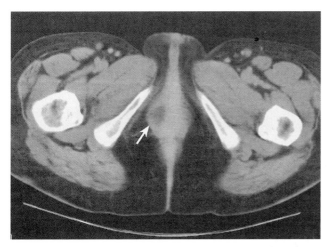

Fig. 29.45   Bartholin cyst. Young woman with a cyst in the right Bartholin gland (arrow).

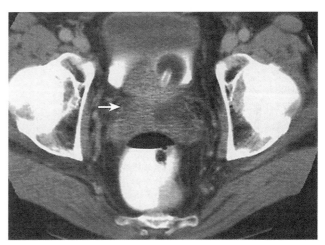

Fig. 29.46   Prostate carcinoma. The tumor invaded the extraprostatic fat at the angle of the right seminal vesicle (arrow), as well as the right seminal vesicle.

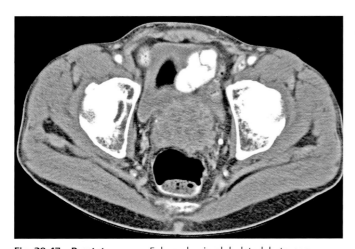

Fig. 29.47   Prostate cancer. Enlarged, microlobulated, heterogeneously enhancing prostate gland.

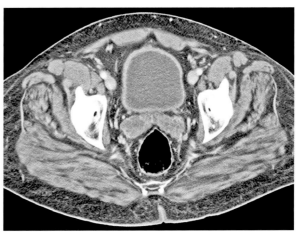

Fig. 29.48   Cystic seminal vesicles. Enlarged, low-attenuation seminal vesicles.

Table 29.3 Bladder lesions

Disease	CT Findings	Comments
Focal lesions		
Carcinoma ▷ *Fig. 29.49a, b* ▷ *Fig. 29.50a–c*	Polypoid or plaquelike areas of wall thickening. Perivesicle fat involvement manifests as irregular projections from bladder tumor margins.	Urachal remnant tumors (see also **Fig. 29.58, p. 831**) may be bilobed with intra- and extravesicle involvement of the bladder dome. Most commonly transitional cell carcinoma (~90%). Other types include squamous cell carcinoma (can be associated with schistosomiasis or bladder diverticula) and adenocarcinoma (associated with urachal remnant at the bladder dome).
Mesenchymal neoplasms ▷ *Fig. 29.51*	Polypoid or plaquelike focal masses.	Uncommon; includes leiomyomas, leiomyosarcomas, and rhabdomyosarcomas.
Lymphoma	Polypoid or plaque like focal masses; may present as diffuse wall thickening.	
Metastases/direct tumor extension ▷ *Fig. 29.52*	Focal bladder mass, often associated with other pelvic/abdominal lesions or confluent extension from an adjacent tumor (e.g., prostate, rectal, or cervicouterine origin).	When viewed cystoscopically, extrinsic masses from invading tumor or perivesicle infections are referred to as "herald" lesions.
Paraganglioma ▷ *Fig. 29.53*	Focal mass, most often at the bladder base; may also occur along the pelvic sidewall.	Uncommon site of extra-adrenal pheochromocytoma; search for lesions in other retroperitoneal locations. Multiple endocrine neoplasia (MEN) II association.
Endometriosis ▷ *Fig. 29.54*	Focal mass with intra- and/or extravesicle components.	May be indistinguishable from neoplasm. High-attenuation adnexal masses with fluid–fluid levels on nonenhanced scans may be an associated finding.

(continues on page 830)

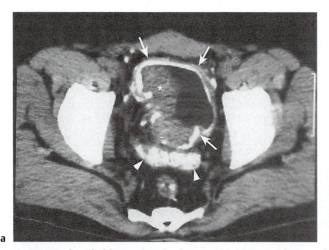
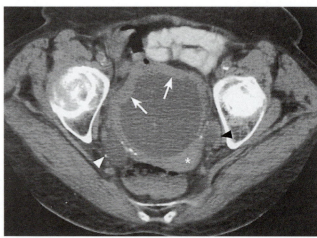

a   b

Fig. 29.49a, b **Bladder carcinomas (two cases).** (**a**) Typical pattern of **squamous cell carcinoma** (asterisk) arising in a bladder with extensive wall calcifications (arrows) from schistosomiasis. There are associated seminal vesicles calcifications. (**b**) **Transitional cell carcinoma** that involves most of the bladder wall (arrows). The atrophic uterus (asterisk) and adnexa (arrowheads) lie posteriorly in this postmenopausal woman.

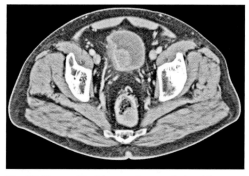
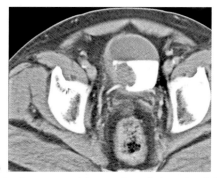
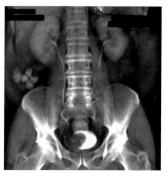

a   b   c

Fig. 29.50a–c   Bladder carcinoma. Polypoid transitional cell carcinoma (**a**). Note the right lateral wall thickening with intraluminal mildly lobulated mass (**b**), seen as a filling defect on the maximum intensity projection (MIP) reconstruction (**c**).

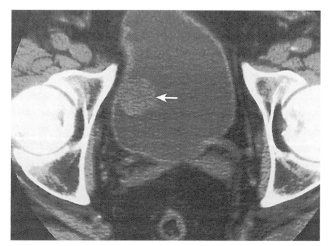

Fig. 29.51   Bladder leiomyosarcoma. This tumor (arrow) is indistinguishable from a polypoid transitional cell carcinoma.

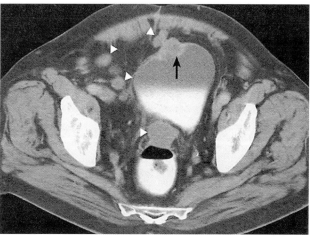

Fig. 29.52   Metastatic colon carcinoma. This patient's recurrence presented with hematuria. The tumor involves the bladder wall (arrow), as well as several other sites (arrowheads) in the pelvic cavity.

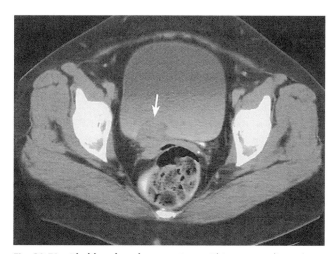

Fig. 29.53   Bladder pheochromocytoma. This paraganglioma (arrow) was an isolated occurrence of the disease in this patient.

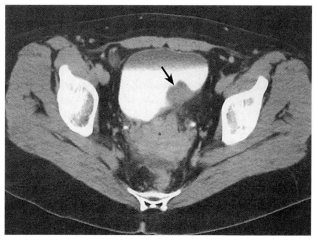

Fig. 29.54   Bladder wall endometriosis. Large implant of endometriosis (arrow) that is both intra- and extravesicular.

Table 29.3 (Cont.) Bladder lesions

Disease	CT Findings	Comments
Hematoma trauma ▷ *Fig. 29.55* ▷ *Fig. 29.56*	Focal wall thickening or discontinuity with bladder contrast and/or fluid in an intra- or extraperitoneal location with or without pelvic fractures. Interstitial (mural) extravasation should be distinguished from diverticula. Diverticula are typically associated with other signs of outlet obstruction.	In the setting of blunt trauma, extraperitoneal bladder rupture often associated with pelvic fractures and intraperitoneal bladder rupture typically occurs with a full bladder. Delayed images, to allow bladder filling, may be needed to document bladder injury.
Bladder diverticula ▷ *Fig. 29.57a, b*	Intra- or extramural outpouching of bladder lumen, single or multiple. Often vary in size.	More commonly acquired, due to bladder outlet obstruction. Congenital diverticula most common at the bladder base.
Urachal remnants ▷ *Fig. 29.58a, b*	Focal mass at bladder dome aligned with umbilicus with or without communication with bladder lumen.	Spectrum of benign urachal remnant findings includes cysts, diverticula, and sinuses.
Calculi	Single or multiple rounded or elliptical foci, typically in a dependent location.	Frequently associated with signs of bladder outlet obstruction, such as diverticula and thick wall bladder.
Inflammation	Malacoplakia may present as a mass in a setting of recurrent infections and may extend outside the bladder wall. Wall calcifications described in alkaline encrustation cystitis, tuberculosis (TB), schistosomiasis, and, rarely, with tumors.	Focal inflammatory bladder masses, such as malacoplakia, occur as a response to bladder infection or secondary to bladder involvement from the sigmoid colon (e.g., diverticulitis) or adnexal (e.g., TOA) inflammatory processes adjacent to the bladder.
Ureterocele	Cystic focus most commonly at the ureterovesicle junction with or without distal ureteral dilation.	Intra- or extramural ureteroceles can mimic diverticula. Ectopic ureteroceles extend into the bladder neck and/or urethra.
Diffuse lesions		
Bladder outlet obstruction	Most commonly associated with diffuse wall thickening, bladder diverticula, and enlarged prostate gland in men.	
Inflammation ▷ *Fig. 29.59*	Typically uniform, diffuse, smooth or irregular wall thickening with or without perivesical fat infiltrative changes.	Includes infectious causes as well as mechanical or chemical irritation (e.g., Foley catheter or cyclophosphamide) and radiation changes. Emphysematous cystitis most commonly occurs in diabetics secondary to *Escherichia coli*. In hemorrhagic cystitis, high-attenuation bladder contents due to blood may be seen.
Carcinoma and lymphoma	Focal or diffuse process.	Primary bladder lymphoma is uncommon. Uniform, circumferential transitional cell carcinoma is uncommon, and there is often variable wall thickening when there is widespread mural tumor (see also **Fig. 29.49 p. 828**).

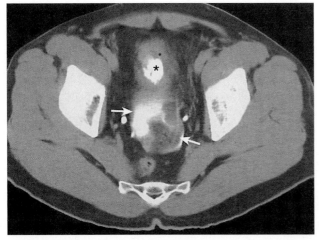

Fig. 29.55 Intraperitoneal bladder rupture. Extravasated intraperitoneal bladder contrast (arrows) outlines the distal sigmoid colon. The decompressed bladder lies anteriorly (star).

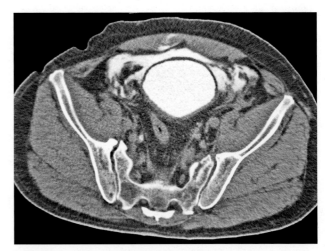

Fig 29.56 Extraperitoneal bladder rupture. Spillage of contrast into the extraperitoneal anterior vesical space (space of Retzius), with some contrast also insinuated within the right rectus muscle.

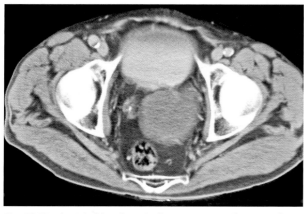
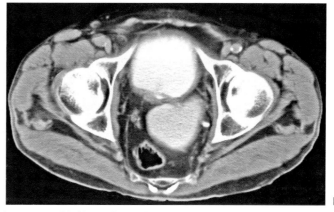

a   b

Fig. 29.57a, b   Bladder diverticulum. Narrow neck outpouching of the posterior bladder wall near the ureteral insertion (**a**) eventually fills with contrast on delayed imaging (**b**): a Hutch diverticulum.

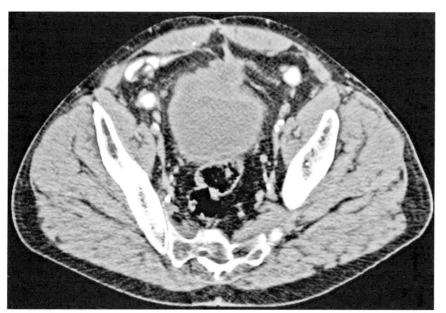
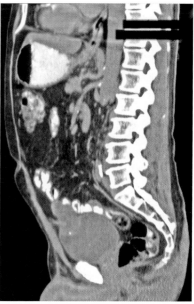

a   b

Fig. 29.58a, b   Urachal remnant (carcinoma). Axial (**a**) and sagittal (**b**) views of a midline exophytic mass of somewhat heterogeneous attenuation (with calcific focus) from the anterior bladder dome.

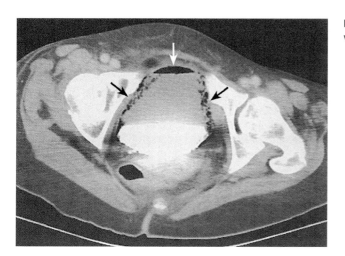

Fig. 29.59   Emphysematous cystitis. Air outlines the entire bladder wall (arrows).

Table 29.4 Pelvic peritoneal and extraperitoneal lesions

Disease	CT Findings	Comments
Peritoneal lesions		
Metastases ▷ *Fig. 29.60* ▷ *Fig. 29.61*	Peritoneal margin, mesenteric or omental solid and/or cystic masses, with or without calcifications, with or without ascites.	Common origins include ovarian and gastrointestinal (GI) primary sites, such as stomach, colon, and pancreas. Less commonly, lymphoma or sarcoma disseminates in the peritoneum.
Pseudomyxoma peritonei ▷ *Fig. 29.62*	Low-attenuation pelvic cavity material with mass effect with or without septations or calcifications. May be of higher attenuation than water.	This is a special form of peritoneal dissemination of disease with gelatinous material distributed in the peritoneal cavity. Etiologies for the mucinous material include cystadenomas and cystadenocarcinomas of the appendix or ovary.
Mesothelioma ▷ *Fig. 29.63a, b*	Solid or cystic masses or plaques involving peritoneal margins, mesentery, or omentum with or without ascites.	Malignant peritoneal mesothelioma is an extremely rare cancer, accounting for < 30% of all mesothelioma cases. Because pleural mesothelioma is more common and often spreads to the peritoneal cavity, it is important to determine if pleural mesothelioma is the primary cancer.
Peritonitis ▷ *Fig. 29.64*	Appearance may mimic metastases or uncomplicated ascites.	Tuberculous peritonitis may mimic neoplastic involvement of the peritoneum.
Abscess	Fluid- and/or air-containing collections. Large amounts of air often indicate an enteric communication (see **Fig. 29.16, p. 818**).	Most commonly follows surgery or as a result of diverticulitis or appendicitis.
Hematoma	Mixed low- to high-attenuation, often amorphous masses. Fluid–fluid levels with dependent high-attenuation collections are sometimes seen.	In premenopausal women, considerations include ectopic pregnancy, ruptured functional cysts, and endometriosis.
Urinoma	Collections containing fluid or extravasated urinary contrast agents.	Typically follows trauma or recent surgery, such as radical prostatectomy.
Urinary conduits	Ileal loops and segmental colonic pouches may contain fluid or excreted IV contrast.	
Extraperitoneal lesions		
Lymphadenopathy ▷ *Fig. 29.65* ▷ *Fig. 29.66* ▷ *Fig. 29.67a, b*	Intermediate- or low-attenuation masses along the course of the pelvic vessels, with or without central necrosis (see also **Fig. 29.38, p. 825**).	Most common sidewall mass. Lymphoma and nodal metastases from pelvic organ and lower extremity malignancies account for most lesions.

(continues on page 834)

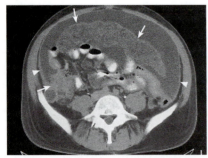

Fig. 29.60 Colonic carcinoma metastases. Large amounts of ascites with omental and right paracolic gutter tumor implants (arrows). There are also tumor implants that thicken the lateral peritoneal margins (arrowheads).

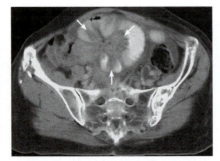

Fig. 29.61 Metastatic breast carcinoma. Small bowel mesentery tumor implants (arrows), as well as a small amount of ascites.

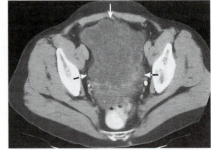

Fig. 29.62 Pseudomyxoma peritonei. Confluent disease with multiple septations (arrows) is seen in this patient with a primary ovarian malignancy.

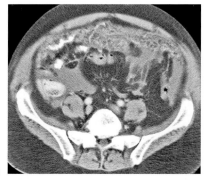
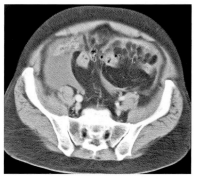

a   b

Fig 29.63a, b   Malignant peritoneal mesothelioma. "Cystic" masses distributed along the expected location of the peritoneal lining of the greater omentum with concomitant ascites.

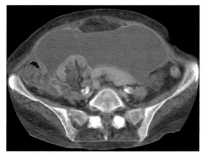
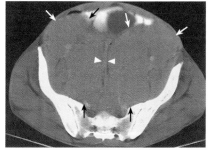
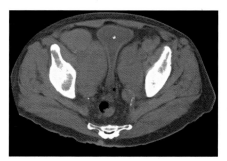

Fig 29.64   Peritonitis (tension ascites). Enhancing smoothly thickened peritoneal lining and ascites causing mass effect on the neighboring hollow viscus.

Fig. 29.65   Adenopathy. Massive confluent external and internal iliac adenopathy (arrows) due to chronic lymphocytic leukemia compresses the rectosigmoid colon (arrowheads) in the midline.

Fig. 29.66   Lymphoma. Markedly enlarged bilateral internal iliac nodes compressing the bladder (*).

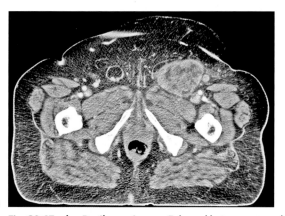
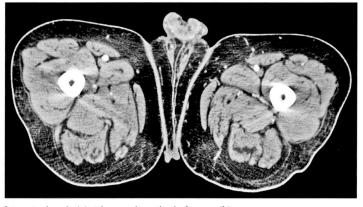

a   b

Fig. 29.67a, b   Penile carcinoma. Enlarged heterogeneous left inguinal node (**a**). Ulcerated penile shaft mass (**b**).

Table 29.4 (Cont.) Pelvic peritoneal and extraperitoneal lesions

Disease	CT Findings	Comments
Aneurysm or pseudoaneurysm ▷ *Fig. 29.68* ▷ *Fig. 29.69* ▷ *Fig. 29.70*	Focal increase in arterial caliber with or without mural plaque or thrombus.	True aneurysms are most commonly atherosclerotic in origin. Pseudoaneurysms are not uncommon following catheter procedures.
Venous thrombi and other venous lesions ▷ *Fig. 29.71* ▷ *Fig. 29.72a, b*	Venous thrombi typically are of lower attenuation than enhanced blood; however, acute thrombus can also be iso- or hyperattenuating. A varix is a focal dilation of a vein.	A varix is often idiopathic or may result from more cephalad vascular obstructions, such as IVC thrombosis and left common iliac artery compression of vein. Uncommonly, a varix is due to arteriovenous fistula where venous distention results from shunting of arterial pressures.
Neural lesions ▷ *Fig. 29.73* ▷ *Fig. 29.74*	Masses of variable attenuation along neural pathways, such as the sacral foramina and sciatic notch.	Types include nerve root sleeve cysts, as well as neoplasms, such as schwannomas and neurofibromas.
Infection ▷ *Fig. 29.75* ▷ *Fig. 29.76a, b*	Most commonly musculoskeletal or GI origin fluid and/or air collections. Lymphoceles, urinomas, and hematomas may become secondarily infected.	Most commonly result of trauma or GI fistulas, such as Crohn disease.
Hematoma	Mixed attenuation masses with or without associated pelvic fractures. Rectus sheath hematomas may track into retropubic space or pelvic sidewall tissue planes.	May follow minor trauma in anticoagulated patients. May see typical "molar tooth" configuration in retropubic space of Retzius. Hemophiliacs may present with pelvic musculoskeletal pseudotumors secondary to hemorrhage.
Urinoma	Fluid or higher attenuation collection (with or without iodinated contrast) adjacent to ureters or bladder. Delayed scans following IV contrast administration may be helpful.	Etiologies include blunt and penetrating trauma and from surgical procedures, such as abdominoperineal resections, urinary diversions, and prostatectomies.

(continues on page 836)

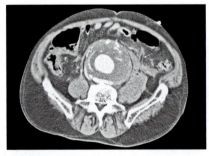

Fig. 29.68 Leaking aortic aneurysm. Large infrarenal aortic aneurysm with intraluminal thrombus and contrast streaks within the thrombus. Note the periaortic stranding representing hemorrhage (arrow), as well as a few foci of intimal calcifications.

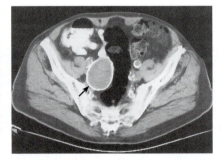

Fig. 29.69 Iliac artery aneurysm. Typical rim calcification of an atherosclerotic internal iliac artery aneurysm (arrow).

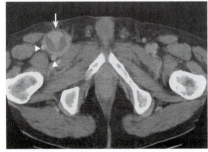

Fig. 29.70 Pseudoaneurysm. A right deep femoral artery pseudoaneurysm (arrow) is present following an arterial catheterization procedure. The native arteries are displaced (arrowheads).

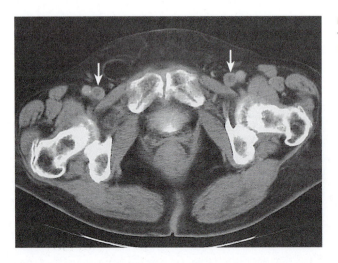

Fig. 29.71 Deep venous thrombosis. Bilateral common femoral vein thrombi are present in this patient with cryoglobulinemia due to lymphoma (arrows).

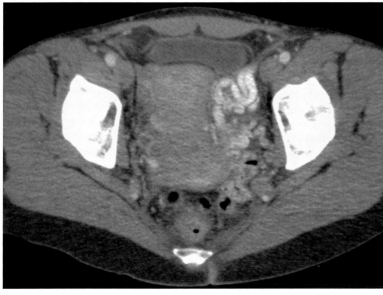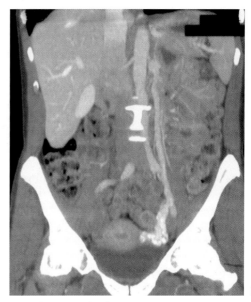

a   b

Fig. 29.72a, b Pelvic congestion syndrome. Dilated, mildly tortuous venous channels arising from the left adnexal region.

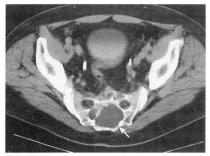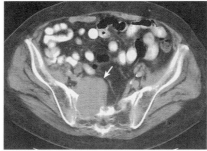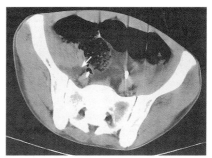

Fig. 29.73 Sacral cyst. Large incidental asymptomatic sacral thecal sac cyst (arrow).

Fig. 29.74 Schwannoma. Large right sacral nerve schwannoma (arrow) enlarging the sacral foramen.

Fig. 29.75 Abscess. Right iliacus abscess (arrow) due to a sacroiliac joint infection.

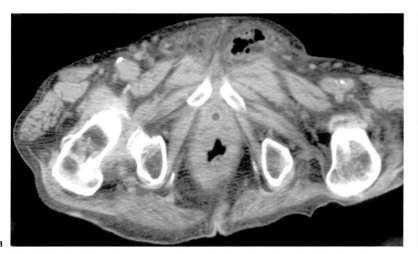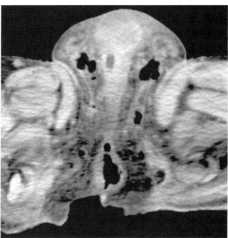

a   b

Fig. 29.76a, b Fournier gangrene. Gas collections interspersed within the subcutaneous fat adjacent to the spermatic cords, migrated from the scrotum (not shown). Note the Foley catheter within the corpus and bulbus spongiosus.

Table 29.4   (Cont.) Pelvic peritoneal and extraperitoneal lesions

Disease	CT Findings	Comments
Lymphocele ▷ *Fig. 29.77*	Fluid-filled mass with or without septations with or without nearby surgical clips.	Most commonly postoperative following nodal dissection or organ transplantation (e.g., renal transplants).
Retroperitoneal fibrosis ▷ *Fig. 29.78*	Soft tissue attenuation mass(es). Most commonly affects area of lower lumbar spine/lumbosacral junction. May cause vascular or urinary tract obstructions. Most commonly idiopathic, but may occur as a desmoplastic response to tumors.	
Pelvic lipomatosis ▷ *Fig. 29.79*	Bilateral, symmetric, fat-attenuation masses displacing and compressing central and lateral pelvic structures.	May cause vascular or urinary tract obstructions.
Neoplasms	Typically arise from pelvic musculoskeletal framework or supporting tissues.	Uncommon; most pelvic sidewall masses are of lymph node or vascular origin. Anterior pelvic wall tumors include desmoids (especially in the rectus sheath; see **Fig. 29.1, p. 814**). These show intense contrast enhancement. They may enlarge during pregnancy. Desmoids are sometimes seen in Gardner syndrome. Posterior midline lesions include chordomas, sacrococcygeal teratomas, and metastases or local recurrence of rectal carcinomas.
Hernia ▷ *Fig. 29.80* ▷ *Fig. 29.81* ▷ *Fig. 29.82a, b* ▷ *Fig. 29.83a–d*	Bowel and abdominal/pelvic fat herniate via neurovascular canals or areas of pelvic musculature weaknesses.	Pelvic hernias include inguinal, femoral, obturator, and perineal, as well as anterior pelvic wall.
Iatrogenic pseudolesions	Transposed ovaries: cystic and solid foci, typically in iliac fossa with or without surgical clips. Presacral masses after abdominoperineal resection: in women, the uterus and in men, the prostate and seminal vesicles may lie in this location (see also **Figs. 29.7, 29.8, 29.9, [all on p. 816]**).	See text in this chapter; must distinguish from recurrent tumor.
Extramedullary hematopoiesis	Typically associated with evidence of marrow expansion in pelvic skeletal structures.	

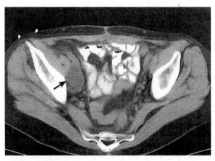

Fig. 29.77   Lymphocele. Right sidewall lymphocele following node dissection for a gynecologic malignancy (arrow).

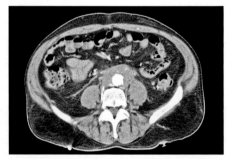

Fig. 29.78   Retroperitoneal fibrosis. Thick soft tissue rind almost completely encircling the aorta, rendering the IVC indistinct. Absence of venous collateral circulation suggests that substantial IVC flow obstruction is not present.

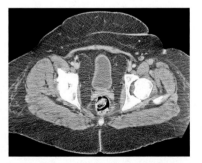

Fig. 29.79   Pelvic lipomatosis. Displacement of lateral bladder walls toward the midline from increased pelvic fat.

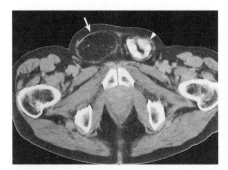

Fig. 29.80   Bilateral inguinal hernias. The right hernia contains omental fat (arrow), and the left hernia contains small bowel (arrowhead).

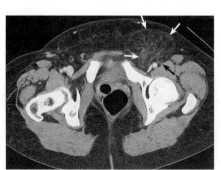

Fig. 29.81   Femoral canal hernia. This left-sided femoral canal hernia of omental fat (arrows) compresses the left common femoral vein and tracks into the anterior pelvic wall.

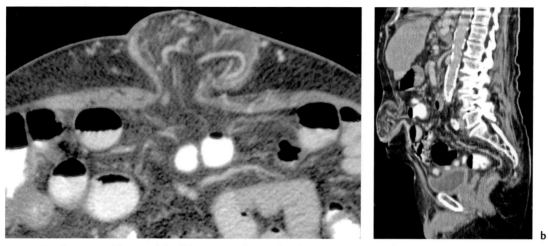

Fig. 29.82a, b   Ventral (periumbilical) hernia. Axial (**a**) and midsagittal (**b**) views of herniation of omental fat and vessels through a defect between the recti abdomini (within the linea alba).

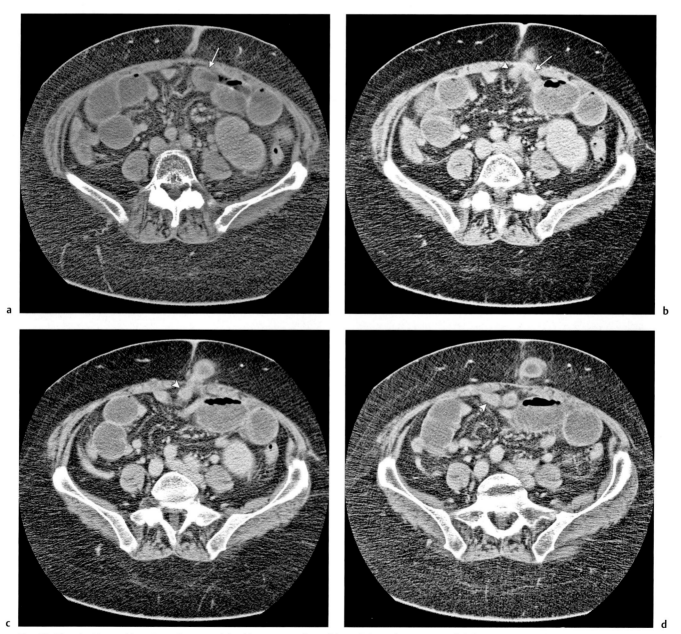

Fig. 29.83a–d   Ventral hernia. Left paraumbilical herniation of small bowel through anterior wall defect causing small bowel obstruction. Afferent dilated segment (arrow); efferent collapsed segment (arrowhead).

References

Atlas SW. Resonance Imaging of the Brain and Spine. 4th ed. Philadelphia: Lippincott Williams & Wilkins; 2008

Barkovich AJ. Pediatric Neuroimaging. 4th ed. Philadelphia: Lippincott Williams & Wilkins; 2005

Budoff MMJ. Cardiac CT Imaging: Diagnosis of Cardiovascular Disease. Berlin: Springer; 2006

Burgener FA, Meyers SP, Tan RK, Zaunbauer W. Differential Diagnosis in Magnetic Resonance Imaging. Stuttgart: Thieme; 2002

Burgener FA, Kormano M, Pudas T. Differential Diagnosis in Conventional Radiology. 3rd ed. Stuttgart: Thieme; 2008

Dähnert W. Radiology Review Manual. 6th ed. Philadelphia: Lippincott Williams & Wilkins; 2007

Federle MP, Jeffrey RB, Woodward PJ, et al. Diagnostic Imaging: Abdomen. Philadelphia: Lippincott Williams & Wilkins; 2009

Fraser RS, Müller NL, Coleman NC, Paré PD. Fraser and Paré's Diagnosis of Diseases of the Chest. 4th ed. Philadelphia: Saunders; 1999

Freyschmidt J, Sternberg A, Brossmann J, et al. Koehler/Zimmer's Borderlands of Normal and Early Pathological Findings in Skeletal Radiography. 5th ed. Stuttgart: Thieme; 2002

Goering R, Dockrell H, Roitt I, et al. Mim's Medical Microbiology. 4th ed. London: Elsevier; 2007

Goldman L. Cecil's Textbook of Medicine. 23rd ed. Philadelphia: Saunders; 2010

Gray HL, Bannister LH, William PL. Gray's Anatomy. 40th ed. Edinburgh: Churchill Livingstone; 2008

Greenspan A. Orthopedic Imaging. 5th ed. Philadelphia: Lippincott Williams & Wilkins; 2006

Gurney JW, Stern EJ, Franquet T. Diagnostic Imaging: Chest. Philadelphia: Saunders; 2009

Harnsberger HR, Osborn AG, Ross J, et al. Diagnostic and Surgical Imaging Anatomy: Brain, Head and Neck, Spine. Salt Lake City, UT: Amirsys; 2004

Harnsberger HR, Wiggins RH, Hudgins PA, et al. Diagnostic Imaging: Head and Neck. Salt Lake City, UT: Amirsys; 2004

Harnsberger HR, Koch BL, Philips CD, et al. Expertddx: Head and Neck. Salt Lake City, UT: Amirsys; 2009

Kasper D. Harrison's Principles of Internal Medicine. 18th ed. New York: McGraw-Hill; 2011

Kleihues P, Cavenee WK. Pathology and Genetics of Tumours of the Nervous System. World Health Organization Classification of Tumours. Lyon: IARC Press; 2000

Kuhn JP, Slovis TL, Haller JO. Caffey's Pediatric Diagnostic Imaging. Chicago: Year Book Medical; 2003

Kumar V, Abbas AK, Fausto N. Aster J. Robbins and Cotran's Pathologic Basis of Disease. 8th ed. Philadelphia: Saunders; 2010

Lachman RS. Taybi and Lachman's Radiology of Syndromes, Metabolic Disorders and Skeletal Dysplasias. 5th ed. Chicago: Year Book Medical; 2006

Lang S, Walsh G, Montag M. Radiology of Chest Diseases. New York: Thieme Medical Publishers; 2007

Lee JKT, Stanley RJ, Heiken JP. Computed Body Tomography with MRI Correlation. Philadelphia: Lippincott Williams & Wilkins; 2005

Lenz M. Computed Tomography and Magnetic Resonance Imaging of Head Tumors: Methods, Guidelines, Differential Diagnosis and Clinical Results. Stuttgart: Thieme; 1993

Mafee MF, Valvassori GE, Becker M. Valvassori's Imaging of the Head and Neck. 2nd ed. Stuttgart: Thieme; 2005

Mafee MF. Ophthalmologic Neuro-imaging. Neuroimaging Clinics of North America. Philadelphia: Elsevier; 2005

Meyers MA. Dynamic Radiology of the Abdomen: Normal and Pathologic Anatomy. Heidelberg: Springer; 2000

Meyers SP. MRI of Bone and Soft Tissue Tumors and Tumor like Lesions: Differential Diagnosis and Atlas. Stuttgart: Thieme; 2008

Moss AA, Gamsu G, Genant HK. Computed Tomography of the Body. 2nd ed. Philadelphia: Saunders; 1992

Müller-Forell WS. Imaging of Orbital and Visual Pathway Pathology: Medical Radiology, Diagnostic Imaging. Berlin: Springer; 2006

Müller NL, Fraser RS, Coleman NC, Paré PD. Radiologic Diagnosis of Diseases of the Chest. Philadelphia: Saunders; 2001

Naidich DP, Webb WR, Müller NL, Vlahos I, Krinsky GA. Computed Tomography and Magnetic Resonance of the Thorax. 4th ed. Philadelphia: Lippincott Williams & Wilkins; 2007

Ney C, Friedenberg RM. Radiographic Atlas of the Genitourinary System. Philadelphia: Lippincott Williams & Wilkins; 1981

Osborn AG, Salzman KL, Barkovich AJ. Diagnostic Imaging: Brain. 2nd ed. Salt Lake City, UT: Amirsys; 2008

Oudkerk M, Reiser MF. Coronary Radiology (Medical Radiology: Diagnostic Imaging). Berlin: Springer; 2008

Pollack HM, McClennan BL, Dyer RB, Kenney PJ. Clinical Urography. Philadelphia: Saunders; 2001

Prokop CM. Spiral and Multislice Computed Tomography of the Body. Stuttgart: Thieme; 2010

Reed JC. Chest Radiology: Patterns and Differential Diagnosis. Chicago: Year Book Medical; 2003

Reeder MM. Reeder and Felson's Gamuts in Radiology. 4th ed. New York: Springer; 2003

Resnick D. Diagnosis of Bone and Joint Disorders. 4th ed. Philadelphia: Saunders; 2002

Resnick D, Kransdorf MJ. Bone and Joint Imaging. 3rd ed. Philadelphia: Saunders; 2005

Sahani D, Samir A. Abdominal Imaging: Expert Consult- Online and Print (Expert Radiology). Philadelphia: Saunders; 2010

Saini S, Rubin GD, Kalra MK. MDCT: A Practical Approach. Berlin: Springer; 2006

Schoepf UJ. CT of the Heart: Principles and Applications (Contemporary Cardiology). Berlin: Springer; 2004

Semelka RC. Abdominal-Pelvic MRI. Philadelphia: John Wiley & Sons; 2010

Skucas J. Advanced Imaging of the Abdomen. Heidelberg: Springer; 2006

Slovis TL. Caffey's Pediatric Diagnostic Imaging. 11th ed. Chicago: Mosby; 2007

Som PM, Curtin HD. Head and Neck Imaging. 4th ed. Chicago: Mosby; 2002

Stoller DW, Tirman PF, Bredella M. Diagnostic Imaging: Orthopaedics. Salt Lake City, UT: Amirsys; 2004

Sutton D. Textbook of Radiology and Imaging. 7th ed. Edinburgh: Churchill Livingstone; 2003

Swischuk LE. Imaging of the Newborn, Infant and Young Child. Baltimore: Williams and Wilkins; 2003

Tortori-Donati P. Pediatric Neuroradiology: Brain: Head and Neck, Spine. Heidelberg: Springer; 2005

van der Knapp MS, Vaalk J. Magnetic Resonance of Myelination and Myelin Disorders. 3rd ed. Heidelberg: Springer; 2005

Van Rijn RR, Blickman JG. Differential Diagnosis in Pediatric Radiology. Stuttgart: Thieme; 2011

Webb WR, Brant WE, Helms CA. Fundamentals of Body CT. 2nd ed. Philadelphia: Saunders; 1998

Webb WR, Müller NL, Naidich DF. High Resolution CT of the Lung. 3rd ed. Philadelphia: Lippincott Williams & Wilkins; 2009

Weber AL. Radiologic Evaluation of the Neck. The Radiologic Clinics of North America. Philadelphia: Elsevier; 2000

Weber AL. Imaging of the Mandible, Maxilla and Pharynx. Neuroimaging Clinics of North America. Philadelphia: Elsevier; 2003

Yousem DM. Head and Neck Imaging. The Radiologic Clinics of North America. Philadelphia: Elsevier; 1998

Index

Page numbers in *italics* refer to illustrations